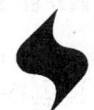

Stedman's

RADIOLOGY

WORDS

INCLUDES
NUCLEAR MEDICINE
& OTHER IMAGING
Sixth Edition

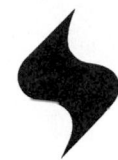

Stedman's

RADIOLOGY
WORDS

INCLUDES
NUCLEAR MEDICINE
& OTHER IMAGING
Sixth Edition

Wolters Kluwer | Lippincott Williams & Wilkins
Health

Philadelphia · Baltimore · New York · London
Buenos Aires · Hong Kong · Sydney · Tokyo

Publisher: Julie K. Stegman
Editorial Manager: Eric Branger
Associate Managing Editor: Erin M. Cosyn
Typesetter: Aptara, Inc.
Printer & Binder: Data Reproductions Corporation

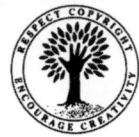

Printed in the United States of America

Sixth Edition, 2009

Library of Congress Cataloging-in-Publication Data

Stedman's radiology words: includes nuclear medicine & other imaging. — 6th ed.
     p. ; cm. — (Stedman's word books)
   Includes bibliographical references.
   ISBN 978-0-7817-9731-3
   1. Radiology—Terminology.   2. Radiography, Medical—Terminology.
3. Diagnosis, Radioscopic—Terminology.   4. Diagnostic imaging—Terminology.
5. Radioisotope scanning—Terminology.   I. Stedman, Thomas Lathrop, 1853–1938.
II. Title: Radiology words.   III. Series: Stedman's word books.
   [DNLM: 1. Diagnostic Imaging—Terminology—English. WN 15 S812 2009]
RC78.A3S74 2009
616.07′57014—dc22

                                                      2009001582

                                             09 10 11 12
                                    1 2 3 4 5 6 7 8 9 10

Contents

ACKNOWLEDGMENTS vii

EDITOR'S PREFACE ix

PUBLISHER'S PREFACE xi

EXPLANATORY NOTES xiii

REFERENCES xvii

A-Z WORD LIST 1

APPENDICES

    1. Anatomical Illustrations A1

    2. Contrast Media, Imaging Agents, and Related
       Substances A25

    3. Common Radiation Oncology Terms A29

    4. Sample Reports A34

    5. Common Terms by Procedure A49

    6. Common Breast Imaging Terms A55

    7. Common Radiographic Imaging Techniques A59

Acknowledgments

An important part of our editorial process is the involvement of medical language specialists and other health professionals—as advisors, reviewers, and/or editors.

We extend special thanks to Kathy Hess, CMT and Janet West for editing the manuscript and helping to resolve many difficult questions. We are grateful to the members of our Editorial Advisory Board, Robin Koza and Robin Snider, who were instrumental in shaping the direction of this revision. They shared their valuable judgment, insight, and perspective.

We also extend our gratitude to Janet West for developing and revising the appendices; to Susan Caldwell for her assistance with the anatomical illustrations; to Jeanne Bock, CSR, MT for her contributions to the sample reports and her exceptional research skills.

Our appreciation goes to the following reviewers who helped to enhance the A-to-Z content for this edition: Susan Bartolucci, CMT, FAAMT; Jeanne Bock, CSR, MT; Shemah Fletcher; Paula Graham; Rhonda S. Hase; Robin Koza; and Jenifer Walker, MA. Additional thanks to Jeanne Bock for performing the final prepublication review.

As with all our *Stedman's* word references, this resource incorporates the suggestions and expertise of our many contacts in the medical community. Thanks to all of our advisory board participants, reviewers, and editors; AAMT meeting attendees; and others who have written us with requests and comments—keep talking, and we'll keep listening.

Editor's Preface

Writing this Editor's Preface is by far the most difficult part of the editing process for me. I usually look back at prefaces written by editors from prior books for some direction but then I'm really intimidated! I feel that my words should at least be inspiring if not profound, and sometimes it takes me a really long time to even get to the point of inspiration, never mind getting to profound. Be that as it may, the editing process can be an arduous task at times, given the size of the projects combined with so many things to watch for in an effort to maintain consistency within the current book and between other word books published by Stedman's.

Consistency—that's one of those double-edged swords—at least for me. It's something I used to strive for in disciplining my children but seldom achieved—at least much of the time I was not as consistent as I would like to have been! But I'm happy when things are consistent. Consistency gives me a sense of safety and security—maybe that's just code for control! But it's more than that—it's important that Stedman's word books be consistent in order to be as beneficial to the user as possible. And consistency is important in the production of an accurate medical document to assist in and document patient care. Rest assured that I have tried to be as consistent as possible within the covers of this book, but thankfully, I had the very capable assistance of Janet West as second editor. This was Janet's maiden adventure as a word book editor but I foresee many future journeys ahead for her! I was also incredibly fortunate to have worked with Erin Cosyn again. Erin is a gifted writer with a discerning eye toward, yes, consistency!

Despite the intense nature of these editing projects, I continue to accept the challenge in hopes of expanding my own knowledge while creating a valuable—and consistent—resource for all medical language specialists. I continue to marvel at the professionalism and dedication of everyone at Lippincott Williams & Wilkins/Stedman's. A valuable, useful product is the ultimate goal for all involved.

Kathy Hess, CMT
Editor

Publisher's Preface

Stedman's Radiology Words, Includes Nuclear Medicine & Other Imaging, Sixth Edition offers an up-to-date, authoritative reference for the wordsmiths of the healthcare professions—medical transcriptionists, medical editors and copyeditors, health information management personnel, court reporters, medical coders, and the many other users and producers of medical documentation.

With the rapid rate of technological advancement, we realized the need to develop a comprehensive reference that reflects the changes that have taken place within radiology, nuclear medicine, and imaging since the Fifth Edition published. With this revised edition, we have focused on incorporating new developments in technology, including thorough coverage of the equipment and contrast materials used in imaging today, as well as techniques, procedures, tests, and phrases.

Stedman's Radiology Words, Includes Nuclear Medicine & Other Imaging, Sixth Edition provides users with tens of thousands of words and phrases encompassing various aspects of imaging and nuclear medicine, including: diagnostic, therapeutic, and interventional radiology; abdominal, chest, gastrointestinal, genitourinary, and skeletal imaging; CT, MRI, PET and SPECT imaging; mammography, ultrasonography, x-ray, neuroradiology, roentgenology, investigational radiology, radiographics, and radiologic technology terminology, as well as various contrast materials. Users will also find terms for diagnostic and therapeutic procedures, new techniques, and equipment names, plus abbreviations with their expansions. The appendix sections provide labeled anatomical illustrations, contrast media and other related materials, sample reports, and common terms by procedure.

This compilation of more than 100,000 entries, fully cross-indexed for quick access, was built from a base vocabulary of approximately 66,000 medical words, phrases, abbreviations and acronyms. The extensive A-Z list was developed from the lexicon of *Stedman's Medical Dictionary, 28th Edition,* and supplemented by terminology found in current medical books, journals, newsletters, and websites (please see list of References on page xvii).

We at Lippincott Williams & Wilkins strive to provide you with the most up-to-date and accurate word references available. Your use of this word book will prompt new editions, which we will publish as often as updates and revisions justify. We welcome your suggestions for improvements, changes, corrections, and additions—whatever will make this *Stedman's* product more useful to you.

Explanatory Notes

Medical transcription is an art as well as a science. Both approaches are needed to correctly interpret the dictation of a physician, whose language is a product of education, training, and experience. This variety in medical language means that there are several acceptable ways to express certain terms, including jargon. *Stedman's Radiology Words, Includes Nuclear Medicine & Other Imaging, Sixth Edition,* seeks to reflect current usage of medical language and provides variant spellings and phrasings for many terms. These elements, in addition to complete cross-indexing, make *Stedman's Radiology Words, Includes Nuclear Medicine & Other Imaging, Sixth Edition* a valuable resource for determining the validity of terms as they are encountered.

Alphabetical Organization

Alphabetization of main entries is letter by letter as spelled, ignoring punctuation, spaces, prefixed numbers, Greek letters, or other characters. For example:

> hydrops
> hydropyonephrosis
> 5-hydroxyindoleacetic acid (5-HIAA)
> Hypaque
> Hypaque-76 imaging agent

In subentry alphabetization, the abbreviated singular form or the spelled-out plural form of the noun main entry word is ignored.

Format and Style

All main entries are in **boldface** to expedite locating a sought-after term, to enhance distinction between main entries and subentries, and to relieve the textual density of the pages.

Irregular plurals and variant spellings are shown on the same line as the singular or preferred form of the word. For example:

index, indices
mammoplasty, mammaplasty

Hyphenation

As a rule of style, multiple eponyms (e.g., Mears-Rubash approach) are hyphenated. Also, hyphens have been added between a manufacturer and one or more eponyms (e.g., Vital-Metzenbaum dissecting scissors). Please note that in many cases, hyphenation is a question of style, not of accuracy, and thus is a matter of choice.

Possessives

Possessive forms have been dropped in this reference for the sake of consistency and conformance with the guidelines of the American Medical Association (AMA), Association for Healthcare Documentation Integrity (AHDI) (formerly AAMT), and other groups. Please note, however, that in many cases, retaining the possessive, like hyphenating, is a question of style, not of accuracy, and thus is a matter of choice. To form the possessive of a word, simply add the apostrophe or apostrophe "s" to the end of the word.

Cross-indexing

The word list is in an index-like main entry-subentry format that contains two combined alphabetical listings:

(1) A *noun* main entry-subentry organization, which is typical of the A-Z section of medical dictionaries like *Stedman's*:

image
  acoustic i.
  delayed phase i.

table
  binary opacity t.
  radionuclide t.

(2) An *adjective* main entry-subentry organization, which lists words and phrases as you hear them. The main entries are the adjectives or modifiers in a multiword term. The subentries are the nouns around which the terms are constructed and to which the adjectives or modifiers pertain:

magnetic
  m. anisotropy
  m. dipole

bright
  b. echo
  b. signal intensity

This format provides the user with more than one way to locate and identify a multiword term. For example:

gradient
  diastolic g.

diastolic
  d. gradient

assessment
  sonographic a.

sonographic
  s. assessment

It also allows the user to see together all terms that contain a particular descriptor, as well as all types, kinds, or variations of a noun entity. For example:

fracture
  abduction f
  basal neck f.
  f. bracing

valve
  v. area
  atrioventricular nodal v.
  v. attenuation

Wherever possible, abbreviations are separately defined and cross-referenced. For example:

BI-RADS
  Breast Imaging Reporting and Data System

breast
  B. Imaging Reporting and Data System (BI-RADS)

system
  Breast Imaging Reporting and Data S. (BI-RADS)

References

In addition to the manufacturers' literature we gather at various medical meetings, scientific reports from hospitals, and the lists of our MT Editorial Advisory Board members (from their daily transcription work), we used the following resources in the development of *Stedman's Radiology Words, Includes Nuclear Medicine & Other Imaging, Sixth Edition*.

Books

The AAMT Book of Style, Second Edition. Modesto, CA: AAMT, 2002.

Brant, William E. and Clyde E. Helms. *Fundamentals of Diagnostic Radiology, Third Edition*. Baltimore: Lippincott Williams & Wilkins, 2007.

Billups, N.F. *American Drug Index 2003, 47th Edition*. St. Louis, Missouri: Facts & Comparisons, 2002.

Collins, Jannette and Eric J. Stern. *Chest Radiology: The Essentials, Second Edition*. Baltimore: Lippincott Williams & Wilkins, 2007.

Daffner, Richard H. *Clinical Radiology: The Essentials, Third Edition*. Baltimore: Lippincott Williams & Wilkins, 2007.

Dorland's Radiology/Oncology Word Book for Medical Transcriptionists. Philadelphia: WB Saunders, 2001.

Drake E. Sloane's Medical Word Book, Fourth Edition. Philadelphia: WB Saunders, 2002.

Drake, E. and R. Drake *Drake and Drake Pharmaceutical Word Book 2002*. Philadelphia: WB Saunders, 2002.

Eng, John and Clifford Weiss. *Manual of Radiology: Acute Problems and Essential Procedures, Second Edition*. Baltimore: Lippincott Williams & Wilkins, 2007.

Freeman, L.M. *Nuclear Medicine Annual 2001*. Philadelphia: Lippincott Williams & Wilkins, 2001.

Kandarpa K. and J.E. Aruny. *Handbook of Interventional Radiologic Procedures, Third Edition*. Philadelphia: Lippincott Williams & Wilkins, 2002.

Keats T.E. and C. Sistrom. *Atlas of Radiologic Measurement, Seventh Edition*. St. Louis, MO: Mosby, 2001.

Miller W.T. and W.T Miller, Jr. *Field Guide to the Chest X-Ray*. Baltimore: Lippincott Williams & Wilkins, 1999.

Silverman, P.M., ed. *Multislice Computed Tomography: A Practical Approach to Clinical Protocols*. Philadelphia: Lippincott Williams & Wilkins, 2002.

Grainger, R.G., D.J. Allison, A. Adam, and A.K. Dixon. *Grainger & Allison's Diagnostic Radiology: A Textbook of Medical Imaging, Fourth Edition*. Vols 1–3. London: Churchill Livingstone, 2001.

Lance, L.L. *Quick Look Drug Book 2003*. Baltimore: Lippincott Williams & Wilkins, 2003.

Stedman's Medical Dictionary, 28th Edition. Baltimore: Lippincott Williams & Wilkins, 2006.

Stedman's Radiology Words, Fifth Edition. Baltimore: Lippincott Williams & Wilkins, 2006.

Van Heertum, R.L. and R.S. Tikofsky. *Functional Cerebral SPECT and PET Imaging, Third Edition*. Philadelphia: Lippincott Williams & Wilkins, 2000.

Vera Pyle's Current Medical Terminology, Eighth Edition. Modesto, CA: Health Professions Institute, 2000.

Wahl, R.L. and J.W. Buchanan. *Principles and Practice of Positron Emission Tomography*. Philadelphia: Lippincott Williams & Wilkins, 2002.

Images

Agur, A.M.R. and M.J. Lee. *Grant's Atlas of Anatomy, 10th edition*. Baltimore: Lippincott Williams & Wilkins, 1999.

Hardy, Neil O. Westport, CT. From *Stedman's Medical Dictionary, 27th edition*. Baltimore: Lippincott Williams & Wilkins, 2000.

MediClip Human Anatomy 1–3, CD-ROM. Baltimore: Lippincott Williams & Wilkins.

Senkarik, Mikki. San Antonio, TX. From *Stedman's Medical Dictionary, 27th edition*. Baltimore: Lippincott Williams & Wilkins, 2000.

Journals

American Journal of Neuroradiology. Oak Brook, IL: American Society of Neuroradiology, 2002.

American Journal of Roentgenology. Leesburg, VA: American Roentgen Ray Society, 2002.

Clinical Nuclear Medicine. Philadelphia: Lippincott Williams & Wilkins, 2001–2008.

Contemporary Diagnostic Radiology. Baltimore: Lippincott Williams & Wilkins, 2001–2002.

Investigative Radiology. Philadelphia: Lippincott Williams & Wilkins, 2001–2008.

JAAMT. Modesto, CA: American Association for Medical Transcription, 2001–2002.

Journal of Computer Assisted Tomography. Philadelphia: Lippincott Williams & Wilkins, 2001–2008.

Journal of Thoracic Imaging. Philadelphia: Lippincott Williams & Wilkins, 2001–2002.

Journal of Vascular and Interventional Radiology. Philadelphia: Lippincott Williams & Wilkins, 2001–2002.

Journal of Women's Imaging. Philadelphia: Lippincott Williams & Wilkins, 2001–2002.

Latest Word. Philadelphia: Saunders, 1999–2002.

Perspectives on the Medical Transcription Profession. Modesto, CA: Health Professions Institute, 1999–2002.

Radiographics. Oak Brook, IL: Radiological Society of North America, 2001–2002.

Radiologic Technology. Albuquerque, NM: American Society of Radiologic Technologists, 2001–2002.

The Radiologist. Philadelphia: Lippincott Williams & Wilkins, 2001–2002.

Radiology. Richmond, VA: Radiological Society of North America, Inc., 2002.

Topics in Magnetic Resonance Imaging. Philadelphia: Lippincott Williams & Wilkins, 2001–2008.

Ultrasound Quarterly. Philadelphia: Lippincott Williams & Wilkins, 2001–2002.

Websites

http://gentili.net

http://radiology.rsnajnls.org

http://www.accessdata.fda.gov

http://www.ajnr.org

http://www.amershamhealth.com

http://www.bms.com

http://www.bracco.com

http://www.carpe-edatum.com

http://www.diagnosticimaging.com

http://www.drugs.com

http://www.egal.com

http://www.elsevier.com/wps/find/journaldescription.cws_home/623249/description#description

http://www.ezem.com

http://www.gemedicalsystems.com

http://www.hpisum.com/terms.html

References

http://www.iatrics.com
http://www.imageanalysis.com
http://www.link.springer.de
http://www.mallinckrodt.com
http://www.mtdesk.com
http://www.neurophysics.com
http://www.radiographics.org
http://www.rtstudents.com/radiology/radiology-abbreviations.htm

Å
  Angström
A
  amyloid A
  A level of esophagus
  mycalamide A
  A point
  psoralen and ultraviolet A (PUVA)
  A ring of esophagus
  A scan
AA
  acetabular anteversion
  aortic aneurysm
  ascending aorta
AAA
  abdominal aortic aneurysm
AAI
  ankle-arm index
  atlantoaxial instability
  axial acetabular index
    AAI rate-responsive mode
AAL
  anterior axillary line
AAN
  American Academy of Neurology
AAOS
  American Academy of Orthopaedic
  Surgeons
    AAOS acetabular abnormality
    classification
Aaron sign
AAS
  acute abdominal series
A1-A5 segment of anterior cerebral
  artery
ab
    a. externo laser sclerotomy
    a. interno laser sclerotomy
abampere
abandonment
    mode a.
abapical pole
ABBI
  advanced breast biopsy instrumentation
    ABBI system
Abbokinase
Abbott artery
abbreviated injury scale (AIS)
ABC
  aneurysmal bone cyst
  aortic-brachiocephalic
  argon beam coagulator
  automatic brightness control
abciximab

ABCS
  anatomic appearance and alignment,
  bony mineralization and texture,
  cartilage, and soft tissue
  abnormalities
    ABCS joint and bone lesions
abdomen
  distended a.
  flat plate of a.
  gasless a.
abdominal
  a. abscess
  a. adenopathy
  a. adhesion
  a. air collection
  a. aorta
  a. aorta thrombosis
  a. aortic aneurysm (AAA)
  a. aortic artery
  a. aortic coarctation
  a. aortic dissection
  a. aortic plexus
  a. aortography
  a. apron
  a. blunt trauma
  a. canal
  a. carcinomatosis
  a. cavity
  a. circumference
  a. collection of fluid
  a. compression cylinder
  a. contents
  a. CT scan
  a. distention
  a. ectopic pregnancy
  a. fat
  a. fibromatosis
  a. fissure
  a. fistula
  a. fluid wave
  a. gas
  a. girth
  a. great vessel
  a. heart
  a. hemorrhage
  a. heterotaxia
  a. hysterectomy
  a. inflammation
  a. irradiation
  a. kidney
  a. left ventricular assist device
    (ALVAD)
  a. lymph node
  a. lymphoma

abdominal (*continued*)
a. muscle deficiency syndrome
a. neurilemoma
a. paracentesis
a. pseudotumor
a. radiography
a. raphe
a. rhabdomyosarcoma
a. ring
a. sac
a. series
a. situs inversus
a. situs solitus
a. sonography
a. space
a. splenosis
a. stoma
a. tuberculosis
a. ultrasound
a. vascular accident
a. vertebra
a. view
a. visceral arteriography
a. viscus
a. wall calcification
a. wall defect
a. wall desmoid tumor
a. wall hernia
abdominogenital
abdominopelvic
a. actinomycosis
a. cavity
a. mass
a. viscus
abdominoperineal resection (APR)
abdominoscrotal
abdominothoracic
abdominovaginal
abdominovesical
abducens
abducted and externally rotated (ABER)
abduction
a. fracture
a. position
a. stress test
abduction-external
a.-e. rotation fracture
a.-e. rotation position
abductor
a. digiti quinti (ADQ)
a. digiti quinti muscle
a. digiti quinti tendon
a. hallucis muscle
a. hallucis tendon
a. pollicis brevis (APB)
a. pollicis brevis muscle
a. pollicis brevis tendon
a. pollicis longus (APL)
a. pollicis longus tendon

abductovalgus
hallux a.
abductus
pes a.
ABER
abducted and externally rotated
ABER position
aberrant
a. artery
a. band
a. bone marrow
a. bundle
a. ganglion
a. intrahepatic bile duct
a. origin
a. pancreas
a. papilla
a. right subclavian artery
a. spleen
a. tissue
a. umbilical
a. vascular channel
a. venous drainage
a. vessel
aberration
chromatid-type a.
intersegmental a.
intraventricular a.
ventricular a.
ABI
ankle-brachial index
ability
cardiac pumping a.
Ablatherm HIFU system
ablation
acetic acid injectable for tumor a.
Amazr radiofrequency catheter a.
ethanol a.
image-guided radiofrequency tumor a.
laparoscopic uterosacral nerve a. (LUNA)
laser thermal a. (LTA)
microwave endometrial a. (MEA)
MRI-guided laser thermal a.
percutaneous chemical a.
percutaneous radiofrequency catheter a.
percutaneous transluminal septal myocardial a. (PTSMA)
radioactive iodine a.
radiofrequency a. (RFA)
radiofrequency catheter a. (RFCA)
radiofrequency thermal a.
radiopharmaceutical a.
remnant a.
saline-enhanced radiofrequency tissue a.
small-volume tissue a.

A

soft tissue a.
stereotactic a.
thermal a.
total a.
transaortic radiofrequency a.
transapical endocardial a.
transcatheter a.
transseptal radiofrequency a.
transurethral needle a. (TUNA)
tumor a.
ultrasound-guided percutaneous
   interstitial laser a.
Urolase fiber laser a.

ablative laser therapy
abluminal
**AbMap electrophysiologic imaging
   system**
ABMMN
   autologous bone marrow mononuclear
      ABMMN cell
      ABMMN cell-based therapy
ABMT
   autologous bone marrow transplant
abnormal
   a. adherence of placenta
   a. bright signal
   a. cisterna magna
   a. dimension of cardiac chamber
   a. ejection fraction response
   a. esophageal fold
   a. esophageal peristalsis
   a. heart chamber dimension
   a. lung opacity
   a. lung pattern
   a. ossification
   a. pancreatobiliary junction (APBJ)
   a. peristaltic esophagus
   a. placenta size
   a. position of foot
   a. small bowel fold
   a. tissue
   a. tissue uptake
   a. tracer accumulation
   a. tracking
   a. tubular function
   a. umbilical cord attachment
abnormality
   accumulation a.
   anatomic appearance and alignment,
      bony mineralization and texture,
      cartilage, and soft tissue a.'s
      (ABCS)
   arch of aorta a.
   bony a.
   bulbar a.
   calyceal a.
   cardiopulmonary a.
   congenital a.
   congruent signal intensity a.

definitive a.
drug-induced brain a.
dyskinetic segmental wall motion a.
facial a.
fetal a.
focal limb a.
focal metabolic a.
focal wall motion a.
focal white matter signal a.
functional a.
gestational sac a.
global wall motion a.
gray matter a.
gyral a.
high-signal a.
hyperkinetic segmental wall motion
   a.
hypokinetic segmental wall motion
   a.
ileocecal valve a.
interstitial a.
intracranial vascular a.
labeling a.
left ventricular regional wall motion
   a.
limb reduction a.
mesenchymal a.
microcirculation a.
migration a.
mucosal a.
obstructive a.
osseous a.
paraspinal a.
perfusion a.
placentation a.
pulmonary interstitial a.
regional perfusion a.
restrictive a.
reticular a.
rostrocaudal extent signal a.
screening-detected a.
segmental bronchus perfusion a.
snowman a.
soft tissue a.
spinal cord injury without
   radiographic a. (SCIWORA)
stellate a.
structural a.
subsegmental perfusion a.
torsion a.
tracer a.
ultrastructural a.
urachal a.
vascular a.
vertebral border a.
vertebral endplate a.
vessel wall a.
wall motion a. (WMA)
white matter a.

abnormally thin skull
aborad, aboral
    a. direction
aboral (*var. of* aborad)
abortive neurofibromatosis
above
    a. diaphragm
    a. elbow (AE)
    a. selected threshold (AST)
above-knee amputation (AKA)
ABPA
    allergic bronchopulmonary aspergillosis
ABR
    artery-bronchus ratio
Abrahams sign
Abrams biopsy needle
abrasion
    cortical a.
    subperiosteal cortical a.
abrasor
Abrikosov tumor
abruption
    placental a.
abruptio placentae
abrupt vessel closure
abscess
    abdominal a.
    actinomycotic brain a.
    acute a.
    amebic a.
    anaerobic lung a.
    anular a.
    aortic anulus a.
    appendiceal a.
    Aspergillus cerebral a.
    atheromatous a.
    bilateral iliopsoas a.'s
    bone a.
    brain a.
    breast a.
    Brodie metaphysial a.
    cerebral a.
    chronic breast a.
    cold breast a.
    cold spine a.
    collagen brain a.
    collar-button a.
    Corynebacterium brain a.
    crypt a.
    cuff a.
    daughter a.
    deep interloop a.
    deep pelvic a.
    diverticular a.
    a. drainage catheter
    echinococcal a.
    encapsulated brain a.
    enteroperitoneal a.
    epidural a.

    extradural a.
    a. formation
    frontal a.
    gallbladder wall a.
    granulomatous brain a.
    growth plate a.
    hepatic a.
    horseshoe a.
    iliac fossa a.
    iliopsoas a.
    interloop a.
    intermesenteric a.
    intersphincteric a.
    intraabdominal a.
    intradural a.
    intrahepatic a.
    intramesenteric a.
    intraosseous a.
    intraperitoneal a.
    intrascrotal a.
    ischiorectal a.
    kidney a.
    lacunar a.
    lesser sac a.
    liver a.
    lung a.
    mediastinal a.
    metaphysial a.
    midpalmar a.
    Nocardia brain a.
    orbital a.
    ovarian a.
    Paget a.
    pancreatic a.
    paracolic a.
    parapharyngeal a.
    pararectal a.
    pararenal a.
    paraspinal a.
    parotid a.
    partial pericardial a.
    pelvic a.
    perianal a.
    periappendiceal a.
    pericecal a.
    pericholecystic a.
    pericolic a.
    pericolonic a.
    perihepatic a.
    perinephritic a.
    periprosthetic a.
    perirectal a.
    perirenal a.
    peritoneal a.
    pharyngeal a.
    phlegmonous a.
    postchemoembolization liver a.
    Pott a.
    premasseteric space a.

prevertebral a.
prostate a.
psoas a.
pulmonary a.
pulp a.
pyogenic brain a.
pyogenic liver a.
renal a.
retropharyngeal a.
scrotal a.
soft tissue a.
space of Retzius a.
spinal epidural a. (SEA)
splenic a.
Staphylococcus brain a.
sternal a.
subaponeurotic a.
subdiaphragmatic a.
subdural a.
subgalcal a.
subhepatic a.
subperiosteal a.
subphrenic a.
subungual a.
testicular a.
thecal a.
thenar space a.
thyroid a.
tuberculous a.
tuboovarian a. (TOA)
ventral epidural a.
walled-off a.
Abscession drainage catheter
abscessogram
abscissa
abscission needle
absconsio
abscopal effect
absence
congenital pericardial a.
limb a.
a. of haustral marking
a. of innominate line
a. of outer end of clavicle
a. of primary peristalsis
a. of spleen
a. of uptake
a. of vascular marking
partial pericardial a.
a. seizure
absent
a. aortic knob
a. bow-tie sign
a. bronchial cartilage
a. diaphragm sign
a. greater sphenoid wing
a. kidney
a. kidney outline

a. lower esophageal sphincter
relaxation
a. peripheral vein
a. peristalsis
a. radiotracer uptake
a. runoff
a. valve
a. ventricle
absolute
a. artery dimension
a. blood flow
a. curative resection
a. dose intensity (ADI)
a. efficiency
a. emission probability
a. function quantitation
a. granulocyte count
a. linearity
a. noncurative resection
a. peak efficiency calibration
a. percentage loss of enhancement
(APLE)
absorb
absorbance, absorbancy, absorbency
absorbancy (*var. of* absorbance)
absorbed
a. dose
a. dose range
a. fraction
absorbency (*var. of* absorbance)
absorbent
a. gland
a. vessel
absorptiometer
single-energy x-ray a. (SXA)
absorptiometry
dual-energy x-ray a. (DEXA,
DXA)
dual-photon a. (DPA)
morphometric x-ray a.
peripheral dual-energy x-ray a.
(pDEXA)
single-photon a. (SPA)
absorption
a. atelectasis
a. band
bone radiation a.
broad-beam a.
a. cavity
a. cell
a. chromatography
a. coefficient
a. collapse
electromagnetic a.
external a.
interstitial a.
laser energy a.
a. line
a. of radionuclide

absorption (*continued*)
    photoelectric a.
    radiofrequency a.
    radioiron oral a.
    ratio of photoelectric to Compton a.
    a. spectrophotometer
    a. unsharpness
    a. x-ray spectrum
absorptive
absorptivity
abut
abutment
abutting
AC
    acromioclavicular
    alternating current
    anterior commissure
ACA
    anterior cerebral artery
ACAD
    atherosclerotic carotid artery
    disease
**Academy of Radiology Research
(ARR)**
acalculia
acalculous
    a. biliary disease
    a. cholecystitis
acallosal
acanthocytosis
acantholysis
acanthomeatal line
acanthosis
    glycogenic a.
    a. nigricans
acanthotic
acardia
ACAT
    automated computed axial tomography
ACBE
    air-contrast barium enema
accelerated
    a. atherosclerosis
    a. fractionation
    a. hyperfractionation
    a. particle
    a. peristalsis
    a. phase
    a. phase gain
    a. silicosis
acceleration
    fetal growth a.
    flow a.
    growth a.
    a. index (AI)
    a. map
    a. time
accelerator
    alpha-particle a.

    dedicated linear a.
    dual-energy linear a.
    electron linear a.
    a. factor
    high-energy bent-beam linear a.
    linear a. (LINAC)
    a. mass spectrometry (AMS)
    microtron a.
    modified linear a.
    particle a.
    Philips linear a.
    racetrack microtron a.
    Siemens Mevatron 74 linear a.
    University of Florida linear a.
    Varian a.
Accel stopcock
accentuation
    a. of marking
    paramagnetic enhancement a.
access
    arterial a.
    central venous a.
    femoral a.
    intravenous a.
    jugular venous a.
    a. loop
    a. set
accessory
    a. adhesion molecule
    a. atlantoaxial ligament
    a. atrium
    a. azygos fissure
    BabyFace 3D surface rendering a.
    a. bile duct
    a. blood supply
    a. breast
    a. cephalic vein
    a. communicating tendon
    a. cusp
    a. diaphragm
    a. digit
    extravasation detection a.
    a. hemiazygos vein
    a. hemidiaphragm
    a. hepatic duct
    a. hepatic vein
    a. lobe
    a. lymph node
    a. middle cerebral artery
    a. multangular bone
    a. muscle
    a. nasal cartilage
    a. navicular bone
    a. nerve
    a. neuroenteric canal
    a. organ
    a. ossicle
    a. ossification center
    a. pancreas

a. pancreatic duct
a. placenta
a. process
a. right renal artery
a. right uterine artery
a. saphenous vein
a. sesamoid bone
a. sinus
a. spleen
a. thyroid gland
a. tubercle
a. ureteral bud
a. vertebral vein

accident
abdominal vascular a.
cardiovascular a. (CVA)
cerebrovascular a. (CVA)

accidental
a. correction
a. intradural injection

accompanying vein

accordion
a. fold
a. sign
a. vertebra

accordion-shaped pleat

accreta
placenta a.

Accuclot D-dimer assay

Accucore II biopsy needle

accuDEXA
a. bone densitometer
a. bone mineral density assessment
system

AccuLase excimer laser

**AccuLength arthroplasty measuring
system**

Acculink stent

accumulation
a. abnormality
abnormal tracer a.
dependent extracellular
fluid a.
fluid a.
intratumoral a.
nonspecific a.
a. of gas
parenchymatous tracer a.
a. phase
radioactive a.
radiotracer a.
residual urine a.
Thorotrast a.
tracer a.

Accunet distal protection device

AccuProbe

accuracy calibrator

AccuView computer workstation

Accu-Vu sizing catheter

ACD
annihilation coincidence detection
anterior capsular distance

ACE
angiotensin-converting enzyme
ACE inhibition renography
ACE inhibition scintigraphy

aceruloplasminemia

acetabula (*pl. of* acetabulum)

acetabular
a. anteversion (AA)
a. bone
a. cavity
a. cup
a. depth
a. depth to femoral head diameter
(AD/FHD)
a. fossa
a. head index (AIII)
a. labrum
a. line
a. posterior wall fracture
a. protrusion
a. reconstruction plate
a. residual dysplasia
a. rim fracture
a. roof
a. sector angle
a. shell
a. teardrop figure

acetabular-prosthetic interface

acetabuli
protrusio a.

acetabulum (*pl.* acetabula)
cartilaginous a.
deep-shelled a.
os a.
Y-shaped a.

acetazolamide
a. challenge brain SPECT imaging
a. dual-isotope image
a. renography
a. vasodilator test

acetazolamide-enhanced SPECT

acetic acid injectable for tumor ablation

acetrizoate
a. contrast agent
meglumine a.
a. sodium

acetylated

acetylation

acetylator

acetylsalicylic acid

ACF
anterior cervical fusion

ACG
angiocardiogram
angiocardiography
apexcardiogram

achalasia
> cricopharyngeal a.
> megaesophagus of a.
> a. of esophagus
> primary a.
> secondary a.
> ureteral a.
> vigorous a.

acheiria

achievable
> as low as reasonably a.
> (ALARA)

Achiever balloon dilation catheter

Achilles
> A. bursa
> A. densitometer
> A. tendinitis
> A. tendon
> A. tendon rupture
> A. tendon shortening
> A. tendon xanthoma

Achillis
> tendo A.

acholangic biliary cirrhosis

achondrogenesis

achondroplasia

achondroplastic dwarfism

achoresis

acid
> acetylsalicylic a.
> ametriodinic a.
> amidotrizoic a.
> azelaic a.
> benzoic a.
> betamethyliodophenyl pentadecanoic a. (BMIPP)
> beta-oxybutyric a.
> butyl iminodiacetic a.
> chenodeoxycholic a.
> chromium-hepatic dimethyl iminodiacetic a. (Cr-HIDA)
> deoxyribonucleic a. (DNA)
> diethylenetriamine pentaacetic a. (DTPA)
> diisopropyl iminodiacetic a. (DISIDA)
> dimercaptosuccinic a. (DMSA)
> dimethyl iminodiacetic a. (DIDA)
> dimethylsuccinic a.
> ethylenediamine tetramethylene phosphoric a. (EDTMP)
> ^{18}F-fluoro-6-thia-heptadecanoic a. (FTHA)
> ^{18}F-labeled fatty a.
> flavone acetic a. (FAA)
> free fatty a. (FFA)
> gadolinium-diethylenetriamine pentaacetic a. (Gd-DTPA)
> gadolinium-ethoxybenzyl-diethylenetriamine pentaacetic a. (Gd-EOB-DTPA)
> gadolinium ethylenediamine tetraacetic a.
> gadolinium-hepatoiminodiacetic a. (Gd-HIDA)
> gadolinium tetraazacyclododecanetetraacetic a. (Gd-DOTA)
> gadopentetic a.
> gadoxetic a.
> gamma-aminobutyric a. (GABA)
> glacial acetic a.
> glucoheptanoic a. (GHA)
> hepatoiminodiacetic a. (HIDA)
> homovanillic a. (HVA)
> hydroxyethylidene-1,1-diphosphonic a.
> 5-hydroxyindoleacetic a. (5-HIAA)
> ^{123}I heptadecanoic a.
> iminodiacetic a. (IDA)
> iobenzamic a.
> iocarmic a.
> iocetamic a.
> iodine-123 iodophenyl pentadecanoic a. (^{123}I-IPPA, I-123 IPPA)
> iodoalphionic a.
> iodopanoic a.
> iodophenyl pentadecanoic a.
> ioglycamic a.
> iopanoic a.
> iophenoxic a.
> iothalamic a.
> ioxaglic a.
> long-chain fatty a.
> meclofenamic a.
> mefenamic a.
> metrizoic a.
> ^{99m}Tc-labeled iminodiacetic a.
> mycophenolic a.
> nonesterified fatty a. (NEFA)
> okadaic a.
> ophenoxic a.
> palmitic a.
> paraaminobenzoic a.
> paraaminohippuric a.
> paraaminosalicylic a. (PAS)
> paraisopropyliminodiacetic a. (PIPIDA)
> phenoxyacetic a.
> polylactic a.
> a. reflux
> ribonucleic a. (RNA)
> technetium hepatoiminodiacetic a. (TcHIDA)
> technetium 99m diethylenetriamine pentaacetic a. (^{99m}Tc-DTPA)

technetium 99m dimercaptosuccinic
a. (^{99m}Tc-DMSA)
tetraazacyclododecanetetraacetic a.
(DOTA)
tricarboxylic a. (TCA)
trichloroacetic a.
triiodobenzoic a.

acid-bismethylamide
dysprosium-diethylenetriamine
pentaacetic a.-b.
gadolinium-diethylenetriamine
pentaacetic a.-b. (Gd-DTPA-BMA)

acidemia
organic a.

acidophilic
a. adenoma
a. pituitary tumor

acid-peptic ulcer
acid-Schiff
periodic a.-S.

acid-Schiff-positive
aciduria
glutaric a. (type I, II)

acinar
a. adenocarcinoma
a. airspace disease
a. collapse
a. nodule
a. pancreatic cell carcinoma
a. pattern
a. sarcoidosis
a. tuberculosis

acinarization
acini (*pl. of* acinus)
acinic
a. cell adenocarcinoma
a. cell carcinoma
a. cell tumor

acinous adenoma
acinus, *pl.* **acini**
pulmonary a.

ACIS
adenocarcinoma in situ
automated cellular imaging
system

ACIST
angiographic contrast injection
system technology

ACJ
acromioclavicular joint

Ackerman
A. bone biopsy set
A. criteria for osteomyelitis

Ackrad balloon-bearing catheter
ACL
anterior cruciate ligament

aclasis
diaphysial a.
tarsoepiphysial a.

ACM
automated cardiac flow measurement
ACM ultrasound

Acoma portable x-ray machine
acoprosis
acoustic, acoustical
a. artifact
a. canal
a. crest
a. cyst
a. enhancement
a. gel
a. imaging
a. impedance
a. interface
a. lens
a. meatus
a. nerve
a. nerve sheath tumor
a. neuroma
a. papilla
a. penetration
a. pressure
a. pressure amplitude
a. quantification
a. reflection method
a. response technology
a. schwannoma
a. shadow
a. standoff
a. trauma
a. tubercle
a. velocity
a. vesicle
a. wave
a. window

acoustical (*var. of* acoustic)
acousticofacial
a. crest
a. ganglion

AC-PC
anterior commissure-posterior
commissure
AC-PC line
AC-PC plane
AC-PC referenced MR imaging

ACPL
antibody-conjugated paramagnetic
liposome

AC 3 plate reader
AcQsim CT simulator
acquired
a. acroosteolysis
a. adult Fanconi syndrome
a. aortic valve stenosis
a. atelectasis
a. bronchiectasis
a. cystic kidney disease
a. epidermoid

acquired (*continued*)
- a. fragility
- a. hepatic cyst
- a. hepatocerebral degeneration
- a. hydrocephalus
- a. immunity
- a. immunodeficiency syndrome (AIDS)
- a. intestinal lymphangiectasis
- a. left ventricular aneurysm
- a. lobar emphysema
- a. megacolon
- a. mitral stenosis
- a. occupational lung disease
- a. porencephaly
- a. radiation resistance
- a. renal cystic disease
- a. spinal stenosis
- a. tracheobronchomalacia
- a. unilateral hyperlucent lung
- a. uremic cystic kidney disease
- a. urethral diverticulum

acquisition
- biphasic a.
- cine a.
- combined dynamic 2D and bolus-chase 3D a.
- continuous volumetric a.
- data a.
- 3D fast low-angle shot a.
- 2D fast spin-echo a.
- 3D fast spin-echo a.
- 3D FLASH a.
- double-helix a.
- dynamic a.
- electronic picture a.
- elliptic centric a.
- fast imaging employing steady-state a. (FIESTA)
- fast spin-echo a.
- FLASH a.
- generalized autocalibrating partial parallel a. (GRAPPA)
- gradient a.
- image a.
- interleaved image a.
- long-axis a.
- a. matrix
- multigated a. (MUGA)
- multiple overlapping thin-slab a. (MOTSA)
- multiple-slice a.
- multiple thin-slab a. (MTSA)
- multisection multirepetition a.
- multislice a.
- off-axis rotational a.
- a. optimization
- polarity-altered spectral-selective a.
- primary digital a.
- prone PET breast a.
- reduced a.
- rest image a.
- segmented k-space data a.
- sequential image a.
- short-axis a.
- signal a.
- simultaneous multislice a.
- 4-slice a.
- small-voxel a.
- spirometric a.
- 1st-pass a.
- stress image a.
- a. technique
- thin-slab coronal a.
- a. time
- T1-weighted a.
- volume a.
- volumetric a.
- whole-brain a.
- a. window

acquisitions
- multiple gated a. (MUGA)

ACR
- American College of Radiology
- ACR rate
- ACR teleradiology standard

acrania

Acrel ganglion

acridine orange

acrocephalosyndactylia (*var. of* acrocephalosyndactyly)

acrocephalosyndactyly, acrocephalosyndactylia
- Pfeiffer a.
- Saethre-Chotzen a.

acrodermatitis enteropathica

acrodysostosis

acrofacial

acrokeratosis

acromegalia (*var. of* acromegaly)

acromegaly, acromegalia

acromelia

acromelic
- a. dwarfism
- a. dysplasia

acromesomelic dysplasia

acromial
- a. angle
- a. articular surface
- a. bone
- a. slope
- a. spur

acromiale
- os a.

acromicria

acromioclavicular (AC)
- a. articulation
- a. injury classification

a. joint (ACJ)
a. joint disc
a. joint separation
a. ligament
a. space
acromiocoracoid ligament
acromiohumeral
a. distance
a. interval (AHI)
acromion
cupping of a.
hooked a.
a. process
acromutilation
acroosteolysis
acquired a.
acroosteosclerosis
acropachy
thyroid a.
acropachyderma
acroparesthesia
acropectorovertebral dysplasia
acrosomal vesicle
acrosyndactyly
acrylic
a. microsphere
a. syringe shield
ACS
Advanced Cardiovascular Systems
American Cancer Society
ACS balloon catheter
ACS Concorde catheter
ACS Endura coronary dilation
catheter
ACS OTW Photon coronary
dilation catheter
ACS RX Comet coronary dilation
catheter
ACS Tourguide II guiding catheter
ACS-grade pyridine
ACS-NT
Gyroscan ACS-NT
act
Mammography Quality Standards A.
(MQSA)
ACTH
adrenocorticotropic hormone
ACTH-producing tumor
actinic
a. granuloma
a. ray
a. reticuloid
actinium emanation
Actinomyces israelii
actinomycetes
thermophilic a.
actinomycosis
abdominopelvic a.
retroperitoneal a.

actinomycotic
a. brain abscess
a. infection
action
phase-specific a.
a. space
Activase
Cathflo A.
activated
a. atom
a. partial thromboplastin time
a. voxel cluster
activation
a. analysis
compensatory cortical a.
a. factor
a. pattern
PMC a.
premotor coret a.
region of a.
a. sequence mapping
activation-induced uncoupling of cerebral oxygen
activator
alteplase recombinant tissue
plasminogen a.
recombinant tissue plasminogen a.
tissue plasminogen a.
tissue-type plasminogen a.
active
a. acquired immunity
a. biplanar MR imaging guidance
a. congestion
a. duodenal ulcer
a. emptying fraction
a. hyperemia
a. infiltrate
a. mode
a. MRI stent (AMRIS)
a. needle tip
a. osteomyelitis
a. parenchymal disease
a. precordium
a. shielding
a. shimming
activity
ankylosing spondylitis spine MRI
score for a.
a. assessment
background a.
biliary excretion bowel a.
blood pool a.
body background a.
bone morphogenetic a.
brain a.
colonic a.
cortical a.
crossover of a.
decreased a.

activity (*continued*)
dihydropyrimidine dehydrogenase a.
early bladder a.
electrical a.
extrapulmonary a.
increased tracer a.
lung-heart ratio of thallium-201 a.
mast cell-enhancing a.
normalized to plasma a.
osseous a.
osteoblastic a.
peak parenchymatous a.
peristaltic a.
physiologic high a.
problematic abdominal a.
radiotracer a.
reflux a.
retained cortical a. (RCA)
scatter a.
slow-wave a.
specific a.
time to peak a.
tracer a.
ventricular ectopic a. (VEA)
actocardiotocograph monitor
actuator
linear a.
acuminatum
papilloma a.
urethral condyloma a.
AcuNav ultrasound catheter
acupuncture laser
Acuson
A. 128 apparatus
A. computed sonography
A. 128 Doppler ultrasound
A. 128EP imager
A. 128EP scanner
A. linear-array transducer
A. 5-MHz linear array
A. P10 handheld diagnostic
ultrasound system
A. Sequoia 512 scanner
A. transvaginal sonography
A. V5M monitor
A. V5M multiplane transesophageal
echocardiographic transducer
A. XP 10 scanner
A. 128XP transducer
A. 128XP ultrasound system
acute
a. abdominal obstruction
a. abdominal series (AAS)
a. abscess
a. alveolar hypoperfusion
a. alveolar infiltrate
a. aortic pathology
a. atelectasis
a. atherothrombotic event

a. avulsion fracture
a. basophilic leukemia
a. berylliosis
a. central cord syndrome
a. cerebellar hemispheric lesions
a. cerebral infarct imaging
a. cerebrovascular insufficiency
a. chest syndrome
a. cholecystitis
a. compartment syndrome
a. compression triad
a. cortical necrosis
a. diffuse bacterial nephritis
a. diffuse interstitial fibrosis
a. disease
a. disseminated encephalomyelitis
(ADEM)
a. diverticulitis
a. eosinophilic pneumonia
a. erosive gastritis (AEG)
a. esophagitis
a. extrinsic allergic alveolitis
a. focal bacterial nephritis
a. focal bacterial pyelonephritis
a. glomerulonephritis
a. heart failure
a. hematogenous osteomyelitis
(AHO)
a. hemodynamic overload
a. hemorrhagic leukoencephalitis
a. hepatitis
a. hydrocephalus
a. hydronephrosis
a. idiopathic hemorrhage (AIPH)
a. inflammatory demyelinating
polyradiculopathy
a. interosseous disc herniation
a. interstitial lung edema
a. interstitial nephritis (AIN)
a. interstitial pneumonia (AIP)
a. interstitial pneumonitis
a. intramural hematoma
a. ischemic brain infarct
a. juvenile cirrhosis
a. laminar necrosis
a. leg ischemia
a. lethal carditis
a. lung stiffness
a. lymphoblastic leukemia
a. lymphoblastic lymphoma
a. lymphocytic leukemia
a. marginal branch
a. mediastinal widening
a. mediastinitis
a. mesenteric ischemia (AMI)
a. monoblastic leukemia
a. myeloblastic leukemia
a. myelocytic leukemia
a. myelofibrosis

a. myelogenous leukemia (AML)
a. myeloid leukemia
a. myocardial infarct
a. native kidney tubular necrosis
a. nonhemorrhagic infarct
a. nonsuppurative ascending
  cholangitis
a. obstructive cholangitis
a. on chronic fracture
a. pancreatitis
a. peptic ulcer
a. phase of inflammation
a. pleurisy
a. posttraumatic myelopathy
a. promyelocytic leukemia
a. pulmonary edema
a. pyogenic spondylitis
a. radiation injury
a. radiation pneumonitis
a. radiation syndrome (ARS)
a. renal failure (ARF)
a. renal infarct
a. renal transplant tubular necrosis
a. renal vein thrombosis
a. respiratory distress syndrome
  (ARDS)
a. respiratory failure (ARF)
a. retroviral syndrome
a. sclerosing hyaline necrosis
  (ASHN)
a. silicoproteinosis
a. sinusitis
a. splenic tumor
a. sprain
a. stretch injury
a. subarachnoid hemorrhage
a. subdural hematoma
a. suppurative appendicitis
a. suppurative ascending cholangitis
a. suppurative pyelonephritis
a. suppurative sialadenitis
a. suppurative thyroiditis
a. testicular torsion
a. thoracic aortic injury
a. thromboembolic pulmonary
  arterial hypertension
a. transverse myelitis
a. traumatic aortic injury (ATAI)
a. tubular necrosis (ATN)
a. tumor lysis
a. varicella infection
a. vertebral collapse
AcuTect imaging agent
acutely symptomatic scrotum
ACV
  adaptive cardiac volume
    ACV reconstruction
acyanotic congenital heart disease
acyl CoA oxidase deficiency

ADAC MCD Vertex Plus MCD gamma
  camera
adactylia (*var. of* adactyly)
adactyly, adactylia
adamantinoma of long bone
adamantinomatous craniopharyngioma
Adamkiewicz
  arteria radicularis magna of A.
  A. artery
Adams-Stokes syndrome
adapted standard mammography unit
adapter, adaptor
  ventricle impedance a.
adaptic detector configuration
adaptive
  a. cardiac volume (ACV)
  a. cardiac volume reconstruction
  a. carpus
  a. correction
  a. focusing technology (AFT)
  a. hyperplasia
  a. hypertrophy
  a. noise reduction filter
adaptor
  Tuohy-Borst a.
ADC
  analogue-to-digital converter
  apparent diffusion coefficient
  ADC decline
  ADC map
  ADC quantization error
ADCav value
Addison
  A. disease
  A. point
additive solution
add-on
  A.-O. Bucky direct x-ray detector
  A.-O. Bucky image acquisition
    system
  A.-O. Bucky radiographer detector
    image
  a.-o. stereotactic unit
  a.-o. technique
adducta
  coxa a.
adducted thumb
adduction
  a. fracture
  a. frame
  a. position
  a. stress
  a. to neutral
adductor
  a. canal
  a. canal syndrome
  a. hallucis
  a. hallucis tendon
  a. hiatus

adductor (*continued*)
    a. insertion avulsion syndrome
    a. longus
    a. magnus
    a. magnus muscle
    a. muscle strain
    a. pollicis
    a. pollicis brevis tendon
    a. sweep of thumb
    a. tubercle
adductus
    metatarsus a.
    pes a.
    true metatarsus a. (TMA)
ADEM
    acute disseminated encephalomyelitis
adenitis
    cervical lymph node tuberculous a.
    mesenteric a.
    sclerosing a.
adenoacanthoma
    endometrial a.
adenocarcinoma
    acinar a.
    acinic cell a.
    ampullary a.
    bronchiolar a.
    cervical a.
    colloid a.
    colorectal a.
    cystic a.
    distal rectal a. (DRA)
    ductal pancreatic a.
    duct cell a.
    duodenal a.
    endometrial secretory a.
    esophageal a.
    exophytic a.
    fetal a.
    gastric a.
    gastrointestinal tract a.
    giant cell a.
    hepatoid a.
    infiltrating a.
    a. in situ (ACIS)
    intraluminal a.
    kidney a.
    lung a.
    medullary-type a.
    metastatic a.
    moderately differentiated a.
    mucinous a.
    mucinous cyst a.
    mucin-producing a.
    nonmucinous a.
    a. of unknown primary syndrome
    a. of uterus
    pancreatic ductal a.
    papillary serous a.

    poorly differentiated a. (PDA)
    renal a.
    scarring a.
    scirrhous infiltrating a.
    secretory a.
    serous a.
    sinonasal a.
    small bowel a.
    stomach a.
    ulcerating a.
    urinary bladder a.
    vulvar adenoid cystic a.
    well-differentiated fetal a. (WDFA)
adenocystic carcinoma
adenofibroma
adenofibromyoma
adenography
adenohypophyseal (*var. of* adenohypophysial)
adenohypophysial, adenohypophyseal
adenohypophysis
adenoid
    a. cystic carcinoma parotitis
    a. cystic lung carcinoma
    a. hypertrophy
    a. squamous cell carcinoma
    a. tonsil
    a. tumor
adenoidal-nasopharyngeal ratio
adenoleiomyofibroma
adenolipoma
adenolymphoma
adenoma, *pl.* **adenomas,** *pl.* **adenomata**
    acidophilic a.
    acinous a.
    adnexal a.
    adrenal a.
    adrenocortical a.
    apocrine a.
    autonomous thyroid a.
    basal cell a.
    basophilic brain a.
    benign oxyphilic a.
    bile duct a. (BDA)
    bronchial a.
    bronchoalveolar cell a.
    bronchogenic a.
    Brunner gland a.
    carcinoma ex pleomorphic a.
    carotid sheath a.
    colloid a.
    colonic a.
    colorectal a.
    cortical a.
    cutaneous a.
    cystic a.
    descended superior parathyroid a.
    ductal a.
    ectopic parathyroid a.
    embryonal a.

eosinophilic brain a.
fetal a.
fibroid a.
flat a.
follicular thyroid a.
Fuchs a.
functioning pituitary a.
gallbladder a.
giant cervical parathyroid a.
giant parathyroid a.
giant villous a.
glycoprotein-secreting a.
gonadotroph cell a.
gonadotropin-secreting a.
growth hormone-producing a.
hepatic a.
hepatocellular a.
Hürthle cell a.
inferior parathyroid a.
intraspinal a.
intrathymic parathyroid a.
intrathyroid superior parathyroid a.
kidney a.
lactating a.
Leydig cell a.
liver cell a.
macrocystic a.
malignant pleomorphic a.
a. malignum
mediastinal parathyroid a.
microcystic a.
mucinous a.
multifocal autonomic a.
nephrogenic bladder a.
nonfunctioning pituitary a.
nonhyperfunctioning adrenal a.
a. of breast
a. of nipple
oncocytic thyroid a.
oxyphilic a.
pancreatic macrocystic a.
pancreatic microcystic a.
papillary cystic a.
parathyroid a.
parotid pleomorphic a.
Pick tubular a.
pituitary a.
pleomorphic lung a.
polypoid a.
prostatic a.
proximal tubular a.
renal cortical a.
retrotracheal a.
sebaceous a.
a. sebaceum
sessile a.
silent parathyroid a.
small bowel a.
solitary a.

superior parathyroid a. (SPA)
supernumerary parathyroid a.
suprasellar a.
sweat duct a.
testicular tubular a.
thyroid a.
thyrotroph cell a.
toxic a.
tubulovillous colon a.
villotubular a.
villous a.
well-differentiated a.
adenoma-associated calcification
adenomas (*pl. of* adenoma)
adenomata (*pl. of* adenoma)
adenomatoid
    a. malformation
    a. odontogenic tumor
adenomatosis
adenomatous
    a. goiter
    a. hyperplasia
    a. nodule
    a. polyp
adenomyoma
adenomyomatosis
adenomyosarcoma
adenomyosis
    diffuse a.
    ureteral a.
    uterine a.
adenopapillomatosis
    gastric a.
adenopathy
    abdominal a.
    axillary a.
    bilateral hilar a.
    cervical a.
    hemorrhagic mediastinal a.
    hilar a.
    hypermetabolic a.
    infradiaphragmatic a.
    jugular chain a.
    mediastinal a.
    mesenteric a.
    metastatic a.
    paratracheal a.
    postinflammatory a.
    pulmonary a.
    reticulation with hilar a.
    retrocrural a.
    retroperitoneal a.
    sandwich configuration a.
    secondary axillary a.
    supradiaphragmatic a.
    thoracic a.
    tuberculous mediastinal a.
    widespread hyperattenuating
      mediastinal a.

adenosarcoma
  breast a.
Adenoscan imaging agent
adenosine
  a. echocardiogram
  a. echocardiography
  a. stress imaging
  a. stress imaging agent
  a. triphosphate
adenosis
  breast a.
  microglandular a.
  radiation-induced sclerosing a.
  sclerosing a.
adenosquamous carcinoma
adenovirus
  genetically engineered oncolytic a.
  Onyx-015 genetically engineered a.
  a. pneumonia
adequate
  a. cardiac output
  a. contention
  a. coronary perfusion
  a. stroke volume
AD/FHD
  acetabular depth to femoral head
    diameter
adherence factor
adherent
  a. pericardium
  a. placenta
  a. profundus tendon
  a. thrombus
adhesed
adhesion
  abdominal a.
  attic a.
  bandlike a.
  fibrous pleural a.
  inflammatory a.
  intraarticular a.
  pericardial diaphragmatic a.
  peritendinous a.
  pleuropericardial a.
  pleuropulmonary a.
  subacromial bursa a.
  subdeltoid bursa a.
adhesive
  a. arachnoiditis
  a. atelectasis
  a. bursitis
  a. capsulitis
  cyanoacrylate tissue a.
  a. ileus
  a. inflammation
  Neuroacryl tissue a.
  a. periarthritis
  a. platelet
  tissue a.

ADI
  absolute dose intensity
  atlantodens interval
adiabatic
  a. demagnetization
  a. demagnetization in rotating frame
    (ADRF)
  a. fast passage
  a. fast scanning technique
  a. inversion pulse
  a. off-resonance spin locking
  a. rapid passage (ARP)
  a. slice-selective radiofrequency
    pulse
adiadochokinesia
adipiodone
adipose
  a. fold
  a. fossa
  a. ligament
  a. tissue
  a. tumor
  uptake in supraclavicular a. (USA)
adiposogenital dystrophy
adiposum
  cor a.
aditus (*pl.* **aditus**)
  a. ad antrum
  a. ad pelvem
  a. orbitae
  a. pelvis
  a. vaginae
adjacent
  a. edema
  a. field x-ray dosimetry
  a. organ
  a. voxel
adjunctive
  a. mechanical thrombectomy
  a. surgical bypass
  a. therapy
adjustment
  Bonferroni a.
  photomultiplier gain a.
adjuvant
  a. analgesic drug
  a. chronotherapy
  a. irradiation
  a. radiation
  a. therapy
adjuvanticity
admaxillary gland
admedial, admedian
admedian (*var. of* admedial)
adminicula (*pl. of* adminiculum)
adminiculum, *pl.* **adminicula**
  a. lineae albae
administration
  competitive iron a.

contrast a.
drug a.
Food and Drug A. (FDA)
intralymphatic radioactivity a.
intraperitoneal drug a.
A. of Radioactive Substances
  Advisory Committee (ARSAC)
vasodilator a.

admixture lesion

adnexa
ocular a.
transposed a.

adnexal
a. adenoma
a. carcinoma
a. condition
a. cyst
a. embryo
a. metastasis
a. torsion

adolescent
a. hallux valgus
a. idiopathic scoliosis (AIS)
a. tibia vara

ADPKD
autosomal dominant polycystic kidney
disease

ADQ
abductor digiti quinti

ADR
Advanced Diagnostic Research
  ADR Ultramark 4 ultrasound

ADRDA
Alzheimer's Disease and Related
Disorders Association

adrenal
a. adenoma
a. angiography
a. artery
bilateral large a.'s
a. calcification
a. capsule
a. carcinoma
a. cortex
a. cyst
a. cystic mass
a. failure
a. ganglioneuroma
a. gland
a. hematoma
a. hemorrhage
a. hyperplasia
a. imaging
a. incidentaloma
a. insufficiency
a. lesion
a. leukodystrophy
a. malignancy
a. mass

a. medulla
a. medullary disease
a. metastasis
a. myelolipoma
a. neuroblastoma
a. paraganglioma
a. pheochromocytoma
a. pseudocyst
a. scan
a. scintigraphy
a. tuberculosis
a. tumor
a. vein
a. venography

adrenal-spleen ratio (ASR)
adrenergic drug
adrenocortical
a. adenoma
a. carcinoma
a. hyperfunction
a. hyperplasia
a. macrocyst
a. neoplasia
a. secretion
a. tumor

adrenocorticosteroid
adrenocorticotropic hormone (ACTH)
adrenocorticotropin microadenoma
adrenogenital syndrome
adrenogram
adrenoleukodystrophy
X-linked a.
adrenoleukodystrophy-
adrenomyeloneuropathy
(ALD-AMN)
ADRF
adiabatic demagnetization in rotating
frame
Adrian-Crooks cassette
Adson maneuver
adsorption
competitive a.
adsternal
adult
a. coarctation
a. dose
a. herpes encephalitis
a. polycystic kidney disease
a. progeria
a. respiratory distress syndrome
(ARDS)
a. rheumatoid arthritis
a. T-cell lymphoma
a. type III TIE fracture
adult-to-adult
a. t. a. liver transplant
a.-t.-a. living related liver transplant
donor
adumbration

advanced
- a. breast biopsy instrumentation (ABBI)
- a. cardiac mapping
- A. Cardiovascular Systems (ACS)
- A. Diagnostic Research (ADR)
- a. hepatocellular carcinoma
- A. Interventional Systems
- a. life support technique
- a. multiple-beam equalization radiography (AMBER)
- A. NMR Systems scanner
- a. nuclear medical resonance (ANMR)
- a. real-time motion analysis (ARTMA)
- a. ultrasonography
- a. vessel analysis (AVA)

advance directive

advancement
- frontoorbital a.
- vastus medialis a. (VMA)

Advantage Workstation

AdvanTeq II TENS unit

Advantx-E Legacy system

Advantx LC + cardiovascular imaging system

adventitial
- a. fibroplasia
- a. tissue

adventitia of artery

adventitious bursa

adverse effect

adynamic
- a. ileus
- a. intestinal obstruction

adynamic/paralytic ileus

AE
- above elbow
- AE amputation

Aeby
- A. muscle
- A. plane

AEC
- Atomic Energy Commission
- automatic exposure control
- AEC technique

AED
- automatic external defibrillator

AEG
- acute erosive gastritis

Aegis sonography management system

AER
- apical ectodermal ridge

aerated tissue

aeration
- regional difference in a.

aerobilia

aerocele

AeroChamber

aerodigestive
- a. carcinoma
- a. fistula
- a. tract

aerophagia, aerophagy

aerophagy (*var. of* aerophagia)

aerosol
- radioactive a.
- technetium 99m DTPA a.
- a. ventilation scan

aerosolized ^{99m}Tc DTPA imaging agent

AESOP
- automatic endoscopic system for optimal positioning
- AESOP Hermes-Ready system

Aestiva/5 MRI anesthesia machine

A-FAIR
- arrhythmia-insensitive flow-sensitive alternating inversion recovery
- A-FAIR imaging
- A-FAIR MRI

AFBG
- aortofemoral bypass graft

affect
- pseudobulbar a.

afferent
- a. digital nerve
- a. loop
- a. loop syndrome
- a. lymph vessel
- a. nerve lesion
- a. nipple valve
- a. view

AFI
- amnionic fluid index

AFP
- alpha-fetoprotein

African
- A. Burkitt lymphoma
- A. Kaposi sarcoma

AFROC
- alternative free-response receiver operating characteristic

AFT
- adaptive focusing technology

afterglow

afterload
- increased ventricular a.
- left ventricular a.

afterloader
- Fletcher a.
- Henschke a.
- Nucletron MicroSelectron/LDR remote a.

afterloading
- a. brachytherapy
- high dose-rate remote a.

a. radiation
a. tandem and ovoid
a. technique

Ag
silver

aganglionic
a. bowel
a. megacolon
a. segment

aganglionosis
skip a.

Agatston
A. calcium scoring method
A. score

AGC
anatomically graduated component
automatic gain control

age
anatomic a.
biologic a.
bone a.
chronologic a.
delayed bone a.
fetal a.
gestational a.
indeterminate a.
large for gestational a.

AGE
angle of greatest extension

age-indeterminate infarct

agenesis
Bayne classification of radial a.
(I-IV)
callosal a.
corpus callosum a.
gallbladder a.
liver a.
lumbosacral a.
lung a.
partial corpus callosum a.
pulmonary artery a.
renal a.
sacral a.
thymic a.
unilateral pulmonary a.
uterine a.
vaginal a.
vermian a.

agenetic
a. fracture
a. porencephaly

agent
acetrizoate contrast a.
AcuTect imaging a.
Adenoscan imaging a.
adenosine stress imaging a.
aerosolized ^{99m}Tc DTPA imaging
a.
air imaging a.

alkylating a.
Altropane radioimaging a.
AMI 121, 227 contrast a.
amidotrizoic acid contrast a.
Amipaque imaging a.
Amiscan imaging a.
Angio-Conray imaging a.
Angiografin imaging a.
AngioMARK contrast a.
antifibrin antibody imaging a.
antimyosin monoclonal antibody
imaging a.
antiplatelet a.
Apomate radiopharmaceutical
imaging a.
baby formula with ferrous sulfate
contrast a.
Baricon imaging a.
barium sulfate imaging a.
Baro-CAT imaging a.
Barosperse imaging a.
benzamide imaging a.
Biliscopin imaging a.
Bilopaque imaging a.
Biloptin imaging a.
bioreductive a.
bis-Gd-MP imaging a.
blood oxygenation level-dependent
contrast a.
blood pool contrast a.
bone marrow a.
bone-seeking a.
bromodeoxyuridine imaging a.
bromophenol blue imaging a.
^{11}C acetate imaging a.
^{45}Ca imaging a.
calcium-45 imaging a.
calcium ipodate imaging a.
carbon imaging a.
Cardiolite imaging a.
cardioselective a.
^{11}C butanol imaging a.
^{11}C carfentanil imaging a.
CEA-Scan imaging a.
Ceretec radioisotope imaging a.
cerium silicate imaging a.
cesium chloride imaging a.
^{11}C flumazenil imaging a.
CheeTah radiopaque contrast a.
chelating a.
Cholebrine imaging a.
Choletec radionuclide imaging a.
Cholografin meglumine imaging a.
chromated Cr-51 serum albumin
imaging a.
chromium imaging a.
^{11}C imaging a.
^{11}C-labeled cocaine imaging a.
^{11}C-labeled fatty acid imaging a.

agent (*continued*)
Clariscan imaging a.
^{11}C N-methylspiperone imaging a.
^{11}C nomifensine imaging a.
Combidex MRI contrast a.
CO_2-negative imaging a.
Conray 30, 43, 400 imaging a.
contrast a.
copper imaging a.
copper-zinc superoxide dismutase
  imaging a.
^{11}C raclopride imaging a.
^{11}C thymidine imaging a.
^{64}Cu imaging a.
^{67}Cu imaging a.
^{62}Cu PTSM imaging a.
^{64}Cu-TETA-octreotide imaging a.
Cu/Zn-SOD imaging a.
cyanocobalamin imaging a.
Cysto-Conray contrast a.
Cysto-Conray II imaging a.
Cystografin-Dilute imaging a.
DaTSCAN imaging a.
Definity contrast a.
denatured ^{99m}Tc-RBC imaging a.
depilatory a.
a. detection imaging
deuterium imaging a.
dextrose 5% in water imaging a.
diethylenetriamine pentaacetic acid
  imaging a.
Digibar 190 contrast a.
dihydroxyphenylalanine imaging a.
Dionosil imaging a.
dispersing a.
d, l-HMPAO imaging a.
dodecafluoropentane imaging a.
DOPA imaging a.
Dopascan radiopharmaceutical
  imaging a.
DTPA imaging a.
Dy-DTPA-BMA imaging a.
dysprosium HP-DO3A imaging a.
echo contrast a.
echo-enhancing a.
EchoGen ultrasound imaging a.
Echovist imaging a.
EDTMP imaging a.
effervescent a.
endogenous contrast a.
Eovist contrast a.
Ethiodol imaging a.
etidronate disodium imaging a.
Evans blue imaging a.
exametazime imaging a.
extracellular contrast a.
extravasated contrast a.
extravasation of contrast a.
E-Z-CAT Dry contrast a.

Feridex IV MRI contrast a.
ferucarbotran MR imaging a.
feruglose contrast a.
ferumoxide imaging a.
ferumoxsil imaging a.
ferumoxtran imaging a.
^{18}F estradiol imaging a.
^{18}F fludeoxyglucose imaging a.
^{18}F fluorodeoxyglucose imaging a.
^{18}F fluoro-DOPA imaging a.
^{18}F fluoroisonidazole imaging a.
^{18}F fluorotamoxifen imaging a.
Fibrimage diagnostic imaging a.
fibrin-specific contrast a.
^{18}Fl-DOPA imaging a.
Fluoratec imaging a.
fluorine-18 fluoro-2-deoxyglucose
  imaging a. (F-18 FDG)
fluorine imaging a.
fluorocarbon-based ultrasound
  contrast a.
fluorodeoxyglucose imaging a.
^{18}FN-methylspiperone imaging a.
^{18}F sodium fluoride imaging a.
^{18}F spiperone imaging a.
FS-069 sterile injectable sonography
  contrast a.
furosemide imaging a.
gadobenate dimeglumine contrast a.
gadobenic acid imaging a.
gadobutrol imaging a.
gadodiamide imaging a.
gadolinium-based contrast a.
gadolinium oxide imaging a.
Gadolite oral suspension contrast a.
gadopentetate contrast a.
gadopentetate dimeglumine imaging
  a.
gadoteridol imaging a.
gadoversetamide contrast a.
gadoversetamide imaging a.
gallium imaging a.
Gastrografin imaging a.
GastroMARK oral imaging a.
Gastroview imaging a.
Gastrovist imaging a.
Gd-BOPTA/Dimeg imaging a.
Gd-DTPA PGTM imaging a.
Gd-DTPA with mannitol contrast a.
Gd-enhanced imaging a.
Gd-EOB-DTPA imaging a.
Gd-HP-DO3A imaging a.
Gd-153 imaging a.
glomerular filtration a.
glucagon imaging a.
glucarate imaging a.
gold imaging a.
GSA imaging a.
hand-agitated imaging a.

hepatobiliary contrast a.
Hepatolite imaging a.
Hexabrix imaging a.
high-density barium imaging a.
high-osmolar contrast a. (HOCA)
hippuran imaging a.
Histoacryl embolic a.
holmium imaging a.
HpD photosensitizing a.
human serum albumin imaging a.
HumaSPECT imaging a.
hybrid MRI imaging a.
hydrogen peroxide imaging a.
hydrophilic contrast a
hydrosoluble contrast a.
hyoscine butylbromide imaging a.
Hypaque-Cysto imaging a.
Hypaque-76 imaging a.
Hypaque meglumine imaging a.
Hypaque-M imaging a.
Hypaque sodium imaging a.
hyperpolarized ^{3}He imaging a.
hyperpolarized ^{129}Xe imaging a.
Imagent GI US imaging a.
imaging a.
imidoacetic acid imaging a.
ImmuRAID antibody imaging a.
indium imaging a.
indocyanine green imaging a.
inhaled oxygen imaging a.
intercalating a.
intratumoral a.
intravenous microbubble contrast a.
in vivo imaging a.
iobitridol imaging a.
iocetamic acid imaging a.
iodamine imaging a.
iodinated imaging a.
iodine-123 MIBG radioactive
  imaging a.
iodine-131 MIBG radioactive
  imaging a.
iodipamide meglumine imaging a.
iodized oil imaging a.
5-iodo-2-deoxyuridine imaging a.
Iodo-gen imaging a.
iodohippurate sodium imaging a.
Iodotope imaging a.
iohexol imaging a.
ionic contrast a.
ionic paramagnetic imaging a.
iopamidol imaging a.
Iopamiron 310, 370 imaging a.
iopanoic acid imaging a.
iopentol nonionic imaging a.
iophendylate imaging a.
iopromide nonionic imaging a.
iosefamic acid imaging a.
iothalamate meglumine imaging a.

iothalamate sodium imaging a.
iotroxic acid imaging a.
ioversol imaging a.
ioxaglate meglumine imaging a.
ioxaglate sodium imaging a.
ioxilan imaging a.
ioxithalamic acid contrast a.
ipodate calcium imaging a.
ipodate sodium imaging a.
ipodic acid contrast a.
iridium imaging a.
Isovue-200, -250, -300, -370
  imaging a.
Isovue-M 200, 300 imaging a.
Isovue nonionic imaging a.
kinase C antiglioma monoclonal
  antibody imaging a.
Kinevac imaging a.
LeukoScan imaging a.
LeuTech radiolabeled imaging a.
Levovist imaging a.
ligand a.
Lipiodol myelographic imaging a.
lipophilic imaging a.
liposome-based contrast a.
liquid embolic a.
litholytic a.
liver-specific MRI contrast a.
long-scale imaging a.
low-osmolality contrast a.
low-osmolar contrast a. (LOCA)
l-tyrosine imaging a.
lymphangiographic imaging a.
Lymphazurin imaging a.
LymphoScan imaging a.
macroaggregated albumin imaging a.
macromolecular imaging a.
Macrotec imaging a.
magnetic resonance receptor a.
magnetite albumin imaging a.
  (Fe_3O_4)
Magnevist imaging a.
mangafodipir trisodium a.
manganese-containing contrast a.
manganese imaging a.
mannitol and saline imaging a.
MD-Gastroview imaging a.
meglumine diatrizoate imaging a.
meglumine iodipamide imaging a.
meglumine iotroxate imaging a.
methiodal sodium imaging a.
methyl methacrylate imaging a.
metrizamide imaging a.
metrizoate imaging a.
microbubble-based contrast a.
mineral oil imaging a.
monoclonal antibody imaging a.
monodisperse iodinated
  macromolecular blood pool a.

agent (*continued*)
MS-325 contrast a.
^{99m}Tc aggregated albumin imaging a.
^{99m}Tc albumin colloid imaging a.
^{99m}Tc albumin microsphere imaging a.
^{99m}Tc biciromab imaging a.
^{99m}Tc bicisate imaging a.
^{99m}Tc dimer captosuccinic acid imaging a.
^{99m}Tc disofenin imaging a.
^{99m}Tc exametazime imaging a.
^{99m}Tc furifosmin imaging a.
^{99m}Tc galactosyl human serum albumin imaging a.
^{99m}Tc glucarate imaging a.
^{99m}Tc gluceptate imaging a.
^{99m}Tc GSA imaging a.
^{99m}Tc human serum albumin imaging a.
^{99m}Tc-labeled cerebral perfusion imaging a.
^{99m}Tc lidofenin imaging a.
^{99m}Tc mebrofenin imaging a.
^{99m}Tc medronate imaging a.
^{99m}Tc mertiatide imaging a.
^{99m}Tc microaggregated albumin imaging a.
^{99m}Tc-N-NOEt neutral myocardial perfusion imaging a.
^{99m}Tc oxidronate imaging a.
^{99m}Tc pentetate calcium trisodium imaging a.
^{99m}Tc pentetate sodium imaging a.
^{99m}Tc polyphosphate imaging a.
^{99m}Tc pyrophosphate imaging a.
^{99m}Tc sestamibi imaging a.
^{99m}Tc sodium pertechnetate imaging a.
^{99m}Tc succimer imaging a.
^{99m}Tc sulfur colloid imaging a.
^{99m}Tc teboroxime imaging a.
^{99m}Tc tetrofosmin imaging a.
MultiHance imaging a.
myelographic imaging a.
Myoscint imaging a.
Myoview imaging a.
naloxone imaging a.
nanoparticulate imaging a.
negative-contrast imaging a.
NeoSpect diagnostic imaging a.
NeoTect imaging a.
Neurolite imaging a.
neurotrophic imaging a.
nicotinamide imaging a.
nimodipine imaging a.
Niopam imaging a.
NIR contrast a.

nitrogen-13 ammonia imaging a.
no-carrier-added ^{18}F imaging a.
nofetumomab diagnostic imaging a.
nonionic iodinated contrast a.
nonionic paramagnetic contrast imaging a.
nonnephrotoxic contrast a.
novel a.
occluding a.
OctreoScan 111 radioactive imaging a.
octreotide imaging a.
oil emulsion imaging a.
oily contrast a.
Omnipaque 140, 180, 240, 300, 350 imaging a.
Omniscan imaging a.
OncoScint CR/OV breast imaging a.
OptiMARK contrast a.
Optiray 10, 240, 300, 320, 350 imaging a.
Optison sterile injectable sonography contrast a.
Oragrafin calcium imaging a.
Oragrafin sodium imaging a.
oral contrast imaging a.
Oxilan imaging a.
oxygen imaging a.
palladium imaging a.
Pantopaque imaging a.
paramagnetic contrast a.
particulate embolic a.
pentagastrin imaging a.
pentavalent DMSA imaging a.
pentetic acid imaging a.
pentetreotide imaging a.
peppermint oil imaging a.
peptide imaging a.
perflubron imaging a.
perfluorocarbon imaging a.
perfusion a.
Persantine imaging a.
phenobarbital imaging a.
phosphoric acid imaging a.
phosphorus imaging a.
PIB imaging a.
Pittsburgh Compound B imaging a.
pixel-specific contrast a.
PMT imaging a.
polidocanol sclerosing a.
polymerizing a.
positive-contrast a.
potassium imaging a.
ProHance imaging a.
propyliodone imaging a.
ProstaScint monoclonal antibody imaging a.
protein-interacting contrast a.
pulmonary perfusion MRI contrast a.

radioactive cancer-specific targeting a.
radioactive isotope imaging a.
radiolabeled MoAb imaging a.
radiopaque imaging a.
radiopharmaceutical a.
radioprotective a.
radiotherapeutic a.
recombinant thyrotropin contrast a.
renal cortical isotope scanning a.
Renografin-60, -76 imaging a.
Renovist II imaging a.
Renovue-Dip imaging a.
Renovue-65 imaging a.
residual imaging a.
reticuloendothelial imaging a.
rhenium imaging a.
RIGScan CR49 imaging a.
rose bengal ^{131}I radioactive a.
rubidium chloride imaging a.
Rubratope-57 imaging a.
samarium imaging a.
satumomab pendetide imaging a.
sclerosing a.
selenium imaging a.
[75]Se selenomethionine radioactive a.
sestamibi imaging a.
Sethotope radioactive imaging a.
SH U 508A contrast a.
sincalide imaging a.
Sinografin imaging a.
SmartPrep imaging a.
sodium and/or methylglucamine diatrizoate contrast a.
sodium bicarbonate imaging a.
sodium chloride imaging a.
sodium diatrizoate imaging a.
sodium iodide ring imaging a.
sodium iodohippurate imaging a.
sodium iothalamate imaging a.
sodium ipodate imaging a
sodium meglumine ioxaglate contrast a.
sodium metrizoate acid contrast a.
sodium pertechnetate imaging a.
sodium tyropanoate imaging a.
solidifying a.
somatostatin imaging a.
Sonazoid contrast a.
sonicated dextrose albumin imaging a.
SonoRx oral ultrasound contrast a.
sorbitol 70% imaging a.
sprodiamide imaging a.
stool-tagging a.
strontium-89 imaging a.
sucrose polyester imaging a.
sulfobromophthalein imaging a.
sulfur colloid imaging a.

superparamagnetic iron oxide blood pool a.
superparamagnetic iron oxide imaging a.
tantalum imaging a.
targeted contrast a.
teboroxime imaging a.
Techneplex imaging a.
TechneScan HDP, MAA, MAG3, PYP imaging a.
technetium imaging a.
Telepaque imaging a.
teratogenicity of contrast a.
thullium imaging a.
thallous chloride imaging a.
TheraSeed imaging a.
thorium dioxide imaging a.
Thorotrast imaging a.
ThromboView imaging a.
tissue-specific imaging a.
Tomocat imaging a.
triiodinated imaging a.
Tyropaque imaging a.
Ultravist 150, 240, 300, 370 contrast a.
uniphasic imaging a.
uranium imaging a.
Urografin imaging a.
urokinase imaging a.
Urovist Cysto imaging a.
Urovist meglumine Diu/CT imaging a.
Urovist sodium 300 imaging a.
USPIO imaging a.
Varibar oral contrast a.
vasodilating a.
Verluma diagnostic imaging a.
Visipaque 270, 320 contrast a.
water-soluble iodinated imaging a.
water-soluble nonionic imaging a.
xenon imaging a.
xylenol orange imaging a.

age-related
   a.-r. change
   a.-r. demyelination

AGF
   angle of greatest flexion

Agfa
   A. ADC 70 storage phosphor system
   A. CR PACS system
   A. LR 3300 laser imager
   A. Medical scanner

agger nasi

aggregated
   a. lymphatic follicle
   a. sludge

aggregation
   nuclear a.

aggregometer
aggregometry
aggressive
    a. angiomyxoma
    a. good prognosis non-Hodgkin
    lymphoma
    a. histology lymphoma
    a. infantile fibromatosis
    a. interstitial infiltrate
    a. malignancy
    a. metastasis
    a. osteoporosis
    a. perivascular infiltrate
    a. tissue-protective therapy
aggressiveness
    bone tumor a.
aging gut
AGL
    anterior glenoid labrum
agnogenic
    a. myeloid metaphysis
    a. myeloid metaplasia
agnosia
    visual object a.
agonal clot
agonist
agranular leukocyte
agretope
agyria-pachygria complex
ahaustral
AHI
    acetabular head index
    acromiohumeral interval
    apnea-hypopnea index
Ahmed glaucoma valve
Ahn thrombectomy catheter
AHO
    acute hematogenous osteomyelitis
AHQ
    amnionic head quotient
AHR
    airway hyperreactivity
AHS
    Alpers-Huttenlocher syndrome
AI
    acceleration index
AICA
    anteroinferior cerebellar artery
    anteroinferior cerebral artery
    anteroinferior communicating
    artery
Aicardi-Goutières syndrome
Aicardi syndrome
AICD
    automatic implantable
    cardioverter-defibrillator
AICS
    artery of inferior cavernous sinus
AI 5200 diagnostic ultrasound

AIDS
    acquired immunodeficiency syndrome
    AIDS cholangitis
    AIDS encephalopathy
    AIDS service organization
AIDS-related esophagitis
AIF
    arterial input function
AIN
    acute interstitial nephritis
AIOD
    aortoiliac occlusive disease
AIP
    acute interstitial pneumonia
    autoimmune pancreatitis
AIPC
    androgen-independent prostate
    carcinoma
AIPH
    acute idiopathic hemorrhage
    attenuation in phantom
    AIPH method
air
    ambient a.
    a. arthrography
    a. block
    a. bolus
    bowel loop a.
    a. bronchogram
    a. bronchogram sign
    a. cavity
    a. cisternography
    a. collection
    colonic a.
    a. conditioner lung
    a. crescent
    a. cyst
    a. cystogram
    a. density
    a. dose
    a. embolus
    a. encephalography
    a. enema fluoroscopic imaging
    a. esophagram
    a. exchange
    a. expansion
    extraalveolar a. (EAA)
    extraluminal a.
    flail a.
    free intraperitoneal a.
    free peritoneal a.
    a. gap
    a. hunger
    a. imaging agent
    a. inflation
    a. injection
    inspired a.
    a. insufflation
    a. interface

intracranial a.
intraluminal a.
intramural colonic a.
intraorbital a.
intraperitoneal a.
a. Kerma
a. Kerma rate constant
a. Kerma strength
a. leak
a. leak complication
a. lock
a. luminogram
mediastinal a.
a. monitor
a. myelography
a. plasma spray hydroxyapatite
a. plethysmography
a. pocket
a. pyelography
retrocrural a.
retroperitoneal a.
a. sac
subcutaneous a.
transradiant a.
a. trapping
a. vesicle

AIR
automatic image registration
air-bone-tissue boundary
airborne
a. precaution
a. transmission
air-containing neck mass
air-contrast
a.-c. barium enema (ACBE)
a.-c. imaging
a.-c. study
a.-c. view
a.-c. view of stomach
air-core magnet
air-crescent sign
air-driven artificial heart
air-filled
a.-f. cyst
a.-f. loop
a.-f. lung
air-filtration system
airflow obstruction disease (AOD)
air-fluid
a.-f. level
a.-f. line
air-gap
a.-g. radiography
a.-g. technique
Airis II MR system
airless
a. lung
a. mass
air-meniscus sign

air-soft tissue interface
airspace
a. consolidation
a. disease
a. edema
a. enlargement
a. filling pattern
lung a.
a. nodule
a. opacity
retrosternal a.
terminal a.
volumetry of ventilated a.
airtrapping zone
airway
a. anatomy
asthmatic a.
bronchiectatic a.
a. constriction
dilated small a.
a. disease
a. embryology
esophageal obturator a.
a. fluoroscopy
a. hyperreactivity (AHR)
hypertonic a.
increased a.
large a.
mucoid plugging of a.
mucus-filled small a.
a. narrowing
a. obstruction
oropharyngeal a.
a. pattern
a. pressure
a. pressure release ventilation
a. resistance (RAW, ^{R}AW)
a. responsiveness
small a.
a. tree
a. tuberculosis
AIS
abbreviated injury scale
adolescent idiopathic scoliosis
Aitken
A. acromioclavicular injury
classification
A. classification of epiphysial
fracture
A. femoral deficiency
AIVV
anterior internal vertebral vein
AJCC
American Joint Committee on Cancer
AJCC-UICC
American Joint Committee on Cancer-
Union Internationale Contre le Cancer
AJCC-UICC mediastinal lymph node
classification

AKA
  above-knee amputation
Åkerlund deformity
akinesia, akinesis
akinesic (*var. of* akinetic)
akinesis (*var. of* akinesia)
  inferior wall a.
akinetic, akinesic
  a. left ventricle
  a. segment
  a. segmental wall motion
ala, *pl.* **alae**
  collagenous perivascular a.
  a. cristae galli
  a. lobuli centralis
  sacral a.
alae (*pl. of* ala)
Alagille syndrome
alanine-silicone pellet
Alanson amputation
alar
  a. bone
  a. cartilage
  a. chest
  a. dysgenesis
  a. fold
  a. ligament
  a. plate
  a. process
  a. spine
ALARA
  as low as reasonably achievable
  ALARA radiation dose
ALARP
  as low as readily practicable
alba, *pl.* **albae**
  adminiculum lineae albae
  linea a.
albae (*pl. of* alba)
Albarran gland
Albers-Schönberg
  A.-S. disease
  A.-S. position
Albert position
Albini nodule
Albinus muscle
Albrecht bone
Albright
  A. hereditary osteodystrophy
  A. syndrome
Albright-McCune-Sternberg syndrome
albuginea
  tunica a.
albumin
  a. calculus
  chromium CR-51 serum a.
  Evans blue a.
  galactosyl human serum a. (GSA)
  Gd-DTPA-labeled a.

human serum a. (HSA, HuSA)
I-labeled macroaggregated a.
iodinated human serum a. (IHSA)
iodinated I-131 aggregated a.
iodinated I-125 serum a.
iodinated I-131 serum a.
macroaggregated a. (MAA)
microaggregated a.
neogalactosyl a.
perfluorocarbon-exposed sonicated
  dextrose a. (PESDA)
radioactive iodinated serum a. (RISA)
radioiodinated serum a. (RISA)
technetium 99m macroaggregated a.
  (Tc-99m MAA)
technetium 99m
  mini-microaggregated a.
ALCAPA
  anomalous origin of left coronary
  artery from pulmonary artery
ALCL
  anaplastic large cell lymphoma
Alcock
  A. canal
  A. test
alcohol
  polyvinyl a. (PVA)
alcoholic
  a. avascular necrosis
  a. cirrhosis
  a. fatty liver
  a. fibrosis
  a. heart
  a. liver disease (ALD)
  a. myopathy
  a. pneumonia
ALD
  alcoholic liver disease
  alveolar lung disease
ALD-AMN
  adrenoleukodystrophy-
    adrenomyeloneuropathy
aldehyde
Alder constitutional granulation anomaly
Alder-Reilly anomaly
Alderson anthropomorphic phantom
aldolase
aldosterone-producing carcinoma
aldosterone-secreting carcinoma
Alert catheter
Alexander
  A. acromioclavicular joint view
  A. disease
alexandrite laser
Alexa 1000 system
alexia
  motor a.
  optic a.
  pure word a.

sensory a.
visual a.
AlexLAZR laser
algebraic reconstruction technique (ART)
algorithm
3D reconstruction a.
3D surface detection a.
dual-lookup table a.
iterative a.
ALH
atypical lobular hyperplasia
aliased
a. flow
a. pixel
aliasing
a. artifact
image a.
temporal a.
Alibert-Bazin syndrome
alignment
anatomic a.
a. and registration of 3D image
angular a.
bony a.
Cooley-Tukcy a.
field a.
a. of fracture fragments
rotational a.
torsion a.
transverse plane a.
vertebral body a.
alimentary
a. canal
a. tract
a. tract calcification
aliquorrhea
aliquot
alkalinity
Engel a.
alkali reflux
Alken-Marberger nephroscope
alkylating agent
allantoic
a. circulation
a. cyst
a. vesicle
allergic
a. bronchopulmonary aspergillosis (ABPA)
a. granulomatosis
a. pneumonia
a. reaction
a. sinusitis
allergy
iodine a.
Allis sign
Allman classification
allocation
bit-rate a.
a. of treatment

allocortex
allodynia
alloesthesia
allogeneic
a. bone marrow transplant
a. peripheral cell transplant
a. stem cell transplant
allograft
aortic a.
bone a.
bone-chip a.
a. nephropathy
renal a.
alloimmune disease
allowed beta transition
alloxan-Schiff staining
all-purpose
low-energy a.-p. (LEAP)
All-Terrain Balloon (ATB)
All-Tronics scanner
ALN
axillary lymph node
ALND
axillary lymph node dissection
alobar holoprosencephaly
Aloka
A. color Doppler real-time 2D blood flow imaging with cine memory
A. imaging
A. linear ultrasound
A. sector ultrasound
A. SSD-1700 transducer
A. SSD ultrasound system
A. SSD ultrasound system and probe
A. ultrasound linear scanner
A. ultrasound sector scanner
Alouette amputation
Alpers disease
Alpers-Huttenlocher syndrome (AHS)
alpha
a. angle
a. chamber
a. cradle
a. decay
a. frequency band
a. heavy-chain disease
A. 21064 microprocessor workstation
a. particle
a. radiation
a. ray
a. sigmoid loop
a. threshold
a. tocopherol
alpha-1-antitrypsin deficiency
alpha-fetoprotein (AFP)
alpha-M2
radiolabeled peptide a.-M2

alpha-particle
    a.-p. accelerator
    a.-p. bombardment
    a.-p. emitter
alpine hunter's cap deformity
ALPSA
    anterior labroligamentous periosteal
    sleeve avulsion
        ALPSA lesion
ALS
    amyotrophic lateral sclerosis
alta
    patella a.
    A. reconstruction rod
    A. tibial/humeral rod
alteplase recombinant tissue plasminogen
activator
alteration
    bilateral a.
    hemodynamic a.
    metabolic a.
altered
    a. aortic contour
    a. blood flow
    a. mediastinal contour
alternans
    pulsus a.
    strabismus convergens a.
alternating
    a. calculi
    a. current (AC)
    a. hemifield stimulation
    a. sinus
alternative free-response receiver
operating characteristic (AFROC)
alternator
    film a.
altitudinal hemianopsia
Altman classification
Altropane radioimaging agent
altus
    calcaneus a.
aluminum
    a. ion breakthrough test
    a. pneumoconiosis
ALVAD
    abdominal left ventricular assist device
alveodental ridge
alveolar
    a. atrophy
    a. basal cell carcinoma
    a. bone fracture
    a. border of mandible
    a. bronchiole
    a. canal
    a. clouding
    a. collapse
    a. consolidation
    a. consolidative process

    a. crest
    a. dead space
    a. dilation
    a. distention
    a. duct
    a. duct emphysema
    a. echinococcosis
    a. ectasia
    a. epithelial hyperplasia
    a. foramen
    a. gland
    a. hemorrhage
    a. hydatid
    a. hypersensitivity
    a. infection
    a. infiltrate
    a. instability
    a. interstitium
    a. lung disease (ALD)
    a. microlithiasis
    a. mucosal carcinoma
    a. overdistention
    a. overventilation
    a. pattern
    a. paucity
    a. pneumonia
    a. point
    a. pressure
    a. proteinosis
    a. pulmonary edema
    a. rhabdomyosarcoma
    a. ridge
    a. sac
    a. sarcoidosis
    a. septal amyloidosis
    a. septal inflammation
    a. septal necrosis
    a. septum
    a. soft part sarcoma (ASPS)
    a. supporting bone
    a. ventilation
    a. volume
alveolar-capillary block
alveolarization
alveoli (*pl. of* alveolus)
alveolingual groove
alveolitis
    acute extrinsic allergic a.
    chronic diffuse sclerosing a.
    chronic extrinsic allergic a.
    chronic fibrosing a.
    cryptogenic fibrosing a.
    desquamative fibrosing a.
    diffuse sclerosing a.
    extrinsic allergic a.
    fibrosing cryptogenic a.
    mural fibrosing a.
    subacute extrinsic allergic a.
alveolobuccal groove

alveolodental canal
alveologram
alveololabial groove
alveolus, *pl.* alveoli
    pulmonary a.
alvine calculus
alymphocytosis
alymphoplasia
Alzheimer disease
Alzheimer's Disease and Related
  Disorders Association (ADRDA)
^{241}Am
    americium 241
Am
    americium
AMA
    American Medical Association
amastia
AMATC
    Amplatz maceration-aspiration
      thrombectomy catheter
amaurosis
    central a.
    cerebral a.
    a. fugax
    uremic a.
Amazr radiofrequency catheter
  ablation
AMBER
    advanced multiple-beam equalization
      radiography
ambient
    a. air
    a. segment of posterior cerebral
      artery
    a. wing of quadrigeminal cistern
ambiguous genitalia
ambilevous
AMBRI
    atraumatic multidirectional bilateral
      radial instability
ambulant (*var. of* ambulatory)
ambulatory, ambulant
    a. equilibrium angiocardiography
    a. equilibrium angiography
    a. Holter echocardiography
AME
    Austin Medical Equipment
      AME bone growth stimulator
      AME PinSite shield
amebiasis
amebic abscess
amelanotic tumor
ameloblastic
    a. adenomatoid tumor
    a. carcinoma
    a. fibroma
    a. fibrosarcoma
    a. sarcoma

ameloblastoma of jaw
amelogenesis imperfecta
amenorrhea
    secondary a.
amentia
America
    Radiological Society of North A.
      (RSNA)
American
    A. Academy of Neurology (AAN)
    A. Academy of Orthopaedic
      Surgeons (AAOS)
    A. Academy of Pediatrics guideline
    A. Board of Radiology
    A. Cancer Society (ACS)
    A. College of Radiology (ACR)
    A. College of Rheumatology
      criterion
    A. Diabetes Association
    A. Joint Committee on Cancer
      (AJCC)
    A. Joint Committee on
      Cancer/Union International Contre
      le Cancer
    A. Medical Association (AMA)
    A. Medical Association ligament
      injury classification system
    A. Radiological Nurses Association
      (ARNA)
    A. Registry of Diagnostic Medical
      Sonographers
    A. Registry of Radiologic
      Technology (ARRT)
    A. Rheumatism Association (ARA)
    A. Roentgen Ray Society (ARRS)
    A. Shared-CuraCare scanner
    A. Society of Echocardiography
    A. Society of Neuroradiology
    A. Society of Radiologic
      Technologists (ASRT)
    A. Society of Registered
      Technologists
    A. Spinal Cord Injury Association
    A. Spinal Cord Injury Association
      classification
    A. Standards Association (ASA)
    A. Thoracic Society
    A. Thoracic Society node station
    A. Thyroid Association
    A. Urological Association
americium (Am)
    a. 241 (^{241}Am)
    a. radioactive source
ameroid occluder
ametriodinic acid
AMI
    acute mesenteric ischemia
      AMI 121, 227 contrast agent
amiculum of olive

amidotrizoic
    a. acid
    a. acid contrast agent
amine
    heterocyclic aromatic a.
    a. precursor uptake and
      decarboxylation (APUD)
aminobutyrate
    gamma a.
5-aminolevulinic acid photodynamic therapy
aminooxypentane
amiodarone
    a. liver
    a. lung
Amipaque imaging agent
Amiscan imaging agent
AML
    acute myelogenous leukemia
    angiomyolipoma
ammeter
Ammon horn
ammonia
    anhydrous a.
ammonium excretion
amniocentesis
    therapeutic a.
amniodrainage
amniography
amnioinfusion
amnion
    a. ring
    a. rupture
    a. rupture sequence
amnionic, amniotic
    a. band
    a. band syndrome
    a. cavity
    a. duct
    a. fluid
    a. fluid embolus
    a. fluid index (AFI)
    a. fluid volume
    a. fold
    a. head quotient (AHQ)
    a. inclusion cyst
    a. membrane
    a. raphe
    a. sac
    a. sheet
amnionicity
amniotic (*var. of* amnionic)
A-mode
    A-m. amplitude modulation scan
    A-m. display
    A-m. echocardiography
    A-m. encephalography
amorphous
    a. fetus

    a. high signal intensity
    a. selenium
    a. selenium plate
    a. silicon (a-Si)
    a. silicon filmless digital x-ray
      detection technology
    a. silicon filmless digital x-ray
      detection technology device
amosite
Amoss sign
amp
    amplification
    low-pressure mercury arc amp
ampere
amphiarthrodial
amphiarthrosis
amphibole asbestos
amphoric echo
amphoteric dipolar ion
Amplatz
    A. anchor system
    A. angiography needle
    A. Clot Buster
    A. coronary catheterization technique
    A. dilator set
    A. gooseneck snare
    A. left coronary catheter
    A. maceration-aspiration
      thrombectomy catheter (AMATC)
    A. radiolucent handle
    A. right coronary catheter
    A. Super Stiff catheter
    A. Super Stiff guidewire
    A. Teflon sheath
    A. thrombectomy device
Amplatzer septal occluder device
amplification (amp)
    multiscale image detail contrast a.
      (Musica)
amplifier
    buffer a.
    gradient a.
    image a.
    linear a.
    log a.
    nuclear pulse a.
    pulse a.
    servo power a.
    Servox a.
    voltage a.
amplitude
    acoustic pressure a.
    a. asymmetry
    deformation a.
    gradient a.
    a. image
    a. imaging
    a. modulation
    a. of phase encoding

output a.
peak a.
pressure a.
septal a.
ampoule (*var. of* ampule)
ampul (*var. of* ampule)
ampule, ampul, ampoule
ampulla, *pl.* **ampullae**
    a. biliaropancreatica
    a. canaliculi lacrimalis
    a. chyli
    a. ductus deferentis
    duodenal a.
    a. duodeni
    hepatopancreatic a.
    a. hepatopancreatica
    a. membranacea anterior
    a. of semicircular canal
    a. of Vater
    a. ossea anterior
    a. ossea lateralis
    a. ossea posterior
    phrenic a.
    rectal a.
    a. recti
    a. tubae uterinae
    a. tumor
ampullae (*pl. of* ampulla)
ampullar pregnancy
ampullary
    a. adenocarcinoma
    a. aneurysm
    a. carcinoma
    a. crest
    a. stenosis
amputated foot view
amputation
    above-knee a. (AKA)
    AE a.
    Alanson a.
    Alouette a.
    Béclard a.
    below-knee a. (BKA)
    Berger interscapular a.
    Bier a.
    Boyd ankle a.
    Bunge a.
    Burgess below-knee a.
    button toe a.
    Callander a.
    Carden a.
    chop a.
    Chopart hindfoot a.
    circular supracondylar a.
    closed flap a.
    congenital a.
    digital a.
    femoral head a.
    fetal a.

fingertip a.
fishmouth a.
forearm a.
Guyon a.
Hey a.
interscapulothoracic a.
Jaboulay a.
Kirk distal thigh a.
Le Fort a.
Lisfranc a.
midthigh a.
nonreplantable a.
Pirogoff a.
ray a.
replantable a.
1-stage a.
2-stage a.
supramalleolar open a.
Syme ankle disarticulation a.
Teale a.
transcarpal a.
transcondylar a.
translumbar a.
transmetatarsal a. (TMA)
traumatic a.
Vladimiroff-Mikulicz a.
AMRIS
    active MRI stent
AMS
    accelerator mass spectrometry
Amsterdam dwarfism
Amstutz classification
AMT-25-enhanced MR imaging
amu
    atomic mass unit
amygdala, *pl.* **amygdalae**
    a. of cerebellum
    a. volume
amygdalae (*pl. of* amygdala)
amygdaline
amygdalofugal pathway
amygdaloid
    a. area
    a. fossa
    a. nuclear complex
    a. tubercle
amylacea (*pl. of* amylaceum)
amylaceum, *pl.* **amylacea**
    corpora amylacea
    corpus a.
amyloid
    a. A
    a. angiopathy
    a. deposit
    a. L
    a. lymphadenopathy
    a. tumor
amyloidoma
    pulmonary a.

amyloidosis
    alveolar septal a.
    chronic renal failure a.
    CNS a.
    GI tract a.
    heart a.
    hereditary a.
    idiopathic a.
    immunocytic a.
    kidney a.
    lung a.
    lymph node a.
    a. of multiple myeloma
    a. of small bowel
    orbital a.
    primary a.
    pulmonary a.
    renal a.
    secondary a.
    senile a.
    skeletal a.
    splenic a.
    urethral a.
amyloidotic cardiomyopathy
amyotonia congenita
amyotrophic lateral sclerosis (ALS)
anacrotic notch
anaerobic
    a. bacterial infection
    a. lung abscess
anal
    a. apparatus
    a. atresia
    a. bulge
    a. canal
    a. cleft
    a. column
    a. crypt
    a. disc
    a. fascia
    a. fissure
    a. fistula
    a. intermuscular septum
    a. intersphincteric groove
    a. manometry
    a. orifice
    a. pit
    a. plate
    a. protrusion
    a. stenosis
    a. stricture
    a. vein
    a. verge
analeptic enema
analgesic nephropathy
analog (*var. of* analogue)
analogous
analogue, analog
    a. computation

    dysprosium a.
    halogenated thymidine a.
    ^{99m}Tc-labeled phosphate a.
    a. photo
    pyrimidine a.
    radiolabeled estrogen a.
    a. rate meter
    technetium 99m IDA a.
analogue-to-digital
    a.-t.-d. conversion quantization error
    a.-t.-d. converter (ADC)
analyses (*pl. of* analysis)
analysis, *pl.* **analyses**
    activation a.
    advanced real-time motion a.
      (ARTMA)
    advanced vessel a. (AVA)
    basic volume image a.
    bayesian a.
    5-bromodeoxyuridine a.
    calvarial volume a.
    cephalometric a.
    CEqual quantitative a.
    Cerenkov scintillation a.
    clinicopathologic a.
    compartmental a.
    computer-aided image a.
    computer-aided joint space a.
      (CAJSA)
    computer-assisted joint motion a.
    correlation a.
    cue-based image a.
    deconvolution a.
    deformation-based hippocampal
      segmentation and shape a.
    diagnostic efficacy a.
    digital frequency a.
    3-dimensional a.
    direct immunofluorescence a.
    discriminant a.
    Doppler spectral a.
    Doppler waveform a.
    duplex Doppler signal a. (DDSA)
    duplex ultrasound a.
    eigenvector a.
    electrooculographic a.
    energy a.
    fast Fourier spectral a.
    field-fitting a.
    fission track a.
    focal and diffuse lung texture a.
    folding potential a.
    footprint a.
    Fourier a.
    fractal a.
    fractional volumetric a.
    frequency a.
    gamma spectrometric a.
    high-definition 3-dimensional a.

image display and a. (IDA)
intracardiac pressure waveform a.
iodine-131 outcome a.
isotope dilution a.
kinetic parameter a.
late-effect a.
linear regression a.
liquid scintillation a.
multielemental neutron activation a.
multivariant regressional a.
myocardial texture a.
neutron activation a.
nuclide a.
phase a.
planar thallium with quantitative a.
pole figure texture a.
power spectral a. (PSA)
prospective a.
pulse-height spectral a.
quadratic discriminant a. (QDA)
qualitative a.
quantitative a.
radiometric a.
range-gated Doppler spectral flow a.
rate a.
recursive partitioning a.
regression a.
residual stress a.
roentgen stereophotogrammetric a.
  (RSA)
Sassouni a.
saturation a.
sensitivity a.
signal sonographic feature a.
slope blot a.
sonographic feature a.
spectral a.
S-phase a.
stepwise regression a.
thin-film a.
time-action a.
volume a.
volumetric a.
voxel-by-voxel a.
x-ray diffraction a.

analytic reconstruction
analyzer, analyzor
automated biochemical a.
automated cerebral blood flow a.
ChromaVision digital a.
Dow hollow-fiber a.
Gammex RBA-5 radiation beam a.
Medigraphics a.
multichannel a. (MCA)
platelet function a. (PFA)
pulse height a. (PHA)
Readia COR a. (I, II)
single-channel a. (SCA)
analyzor (*var. of* analyzer)

ANAP
anionic neutrophil-activating peptide
anaphylactic
a. reaction
a. shock
anaphylactoid reaction
anaplasia
cancer cell a.
cerebellar a.
anaplastic
a. astrocytoma
a. cerebral glioma
a. ependymoma
a. large cell lymphoma (ALCL)
a. mixed oligoastrocytoma
a. plasmacytoma
a. thyroid carcinoma
a. tumor
anastomoses (*pl. of* anastomosis)
anastomosis, *pl.* **anastomoses**
arterial a.
arterial brain a.
arteriovenous a. (AVA)
Baffe a.
bidirectional cavopulmonary a.
bile duct a.
biliary-enteric a.
Billroth I, II a.
Blalock-Taussig, Waterston, Potts,
  and Glenn a.
bowel-to-bowel a.
cholecystenteric a.
cobra-head a.
coiling of a.
colocolic a.
colorectal a.
embryonic a.
end-to-end a.
end-to-side biliary-enteric a.
extradural a.
gastroenteric a.
Glenn a.
hepatic arterial a.
hepatojejunal a.
heterocladic a.
Hofmeister a.
Horsley a.
ileal pouch-anal a.
ileocolic a.
ileorectal a. (IRA)
ileotransverse colon a.
infrahepatic inferior vena cava a.
intercavernous a.
J-shaped a.
Kocher a.
Kugel a.
laser-assisted microvascular a.
left internal mammary artery a.
leptomeningeal a.

anastomosis (*continued*)
    LIMA a.
    magnet compression a.
    portal venous a.
    portosystemic a.
    splenorenal a.
    stenotic esophagogastric a.
    Sucquet-Hoyer a.
    suprahepatic inferior vena cava a.
    tracheal a.
    UA to OA a.
    ureteroureteral a.
    ureterovesical a.

anastomotic
    a. aneurysm
    a. arch
    a. arterial circle
    a. dehiscence
    a. disruption
    a. hemorrhage
    a. leakage
    a. pseudoaneurysm
    a. site
    a. stenosis
    a. stoma
    a. stricture
    a. ulcer
    a. vein

anatomic, anatomical
    a. age
    a. alignment
    a. appearance and alignment, bony
      mineralization and texture,
      cartilage, and soft tissue
      abnormalities (ABCS)
    a. axis
    a. barrier
    a. bile duct variant
    a. brain classification
    a. configuration
    a. dead space
    a. distribution
    a. esophageal vestibule
    a. fracture
    a. genu valgus
    a. image
    a. landmark
    a. landscape
    a. localization
    a. marker
    a. misregistration
    a. neck
    a. overlay
    a. plane
    a. position
    a. programmed radiography (APR)
    a. reduction
    a. resolution
    a. root

    a. shunt flow
    a. snuffbox
    a. variability
    a. variation

anatomical (*var. of* anatomic)

anatomically
    a. dominant
    a. graduated component (AGC)

anatomometabolic image

anatomopathologic study

anatomy
    airway a.
    anomalous a.
    arterial a.
    basal ganglion a.
    breast a.
    bronchopulmonary lung segment a.
    bulbourethral gland a.
    carpal bone a.
    chain-of-lakes a.
    cochlear a.
    computational a.
    coronary artery a.
    craniovertebral junction a.
    cross-sectional lung segment a.
    Daseler-Anson classification of
      plantaris muscle a.
    distorted a.
    donor-recipient a.
    endometrial a.
    a. exclusion artifact
    facial nerve a.
    hepatic artery a.
    inner ear a.
    internal auditory canal a.
    kidney a.
    left-dominant coronary a.
    lobar breast a.
    Lowsley lobar a.
    maxillary nerve a.
    medullary venous a.
    neck-space a.
    normal planar MR a.
    ovarian a.
    pituitary gland a.
    plantar compartmental a.
    prostate a.
    radiologic a.
    renal vascular a.
    renovascular a.
    right-dominant coronary a.
    Saltzman a.
    scrotal a.
    sectional segmental a.
    segmental liver a.
    small bowel fold a.
    stapedial nerve a.
    superior orbital fissure a.
    teardrop pelvic a.

temporal bone a.
thoracic spine a.
trigeminal nerve a.
umbilical cord a.
uterine a.
vascular kidney a.
vascular renal a.
venous a.
zonal prostate a.
zonal uterine a.
anatomy-based extraction
anatomy-oriented colon segmentation (AOCS)
anchor
Mitek bone a.
a. plate
traction a.
anchoring
a. tendon
a. villus
ancillary imaging finding
anconal, anconeal
a. fossa
anconeal (*var. of* anconal)
anconeus muscle
anconoid
Ancure tube graft
ancyroid, ankyroid
a. cavity
Anderson-Hutchins tibial fracture
Andren method
Andren-von Rosen line
androblastoma
androgen deprivation therapy
androgen-independent prostate carcinoma (AIPC)
androgen-producing tumor
android pelvis
anechoic
a. area
a. center
a. cyst
a. fluid
a. fluid collection
a. lesion
a. mantle
a. mass
a. thrombus
anembryonic pregnancy
anemia
Fanconi a.
hemolytic autoimmune a.
macrocytic a.
nutritional a.
radiation a.
sickle cell a.
anemic infarct
anencephalia (*var. of* anencephaly)
anencephaly, anencephalia

aneroid manometry
anesthetic drug
aneuploid cell line
AneuRx
A. bifurcated stent-graft system
A. endograft
A. stent
A. stent-graft
aneurysm
abdominal aortic a. (AAA)
acquired left ventricular a.
ampullary a.
anastomotic a.
anterior communicating artery a.
aortic a. (AA)
aortic arch a.
aortic sinus a.
aortoiliac a.
arterial a.
arteriosclerotic intracranial a.
arteriosclerotic thoracoabdominal
  aortic a.
arteriovenous pulmonary a.
ascending aortic a.
aspergillotic a.
atherosclerotic aortic a.
atrial septal a.
axillary a.
bacterial a.
basilar artery a.
basilar tip a.
bifurcation a.
bland aortic a.
brachiocephalic arterial a.
brain a.
bulging a.
calcified wall of a.
cardiac ventricle a.
carotid artery a.
carotid-ophthalmic a.
cavernous sinus a.
cavity of a.
celiac artery a.
cerebral a.
circumscript a.
cirsoid a.
clinoid a.
clip ligation of a.
clipping of a.
coating of a.
coiling of a.
communicating artery a.
compound a.
congenital aortic sinus a.
congenital arteriosclerotic a.
congenital cerebral a.
congenital intracranial a.
congenital left ventricular a.
congenital pulmonary artery a.

aneurysm (*continued*)

congenital renal a.
contained leak of aortic a.
coronary artery a.
coronary vessel a.
cranial a.
cylindroid a.
degenerative aortic a.
de novo a.
dilation of a.
dissecting abdominal a.
dissecting aortic a.
dissecting basilar artery a.
dissecting intracranial a.
distal aortic arch a.
dome of a.
Dorendorf sign of aortic arch a.
Drummond sign of aortic a.
ductal a.
ductus arteriosus a.
ectatic a.
eggshell border of a.
embolic a.
extracerebral a.
extracranial a.
false a.
feeding artery of a.
fenestration of dissecting a.
fundus of a.
fusiform a.
Galen vein a.
giant brain a.
giant saccular a.
giant serpentine a.
hepatic artery a.
hernial a.
Hunt and Hess a. (grade I–V)
Hunt and Kosnik a. (grade 0–V)
hunterian ligation of a.
Hunt-Kosnik classification of a.
  (grade 0–4)
IC-PC artery a.
iliac artery a.
induced thrombosis of aortic a.
infected a.
inflammatory aortic a.
infrarenal abdominal aortic a.
innominate a.
internal carotid artery a.
intracerebral a.
intracranial a. (ICA)
intracranial berry a.
intracranial saccular a.
intramural coronary artery a.
juxtarenal aortic a.
kidney a.
Kommerell a.
late false a.
lateral a.

leaking abdominal aortic a.
left ventricular a. (LVA)
lower basilar a.
luetic aortic a.
malignant bone a.
miliary a.
mirror-image a.
mixed a.
M1-segment a.
mural a.
mycotic aortic a.
mycotic brain a.
mycotic intracranial a.
neck of a.
neoplastic a.
nodular a.
orbital a.
oval a.
pararenal aortic a.
pelvic a.
perforating a.
peripheral artery a.
popliteal artery a.
portal vein a.
posterior communicating artery a.
postinfarction ventricular a.
Pott a.
precursor sign to rupture of a.
prerenal aortic a.
prerupture of a.
P2-segment a.
pulmonary arteriovenous a.
pulmonary artery a.
pulmonary artery compression
  ascending aortic a.
racemose a.
Rasmussen mycotic a.
rebleeding of a.
a. remnant neck
renal artery a.
ruptured a.
sacciform a.
saccular cerebral a.
sac of a.
sacral a.
a. sac shrinkage
serpentine a.
sinus of Valsalva a.
slow-flow giant saccular a.
spindle-shaped a.
splanchnic a.
splenic artery a.
spontaneous infantile ductal a.
spurious a.
subarachnoid a.
subclavian a.
subvalvular a.
supraclinoid carotid a.
suprarenal aortic a.

suprarenal extension of a.
suprasellar a.
syphilitic aortic a.
thoracic aortic a.
thoracoabdominal aortic a.
thrombosed giant vertebral artery a.
thrombotic a.
trapping of a.
traumatic intracranial a. (TICA)
true aortic a.
true heart a.
true ventricular a.
tubular a.
uterine cirsoid a.
varicose a.
varix of a.
vascular a.
venous a.
ventricular septal a.
verminous a.
wide-neck carotid cavernous a.
windsock a.
a. with simple shape
worm a.

aneurysmal, aneurysmatic
a. bone cyst (ABC)
a. cavity
a. clip
a. coil
a. dilation
a. disease
a. dissection
a. fundus
a. hematoma
a. hemorrhage
a. neck
a. ostium
a. outpouching
a. proportion
a. rupture
a. sac
a. vein
a. wall
a. wall calcification
a. wall gas
a. widening of aorta
a. wrap

aneurysmatic (*var. of* aneurysmal)
aneurysmogram
aneurysmograph
aneurysmography
AngeLase combined mapping-laser probe
Angelchik reflux prosthesis
Angeles
University of California Los A. (UCLA)
angel-wing sign
Anger scintillation camera

angiitis-granulomatosis disorder
angina
Ludwig a.
a. pectoris
angioarchitecture
angioblastic lymphadenopathy
angioblastoma
bone a.
cord a.
angiocardiogram (ACG)
angiocardiography (ACG)
ambulatory equilibrium a.
biplane a.
equilibrium radionuclide a.
exercise radionuclide a.
gas a.
gated radionuclide a.
intravenous a.
radionuclide a.
rapid biplane a.
retrograde a.
right-sided a.
selective a.
1st-pass radionuclide exercise a.
transseptal a.
venous a.
Angiocath
A. Autoguard Shielded IV catheter
A. PRN catheter
angiocatheter
angiocentric
a. immunoproliferative disorder
a. immunoproliferative lesion
a. lymphoproliferative lesion
angiocholitis
Angio-Conray imaging agent
angio-CT
superselective angio-CT
AngioDynamics
angiodynography
angiodysplasia
colonic a.
a. of colon
angioedema
angiofibroblastic
a. hyperplasia
a. proliferation
a. tendinosis
angiofibroma
juvenile nasopharyngeal a. (JNPA)
Angioflow meter system
angiofollicular
a. and plasmacytic polyadenopathy
a. lymph node hyperplasia
angiogenesis
a. gene delivery
a. tumor
angiogenic factor
Angiografin imaging agent

angiogram
balloon occlusion pulmonary a.
biplane left ventricular a.
computed tomography a.
control a.
dynamic subtraction magnetic
  resonance a.
fluorescein a.
flush a.
interventional vascular a.
noninvasive a.
overview a.
projection a.
radionuclide a. (RNA)
radionuclide cerebral a.
small-angle double-incidence a.
spinal a.
triple-dose MR a.
volume-rendered CT a.
volume-rendered MR a.

angiographic
a. blush
a. catheter
a. contrast injection system
  technology (ACIST)
a. corkscrew artery
a. finding
a. guidewire
a. muscle mass index
a. occlusion
a. system for unlimited rolling field
  of view (AngioSURF)
a. target
a. targeting
a. Teflon dilator

angiographically
a. occult intracranial vascular
  malformation (AOIVM)
a. occult vascular malformation
  (AOVM)
a. occult vessel
a. visualized vascular malformation
  (AVVM)

angiography
adrenal a.
ambulatory equilibrium a.
aortic arch a.
axial a.
basilar a.
biliary a.
biplane a.
black blood magnetic resonance a.
blood pool radionuclide a.
blush of dye on a.
brachial a.
brain capillary a.
breath-hold contrast-enhanced
  3-dimensional MR a.
bronchial a.

Brown-Dodge method for a.
cardiac computed tomographic a.
cardiac gated MR a.
carotid a.
catheter a.
catheter coronary a.
cavernous brain a.
celiac a.
cerebral a.
CO_2 a.
color power a.
3-compartment wrist a.
computed tomographic a. (CTA)
computed tomographic pulmonary a.
computerized tomographic hepatic a.
  (CTHA)
contrast a.
contrast-enhanced magnetic resonance
  a. (CEMRA)
contrast-enhanced MR a.
contrast x-ray a.
conventional a.
coronary a.
coronary electron beam a.
CT a.
cut-film a. (CFA)
cystic duct a.
3D contrast-enhanced MR a.
3D coronary magnetic resonance a.
3DFT magnetic resonance a.
2DFT time-of-flight MR a.
3D gadolinium-enhanced magnetic
  resonance a.
3D helical CT a.
diagnostic a.
digital celiac trunk a.
digital rotational a. (DRA)
digital subtraction a. (DSA)
digital subtraction rotational a.
3-dimensional contrast-enhanced MR
  a.
3-dimensional digital subtraction a.
3-dimensional magnetic resonance a.
2-dimensional magnetic resonance
  digital subtraction a.
3D inflow MR a.
directional color a. (DCA)
dobutamine thallium a.
3D phase-contrast magnetic
  resonance a.
3D rotational a.
dual-detector helical CT a.
3D volume-rendered helical CT a.
3D volume-rendering CT a.
dynamic tagging magnetic resonance
  a.
EBCT IV a.
ECG-synchronized digital subtraction
  a.

edge-detection a.
elastic subtraction spiral CT a.
electrocardiogram-synchronized digital
  subtraction a.
electron beam a. (EBA)
emission a.
Epistar subtraction a.
equilibrium radionuclide a.
extremity CT a.
femoral runoff a.
femorocerebral catheter a.
fluorescein indocyanine green a.
FluoroPlus a.
frameless stereotactic digital
  subtraction a.
functional magnetic resonance a.
  (fMRA)
gadolinium-enhanced elliptically
  reordered 3-dimensional MR a.
gadolinium-enhanced subtracted MR
  a.
gadoterate-enhanced digital
  subtraction a.
gated blood pool a.
gated equilibrium radionuclide a.
gated nuclear a.
Gd-enhanced MR a.
hand a.
helical computed tomographic a.
  (HCTA)
helical CT a.
hepatic arterial a.
a. imaging
indocyanine green a.
innominate a.
intercostal artery a.
internal carotid a.
interventional a.
intraarterial digital subtraction a.
  (IADSA)
intraarterial stereotactic digital
  subtraction a.
intracranial MR a.
intraoperative digital subtraction a.
  (IDSA)
intravenous digital subtraction a.
  (IVDSA)
intravenous fluorescein a. (IVFA)
intravenous renal a.
intravenous stereotactic digital
  subtraction a.
left coronary a. (LCA)
left ventricular a.
low-field MR a.
magnetic resonance a. (MRA)
magnetic resonance digital
  subtraction a. (MRDSA)
magnification a.
mesenteric a.

minimum basis set magnetic
  resonance a. (MBS-MRA)
multigated a.
multiple-projection biplane a.
multislab magnetic resonance a.
multislice computed tomographic a.
  (MSCTA)
noncardiac a.
noncontrast-enhanced a.
nonselective a.
nontriggered phase-contrast MR a.
nuclear a.
occlusion a.
orbital a.
orthogonal view on a.
pancreatic a.
PC MR a.
peripheral MR a.
phase-contrast a.
postangioplasty a.
postembolization a.
postoperative a.
posttourniquet occlusion a.
preoperative a.
pulmonary artery wedge a.
pulmonary magnetic resonance a.
  (PMRA)
pulmonary vein wedge a.
quantitative coronary a. (QCA)
radionuclide a.
renal a.
resistive index a.
rest and exercise gated nuclear a.
right coronary a. (RCA)
rotational a. (RA)
scintigraphic a.
segmented k-space time-of-flight MR
  a.
Seldinger a.
selective arterial magnetic resonance a.
selective presaturation MR a.
selective venous magnetic resonance
  a.
semiautomated computed tomography
  a.
single-plane a.
sitting-up view a.
spinal cord a.
spiral CT a.
splenic a.
stereotactic cerebral a.
1st-pass radionuclide a. (FPRNA)
subtraction a.
superselective magnified digital a.
Tagarno 3SD cine projector for a.
therapeutic a.
thoracic a.
time-of-flight magnetic resonance a.
  (TOF-MRA)

A

angiography (*continued*)
> transfemoral cerebral a.
> transseptal a.
> transvenous digital subtraction a.
> tumor blush on a.
> ultrafast 3D MR digital subtraction a.
> velocity encoding on brain MR a.
> venous brain a.
> vertebral a.
> 4-vessel cerebral a.
> 3-vessel multiple-projection biplane a.
> 4-vessel multiple-projection biplane a.
> visceral a.

AngioGuard-EX distal protection device
angioimmunoblastic
> a. lymphadenopathy
> a. lymphadenopathy-like T-cell lymphoma
> a. T-cell lymphoma (ATCL)

angioinfarction
angioinvasion
AngioJet
> A. thrombectomy device
> A. Xpeedior catheter

angiokeratoma
angioleiomyoma
Angiolink EVS closure device
angiolipofibroma
angiolipoma
> epidural a.
> mediastinal a.

angiolithic
> a. degeneration
> a. sarcoma

angiolymphangioma
angiolymphoid hyperplasia
angioma, *pl.* **angiomata, angiomas**
> arterial a.
> arteriovenous interhemispheric a.
> capillary a.
> cavernous a.
> cutaneous a.
> encephalic a.
> extracerebral cavernous a.
> extraosseous a.
> intracranial cavernous a.
> intradermal a.
> littoral cell a.
> a. lymphaticum
> pulmonary a.
> a. serpiginosum
> spider a.
> superficial a.
> telangiectatic a.
> a. venosum racemosum
> venous a.

AngioMARK contrast agent
angiomas (*pl. of* angioma)
Angiomat
> A. 3000, 6000 contrast delivery system
> A. Illumena injector system

angiomata (*pl. of* angioma)
angiomatoid
> a. malignant fibrous histiocytoma
> a. tumor

angiomatous
> a. disease
> a. lymphoid hamartoma
> a. nasal polyp
> a. syndrome

angiomyofibroma
angiomyolipoma (AML)
> hepatic a.
> kidney a.
> renal a.

angiomyoma
angiomyosarcoma
angiomyxoma
> aggressive a.
> umbilical cord a.

angioneuromyoma
angioneurotic edema
angioosteohypertrophy syndrome
angiopathy
> amyloid a.
> cardiac a.
> cerebral amyloid a.
> congophilic a.
> diabetic a.

angioplastic meningioma
angioplasty
> cardiac a.
> excimer laser coronary a.
> infrainguinal percutaneous transluminal a.
> laser-assisted balloon a. (LABA)
> percutaneous excimer laser coronary a.
> percutaneous transluminal a. (PTA)
> percutaneous transluminal coronary a. (PTCA)
> percutaneous transluminal renal a. (PTRA)
> peripheral excimer laser a. (PELA)
> peripheral laser a.
> a. sheath
> smooth excimer laser coronary a. (SELCA)
> transluminal balloon a.
> venous a.
> vessel reshaping by a.

angiopneumography
AngiOptic microcatheter
AngioRad radiation system

angioreticuloendothelioma of heart
angioreticuloma
    spine a.
angiosarcoma
    bone a.
    breast a.
    cardiac a.
    cavernous a.
    cutaneous a.
    hepatic a.
    liver a.
    a. of heart
    parosteal soft tissue a.
    spleen a.
    venous a.
angioscintigraphy
angioscopic guidance
angioscopy
    virtual a.
Angio-Seal
    A.-S. carrier tube
    A.-S. closure device
    A.-S. diagnostic device
    A.-S. system
    A.-S. therapeutic device
angiosome
AngioSURF
    angiographic system for unlimited
    rolling field of view
    AngioSURF system
angiotensin-converting enzyme (ACE)
angiotensin (II) (AT II)
angiotherapy
    vasoocclusive a. (VAT)
angiotomomyelography
angiotropic large cell lymphoma
angle
    acetabular sector a.
    acromial a.
    alpha a.
    anorectal a. (ARA)
    antegonial a.
    anterior angulation a.
    anterior talocalcaneal a.
    arch a.
    basal a.
    Baumann supracondylar fracture a.
    Beatson radiographic combined
      talocalcaneal a.
    beta a.
    bimalleolar a.
    blunting of costovertebral a.
    blurring of costophrenic a.
    board a.
    Böhler a.
    Bragg x-ray a.
    brain tumor at cerebellopontine a.
    C a.
    calcaneal inclination a. (CIA)

calcaneal pitch a.
calcaneoplantar a.
capital epiphysis a.
capitolunate a.
cardiodiaphragmatic a.
cardiohepatic a.
cardiophrenic a.
carinal a.
carpal wrist a.
carrying a.
CCD a.
central collodiaphysial a.
cephalic a.
cephalometric a.
cerebellopontine a. (CPA)
Clarke arch a.
clivus-canal a.
Cobb scoliosis a.
Codman a.
condylar a.
congruence a.
costal a.
costolumbar a.
costophrenic a.
costosternal a.
costovertebral a. (CVA)
CP a.
craniofacial a.
craniovertebral a.
de Seze a.
distal articular set a. (DASA)
distal metatarsal articular a. (DMAA)
Doppler a.
dorsiflexion a. (DFA)
dorsoplantar talometatarsal a.
dorsoplantar talonavicular a.
Drennan metaphysial-epiphysial a.
duodenojejunal a.
Ebstein a.
epigastric a.
Ernst a.
exposure a.
fan a.
femoral torsion V a.
femorotibial a. (FTA)
Ferguson a.
flip a.
focal spot-to-film a.
foot-progression a. (FPA)
Frankfort mandibular incisor a.
Garden femoral neck fracture a.
gastroesophageal a.
Gissane calcaneal x-ray a.
gonial a.
Graf alpha a.
Graf beta a.
hallux dorsiflexion a.
hallux interphalangeus a. (HIA)
hallux valgus a. (HVA)

angle (*continued*)

hallux valgus interphalangeus a.
hepatic a.
hepatorenal a.
Hibbs metatarsocalcaneal a.
Hilgenreiner epiphysial a.
His a.
horizontal toit externe a.
HTE a.
incident a.
increased carrying a.
infrasternal a.
interbronchial a.
intercarpal a.
intermetatarsal a. (IMA)
kite a.
Konstram a.
lateral divergence a. (LDA)
lateral patellofemoral a.
lateral plantar metatarsal a.
lateral talocalcaneal a.
lateral talometatarsal a.
lateral tarsometatarsal a.
Laurin a.
Lewis a.
Lippman-Cobb a.
Louis a.
Ludovici a.
Ludwig a.
lumbar facet a.
lumbosacral joint a.
magnetization precession a.
mandibular a.
Meary metatarsotalar a.
medial a.
mediolateral radiocarpal a.
Merchant a.
metaphysial-diaphysial a.
metaphysial-epiphysial a.
metatarsal a.
metatarsocalcaneal a.
metatarsotalar a.
metatarsus adductus a.
metatarsus primus varus a. (MPVA)
Mikulicz a.
navicular to 1st metatarsal a.
neck-shaft a. (NSA)
nidus a.
nutation a.
obliterated costophrenic a.
occipitocervical a.
a. of anteversion
a. of declination of metatarsal
a. of greatest extension (AGE)
a. of greatest flexion (AGF)
a. of inclination of urethra
a. of incongruity
a. of insonation
a.'s of Lequesne and de Seze

a. of orientation
a. of rib
a. of trigone
patellofemoral a.
Pauwel a.
pelvic femoral a.
phase a.
phrenopericardial a.
Pirogoff a.
plantar metatarsal a.
pontile a.
posterior urethrovesical a. (PUVA)
precession a.
proximal articular set a.
psoas shadow a.
pulse flip a.
Q a.
QRS-T a.
radiocarpal a.
Ranke a.
resting forefoot supination a.
Rolando a.
rotation a.
sacrohorizontal a.
sacrovertebral a.
scapular a.
set a.
Sharp a.
slip a.
sphenoid a.
spinographic a.
splenic a.
splenorenal a.
sternal a.
sternoclavicular a.
1st metatarsal a.
1st-2nd intermetatarsal a.
1st-5th intermetatarsal a.
subcarinal a.
substernal a.
subtalar a.
sulcus a.
surgical a.
talar tilt a.
talocalcaneal a.
talocrural a.
talohorizontal a.
talometatarsal a.
talonavicular a.
tarsometatarsal a.
thigh-foot a. (TFA)
tibiocalcaneal a.
tibiofemoral a. (TFA)
tibiotalar a.
tip a.
tracheal bifurcation a.
tracheobronchial a.
transmalleolar axis-thigh a.
transmetatarsal-thigh a.

A

urethral a.
urethrovesical a. (UVA)
valgus carrying a.
a. variation resolution
varus metatarsophalangeal a.
venous brain a.
venous neck a.
vertebrophrenic a.
vertical-center-anterior a.
vesicourethral a.
wedge isodose a.
Welcher basal a.
Welcker a.
Wiberg a.
Wiltse a.
xiphoid a.

angled
    a. craniocaudal view
    a. Glidewire
    a. pleural tube
    a. slice
angled-tip catheter
Angle-Iron skull immobilizer
Angström (Å)
    A. law
    A. unit
angular
    a. alignment
    a. artery
    a. bolster
    a. curvature
    a. deformity
    a. deviation
    a. frequency
    a. gyrus
    a. momentum
    a. notch
    a. process of orbit
    a. sampling
    a. vein
    a. velocity
angularis
    a. body
    incisura a.
    sulcus a.
angulated
    a. catheter
    a. fracture
    a. hydrophilic guidewire
    a. lesion
    a. segment
angulation
    anterior a.
    bowel loop a.
    caudocranial a.
    cephalic a.
    coronal a.
    cranial a.
    craniocaudal needle a.

forefoot a.
gantry a.
kyphotic a.
a. of spine
palmar a.
posttraumatic a.
spinal a.
valgus a.
varus a.
volar a.
angulator
angulus of stomach
anhaustral colonic gas pattern
anhydrous ammonia
ani (*pl. of* anus)
aniline carcinoma
anionic neutrophil-activating peptide
  (ANAP)
anisotropic
    a. diffusion
    a. 3D imaging
    a. resolution
    a. rotation
    a. tissue
    a. volume study
anisotropically
    a. rotational diffusion (ARD)
    a. rotational diffusion imaging
anisotropy
    brain diffusion a.
    curvature a.
    decreased diffusion a.
    diffusion a.
    a. factor
    fractional a.
    functional diffusion a.
    magnetic a.
    a. map
ankle
    athlete's a.
    a. bone
    disc of a.
    eccentric axis of rotation of a.
    eversion of a.
    fused a.
    a. fusion
    a. instability
    a. inversion injury
    inversion injury of a.
    a. joint
    a. joint complex
    laciniate ligament of a.
    a. mortise
    a. mortise axis
    a. mortise fracture
    a. mortise widening
    neuropathic a.
    a. swelling
    synthetic graft bypass to a.

ankle (*continued*)
  a. systolic pressure
  tailor's a.
  transmalleolar a.
  twisted a.
ankle-arm
  a.-a. index (AAI)
  a.-a. pressure
ankle-brachial
  a.-b. index (ABI)
  a.-b. pressure measurement
  a.-b. pressure ratio
ankylosing
  a. hyperostosis
  a. spondylitis
  a. spondylitis spine MRI score for
    activity
ankylosis
  bony a.
  extracapsular a.
  false a.
  fibrous a.
  intracapsular a.
  joint a.
  ligamentous a.
  shoulder a.
  spurious a.
  vertebral a.
ankyroid (*var. of* ancyroid)
anlage, *pl.* **anlagen**
  cartilaginous a.
  pancreatic dorsal a.
  ventral pancreatic a.
anlagen (*pl. of* anlage)
ANMR
  advanced nuclear medical resonance
    ANMR Insta-scan MR scanner
Ann
  A. Arbor Hodgkin disease
    classification
  A. Arbor staging system
annealing
  simulated a.
annihilation
  a. coincidence detection (ACD)
  a. photon
  a. radiation
  a. reaction
annotated imaging
annotation
annular (*var. of* anular)
annularis
  digitus a.
annulus (*var. of* anulus)
ano
  fissure in a.
  fistula in a.
anococcygeal
  a. body

  a. ligament
  a. raphe
anodal block
anode
  molybdenum a.
  a. ray
  rhodium a.
  rotating a.
  stationary a.
  a. tube
  a. tube reloading
  tungsten a.
anode-cathode axis
anodontia
anogenital
  a. band
  a. raphe
anomalad
  Robin a.
anomalous
  a. anatomy
  a. branching
  a. bronchus
  a. craniovertebral junction
  a. development
  a. distribution
  a. insertion
  a. left coronary artery
  a. left pulmonary artery
  a. muscle
  a. origin
  a. origin of artery
  a. origin of left coronary artery
    from pulmonary artery (ALCAPA)
  a. pathway
  a. pulmonary venous connection
  a. pulmonary venous return
  a. right coronary artery
  a. right subclavian artery
  a. vessel
anomaly
  Alder constitutional granulation a.
  Alder-Reilly a.
  anorectal a.
  aortic arch a.
  associated a.
  atlas a.
  atrioventricular junction a.
  axis a.
  back-angle a.
  bell-clapper a. (BCA)
  cardiac a.
  cardiovascular a.
  cervical rib a.
  cloacal a.
  conjoined nerve roots a.
  conotruncal congenital a.
  cranial a.
  craniofacial a.

craniovertebral a.
Cruveilhier-Baumgarten a.
cutaneous vascular a.
double-inlet ventricle a.
duplication a.
Ebstein a.
extracardiac a.
fast-flow vascular a.
fetal cardiac a.
fetal chest a.
fetal CNS a.
fetal gastrointestinal a.
fetal heart a.
fetal neck a
fetal urinary tract a.
Freund a.
genitourinary a.
heart a.
intracranial leptomeningeal vascular
 a.
in utero detection of cardiac a.
jugular bulb a.
kidney a.
limb reduction a.
May-Hegglin a.
Michel a.
migrational a.
Mondini a.
müllerian duct a.
multiple congenital a.'s (MCA)
numerary renal a.
occipitoatlantoaxial a.
portal vein a. (type I-V)
presacral a.
radial ray a.
renal a.
rotation a.
segmentation a.
Shone a.
slow-flow vascular a.
spinal a.
structural a.
Taussig-Bing a.
tricuspid valve a.
Uhl a.
Undritz a.
urachal a.
urinary tract a.
uterine duplication a.
vascular a.
vena cava a.
venous a.
vertebral segmentation a.
Zahn a.
anonymous vein
anophthalmia, anophthalmos
anophthalmos (*var. of* anophthalmia)
anorectal
 a. angle (ARA)

 a. anomaly
 a. atresia
 a. dysgenesis
 a. fistula
 a. junction (ARJ)
 a. line
 a. lymph node
 a. malformation
 a. manometry
 a. ring
 a. tuberculosis
anorectum
anosmia
anovaginal fistula
anovular ovarian follicle
anoxia
 brain a.
 cerebral a.
 perinatal a.
anoxic
 a. encephalopathy
 a. ischemia
Anrep effect
ansa, *pl.* **ansae**
 a. of Vieussens
ansae (*pl. of* ansa)
anserine
 a. bursa
 a. bursitis
anserinus
 pes a.
antacid
antagonist
Antares ultrasound platform
anteater
 a. nose
 a. nose sign
antebrachial
 a. fascia
 a. vein
antebrachium
antecedent sign
antecolic
antecubital
 a. fossa
 a. space
 a. vein
anteflexed uterus
anteflexion
antegonial
 a. angle
 a. notch
antegrade
 a. aortography
 a. aspiration
 a. bile flow
 a. block
 a. blood flow
 a. cystography

antegrade (*continued*)
a. diastolic flow
a. fast pathway
a. femoral artery catheterization
a. filling of vessel
a. perfusion
a. perfusion pressure measurement (APPM)
a. peristalsis
a. pressure study
a. puncture
a. pyelography
a. pyelography imaging
a. refractory period
a. transluminal balloon dilation
a. ureteral stenting
a. urography
a. venography

antenna
loopless a.

antepartum hemorrhage

anteprostatic gland

anterior
a. abdominal wall
ampulla membranacea a.
ampulla ossea a.
a. angulation
a. angulation angle
a. aspect
a. atlas arch
a. atrial myocardial bundle
a. axillary line (AAL)
a. band
a. band of colon
a. border
a. border of heart
a. bowing of sternum
a. bowing of tibia
a. capsular distance (ACD)
a. capsular shift
a. cardiac vein
a. carotid circulation
a. central beaking
a. central indentation
a. cerebral artery (ACA)
a. cerebral artery crawling under skull
a. cervical fusion (ACF)
a. choroidal artery
a. clear space
a. colliculus
a. column fracture
a. column of spine
a. commissure (AC)
a. commissure-posterior commissure (AC-PC)
a. communicating artery
a. communicating artery aneurysm
a. communicating artery complex
a. communicating artery distribution infarct
a. compartment syndrome
a. condylar canal
a. condyloid foramen
a. cord syndrome
a. coronary plexus
a. corpus
a. corticospinal tract
a. cranial base lesion
a. cruciate deficit of knee
a. cruciate ligament (ACL)
a. cruciate ligament injury
a. current generator
a. curvature
a. cusp
a. cutaneous branch
a. descending artery
a. dislocation
a. drawer sign
a. epidural fat
a. exenteration
a. fascicular block
a. fibular ligament
a. fontanelle
a. foot view
a. fornix of vagina
a. glenoid labrum (AGL)
a. gray column
a. gray column of cord
a. horn
a. horn cell disease
a. horn of spinal cord
a. humeral line
a. hypothalamus
a. iliac crest
a. impingement syndrome
a. intercostal artery
a. interhemispheric cistern
a. interhemispheric fissure
a. internal vertebral vein (AIVV)
a. internodal pathway
a. internodal tract of Bachmann
a. interventricular groove
a. intervertebral disc
a. intraoccipital synchondrosis
a. joint capsule thickening
a. jugular vein
a. junction line
a. labral avulsion
a. labral disruption
a. labroligamentous periosteal sleeve avulsion (ALPSA)
a. labroligamentous periosteal sleeve avulsion lesion
a. leaflet prolapse
a. maxillary spine
a. median fissure
a. mediastinal compartment

a. mediastinal mass
a. mediastinum
a. meningeal artery
a. metatarsal arch
a. midbody of corpus callosum
a. motion of posterior mitral valve
  leaflet
a. nasal spine of maxilla
a. oblique position
a. oblique view
a. osteophyte
a. palatine foramen
a. palatine suture
a. papillary muscle (APM)
a. pararenal space (APS)
a. parietal lesion
a. pillar of fauces
a. precordium
a. predominance
a. projection
a. pulmonary plexus
a. recess of ischiorectal fossa
a. rectus fascia
a. rectus sheath
a. sacral foramen
a. sacral meningocele
a. sagittal diameter (ASD)
scalenus a.
a. scalloping of vertebra
a. semicircular canal
a. semilunar valve
a. septal myocardial infarct
serratus a.
a. spinal artery
a. spinal artery stroke
a. spinal artery syndrome
a. spinal ligament calcification
a. spine fusion (ASF)
a. spinocerebellar tract
a. spinothalamic tract
a. spur
a. surface of pancreas
a. talar dome
a. talocalcaneal angle
a. talofibular (ATF)
a. talofibular ligament
a. tarsal tunnel syndrome
a. temporal branch of posterior
  cerebral artery
a. temporal lobectomy (ATL)
a. terminal vein (ATV)
a. thalamotomy
a. thoracic meningocele
a. tibial artery
a. tibial bowing
a. tibial compartment
tibialis a.
a. tibial subluxation
a. tibial tendon (ATT)

a. tibiofibular ligament
a. tibiotalar ligament
a. tip of temporal lobe
a. tracheal displacement
a. tracking
a. tricuspid valve leaflet
a. urethra
a. urethral injury
a. vertebral body margin
a. wall antral ulcer
a. wall motion
a. wall myocardial infarct
a. wedge compression fracture
a. wedge compression fracture
a. wedging
anterior-inferior (*var. of* anteroinferior)
anterior-posterior (*var. of*
  anteroposterior)
**anterior-to-posterior sagittal canal
  diameter**
anteroapical
  a. defect
  a. trabecular septum
anterobasal
  a. bronchus
  a. segment
anterochiasmatic lesion
anterofundal placenta
anteroinferior, anterior-inferior
  a. cerebellar artery (AICA)
  a. cerebral artery (AICA)
  a. communicating artery (AICA)
  a. corner fracture
  a. dislocation
  a. iliac spine
  a. myocardial infarct
  a. tibiofibular ligament
  a. triangular fragment
anterolateral
  a. abdominal wall
  a. aspect
  a. compression fracture
  a. fontanelle
  a. groove
  a. gutter
  a. impingement
  a. impingement syndrome
  a. myocardial infarct
  a. osteoplasty
  a. rotary knee instability
  a. segment
  a. surface
  a. system
  a. white matter of cord
anterolisthesis
anteromedial
  a. superior humeral head impaction
  a. surface
anteromedian groove

anteroposterior (AP), anterior-posterior
a. aspect
a. axis
a. diameter
a. dimension
a. film
a. flow direction
a. iliac spine
a. lordotic projection
a. position
a. talocalcaneal (APTC)
a. tube
a. view
anteroposterior-posteroanterior (AP-PA)
a.-p. view
anteroseptal
a. commissure
a. myocardial infarct
anterosuperior iliac spine (ASIS)
antetorsion
femoral a.
anteversion
acetabular a. (AA)
angle of a.
femoral a.
Magilligan technique for measuring
neutral a.
anteverted uterus
anthracis
Bacillus a.
anthracosilicosis
anthracosis
anthracotic
a. material
a. tuberculosis
anthracycline-induced myocardial damage
anthrax
a. exposure
inhalation a.
a. pneumonia
Anthron heparinized catheter
anthropoid pelvis
anthropologic baseline
anthropometric imaging
anthropometry
3D surface a.
anthropomorphic
a. baseline
a. phantom
antiadrenergic drug
antiaggregant therapy
antiaggregation
antialiasing technique
antiangiogenic
a. chemotherapy
a. therapy
antibody
a. half-life
human antimouse a. (HAMA)

humanized anti-human IL-2 receptor
a.
immunofluorescence a.
a. labeling
Lewis a.
monoclonal a. (MoAb, MoAb)
^{99m}Tc-labeled antigranulocyte a.
polyclonal a.
radiolabeled a.
recombinant anti-p185HER2
monoclonal a.
a. to Epstein-Barr virus
transactivator protein
antibody-conjugated paramagnetic
liposome (ACPL)
antibody-labeled circulating granulocyte
anti-CEA
radiolabeled anti-CEA
anticoagulant bleed
anticoagulant-related bleed
anticoagulation
anticoincidence circuit
anticonvulsant drug
antidepressant drug
antidysrhythmic
antiemetic
antiestrogen radiologic therapy
antiferromagnetism
antifibrin
a. antibody imaging
a. antibody imaging agent
a. scintigraphy
antifolate
multitargeted a.
antigen
cancer a.
a. expression
HLA-A3 histocompatibility a.
HLA-B7 histocompatibility a.
HLA-B14 histocompatibility a.
human leukocyte a. (HLA)
prostate-specific a. (PSA)
prostate-specific membrane a.
(PSMA)
antigen-induced arthritis
antigen-modulated mini-stem cell
transplant
antigravity muscle
antihyperlipidemic
antiidiotypic affinity chromatography
Anti-Lung Cancer Association
antimesenteric
a. border
a. border of distal ileum
a. fat-pad
antimesocolic side of cecum
antimuscarinic drug
antimyosin monoclonal antibody imaging
agent

A

antineoplastic drug
antineutrino
antiparticle
antiphospholid antibody syndrome
antiplatelet agent
antiproton
antipsychotic drug
antipyretic
antiradial technique
antireflection coating
antiscatter grid
antisense oligonucleotide
antisiphon device
antitragohelicine fissure
antitubercular therapy
antivascular therapy
Antopol-Goldman lesion
antra (*pl. of* antrum)
antral
- a. beaking
- a. edema
- a. gastritis
- a. G-cell hyperplasia
- a. mucosal diaphragm
- a. mucosal thickening
- a. padding
- a. polyp
- a. pouch
- a. sphincter
- a. stasis
- a. stenosis
- a. stomach narrowing
- a. stricture
- a. ulcer
- a. web

antrochoanal polyp
antroduodenal motility
antropyloric
- a. canal
- a. muscle thickness

antrum, *pl.* **antra**
- aditus ad a.
- cardiac a.
- gastric a.
- Highmore a.
- Malacarne a.
- mastoid a.
- maxillary a.
- a. of Highmore
- a. of stomach
- prepyloric a.
- pyloric a.
- retained gastric a.
- Willis a.

anular, annular
- a. abscess
- a. appearance
- a. array
- a. array transducer

- a. calcification
- a. constricting lesion
- a. detector
- a. dilation
- a. disc bulge
- a. disruption
- a. epiphysis
- a. esophageal stricture
- a. fiber
- a. fibrosis
- a. foreshortening
- a. fracture
- a. hypoplasia
- a. lamella
- a. ligament
- a. ligament of trachea
- a. pancreas
- a. phased-array hyperthermia
- a. placement
- a. placenta
- a. rim of cartilage
- a. tear
- a. tear classification
- a. tear extent
- a. tear pattern

anuli (*pl. of* anulus)
anuloaortic ectasia
anulospiral organ
anulus, annulus, *pl.* **anuli**
- aortic valve a.
- atrioventricular a.
- bulging a.
- calcified a.
- a. fibrosus
- fissure of a.
- friable a.
- mitral valve a.
- a. ovalis
- periphery of a.
- posterior a.
- pulmonary valve a.
- redundant scallop of posterior a.
- septal tricuspid a.
- tricuspid valve a.
- a. umbilicalis
- valve a.
- Vieussens a.
- Zinn a.

anus, *pl.* **ani**
- ectopic a.
- imperforate a.
- levator ani

anvil bone
AO
- Arbeitsgemeinschaft für Osteosynthesefragen
- AO and Danis-Weber ankle fracture classification
- AO ankle fracture classification

AO (*continued*)
  AO classification of ankle fracture
  AO tension band
AO/AC
  aortic valve opening to aortic valve
  closing ratio
AOCS
  anatomy-oriented colon segmentation
AOD
  airflow obstruction disease
AOIVM
  angiographically occult intracranial
  vascular malformation
aorta, *pl.* **aortae**
  abdominal a.
  aneurysmal widening of a.
  ascending a. (AA)
  ascending hypoplasia of a.
  bifurcatio aortae
  bifurcation of a.
  biventricular origin of a.
  biventricular transposed a.
  brachiocephalic trunk of a.
  calcified a.
  central a.
  cervical a.
  coarctation of a.
  descending thoracic a.
  dextropositioned a.
  dilated descending a.
  distal a.
  D-malposition of a.
  double-arch a.
  double-barrel a.
  draped a.
  dynamic a.
  ectasia of a.
  elongated a.
  feminine a.
  Hodgson aneurysmal dilation of a.
  infantile coarctation of a.
  infrarenal abdominal a.
  intramural hematoma of a.
  juxtaductal coarctation of a.
  kinked a.
  L-malposition of a.
  native a.
  overriding a.
  pericardial a.
  porcelain a.
  postductal coarctation of a.
  proximal a.
  pseudocoarctation of a.
  recoarctation of a.
  reconstruction of a.
  retroesophageal a.
  reversed coarctation of a.
  small feminine a.

stenosis of a.
supraceliac a.
supradiaphragmatic a.
symptomatic coarctation of a.
terminal a.
thoracic a.
thoracoabdominal a.
tortuous a.
transposed a.
tulip bulb a.
uncoiling ascending a.
uncoiling descending a.
unwinding of a.
ventral a.
widening of a.
wide tortuous a.
aortae (*pl. of* aorta)
aortic
  a. allograft
  a. aneurysm (AA)
  a. anulus abscess
  a. aperture
  a. arch
  a. arch aneurysm
  a. arch angiography
  a. arch anomaly
  a. arch atresia
  a. arch calcification
  a. arch interruption
  a. arch lesion
  a. arch malformation
  a. arch obstruction
  a. atherosclerosis
  a. attenuation
  a. bifurcation
  a. body tumor
  a. bulb
  a. button
  a. cannulation
  a. cartilage
  a. closure
  a. coarctation
  a. cuff
  a. cusp
  a. cusp separation
  a. deviation
  a. dissection
  a. distensibility
  a. elongation
  a. flow
  a. flow volume
  a. foramen
  a. gland
  a. graft infection
  a. hiatus
  a. idiopathic necrosis
  a. impedance
  a. incisura

a. inflammation
a. inflow
a. insult
a. intimal dehiscence
a. intramural hematoma
a. isthmus
a. kinking
a. knob
a. knuckle
a. lumen
a. lymph node
a. motion artifact
a. nipple
a. nipple sign
a. node metastasis
a. notch
a. opening
a. opening of heart
a. orifice
a. ostium
a. outflow gradient
a. outflow obstruction
a. override
a. oxygen saturation
a. paravalvular leak
a. penetrating ulcer
a. plexus
a. prominence
a. pseudoaneurysm
a. pullback
a. reconstruction
a. regurgitation
a. root
a. root cineangiography
a. root diameter
a. root dilation
a. root dimension
a. root echocardiography
a. root homograft
a. root pressure
a. root ratio
a. root replacement
a. runoff
a. rupture
a. sac
a. sclerosis
a. segment
a. septal defect
a. septum
a. shag
a. sinotubular junction
a. sinus aneurysm
a. sinus to right ventricle fistula
a. spindle
a. stenosis
a. stiffness
a. stump blowout
a. syndrome

a. thromboembolism
a. thrombosis
a. tract complex hypoplasia
a. transection
a. tube graft
a. valve
a. valve anulus
a. valve area (AVA)
a. valve atresia
a. valve calcification
a. valve calcium quantification with MSCT
a. valve calcium score
a. valve deformity
a. valve echocardiography (AVE)
a. valve endocarditis
a. valve gradient (AVG)
a. valve lesion
a. valve nodule
a. valve obstruction
a. valve opening
a. valve opening to aortic valve closing ratio (AO/AC)
a. valve peak instantaneous gradient
a. valve pressure gradient
a. valve replacement (AVR)
a. valve sinus
a. valve stenosis
a. valve thickening
a. valvular disease (AVD)
a. valvular incompetence
a. valvular insufficiency
a. vasa vasorum
a. vent suction line
a. vestibule of ventricle
a. wall thickening
a. window
a. window node
a. wrap

aortica
  bifurcatio a.
aortic-brachiocephalic (ABC)
  a.-b. injury
aortic-enteric fistula
aortic-left
  a.-l. ventricular fistula
  a.-l. ventricular tunnel
aorticopulmonary (*var. of* aortopulmonary)
aorticorenal
  a. ganglion
  a. graft
aortic-right ventricular fistula
aortitis
  infectious a.
  luetic a.
  a. syndrome
  syphilitic a.
  Takayasu a.

aortoaortic bypass grafting
aortobifemoral
    a. graft
    a. reconstruction
aortocaval fistula
aortocoronary valve
aortoduodenal fistula
aortoenteric fistula
aortoesophageal fistula
aortofemoral
    a. arteriography
    a. bypass graft (AFBG)
    a. runoff
aortogastric
aortogram
    arch a.
    transbrachial arch a.
aortography
    abdominal a.
    antegrade a.
    arch a.
    ascending a.
    balloon occlusive a.
    biplanar a.
    catheter a.
    contrast a.
    countercurrent a.
    digital subtraction a.
    flush a.
    a. imaging
    intravenous a.
    lumbar a.
    postangioplasty a.
    preembolization a.
    renal a.
    retrograde femoral a.
    retrograde transaxillary a.
    retrograde transfemoral a.
    retrograde translumbar a.
    selective visceral a.
    supravalvular a.
    thoracic arch a.
    translumbar a. (TLA)
    ultrasonic a.
    venous a.
    visceral a.
aortoiliac
    a. aneurysm
    a. bypass
    a. bypass graft
    a. inflow assessment
    a. inflow system
    a. obstruction
    a. occlusive disease
     (AIOD)
    a. stenosis
    a. thrombosis
aortoiliofemoral artery
aortojejunal fistula

aortomegaly
    diffuse a.
aortoplasty
    balloon a.
    patch-graft a.
    posterior patch a.
    subclavian flap a.
    a. with patch graft
aortopulmonary, aorticopulmonary
    a. fenestration
    a. fistula
    a. mediastinal stripe
    a. septal defect
    a. septum
    a. trunk
    a. window
    a. window mass
aortosclerosis
aortoseptal continuity
aortosigmoid fistula
aortovelography
    transcutaneous a. (TAV)
aortoventriculoplasty
AOVM
    angiographically occult vascular
    malformation
AP
    anteroposterior
     AP inversion stress vaginal view
     AP malleolar bisection
     AP projection
     AP supine portable view
apallic syndrome
APB
    abductor pollicis brevis
APBJ
    abnormal pancreatobiliary junction
APC-3, APC-4 collimator
ape hand of syringomyelia
apelike hand
aperiodic
    a. complex
    a. functional MR imaging
    a. wave
aperistalsis
    esophageal a.
aperistaltic
    a. distal ureteral segment
    a. esophagus
aperta
    spina bifida a.
apertura, *pl.* **aperturae**
    a. externa aqueductus vestibuli
    a. externa canaliculi cochleae
    a. lateralis ventriculi quarti
    a. mediana ventriculi quarti
    a. pelvis inferior
    a. pelvis superior
    a. piriformis

a. sinus frontalis
a. sinus sphenoidalis
aperturae superior et inferior fossae
  axillaris
a. thoracis inferior
a. thoracis superior
a. tympanica canaliculi chordae
  tympani
aperturae (*pl. of* apertura)
aperture
  aortic a.
  coded-image a.
  a. diaphragm
  superior thoracic a.
apex, *pl.* **apices**
  a. beat
  A. 409, 415 camera
  cardiac a.
  a. cordis
  displaced left ventricular a.
  duodenal bulb a. (DBA)
  external ring a.
  F point of cardiac a.
  Koch triangle a.
  left ventricular a.
  lung a.
  a. of bladder
  a. of femur
  a. of fibula
  a. of head of patella
  a. of heart
  a. of petrous portion of temporal
   bone
  a. of prostate
  orbital a.
  petrous a.
  A. Plus excimer laser
  prostate a.
  right ventricular a. (RVA)
  sternal a.
  systolic retraction of a.
  true a.
  uptilted cardiac a.
  ventricular a.
apexcardiogram (ACG)
  derived value on a. (dD/dt)
  upstroke pattern on a. (dP/dt)
aphalangia
aphasia
apheresis catheter
aphtha, *pl.* **aphthae**
aphthae (*pl. of* aphtha)
aphthoid ulcer
aphthous stomach ulcer
apical
  a. and subcostal 4-chamber views
  a. aspect
  a. atelectasis
  a. bronchus

a. canaliculus
a. cap
a. capping
a. cap sign
a. 2-chamber view echocardiography
a. 5-chamber view echocardiography
a. complex
a. corn
a. defect
a. dip
a. duodenal ulcer
a. ectodermal ridge (AER)
a. fenestration
a. foramen
a. gland
a. granuloma
a. hypertrophy
a. hypokinesis
a. hypoperfusion
a. impulse
a. infiltrate
a. lesion
a. ligament
a. lordotic projection
a. lordotic view
a. lymph node
a. myocardial infarct
a. notch
a. petrositis
a. pleural thickening
a. posterior artery
a. process
a. pulse
a. scarring
a. segment
a. short-axis slice
a. surface of heart
a. suture
a. thinning
a. tissue
a. wall
a. wall motion
a. window
apical-lateral wall myocardial infarct
apically directed chest tube
apices (*pl. of* apex)
apicoposterior
  a. bronchus
  a. segment
apiculate waveform
APL
  abductor pollicis longus
aplasia
  bilateral semicircular canal a.
  cerebellar a.
  cochlea a.
  deep venous a.
  lung a.
  Michel a.

aplasia (*continued*)
    a. of deep vein
    pulmonary a.
    radial a.
    red cell a.
aplastic uterus
APLD
    automated percutaneous lumbar
    discectomy
APLE
    absolute percentage loss of
    enhancement
APM
    anterior papillary muscle
apnea-bradycardia ratio
apnea-hypopnea index (AHI)
apocrine
    a. adenoma
    a. carcinoma
    a. cyst
    a. metaplasia
    a. sweat gland
Apogee
    A. CX100, CX200 echocardiography
    system
    A. RX400 diagnostic ultrasound
    system
Apollo DXA bone densitometry system
Apomate radiopharmaceutical imaging
  agent
aponeuroses (*pl. of* aponeurosis)
aponeurosis, *pl.* **aponeuroses**
    bicipital a.
    digital a.
    epicranial a.
    external oblique a.
    flexor carpi ulnaris a.
    internal oblique a.
    palmar a.
    plantar a.
    tendon a.
aponeurosisbicipitalis (*var. of* bicipital
  aponeurosis)
aponeurotic
    a. band
    a. fibroma
    a. portion of diaphragm
    a. tendon
    a. triangle
    a. troika
aponeurotica
    galea a.
apophysary (*var. of* apophysial)
apophyseal (*var. of* apophysial)
apophyses (*pl. of* apophysis)
apophysial, apophyseal, apophysary
    a. fracture
    a. injury
    a. joint

    a. lesion
    a. point
    a. pouch
apophysis, *pl.* **apophyses**
    bone lesion a.
    calcaneal a.
    fragmentation of a.
    a. of Rau
    rim a.
    ring a.
apophysitis
    calcaneal a.
    iliac a.
apoplexy
    cerebellar a.
    delayed pineal a.
    mesenteric a.
    pineal a.
    pituitary a.
    postpartum pituitary a.
    pulmonary artery a.
    pulmonary vein a.
apoptic
    a. body
    a. nuclear fragment
aporic gland
apotentiality
    cerebral a.
APP
    average pixel projection
AP-PA
    anteroposterior-posteroanterior
    AP-PA skull block
    AP-PA skull immobilizer
apparatus (*pl.* **apparatus**)
    Acuson 128 a.
    anal a.
    electrooculogram a.
    extensor a.
    Hilal embolization a.
    Jaquet a.
    juxtaglomerular a. (JGA)
    mammoPET breast a.
    mitral a.
    oculomotor a.
    stereotactic a.
    valvular a.
    vestibular a.
    zero time of x-ray a.
apparent
    a. diffusion coefficient (ADC)
    a. paramagnetism
    a. volume of distribution
appearance
    anular a.
    apple-core a.
    apple-peel a.
    applesauce a.
    asymmetric target a.

ball-in-hand a.
ball-on-spoon a.
banding a.
batwing a.
beaded necklace a.
beaked a.
beaten brass a.
beaten silver a.
beaver-tail a.
bilaminar a.
birdlike a.
blade-of-grass a.
blown-out a.
bone-within-bone a.
bubblelike a.
bull-neck a.
bull's-eye a.
bunch-of-grapes a.
butterfly a.
candle dripping a.
catheter tip hockey-stick a.
cauliflower a.
chisellike truncated a.
Christmas tree a.
cobblestone a.
cobra-head a.
cobweb a.
cockscomb a.
coffee-bean a.
coiled spring a.
collar-button a.
colonic lead-pipe a.
constant level a.
corkscrew a.
cottage loaf a.
cotton ball a.
cotton-wool a.
crabmeatlike a.
crazy paving a.
cystic a.
double-bubble a.
double-bulb a.
double decidual ring a.
double-halo a.
dripping candle-wax a.
drooping lily a.
drumstick a.
dumbbell a.
duodenal teardrop a.
echogenic a.
Erlenmeyer flask a.
feathery a.
featureless a.
figure-8 a.
fine speckled a.
fish flesh a.
fishnet a.
flame a.
frayed-string a.

froglike a.
frondlike a.
ground-glass a.
hair-on-end a.
hammered brass a.
hammered silver a.
heterogeneous a.
hole-within-hole a.
holly leaf a.
homogeneous a.
Honda sign a.
honeycomb a.
horseshoe a.
hot-cross bun a.
hourglass a.
ill-defined a.
inner isoattenuated a.
inverse comma a.
inverted-T a.
irregular tapered a.
isodense a.
jail-bar a.
jelly-belly a.
kernel-of-corn a.
lacelike a.
leafless tree a.
light bulb a.
lobulated saccular a.
lollipop tree a.
Mickey Mouse a.
middle hypoattenuated a.
mixed-echo a.
molar tooth a.
moth-eaten a.
mottled a.
mouse-ear a.
multiseptate a.
mushroom a.
Neptune trident a.
nodular a.
nodule-in-nodule a.
onion peel a.
onionskin a.
outer isoattenuated striated mural a.
owl's-eye a.
pancake a.
panda a.
partial tubular a.
pencil-in-cup a.
picket fence a.
picture-frame a.
pistol-grip a.
pluglike a.
polka-dot a.
popcornlike a.
pruned-tree a.
pseudokidney a.
pseudo-post Billroth I a.
pseudotumor a.

A

appearance (*continued*)
    punched-out a.
    radial scarlike mammographic a.
    railroad track a.
    reticulogranular a.
    ringlike a.
    rounded a.
    rugger jersey a.
    saber-shin a.
    sandwich a.
    sausage-shaped a.
    sawtooth a.
    scalloped a.
    scotty dog a.
    septate a.
    serpentine a.
    serrated a.
    shading a.
    shell-of-bone a.
    smooth tapered a.
    snake's head a.
    snowstorm a.
    soap-bubble a.
    spadelike a.
    spiderweb a.
    spiral a.
    spongy a.
    stacked-coins a.
    stained-glass a.
    stepladder a.
    stippled a.
    string-of-beads a.
    string-of-pearls a.
    stumped-off a.
    sunburst a.
    sun-ray a.
    swirl a.
    Swiss Alps a.
    Swiss cheese a.
    tam-o-shanter a.
    target a.
    teardrop a.
    thumbprint a.
    tram-track a.
    tree-in-winter bile duct a.
    trefoil a.
    trilaminar a.
    trilayer a.
    twisted small bowel ribbon a.
    violin string a.
    waferlike a.
    walking-stick a.
    waterfall a.
    weblike a.
    well-defined a.
    whirl a.
    whirlpool a.
    whorled a.
    windsock a.

    wine glass a.
    wormy a.
    yin-yang a.
    zebra stripe a.

appendage
    atrial a.
    cecal a.
    coccygeal a.
    epiploic a.
    inverted left atrial a.
    left atrial a. (LAA)
    left auricular a.
    right atrial a. (RAA)
    testicular torsion a.
    truncated atrial a.
    vermicular a.
    wide-based, blunt-ended, right-sided
      atrial a.

appendical (*var. of* appendiceal)

appendiceal, appendical
    a. abscess
    a. carcinoma
    a. intussusception
    a. lesion
    a. mass
    a. stump

appendices (*pl. of* appendix)

appendicitis
    acute suppurative a.
    perforated a.

appendicular
    a. bone mass measurement
    a. lymph node
    a. skeleton
    a. vein

appendiculare
    skeleton a.

appendix, *pl.* **appendixes,**
  pl. **appendices**
    cecal a.
    double a.
    ensiform a.
    epiploic a.
    a. epiploica
    appendices epiploicae
    filiform a.
    Morgagni a.
    a. mucocele
    a. of epididymis
    a. of testis
    a. of ventricle of larynx
    paracecal a.
    perforated gangrenous a.
    retrocecal a.
    retroileal a.
    a. rupture
    subcecal a.
    vermicular a.
    vermiform a.

a. vesiculosa
xiphoid a.
appendixes (*pl. of* appendix)
apperceptive mass
apple-core
a.-c. appearance
a.-c. carcinoma
a.-c. lesion
a.-c. tumor
apple-peel
a.-p. appearance
a.-p. appearance of GI tract
a.-p. bowel
a.-p. syndrome
applesauce appearance
application
infradiaphragmatic a.
interstitial radioelement a.
intracavitary radioelement a.
ribbon a.
surface radioelement a.
application-specific integrated circuit (ASIC)
applicator
beam-therapy a.
beta ray a.
Burnett a.
colpostat a.
Henschke seed a.
intracavitary afterloading a.
LITT a.
Mick seed a.
Nucletron a.
perfused needle a.
RFA with perfused needle a.
small LITT a.
^{90}Sr-loaded eye a.
standard LITT a.
Syed-Puthawala-Hedger esophageal a.
tandem a.
Wang a.
APPM
antegrade perfusion pressure measurement
apposing articular surfaces
apposition
bone-to-bone a.
bony a.
close a.
fracture in close a.
margin of a.
a. of leaflets
Appraise monitor
approach
axillofemoral a.
Bartko-Carpenter a.
bipediculate a.
black box a.
brachial artery a.

catheter-directed a.
direct transtorcular a.
endovascular embolization femoral a.
femoral artery a.
femoral venous a.
flow-directed a.
hybrid a.
interscalene a.
mask-based a.
organ-sparing treatment a.
palpation-guided a.
particle a.
pencil-beam a.
posterior retrocrural a.
posterior transcaval a.
pterional transsylvian a.
retrograde femoral artery a.
skull base a.
sliding thin-slab a.
tourniquet-directed a.
unipediculate a.
approximation
Born a.
APR
abdominoperineal resection
anatomic programmed radiography
apraxia
apron
abdominal a.
lead-rubber a.
quadriceps a.
a. shield
APS
anterior pararenal space
APT
attached proton test
automatic peak tracking
APTC
anteroposterior talocalcaneal
APUD
amine precursor uptake and decarboxylation
AQ
aqueous
AQP4 expression
aquagenic
AquariusBLUE 3D imaging
AquariusNET 2D/3D medical imaging server
AquaSens fluid monitoring system
aqueduct
cerebral a.
cochlear a.
a. compression
forking of sylvian a.
gliosis of sylvian a.
mesencephalon a.
midbrain a.
Monro a.

aqueduct (*continued*)
   a. of Sylvius
   a. stenosis
   sylvian a.
   ventricular a.
   vestibular a.
aqueductal
   a. CSF stroke volume
   a. forking
   a. jet
   a. obstruction
   a. occlusion
   a. stenosis
aqueous (AQ)
   a. solution
   a. vein
Aquilion
   A. combined CT-fluoroscopy scanner
   A. Plus V-detector CT scanner
ARA
   American Rheumatism Association
   anorectal angle
arabinoside
   cytosine a.
arabinsylguanosine triphosphate
arachnodactylia (*var. of* arachnodactyly)
arachnodactyly, arachnodactylia
   a. CHD
arachnoid
   a. brain cyst
   a. canal
   a. diverticulum
   a. fibrosis
   a. granulation
   a. granulation calcification
   a. hyperplasia
   a. loculation of spine
   a. of uncus
   pia a.
   a. retrocerebellar pouch
   a. space
   a. spine cyst
   a. villus
   a. villus obstruction
arachnoidal
   a. foramen
   a. gliomatosis
arachnoidea mater encephali
arachnoiditis
   adhesive a.
   cystic a.
   fibrosing a.
Arantius
   A. canal
   A. ligament
   A. nodule
   A. ventricle
Arbeitsgemeinschaft für Osteosynthesefragen (AO)

arborescens
   lipoma a.
arborescent
arborization
   a. block
   cervical mucus a.
   a. of duct
   a. pattern
   pulmonary a.
arborize
arboroid
arc
   bregmatolambdoid a.
   nasobregmatic a.
   nasooccipital a.
   pulmonary a.
   a. radiotherapy
   reflex a.
   a. ring
   a. therapy
   a. welder's lung
arcade
   collateral a.
   Frohse ligamentous a.
   gastroepiploic a.
   mitral a.
   a. of Frohse
   septal a.
   Struthers a.
   subpleural pulmonary a.
   superficialis a.
Arcelin petrous temporal view
arch
   anastomotic a.
   a. angle
   anterior atlas a.
   anterior metatarsal a.
   aortic a.
   a. aortogram
   a. aortography
   articular a.
   atlas a.
   azygos a.
   a. bar
   carpal a.
   cervical aortic a.
   chimney-shaped high aortic a.
   circumflex retroesophageal a.
   congenital interruption of aortic a.
   coracoacromial a.
   cortical kidney a.
   deep a.
   distal aortic a.
   double aortic a.
   ductal a.
   embryonic aortic a.
   embryonic branchial a.
   flattened a.
   a. fracture

Hapad metatarsal a.
hemal a.
high a.
Hillock a.
hyoid a.
hypochordal a.
hypoplastic aortic a.
keystone of calcar a.
a. length index
longitudinal a.
lung a.
medial a.
midaortic a.
mural a.
2nd branchial a.
neural vertebral a.
a. of aorta abnormality
a. of bone
a. of fauces
a. of foot
osseocartilaginous a.
osseoligamentous a.
palmar arterial a.
plantar arterial a.
posterior metatarsal a.
posterior neural a.
posterior turn of aortic a.
pubic a.
3rd branchial a.
retroesophageal a.
right aortic a.
right-sided aortic a.
Riolan a.
a. rupture
1st branchial a.
subpubic a.
superciliary a.
superficial palmar arterial a.
target a.
tarsal a.
4th branchial a.
tortuous aortic a.
transverse aortic a.
vertebral a.
Zimmerman a.
zygomatic a.

arched crest
archenteric canal
archicortex
arching of mitral valve leaflet
arch-isthmic junction
architectural
a. alteration of bone
a. disorder of breast
a. distortion
a. disturbance
a. effacement
a. pattern
a. symmetry

architecture
bony a.
brain a.
disorganized a.
ductal a.
foot a.
hepatic a.
internal a.
intestinal villous a.
intranodal a.
lobular a.
lung a.
microstructural a.
mural a.
trabecular a.
archival system
arciform (*var. of* arcuate)
ARCO
Association Research Circulation
Osseous
ARCO osteonecrosis classification
arcuate, arciform
a. artery
a. complex
a. crest
a. eminence
a. fasciculus
a. fiber involvement
a. ligament
a. movement
a. nucleus
a. uterus
a. vein
a. vessel
arcuatus
pes a.
talipes a.
uterus a.
ARD
anisotropically rotational diffusion
ARDS
acute respiratory distress syndrome
adult respiratory distress syndrome
area
amygdaloid a.
anechoic a.
aortic valve a. (AVA)
arrhythmogenic a.
Bamberger a.
bare a.
body surface a. (BSA)
Broca a.
Brodmann a.
callosal a.
cardiac frontal a.
cluster of radiolucent a.'s (CORLA)
cortical motor a.
cross-sectional a. (CSA)
cystic-malacic a.

area (*continued*)
    denervated a.
    echo-free a.
    echo-poor a.
    effective balloon-dilated a. (EBDA)
    fat-density a.
    fractional a.
    a. gastrica
    gastrohepatic bare a.
    Gorlin formula for aortic valve
      a.
    Gorlin formula for mitral valve
      a.
    Hatle method to calculate mitral
      valve a.
    hilar a.
    hot a.
    hyperechoic a.
    hypodense a.
    hypoechoic a.
    hypoenhanced a.
    hypometabolic a.
    infraclavicular a.
    infrahilar a.
    ischemic a.
    jet a.
    lenticular a.
    luminal a.
    lytic a.
    metabolically inert a.
    midsternal a.
    mitral regurgitant signal a.
    mitral valve a. (MVA)
    motor a.
    a. of abnormal density
    a. of denudation
    a. of increased radiolabeling
    a. of lucency
    olfactory a.
    parietal association a.
    parietooccipital a.
    parietotemporal a.
    peak a.
    periaortic a.
    perihilar a.
    periportal a.
    pharyngeal a.
    photon-deficient a.
    photopenic a.
    postcricoid a.
    premotor a.
    primary somesthetic a.
    proliferation a.
    a. prostrema
    proximal isovelocity surface a.
      (PISA)
    puboischial a.
    pulmonary a.
    pulmonary valve a.

    punched-out a.
    radiodensity a.
    radiolucent a.
    rarefied a.
    regurgitant orifice a. (ROA)
    retrocardiac a.
    retroperitoneal a.
    retrosternal a.
    Rolando a.
    sclerotic a.
    scrotal a.
    septal a.
    skip a.
    sonolucent a.
    speech a.
    stenosis a.
    subglottic a.
    subhepatic a.
    suprapubic a.
    transverse cranial a.
    tricuspid valve a.
    a. under curve (AUC)
    valve a.
    visual word form a.
    water density a.
    watershed a.
    Wernicke a.
    xiphopubic a.
    zygomaticomalar a.
area/hemidiameter variation
area-length
    a.-l. method
    a.-l. method for ejection fraction
Arelin method
areola, *pl.* **areolae**
    a. of bone
areolae (*pl. of* areola)
areolar
    a. connective tissue
    a. plane
ARF
    acute renal failure
    acute respiratory failure
ArF
    argon fluoride
    ArF excimer laser
argentaffinoma
argon
    a. beam coagulator (ABC)
    a. fluoride (ArF)
    a. laser
    a. laser trabeculectomy
    a. pumped-dye laser
argon/krypton laser
Argus
    A. camera
    A. image processing workstation
ARJ
    anorectal junction

arm
Leyla a.
linebacker's a.
outrigger a.
PinPoint stereotactic a.
scanning a.
Armanni-Ebstein lesion
arm-down image
arm-lung time
armored heart
arm-up
a.-u. image
a.-u. positioning
ARNA
American Radiological Nurses Association
Arnold
A. canal
A. convolution
Arnold-Chiari
A.-C. deformity
A.-C. malformation
A.-C. syndrome
aromatic solvent-induced shift (ASIS)
ARP
adiabatic rapid passage
ARPKD
autosomal recessive polycystic kidney disease
ARR
Academy of Radiology Research
arrangement
string-of-pearls nuclear a.
array
Acuson 5-MHz linear a.
anular a.
coil a.
convex linear a.
detector a.
electrode a.
gate a.
high-density linear a.
linear electrode a.
linear phased a.
multiple-coil a.
NMR quadrature detection a.
parallel a.
a. processor
satellite-borne phased a. (SBPA)
silicon diode a.
a. spatial sensitivity encoding technique (ASSET)
symmetric phased a.
thin-film transistor a.
virtual a.
voxel a.
arrest
circulatory a.
electrical circulatory a.

epiphysial a.
flow a.
growth plate a.
intermittent sinus a.
profound hypothermic circulatory a.
a. reaction
sinus a.
transient sinus a.
arrested circulation
arrhenoblastoma
arrhinencephalia (*var. of* arrhinencephaly)
arrhinencephaly, arrhinencephalia
arrhythmia
a. circuit
a. mapping system
a. mapping system catheter
venography-related a.
arrhythmia-insensitive
a.-i. flow-sensitive alternating inversion recovery (A-FAIR)
a.-i. flow-sensitive alternating IR
arrhythmic myocardial infarct
arrhythmogenic
a. area
a. border zone
a. myocardial tissue ablation catheter
a. right ventricular cardiomyopathy (ARVC)
a. right ventricular dysplasia (ARVD)
arrow
A. catheter
A. Fischell EVAN Needle
A. PICC line
A. TwinCath
ArrowFlex sheath
ARROWgard
A. Blue Line catheter
A. Blue Plus multilumen central venous catheter kit
arrowhead sign
Arrow-Howes multilumen catheter
Arrow-Trerotola
A.-T. percutaneous thrombectomy device
A.-T. percutaneous thrombolytic device
ARRS
American Roentgen Ray Society
ARRT
American Registry of Radiologic Technology
ARS
acute radiation syndrome
ARSAC
Administration of Radioactive Substances Advisory Committee
ART
algebraic reconstruction technique
ART transducer

artefact (*var. of* artifact)
arteria, *pl.* **arteriae**
  a. lusoria
  a. radicularis anterior magna
  a. radicularis magna of
    Adamkiewicz
arteriae (*pl. of* arteria)
arterial
  a. access
  a. anastomosis
  a. anatomy
  a. aneurysm
  a. angioma
  a. avulsion
  a. blockage
  a. brachiocephalic trunk
  a. brain anastomosis
  a. brain displacement
  a. branch
  a. bulb
  a. bypass graft
  a. calcification
  a. canal
  a. cannulation
  a. capillary
  a. circle
  a. circle of Willis
  a. collateral
  a. cone
  a. cutoff
  a. deficiency pattern
  a. degenerative disease
  a. dilation
  a. dilation and rupture
  a. dimension
  a. duct
  a. embolus
  a. endothelium
  a. fenestration
  a. flow-phase image
  a. gland
  a. groove
  a. hemorrhage
  a. hyperemia
  a. hypertension
  a. hypotension
  a. hypoxemia
  a. infusion
  a. input function (AIF)
  a. insufficiency
  a. intima
  a. invasion
  a. kinking
  a. ligament
  a. linear density
  a. lumen
  a. malformation
  a. narrowing
  a. nephrosclerosis

  a. obstruction
  a. occlusion
  a. opacification
  a. oxygen saturation
  a. patency
  a. peak systolic pressure
  a. phase
  a. plaque
  a. port catheter system
  a. portography
  a. pseudoaneurysm
  a. pulsatility
  a. pulsation artifact
  a. puncture site closure device
  a. return
  a. runoff
  a. sclerosis
  a. scrotum supply
  a. segment
  a. sheath
  a. spasm
  a. spin-labeling (ASL)
  a. steal
  a. stenosis
  a. stiffness
  a. sump effect
  a. thrombosis
  a. tonus
  a. topography
  a. tree
  a. varix
  a. vein
  a. wall
  a. wall dissection
  a. wall thickness
  a. waveform
arterial-arterial fistula
arterialization
  hypervascular a.
  a. of venous blood
arterial-portal fistula
arteriobiliary fistula
arteriocapillary sclerosis
arteriococcygeal gland
arteriogenic impotence
arteriogram
arteriography
  abdominal visceral a.
  aortofemoral a.
  axillary a.
  balloon occlusion a.
  bilateral carotid a.
  biplane pelvic a.
  biplane quantitative coronary a.
  brachial a.
  brachiocephalic a.
  bronchial a.
  carotid cerebral a.
  catheter a.

celiac a.
cerebral a.
cine coronary a.
completion a.
contrast a.
coronary a.
cortical kidney a.
CT a.
delayed phase of a.
3D hepatic a.
diagnostic a.
digital subtraction a. (DSA)
documentary a.
femoral runoff a.
hepatic a.
infrahepatic a.
intraoperative a.
ipsilateral antegrade a.
Judkins coronary a.
longitudinal a.
lumbar a.
mesenteric a.
operative a.
pancreatic a.
pelvic a.
percutaneous femoral a.
peripheral a.
postdilation a.
proximity a.
pulmonary a.
quantitative coronary a.
 (QCA)
renal a.
retrograde a.
ring blush on cerebral a.
runoff a.
selective cerebral a.
selective coronary a.
selective visceral a.
Sones selective coronary a.
spinal a.
spiral computed tomography a.
 (SCTA)
splenic a.
subclavian a.
superior mesenteric a.
transfemoral a.
vertebral a.
4-vessel a.
visceral a.
wedge a.
x-ray a. (XRA)
arteriohepatic dysplasia
arteriolar
  a. ischemic ulcer
  a. narrowing
  a. necrosis
  a. resistance
  a. sclerosis

arteriole
  pulmonary precapillary a.
  reactive a.
arteriole-capillary-venous bed
arteriolovenular bridge
arteriomyomatosis
arteriopathy
  plexogenic pulmonary a.
arterioportobiliary fistula
arterioportography
  computed tomography with a.
  (CTAP)
arteriorenal
arteriosclerosis
  calcific a.
  cerebral a.
  coronary a.
  generalized a.
  hyaline a.
  hypertensive a.
  idiopathic pulmonary a. (IPA)
  infantile a.
  intimal a.
  kidney a.
  medial a.
  Mönckeberg a.
  a. obliterans (ASO)
  obliterative a.
  obscuration a.
  obstructing embolus a.
  peripheral a.
  presenile a.
  pulmonary a.
  renal a.
  senile a.
arteriosclerotic
  a. cardiovascular disease (ASCVD)
  a. deposit
  a. heart disease (ASHD)
  a. intracranial aneurysm
  a. kidney
  a. occlusive disease
  a. peripheral vascular disease
  a. plaque
  a. thoracoabdominal aortic aneurysm
arteriosinusoidal penile fistula
arteriostenosis
arteriosum
  cor a.
  ligamentum a.
arteriosus
  calcified ductus a.
  Collet-Edwards type IV truncus a.
  ductus a.
  embryonic truncus a.
  patent ductus a. (PDA)
  persistent ductus a.
  persistent truncus a. (PTA)
  premature closure of ductus a.

arteriosus (*continued*)
    pseudotruncus a.
    railroad track ductus a.
    reversed ductus a.
    silent patent ductus a.
    truncus a.
arteriovascular calcification
arteriovenous (AV, A-V)
    a. anastomosis (AVA)
    a. brain malformation
    a. colon malformation
    a. cord malformation
    a. fistula (AVF)
    a. fistula transplant
    a. hemangioma
    a. interhemispheric angioma
    a. kidney malformation
    a. malformation (AVM)
    a. malformation nidus
    a. pressure gradient
    a. pulmonary aneurysm
    a. shunt imaging
    a. varix
arteritis
    carotid artery a.
    cranial granulomatous a.
    giant cell a.
    luetic a.
    radiation a.
    Takayasu a.
    temporal a.
    temporal granulomatous a.
artery, arteria
    A1-A5 segment of anterior cerebral a.
    Abbott a.
    abdominal aortic a.
    aberrant a.
    aberrant right subclavian a.
    accessory middle cerebral a.
    accessory right renal a.
    accessory right uterine a.
    Adamkiewicz a.
    adrenal a.
    adventitia of a.
    ambient segment of posterior cerebral a.
    angiographic corkscrew a.
    angular a.
    anomalous left coronary a.
    anomalous left pulmonary a.
    anomalous origin of a.
    anomalous origin of left coronary artery from pulmonary a. (ALCAPA)
    anomalous right coronary a.
    anomalous right subclavian a.
    anterior cerebral a. (ACA)
    anterior choroidal a.

anterior communicating a.
anterior descending a.
anterior intercostal a.
anterior meningeal a.
anterior spinal a.
anterior temporal branch of posterior cerebral a.
anterior tibial a.
anteroinferior cerebellar a. (AICA)
anteroinferior cerebral a. (AICA)
anteroinferior communicating a. (AICA)
aortoiliofemoral a.
apical posterior a.
arcuate a.
ascending frontoparietal a.
ascending pharyngeal a.
atrial circumflex a.
atrioventricular node a. (AVNA)
auricular a.
axillary a.
azygos anterior cerebral a.
basal cerebral a.
basal perforating a.
basilar a.
beading of a.
bifurcation of anterior communicating a.
bifurcation of internal carotid a.
blocked a.
brachial a.
brachiocephalic a.
branch of a.
bronchial a.
buckled innominate a.
bulbourethral a.
calcarine a.
calcific a.
callosomarginal a.
candelabrum a.
cannulated a.
caroticotympanic a.
carotid a.
cavernous segment of internal carotid a.
C1-C5 segment of internal carotid a.
celiac branch a.
central a.
cerebellar a.
cerebellolabyrinthine a.
cerebral a.
cervical segment of internal carotid a.
choroidal pericallosal a.
circumflex coronary a.
circumflex groove a.
colic a.

collateral circulation in compression
of a.
common carotid a. (CCA)
common femoral a.
common hepatic a.
common iliac a.
common peroneal a.
communicating a.
complete transposition of great a.'s
computed tomographic angiography
of pulmonary a.
congenital absence of pulmonary a.
congenital aneurysm of pulmonary
a.
congenitally corrected transposition
of great a.'s
contralateral a.
conus a.
corduroy a.
corkscrew appearance of hepatic a.
coronary a.
corrected transposition of great
a.'s
cortical a.
costocervical a.
course of a.
cremasteric a.
cystic a.
deep a.
deferential a.
deltoid branch of posterior tibial a.
descending septal a.
dextrotransposition of great a.'s
diagonal branch of a.
a. diameter
dilated pulmonary a.
diminutive interlobar right pulmonary
a.
dissection of a.
distal circumflex marginal a.
dominant left coronary a.
dominant right coronary a.
dorsal a.
Drummond marginal a.
ductus deferens a.
duodenal a.
duplex ultrasound of carotid a.
dural a.
dynamic entrapment of vertebral a.
eccentric coronary a.
ectatic carotid a.
elastic recoil of a.
en passage feeder a.
a. entrapment
epicardial coronary a
ethmoidal a.
external carotid a. (ECA)
external iliac a.
extracranial vertebral a.

extradural a.
facial a.
falx a.
familial fibromuscular dysplasia of
a.
feeder a.
feeding branch of a.
femoral a.
femoropopliteal a.
fenestration of basilar a.
FP a.
friable a.
frontal a.
frontopolar a.
fusiform narrowing of a.
gastric a.
gastroduodenal a.
gastroepiploic a.
gonadal a.
helicine a.
hepatic a.
Heubner a.
high left main diagonal a.
hilar a.
horizontal segment of middle
cerebral a.
hyaloid a.
hypogastric a.
IC-PC a.
idiopathic dilated pulmonary a.
ileocolic a.
iliac a.
iliofemoral a.
infarct-related a.
inferior epigastric a.
inferior mesenteric a. (IMA)
infragastric infragenicular popliteal
a.
infragenicular popliteal a.
innominate a.
insular segment of middle cerebral
a.
intercostal a.
interlobar a.
intermediate coronary a.
internal aberrant carotid a.
internal carotid a. (ICA)
internal carotid-posterior
communicating a.
internal iliac a.
internal mammary a. (IMA)
internal pudendal a.
internal thoracic a. (ITA)
intraacinar pulmonary a.
intracavernous internal carotid a.
intracerebral a.
intracranial vertebral a.
invisible main pulmonary a.
ipsilateral downstream a.

artery (*continued*)
  Kugel a.
  labyrinthine a.
  lacrimal a.
  left anterior descending a.
  left atrioventricular groove a.
  left circumflex coronary a.
  left common carotid a.
  left common femoral a.
  left coronary a. (LCA)
  left descending a. (LDA)
  left gastric a.
  left internal carotid a. (LICA)
  left internal mammary a. (LIMA)
  left main coronary a. (LMCA)
  left pulmonary a. (LPA)
  lenticulostriate a.
  leptomeningeal a.
  lingual a.
  lumbar a.
  main pulmonary a. (MPA)
  mainstem coronary a.
  major aortopulmonary collateral a.
  malposition of branch pulmonary a.
  mammary a.
  marginal branch of left circumflex coronary a.
  marginal branch of right coronary a.
  marginal circumflex a.
  maxillary a.
  medial plantar a.
  median sacral a.
  medullary a.
  meningeal a.
  meningohypophysial a.
  mesencephalic a.
  mesenteric a.
  middle cerebral a. (MCA)
  middle meningeal a.
  M1-M5 segment of middle cerebral a.
  multiple aortopulmonary collateral a.'s (MAPCA)
  musculophrenic a.
  narrowing of a.
  native coronary a.
  nodular induration of temporal a.
  obtuse marginal coronary a.
  occipital a.
  occlusion of a.
  a. of conus medullaris
  a. of inferior cavernous sinus (AICS)
  a. of labyrinth
  a. of Percheron
  a. of Willis
  OM a.
  omphalomesenteric a.

  opercular segment of middle cerebral a.
  operculofrontal a.
  ophthalmic a.
  origin of a.
  a. ostium
  ovarian a.
  overriding great a.
  pancreaticoduodenal a.
  paracentral a.
  paramalleolar a.
  paramedian thalamic a.
  paramedian thalamopeduncular a.
  parietal middle cerebral a.
  parietooccipital branch of posterior cerebellar a.
  partial transposition of great a.
  patency of a.
  peduncular segment of superior cerebellar a.
  pelvic a.
  penile a.
  perforating a.
  pericallosal a.
  periosteal a.
  peripancreatic a.
  peripheral a.
  peroneal a.
  persistent primitive trigeminal a.
  persistent sciatic a.
  petrous segment of internal carotid a.
  pharyngeal a.
  phrenic a.
  pipestem a.
  plantar metatarsal a.
  plaque-containing a.
  pontile a.
  popliteal a.
  posterior aorta transposition of great arteries
  posterior cerebral a. (PCA)
  posterior choroidal a.
  posterior circumflex humeral a.
  posterior communicating a. (PCA)
  posterior descending a. (PDA)
  posterior intercostal a.
  posterior spinal a.
  posterior temporal a.
  posterior tibial a.
  posteroinferior cerebellar a. (PICA)
  posterolateral spinal a.
  posteroparietal a.
  posttemporal middle cerebral a.
  P1-P4 segment of posterior cerebral a.
  precentral a.
  precommunicating segment of anterior cerebral a.

precommunicating segment of
  posterior cerebral a.
prefrontal a.
premammillary a.
primitive acoustic a.
primitive hypoglossal a.
primitive trigeminal a. (PTA)
profunda femoris a.
proper hepatic a. (PHA)
proximal anterior tibial a.
proximal circumflex a.
proximal digital a.
proximal left anterior descending a.
proximal popliteal a.
pterygoid a.
pulmonary a.
quadrigeminal segment of posterior
  cerebral a.
radial digital a.
radicular a.
radiculomedullary a.
radiculospinal a.
radiomedullary a.
ramus intermedius a.
ramus medialis a.
recanalized a.
a. reconstitution
reconstitution of blood flow in a.
reconstitution via profunda a.
redundant carotid a.
renal a.
reperfused a.
resilient a.
retinal a.
retroesophageal right subclavian a.
right coronary a. (RCA)
right descending pulmonary a.
  (RDPA)
right femoral a.
right ileocolic a.
right inferior epigastric a.
right internal iliac a.
right internal jugular a.
right ovarian a.
right pulmonary a. (RPA)
right ventricular branch of right
  coronary a.
Riolan a.
rolandic a.
round ligament a.
scalp branch of external carotid a.
sclerotic coronary a.
segmental branch of a.
septal perforator a.
shared coronary a.
side-by-side transposition of great
  a.'s
single umbilical a.
sinuatrial node a.

sinus node a.
a. spectrum
spermatic a.
spinal a.
splenial branch of posterior cerebral
  a.
splenic a.
stapedial a.
1st diagonal branch a.
stenotic coronary a.
1st obtuse marginal a.
subclavian a.
subcostal a.
subscapular a.
sudden blockage of coronary a.
sulcocommissural a.
superdominant left anterior
  descending a.
superficial external pudendal a.
superficial femoral a. (SFA)
superficial temporal a.
superior bronchial a.
superior cerebellar a. (SCA)
superior epigastric a.
superior genicular a.
superior intercostal a.
superior mesenteric a. (SMA)
superior pulmonary a.
superior thyroid a.
supernormal a.
supraclinoid segment of internal
  carotid a.
supraorbital a.
supratrochlear a.
surgically corrected transposition of
  great a.'s
takeoff of a.
telencephalic ventriculofugal a.
temporal a.
temporooccipital a.
terminal segment of posterior
  cerebral a.
testicular a.
thalamocaudate a.
thalamogeniculate a.
thalamoperforating a.
thoracoacromial a.
thoracodorsal a.
thrombosed intraaortic a.
thrombotic pulmonary a. (TPA)
thyrocervical trunk of subclavian a.
thyroid a.
tibial a.
translocation of coronary a.
transposition of great a.'s (TGA)
trifurcation of a.
truncal a.
twig of a.
ulnar digital a.

artery (*continued*)
 umbilical a. (UA)
 ureteral a.
 uterine a. (UA)
 ventriculofugal a.
 vertebral a.
 vertebrobasilar a.
 vidian a.
 visceral a.
 weakened a.
artery-aortic velocity ratio
artery-bronchus ratio (ABR)
artery-like pattern of enhancement
artery-vein-nerve bundle
arthritic talonavicular change
arthritides (*pl. of* arthritis)
arthritis, *pl.* **arthritides**
 adult rheumatoid a.
 antigen-induced a.
 a. arthrogram
 Bekhterev a.
 Cedell-Magnusson classification
  of a.
 crystal-induced a.
 cystic rheumatoid a.
 degenerative a.
 destructive brucellar a.
 elderly onset rheumatoid a.
 facet joint a.
 gouty a.
 hand/wrist a.
 infectious a.
 inflammatory bowel disease a.
 Jaccoud a.
 juvenile rheumatoid a. (JRA)
 Kellgren a.
 lunohamate a.
 metatarsophalangeal joint a.
 mixed rheumatoid and degenerative
  a.
 a. mutilans
 pancarpal destructive a.
 posttraumatic a.
 psoriatic a.
 reactive a.
 Reiter syndrome a.
 rheumatoid a.
 septic a.
 seronegative rheumatoid a.
 a. syphilitica deformans (ASD)
 systemic juvenile rheumatoid a.
  (S-JRA)
 traumatic a.
 tuberculous a.
arthrodesed digit
arthrodial cartilage
arthroempyesis
arthrogram
 arthritis a.

arthrography
 air a.
 3-compartment a.
 coronal computed tomographic a.
  (CCTA)
 CT a.
 double-contrast a.
 Gordon-Bröstrom single-contrast a.
 a. imaging
 indirect MR a.
 joint a.
 magnetic resonance a.
 MR a.
 opaque a.
 saline-enhanced MR a.
 single-contrast a.
 temporomandibular joint a.
 vacuum a.
arthrogryposis multiplex congenita
arthroosteitis
 pustulotic a.
arthropathy
 Charcot a.
 crystal deposition a.
 dialysis a.
 facet degenerative a.
 gouty a.
 Jaccoud a.
 neuropathic a.
 pyrophosphate a.
 rotator cuff a.
 urate a.
arthrophyte
arthroplasty
 shoulder a.
 total knee a. (TKA)
arthropneumoradiography,
 arthropneumoroentgenography
arthropneumoroentgenography (*var. of*
 arthropneumoradiography)
ArthroProbe laser system
arthropyosis
arthroscintigraphy
arthroscope
 Citscope disposable a.
arthroscopic decompression
arthroscopy
 2nd-look a.
arthroses (*pl. of* arthrosis)
arthrosis, *pl.* **arthroses**
 crystal-induced a.
 a. deformans
 degenerative a.
 spiral a.
arthrotomography
 contrast computed a.
 a. of shoulder
articular
 a. arch

a. calculus
a. capsule
a. cartilage
a. cartilage attenuation
a. cartilage degeneration
a. cartilage violation
a. cartilage volume
a. cortex
a. crest
a. derangement
a. disc
a. eminence
a. erosion
a. facet
a. fluid
a. fossa
a. fragment
a. gout
a. hand disorder
a. instability
a. labrum
a. lamella
a. lamella of bone
a. mass separation fracture
a. meniscus
a. metaplasia
a. network
a. pillar fracture
a. pit
a. process
a. process of vertebra
a. rheumatism
a. surface
a. tubercle
a. tubercle of temporal bone
a. vascular circle
a. wrist disorder

articularis
meniscus a.
articulated skeleton
articulating surface
articulation
acromioclavicular a.
atlantoaxial a.
calcaneocuboid a.
carpometacarpal a.
carporadial a.
condylar a.
congruent a.
costovertebral a.
DIP a.
disturbance of a.
femoral a.
fixation a.
humeroradial a.
humeroulnar a.
intercarpal a.
intermetacarpal a.
interphalangeal a.

interval a.
joint a.
metacarpophalangeal a.
occipitocervical a.
patellofemoral a.
pisotriquetral a.
posterior membrane a.
proximal interphalangeal a.
proximal interphalangeal joint a.
radiocapitellar a.
radiocarpal a.
radiohumeral a.
radiolunate a.
radioscaphoid a.
radioulnar a.
sacroiliac a.
scapuloclavicular a.
subluxation a.
subtalar a.
talocalcaneal a.
talocalcaneonavicular a.
talonavicular a.
tarsometatarsal a.
thorax a.
tibiofibular a.
triquetropisiform a.
zygapophysial a.
articulography
electromagnetic a. (EMA)
artifact, artefact
acoustic a.
aliasing a.
anatomy exclusion a.
aortic motion a.
arterial pulsation a.
asymmetric a.
attenuation a.
barium a.
baseline a.
beam-hardening a.
beamlike a.
black boundary a.
black comet a.
blooming a.
blur a.
bone-hardening a.
bounce-point a.
bowel gas a.
brace a.
breast a.
breathing a.
broadband noise detection error a.
bulk susceptibility a.
calibration failure a.
catheter impact a.
catheter tip motion a.
catheter tip position a.
catheter whip a.
center line a.

artifact (*continued*)
    central point a.
    chastity ring a.
    chemical-shift a.
    clothing a.
    coin a.
    color Doppler twinkling a.
    comet-tail a.
    computed tomography truncation a.
    computer-generated a.
    construction a.
    corduroy a.
    crescent a.
    crinkle a.
    crosstalk effect a.
    crush a.
    CSF pulsation a.
    data-clipping detection error a.
    data spike detection error a.
    DC offset a.
    developer a.
    dielectric a.
    direct current offset a.
    dirty film a.
    Doppler a.
    double-exposure drift a.
    eddy current a.
    eddy ringing a.
    edge-boundary a.
    edge misalignment a.
    edge ringing a.
    a. effect
    effusion a.
    end-pressure a.
    entry slice phenomenon a.
    equipment a.
    external a.
    eyebrow ring a.
    faulty radiofrequency shielding a.
    ferromagnetic a.
    fingerprint mark a.
    flow effect a.
    flow-induced a.
    flow-related a.
    fluid-flow a.
    fog a.
    foldover a.
    foreign material a.
    foreshortening a.
    gaseous oxygen a.
    geophagia a.
    ghosting a.
    glass eye a.
    glove phenomenon a.
    hair a.
    half-moon a.
    hardening a.
    hot-spot a.

    iatrogenically induced a.
    a. image
    image postprocessing error a.
    image wraparound a.
    imaging timing a.
    imbalance of gain a.
    imbalance of phase a.
    India ink a.
    intensifying screen a.
    intravascular stent a.
    iron overload a.
    kink a.
    kissing a.'s
    large clothing a.
    large susceptibility a.
    lettering a.
    line a.
    linear a.
    lipid a.
    lip ring a.
    low-attenuation pulsation a.
    low signal-intensity a.
    magic angle effect a.
    magnetic susceptibility a.
    main magnetic field inhomogeneity a.
    mercury a.
    metallic a.
    micrometallic a.
    minus-density a.
    mirror-image a.
    misregistration a.
    mitral regurgitation a.
    moiré fringe a.
    mosaic a.
    motion a.
    movement a.
    muscle a.
    navel ring a.
    nipple ring a.
    noise spike a.
    nose ring a.
    orbit a.
    out-of-slice a.
    overlying attenuation a.
    pacemaker a.
    pacing a.
    paramagnetic a.
    partial volume effect a.
    patient motion a.
    pellet a.
    phase discontinuity a.
    phase-encoding motion a.
    phase-shift a.
    pica a.
    pick-off a.
    plus-density a.
    popliteal artery pulsation a.
    posterior ghosting a.

processor-related a.
a. pronunciation
propagation speed a.
pseudofracture a.
pulsation a.
quadrature phase detector a.
radiofrequency overflow a.
radiofrequency spatial distribution problem reconstruction a.
range ambiguity a.
reconstruction a.
respiratory motion a.
reticulation a.
reverberation a.
ring-down a.
roller mark a.
scintigraphy a.
screen craze a.
side lobe a.
signal dropout a.
skin crease a.
skinfold a.
skin lesion a.
slice overlap a.
slice profile a.
spatial misregistration a.
spatial offset image a.
split image a.
stairstep a.
star a.
stent-related a.
stimulated echo a.
streak a.
streaklike a.
subcutaneous injection of contrast a.
summation shadow a.
superimposition a.
suppression of heart pulsation a.
surgical a.
susceptibility a.
swallowing a.
swamp-static a.
T a.
T1-contamination a.
technically induced a.
temporal instability a.
tongue stud a.
tree a.
truncation band a.
twinkling a.
velocity a.
venetian blind a.
view insufficiency a.
volume a.
wheelchair a.
white noise a.
wraparound ghosting a.
wrapped a.
wrinkle a.
zebra stripe a.
zipper a.

artifactitious (*var. of* artifactual)
artifactual, artifactitious
    a. gap
    a. lucency
artificial
    a. active acquired immunity
    a. cardiac valve
    a. eye
    a. fracture
    a. heart
    a. lumen narrowing
    a. lung
    a. neural network
    a. passive acquired immunity
    a. pleural effusion procedure
    a. pneumothorax
    a. radioactivity
ARTMA
    advanced real-time motion analysis
    ARTMA virtual patient technology
Artoscan
    A. M
    A. MRI imaging
    A. MRI scanner
    A. MRI system
ARVC
    arrhythmogenic right ventricular cardiomyopathy
ARVD
    arrhythmogenic right ventricular dysplasia
Arvidsson dimension-length method for ventricular volume
aryepiglottic
    a. cyst
    a. fold
    a. fold carcinoma
    a. fold neurofibroma
    a. fold width
arytenoepiglottidean fold
arytenoid
    a. articular surface
    a. cartilage
    a. sparing
as
    a. low as readily practicable (ALARP)
    a. low as reasonably achievable (ALARA)
ASA
    American Standards Association
asbestos
    amphibole a.
    blue a.

asbestos (*continued*)
   a. body
   brown a.
   chrysotile a.
   crocidolite a.
   a. exposure
   a. fiber
   a. pleural plaque
   serpentine a.
   white a.
asbestos-induced pleural fibrosis
asbestosis
   pulmonary a.
asbestos-related
   a.-r. lung carcinoma
   a.-r. mesothelioma
   a.-r. pleural disease
   a.-r. pleural effusion
   a.-r. pleural thickening
A-scan
   A-s. imaging
   A-s. ultrasound
ascariasis, ascaridiasis, ascaridosis, ascariosis
   biliary a.
ascaridiasis (*var. of* ascariasis)
ascaridosis (*var. of* ascariasis)
ascariosis (*var. of* ascariasis)
Ascaris lumbricoides
ascendant follicle
ascending
   a. aorta (AA)
   a. aorta dilation
   a. aorta hypoplasia
   a. aortic aneurysm
   a. aortography
   a. cholangitis
   a. colon
   a. contrast MR phlebogram
   a. contrast phlebography
   a. contrast phlebography
     imaging
   a. contrast venography
   a. dynamic flow image
   a. frontal convolution
   a. frontoparietal artery
   a. hypoplasia of aorta
   a. lumbar vein
   a. medullary vein thrombosis
   a. parietal convolution
   a. parietal gyrus
   a. pharyngeal artery
   a. process
   a. pyelography
   a. ramus of ischium
   a. ramus of mandible
   a. tract
   a. urography
Ascent guiding catheter

Aschoff
   A. node
   A. nodule
Aschoff-Tawara node
ascites
   biliary a.
   chylous a.
   a. due to bile leak
   fetal a.
   gelatinous a.
   malignant a.
   massive a.
   neonatal a.
   pancreatic a.
   urine a.
ascitic fluid
ASCVD
   arteriosclerotic cardiovascular disease
   atherosclerotic cardiovascular
     disease
ASD
   anterior sagittal diameter
   arthritis syphilitica deformans
   atrial septal defect
Aselli pancreas
asepsis
   medical a.
   surgical a.
aseptic
   a. gossypiboma
   a. granulomatous foreign body
     reaction
   a. necrosis
   a. technique
ASF
   anterior spine fusion
ASH
   asymmetric septal hypertrophy
ASHD
   arteriosclerotic heart disease
   atherosclerotic heart disease
Asherson syndrome
Ashhurst-Bromer classification of ankle fracture
Ashhurst transcondylar humeral fracture classification (I, II)
ash leaf patch
Ashman
   A. index
   A. phenomenon
ASHN
   acute sclerosing hyaline necrosis
a-Si
   amorphous silicon
ASIC
   application-specific integrated circuit
ASIS
   anterosuperior iliac spine
   aromatic solvent-induced shift

Askin thoracopulmonary neuroepithelial tumor
A·S·KMerit safety access kit
Ask-Upmark kidney
ASL
 arterial spin-labeling
ASO
 arteriosclerosis obliterans
asoma, *pl.* **asomata**
asomata (*pl. of* asoma)
aspartate
 N-acetyl a. (NAA)
aspecific lymphocytic thyroiditis
aspect
 anterior a.
 anterolateral a.
 anteroposterior a.
 apical a.
 axial a.
 dorsal a.
 dorsolateral a.
 dorsoplantar a.
 inferior a.
 infrapatellar a.
 lateral a.
 lordotic a.
 medial a.
 mediolateral a.
 mesial a.
 plantar a.
 posterior a.
 posterolateral a.
 proximal a.
 superior a.
 superolateral a.
 ventral a.
Aspen
 A. digital ultrasound system
 A. sonography unit
aspergilloma
aspergillosis
 allergic bronchopulmonary a. (ABPA)
 bronchopulmonary a.
 chronic necrotizing a.
 disseminated a.
 invasive pulmonary a. (IPA)
 necrotizing a.
 noninvasive a.
 primary a.
 pulmonary a.
 saprophytic a.
 semiinvasive a.
aspergillotic
 a. aneurysm
 a. granuloma
Aspergillus **cerebral abscess**

asphyxia
 fetal a.
 perinatal a.
asphyxial renal trauma
asphyxia-related renal necrosis
asphyxiating
 a. thoracic dysplasia
 a. thoracic dystrophy
aspiration
 antegrade a.
 barium a.
 a. biopsy
 a. biopsy needle
 breast cyst a.
 Cosman-Roberts-Wells guided stereotactic a.
 CT-guided needle a.
 endoscopic ultrasound-guided fine-needle a. (EUS-FNA)
 fine-needle a. (FNA)
 hydrocarbon a.
 intraswallowing a.
 meconium a.
 a. of ova
 pleural fluid a.
 a. pneumonia
 a. pneumonitis
 pulmonary a.
 stereotactic needle a.
 tracheal a.
 tracheobronchial a.
 tracheopulmonary a.
 transbronchial needle a. (TBNA)
 transtracheal a.
 ultrasonic a.
 ultrasound-guided cyst a.
 ultrasound-guided transthoracic needle a.
aspirator
 Cavitron ultrasonic surgical a. (CUSA)
 Sonocut ultrasonic a.
aspire
 A. continuous imaging system
 A. covered stent
asplenia syndrome R
asplenic
ASPS
 alveolar soft part sarcoma
ASPVD
 atherosclerotic peripheral vascular disease
ASR
 adrenal-spleen ratio
ASRT
 American Society of Radiologic Technologists
assay
 Accuclot D-dimer a.
 Clauss a.

assay (*continued*)
    enzyme-linked immunoabsorbent a.
    erythropoietin a.
    immunofluorimetric a.
    radiometric a.
    renal vein renin a.
assembly
    linear-array hydrophone a.
assessment
    activity a.
    aortoiliac inflow a.
    BFM stroke impairment a.
    Brunnstrom-Fugl-Meyer arm
      impairment a.
    diagnostic and therapeutic
      technology a.
    Doppler a.
    hemodynamic a.
    indicator dilution method of
      perfusion a.
    individualized functional status a.
    invasive a.
    in vivo stereologic a.
    lumen a.
    multireader E-MRI a.
    myocardial function a.
    noninvasive vascular a.
    qualitative a.
    quantitative Doppler a.
    real-time a.
    regional wall motion a.
    sonographic a.
    transmetallation a.
    ultrasonic a.
    vascular a.
ASSET
    array spatial sensitivity encoding
    technique
assimilation
    atlantooccipital a.
    a. pelvis
assist
    intraaortic balloon a.
assistance
    fluoroscopic a.
Assmann
    A. focus
    A. tuberculous infiltrate
associated
    a. anomaly
    a. imaging characteristic
    a. sequestrum
association
    Alzheimer's Disease and Related
      Disorders A. (ADRDA)
    American Diabetes A.
    American Medical A. (AMA)
    American Radiological Nurses A.
      (ARNA)

    American Rheumatism A. (ARA)
    American Spinal Cord Injury A.
    American Standards A. (ASA)
    American Thyroid A.
    American Urological A.
    Anti-Lung Cancer A.
    a. cortex of parietal lobe
    a. fiber
    Japanese Gastric Cancer A.
    New York Heart A. (NYHA)
    A. of University Radiologic
      Technicians (AURT)
    Takayasu Arteritis A.
    VATER a.
Assurant balloon-expanded stent
AST
    above selected threshold
astatine
asterixis
asteroid body
asthenia
asthma
    cardiac a.
asthmatic
    a. airway
    a. bronchitis
    a. pneumonia
astragalar bone
astragalocalcanean bone
astragalocrural bone
astragaloscaphoid bone
astragalotibial bone
astragalus
    aviator's a.
    a. bone
    fracture of a.
astroblastoma
astrocytic
    a. gliosis
    a. hamartoma
    a. proliferation
    a. tumor
astrocytoma
    anaplastic a.
    calcified a.
    cerebellar a.
    cerebral a.
    chiasmatic-hypothalamic pilocytic
      a.
    CNS juvenile pilocytic a.
    a. cord
    cystic pilocytic a.
    desmoplastic infantile a.
    fibrillary a.
    gemistocytic a.
    giant cell a.
    high-grade infiltrative a.
    infiltrative a.
    juvenile orbital pilocytic a.

juvenile pilocytic a. (JPA)
low-grade a.
macrocystic pilocytic cerebellar a.
microcystic pilocytic cerebellar a.
multifocal anaplastic a.
orbital juvenile pilocytic a.
pilocytic a.
protoplasmic a.
radiation-treated a.
retinal a.
solid pilocytic a.
subependymal giant cell a.
supratentorial a.
temporoinsular a.
well-differentiated a.
astroglial tumor
asymmetric, asymmetrical
a. appearance time
a. artifact
a. bile duct
a. breast density
a. closure of cusp
a. collimation
a. data sampling
a. echo
a. intrauterine growth retardation
a. IUGR
a. limb uptake
a. lookup table
a. lung opacity
a. negative T-wave
a. pulmonary congestion
a. septal hypertrophy (ASH)
a. signal change
a. target appearance
a. thorax
asymmetrical (*var. of* asymmetric)
asymmetry
amplitude a.
congestive a.
facial a.
focal a.
frontal horn a.
hypertrophic a.
interhemispheric a.
left-right a.
limb-length a.
narrowing a.
septal a.
skull a.
thoracic a.
asymptomatic
a. coarctation
a. gallstone
a. hydrocephalus
a. hypertrophy
asynchronous transfer mode (ATM)
asynergia (*var. of* asynergy)

asynergic myocardium
asynergy, asynergia
infarct-localized a.
left ventricular a.
regional a.
segmental a.
asystolic pause
ATAI
acute traumatic aortic injury
atavistic epiphysis
ataxia, ataxy
a., autosomal recessive, with
deafness and optic atrophy
Friedreich a.
a. telangiectasia
ataxy (*var. of* ataxia)
ATB
All-Terrain Balloon
ATB PTA ablation catheter
ATCL
angioimmunoblastic T-cell lymphoma
atelectasis
absorption a.
acquired a.
acute a.
adhesive a.
apical a.
band of a.
basilar a.
bibasilar discoid a.
bronchopulmonary a.
chronic intermittent a.
cicatricial a.
cicatrization a.
combined middle and right lower
lobe a.
compressive a.
confluent areas of a.
congenital a.
congestive a.
dependent a.
diffuse a.
disclike a.
discoid a.
gravity-dependent a.
initial a.
linear a.
lobar resorption a.
lobular a.
lower pulmonary lobe a.
middle pulmonary lobe a.
nonobstructive a.
obstructive a.
passive a.
patchy a.
peripheral parenchymatous a.
platelike a.
postobstructive a.
postoperative resorption a.

atelectasis (*continued*)
    primary a.
    pulmonary a.
    reabsorption a.
    relaxation a.
    resorption a.
    resorptive a.
    right lower lobe a.
    round a.
    rounded a.
    secondary a.
    segmental resorption a.
    slowly developing a.
    streak of a.
    subsegmental a. (SSA)
    subsegmental bibasilar a.
    subsegmental lower lobe a.
    upper pulmonary lobe a.
atelectatic
    a. asbestos pseudotumor
    a. lung
atelosteogenesis
ateriography
    MR coronary a.
ateriomegaly
ATF
    anterior talofibular
    ATF ligament
atherectomy
    directional coronary a. (DCA)
    extraction catheter a.
    percutaneous coronary rotational a.
      (PCRA)
    peripheral directional a.
    retrograde a.
    rotational coronary a. (RCA)
    Simpson a.
    transcutaneous extraction catheter a.
    transluminal a.
AtheroCath
    A. Bantam coronary atherectomy
      catheter
    DVI Simpson A.
    Simpson Coronary A. (SCA)
atheroembolic renal disease
atheroembolism
atherogenesis
atherolysis
    ultrasonic a.
atherolytic
atheroma
    carotid bifurcation a.
    coral reef a.
    a. molding
    protruding a.
    resection of mobile aortic arch a.
atheromatosis
atheromatous
    a. abscess

    a. debris
    a. degeneration
    a. embolus
    a. lesion
    a. material
    a. plaque
    a. stenosis
    a. ulcer
atherosclerosis
    accelerated a.
    aortic a.
    carotid a.
    coronary a.
    extracranial carotid artery a.
    fatty streak a.
    fibrous plaque a.
    intimal a.
    intracranial carotid artery a.
    juxtarenal aortic a.
    native a.
    pararenal aortic a.
    premature a.
    Stroke Outcome and Neuroimaging
      of Intracranial A. (SONIA)
    virulent a.
atherosclerotic
    a. aortic aneurysm
    a. aortic ulcer
    a. calcification
    a. cardiovascular disease
      (ASCVD)
    a. carotid artery disease (ACAD)
    a. change
    a. debris
    a. fatty streak
    a. heart disease (ASHD)
    a. lesion
    a. narrowing
    a. occlusive syndrome
    a. peripheral vascular disease
      (ASPVD)
    a. pulmonary vascular disease
    a. renal occlusive disease
    a. stenosis
    a. uptake
atherostenosis
atherothrombotic brain infarct
AtheroTrack catheter
Athlete GT coronary guidewire
athlete's
    a. ankle
    a. heart
    a. pseudonephritis
Atkin epiphysial fracture
ATL
    anterior temporal lobectomy
    ATL HDI 5000 color Doppler
    ATL HDI 3000, 3500, 4000, 5000
      ultrasound system

A

ATL Mark 600 real-time sector scanner
ATL Neurosector real-time scanner
ATL Ultramark 8, 9
atlantal ligament
Atlantis SR IVUS catheter
atlantoaxial, atloaxoid
  a. articulation
  a. instability (AAI)
  a. interval
  a. joint
  a. relationship
  a. rotary displacement
  a. rotary fixation
  a. separation
  a. subluxation
atlantodens interval (ADI)
atlantodental
atlantomastoid
atlantooccipital, atlooccipital
  a. assimilation
  a. dislocation
  a. fusion
  a. joint
  a. junction
  a. membrane
  a. separation
atlantoodontoid
atlas
  a. anomaly
  a. arch
  bifid a.
  Cerefy neuroradiology a.
  A. diagnostic ultrasound system
  a. facet
  a. fracture
  Greulich and Pyle a.
  a. matching
  a. occipitalization
  a. odontoid distance
  rachischisis of a.
  split a.
  standard a.
  Talairach-Tournoux a.
  transverse ligament of a.
  a. warping
atloaxoid (*var. of* atlantoaxial)
atlooccipital (*var. of* atlantooccipital)
ATM
  asynchronous transfer mode
atmospheric pressure
ATN
  acute tubular necrosis
  autonomous thyroid nodule
atom
  activated a.
  Bohr a.
  excited a.
  ionized a.

  labeled a.
  nuclear a.
  radioactive a.
  recoil a.
  stripped a.
  tagged a.
atomic
  a. absorption spectrophotometry
  a. absorption spectroscopy
  a. energy
  A. Energy Commission (AEC)
  a. mass unit (amu)
  a. volume
atomization
atonia (*var. of* atony)
atonic
  a. esophagus
  a. ureter
  a. urinary bladder
atony, atonia
  chronic gastric a.
  collecting system a.
  gastric a.
  intestinal a.
  renal collecting system a.
  sphincter a.
  stomach a.
  urinary bladder a.
atopic
atopy
ATP
  adenosine triphosphate
ATP-binding cassette transporter
atraumatic
  a. multidirectional bilateral radial instability (AMBRI)
  a. occlusion of vessel
atresia
  anal a.
  anorectal a.
  aortic arch a.
  aortic valve a.
  bile duct a.
  biliary a.
  bowel a.
  bronchial a.
  choanal a.
  colonic a.
  congenital biliary a.
  congenital intestinal a.
  congenital laryngeal a.
  diffuse aortic a.
  duodenal a.
  esophageal a.
  external auditory canal a.
  extrahepatic biliary a. (EBA)
  familial a.
  gastric a.
  ileal a.

atresia (*continued*)
    infundibular a.
    inner ear a.
    intrahepatic a. (IHA)
    intrahepatic biliary a.
    jejunal a.
    laryngeal a.
    mitral valve a.
    nasopharyngeal a.
    phenobarbital biliary a.
    prepyloric a.
    pulmonary a.
    pulmonary artery a.
    pulmonary valve a.
    pulmonary vein a.
    small bowel a.
    tricuspid a.
    tricuspid valve a.
    unilateral pulmonary vein a.
    urethral a.
    valvular a.
    ventricular a.
atresic (*var. of* atretic)
atretic, atresic
    a. aortic segment
    a. cephalocele
    a. ovarian follicle
    a. tube
atria (*pl. of* atrium)
atrial
    a. activation time
    a. appendage
    a. appendage juxtaposition
    a. bigeminal rhythm
    a. canal
    a. cannulation
    a. circumflex artery
    a. complex
    a. cuff
    a. disc
    a. diverticulum of brain
    a. dome
    a. echo
    a. ectopic automatic tachycardia
    a. electrogram
    a. emptying volume
    a. fetal flutter
    a. fibrillation
    a. focus
    a. infarct
    a. irritability
    a. isomerism
    a. kick
    a. mesenchymoma
    a. metastasis
    a. myxoma
    a. ostium primum defect
    a. partition
    a. pressure

    a. rate
    a. septal aneurysm
    a. septal defect (ASD)
    a. septal defect occlusion
    a. septal resection
    a. septostomy
    a. septum
    a. situs
    a. situs solitus
    a. standstill
    a. systole
    a. thrombosis
    a. transposition
atrialized ventricle
atrial-phase volumetric function
atriocaval junction
atriofascicular tract
atriography
    contrast left a.
    negative-contrast left a.
atrio-His
    a.-H. bypass tract
    a.-H. fiber
    a.-H. pathway
atriohisian
atrioventricular (AV), auriculoventricular
    a. anulus
    a. band
    a. block
    a. bundle
    a. canal
    a. canal defect
    a. connection
    a. gradient
    a. groove
    a. groove branch
    a. junction
    a. junction anomaly
    a. nodal bypass tract
    a. nodal orifice
    a. nodal ostium
    a. nodal reentry tachycardia
    a. nodal rhythm
    a. nodal septal defect
    a. nodal septum
    a. nodal valve
    a. node
    a. node artery (AVNA)
    a. node mesothelioma
    a. septal defect (AVSD)
    a. sulcus
    a. time
    a. trunk
atrium, *pl.* **atria**
    accessory a.
    common a.
    a. dextrum cordis
    giant left a. (GLA)
    high right a. (HRA)

left a.
low right a. (LRA)
low septal right a.
maximum volume of left a.
nontrabeculated a.
oblique vein of left a.
a. pulmonale
pulmonary a.
respiratory a.
right a.
shunt with normal left a.
single a.
a. sinistrum
a. sinistrum cordis
stenosing ring of left a.
thin-walled a.
trabeculated a.
ventricular a.

atrophia (*var. of* atrophy)
a. cutis
a. cutis senilis
a. maculosa

atrophic
a. brain lesion
a. breast
a. cirrhosis
a. degeneration
a. emphysema
a. fracture
a. gastritis
a. inflammation
a. kidney
a. nonunion
a. pyelonephritis
a. thrombosis
a. villus

atrophie
a. blanche
a. noire

atrophied ovary
atrophy, atrophia
alveolar a.
back pressure a.
bone a.
brachial a.
brain a.
brown a.
cerebellar a.
cerebral surface a.
compensatory a.
compression a.
cord a.
cortical a.
degenerative a.
denervation a.
dentatorubral pallidoluysian a.
divopontocerebellar a.
dorsum sellae a.
eccentric a.

endometrial a.
focal a.
frontotemporal a.
gastric a.
hemisphere a.
hippocampal a.
Hoffmann a.
interstitial a.
kidney a.
lesser a.
lobar lung a.
multiple-system a. (MSA)
olivopontocerebellar a.
optic nerve a.
pancreatic a.
parenchymatous a.
physiologic a.
postinflammatory renal a.
postischemic a.
postmenopausal uterine a.
postobstructive renal a.
primary optic a.
progressive encephalopathy with
    edema, hypsarrhythmia, and optic
    a. (PEHO)
progressive postpolio muscle a.
radiation-induced cerebral a.
reflux a.
renal reflux a.
seminal vesicle a.
small bowel fold a.
spinal cord a.
spinal muscular a. (SMA)
subacute denervation a.
subcortical Sudeck osteoporotic a.
Sudeck a.
sulcal a.
temporal horn a.
vascular villous a.
villous a.

ATRT
atypical teratoid/rhabdoid tumor
ATT
anterior tibial tendon
attached proton test (APT)
attachment
abnormal umbilical cord a.
biopsy-guided a.
capsular a.
central rhomboid a.
cerebellar a.
commissural a.
dural a.
epicardial a.
fibroosseous a.
fibrous a.
Hudson a.
intimate a.
lateral pterygoid tendinous a.

attachment (*continued*)
    ligamentous a.
    meniscocapsular a.
    meniscofemoral a.
    meniscotibial a.
    mesenteric a.
    Pearson a.
    peritoneal a.
    tendinous a.
    tendon-to-bone a.
    tentorium cerebelli a. (TCA)
    vascular pterygoid a.

attack
    transient ischemic a. (TIA)

attenuate

attenuated
    a. adenomatous polyposis
    a. cortical surface
    a. dura
    a. image
    a. intercarpal articular cartilage
    a. ligament
    a. lumen

attenuating

attenuation
    aortic a.
    articular cartilage a.
    a. artifact
    beam a.
    breast a.
    a. coefficient
    a. compensation
    a. correction
    CT correction a.
    decreased a.
    diaphragmatic a.
    diffuse low a.
    digital beam a.
    a. effect
    expiratory a.
    focal a.
    gamma ray a.
    ground-glass a.
    hemidiaphragm a.
    a. imaging
    increased a.
    inhomogeneous a.
    a. in phantom (AIPH)
    a. in phantom meter
    a. level
    linear a.
    low a.
    a. measurement
    mosaic pattern of
      lung a.
    near-water a.
    nonuniform a.
    a. pattern
    photon a.

    a. scan
    signal a.
    tendon a.
    theophylline a.
    a. threshold
    ultrasonic a.
    a. value
    valve a.
    vascular a.
    x-ray a.

attenuation-based online modulation of tube current

attenuation-corrected image

attenuation-correction coefficient

attenuator

attic
    a. adhesion
    a. cholesteatoma
    a. recess
    a. temporal bone

attitude
    fetal a.

attritional
    a. pattern change
    a. tear

attrition rupture of tendon

ATV
    anterior terminal vein

atypical
    a. angiomyolipoma of kidney
    a. aortic valve stenosis
    a. benign fibrous histiocytoma
    a. brain teratoma
    a. bronchial pneumonia
    a. carcinoid
    a. chondrocyte
    a. ductal hyperplasia
    a. epithelium
    a. finding
    a. interstitial pneumonia
    a. lobular breast hyperplasia
    a. lobular hyperplasia (ALH)
    a. measles pneumonia
    a. medullary carcinoma
    a. meningioma
    a. parkinsonian disorder
    a. primary pneumonia
    a. regenerative hyperplasia
    a. renal cyst
    a. subisthmic coarctation
    a. teratoid/rhabdoid tumor (ATRT)
    a. tuberculosis
    a. verrucous endocarditis
    a. vessel colposcopic pattern

Au
    gold

AUC
    area under curve

^{198}Au colloid

auditory
- a. canal
- a. capsule
- a. cartilage
- a. cortex
- a. ganglion
- a. pit
- a. plate
- a. process
- a. tube
- a. vein
- a. vesicle

Auerbach
- myenteric plexus of A.

Auer body

auger
- A. effect
- A. electron
- A. electron emitter

augmentation
- bladder a.
- a. mammaplasty
- mechanical a.
- simultaneous areolar mastopexy and breast a. (SAMBA)
- thiol a.

augmented
- a. breast
- a. cardiac output
- a. filling
- a. filling of right ventricle
- a. pressure colostogram
- a. stroke volume

Aunt Minnie sign

aura, *pl.* **aurae**
- A. desktop laser
- A. Laser helical scanner
- uncinate a.

aurae (*pl. of* aura)

aural thermometer

aureus
- *Staphylococcus a.*

auricle, auricula
- left a.
- right a.

auricula (*var. of* auricle)

auricular
- a. artery
- a. canaliculus
- a. cartilage
- a. complex
- a. fissure
- a. ganglion
- a. ligament
- a. line
- a. lymph node
- a. muscle
- a. notch
- a. point

- a. surface
- a. triangle
- a. tubercle
- a. vein

auriculoventricular (*var. of* atrioventricular)

Aurora
- A. dedicated breast MRI system
- A. diode-based dental laser system
- A. diode soft tissue laser
- A. MR breast imaging system scanner

AURT
- Association of University Radiologic Technicians

auscultatory finding

Aussies-Isseis unstable scoliosis

Austin
- A. Flint phenomenon
- A. Medical Equipment (AME)

Auth Rotablator atherectomy catheter

autoattenuation correction method

autocalibration k-space profile

autocancellation

AutoCAT intraaortic balloon pump

autocorrelation function

Autocorrelator

autoerythrocyte sensitization syndrome

autofluorescence

autofluoroscope
- digital a.

autofusion

autogenous
- a. bone
- a. hemodialysis fistula
- a. vein
- a. vein bypass graft

autograft
- bridge a.
- double a.

autohistoradiograph

autoimmune
- a. disorder
- a. pancreatitis (AIP)
- a. phenomenon
- a. response
- a. sialadenitis

autologous
- a. blood clot
- a. bone marrow mononuclear (ABMMN)
- a. bone marrow rescue
- a. bone marrow transplant (ABMT)
- a. hematopoietic progenitor cell transplant
- a. labeled leukocyte
- a. patch graft

autologous (*continued*)
   a. pericardium
   a. peripheral blood stem cell transplant
   a. stem
   a. stem cell transplant
   a. vein graft
   a. white cell localization

automated
   a. airway tree segmentation method
   a. angle-encoder system
   a. biochemical analyzer
   a. biopsy gun
   a. biopsy needle
   a. biopsy system
   a. border detection by echocardiography
   a. cardiac flow measurement (ACM)
   a. cardiac flow measurement ultrasound
   a. cellular imaging system (ACIS)
   a. cerebral blood flow analyzer
   a. computed axial tomography (ACAT)
   a. gamma counter
   a. gun-needle device
   a. Hough transform
   a. infusion system
   a. large-core breast biopsy
   a. percutaneous lumbar discectomy (APLD)
   a. polyp detection
   a. quantification

automatic
   a. bladder
   a. brightness control (ABC)
   a. collimator
   a. endoscopic system for optimal positioning (AESOP)
   a. exposure control (AEC)
   a. external defibrillator (AED)
   a. extraction
   a. gain control (AGC)
   a. image registration (AIR)
   a. implantable cardioverter-defibrillator (AICD)
   a. lumen edge segmentation
   a. lung nodule segmentation
   a. motion correction
   a. peak tracking (APT)
   a. registration tool
   a. spring-loaded biopsy device
   a. vessel tracking technique

automaticity
   sinus node a.

automotility factor

autonephrectomy

autonomic
   a. denervation
   a. insufficiency
   a. nerve block
   a. nervous system
   a. neuropathy
   a. plexus

autonomous
   a. thyroid adenoma
   a. thyroid nodule (ATN)

autoparenchymatous metaphysis

autoprescanning

autopsy
   digital a.
   a. protocol

autoradiogram

autoradiograph

autoradiographic
   a. localization
   a. technique

autoradiography
   quantitative track etch a.

autoregressive moving average

autoregulation of cerebral blood flow

autosomal
   a. dominant benign form of osteopetrosis
   a. dominant leukodystrophy
   a. dominant polycystic kidney disease (ADPKD)
   a. recessive polycystic kidney disease (ARPKD)

AutoSPECT

autosplenectomy

autostereoscopic

autotomogram

autotomographic

autotomography

autotopagnosia

autotransformer formula

autotransplantation

autotriggering software

auxiliary
   a. CT tabletop
   a. ventricle

A-V
   arteriovenous
   A-V nodal rhythm

AV
   arteriovenous
   atrioventricular
   AV block
   AV node
   AV Wenckebach heart block

AVA
   advanced vessel analysis
   aortic valve area
   arteriovenous anastomosis

availability
> PET measurement of dopamine receptor a.

Avantx LC angiography suite

avascular
> a. bone necrosis
> a. brain mass
> a. cortical infarction necrosis
> a. femoral head necrosis
> a. fibrocartilage
> a. kidney mass
> a. necrosis (AVN)
> a. necrosis of lunate
> a. renal mass
> a. tarsal scaphoid necrosis
> a. vertebral body necrosis

avascularity

AVD
> aortic valvular disease

AVE
> aortic valve echocardiography
> AVE Bridge flexible balloon-expanded stent
> AVE Bridge SE self-expanding stent
> AVE Bridge stainless steel balloon-expandable stent

Avellis syndrome

Avera breast imaging system

average
> autoregressive moving a.
> a. diffusivity histogram
> a. gradient number
> a. peak velocity
> a. pixel projection (APP)
> a. positron energy
> a. radiation dose
> signal a.
> spatial average-pulse a. (SAPA)
> spatial average-temporal a.
> spatial peak-temporal a. (SPTA)
> time-weighted a.

averaged
> number of signals averaged (NSA)

averaging
> motion a.
> multiple a.
> partial volume a.
> spike a.
> volume a.

AVF
> arteriovenous fistula
> spinal dural AVF

AVG
> aortic valve gradient

aviator's astragalus

avis
> calcar a.

avium-intracellulare
> *Mycobacterium a.-i.* (MAI)

Aviva mammography system

AVM
> arteriovenous malformation
> intradural spinal AVM
> pial AVM
> AVM radiotherapy

AVN
> avascular necrosis

AVNA
> atrioventricular node artery

Avogadro
> A. constant
> A. law
> A. postulate

Avotec
> A. MR-compatible headphones
> A. MR-compatible liquid crystal display goggles

AVR
> aortic valve replacement

AVSD
> atrioventricular septal defect

avulse

avulsed
> a. fracture fragment
> a. ligament
> a. retinaculum

avulsion
> anterior labral a.
> anterior labroligamentous periosteal sleeve a. (ALPSA)
> arterial a.
> bony humeral a.
> a. chip fracture
> coracoid tip a.
> epiphysis a.
> iatrogenic a.
> a. injury
> lumbar root a.
> nail plate a.
> nerve root a.
> peroneus longus muscle a.
> posterior labroscapular periosteal a. (POLPSA)
> spinal nerve root a.
> spinous process a.
> a. stress fracture
> testicular artery a.
> traumatic a.
> venous a.

avulsive cortical irregularity

AVVM
> angiographically visualized vascular malformation

A-wave pressure

awl
> Kodros radiolucent a.

axes (*pl. of* axis)
axial, axile
    a. acetabular index (AAI)
    a. angiography
    a. aspect
    a. BMD center with agreed joint protocol
    a. carpal dislocation
    a. celloidin section
    a. cineangiography
    a. compression fracture
    a. compression injury
    a. dimension
    a. echo-planar diffusion-weighted imaging
    a. fat-suppressed T2-weighted image
    a. gradient-echo image
    a. gradient-echo imaging
    a. hiatal hernia
    a. interstitium
    a. joint dissection
    a. left anterior oblique ventriculogram
    a. loading injury
    a. load 3-part 2-plane fracture
    a. load teardrop fracture
    a. localizer
    a. manual traction test
    a. multiplanar reformation technique
    a. musculature
    a. neuritis
    a. orientation
    a. osteomalacia
    a. plane
    a. plane imaging
    a. plate
    a. pressure
    a. projection
    a. proton density-weighted image
    a. radiograph
    a. resolution
    a. rotation
    a. scan
    a. sesamoid view
    a. single-shot fast spin-echo
    a. skeleton
    a. slice
    a. spin density
    a. surface
    a. transabdominal image
    a. transverse tomography
    a. T1-SE protocol
    a. T1-weighted spin-echo imaging
    a. unenhanced CT scan
    a. wall
    a. weight loading
axiale
    skeleton a.
axile (*var. of* axial)

axilla, *pl.* **axillae**
axillae (*pl. of* axilla)
axillaris
    aperturae superior et inferior fossae a.
axillary
    a. adenopathy
    a. aneurysm
    a. arteriography
    a. artery
    a. bed
    a. cavity
    a. fascia
    a. fold
    a. fossa
    a. hematoma
    a. irradiation
    a. line
    a. lymphadenopathy
    a. lymph node (ALN)
    a. lymph node dissection (ALND)
    a. muscle
    a. node involvement
    a. node metastasis
    a. plexus
    a. pouch
    a. projection
    a. sheath
    a. space
    a. sweat gland
    a. tail of Spence
    a. tail view
    a. triangle
    a. tumor downstaging
    a. ultrasonography
    a. vein
    a. vein traumatic thrombosis
    a. vessel
axillary-axillary bypass graft
axillary-brachial bypass graft
axillary-femoral bypass graft
axillary-femorofemoral bypass graft
axillobifemoral bypass graft
axillofemoral approach
axillosubclavian vein thrombosis
axiolabiolingual plane
Axiom Artis dBC magnetic navigation system
axiomesiodistal plane
axipetal
axis, *pl.* **axes**
    anatomic a.
    ankle mortise a.
    anode-cathode a.
    a. anomaly
    anteroposterior a.
    basibregmatic a.
    basicranial a.
    bimalleolar foot a.

A

a. body
bowel a.
carpal a.
celiac a.
condylar a.
coordinate a.
cortical hinge a.
craniocaudal a.
craniospinal a.
distal reference a. (DRA)
enteroinsular a.
femoral shaft a.
a. fracture
horizontal long a.
hypothalamic-pituitary a.
hypothalamic-pituitary-adrenal a.
hypothalamic-pituitary-gonadal a.
hypothalamoneurohypophysial a.
hypothalamopituitary a.
leg a.
a. ligament
long a.
longitudinal a.
mechanical a.
metatarsal a.
midpapillary short a.
normal a.
a. of heart
pendulous reference a. (PRA)
proximal reference a.
renal a.
single a.
spinal a.
subtalar a.
T a.
transcondylar a. (TCA)
transporionic a.
vertical a.
vertical long a.
weightbearing a.

X a.
Y a.
Z a.
3-axis gradient coil
axon
obliquely oriented a.
axonal
a. bouton
a. cylinder
a. membrane
a. shearing
a. transport impairment
axonopathic neurogenic thoracic outlet syndrome
Ayerza syndrome
azelaic acid
azotemic osteodystrophy
azygoesophageal
a. line
a. recess
azygogram
azygography
azygos
a. anterior cerebral artery
a. arch
a. artery of vagina
a. blood flow
a. continuation
a. continuation of inferior vena cava
a. fissure
a. hematoma cap
a. lobe of lung
a. lymph node
nodus arcus venae a.
a. vein
a. vein distention
a. vein enlargement
azygos-hemiazygos complex
Azzopardi tumor

B

B level of esophagus
Pittsburgh Compound B (PIB)
B ring of esophagus
B scan

Ba

basion
point Ba

Baastrup disease
BabyFace

B. 3D surface rendering accessory
B. 3D surface rendering accessory device

baby formula with ferrous sulfate contrast agent
babyPAC ventilator
BAC

bacterial artificial chromosome

Baccelli sign of pleural effusion
Bachmann

anterior internodal tract of B.
B. bundle

bacillary embolus
Bacillus anthracis
back

b. crease
b. pressure atrophy
b. projection
b. stroke volume

back-angle anomaly
backbleeding
backfire fracture
backflow

b. of blood
pyelolymphatic b.
pyelorenal b.
pyelotubular b.
pyelovenous b.
venous b.

backflux
background

b. activity
b. count
b. density
b. erase
b. radiation
b. slowing
b. subtraction
b. subtraction technique

back-knee deformity
backlit digitizer
backprojection
backrush of blood into left ventricle
backscatter

b. electron

b. factor (BSF)
b. of blood
b. peak

backscattered

b. power
b. radiation

back-to-back configuration
backup of blood
backward

b. curvature
b. flow
b. heart failure

backwash ileitis
bacterial

b. aneurysm
b. artificial chromosome (BAC)
b. cholangitis
b. endocarditis
b. ependymitis
b. epiglottitis
b. meningitis
b. nephritis
b. osteomyelitis
b. peritonitis
b. pneumonia
b. pneumonitis
b. sinusitis
b. spondylitis
b. superinfection
b. toxin

Bacteroides
badge

film b.
ring b.

BAE

bronchial artery embolization

Baehr-Lohlein lesion
Baer plane
Baerveldt glaucoma drainage implant
Baeyer-Villiger oxidation
Baffe anastomosis
baffle

intrapulmonary b.
b. leak

baffled tunnel
Bäfverstedt syndrome
bag

balloon b.
bile b.
nephrostomy b.
b. of bagassosis
Tedlar b.

bagasse
bagassosis

bag of b.

Bagby and Kuslich (BAK)
BAI
    basion axial interval
Baillinger
    inner stripe of B.
bail-lock knee joint
baja
    patella b.
BAK
    Bagby and Kuslich
    BAK interbody fusion system
Baker cyst
baker's leg
BAL
    bronchoalveolar lavage
balance
    mass b.
    b. pattern
balanced
    b. circulation
    b. fast field-echo pulse
    b. gradient
    b. gradient technique
    b. hemivertebra
    b. ischemia
    b. pneumoperitoneum
balancing subdural hematoma
bald gastric fundus
Balint syndrome
Balkan
    B. fracture frame
    B. nephritis
    B. nephropathy
ball
    fungus b.
    keratin urinary tract b.
    kidney fungus b.
    lung fungus b.
    B. method
    mobile fat b.
    myelin b.
    b. occluder valve
    b. of foot
    renal fungus b.
    sludge b.
ball-and-socket
    b.-a.-s. ankle mortise
    b.-a.-s. epiphysis
    b.-a.-s. joint
ball-catcher
    b.-c. projection
    b.-c. view
ballerina-foot pattern
8-ball hemorrhage
ball-in-hand appearance
ballistic
    b. injury
    b. material
ballistocardiography

ball-on-spoon appearance
balloon
    All-Terrain B. (ATB)
    b. aortoplasty
    b. atrial septostomy
    b. bag
    Bardex b.
    barium enema retention b.
    b. biliary catheter
    Blue Max high-pressure b.
    b. bronchoplasty
    b. catheter fenestration
    b. catheterization
    b. cholangiogram
    b. coil
    b. counterpulsation
    cryoplasty b.
    cutting b.
    b. dilation
    b. dilator
    b. dissector
    Duralyn b.
    b. embolectomy catheter
    b. epiphysis
    b. expulsion imaging
    b. fenestration
    GuardWire distal b.
    high-pressure Blue Max b.
    b. inflation
    kissing b.'s
    low-compliance fixed-diameter b.
    b. mitral valvoplasty
    nondetachable b.
    b. occlusion
    b. occlusion arteriography
    b. occlusion pulmonary angiogram
    b. occlusion tolerance test
    b. occlusive aortography
    Opta 5 angioplasty b.
    Optiplast Centurion b.
    Penta b.
    percutaneous intraaortic b.
    percutaneous transluminal
      angioplasty b.
    PET b.
    pressure-detachable silicone b.
    b. proctogram
    b. PTA catheter
    b. pump
    radiofrequency b.
    rectal b.
    b. remodeling
    scintigraphic b.
    self-sealing latex b.
    b. tamponade
    b. test occlusion
    b. test occlusion imaging
    b. topography
    b. tuboplasty

Ultrathin Diamond b.
USCI PET b.
b. valvotomy
waist in b.
windowed b.
ballooned
b. floor of ventricle
b. sella
balloon-expandable stent
ballooning
b. degeneration
disc b.
b. mitral cusp
b. of vertebral interspace
balloon-occluded
b.-o. arterial infusion
b.-o. transvenous obliteration
balloon-related trauma
balloon-retriever technique
balloon-shaped heart
2-balloon technique
balloon-tipped angiographic catheter
ball-tip microcatheter
ball-type valve
ball-valve
b.-v. obstruction
b.-v. thrombus
b.-v. tumor
Baló concentric sclerosis
BALT
bronchus-associated lymphoid tissue
Bamberger area
Bamberger-Marie disease
bamboo
b. spine
b. spine sign
banana
b. fracture
b. sign
banana-shaped uterine cavity
Bancaud phenomenon
bancrofti
Wuchereria b.
band
aberrant b.
absorption b.
alpha frequency b.
amnionic b.
anogenital b.
anterior b.
AO tension b.
aponeurotic b.
atrioventricular b.
Broca diagonal b.
calf b.
Clado b.
conduction b.
constriction b.
dark Mach b.

dense metaphysial b.
echogenic b.
external b.
fascial b.
fibroelastic b.
fibromuscular b.
fibrous b.
Gennari b.
H b.
Harris b.
b. heterotopia
His b.
Hunter-Schreger b.
hypoechoic b.
iliotibial b.
intercaval b.
internal b.
intratesticular b.
IT b.
Ladd b.
Lane b.
lateral b.
longitudinal b.
low signal intensity fibrous b.
low signal intensity peripheral b.
lucent b.
Mach b.
Maissiat b.
Marlex b.
Meckel b.
mesocolic b.
metaphysial lucent b.
moderator b.
myocardial b.
negative Mach b.
b. of atelectasis
b. of Broca
b. of density
b. of deossification
omental b.
parenchymatous fibrous b.
parenchymatous lung b.
Parham-Martin b.
parietal b.
peritoneal b.
posterior tracheal b.
pretendinous b.
radiofrequency saturation b.
Reil b.
saturation b.
scar b.
sclerotic b.
septal b.
septomarginal b.
serpiginous b.
silicone elastomer b.
Simonart b.
spatial presaturation b.
tendinous b.

band (*continued*)
    b. tenodesis
    tracheal b.
    transverse b.
    valence b.
    vascular b.
    walking saturation b.
    Z b.
bandage
    Esmarch b.
bandbox resonance
bandelette
banding
    b. appearance
    halftone b.
bandlike
    b. adhesion
    b. margin
    b. shadow
bandpass filter
bandwidth
    receive b.
Bankart
    B. deformity
    B. dislocation
    B. fracture
    B. lesion
Bannayan-Riley-Ruvalcaba syndrome
Banti syndrome
Banyan emergency kit
BAP
    brightness area product
bar
    arch b.
    Bill b.
    bony b.
    cartilaginous b.
    cecal b.
    congenital b.
    coracoclavicular b.
    cricopharyngeal b.
    b. defect
    fibrous b.
    hyoid b.
    median b.
    Passavant b.
    physial b.
    PLES b.
    unsegmented vertebral b.
barber-chair position
Bard
    B. CPS system
    B. Monoply reusable core biopsy
      instrument
    B. percutaneous cardiopulmonary
      support system
    B. rotary atherectomy device
    B. Safety Excalibur catheter
    B. Saxx stent

Bardeleben
    prefrontal bone of von B.
Bardex
    B. balloon
    B. Lubricath catheter
Bardinet ligament
BardPort
    B. low-profile port
    B. MRI full-size port
bare area
bare-metal stent
Baricon imaging agent
baritosis
barium
    b. artifact
    b. aspiration
    b. bolus
    cesium with b. 137m
    double tracking of b.
    b. enema (BE)
    b. enema imaging
    b. enema retention balloon
    b. enema through colostomy
    b. enema with air contrast
    b. esophagram
    flocculation of b.
    b. fluoride
    b. fluorochloride
    b. followthrough examination
    fragmentation of b.
    b. GI series
    high-density b.
    holdup in flow of b.
    hydrophilic nonflocculating b.
    b. injection
    b. injection through colostomy
    b. lead sulfate
    low-concentration b. (LCB)
    b. meal
    b. meal and followthrough
    b. meal study
    b. mixture
    b. pill
    b. platinocyanoide
    b. pneumoconiosis
    pocketing of b.
    b. powder
    b. radiography
    reflux of b.
    residual b.
    retained b.
    retention of b.
    b. segmentation
    sterile b.
    b. strontium sulfate
    b. sulfate (BaSO$_4$)
    b. sulfate contrast medium
    b. sulfate imaging agent
    b. sulfate-impregnated shunt

b. suspension
b. swallow
b. swallow imaging
b. titanate
b. vaginography
barium-based fecal tagging
barium-filled colon
barium-impregnated poppet
barium-water esophagram
barked injury
Barkow ligament
Barlow
    B. pediatric hip instability test
    B. syndrome
Baro-CAT imaging agent
baroreceptor
    b. bulb
    carotid bulb b.
Barosperse imaging agent
barotrauma
    intrapulmonary b.
    pulmonary b. (PBT)
barrel chest
Barré-Lieou syndrome
barreling distortion
barrel-shaped
    b.-s. lesion
    b.-s. stone
Barrett
    B. epithelium
    B. esophagus
    B. ulcer
barrier
    anatomic b.
    b. beam
    blood-brain b. (BBB)
    blood-spinal cord b. (BSCB)
    blood-thymus b.
    brain-blood b.
    contrast absorption b.
    incompetent blood-brain b.
    radiation b.
Bart abdominoperipheral angiography unit
Barth hernia
Bartholin
    B. duct
    B. gland
    B. gland carcinoma (BGC)
Bartko-Carpenter approach
Bartonella
Barton fracture
Barton-Smith fracture
Bartter syndrome
basal
    b. angle
    b. arachnoid cistern
    b. bone
    b. cell adenoma

b. cell carcinoma
b. cell nevus syndrome
b. cell papilloma
b. cerebral artery
b. chorda
b. cistern of brain
b. descent
b. extension
b. forebrain cholinergic structure
b. ganglion
b. ganglion anatomy
b. ganglion calcification
b. ganglion echogenic focus
b. ganglion hematoma
b. ganglionic change
b. ganglion infarct
b. ganglion of cerebellum
b. joint
b. joint of thumb
b. lamella
b. layer
b. neck fracture
b. nucleus
b. perforating artery
b. placenta vein
b. plate
b. ridge
b. segmental bronchus
b. short-axis slice
b. short-axis view
b. skull fracture
b. sphincter
b. surface
b. tuberculosis
b. vein of Rosenthal (BVR)
b. zone
bascule
    cecal b.
base
    cranial b.
    b. deficit
    b. density
    Dycal b.
    b. fog
    invagination of skull b.
    lung b.
    b. of bladder
    b. of brain
    b. of finger
    b. of heart
    b. of metacarpal
    b. of phalanx
    b. of skull (BOS)
    b. of skull foramen
    b. of thumb
    b. of toe
    orbital b.
    b. projection
    respiratory disturbance of acid b.

base (*continued*)
    skull b.
    ulcer b.
    b. view
baseball
    b. bat shape
    b. finger
    b. finger fracture
    b. pitcher's elbow
    b. shoulder
Basedow goiter
baseline
    anthropologic b.
    anthropomorphic b.
    b. artifact
    b. chest x-ray
    b. correction
    b. mammography
    b. of bulb
    radiographic b.
    Reid b.
    reproducible b.
    return to b.
    b. tenting
    b. view
basialis
basibregmatic axis
basic
    b. cycle length (BCL)
    b. drive cycle length (BDCL)
    b. life support (BLS)
    b. volume image analysis
basicervical fracture
basicranial axis
basicranium
basilar, basilaris
    b. angiography
    b. artery
    b. artery aneurysm
    b. artery bifurcation
    b. artery ectasia
    b. artery insufficiency
    b. artery syndrome
    b. atelectasis
    b. block skull positioner
    b. cartilage
    b. cistern
    b. crest
    b. femoral neck fracture
    b. fibrosis
    b. groove
    b. impression
    b. intracerebral hemorrhage
    b. invagination
    b. line
    b. occlusion
    b. part of occipital bone
    b. pleural scarring
    b. plexus

    b. pneumonitis
    b. pneumothorax
    b. predominance
    b. process
    b. projection
    b. reticular opacity
    b. sinus
    b. skull fracture
    b. spine
    b. sulcus
    b. suture
    b. tip aneurysm
    b. vertebra
    b. zone infiltrate
basilaris (*var. of* basilar)
basilic vein
basin
    positive node b.
basioccipital bone
basiocciput
    b. hypoplasia
    b. tumor
basion (Ba)
    b. axial interval (BAI)
    b. dens interval (BDI)
basipharyngeal canal
basisphenoid bone
basis pontis
basivertebral
    b. vein
    b. venous complex
basket
    b. cell
    double b.
    b. guidewire
    Highflex large stone retrieval b.
basketlike calcification
basket-weave pattern
BaSO$_4$
    barium sulfate
basophil (*var. of* basophilic)
basophilic, basophil
    b. brain adenoma
    b. leukocyte
    b. series
basovertical projection
BAT
    B-mode acquisition and targeting
    bolus arrival time
    brown adipose tissue
    BAT system
Bateman classification of full-thickness tear
batimastat
Batson
    B. plexus
    B. vertebral brain system
bat's-wing pattern
battered child syndrome

battledore placenta
Battle sign
batwing
>   b. appearance
>   b. appearance of ventricle
>   b. configuration
>   b. configuration of ventricle
>   b. distribution
>   b. edema
>   b. formation
>   b. lung consolidation
>   b. shadow

Baudelocque diameter
Bauer-Kirby disc diffusion method
Bauer-Temno biopsy needle
Bauhin valve
Baumann supracondylar fracture angle
Baumgarten recess
bauxite
>   b. fibrosis of lung
>   b. pneumoconiosis

Baxter PMT device
bayesian
>   b. analysis
>   b. calculation
>   b. formula
>   b. image estimation (BIE)
>   b. technique

Bayes theorem
Bayle granulation
Bayler-Pinneau method
Bayliss effect
Baylor total artificial heart
Bayne
>   B. classification
>   B. classification of radial agenesis (I-IV)

bayonet
>   b. deformity
>   b. dislocation
>   b. fracture
>   b. fracture position
>   b. leg

bayoneting of fracture fragment
Bazex syndrome
BBB
>   blood-brain barrier
>   BBB breakdown

BBBB
>   bilateral bundle-branch block

BBC
>   biceps, brachialis, coracobrachialis
>   BBC muscles

BBD
>   benign breast disease
>   brittle bone disease

BBO
>   benign biliary obstruction

BBR
>   bundle-branch reentry

B6 bronchus sign
BCA
>   bell-clapper anomaly

B-cell
>   B-c. monocytoid lymphoma
>   B-c. non-Hodkin lymphoma
>   B-c. tumor

BCI
>   bicaudate index
>   brain-computer interface

BCL
>   basic cycle length

B-D
>   Becton-Dickinson
>   B-D bone marrow biopsy needle
>   B-D Insyte Autoguard shielded intravenous catheter

BDA
>   bile duct adenoma

BDCL
>   basic drive cycle length

BDI
>   basion dens interval

BDM
>   border detection method

BE
>   barium enema

Be
>   beryllium

beach-chair position
bead
>   b. block
>   b. image
>   immunomagnetic b.
>   methyl methacrylate b.
>   packed b.'s
>   Sephadex b.
>   targeting b.
>   tungsten b.

bead-chain
>   b.-c. cystogram
>   b.-c. cystography

beaded
>   b. bile duct
>   b. bronchus
>   b. ductal dilation
>   b. hepatic duct
>   b. necklace appearance
>   b. pancreatic duct
>   b. rib
>   b. septal thickening
>   b. septum sign
>   b. ureter

beading
>   b. of artery
>   b. of vessel
>   rosary b.

B

beak
dorsal talar b.
b. fracture
b. ligament
b. sign
beaked
b. appearance
b. cervicomedullary junction
b. pelvis
b. vertebra
beaking
anterior central b.
antral b.
central b.
inferior b.
b. of head of talus
talar b.
talonavicular b.
tectal b.
beaklike
b. configuration
b. narrowing
b. osteophyte formation
beak-shaped nose
Beall valve
beam
b. attenuation
barrier b.
blended b.
broad b.
cobalt-60 b.
cone b.
coplanar b.
CT scanner b.
b. current
b. diffraction
electron b.
b. energy
b. filtration
flattening filter b.
gaussian-mode profile laser b.
b. geometry
b. hardening
helium ion b.
b. intensity
intensity-modulated photon b.
laser b.
lateral opposed b.
b. limitation
Lucite b.
megavoltage treatment b.
b. monitor
monochromatic x-ray b.
multifield b.
narrow b.
neutron b.
noncoplanar therapy b.
offset fan b.

open b.
parallel-opposed b.'s
b. pattern
pencil electron b.
pion b.
b. pitch
primary b.
proton b.
b. quality comparison
radiation b.
b. restrictor
b. shaper
sound b.
b. splitter
b. steering
b. therapy
useful b.
wedged-pair b.
x-ray b.
BEAM
brain electrical activity mapping
beam-bending magnet
beam-hardening
b.-h. artifact
b.-h. effect
beam-indicating device
beamlike artifact
beam-modifying device
beam's-eye
b.-e. view
b.-e. view dosimetry
beam-splitting mirror
beam-therapy applicator
bear's
b. claw ulcer
b. paw hand
beat
apex b.
ectopic b.
escape b.
inferolateral displacement of apical
  b.
ventricular capture b. (VCB)
ventricular ectopic b. (VEB)
ventricular premature b. (VPB)
ventricular pseudoperfusion b.
beaten
b. brass appearance
b. brass skull
b. silver appearance
b. silver appearance of skull
Beath view
beat-knee syndrome
Beatson
B. combined ankle length
B. radiographic combined
  talocalcaneal angle
beat-to-beat variability

B

beaver-tail appearance
Bechterew (*var. of* Bekhterev)
Beck triad
Beckwith-Wiedemann syndrome
Béclard
    B. amputation
    B. hernia
Beclere position
Becquerel (Bq)
    B. ray
Becton-Dickinson (B-D)
    B.-D. FAC scan
bed
    arteriole-capillary-venous b.
    axillary b.
    bladder b.
    distal tissue b.
    draining lymphatic b.
    gallbladder b.
    hepatic b.
    ipsilateral jugular lymphatic b.
    liver b.
    lumpectomy b.
    nodal b.
    b. of rib
    peritubular vascular b.
    portal vascular b.
    precapillary b.
    primary tumor b.
    prostatic b.
    pulmonary vascular b.
    skeletal b.
    stomach b.
    thyroid b.
    tumor b.
    vascular b.
BED
    bioeffect dose
    biologically equivalent dose
    biologic effective dose
Bednar tumor
bedroom fracture
bedside radiography
beer
    b. heart
    B. law
Beevor sign
Behçet
    B. disease
    B. syndrome
    B. syndrome
Behnken unit
Behr syndrome
BEI
    butanol-extractable iodine
Bekhterev, Bechterew
    B. arthritis
    B. layer

bell
    B. brachydactyly
    B. phenomenon
bell-and-clapper deformity
bell-clapper anomaly (BCA)
2-bellied muscle
Bellini
    duct of B.
    B. ligament
    papillary duct of B.
bellomedullary
bell-shaped thorax
belly
    bubble of b.
    b. of muscle
below diaphragm
below-knee amputation (BKA)
Benassi
    B. method
    B. position
bend
    dorsal b.
    hand-shaped b.
    kneelike b.
bending fracture
Bends asbestos pleurisy
benediction posture
Benedict-Talbot body surface area method
beneficial atrial septal defect
bengal
    I-labeled rose b.
benign
    b. adrenal mass
    b. asbestos-related pleural disease
    b. biliary obstruction (BBO)
    b. biliary stricture
    b. breast calcification
    b. breast disease (BBD)
    b. cerebellar ectopia
    b. chondroblastoma
    b. conal cyst
    b. congenital Wilms tumor
    b. cortical defect
    b. cystic teratoma
    b. duct ectasia
    b. duodenal tumor
    b. fetal hamartoma
    b. fibrous bone lesion
    b. fibrous bone tumor
    b. fibrous histiocytoma
    b. gastric ulcer
    b. hepatic cyst
    b. infiltrate
    b. intracranial hypertension
    b. intraductal papilloma
    b. lung tumor
    b. lymphadenopathy

benign (*continued*)
   b. lymphoepithelial lesion
   b. lymphoepithelial parotid tumor
   b. lymphoma of rectum
   b. lymphoproliferative lesion
   b. meningeal fibrosis
   b. mesenchymoma
   b. mesothelioma
   b. metastasizing leiomyoma
   b. mixed tumor parotitis
   b. neoplasia
   b. nephrosclerosis
   b. node
   b. osteoblastoma
   b. osteochondroma
   b. osteogenic tumor
   b. ovarian cystic disease
   b. ovarian tumor
   b. oxyphilic adenoma
   b. papillary stenosis
   b. peptic stricture
   b. pleural fibroma
   b. postoperative meningeal
     enhancement
   b. prostatic hyperplasia (BPH)
   b. prostatic hypertrophy (BPH)
   b. schwannoma
   b. sclerosing ductal proliferation
   b. small bowel tumor
   b. subdural effusion
   b. teratoid mediastinal tumor
   b. teratoma
   b. thymoma
   b. tracheobronchial stenosis
   b. transient synovitis
   b. urethral tumor
   b. vascular lesion
benign-appearing pattern
Benink tarsal index
Benjamin
   B. binocular slimline laryngoscope
   B. pediatric laryngoscope
Bennett
   B. dislocation
   B. fracture
   B. lesion
Benoist penetrometer
bent-knee pelvic tilt
benzamide imaging agent
benzocaine
benzoic
   b. acid
   b. acid contrast medium
Berdon syndrome
Berenstein catheter
Berger interscapular amputation
Bergman
   B. fiber
   B. sign

Bergonie-Tribondeau law
beriberi heart
berkelium
Berman angiographic catheter
Bernard canal
Bernard-Horner syndrome
Bernard-Soulier syndrome
Berndt-Hardy talar dome classification
Bernoulli
   B. effect
   B. equation
Bernstein catheter
berry
   B. aneurysm rupture
   B. ligament
Bertel
   B. method
   B. position
Bertillon cephalometer
Bertin
   column of B.
   B. ligament
   septum of B.
Bertolotti syndrome
berylliosis
   acute b.
   chronic b.
beryllium (Be)
   b. granuloma
   b. mammography x-ray tube
     window
best-guess technique
beta
   b. amyloid senile plaque
   b. angle
   b. decay
   b. detection
   b. emission
   b. emitter
   b. particle
   b. radiation
   b. ray
   b. ray applicator
   b. ray ophthalmic plaque therapy
   b. ray spectrometer
   b. transition
Beta-Cath
   B.-C. system
   B.-C. system catheter
beta-emitting isotope
**betamethyliodophenyl pentadecanoic acid
 (BMIPP)**
beta-minus decay
beta-oxybutyric acid
beta-plus decay
beta-thalassemia intermedia
betatron
Bethesda unit
Beuren syndrome

BeV
    billion electron volts
beveled
    b. electron beam cone
    b. margin
    b. needle
Bextra
bezoar
    gastric b.
BFI
    bifrontal index
BFM
    Brunnstrom Fugl Meyer
    BFM stroke impairment assessment
BGC
    Bartholin gland carcinoma
BGO
    bismuth germanate
    BGO crystal
BH4 precursor
Biad
    B. camera
    B. SPECT imaging system
Biafine RE
Bianchi nodule
bias
    lead-time b.
    length-time b.
    minimizing b.
    overdiagnostic b.
    selection b.
    self-selection b.
    time-to-treatment b.
biatrial
    b. hypertrophy
    b. myxoma
biaxial
BIB
    biliointestinal bypass
bibasally
bibasilar
    b. bronchopneumonia
    b. discoid atelectasis
Bible printer's lung
bicameral uterus
bicanalicular sphincter
BICAP
    bipolar circumactive probe
    BICAP unit
bicaudate
    b. index (BCI)
    b. ratio
bicaval cannulation
biceps (*pl.* **biceps, bicepses**)
    b., brachialis, coracobrachialis (BBC)
    b., brachialis, coracobrachialis
      muscles
    b. brachialis tendon
    b. brachii tendon

    b. femoris muscle
    b. femoris tendon
    long head of b.
    short head of b.
bicepses (*pl. of* biceps)
biceps-labral complex
bicerebral infarct
Bichat
    B. canal
    B. foramen
    B. ligament
    B. membrane
bicipital
    b. aponeurosis
    b. bursitis
    b. fascia
    b. groove
    b. groove view
    b. rib
    b. synovial sheath
    b. tendon
    b. tendon sheath
    b. tuberosity
bicipitalis
bicisate
    technetium 99m b.
bicollis
    bicornuate b.
bicommissural aortic valve
biconcave
    b. deformity
    b. depression
    b. disc
    b. vertebra
biconcavity
bicondylar
    b. T-shaped fracture
    b. Y-shaped fracture
biconvex
bicornuate
    b. bicollis
    b. uterus
bicoronal synostosis
bicortical
    b. iliac bone
    b. screw
Bicor Top
bicristal diameter
bicuspid
    b. aortic valve
    b. atrioventricular valve
    b. valvular aortic stenosis
bicycle, bike
    b. ergometer
    b. exercise radionuclide
      ventriculogram
    b. exercise stress test
    b. spoke fracture
Bid-Gd mesoporphyrine

B

bidirectional
    b. cavopulmonary anastomosis
    b. interface
    b. shunt
BIE
    bayesian image estimation
Biello criterion
Bielschowsky stain
Bier amputation
Bierman needle
**biexponential fitting of left ventricular
  curve**
bifascicular bundle-branch block
bifemoral graft
bifid
    b. aortic branch
    b. atlas
    b. biceps tendon
    b. pelvis
    b. pons
    b. precordial impulse
    b. renal pelvis
    b. rib
    b. thumb deformity
    b. ureter
bifida
    spina b.
bifidum
    cranium b.
bifocal manipulation with distraction
biforate uterus
bifrontal
    b. index (BFI)
    b. oligodendrogliomas
bifurcate, bifurcated
    b. ligament
bifurcated (*var. of* bifurcate)
bifurcating branch
bifurcatio
    b. aortae
    b. aortica
    b. carotidis
    b. tracheae
    b. trunci pulmonalis
bifurcation
    b. aneurysm
    aortic b.
    basilar artery b.
    carotid artery b.
    common bile duct b.
    common carotid artery b.
    b. graft
    hepatic duct b.
    iliac b.
    b. lesion
    b. lymph node
    middle cerebral artery b.
    b. of anterior communicating artery
    b. of aorta
    b. of internal carotid artery
    b. of trunk
    patent b.
    pulmonary artery b.
    pulmonary trunk b.
    tracheal b.
    ureteral bud b.
Bigelow ligament
bigeminal
    b. pattern
    b. pregnancy
Bigliani
    B. and Morrison method
    B. classification
big rib sign
bihemispheral insult
biischial diameter
bike (*var. of* bicycle)
bilaminar
    b. appearance
    b. zone
bilateral
    b. alteration
    b. anterior chest bulges
    b. arachnoid cysts
    b. breast coils
    b. bronchograms
    b. bundle-branch block (BBBB)
    b. carotid arteriography
    b. carotid stenoses
    b. choroid plexus cysts
    b. consolidation
    b. cortical necrosis
    b. diaphragmatic elevation
    b. diffuse increased uptake
    b. ductal ectasia
    b. dysplasia epiphysialis
      hemimelia
    b. elevation of diaphragm
    b. fetal chest masses
    b. hallux valgus
    b. hilar adenopathy
    b. hilar enlargement
    b. hydroceles
    b. hydrocephalus
    b. hyperlucent lungs
    b. iliac crests
    b. iliopsoas abscesses
    b. incomplete ureteral injuries
    b. infarcts
    b. interstitial pulmonary infiltrates
    b. intrafacetal dislocation
    b. invasive lobular carcinoma
    b. juxtafoveal telangiectasis
    b. large adrenals
    b. large kidneys
    b. left-sidedness
    b. lesions
    b. locked facets

B

b. lower lobe pneumonia
b. lung hyperinflation
b. myocutaneous graft
b. narrowing of urinary bladder
b. obstruction
b. occlusion
b. orbitofrontal cortices
b. pleural effusions
b. pleural tubes
b. pneumothorax
b. pulmonary artery enlargement
b. reduction of tracer uptake
b. renal masses
b. right-sidedness
b. semicircular canal aplasia
b. serous pleural effusions
b. small kidneys
b. striopallidodentate calcinosis
b. superior parietal hypometabolism
b. superior vena cava
b. symmetry
b. upper lobe cavitary infiltrates
b. vagotomy effect
bilaterality
bilaterally symmetric
bile
b. bag
b. capillary
concentrated b.
b. concretion
b. duct
b. duct adenoma (BDA)
b. duct anastomosis
b. duct atresia
b. duct carcinoma
b. duct cystadenoma
b. duct dilation
b. duct dyskinesia
b. duct filling defect
b. duct gas
b. duct imaging
b. duct infundibulum
b. duct lumen
b. duct narrowing
b. duct pressure
b. duct proliferation
b. duct scan
b. duct stone
b. duct stricture
echogenic b.
b. encrustation
b. esophagitis
b. extravasation
b. flow
b. flow obstruction
gastric reflux of b.
b. lake
b. leakage
lithogenic b.

b. papilla
b. peritonitis
b. plug
b. pulmonary embolus
b. reflux
b. reflux gastritis
b. stasis
sterile b.
b. tree
bileaflet valve
bile-tagged 3D magnetic resonance colonography
bilharzial
b. carcinoma
b. granuloma
bilharziasis, bilharziosis
cardiopulmonary b.
protopulmonary b.
bilharziosis (*var. of* bilharziasis)
biliaropancreatica
ampulla b.
biliary
b. angiography
b. ascariasis
b. ascites
b. atresia
b. calculus
b. canal
b. cirrhosis
b. cirrhotic liver
b. colic
b. cystadenoma
b. decompression
b. dilation
b. drainage
b. drainage catheter
b. duct
b. dyskinesia
b. dyssynergia
b. endoprosthesis
b. excretion bowel activity
b. fistula
b. hypoplasia
b. leak
b. lithotripsy
b. manometry
b. microhamartoma
b. mud
b. obstruction syndrome
b. passage
b. piecemeal necrosis
b. plexus
b. radical
b. saturation index
b. sludge
b. stent
b. stenting
b. stricture
b. structure

biliary (*continued*)
  b. stump
  b. system
  b. tract
  b. tract carcinoma
  b. tract CT scan imaging
  b. tract disease
  b. tract obstruction
  b. tract stone
  b. tree
  b. tree compression
  b. tree gas
  b. tree obstruction
biliary-cutaneous fistula
biliary-duodenal
  b.-d. fistula
  b.-d. pressure gradient
biliary-enteric
  b.-e. anastomosis
  b.-e. bypass
  b.-e. fistula
biliary-gastric fistula
biliary-to-bowel transit
BiliBed phototherapy system
Biligram
bilinear rotation decoupling (BIRD)
bilioenteric fistula
biliointestinal bypass (BIB)
biliopancreatic
  b. bypass
  b. diversion
  b. shunt
biliopleural communication
bilious
  b. bronchial pneumonia
  b. expectoration
  b. gastritis
bilirubinate stone
Biliscopin imaging agent
Bilivistan
Bill bar
billion electron volts (BeV)
billowing
  b. mitral valve
  b. mitral valve prolapse
Billroth
  B. I, II anastomosis
  B. I, II gastroduodenostomy
  B. I, II gastrojejunostomy
bilobate, bilobed
  b. configuration
  b. gallbladder
  b. mass
  b. placenta
  b. polypoid lesion
bilobectomy
bilobed (*var. of* bilobate)
bilobulation

bilocular, biloculate
  b. disc
  b. stomach
  b. uterus
biloculare
  cor b.
biloculate (*var. of* bilocular)
biloma
  b. in gallbladder fossa
  intrahepatic b.
  subphrenic b.
Bilopaque imaging agent
Biloptin imaging agent
bimalleolar
  b. angle
  b. ankle fractures
  b. foot axis
bimastoid line
BimOdal Slice Select (BOSS)
bimolecular
binarized image
binary
  b. digit
  b. image
  b. imaging
  b. opacity table
  b. similarity coefficient
bind
  ^{99m}Tc Ceretec b.
binding
  DAT b.
  b. energy
  fragment antigen b. (Fab)
  ionic b.
  receptor b.
  b. site
Bing-Horton syndrome
binned
binning
  projection b.
binocular stereoscope
Binswanger
  B. disease
  B. encephalopathy
bioabsorbable
  b. Dexon suture
  b. sheath-delivered vascular device
bioassay
  erythropoietin b.
biocavity laser
biodegradable
  b. collagen plug
  b. implant
  b. magnetic microcluster
  b. stent
Biodex Venti-Scan III aerosol delivery system
biodistribution
BiodivYsio stent

bioeffect
    b. dose (BED)
    thermal b.
biograph
    B. Duo LSO PET/CT scanner
    b. molecular imaging system
bioheat equation
bioimpedance
    needle-tip b.
biologic, biological
    b. age
    b. effective dose (BED)
    b. half life
    b. osteosynthesis
    b. target volume
    b. tissue valve
    b. variation
    b. window
biological (*var. of* biologic)
biologically equivalent dose (BED)
biology
    radiation b.
biomagnetometer
    Magnes b.
biomarker
biomechanical
    b. imbalance
    b. stress
biomechanically normal spine
biomechanics of limb-length discrepancy
biomedical radiography
biometry
    fetal b.
    longitudinal ultrasonic b.
biomicroscopy
    slit-lamp b.
    ultrasound b. (UBM)
biomodulator
biomolecular reaction
bionucleonic
biophysical
    b. limitation
    b. profile score (BPS)
BioPince needle
biopotential
    induced b.
bioprosthesis
    ProCol vascular b.
biopsy
    aspiration b.
    automated large-core breast b.
    blind b.
    bone marrow b.
    breast b.
    computerized tomography-guided
      needle b.
    core needle b.
    CT-directed b.
    CT-guided needle b.

    CT-guided percutaneous b.
    CT-guided transsternal core b.
    curved-needle b.
    endocardial b.
    endomyocardial b.
    excisional b.
    fetal liver b.
    fetal skin b.
    fine-needle aspiration b.
    guided b.
    interactive MR-guided b.
    intramedullary tumor b.
    large-core ultrasound-guided b.
    Monopty core b.
    MRI-guided breast b.
    b. needle
    needle b.
    needle-guided excisional b.
    needle-localized breast b. (NLBB)
    percutaneous bone b.
    percutaneous transhepatic
      endoluminal biliary b.
    percutaneous transhepatic liver b.
    percutaneous transthoracic needle b.
      (PTNB)
    placenta b.
    point-in-space stereotactic b.
    punch b.
    sentinel lymph node b. (SLNB)
    sentinel node localization and b.
    skeletal b.
    StereoGuide stereotactic core needle
      b.
    stereotactic core needle b. (SCNB)
    stereotactic percutaneous needle b.
    stereotactic vacuum-assisted breast b.
      (SVABB)
    systematic ultrasound-guided b.
    transbronchial lung b. (TBLB)
    b. transducer
    transjugular liver b. (TJLB, TLD)
    transparietal b.
    transthoracic needle b. (TNB)
    transthoracic needle aspiration b.
      (TTNAB)
    trephine b.
    ultrasound-guided anterior subcostal
      liver b.
    ultrasound-guided core b.
    ultrasound-guided large-core needle
      b.
    ultrasound-guided stereotactic b.
    ultrasound-guided vacuum-assisted
      b.
    vacuum-assisted core b.
    vacuum-assisted imaging-guided b.
    ventricular endomyocardial b.
    virtual bone b.
    Wang b.

B

biopsy-guided attachment
Biopsys Mammotome
bioptome
Biopty
    B. biopsy gun
    B. cut needle
bioreductive agent
Biosense-guided LMR
Biosound AU3, AU4, AU5 system
BioSpec
    B. MR imaging system
    B. MR imaging system scanner
BioSphere Medical
bioterrorism exposure
Biotrack coagulation monitor
biotransformation
BioZ system
biparietal
    b. bossing
    b. diameter (BPD)
    b. lesion
    b. plane
    b. suture
biparietotemporal hypometabolism
bipartite
    b. fracture
    b. patella
    b. sesamoid bone
    b. uterus
bipartition
    facial b.
bipedal lymphangiography
bipediculate approach
bipennate muscle
bipenniform muscle of hand
biperforate
biphasic
    b. acquisition
    b. blastoma
    b. breast tumor
    b. contrast-enhanced helical CT
    b. curve
    b. helical CT scan
    b. injection protocol
    b. magnetic resonance
biplanar
    b. aortography
    b. cineventriculography
    b. MR imaging guidance
    b. transducer
biplane
    b. angiocardiography
    b. angiographic system
    b. angiography
    b. axial film
    b. cineangiography
    b. cinefluorography
    b. DSA unit
    b. fluoroscopy

    b. image intensifier system
    b. left ventricular angiogram
    b. orthogonal view
    b. pelvic arteriography
    b. pelvic oblique study
    b. projection
    b. quantitative coronary arteriography
    b. radiograph
    b. screening
    b. sector probe
    b. sector scanner
    b. transesophageal echocardiography
    b. ventriculogram
bipolar
    b. circumactive probe (BICAP)
    b. gradient
    b. hip replacement
    b. lead
    b. pacemaker
BIR
    British Institute of Radiology
biramous
bird
    b. breeder's lung
    b. fancier's lung
    b. handler's lung
BIRD
    bilinear rotation decoupling
bird-beak
    b.-b. configuration or narrowing
    b.-b. esophagus
    b.-b. taper at esophagogastric
      junction
birdcage
    b. coil designed for wrist imaging
    b. head coil
    b. resonator
    b. splint
bird-headed dwarfism
birdlike appearance
bird-of-prey sign
bird's-eye view
bird's-nest
    b.-n. filter
    b.-n. lesion
birefringent
birhinal phantosmia
birth canal
BIS
    bispectral index sensor
bisacodyl tannex
bisacromial diameter
bisagittal ridge
bisection
    AP malleolar b.
biseptate
bisferious pulse rhythm
bis-gadolinium-mesoporphyrine
  (bis-Gd-MP)

B

bis-Gd-MP
  bis-gadolinium-mesoporphyrine
    bis-Gd-MP imaging agent
bismuth
  b. breast shield
  b. contrast medium
  b. germanate (BGO)
  b. germanate detector
  b. injection
bispectral index sensor (BIS)
1,4-bis(5-phenyloxazol-2-yl)benzene
bisphosphonate-related osteonecrosis
bispinous diameter
bistephanic
bistratal
bit CT
bite
  b. block
  b. jumping
  b. plane
  b. sign
biteblock, bite block
  Oxyguard endoscopy b.
bitemporal diameter
bitewing
  b. film
  b. radiograph
bit-rate allocation
bituberous diameter
biVAD
  biventricular assist device
bivalve
biventricular
  b. assist device (biVAD)
  b. configuration
  b. enlargement
  b. hypertrophy
  b. origin of aorta
  b. support (BVS)
  b. transposed aorta
bizarre
  b. parosteal osteochondromatous
    proliferation
  b. subparosteal osteochondromatous
    proliferation
Björk-Shiley heart valve
BKA
  below-knee amputation
black
  b. and white
  b. blood cardiac image
  b. blood coronary arterial wall MRI
  b. blood effect
  b. blood magnetic resonance angiography
  b. blood method
  b. blood sequence
  b. blood technique
  b. blood T2-weighted
    inversion-recovery MR imaging

  b. boundary artifact
  b. box approach
  b. comet artifact
  b. echo writing
  b. epidermoid
  b. faceted stone
  b. hole
  b. lung
  b. lung disease
  b. pleural line
  b. star breast lesion
black-dot heel
Blackett-Healy method
Blackfan-Diamond syndrome
blackout map
bladder
  apex of b.
  atonic urinary b.
  b. augmentation
  automatic b.
  base of b.
  b. bed
  bilateral narrowing of urinary b.
  b. capacity
  b. carcinoma
  centrally uninhibited b.
  contracted b.
  b. contractility study
  b. contusion trauma
  b. cuff
  b. distention
  b. diverticulitis
  b. diverticulum
  b. dome
  b. dysfunction
  b. endometriosis
  b. exstrophy
  b. fistula
  b. flap hematoma
  flat-top b.
  b. floor
  b. fundus
  b. hemorrhage
  b. hernia
  hourglass b.
  hypertrophic b.
  b. hypertrophy
  hypotonic b.
  b. incarceration
  b. incontinence
  intraperitoneal rupture of b.
  kidneys, ureters, b. (KUB)
  b. laceration
  b. map
  b. neck contracture
  neck of b.
  b. neck position
  neurogenic b.
  b. outlet obstruction

bladder (*continued*)
  papilloma of b.
  pear-shaped urinary b.
  b. perforation
  b. pheochromocytoma
  refluxing spastic neurogenic b.
  b. rupture
  sensory paralytic b.
  shrunken b.
  smooth-walled b.
  b. stasis
  b. stone
  b. strangulation
  teardrop b.
  thickened b.
  transurethral resection of b.
  trigone of b.
  b. tumor
  uninhibited b.
  urinary blunt trauma b.
  uvula of b.
  b. volume
  b. wall
  b. wall calcification
  b. wall thickness
BladderManager ultrasound device
bladder-prostate rhabdomyosarcoma
BladderScan ultrasound
blade
  b. bone
  b. plate
blade-of-grass
  b.-o.-g. appearance
  b.-o.-g. osteolysis
  b.-o.-g. sign
Blake pouch
Blalock shunt
Blalock-Taussig
  B.-T. shunt
  B.-T., Waterston, Potts, and Glenn
    anastomosis
blanche
  atrophie b.
Blancophor (*var. of* Blankophor)
bland
  b. aortic aneurysm
  b. embolus
  b. infarct
  b. thrombus
Bland-Garland-White syndrome
Blankophor, Blancophor
  B. FFG, SV solution
blank scan
blank-to-trues ratio
BLAST
  broad-use linear acquisition speed-up
    technique
    k-t BLAST
blast chest

blastic
  b. infiltration
  b. lesion
  b. metastasis
  b. metastatic prostate carcinoma
  b. phase
  b. transformation
  b. variant
blastocytoma
blastoma
  biphasic b.
  cystic b.
  parenchymatous b.
  pleuropulmonary b.
  pulmonary b.
blastomycosis
BLD
  bullous lung disease
bleb
  emphysematous b.
  oval aneurysm with b.
  pulmonary b.
  ruptured emphysematous b.
  subpleural b.
Bleck metatarsus adductus classification
bleed
  anticoagulant b.
  anticoagulant-related b.
  gel b.
  GI b.
  herald b.
  intraparenchymal b.
  subcapsular b.
  technetium 99m pertechnetate GI b.
  technetium 99m sulfur colloid
    GI b.
  tumor-related spontaneous b.
bleeding
  brisk b.
  gastrointestinal b.
  hepatic b.
  b. into brain parenchyma
  intracystic b.
  intrapericardial b.
  b. lesion
  perirenal b.
  b. point
  b. polyp
  renal anticoagulant-related b.
  b. scintigraphy
  b. site
  splenic b.
  1st-trimester b.
  b. ulcer
  b. uterus
  vaginal b.
blended
  b. beam
  b. beam technique

blennorrhagic swelling
bleomycin
blepharitis
blepharoncus
Blesovsky syndrome
Blessig cyst
blind
    b. biopsy
    b. dimple
    b. enema
    b. foramen
    b. gut
    b. intestine
    b. loop syndrome
    b. percutaneous puncture of
      subclavian vein
    b. pouch syndrome
    b. sac
    b. sac epithelium
    b. segment
    b. upper esophageal pouch
blink mode
blipped echo-planar imaging
blister
    bone b.
    fracture b.
    b. of bone sign
blistering lesion
Bloch
    B. equation
    B. scale
block
    air b.
    alveolar-capillary b.
    anodal b.
    antegrade b.
    anterior fascicular b.
    AP-PA skull b.
    arborization b.
    atrioventricular b
    autonomic nerve b.
    AV Wenckebach heart b.
    bead b.
    bifascicular bundle-branch b.
    bilateral bundle-branch b. (BBBB)
    bite b.
    bone b.
    brachial plexus b.
    bundle-branch heart b.
    celiac ganglion b.
    celiac plexus b.
    Cerrobend b.
    cervical, skull, and shoulder b.
    complete atrioventricular b. (CAVB)
    complete congenital heart b.
    complete fetal heart b.
    complete heart b. (CHB)
    complex b.
    conduction b.

    congenital heart b.
    congenital symptomatic AV b.
    continuous psoas compartment b.
      (CPCB)
    CT-guided superior hypogastric
      plexus b.
    custom shielding b.
    deceleration-dependent b.
    b. detector
    divisional b.
    donor heart-lung b.
    dual lateral skull b.
    entrance b.
    exit b.
    false bundle-branch b.
    fascicular b.
    filler b.
    fixed 3rd-degree AV b.
    ganglion impar b.
    heart b.
    high-grade AV b.
    incomplete atrioventricular b. (IAVB)
    incomplete heart b.
    incomplete left bundle-branch b.
      (ILBBB)
    incomplete right bundle-branch b.
      (IRBBB)
    inflammatory heart b.
    infra-His b.
    intercostal nerve b.
    intermittent 3rd-degree AV b.
    interventricular b.
    intraatrial b.
    intra-His b.
    intrahisian b.
    intranodal b.
    intravenous b.
    intraventricular conduction b.
    intraventricular heart b.
    inverted-Y b.
    ipsilateral bundle-branch b.
    irregular b.
    left anterior fascicular b. (LAFB)
    left bundle-branch b. (LBBB)
    lumbar sympathetic b.
    mantle b.
    midline mucosa-sparing b.
    b. motor task
    mucosa-sparing b.
    multiple b.'s
    2nd-degree AV b.
    2nd-degree heart b.
    b. paradigm
    paroxysmal AV b.
    partial heart b.
    periinfarction b.
    pixel b.
    posterior fascicular b.
    pseudo-AV b.

block (*continued*)
    3rd-degree AV b.
    3rd-degree heart b.
    retrograde b.
    right bundle-branch b. (RBBB)
    S-A b.
    simple b.
    sinuatrial b. (SAB)
    sinuatrial exit b.
    sinus node exit b.
    1st-degree AV b.
    1st-degree heart b.
    stellate ganglion b.
    subarachnoid nerve b.
    subarachnoid phenol b.
    superior hypogastric plexus b.
    suprahisian b.
    sympathetic b.
    transient AV b.
    transmission b.
    trifascicular b.
    unidirectional b.
    unifascicular b.
    ventricular b.
    ventriculoatrial b.
    b. vertebra
    vesicular b.
    Wenckebach AV b.
    Wilson b.
blockade
    celiac plexus b.
    combined androgen b.
    neural b.
    sympathetic b.
blockage
    arterial b.
    bronchus b.
    pulmonary artery b.
    ventricular catheter b.
blocked
    b. artery
    b. bronchus
    b. pleurisy
    b. shunt tube
    b. vertex field
blocker
    calcium channel b.
blocker's exostosis
blocking factor
Blom-Singer tracheoesophageal fistula
blood
    b. activity-time curve
    arterialization of venous b.
    backflow of b.
    backscatter of b.
    backup of b.
    b. channel
    b. clearance half-time
    b. clot

b. clotting mechanism
deoxygenated b.
egress of b.
epidural b.
extravasated b.
b. flow
b. flow extraction fraction
b. flow imaging
b. flow measurement
b. flowmetry
b. flow pattern
b. flow redistribution
b. flow reserve
b. flow response
b. flow study
b. flow velocity
high-attenuation b.
hydrostatic pressure of b.
hyperattenuated b.
b. inflow
intracerebral b.
intraparenchymal b.
intraventricular b.
b. leak
left-to-right shunting of b.
marked shunting of b.
mixed venous b.
occult b.
b. oxygenation level-dependent
  (BOLD)
b. oxygenation level-dependent
  contrast agent
b. oxygenation level-dependent
  effect
b. oxygenation level-dependent
  functional magnetic resonance
  imaging (BOLD-fMRI)
b. oxygenation level-dependent
  magnetic resonance imaging
  (BOLD-MRI)
b. oxygenation level-dependent
  response
b. oxygen level-dependent contrast
  imaging
b. oxygen level-dependent fMRI
  method
parenchymatous b.
b. patch
b. perfusion
b. perfusion monitor (BPM)
peripheral b.
periportal tracking of b.
b. plate thrombus
b. pool
b. pool activity
b. pool contrast agent
b. pool imaging
b. pool phase
b. pool radionuclide angiography

B

b. pool radionuclide
  cardioangiography
b. pool radionuclide
  echocardiography
b. pool radionuclide scan
b. pool scintigraphy
b. pressure
b. pressure response
right-to-left shunting of b.
shunted b.
b. sludge
splanchnic b.
subdural b.
upstream b.
vascular b.
venous b.
b. vessel
b. vessel invasion
b. vessel kinking
b. vessel thermography
b. vessel tumor
b. viscosity reduction
b. volume
b. volume per minute
blood-brain
  b.-b. barrier (BBB)
  b.-b. barrier disruption
blood-containment needle
blood-filled bone sponge
bloodless
  b. fluid
  b. zone of necrosis
blood-spinal cord barrier
  (BSCB)
blood-thymus barrier
blood-to-fat contrast ratio
blood-to-myocardium
  b.-t.-m. contrast of
    trueFISP
  b.-t.-m. contrast ratio
blood-tumor barrier leakage
blooming
  b. artifact
  b. focal spot
  signal b.
Bloom syndrome
Blount
  B. disease
  B. tibia vara
blow-in fracture
blowing pneumothorax
blown-out appearance
blown pupil
blow-on-blow
blowout
  aortic stump b.
  b. bone lesion
  bone lesion b.
  b. fracture

b. lesion of posterior vertebral
  element
b. view projection
BLS
  basic life support
  BLS technique
blue
  b. asbestos
  b. digit syndrome
  b. dye
  B. Max high-pressure balloon
  B. Max high-pressure reinforced
    polyethylene balloon catheter
  b. rubber-bleb nevus syndrome
  b. toe syndrome
blueberry muffin syndrome
Blumberg sign
Blumenbach
  B. clivus
  B. plane
Blumensaat anterior cruciate ligament
  line
Blumenthal lesion
Blumer rectal shelf
blunt
  b. border of lung
  b. chest trauma
  b. gastrointestinal trauma
  b. injury
  b. pancreatic trauma
  b. trauma of gallbladder
  b. trauma of kidney
blunted
  b. ejection fraction
  b. mucosal fold
  b. posterior sulcus
blunt-end sialogram needle
blunting
  calyceal b.
  costophrenic angle b.
  haustral b.
  b. of costovertebral
    angle
  b. of valve
blur
  b. artifact
  focal spot b.
  geometric b.
  image b.
  motion b.
  object-plane b.
blurred-image tomogram
blurring
  motion-related b.
  b. of aortic knob
  b. of costophrenic angle
  b. of disc margin
  radial b.
  radiographic b.

blurting
blush
 angiographic b.
 choroid plexus b.
 cortical b.
 kidney papillary b.
 marrow b.
 myocardial b.
 b. of dye on angiography
 b. on imaging
 periventricular b.
 physiologic uterine b.
 pregnancy-induced uterine b.
 renal parenchymal b.
 b. sign
 static b.
 tumor b.
 uterine b.
 vascular b.
BMC
 bone mineral content
BMD
 bone mineral density
BMI
 body mass index
BMIPP
 betamethyliodophenyl pentadecanoic acid
 BMIPP SPECT scan imaging
B-mode
 B-m. acquisition and targeting (BAT)
 B-m. brightness modulation scan
 B-m. display
 B-m. echocardiography
 B-m. echography
 B-m. imaging
 longitudinal B-m.
 pseudocolor B-m.
 B-m. ultrascan
 B-m. ultrasound
BMP
 bone marrow pressure
BMS
 bulk magnetic susceptibility
BO
 bronchiolitis obliterans
 BO field mapping
 BO field variation
Bo
 Bolton craniometric point
board
 b. angle
 immobilizer b.
 National Radiological Protection B. (NRPB)
 right-angled isosceles triangle b.
boat-shaped heart

Bochdalek
 B. foramen
 B. gap
 B. hernia
 B. muscle
body
 angularis b.
 anococcygeal b.
 apoptic b.
 asbestos b.
 asteroid b.
 b. atomic number
 Auer b.
 axis b.
 b. background activity
 b. box plethysmography
 b. burden
 calcific round b.
 calcified pineal b.
 cancer b.
 carotid b.
 caudate b.
 b. cavity
 coccygeal b.
 b. coil
 b. coil-based contrast-enchanced MRA
 b. composition measurement
 compressed b.
 b. contour orbit
 dense b.
 diffuse low-signal replacement of vertebral b.
 elementary b.
 embryoid b.
 empty vertebral b.
 enlargement of vertebral b.
 esophageal b.
 ferruginous b.
 flat vertebral b.
 foreign b.
 free b.
 geniculate b.
 glenoid labral ovoid b.
 glomus b.
 b. habitus
 H-shaped vertebral b.
 b. interface
 intraarticular loose b.
 intraluminal foreign b.
 intraocular foreign b.
 intravascular foreign b.
 juxtarestiform b.
 ketone b.
 lamellar b.
 lateral geniculate b.
 loose intraarticular b.
 Luys b.
 malpighian b.

mamillary b.
b. mass index (BMI)
Masson b.
b. mechanics
medial geniculate b.
metallic foreign b. (MFB)
Michaelis-Gutmann b.
Mott b.
multilaminar b.
navicular b.
nonradiopaque foreign b.
no-threshold b.
b. of epididymis
b. of femur
b. of gallbladder
b. of nail
b. of pancreas
b. of scapula
b. of stomach
b. of uterus
b. of vertebra
opaque foreign b.
ossified b.
osteochondral loose b.
pacchionian b.
pearly b.
pharmacoradiologic disimpaction of
  esophageal foreign b.
Pick b.
picture-frame pattern of vertebral b.
pineal b.
psammoma b.
radiopaque foreign b.
restiform b.
retained foreign b.
rhinencephalic mamillary b.
rice joint b.
Russell b.
scalloping of margin of vertebral b.
b. scanning
scapular b.
Schaumann b.
Schiller-Duval b.
b. section radiography
b. section radiography imaging
Seidelin b.
small vertebral b.
squared vertebral b.
b. stalk
b. surface area (BSA)
b. surface area calculation
b. surface laplacian mapping
  (BSLM)
b. surface potential mapping
Symington b.
threshold b.
thyroid psammoma b.
tracheobronchial foreign b.
trapezoid b.

uterine b.
Verocay b.
vesalianum of vertebral b.
b. wall
Weibel-Palade b.
b. weight
Zuckerkandl b.
body-coil
  b.-c. imaging
  b.-c. MRI
Boehler (*var. of* Böhler)
Boerhaave syndrome
boggy
  b. synovitis
  b. synovium
Bogros space
Böhler, Boehler
  B. angle
Bohr
  B. atom
  B. effect
  B. equation
  B. magneton
  B. radius
  B. theory
BOLD
  blood oxygenation level-dependent
    BOLD contrast functional MRI
    BOLD contrast imaging
    BOLD effect
    BOLD response
    BOLD signal
    BOLD technique
    BOLD time course change
BOLD-fMRI
  blood oxygenation level-dependent
    functional magnetic resonance
    imaging
BOLD-MRI
  blood oxygenation level-dependent
    magnetic resonance imaging
bolster
  angular b.
  breast b.
  b. finger
  knee arthrography b.
Bolton
  B. craniometric point (Bo)
  B. nasion
  B. nasion line
  B. nasion plane
  B. triangle
Boltzmann
  B. distribution
  B. equation
bolus
  air b.
  b. arrival time (BAT)
  barium b.

bolus (*continued*)
CARE b.
b. challenge imaging
b. challenge test
b. chase
contrast b.
b. contrast enhancement
b. dose
dynamic b.
electron b.
intravenous b.
b. intravenous injection
liquid b.
marshmallow b.
b. passage perfusion measurement
B. Pro Ultra
radioactive b.
saline chaser b.
simple b.
special b.
b. tagging
test b.
b. timing
tracer b.
b. tracking
b. transit
b. triggering technique
water b.

bolus-chase
b.-c. image
b.-c. imaging technique
b.-c. stepping-table 3D MRA

bomb
Teflon b.

bombard

bombardment
alpha-particle b.
end of saturated b. (EOSB)
neutron b.

bond
technetium b.
valence b.
wedge b.

bone
b. abscess
accessory multangular b.
accessory navicular b.
accessory sesamoid b.
acetabular b.
acromial b.
adamantinoma of long b.
b. age
b. age imaging
b. age ratio
alar b.
Albrecht b.
b. allograft
alveolar supporting b.
b. and limb growth velocity ratio

b. aneurysmal cyst
b. angioblastoma
b. angiosarcoma
ankle b.
anvil b.
apex of petrous portion of temporal b.
architectural alteration of b.
arch of b.
areola of b.
articular lamella of b.
articular tubercle of temporal b.
astragalar b.
astragalocalcanean b.
astragalocrural b.
astragaloscaphoid b.
astragalotibial b.
astragalus b.
b. atrophy
attic temporal b.
autogenous b.
basal b.
basilar part of occipital b.
basioccipital b.
basisphenoid b.
bicortical iliac b.
bipartite sesamoid b.
blade b.
b. blister
b. block
bowed long b.
breast b.
bregmatic b.
brittle b.
b. bruise sign
bundle b.
calcaneal b.
calvarial b.
b. canaliculus
cancellated b.
candle-wax appearance of b.
cannon b.
b. capillary hemangioma
capitate b.
b. carcinoma
carpal navicular b.
cartilage b.
cavalry b.
b. cement
b. center
central b.
chalky b.
cheek b.
chevron b.
b. chip
b. chloroma
b. coccidioidomycosis
coccygeal b.
coccyx b.

coffin b.
compact b.
b. computed tomography
condylar part of occipital b.
continuity of b.
b. contusion
convoluted b.
b. core
h. cortex
cortical b.
corticocancellous b.
costal b.
coxal b.
cranial b.
craniofacial b.
cribriform b.
b. crisis
cubital b.
cuboid b.
cuneiform b.
dancer's b.
dead b.
b. debris
b. demineralization
dense structure of b.
b. densitometer
b. densitometry
b. density imaging
b. density measurement
b. density study
depression of nasal b.
dermal b.
detecting Down syndrome by
  ultrasound of nose b.
devitalized allogeneic b.
devitalized portion of b.
diastasis of cranial b.
dimple of b.
displaced fragment of b.
dorsal talonavicular b.
b. dysplasia
b. dystrophy
eburnated b.
b. echinococcosis
b. end
endochondral b.
entrapped plantar sesamoid b.
epactal b.
epihyal b.
epihyoid b.
epiphysis b.
epipteric b.
episternal b.
erosion of epiphysial b.
ethmoid b.
exoccipital part of occipital b.
facial b.
femoral b.
fencer's b.

b. fibrosarcoma
fibular sesamoid b.
b. fixation device
b. fixation plate
flank b.
b. flap
flat b.
b. formation
b. formation cloaca
b. fracture
fracture running length of b.
b. fragment
frontal b.
Goethe b.
gracile b.
b. graft
greater multangular b.
great toe sesamoid b.
growth center of b.
b. growth stimulator
hallux sesamoid b.
hamate b.
b. hardening
heel b.
heterotopic b.
hip b.
b. histology
b. histomorphometry
hollow b.
hooked b.
humeral b.
hyoid b.
hyperplastic b.
b. hypertrophy
iliac cancellous b.
immature b.
b. implant
b. implantation cyst
incisive b.
incomplete fracture of b.
incus b.
b. infarct
infected b.
inferior turbinate b.
inflammation of b.
b. ingrowth
b. injury radiation
inner table of frontal b.
innominate b.
intermaxillary b.
intermediate cuneiform b.
interparietal b.
b. interstitium
intracartilaginous b.
intrachondral b.
intramembranous b.
irregular b.
ischial b.
b. island

bone (*continued*)
jaw b.
knuckle b.
lacrimal b.
b. lacuna
lamellar b.
lateral part of occipital b.
lateral sesamoid b.
b. length imaging
b. length study
lenticular b.
lentiform b.
b. lesion apophysis
b. lesion blowout
b. lesion epiphysis
b. lesion of rib
lingual b.
b. lipoma
long b.
long axis of b.
lunate b.
lunocapitate b.
luxated b.
b. lymphoma
malar b.
malignant fibrous histiocytoma of b. (MFH-B)
malleolus b.
marble b.
b. marrow
b. marrow agent
b. marrow biopsy
b. marrow boundary
b. marrow conversion
b. marrow depression
b. marrow dose
b. marrow edema
b. marrow edema pattern on MR imaging
b. marrow edema syndrome
b. marrow embolus
b. marrow expansion
b. marrow fibrosis
b. marrow hypoplasia
b. marrow infiltrate
b. marrow lesion
b. marrow lymphoid hyperplasia
b. marrow metastasis
b. marrow microenvironment
b. marrow myeloid precursor
b. marrow pressure (BMP)
b. marrow purging
b. marrow reconversion
b. marrow relapse
b. marrow rescue
b. marrow scan
b. marrow scintigraphy
b. marrow stroma
b. marrow toxicity

b. marrow transplant
b. mastocytosis
mastoid b.
b. maturation
mature b.
maxillary b.
medial cuneiform b.
medial sesamoid b.
medullary b.
membrane of b.
mesocuneiform b.
metacarpal b.
metatarsal b.
b. microarchitecture
middle cuneiform b.
middle turbinate b.
b. mineral content (BMC)
b. mineral content imaging
b. mineral content study
b. mineral density (BMD)
b. mineral immobilization
b. mineralization
morcellized b.
b. morphogenetic activity
mortise of b.
multangular b.
nasal b.
navicular b.
2nd cuneiform b.
b. neck
necrotic b.
b. neoplasia
Nicoll b.
occipital b.
odontoid b.
omovertebral b.
orbicular b.
orbital b.
orbitosphenoid b.
os calcis b.
osteonal b.
osteopenic b.
osteoporosis of b.
osteoporotic b.
b. overdevelopment
b. oxalosis
Paget disease of b.
pagetoid b.
palatine b.
parietal b.
b. particle
pedal b.
pelvic b.
perichondral b.
periosteal b.
periotic b.
peroneal b.
petrosal b.
petrous temporal b.

phalangeal b.
phantom b.
b. phase image
b. phase imaging
b. pinhole
Pirie b.
pisiform b.
b. plug
pneumatic b.
pole of scaphoid b.
porous b.
postsphenoid b.
posttraumatic atrophy of b.
postulnar b.
b. powder
preinterparietal b.
premaxillary b.
presphenoid b.
primary non-Hodgkin lymphoma of b.
primitive b.
proliferation of b.
prominence of b.
pterygoid b.
pubic b.
b. pulley
pyramidal b.
quadrilateral b.
b. quantitative CT (BQCT)
radial b.
b. radiation absorption
Recklinghausen disease of b.
refractured b.
b. remodeling
replacement b.
b. resorption
reticulated b.
rider's b.
ring of b.
rudimentary b.
sacral b.
b. sarcoidosis
b. scan
scaphoid b.
scapular b.
b. scintiscan imaging
sclerosed temporal b.
b. screw
scroll b.
b. seeker
semilunar b.
septal b.
sesamoid b.
b. shaft
shank b.
shin b.
short b.
sieve b.
b. sliver
solid b.

sphenoid b.
sphenoid turbinate b.
splintered b.
spoke b.
spongy b.
b. spur
squamous part of frontal b.
squamous part of occipital b.
squamous part of temporal b.
1st cuneiform b.
stirrup b.
b. strut
subchondral b.
subperiosteal new b.
b. substance
b. substitute
superior turbinate b.
supernumerary sesamoid b.
supracollicular spike of cortical b.
suprainterparietal b.
supraoccipital b.
suprapharyngeal b.
suprasternal b.
supreme turbinate b.
b. surface
b. survey
sutural b.
b. syphilis
tail b.
talus b.
target b.
tarsal b.
temporal b.
thick b.
thoracic b.
4th turbinate b.
tibia b.
tibial sesamoid b.
trabecular b.
trabeculated b.
trapezium b.
trapezoid b.
triangular b.
triquetral b.
b. tuberculosis
tuberculous b.
tubular b.
b. tumor
b. tumor aggressiveness
tumor-bearing b.
b. tumor matrix
b. tumor scalloping
turbinate b.
b. turnover
tympanic b.
ulnar sesamoid b.
unciform b.
b. unloading
upper jaw b.

bone (*continued*)
  vascular b.
  vesalianum b.
  vomer b.
  weightbearing b.
  b. window
  wing of sphenoid b.
  wormian b.
  woven b.
  wrist triquetrum b.
  b. xanthogranuloma
  xiphoid b.
  zygomatic b.
bone-air interface
bone-chip allograft
bone-forming
  b.-f. bone tumor
  b.-f. neoplasm
  b.-f. sarcoma
bone-hardening artifact
bone-implant interface
bone-in-bone sign
bonelet
bone-on-bone contact
bone-seeking agent
bone-tendon-bone graft
bone-tendon exposure
bone-to-bone apposition
bone-within-bone
  b.-w.-b. appearance
  b.-w.-b. vertebra
Bonferroni adjustment
bonnet
  gluteal b.
Bonopty needle system
bony
  b. abnormality
  b. alignment
  b. ankylosis
  b. apposition
  b. architecture
  b. bar
  b. bridge
  b. callus
  b. callus formation
  b. change
  b. coalition
  b. contusion
  b. cortex interruption
  b. decompression
  b. defect
  b. deformity
  b. degeneration
  b. deposit
  b. destruction
  b. disruption
  b. eburnation
  b. encroachment
  b. enlargement

  b. erosion
  b. excrescence
  b. exostosis
  b. fossa
  b. fusion
  b. glenoid marrow fat
  b. glenoid rim
  b. healing
  b. heart
  b. humeral avulsion
  b. hyperostosis
  b. island
  b. labyrinth
  b. lysis
  b. necrosis
  b. nonunion
  b. orbit
  b. osteophyte
  b. overgrowth
  b. pelvis
  b. plate
  b. process
  b. projection from vertebra
  b. proliferation
  b. prominence
  b. protuberance
  b. rarefaction
  b. remodeling
  b. resorption
  b. ridge
  b. sclerosis
  b. semicircular canal
  b. sequestrum
  b. shadow
  b. skeleton
  b. skull landmark
  b. spicule
  b. spurring
  b. stability
  b. structure
  b. suture
  b. thoracic cage
  b. thorax
  b. tissue
  b. trabecula
  b. trabecular injury
  b. trabecular pattern
  b. tuft of finger
  b. union
  b. vertebra projection
boomerang tendon
BOOP
  bronchiolitis obliterans with organizing
   pneumonia
Boorman classification of gastric
 carcinoma
boost
  brachytherapy b.
  b. dose

electron beam b.
GK-SRS b.
interstitial b.
b. therapy
booster heart
boot-shaped heart
boot-top fracture
border
anterior b.
antimesenteric b.
cardiac b.
ciliated b.
corticated b.
crescentic b.
b. detection method (BDM)
diaphragmatic b.
echocardiographic automated b.
gradually tapering b.
heart b.
inferior b.
interosseous b.
irregular b.
lateral b.
left sternal b.
lobulated b.
lower sternal b.
medial b.
mediastinal b.
mesenteric b.
mid left sternal b.
overhanging b.
peripheral b.
posterior b.
rounded convex b.
scalloped b.
scapulovertebral b.
sclerotic b.
serpiginous low signal-intensity b.
shagging of cardiac b.
shaggy heart b.
smooth b.
spicular b.
sternal b.
sternocleidomastoid muscle b.
straight anterior vertebral b.
superior b.
tapering b.
thin b.
upper sternal b.
well-defined b.
b. zone
borderline
b. cardiomegaly
b. heart size
b. malignancy
b. normal
Borell and Fernström method
Borg scale of treadmill
 exertion

Born
B. approximation
B. method
boron
b. counter
b. neutron capture
Borrelia buregdorferi
BOS
base of skull
Bosniak renal cystic disease classification
BOSS
BimOdal Slice Select
boss
carpal b.
parietal b.
bosselated
b. stone
b. surface
bosselation
bossing
biparietal b.
frontal b.
occipital b.
Bosworth
B. bone peg insertion
B. fracture
Botallo
B. duct
B. foramen
B. ligament
pervious duct of B.
both-bone fracture
both-column fracture
botryoid
b. rhabdomyosarcoma
b. sarcoma
Böttcher canal
Bouchard
B. disease
B. node
bougienage technique
Bouillaud disease
bounce-point artifact
bouncing
ligamentous b.
bound
Cramer-Rao minimum variance b.
 (CR-MVB)
b. electron
boundary
air-bone-tissue b.
bone marrow b.
b. edge
horizontal b.
b. layer
tumor b.
bouquet
fixed-shaped coplanar or nonplanar
 radiation beam b.

B

Bourgery ligament
Bourneville disease
Bourneville-Pringle disease
Boutin thoracoscope
bouton
    axonal b.
boutonnière
    b. deformity
    b. deformity sign
    b. dislocation
Bouveret syndrome
Bovero muscle
bovine heart xenograft
bovinum
    cor b.
Bowditch effect
bowed
    b. leg
    b. long bone
    b. micromelia
bowel
    aganglionic b.
    amyloidosis of small b.
    b. and bladder dysfunction
    apple-peel b.
    b. atresia
    b. axis
    b. caliber
    b. carcinoma
    b. contents
    b. continuity
    corkscrew appearance of small b.
    dead b.
    dilated dry small b.
    dilated fetal b.
    dilated loop of b.
    dilated wet small b.
    distal small b.
    b. distention
    echogenic fetal b.
    fixed segment of b.
    fluid-filled loop of b.
    free-floating loop of b.
    functional immaturity of b.
    b. gangrene
    b. gas
    b. gas artifact
    b. gas pattern
    herniated b.
    hoop-shaped loop of b.
    b. incontinence
    b. infarct
    b. intussusception
    ischemic b.
    kinked b.
    large b.
    b. loop
    b. loop air
    b. loop angulation

    b. loop dilation
    b. loop fixation
    b. lumen
    b. migration
    b. motion
    b. movement
    b. mucosa
    multiple loops of small b.
    multiple stenotic lesions of small b.
    b. necrosis
    normal-caliber b.
    b. obstruction
    b. perforation
    b. peristalsis
    pleating of small b.
    b. preparation
    proximal small b.
    b. pseudoobstruction
    ribbon b.
    b. secretion
    b. serosal endometrial implant
    shaggy contour to b.
    b. shock
    small b.
    small b.
    b. sounds
    b. spasm
    b. stenosis
    b. stoma
    strangulated small b.
    b. strangulation
    b. wall
    b. wall hematoma
    b. wall penetration
bowel-to-bowel anastomosis
bowing
    anterior tibial b.
    b. deformity
    b. fracture
    b. of mitral valve leaflet
    b. of tendon
bow-leg (*var. of* bowleg)
bowleg, bow-leg
bowler hat sign
bowler's thumb
Bowman
    B. capsule
    B. disc
    B. muscle
    B. probe
    B. space
bowstring
    b. sign
    b. tear
bowstringing
bow-tie sign
box
    carpal b.
    ligamentous b.

mammographic view b.
pacing b.
shadow b.
view b.
virtual reality view b.
box-and-whisker plot
boxer's
b. elbow
b. fracture
b. knuckle
boxlike cardiomegaly
Boyd
B. and Griffin subtrochanteric proximal femur fracture classification (I-IV)
B. ankle amputation
B. formula
B. perforating vein
B. type I-IV fracture
Boyden
B. sphincter
B. test meal
Bozzolo sign
BP
bronchopleural
bronchopulmonary
BP fistula
Imagent BP
BP MR
BPD
biparietal diameter
bronchopulmonary dysplasia
BPFM
bronchopulmonary foregut malformation
BPH
benign prostatic hyperplasia
benign prostatic hypertrophy
BPM
blood perfusion monitor
BPS
biophysical profile score
fetal BPS
Bq
becquerel
BQCT
bone quantitative CT
Bracco A-C-D solution
brace artifact
bracelet
^{89}Sr b. (Sr-89)
brachia (*pl. of* brachium)
brachial
b. angiography
b. arteriography
b. artery
b. artery approach
b. artery compression
b. artery cuff pressure

b. artery end-diastolic pressure
b. artery peak systolic pressure
b. artery pulse pressure
b. atrophy
b. fascia
b. lymph node
b. plexopathy
b. plexus
b. plexus birth injury
b. plexus block
b. plexus compression
b. plexus infiltrate
b. plexus neuritis
b. plexus tendon
b. pulse
b. vein
brachial-basilar insufficiency
brachialis tendon
brachii
triceps b.
brachiocephalic
b. arterial aneurysm
b. arteriography
b. artery
b. artery stenting
b. artery thrombolysis
b. branch
b. ischemia
b. lymph node
b. stent
b. trunk
b. trunk of aorta
b. vein
b. vessel
brachiocephaly
brachiocubital
brachioradialis
b. muscle
b. tendon
brachium, *pl.* **brachia**
b. conjunctivum
b. of colliculus
b. pontis
Bracht-Wachter lesion
brachycephalia (*var. of* brachycephaly)
brachycephalic head shape
brachycephalism (*var. of* brachycephaly)
brachycephaly, brachycephalia, brachycephalism
brachydactylia (*var. of* brachydactyly)
brachydactyly, brachydactylia
Bell b.
Christian b.
Mohn-Wriedt b.
brachymetatarsia
brachypellic pelvis
BrachySeed PD-103 implant
brachytelephalangic type of cystic fibrosis

brachytherapy
> afterloading b.
> b. boost
> endovascular b.
> episcleral plaque b.
> high dose-rate b.
> b. implant removal
> interstitial b.
> intracavitary application b.
> intraluminal b.
> IOHDR b.
> permanent b.
> remote afterloading b. (RAB)
> stereotactic b.
> Ultraseed b.
> vascular b.

bracing
> fracture b.

bradycinesia (*var. of* bradykinesia)
bradykinesia, bradycinesia
bradyphemic
bradyphrenia
Bragard sign
Bragg
> B. curve
> B. equation
> B. ionization peak
> B. law
> B. peak radiosurgery
> B. spectrometer
> B. x-ray angle

Bragg-Gray cavity
braided diagnostic catheter
brain
> b. abscess
> b. activation study
> b. activity
> b. anatomy classification
> b. aneurysm
> b. anoxia
> b. architecture
> b. atlas for functional imaging
> atrial diverticulum of b.
> b. atrophy
> basal cistern of b.
> base of b.
> b. bridging vein
> Broca motor speech area of b.
> buckling cortical b.
> b. calcification hemangioma
> b. candle dripping
> b. capillary angiography
> b. carcinoma
> b. cavernoma
> b. concussion
> b. contusion
> b. convexity
> b. cyst
> b. death

> b. degeneration
> b. diffusion anisotropy
> dura mater of b.
> b. dysfunction
> b. dysgerminoma
> b. edema
> edematous b.
> b. electrical activity mapping (BEAM)
> eloquent area of b.
> b. empyema
> b. ependymoma
> b. fiber tracking
> b. fissure
> b. function
> b. geography
> b. Glx-Cr ratio
> b. hamartoma
> b. hematoma
> herniation of b.
> b. homeostasis
> horseshoe configuration of b.
> B. Imaging Council of the Society of Nuclear Medicine
> b. imaging radiopharmaceutical
> b. incidentaloma
> b. infarct
> b. infection
> inflammation of b.
> insular region of b.
> b. iron
> b. ischemia
> b. laceration
> left b.
> b. lesion
> b. lipoma
> b. lymphoma
> b. mantle
> b. mass
> b. mass in jugular foramen
> meninx of b.
> b. metastasis
> b. paragonimiasis
> b. parenchyma
> b. perfusion
> b. perfusion reserve
> b. perfusion scintigraphy
> b. perfusion SPECT
> b. plasticity
> b. proton magnetic resonance spectroscopy
> quantitative proton MR of neonatal b.
> b. region vesicle
> right b.
> sagging b.
> b. scan
> b. scan imaging
> b. shrinkage

silent area of b.
smooth b.
softening of b.
split b.
b. stem
b. stenosis hemorrhage
b. structure
b. substance
b. surface matching technique
b. swelling
b. tissue herniation
b. trauma
b. tuber
b. tuberculoma
b. tumor
b. tumor at cerebellopontine angle
b. tumor classification
b. tumor vasculature
unicameral b.
Virchow-Robin space of b.
b. volume
B. Voyager
b. warping
b. water content
water on b.
watershed zone in b.
wet b.
b. window
brain-blood barrier
brain-computer interface (BCI)
brain-core gradient
brain-infective lesion
**BrainLAB VectorVision neuronavigation
  system**
Brain-Map
brainstem, brain stem
b. compression
b. demyelination
b. displacement
b. edema
b. encephalitis
b. ependymoma
b. glioma
b. hemorrhage
b. infarct
b. ischemia
b. lesion
b. multiple sclerosis
b. primary injury
b. pyramidal tract
b. reticular formation
reticular formation of b.
b. secondary injury
tegmentum of b.
brain-to-background ratio
BrainVoyager interactive software
braking radiation
branch
acute marginal b.

anterior cutaneous b.
arterial b.
atrioventricular groove b.
bifid aortic b.
bifurcating b.
brachiocephalic b.
bronchial b.
bronchus b.
cardiac b.
caudal b.
circumflex b.
collateral b.
cortical b.
cutaneous lateral b.
b. decay
diagonal b.
digital b.
distal b.
dorsal b.
b. duct
feeding b.
geniculate b.
inferior cardiac b.
inferior wall b.
intrahepatic portal vein b.
large obtuse marginal b.
left bundle b.
marginal b.
mid marginal b.
motor b.
muscular b.
musculophrenic b.
2nd diagonal b.
nonlingular b.
obtuse marginal b. (OMB)
b. of artery
b. of vein
paired parietal b.'s
paired visceral b.'s
pancreatic duct b.
perforating b.
phalangeal b.
b. point
posterior descending b.
posterior intercostal b.
posterior ventricular b.
premammillary b.
proper digital nerve b.
pruning of pancreatic duct b.
pudendal b.
b. pulmonary artery stenosis
ramus intermedius artery b.
ramus medialis artery b.
right bundle b.
segmental renal artery b.
septal perforating b.
side b.
sinuatrial b.
1st major diagonal b.

branch (*continued*)
　1st septal perforator b.
　subcostal b.
　subsegmental renal artery b.
　sulcocommissural b.
　superior phrenic b.
　thalamoperforating b.
　unpaired parietal b.
　unpaired visceral b.
　ventral b.
　ventricular b.
branched
　b. calculus
　b. chain
branchial
　b. cartilage
　b. cleft cyst
　b. cleft development
　b. duct
　b. efferent column
　b. fistula
　b. pouch
　b. sinus
branching
　anomalous b.
　b. calcification
　b. centrilobar opacity
　b. decay
　b. fraction
　b. line
　b. linear structure
　mirror-image brachiocephalic b.
　b. pattern
　b. ratio
　right aortic arch with mirror-image b.
　b. tubular structure
Brasdor method
Brasfield scoring system
Braun
　B. canal
　B. tumor
Braune muscle
Braunwald-Cutter valve
Braunwald sign
BRCA1 gene
BRCA2 gene
bread-and-butter
　b.-a.-b. heart
　b.-a.-b. pericarditis
bread loaf technique
breadth
　photopeak b.
breakdown
　BBB b.
breakpoint
　b. cluster region negative
　b. cluster region positive
breakthrough
　normal perfusion pressure b.

　b. vasodilation
　b. visualization
breast
　b. abscess
　accessory b.
　adenoma of b.
　b. adenosarcoma
　b. adenosis
　b. anatomy
　b. angiosarcoma
　architectural disorder of b.
　b. artifact
　atrophic b.
　b. attenuation
　augmented b.
　b. biopsy
　b. bolster
　b. bone
　b. cancer risk factor
　b. cancer screening
　B. Cancer System 2100
　b. carcinoma
　central solitary papilloma b.
　b. coil
　compression of b.
　b. cup opening
　b. cyst
　b. cyst aspiration
　cystic disease of b.
　b. degeneration
　dense b.
　ductography of b.
　dysplastic b.
　b. edema
　b. embryology
　fascia of b.
　b. fat necrosis
　b. fibroadenolipoma
　b. fibroadenoma
　b. fibroadenomatosis
　fibrocystic b.
　b. fibrosis
　b. hamartoma
　b. hematoma
　b. hyperplasia
　B. Imaging Reporting and Data System
　b. intensity-modulated radiation therapy
　b. irradiation
　b. lesion
　b. lipofibroadenoma
　b. lipoma
　b. lobule
　b. localizer
　b. lymphoma
　b. mammographic technique
　b. metastasis
　b. microcalcification

Miraluma nuclear scan of b.
b. mucocele
b. neoplasia
occult lesion of b.
b. papilloma
b. parenchyma
b. phyllode tumor
b. pneumocystography
b. popcorn calcification
prepubertal female b.
b. prosthesis attenuation pitfall
b. prosthesis rupture
b. pseudolymphoma
radiographic-dense b.
round cancer of b.
b. sarcoidosis
b. sarcoma
b. shadow
shoemaker's b.
b. skin thickening
b. sonography
stromal pattern of b.
tail of b.
b. thrombophlebitis
b. tissue
b. tissue displacement
b. traction
b. trigger point
b. ultrasound
varicocele tumor of b.
breast-conservation treatment
breast-conserving therapy
breast-preserving surgery
BreastScan IR system
breaststroker's knee
breath-hold
b.-h. cine-MR
b.-h. contrast-enhanced 3-dimensional
MR angiography
b.-h. contrast-enhanced MRI
b.-h. cycle
deep inspiratory b.-h. (DIBrH)
b.-h. fast-recovery fast-SE pulse
sequence
b.-h. fast spin-echo image
b.-h. fat saturation sequence
b.-h. gradient-recalled echo sequence
b.-h. MR cholangiography
b.-h. MRCP
b.-h. scanning
b.-h. segmented k-space
gradient-echo imaging
single b.-h.
b.-h. technique
b.-h. turbo spin echo
b.-h. T1-weighted gradient-echo
imaging
b.-h. T1-weighted MP-GRE MR
imaging

b.-h. ungated imaging
b.-h. velocity-encoded cine-MR
imaging
breathing
b. artifact
b. feedback
free b.
tidal b.
breath pentane measurement
breech presentation
breeder reactor
bregma
bregmatic
b. bone
b. fontanelle
bregmatolambdoid arc
bregmatomastoid suture
Bremer
B. AirFlo vest
B. halo crown system
bremsstrahlung
b. process
b. radiation
b. scan
Brenner tumor
Breschet canal
Brescia-Cimino
B.-C. fistula
B.-C. graft
Breslow melanoma thickness classification
Brett sun
Breuerton view of hand
breve
vinculum b.
Brevi-Kath epidural catheter
brevis
abductor pollicis b. (APB)
coxa b.
extensor carpi radialis b. (ECRB)
extensor digitorum b. (EDB)
extensor pollicis b. (EPB)
flexor digiti minimi b.
flexor digiti quinti b. (FDQB)
flexor digitorum b.
flexor hallucis b.
flexor pollicis b.
palmaris b.
split peroneus b.
b. tendon
bridge
arteriolovenular b.
b. autograft
bony b.
b. circuit
interthalamic b.
intraductal b.
loop ostomy b.
mucosal b.
muscular b.

bridge (*continued*)
    myocardial b.
    nasal b.
    osseous b.
    osteophytic b.
    portal-to-portal b.
    skin b.
    transphysial bone b.
    ventral b.
    Wheatstone b.
bridged loop-gap resonator
bridging
    b. callus
    b. defect
    b. necrosis
    b. osteophyte
    physial bony b.
bright
    b. contrast enhancement
    b. cystic focus
    b. echo
    b. fatty marrow
    b. layer
    b. pixel value
    b. signal
    b. signal intensity
    b. signal intensity tumor
bright-blood imaging
bright-field imaging
brightly
    b. echogenic focus
    b. increased renal parenchymal
      echogenicity
brightness
    b. area product (BAP)
    b. gain
    b. mode
    b. modulation
    b. modulation scan
brightness-time curve
brilliance
    B. 109 MP PC monitor
    B. 40 scanner
brim
    b. of pelvis
    pelvic b.
    quadrilateral b.
    b. sign
brimstone liver
brisement therapy
brisk
    b. bleeding
    b. wall motion
Brissaud syndrome
BriteSmile laser
Brite Tip guiding catheter
British
    B. Engineering System
    B. Institute of Radiology (BIR)

    B. Standard (BS)
    B. thermal unit (BTU)
brittle
    b. bone
    b. bone disease (BBD)
broad
    b. beam
    b. fascia
    b. ligament
    b. ligament hernia
    b. ligament pregnancy
    b. maxillary ridge
broadband
    b. noise detection error artifact
    b. transducer
broad-based
    b.-b. disc protrusion
    b.-b. polyp
broad-beam
    b.-b. absorption
    b.-b. scattering
Broadbent-Bolton plane
broadening
    dipolar b.
    quadripolar signal b.
    spectral b.
broad-use linear acquisition speed-up technique (BLAST)
Broca
    B. area
    band of B.
    B. convolution
    B. diagonal band
    B. gyrus
    B. index
    B. motor speech area of brain
    B. pudendal pouch
    B. region
Brockenbrough needle
Brödel bloodless line of incision
Broden
    B. position
    B. subtalar joint (I-II) view
Broders tumor index classification
Brodie
    B. bursa
    B. disease
    B. knee
    B. ligament
    B. metaphysial abscess
Brodmann
    B. area
    B. cytoarchitectonic field
broken bough pattern
bromide
    perfluorooctyl b. (PFOB)
brominated oil
bromine-76 bromospirone
brominized oil contrast medium

bromodeoxyuridine
    b. imaging agent
    b. labeling index
5-bromodeoxyuridine analysis
**bromophenol blue imaging
  agent**
bromospirone
    bromine-76 b.
bronchi (*pl. of* bronchus)
bronchia (*pl. of* bronchium)
bronchial
    b. adenoma
    b. angiography
    b. anular cartilage
    b. arteriography
    b. artery
    b. artery embolization (BAE)
    b. atresia
    b. branch
    b. bud
    b. calculus
    b. caliber
    b. carcinoid tumor
    b. carcinoma
    b. cleft cyst
    b. collateral circulation
    b. cuff sign
    b. dehiscence
    b. diameter
    b. dilation
    b. distortion
    b. embolotherapy
    b. erosion
    b. fracture
    b. groove
    b. inflammation
    b. kinking
    b. lumen
    b. mucocele
    b. mucosa
    b. obstruction
    b. polyp
    b. provocation imaging
    b. provocation testing
    b. reactivity
    b. rupture
    b. septum
    b. sinus
    b. smooth muscle spasm
    b. spur
    b. stenosis
    b. stenting
    b. stricture
    b. tract
    b. tree
    b. tube
    b. vein
    b. vessel
    b. wall thickening

bronchiectasis
    acquired b.
    capillary b.
    central b.
    congenital b.
    cylindrical b.
    cystic b.
    distal b.
    dry b.
    follicular b.
    fusiform b.
    Polynesian b.
    postinfectious b.
    recurrent b.
    reversible b.
    saccular b.
    traction b.
    tuberculous b.
    tubular b.
    varicose b.
bronchiectasis-ethmoid sinusitis
bronchiectatic
    b. airway
    b. cyst
    b. pattern
bronchiolar
    b. adenocarcinoma
    b. carcinoma
    b. dilation
    b. edema
    b. emphysema
    b. narrowing
    b. obstruction
bronchiole
    alveolar b.
    conducting b.
    irreversible narrowing of b.
    lobular b.
    membranous b.
    respiratory b.
    segmental b.
    terminal b.
    tree-in-bud b.
bronchiolectasia (*var. of* bronchiolectasis)
bronchiolectasis, bronchiolectasia
    traction b.
bronchioli (*pl. of* bronchiolus)
bronchiolitis
    cellular b.
    constrictive b.
    diffuse aspiration b.
    exudative b.
    b. fibrosa obliterans
    follicular b.
    b. obliterans (BO)
    b. obliterans with organizing
      pneumonia (BOOP)
    obliterative b.
    pediatric b.

B

bronchiolitis (*continued*)
  proliferative b.
  respiratory b.
  smoker's b.
  vesicular b.
bronchioloalveolar cell carcinoma
bronchiolocentric
bronchiolus, *pl.* **bronchioli**
bronchitis
  asthmatic b.
  chronic b.
  follicular b.
  irritant b.
Bronchitrac L catheter
bronchium, *pl.* **bronchia**
bronchoadenitis
bronchoalveolar
  b. carcinoma
  b. cell adenoma
  b. lavage (BAL)
bronchoarterial bundle
bronchobiliary fistula
bronchocavernous
bronchocavitary fistula
bronchocele
bronchocentric
  b. granulomatosis
  b. inflammatory infiltrate
bronchoconstriction
  exercise-induced b.
  isocapnic hyperventilation-induced
  b.
bronchoconstrictor
bronchocutaneous fistula
bronchodilatation (*var. of*
  bronchodilation)
bronchodilation, bronchodilatation
bronchodilator effect
bronchoesophageal fistula
bronchogenic
  b. adenoma
  b. carcinoma
  b. duplication cyst
bronchogram
  air b.
  bilateral b.'s
  Cope method b.
  fiberoptic b.
  fluid-filled b.
  b. imaging
  mucinous b.
  mucous b.
  scattered air b.
  Swiss cheese air b.
  tantalum b.
  unilateral b.
bronchography
  Cope-method b.
  percutaneous transtracheal b.

broncholith
broncholithiasis
bronchomalacia
bronchomediastinal lymph trunk
bronchomotor effect
bronchoplasty
  balloon b.
bronchoplegia
bronchopleural (BP)
  b. fistula
bronchopleuropneumonia
bronchopneumonia
  bibasilar b.
  hemorrhagic b.
  hypostatic b.
  inhalation b.
  b. pattern
  subacute b.
  tuberculous b.
bronchopneumonitis
bronchopulmonary (BP)
  b. aspergillosis
  b. atelectasis
  b. carcinoid tumor
  b. dysplasia (BPD)
  b. fistula
  b. foregut
  b. foregut malformation (BPFM)
  b. lung segment anatomy
  b. lymph node
  b. marking
  b. neoplasia
  b. segment
  b. sequestration
bronchoradiography
bronchorrhea
bronchoscope
  Storz infant b.
bronchoscopy
  fiberoptic b. (FOB)
  virtual b. (VB)
bronchosinusitis
bronchospasm
  paradoxic b.
bronchospastic effect
bronchostaxis
bronchostenosis
bronchotracheal
bronchovascular
  b. anatomy cross-section
  b. bundle
  b. interstitium
  b. marking
  b. pattern
bronchovesicular marking
bronchus, *pl.* **bronchi**
  anomalous b.
  anterobasal b.
  apical b.

apicoposterior b.
basal segmental b.
beaded b.
b. blockage
blocked b.
b. branch
cardiac segmental b.
contracted b.
depression of left mainstem b.
dilated b.
distended central b.
ectatic b.
edematous b.
eparterial b.
extrapulmonary b.
fractured b.
granulomatous inflammation of b.
hyparterial b.
inferior lobe b.
inflamed b.
intermediate b.
b. intermedius
intrapulmonary b.
inverted-T appearance of mainstem
  b.
lateral basal segmental b.
left mainstem b.
left primary b.
lingular b.
lobar b.
mainstem b.
major b.
medial basal segmental b.
medium-sized b.
middle lobe b.
mucoid impaction of b.
nonlingular branch of upper lobe b.
normal-appearing b.
posterobasal segmental b.
primary left b.
primary right b.
principal b.
right lobe b.
right mainstem b.
right primary b.
secondary b.
secretion-filled b.
segmental b.
b. sign
b. stem
subapical b.
subsegmental b.
superior lobe b.
superior segment b.
tracheal b.

**bronchus-associated lymphoid tissue
  (BALT)**
bronchus-to-pulmonary artery ratio
bronzed sclerosing encephalitis

bronze liver
**Brooker periarticular heterotopic
  ossification classification**
Brooke tumor
Broselow-Luten pediatric system
Broviac long-term catheter
brow-down
  b.-d. position
  b.-d. projection
  b.-d. skull view
brown
  b. adipose tissue (BAT)
  b. asbestos
  b. atrophy
  b. cell cyst
  b. edema
  b. fat
  b. fat origin
  b. induration of lung
  b. tumor
  b. tumor of hyperparathyroidism
Brown-Dodge method for angiography
brownian water motion
Brown-Roberts-Wells (BRW)
  B.-R.-W. CT stereotactic guide
  B.-R.-W. frame
  B.-R.-W. stereotactic system
  B.-R.-W. technique
Brown-Séquard
  B.-S. lesion
  B.-S. syndrome
brow presentation
brow-up
  b.-u. position
  b.-u. projection
  b.-u. skull view
brucellar
  b. myositis
  b. osteomyelitis
  b. synovitis
Bruce treadmill protocol
Bruch gland
Bruck disease
Brücke muscle
Brudzinski sign
Bruel-Kjaer
  B.-K. transvaginal ultrasound probe
  B.-K. ultrasound
  B.-K. ultrasound scanner
Brugada syndrome
Brugia malayi
Bruker
  B. AMX 300 NMR spectrometer
  B. console
  B. CSI Omega MR system
  B. minispec measuring device
  B. PC-10 relaxometer
  B. scanner
  B. TC-10 relaxometer

Brunner
  B. gland
  B. gland adenoma
  B. gland hyperplasia
  B. gland hypertrophy
Brunnstrom-Fugl-Meyer (BFM)
  B.-F.-M. arm impairment
    assessment
brush
  Castaneda thrombolytic b.
  Cragg-Castaneda thrombolytic b.
  Cragg thrombolytic b.
bruxism
BRW
  Brown-Roberts-Wells
  BRW CT stereotactic guide
  BRW stereotactic system
Bryant
  B. sign
  B. triangle
BS
  British Standard
BSA
  body surface area
B-scan imaging
BSCB
  blood-spinal cord barrier
BSF
  backscatter factor
BSLM
  body surface laplacian mapping
BTU
  British thermal unit
bubble
  double b.
  encapsulated gas b.
  free gas b.
  Garren-Edwards gastric b.
  gas b.
  gastric air b.
  GEG b.
  intragastric b.
  microscopic air b.
  b. of belly
  b. oxygenator
  b. sign
  stomach b.
  b. ventriculography
bubblebreaker
bubblelike appearance
bubbling lesion
bubbly
  b. bone lesion
  b. bulb
  b. lung
  b. opacity
  b. pattern
bubonulus
bucca, *pl.* **buccae**

buccae (*pl. of* bucca)
buccal
  b. cavity
  b. groove
  b. mucosa
  b. mucosal carcinoma
  b. shelf
  b. space
  b. space infection
  b. surface
buccinator
  b. crest
  b. lymph node
buccogingival ridge
buccolingual plane
bucconeural duct
buccopharyngeal fascia
buck
  B. extension
  B. fascia
bucket-handle
  b.-h. meniscus tear
  b.-h. pattern of fracture
  b.-h. pelvic fracture
Buckland-Wright macroradiography
buckle
  b. fracture
  wire-fixation b.
buckled innominate artery
buckling
  b. cortical brain
  innominate artery b.
  white matter b.
bucky
  B. abdominal view
  chest B.
  B. diaphragm
  B. digital x-ray device
  B. film
  B. grid
  oscillating B.
  B. ray
  B. tomogram
bud
  accessory ureteral b.
  bronchial b.
  capillary b.
  dorsal pancreatic b.
  end b.
  limb b.
  ureteral b.
  vascular b.
  ventral pancreatic b.
Budd
  B. cirrhosis
  B. syndrome
Budd-Chiari syndrome
budge
  ciliospinal center of B.

budgerigar fancier's lung
Budin-Chandler anteversion determination
Budin joint
Buerger disease
buffalo
> b. chest
> b. hump
> B. malleolar rule

buffer amplifier
Buford complex
Buhl desquamative pneumonia
bulb
> aortic b.
> arterial b.
> baroreceptor b.
> baseline of b.
> bubbly b.
> carotid b.
> dehiscent jugular b.
> dental b.
> duodenal b.
> end b.
> heart b.
> high jugular b. (HJB)
> inferior jugular vein b.
> internal jugular b.
> b. of occipital horn of lateral ventricle
> b. of penis
> b. of posterior horn of lateral ventricle
> b. of vein
> olfactory b.
> penile b.
> sinovaginal b.
> superior jugular vein b.
> b. ureterography

bulbar
> b. abnormality
> b. intracerebral hemorrhage
> b. peptic ulcer
> b. ridge
> b. septum
> b. swelling
> b. tract

bulbi
> phthisis b.

bulbocavernosus muscle
bulbocavernous gland
bulbomembranous urethral rupture
bulbosity
bulbospongiosus muscle of penis
bulbourethral
> b. artery
> b. gland
> b. gland anatomy
> b. gland lesion

bulbous
> b. configuration

> b. costochondral junction
> b. enlargement
> b. stump
> b. urethra

bulbous-tip stiff malleable cannula
bulbus cordis
bulge
> anal b.
> anular disc b.
> bilateral anterior chest b.'s
> disc b.
> epiphrenic b.
> inguinal b.
> late systolic b.
> palpable presystolic b.
> parasternal b.
> precordial b.
> suprasternal b.

bulging
> b. aneurysm
> b. anulus
> b. anulus fibrosus
> b. dura
> b. fissure sign
> b. fontanelle
> b. lung fissure
> b. precordium

bulk
> b. laxative
> b. magnetic susceptibility (BMS)
> b. magnetization vector
> mediastinal b.
> muscle b.
> b. susceptibility artifact
> tumor b.

bulky tumor
bulla, *pl.* **bullae**
> emphysematous b.
> ethmoidal b.
> b. ethmoidalis
> b. formation
> pulmonary b.

bullae (*pl. of* bulla)
Bullard laryngoscope
bullectomy
bullet
> hollow-point b.
> b. kit culture medium
> metallic track of b.
> stabilizing b.
> tripoint b.

bullet-shaped vertebra
Bull method
bull-neck appearance
bullosa
> concha b.
> epidermolysis b.
> junctional epidermolysis b.

B

bullous
    b. disorder
    b. edema
    b. edema of bladder wall
    b. emphysema
    b. emphysema of intestine
    b. lung disease (BLD)
bull's-eye
    b.-e. appearance
    b.-e. configuration
    b.-e. deformity
    b.-e. image
    b.-e. imaging
    b.-e. lesion
    b.-e. polar map
    b.-e. technique
    b.-e. view
bump
    ductus b.
    hip b.
    inion b.
    runner's b.
    splenic b.
bumper fracture
bunamiodyl
bunch-of-grapes appearance
bundle
    aberrant b.
    anterior atrial myocardial b.
    artery-vein-nerve b.
    atrioventricular b.
    Bachmann b.
    b. bone
    bronchoarterial b.
    bronchovascular b.
    b. of His
    central bronchovascular b.
    common b.
    fascicular b.
    fiberoptic b.
    Flechsig b.
    b. function
    Gierke respiratory b.
    Gowers b.
    His b.
    intercostal neuromuscular b.
    James b.
    Keith sinuatrial b.
    Kent-His b.
    Mahaim b.
    main b.
    middle perforating collagen b.
    neurovascular b. (NVB)
    b. of Kent
    b. of Vicq d'Azyr
    Pick b.
    pigmented villonodular b.
    Probst b.
    Probst callosal b.

    Schultze b.
    sinuatrial b.
    Thorel b.
    vascular b.
bundle-branch
    b.-b. heart block
    b.-b. reentry (BBR)
Bunge amputation
bunion formation
bunk-bed fracture
Bunsen-type valve
Burdach
    column of B.
burden
    body b.
    coronary plaque b.
    maximum permissible body b.
    plaque b.
    radiation b.
    tumor b.
buregdorferi
    Borrelia b.
Burger scalene triangle
Burgess below-knee amputation
buried tonsil
Burke-type metaphysial dysplasia
Burkhalter-Reyes method of phalangeal
    fracture
Burkitt-like lymphoma
Burkitt lymphoma
burn
    b. boutonnière deformity
    radiation b.
    x-ray b.
burned-out
    b.-o. colon
    b.-o. mucosa
    b.-o. tabes
    b.-o. tumor
    b.-o. tumor of testis
Burnett
    B. applicator
    B. BiDirectional TMJ device
    B. cylinder
burning
    selective hole b.
burnout
    detail b.
Burns ligament
Burrow vein
bursa, *pl.* **bursae**
    Achilles b.
    adventitious b.
    anserine b.
    Brodie b.
    calcaneal b.
    coracoid b.
    deltoid b.
    b. exostotica

Fleischmann b.
flexor b.
gastrocnemius b.
gastrocnemius-semimembranosus b.
iliopsoas b.
infrapatellar b.
interligamentous b.
intermediate b.
intermetatarsophalangeal b.
intraligamentous b.
intratendinous b.
ischiogluteal b.
lateral epicondylar b.
Luschka b.
MCL b.
medial epicondylar b.
Monro b.
b. of Fabricius
olecranon b.
omental b.
b. omentalis minor
patellar b.
pes anserine b.
plantar b.
popliteus b.
premalleolar b.
prepatellar b.
radial b.
retrocalcaneal b.
semimembranosus b.
semimembranosus-tibial collateral
  ligament b.
subacromial b.
subacromial-subdeltoid b.
subdeltoid b.
subgluteus maximus b.
subgluteus medius b.
submctatarsal b.
subscapular b.
subtendinous b.
superficial tendo Achillis b.
suprapatellar b.
synovial b.
tendo Achillis b.
tibial collateral ligament b.
trochanteric b.
ulnar b.

bursae (*pl. of* bursa)
bursal
  b. calcification
  b. flap
  b. fluid
  b. inflammation
  b. osteochondromatosis
  b. sac
bursitis
  adhesive b.
  anserine b.
  bicipital b.

calcaneal b.
calcific b.
chronic retrocalcaneal b.
cubital b.
distended scapulothoracic b.
iliopsoas b.
infracalcaneal b.
intermetatarsal b.
intermetatarsophalangeal b.
intertubercular b.
ischial b.
ischiogluteal b.
olecranon b.
patellar b.
pes anserinus b.
posterior calcaneal b.
prepatellar b.
pseudotrochanteric b.
radiohumeral b.
retrocalcaneal b.
SA-SD b.
septic b.
subacromial b.
subacromial-subdeltoid septic b.
subcoracoid b.
subdeltoid b.
Tornwaldt b.
trochanteric b.
bursography
bursolith
burst
  b. fracture
  b. injury
  respiratory b.
burst-forming unit
bursting
  b. dislocation
  b. pressure
Buschke-Löwenstein tumor
buster
  Amplatz Clot B.
butanol-extractable iodine (BEI)
Butcher staging classification
butterfly
  b. appearance
  b. breast shadow
  b. coil
  b. configuration
  b. distribution
  b. effect
  b. fracture
  b. fracture fragment
  b. glioblastoma
  b. glioma
  b. lesion
  b. lymphoma
  b. pattern
  b. pattern of infiltrate
  b. vertebra

butterfly-wing vertebra
Butterworth filter
button
    aortic b.
    duodenal b.
    full-thickness Carrel b.
    Kistner tracheal b.
    patellar b.
    b. procedure
    b. sequestrum eosinophilic
      granuloma
    b. sequestrum of skull
    subdural b.
    b. toe amputation
    tracheal b.
buttoned device
buttonhole
    b. deformity
    b. fracture
    b. mitral stenosis
    b. opening
    radiopaque wire of counteroccluder
      b.
    b. rupture
    b. tear
buttressing
    medial femoral b.
buttress plate

butyl iminodiacetic acid
butyral
    polyvinyl b. (PVB)
BV2 needle
BVR
    basal vein of Rosenthal
BVS
    biventricular support
Bx Velocity stent
Byler disease
bypass
    adjunctive surgical b.
    aortoiliac b.
    biliary-enteric b.
    biliointestinal b. (BIB)
    biliopancreatic b.
    b. circuit
    extracranial-intracranial b.
    b. failure
    b. graft
    iliofemoral crossover b.
    jejunoileal b. (JIB)
byproduct material
byssinosis
bystander effect
byte mode
B-zone small lymphocytic
  lymphoma

C
carbon
coulomb
C angle
C loop
C loop of duodenum
C scan
C sign
ultraviolet A, B, C

^{11}C, C-11
carbon 11
^{11}C acetate imaging agent
^{11}C butanol imaging agent
^{11}C carbon monoxide
^{11}C carfentanil imaging agent
^{11}C deoxyglucose
^{11}C flumazenil imaging agent
^{11}C imaging agent
^{11}C L-159
^{11}C L-methylmethionine
^{11}C lumazenil
^{11}C methionine
^{11}C methoxystaurosporine
^{11}C N-methylspiperone imaging agent
^{11}C N-methylspiroperidol
^{11}C nomifensine imaging agent
^{11}C palmitate
^{11}C palmitic acid radioactive
^{11}C raclopride imaging agent
^{11}C thymidine imaging agent

^{12}C, C-12
carbon 12

^{13}C, C-13
carbon 13

^{14}C, C-14
carbon 14
^{14}C lactose breath test

C-150
C-150 LXP EBT scanner
C-150 XP scanner

Ca
calcium

^{45}Ca, Ca-45
calcium 45
^{45}Ca imaging agent

^{47}Ca, Ca-47
calcium 47

CAAS
cardiovascular angiography analysis system
CAAS QCA system

CABBS
computer-assisted blood background subtraction

CABG
coronary artery bypass graft

cable
FlexStrand c.

Cabrol composite graft procedure

CABS
coronary artery bypass surgery

CAC
coronary artery calcification

CACG
cineangiocardiogram

CACS
coronary artery calcium score
CACS threshold

CAD
computer-aided diagnosis
RapidScreen RS-2000 CAD

cadaveric renal transplant

CAD-evaluated mammogram

cadmium (Cd)
c. iodide detector

CADstream

CADx SecondLook system

caecitis (*var. of* cecitis)

Caffey
C. hyperostosis
C. syndrome

Caffey-Kempe syndrome

cage
bony thoracic c.
Faraday c.
Harms c.
metallic c.
osseocartilaginous thoracic c.
threaded fusion c. (TFC)

CAH
congenital adrenal hyperplasia

CaHA
calcium hydroxyapatite

caisson disease

Cajal
nucleus of C.

CAJSA
computer-aided joint space analysis

cake
c. kidney
omental c.

cake-glaze consistency

calamus scriptorius

calcaneal, calcanean
c. apophysis
c. apophysitis
c. articular surface
c. avulsion fracture
c. bone
c. bursa

calcaneal (*continued*)
    c. bursa inflammation
    c. bursitis
    c. displaced fracture
    c. inclination angle (CIA)
    c. pitch
    c. pitch angle
    c. process
    c. spur
    c. stress fracture
    c. tendon
    c. tubercle
    c. tuberosity
    c. tumor
calcanean (*var. of* calcaneal)
calcanei
    sulcus c.
calcaneocavus
    c. foot
    pes c.
    talipes calcaneus c.
    talipes cavus c.
calcaneoclavicular ligament
calcaneocuboid
    c. articulation
    c. joint (CCJ)
    c. ligament (CCL)
calcaneofibular ligament (CFL)
calcaneonavicular
    c. coalition
    c. ligament
calcaneoplantar angle
calcaneotibial
    c. fusion
    c. ligament
calcaneovalgocavus
calcaneovalgus
    c. flatfoot
    pes c.
calcaneovarus deformity
calcaneum (*var. of* calcaneus)
calcaneus, calcaneum
    c. altus
    c. deformity
    pes c.
    talipes c.
    tendo c.
    thalamic fracture of c.
    tongue fracture of c.
calcar
    c. avis
    c. femorale
    c. pedis
    pivot of c.
calcareous
    c. degeneration
    c. deposit
    c. infiltrate

    c. metastasis
    c. renal calculus
calcarine
    c. artery
    c. cortex
    c. fissure
    c. sulcus
calciferous canal
calcific
    c. arteriosclerosis
    c. artery
    c. bicuspid valvular stenosis
    c. bursitis
    c. cochleitis
    c. density
    c. discitis
    c. matrix
    c. myonecrosis
    c. round body
    c. senile aortic valvular stenosis
    c. shadow
    c. spur
    c. tendinitis
    c. tendinosis
calcificans
    chondrodysplasia c.
    chondroplasia c.
    liponecrosis macrocystica c.
    liponecrosis microcystica c.
calcification
    abdominal wall c.
    adenoma-associated c.
    adrenal c.
    alimentary tract c.
    aneurysmal wall c.
    anterior spinal ligament c.
    anular c.
    aortic arch c.
    aortic valve c.
    arachnoid granulation c.
    arterial c.
    arteriovascular c.
    atherosclerotic c.
    basal ganglion c.
    basketlike c.
    benign breast c.
    bladder wall c.
    branching c.
    breast popcorn c.
    bursal c.
    calcium c.
    calcium phosphate c.
    cardiac c.
    carotid artery c.
    cartilage c.
    casting breast c.
    cerebral c.
    chicken-wire c.
    choroid plexus c.

clustered c.
coarse c.
concentric c.
conglomerate c.
coronary artery c. (CAC)
costal cartilage c.
curvilinear c.
defined homogeneous c.
dentate nucleus c.
dermal breast c.
diffuse abdominal c.
diffuse stippled c.
disc c.
displaced intimal c.
dural c.
dystrophic soft tissue c.
eggshell breast c.
eggshell nodal c.
falx c.
female genital tract c.
fetal intraabdominal c.
fine c.
fingertip c.
flaky c.
flocculent focus of c.
fluffy amorphous c.
focal alimentary tract c.
focus of c.
free body c.
genital tract c.
glial tumor c.
granular c.
gyriform c.
habenular commissure c.
heart valve c.
hepatic c.
idiopathic pleural c.
inadequate calvarial c.
inadequate cranial c.
intervertebral cartilage c.
intervertebral disc c.
intraabdominal fetal c.
intracardiac c.
intracranial physiologic c.
intraductal c.
intraocular c.
intratumoral c.
involutional breast c.
inwardly displaced c.
irregular c.
isolated clustered c.'s
kidney c.
laminar c.
layering c.
ligamentous c.
c. line
linear c.
liver c.
lobular breast c.

lucent-centered c.
lung popcorn c.
lymph node eggshell c.
male genital tract c.
malignant breast c.
medial collateral ligament c.
medullary c.
meniscus-shaped c.
mesenteric c.
metastatic soft tissue c.
milk-of-calcium c.
mitral ring c.
mitral valve c.
Mönckeberg c.
mottled c.
mulberry-type c.
multiple pulmonary c.'s
myocardial c.
needle-shaped breast c.
neoplastic c.
node c.
normal c.
c. of basal ganglion
c. of myocardium
oyster-pearl breast c.
pancreatic c.
paraarticular c.
paraspinal c.
parentheses-like c.
parietal pericardial c.
pathologic intracranial c.
pearl-like breast c.
Pellegrini-Stieda c.
periarticular c.
pericardial c.
periductal c.
peritendinous c.
periventricular c.
phlebolith-like c.
pineal gland c.
plaquing c.
pleomorphic c.
pleural c.
popcorn c.
popcornlike c.
poppyseed-like c.
postbiopsy eggshell c.
postradiation c.
premature c.
prostate c.
prostatic c.
psammomatous c.
pulmonary c.
punctate c.
railroad track c.
renal c.
residual c.
retroperitoneal c.
ricelike muscle c.

C

calcification (*continued*)
    ring-and-arc c.
    ring apophysis c.
    rod-shaped c.
    scrotal c.
    sebaceous gland c.
    secondary c.
    secretory c.
    sella turcica c.
    semilunar c.
    skin c.
    snowflake-like c.
    soft tissue c.
    splenic c.
    stippled c.
    subanular c.
    suprasellar mass c.
    sutural c.
    suture c.
    target c.
    teacup breast c.
    teacup-shaped c.
    thrombus c.
    thyroid adenoma c.
    tramline cortical c.
    tram-track ductus arteriosus c.
    tram-track gyral c.
    tram-track renal cortical necrosis c.
    tumoral c.
    urinary bladder wall c.
    valvular leaflet c.
    vasa deferentia c.
    vascular abdominal c.
    venous c.
    visceral pericardial c.
    wall c.

calcified
    c. amorphous tumor
    c. anulus
    c. aorta
    c. aortic valve
    c. astrocytoma
    c. brain mass
    c. cartilage
    c. cysticercus granuloma
    c. density structure
    c. ductus arteriosus
    c. fetus
    c. fibroadenoma
    c. fibroid
    c. fibroma
    c. free fragment
    c. gallbladder
    c. intracranial mass
    c. kidney mass
    c. lesion
    c. lung nodule
    c. lymph node
    c. medullary defect

    c. myocardial tuberculoma
    c. nodularity
    c. osteoid
    c. ovarian metastasis
    c. pancreas
    c. pericardial cyst
    c. pericardium
    c. pineal body
    c. pineal gland
    c. plaque
    c. renal mass
    c. sclerosis
    c. sequestra of low signal intensity
    c. thrombus
    c. tumor
    c. wall of aneurysm

calciform lobe

calcifying
    c. Malherbe epithelioma
    c. metastasis

calcinosis
    bilateral striopallidodentate c.
    c. circumscripta
    cutis c.
    c. cutis, Raynaud phenomenon,
      esophageal motility disorder,
      sclerodactyly, and telangiectasis
      (CREST)
    generalized c.
    interstitial c.
    tumoral c.
    c. universalis

calcis
    os c.
    trigonum c.

calcium (Ca)
    c. 45 (^{45}Ca, Ca-45)
    c. 47 (^{47}Ca, Ca-47)
    c. bile soap
    c. calcification
    c. channel blocker
    c. debris
    c. hydroxyapatite (CaHA)
    c. hydroxyapatite deposition disease
    c. infiltrate
    intracardiac c.
    c. ion
    c. ipodate imaging agent
    c. layering
    liquid c.
    c. metabolism
    milk of c.
    c. phosphate calcification
    c. pyrophosphate dihydrate (CPPD)
    c. pyrophosphate dihydrate crystal
      deposition
    c. pyrophosphate dihydrate
      deposition disease
    c. pyrophosphate dihydrate hand

c. salt deposit
c. score
c. scoring
c. scoring software
sedimented c.
c. sign
c. tungstate
calcium-45 imaging agent
calcium/oxyanion-containing particle
calculated
c. clearance time
c. image
c. resistance
c. splenic index
calculation
bayesian c.
body surface area c.
Cerenkov c.
contrast-to-noise c.
gap c.
magnitude c.
Monte Carlo c.
multiplane dosage c.
radiation dosimetry c.
signal-to-noise c.
spectrophotometric c.
velocity c.
volume implant c.
calculi (*pl. of* calculus)
calculogram
calculography
calculous
c. cholecystitis
c. cirrhosis
calculus, *pl.* **calculi**
albumin c.
alternating calculi
alvine c.
articular c.
biliary c.
branched c.
bronchial c.
calcareous renal c.
cat's-eye c.
colloid c.
coral c.
cystic c.
cystine c.
decubitus c.
dendritic c.
echogenic c.
encysted c.
gallbladder c.
gastric hemic c.
gonecystic c.
hemic c.
hemp seed c.
hepatic c.
impacted c.

indigo c.
intestinal c.
intrahepatic biliary c.
joint c.
kidney c.
lacteal c.
lucent c.
lung c.
mammary c.
matrix c.
metabolic c.
mulberry c.
nephritic c.
noncalcareous renal c.
nonopaque c.
obstructive c.
opaque c.
pancreatic c.
pocketed c.
primary vesical c.
prostatic c.
radiopaque vesical c.
renal c.
salivary c.
spermatic c.
staghorn c.
Steinstrasse c.
stomach c.
stonelike c.
struvite c.
submandibular duct c.
urate c.
ureteral c.
urethral c.
uric acid c.
urinary bladder c.
urinary tract c.
urostealith c.
vesical c.
xanthic c.
Caldani ligament
Caldwell
C. method
C. occipitofrontal view
C. position
C. projection
Caldwell-Moloy classification
calf, *pl.* **calves**
c. band
c. vein thrombosis
calf-foot station
caliber
bowel c.
bronchial c.
internal c.
luminal c.
medium c.
modest c.
narrow c.

caliber (*continued*)
    normal bladder c.
    spinal cord c.
    tracheal c.
    vessel c.
    wide c.
calibrate
calibrated
    c. leak
    c. tris-acryl gelatin microsphere
calibration
    absolute peak efficiency c.
    catheter c.
    E-dial c.
    c. factor
    c. failure artifact
    film density c.
    c. method
    pixel size c.
calibrator
    accuracy c.
    digital isotope c.
    dose c.
    isotope c.
    radioisotope c.
caliceal (*var. of* calyceal)
calicectasis (*var. of* caliectasis)
caliectasis, pyelocaliectasis,
  calicectasis
    focal c.
    localized c.
californium (Cf)
    c. 252 (^{252}Cf, Cf-252)
calipers
    restraint c.
calix (*var. of* calyx)
Callander amputation
callosal
    c. agenesis
    c. area
    c. dysgenesis
    c. formation
    c. gyrus
    c. lesion
    c. sulcus
callosi
    tapetum corporis c.
callosomarginal
    c. artery
    c. fissure
callosum
    anterior midbody of corpus c.
    corpus c.
    genu of corpus c.
    isthmus of corpus c.
    posterior midbody of corpus c.
    rostral body of corpus c.
    rostrum of corpus c.
    splenium of corpus c.

callous
callus
    bony c.
    bridging c.
    central c.
    definitive c.
    c. deposit
    endosteal c.
    ensheathing c.
    external c.
    exuberant c.
    florid c.
    c. formation
    fracture c.
    intermediate c.
    permanent c.
    provisional c.
    tumoral c.
    c. weld
Calot triangle
calvaneovalgus
    pes c.
calvaria, skullcap, *pl.* **calvariae**
    external table of c.
    internal table of c.
calvariae (*pl. of* calvaria)
calvarial
    c. bone
    c. echogenicity
    c. fracture
    c. volume analysis
Calvé
    septal cusp of C.
    C. vertebral plane
Calvé-Legg-Perthes disease
Calvé-Perthes disease
calves (*pl. of* calf)
calyceal, caliceal
    c. abnormality
    c. blunting
    c. clubbing
    c. dilation
    c. diverticulum
    c. nephrostolithotomy
    c. system
calyces (*pl. of* calyx)
Calypso
    C. 4D localization system
    C. Rely catheter
calyx, calix, *pl.* **calyces**
    cupping of c.
    major c.
    minor c.
    renal c.
    spiderlike c.
    c. tube
CAM
    complementary and alternative medicine
    computer-assisted myelography

camera

ADAC MCD Vertex Plus MCD gamma c.
Anger scintillation c.
Apex 409, 415 c.
Argus c.
Biad c.
CerASPECT c.
CFA digital c.
charge-coupled device TV c.
CID c.
Cidtech c.
cine c.
coincidence gamma c.
crystal gamma c.
data c.
Digirad gamma c.
DSI c.
dual-head coincidence c.
dual single-crystal gamma c.
electron diffraction c.
Elscint APEX 409-AG ECT c.
Elscint APEX 009 Precursor c.
Elscint dual-detector cardiac c.
Elscint Dual-Head Helix c.
full-ring dedicated BGO PET/CT c.
gamma c.
gantry-free gamma c.
GE 400AC/T STAR II c.
GE gamma c.
GE Millennium MG c.
Genesys c.
GE Neurocam c.
GE single-detector SPECT-capable c.
GE Starcam single-crystal tomographic scintillation c.
Haifa c.
4-head c.
Helix c.
Hitachi SPECT 2000H-40 c.
hybrid PET/SPECT c.
infrared c.
integral uniformity scintillation c.
Isocon c.
Israel c.
large field-of-view gamma c.
MedX c.
multicrystal gamma c.
multiformat c.
multiple-headed gamma c.
nuclear medicine c.
Orthicon c.
Picker Prism 3000XP gamma c.
PillCam ESO video c.
pinhole c.
Pixsys FlashPoint c.
positron scintillation c.
PULSEcdc compact gamma c.

radioisotope c.
radionuclide c.
R&F c.
rotating gamma c.
Scanditronix 1024-7B c.
Scinticore multicrystal scintillation c.
scintillation c.
Shimadzu HeadTome Set-031 c.
Siemens gamma c.
Siemens Orbiter large field-of-view c.
single-head rotating gamma c.
SKYLight gantry-free nuclear medicine gamma c.
slip-ring c.
Sopha DSX1 c.
Sophy c.
SP6 c.
Starcam c.
Strichman SME-810 c.
Technicare c.
Toshiba GGA 9300 c.
Trionix c.
Trionix-Triad c.
triple head gamma c.
variable-angle gamma c.
Vertex c.
video display c.
video pill c.
Vision c.

cameral fistula
Cameron method
cam impingement
Camino

C. intracranial catheter
C. microventricular bolt catheter

Campbell ligament
Camper

C. chiasm
C. fascia
C. ligament
C. line

Camp grid cassette
camplodactyly (*var. of* camptodactyly)
camptocormia
camptodactylia (*var. of* camptodactyly)
camptodactylism (*var. of* camptodactyly)
camptodactyly, camptodactylia, camplodactyly, camptodactylism, streblodactyly
camptomelic dysplasia
Campylobacter

Campylobacter infection
C. jejuni

Camurati-Engelmann disease
CAMV

congenital anomaly of mitral valve

canal

abdominal c.
accessory neuroenteric c.

canal (*continued*)
acoustic c.
adductor c.
Alcock c.
alimentary c.
alveolar c.
alveolodental c.
ampulla of semicircular c.
anal c.
anterior condylar c.
anterior semicircular c.
antropyloric c.
arachnoid c.
Arantius c.
archenteric c.
Arnold c.
arterial c.
atrial c.
atrioventricular c.
auditory c.
basipharyngeal c.
Bernard c.
Bichat c.
biliary c.
birth c.
bony semicircular c.
Böttcher c.
Braun c.
Breschet c.
calciferous c.
caroticotympanic c.
carotid c.
carpal c.
caudal c.
central spinal c.
cerebrospinal c.
cervical c.
cervicoaxillary c.
ciliary c.
Civinini c.
Cloquet c.
cochlear c.
common atrioventricular c.
complex atrioventricular c.
condylar c.
condyloid c.
connecting c.
Corti c.
Cotunnius c.
craniopharyngeal c.
crural c.
Cuvier c.
c. decompression
deferent c.
diploic c.
Dorello c.
Dupuytren c.
endocervical c.
endometrial fluid in c.

ethmoid c.
eustachian c.
facial nerve c.
fallopian c.
femoral medullary c.
Ferrein c.
flexor c.
Fontana c.
galactophorous c.
ganglionic c.
Gartner c.
gastric c.
genital c.
gray horn in spinal c.
greater palatine c.
gubernacular c.
Guyon c.
gynecophoric c.
Hannover c.
haversian c.
hemal c.
Henle c.
Hensen c.
Hering c.
hernia c.
Hirschfeld c.
His c.
Huguier c.
Hunter c.
Huschke c.
hyaloid c.
hydrops c.
hypoglossal c.
iliac c.
incisive c.
inferior dental c.
infraorbital c.
inguinal c.
interfacial c.
internal auditory c.
intersacral c.
intestinal c.
intramedullary c.
Jacobson c.
Kovalevsky c.
lacrimal c.
Lambert c.
lateral semicircular c.
Löwenberg c.
lumbar spinal c.
lumbosacral c.
lymphatic c.
mandibular c.
marrow c.
mastoid c.
maxillary c.
medullary c.
mental c.
Müller c.

musculotubal c.
narrowing of spinal c.
nasal c.
nasolacrimal c.
nasopalatine c.
neural c.
neurenteric c.
notochordal c.
Nuck c.
c. of Scarpa
c. of stomach
olfactory c.
optic c.
orbital c.
palatine c.
palatomaxillary c.
palatovaginal c.
paraurethral c.
parturient c.
pelvic c.
pericardioperitoneal c.
persistent common atrioventricular c.
petrous carotid c.
pharyngeal c.
pleural c.
pleuropericardial c.
pleuroperitoneal c.
pneumatoenteric c.
portal c.
posterior semicircular c.
principal artery of pterygoid c.
pterygoid c.
pterygopalatine c.
pudendal c.
pulmoaortic c.
pulp c.
pyloric c.
recurrent c.
Reichert c.
retronasal c.
Rivinus c.
Rosenthal c.
sacculocochlear c.
sacculoutricular c.
sacral c.
Santorini c.
Schlemm c.
scleral c.
semicircular c.
c. septum
sheathing c.
small internal auditory c.
sphenopalatine c.
sphenopharyngeal c.
spinal cord c.
squamous cell carcinoma of anal c.
c. stenosis
Stensen c.
Stilling c.

subsartorial c.
Sucquet-Hoyer c.
supraorbital c.
target c.
tarsal c.
temporal c.
Theile c.
tibial medullary c.
tight spinal c.
tubal c.
tubotympanic c.
umbilical c.
uniting c.
urogenital c.
uterine c.
uterocervical c.
uterovaginal c.
utriculosaccular c.
vaginal c.
ventricular c.
Verneuil c.
vertebral c.
vesicourethral c.
vestibular c.
vidian c.
Volkmann c.
vomerine c.
vomerorostral c.
vomerovaginal c.
vulvouterine c.
widened optic c.
zygomaticofacial c.
zygomaticotemporal c.
Canale-Kelly talar neck fracture classification
canalicular
  c. duct
  c. sphincter
canaliculi (*pl. of* canaliculus)
canaliculus, *pl.* **canaliculi**
  apical c.
  auricular c.
  bone c.
  cochlear c.
  haversian c.
  innominate c.
canalization
Canavan disease
Canavan-van Bogaert-Bertrand disease
cancelled bone
cancellation
  fat-water signal c.
  phase c.
cancellous
  c. bone chip
  c. hemopoietic marrow
  c. osteoid osteoma
  c. screw
  c. tissue

C

cancer
American Joint Committee on C. (AJCC)
American Joint Committee on Cancer/Union International Contre le C.
c. antigen
c. body
c. cell anaplasia
cervical c.
c. embolus
European Organization for Research and Treatment of C. (EORTC)
c. free
hereditary nonpolyposis colorectal c. (HNPCC)
high-risk primary breast c.
hormone-resistant prostate c.
inflammatory breast c.
International System for staging lung c.
locally advanced breast c.
locoregional breast c.
multicentric primary breast c.
c. of unknown primary (CUP)
c. of unknown primary site
organ-confined prostate c.
radiation-induced c.
cancerization
field c.
cancriform
cancroid
Candela
C. lithotripsy
C. pulsed dye laser
candelabrum
c. artery
sylvian c.
Candida
C. enteritis
C. esophagitis
candidate lesion
candidiasis
oral c.
pulmonary c.
candle
c. drip disc
c. dripping appearance
candle-flame osteolysis
candle-guttering
candle-wax
c.-w. appearance of bone
c.-w. dripping
candy-wrapper
c.-w. effect
c.-w. stenosis
caniocervical junction
canis
Toxocara c.

cannon
c. bone
C. point
Cannon-Boehm point
cannula, *pl.* **cannulas,** *pl.* **cannulae**
bulbous-tip stiff malleable c.
Fluoro Tip c.
indwelling c.
metallic-tip c.
ultrasonic lithotripter c.
cannulae (*pl. of* cannula)
cannulas (*pl. of* cannula)
cannulated
c. artery
c. central vein
percutaneously c.
cannulation, cannulization
aortic c.
arterial c.
atrial c.
bicaval c.
direct caval c.
endoscopic retrograde pancreatic duct c.
left atrial c.
ostial c.
retrograde c.
selective c.
single-cannula atrial c.
2-stage venous c.
subselective c.
venoarterial c.
venous c.
venovenous c.
cannulization (*var. of* cannulation)
Canon scanner
Cantelli sign
canthi (*pl. of* canthus)
canthomeatal
c. line
c. plane
canthus, *pl.* **canthi**
outer c.
Cantlie line
Cantor tube
Cantrell pentalogy
CAO
carotid artery occlusion
chronic airway obstruction
caoutchouc
silicone c.
cap
apical c.
azygos hematoma c.
cartilaginous c.
duodenal c.
fibrous c.
hilar c.
left pleural apical hematoma c.

phrygian c.
c. plate
pleural apical hematoma c.
pyloric c.
thin fibrous c.
capacious vein
capacitative calcium entry (CCE)
capacitive
c. interaction
c. reactance
capacitor
MOS c.
capacity
bladder c.
closing c.
cranial c.
decreased vital c.
diffusing c.
dye-binding c. (DBC)
functional bladder c.
functional residual c.
gastric c.
limited oxidative c.
lung c.
residual volume/total lung c.
respiratory c.
secretory c.
total lung c.
urinary bladder c.
vasodilatory c.
vital c.
CAPD
continuous ambulatory peritoneal
dialysis
Capener
triangle of C.
capillaritis
capillary
c. angioma
arterial c.
bile c.
c. blockade perfusion C-mode scan
c. blood flow
c. blood volume
c. bronchiectasis
c. bud
c. congestion
continuous c.
c. density
c. embolus
c. endothelium
c. filling
c. filling time
c. hemangioblastoma
c. hemangioendothelioma
c. hemangioma
c. hemorrhage
c. hydrostatic pressure
c. lake

c. leak
c. leak syndrome
c. loop
lymph c.
c. lymphangioma
c. lymphatic space invasion
c. malformation
Meigs c.
c. perfusion
c. permeability
c. pneumonia
c. pulsation
c. refill
ruptured c.
sinusoidal c.
c. telangiectasia
telangiectatic brain c.
c. tube
c. valve
c. vein
venous c.
c. vessel
c. wall
c. wedge pressure
**capillary-lymphatic malformation
(CLM)**
capita (*pl. of* caput)
capital
c. epiphysis angle
c. extension
c. femoral epiphysis
c. flexor
c. fragment
capitate
c. bone
c. facet
c. fracture
c. hamate joint
c. soft spot
capitellar fracture
capitellum
humeral c.
capitis (*gen. of* caput)
capitolunate
c. angle
c. joint
capitula (*pl. of* capitulum)
capitular
c. epiphysis
c. process
capitulum, *pl.* **capitula**
c. humeri
c. humeri fracture
mandibular c.
c. radii
c. ulnae
Caplan
C. nodule
C. syndrome

capping
    apical c.
    c. cyst
capsular
    c. attachment
    c. contracture
    c. drop lesion
    c. imbrication
    c. infarct
    c. insertion
    c. invasion
    c. ligament
    c. plane
    c. reefing
    c. space
    c. thickening
    c. thrombosis
capsulatum
    Histoplasma c.
capsule
    adrenal c.
    articular c.
    auditory c.
    Bowman c.
    cartilage c.
    cricoarytenoid articular c.
    cricothyroid articular c.
    dorsal c.
    c. endoscopy
    external c.
    facet joint c.
    fatty renal c.
    fibrous renal c.
    Gerota c.
    Given imaging capsule/M2A c.
    glenoid labrum c.
    Glisson c.
    hepatic c.
    hip joint c.
    hourglass constriction of hip c.
    hypointense fibrous c.
    internal c.
    joint c.
    limb of anterior c.
    liver c.
    M2A swallowable imaging c.
    medial carpal c.
    metatarsophalangeal c.
    organ c.
    otic c.
    plantar c.
    posterolateral c.
    prostate c.
    redundant c.
    renal c.
    rim of c.
    Sitzmarks c.
    splenic c.
    suprasellar c.

    talonavicular c.
    thyroid c.
    tissue c.
    tumor c.
    volar c.
    wrist c.
capsulitis
    adhesive c.
capsulocaudate infarct
capsulolabral complex
capsuloma
capsuloperiosteal envelope
capsuloputaminal infarct
capsuloputaminocaudate infarct
capsulorrhaphy
captopril
    c. renal scintigraphy
    c. renogram
captopril-enhanced renal scintigraphy
captopril-stimulated renal imaging
capture
    boron neutron c.
    cross-section c.
    electron c.
    gamma ray c.
    K c.
    resonance c.
caput, *pl.* capita, *gen.* capitis
    c. cecum
    c. fibulae
    fovea capitis
    c. medusae
carbogen radiosensitizer
Carbomedics valve
carbon (C)
    c. 11 (^{11}C, C-11)
    c. 12 (^{12}C, C-12)
    c. 13 (^{13}C, C-13)
    c. 14 (^{14}C, C-14)
    c. dioxide (CO_2)
    c. dioxide generator
    c. dioxide laser
    c. dioxide microbubble ultrasound
    double-bonded c.
    c. fiber-reinforced plastic
    c. imaging agent
    c. metabolism
    c. monoxide
    c. monoxide toxicity
carbon-13 spectroscopy
carbon-14 urea breath test
carbovir monophosphate
carbuncle
    renal c.
Carcassonne ligament
carcinoembryonic antigen scan
carcinogenesis
    radiation c.
carcinogenicity

carcinoid
> atypical c.
> colorectal c.
> endobronchial c.
> c. GI tract
> goblet cell c.
> occult bronchial c.
> c. syndrome
> thymic c.
> c. tumor
> typical c.

carcinoma, *pl.* **carcinomas,** *pl.*
carcinomata
> acinar pancreatic cell c.
> acinic cell c.
> adenocystic c.
> adenoid cystic lung c.
> adenoid squamous cell c.
> adenosquamous c.
> adnexal c.
> adrenal c.
> adrenocortical c.
> advanced hepatocellular c.
> aerodigestive c.
> aldosterone-producing c.
> aldosterone-secreting c.
> alveolar basal cell c.
> alveolar mucosal c.
> ameloblastic c.
> ampullary c.
> anaplastic thyroid c.
> androgen-independent prostate c.
>   (AIPC)
> aniline c.
> apocrine c.
> appendiceal c.
> apple-core c.
> aryepiglottic fold c.
> asbestos-related lung c.
> atypical medullary c.
> Bartholin gland c. (BGC)
> basal cell c.
> bilateral invasive lobular c.
> bile duct c.
> bilharzial c.
> biliary tract c.
> bladder c.
> blastic metastatic prostate c.
> bone c.
> Boorman classification of gastric c.
> bowel c.
> brain c.
> breast c.
> bronchial c.
> bronchiolar c.
> bronchioloalveolar cell c.
> bronchoalveolar c.
> bronchogenic c.
> buccal mucosal c.

> cavitary squamous cell c.
> cavitating c.
> cecal c.
> cerebriform c.
> cholangiocellular c.
> chorionic c.
> choroid plexus c.
> clay pipe c.
> clear cell c.
> colloid c.
> colon c.
> colorectal c.
> comedo-basal cell c.
> conjugal c.
> contact c.
> corpus c.
> cortisol-producing c.
> cribriform c.
> cylindrical c.
> cylindromatous c.
> cystic renal cell c.
> dendritic c.
> differentiated c.
> differentiated thyroid c. (DTC)
> distal bile duct c. (DBDC)
> ductal in situ breast c.
> ductal papillary c.
> duct cell c.
> early advanced hepatocellular c.
> embryonal cell c.
> encephaloid c.
> c. en cuirasse
> endobronchial c.
> endometrial c.
> endometrioid ovarian c.
> epidermal c.
> epidermoid lung c.
> epiglottic c.
> epithelial-myoepithelial c.
> epithelial ovarian c.
> esophageal c.
> ethmoid sinus c.
> exophytic c.
> c. ex pleomorphic adenoma
> extensive intraductal c. (EIC)
> extrahepatic bile duct c.
> extrapulmonary small cell c.
> fallopian tube c.
> false cord c.
> fibrolamellar hepatocellular c.
> FIGO stage c.
> flat colorectal c.
> focal lobular c.
> follicular c.
> follicular thyroid c.
> gallbladder c.
> gastric neuroendocrine c.
> gastric remnant c.
> gastric stump c.

C

carcinoma (*continued*)
    gastroesophageal junction c.
    gastrointestinal c.
    gelatinous c.
    genital c.
    genitourinary c.
    giant cell lung c.
    gingival c.
    glandular c.
    glans c.
    glottic c.
    granulosa cell c.
    hard palate c.
    head and neck squamous cell c.
    hepatic c.
    hepatobiliary c.
    hepatocellular c. (HCC)
    hereditary clear cell renal c.
    hereditary nonpolyposis colorectal c. (HNPCC)
    hereditary papillary renal c.
    hormone receptor-negative c.
    hormone-resistant prostate c.
    hyopharyngeal c.
    hypernephroid c.
    hypervascular hepatocellular c.
    hypopharyngeal c.
    infantile embryonal c.
    infiltrating ductal c.
    infiltrating esophageal c.
    infiltrating lobular c.
    inflammatory breast c. (IBC)
    c. in situ
    intracystic breast c.
    intraductal c. (IDC)
    intraductal papillary c.
    intrahepatic biliary c.
    invasive breast c.
    invasive ductal c.
    invasive lobular c.
    Japanese classification of gastric c.
    jugular node metastatic c.
    juvenile embryonal c.
    known primary c.
    Kulchitsky cell c. (KCC)
    large cell neuroendocrine c. (LCNEC)
    large cell undifferentiated c.
    laryngeal c.
    lenticular c.
    leptomeningeal c.
    linitis plastica c.
    lobular c.
    locoregional breast c.
    lung c.
    lymphoepithelial c.
    mammographically occult c.
    maxillary sinus c.
    medullary breast c.
    medullary thyroid c.

    meibomian gland c.
    melanotic c.
    Merkel cell c.
    mesometanephric c.
    metachronous transitional cell c.
    metaplastic c.
    metastatic urothelial c.
    micropapillary c.
    missed bronchogenic c.
    moderately differentiated hepatocellular c. (mHCC)
    mucin-hypersecreting c.
    mucinous breast c.
    mucinous bronchoalveolar c.
    mucin-producing c.
    mucoepidermoid c.
    mucous c.
    multicentric basal cell c.
    multicentric invasive lobular c.
    multifocal breast c.
    multifocal invasive lobular c.
    multifocal papillary thyroid c.
    nasopharyngeal c. (NPC)
    nasopharyngeal squamous cell c.
    2nd primary c.
    necrotic renal cell c.
    neuroendocrine small cell c.
    nevoid basal cell c.
    node-negative c.
    node-positive c.
    noncalcified c.
    non-small-cell c. (NSCC)
    non-small-cell lung c. (NSCLC)
    oat cell c.
    occult papillary c.
    occult thyroid c.
    c. of unknown primary (CUP)
    osteoid c.
    ovarian c.
    Paget c.
    palpatory T-stage prostate c.
    pancreatic c.
    papillary breast c.
    papillary renal cell c.
    papillary serous c.
    papillary thyroid c.
    paranasal sinus c.
    parathyroid c.
    perforating colorectal c.
    periampullary c.
    peripheral bronchogenic c.
    pharyngeal wall c.
    pigmented basal cell c.
    piriform sinus c.
    platinum-resistant ovarian c.
    polypoid c.
    poorly differentiated c.
    poorly differentiated hepatocellular c. (pHCC)

postcricoid c.
posterior pharyngeal wall c.
preinvasive c.
prickle cell c.
primary hepatocellular c.
primary intraosseous c.
primary neuroendocrine small cell c.
prostate c.
prostatic c.
pulmonary squamous cell c.
radiation-induced c.
rectal c.
rectosigmoid c.
renal cell c. (stage I, II, IIIA,
  IIIB, IIIC, IVA, IVB) (RCC)
resectable colorectal c.
retinoblastoma hereditary human c.
retromolar trigone c.
salivary duct c.
salivary gland c.
scar c.
schistosomal bladder c.
schneiderian c.
scirrhous breast c.
sclerosing basal cell c.
sclerosing hepatic c. (SHC)
sebaceous c.
secretory c.
serous c.
sessile nodular c.
sigmoid c.
signet ring cell c.
c. simplex
sinonasal c.
skin c.
small bowel c.
small cell cribriform c.
small cell lung c. (SCLC)
small cell undifferentiated c.
small intestine c.
small round cell c.
soft palate c.
solid and papillary pancreatic c.
solid and pseudopapillary c.
solid circumscribed breast c.
spicular c.
splenic flexure c.
sporadic colorectal c.
sporadic medullary thyroid c.
squamous cell c.
string cell c.
stump c.
subareolar c.
subglottic c.
submandibular gland c.
superficial basal cell c.
superficial depressed c.
superficial spreading esophageal c.
superficial spreading stomach c.

superficial transitional cell c.
supraglottic c.
suture line c.
sweat gland c.
synchronous transitional cell c.
telangiectatic c.
terminal c.
testicular c.
testis c.
thymic c.
thyroid c.
tongue c.
tonsillar c.
trabecular c.
transitional cell c. (TCC)
transitional kidney cell c.
transitional ureteral cell c.
transitional urinary bladder cell c.
transverse colon c.
tripartite duodenal c.
tubular breast c.
typical medullary c.
ulcerative esophageal c.
undifferentiated nasopharyngeal c.
unresectable colorectal c.
urachal c.
ureteral c.
urothelial c.
uterine cervix c.
uterine corpus c.
uterine papillary serous c. (UPSC)
vaginal c.
varicoid esophageal c.
verrucous c.
vesical c.
villous c.
vocal cord c.
vulvar c.
vulvovaginal c.
Walker c.
widely invasive follicular c.
wolffian duct c.
carcinomas (*pl. of* carcinoma)
carcinomata (*pl. of* carcinoma)
carcinomatosa
  peritonitis c.
carcinomatosis
  abdominal c.
  lymphangitic c.
  lymphatic c.
  omental c.
  peritoneal c.
  c. peritonei
  pulmonary lymphangitic c. (PLC)
  regional lymphangitic c.
carcinomatous
  c. cavitary metastasis
  c. implant
  c. meningitis

145

carcinomatous (*continued*)
    c. myelopathy
    c. myopathy
    c. neuromyopathy
    c. subacute cerebellar degeneration
carcinosarcoma
    embryonal c.
    esophageal c.
    renal c.
    Walker c.
carcinostatic
card
    Novus Medical Image C.
Carden amputation
cardia
    crescent of c.
    gastric c.
    patulous c.
cardiac
    c. angiopathy
    c. angioplasty
    c. angiosarcoma
    c. anomaly
    c. antrum
    c. apex
    C. Assist intraaortic balloon catheter
    c. asthma
    c. atrial shunt
    c. blood pool imaging
    c. border
    c. branch
    c. calcification
    c. catheterization
    c. catheterization imaging
    c. chamber
    c. circulation
    c. cirrhosis
    c. compression
    c. computed tomographic angiography
    c. congestion
    c. contractility
    c. creep
    c. decompensation
    c. decompression
    c. decortication
    c. denervation
    c. diameter
    c. dilation
    c. disturbance syndrome
    c. effusion
    c. event
    c. failure
    c. fibroma
    c. fibrosarcoma
    c. filling pressure
    c. fossa
    c. frontal area
    c. ganglion
    c. gated MR angiography

c. gated PGSE sequence
c. gated quantitative computed tomography
c. gated respiration
c. gated study
c. gating
c. gating compensation
c. glycoside
c. hamartoma
c. hemangioma
c. hydatidosis
c. hypertrophy
c. hypokinesis
c. impression
c. impression on liver
c. incisura
c. index (CI)
c. infarct
c. insufficiency
c. inversion
c. irradiation
c. irritability
c. ischemia
c. laminagraphy
c. lipoma
c. long-axis view
c. lymphangioma
c. malposition
c. mapping
c. margin
c. metastasis
c. mogul
c. monitor
c. MRI
c. multidetector row computed tomography
c. muscle
c. muscle fiber
c. muscle inflammation
c. myocyte
c. myxoma
c. node
c. notch
c. oblique reformatting
c. obstruction
c. orifice
c. osteosarcoma
c. output
c. output echocardiography
c. output measurement
c. output video densitometry
c. overload
c. paraganglioma
c. perforation
c. PET
c. phase
c. pheochromocytoma
c. plexus
c. polyp

c. position
c. positron emission tomography imaging
C. Protect
c. pulse duplicator
c. pumping ability
c. radiography
c. radiography imaging
c. recovery
c. repolarization
c. reserve
c. rhabdomyoma
c. rhabdomyosarcoma
c. rupture
c. sarcoidosis
c. sarcoma
c. scan
c. scintigraphy
c. scintigraphy ejection fraction
c. segment
c. segmental bronchus
c. series
c. shadow
c. shape
c. shock
c. shock wave therapy (CSWT)
c. short-axis view
c. shunt detection
c. silhouette
c. silhouette enlargement
c. situs inversus
c. situs solitus
c. skeleton
c. sling
c. sphincter
c. standstill
c. status
c. steady state
c. stomach
c. support device (CSD)
c. tamponade
c. teratoma
c. thrombosis
c. tumor
c. valve
c. valve mucoid degeneration
c. valvular lesion
c. vasculature
c. vegetation
c. vein
c. ventricle aneurysm
c. ventriculography
C. View probe
c. volume
c. waist
c. wall motion
c. wall motion imaging
Cardima Pathfinder microcatheter

cardinal
c. event
c. finding
c. ligament
c. point
c. sign
c. vein
cardioangiography
blood pool radionuclide c.
retrograde c.
CardioBeeper CB-12L cardiac monitor
CardioCard
cardiochalasia
CardioCoil coronary stent
cardiocutaneous syndrome
Cardio Data MK3 Holter scanner
cardiodiaphragmatic angle
cardioesophageal (CE)
c. junction
CardioGen-82
cardiogenesis
cardiogenic
c. embolic stroke
c. embolus
c. plate
c. pulmonary edema
c. shock
c. shock heart
cardiogram
ultrasonic c. (UCG)
cardiographic
cardiography
M-mode c.
radionuclide c.
ultrasonic c.
ultrasound c.
cardiohepatic
c. angle
c. triangle
cardiohepatomegaly
cardioinhibitory response
cardiokymography (CKG)
Cardiolite
C. imaging agent
C. scan imaging
technetium-tagged C.
Cardiomed
C. Bodysoft epidural catheter
C. endotracheal ventilation catheter
cardiomediastinal shadow
cardiomegaly
borderline c.
boxlike c.
funnellike c.
globular c.
iatrogenic c.
cardiomotility
cardiomyopathic degeneration

C

cardiomyopathy
    amyloidotic c.
    arrhythmogenic right ventricular c. (ARVC)
    concentric hypertrophic c.
    congenital dilated c.
    congestive c.
    constrictive c.
    degenerative c.
    diabetic c.
    diffuse symmetric hypertrophied c.
    dilated c. (DCM)
    dystrophinopathic c.
    endstage c.
    familial hypertrophic c. (FHC)
    Friedreich ataxic c.
    hypertrophic c. (HCM)
    hypertrophic obstructive c. (HOC, HOCM)
    idiopathic dilated c. (IDC)
    idiopathic restrictive c.
    infantile c.
    infectious c.
    infiltrative c.
    ischemic congestive c.
    left ventricular c.
    metabolic c.
    nonischemic congestive c.
    nonobstructive c.
    obliterative c.
    obstructive hypertrophic c.
    peripartum dilated c.
    postmyocarditis dilated c.
    postpartum c.
    restrictive c.
    right-sided c.
    right ventricular c.
    tachycardia-induced c.
    toxic c.
cardionecrosis
cardiophrenic
    c. angle
    c. junction
    c. right-angle mass
cardiopneumatic
cardioptosis
    Wenckebach c.
cardiopulmonary
    c. abnormality
    c. bilharziasis
    c. disease
    c. edema
    c. exercise test (CPET)
    c. insufficiency
    c. support system
cardiopyloric
cardiorenal disease
cardiorespiratory sign
cardiorrhexis

cardioscan
Cardioscint
cardiosclerosis
CardioSEAL occluder
cardioselective agent
cardiospasm
cardiosplenic syndrome
cardiosynchronous stimulation
CardioTec scan
cardiothoracic
    c. index
    c. ratio (CTR)
    c. surgery
    c. trauma
cardiothymic
    c. shadow
    c. silhouette
cardiothyrotoxicosis
cardiotocogram
cardiotocography imaging
cardiotopometry
cardiovalvular
cardiovascular
    c. accident (CVA)
    c. angiography analysis system (CAAS)
    c. anomaly
    c. computed tomographic scanner
    c. disease (CVD)
    c. imaging technique
    c. infection
    c. information system (CVIS)
    c. malformation
    c. pressure
    c. radioisotope scan and function imaging
    c. radiology
    c. renal disease
    c. shadow
    c. shunt
    c. silhouette
    c. system
    c. system scintigraphy
cardioverter-defibrillator
    automatic implantable c.-d. (AICD)
cardiovolume
    multislice c. (MSCV)
carditis
    acute lethal c.
    Lyme c.
care
    C. bolus
    home infusion c.
CareGraph skin dose-mapping software
Carey-Coons soft-stent biliary endoprosthesis
CA15-3 RIA
caries
    radiation c.

carina, *pl.* **carinae**
    mainstem c.
    c. of trachea
    sharp c.
carinae (*pl. of* carina)
carinal
    c. angle
    c. angle narrowing
    c. lesion
carinii
    Pneumocystis c.
Carleton spot
C-arm
    C-a. DSA system
    C-a. fluoroscopic control
    C-a. fluoroscopy
    Mini 6000 C-a.
    C-a. portable x-ray unit
    Siremobile Iso-C3d isocentric
      C-a.
Carman sign
Carnesale-Stewart-Barnes hip dislocation classification
Carnett sign
Carncy
    C. syndrome
    C. triad
Carnoy solution
Caroli disease
caroticocavernous fistula
caroticoclinoid ligament
caroticojugular spine
caroticotympanic
    c. artery
    c. canal
carotid
    c. and vertebral artery transluminal angioplasty study (CAVATAS)
    c. angiography
    c. angioplasty with stenting (CAS)
    c. artery
    c. artery aneurysm
    c. artery arteritis
    c. artery bifurcation
    c. artery calcification
    c. artery disease
    c. artery dissection trauma
    c. artery ischemia
    c. artery kinking
    c. artery occlusion (CAO)
    c. artery plaque
    c. artery stenosis
    c. artery stenting
    c. atherosclerosis
    c. atherosclerotic disease
    c. bifurcation atheroma
    c. blowout syndrome
    c. body

c. body tumor
c. bulb
c. bulb baroreceptor
c. canal
c. cerebral arteriography
c. circulation
c. cistern
c. compression tonography
c. disobliteration
c. distribution TIA
c. duct
c. duplex imaging
c. duplex study
c. duplex ultrasound
c. ejection time
c. endarterectomy (CEA)
external c.
c. foramen
c. ganglion
c. gland
c. groove
c. hemorrhage
internal c.
c. lumen
c. occlusive disease
c. phonoangiography
c. plaque hematoma
c. plexus
c. pulse
c. pulse peak
c. pulse tracing
c. pulse upstroke
c. revascularization endarterectomy stent trial
c. sheath
c. sheath adenoma
c. shudder
c. sinus
c. sinus hypersensitivity
c. sinus imaging
c. sinus syndrome (CSS)
c. siphon
c. sonography
c. space
c. space mass
c. stenosis
c. string sign
c. sulcus
c. triangle
c. tubercle
c. vein
c. velocity
c. wall
carotid-carotid venous bypass graft
carotid-cavernous
    c.-c. fistula (CCF)
    c.-c. fistula occlusion
    c.-c. sinus fistula

C

carotid-dural fistula
carotidis
    bifurcatio c.
carotid-jugular fistula
carotid-ophthalmic aneurysm
carotid-subclavian transposition
Carotid-Wallstent Monorail
carpal
    c. arch
    c. articular surface
    c. axis
    c. bone anatomy
    c. bone stress fracture
    c. boss
    c. box
    c. canal
    c. coalition
    c. content ratio
    c. deviation
    c. groove
    c. height index
    c. height ratio
    c. navicular
    c. navicular bone
    c. navicular fracture
    c. row
    c. scaphoid bone fracture
    c. tunnel
    c. tunnel projection
    c. tunnel syndrome
    c. tunnel view
    c. wrist angle
Carpentier-Edwards ring
Carpentier ring
carpet
    c. lesion
    c. lesion of colon
    c. polyp
carpi (*pl. of* carpus)
carpometacarpal (CMC)
    c. articulation
    c. fusion
    c. joint fracture
    c. ligament
carpophalangeal joint
carporadial articulation
carpotarsal osteolysis
carpus, *pl.* carpi
    adaptive c.
    cuneiform bone of c.
    carpi radialis brevis tendon
    carpi radialis longus tendon
    ulnar translocation of c.
carrier
    ^{67}Ga GABA uptake c.
    c. protein
    radionuclide c.
    c. tube
carrier-added radionuclide

carrier-free
    c.-f. isotope
    c.-f. radioisotope
    c.-f. radionuclide
    c.-f. separation
    c.-f. separation process
carrier-mediated transport system
Carrington disease
carrot-shaped trachea
Carr-Purcell (CP)
    C.-P. sequence
Carr-Purcell-Meiboom-Gill (CPMG)
    C.-P.-M.-G. sequence
carrying angle
Carson procedure
Carter
    C. equation
    C. Rowe shoulder view
cartesian reference coordinate system
cartilage
    absent bronchial c.
    accessory nasal c.
    alar c.
    anular rim of c.
    aortic c.
    arthrodial c.
    articular c.
    arytenoid c.
    attenuated intercarpal articular c.
    auditory c.
    auricular c.
    basilar c.
    c. bone
    branchial c.
    bronchial anular c.
    c. calcification
    calcified c.
    c. capsule
    ciliary c.
    circumferential c.
    conchal c.
    connecting c.
    corniculate c.
    costal intraarticular c.
    cricoid c.
    cricothyroid c.
    cuneiform c.
    delayed gadolinium-enhanced
      magnetic resonance imaging of c.
      (dGEMRIC)
    delayed gadolinium-enhanced MRI
      of c.
    elastic c.
    c. endplate
    ensiform c.
    epiglottic c.
    epiphysial c.
    facet c.
    falciform c.

fibroelastic c.
fibrous c.
flaking of c.
floating c.
free flap of c.
hyaline articular c.
interarticular c.
c. island
c. joint space
c. lacuna
laryngeal c.
liplike projection of c.
loss of elasticity of c.
c. matrix
ossified c.
osteoarthritic c.
patellofemoral articular c.
physial c.
pitted c.
pulmonary c.
quadrangle c.
rim of c.
roughened c.
scored c.
semilunar c.
shelling off of c.
softening of c.
sternal c.
c. stroma
swelling of c.
tag of c.
talar dome articular c.
thinned c.
thyroid c.
tracheal c.
triradiate c.
unossified c.
xiphoid c.
Y c.
yellow c.
cartilage-capped exostosis
cartilage-containing giant cell tumor
cartilage-forming bone tumor
cartilage-hair hypoplasia
cartilaginous
c. acetabulum
c. anlage
c. bar
c. cap
c. cap of phalangeal head
c. degeneration
c. disc
c. endplate
c. epiphysis
c. growth plate
c. growth plate disorder
c. hamartoma
c. joint surface

c. lesion
c. metaplasia
c. node
c. nodule
c. ring
c. septum
c. soft tissue tumor
c. synchondrosis
c. tissue
c. viscerocranium
Carto EP navigation system
cartographic projection
cartwheel fracture
Carvallo sign
Cary-Coon biliary stent
CAS
carotid angioplasty with stenting
coronary artery scan
coronary artery spasm
CAS imaging
cascade
diagnostic c.
gamma c.
c. stomach
c. system
time-dependent metabolic c.
caseating granuloma
caseation necrosis
caseous
c. granulomatous osteomyelitis
c. necrosis
c. pneumonia
casium iodide (CsI)
Casser
C. ligament
C. muscle
casserian
c. ligament
c. muscle
cassette
Adrian-Crooks c.
Camp grid c.
Curix film-screen c.
film-screen c.
cassette-based screen-film radiography
CAST
computer automated scan technology
Castaneda thrombolytic brush
casting breast calcification
Castleman
C. disease
C. lymphoma
cast-off x-ray
CAT
computed axial tomography
computerized axial tomography
catadioptric lens
catamenial pneumothorax
catapophysis

C

151

cataract
    radiation c.
catarrhal pneumonia
catastrophe
    vascular c.
catecholamine-producing tumor
catechol-*O*-methyltransferase
category
    iliac PTA c. (1–4)
    Rutherford-Becker claudication c.
      (1-5)
catenary system
caterpillar stomach
cathartic colon
catheter
    abscess drainage c.
    Abscession drainage c.
    Accu-Vu sizing c.
    Achiever balloon dilation c.
    Ackrad balloon-bearing c.
    ACS balloon c.
    ACS Concorde c.
    ACS Endura coronary dilation c.
    ACS OTW Photon coronary dilation
      c.
    ACS RX Comet coronary dilation c.
    ACS Tourguide II guiding c.
    AcuNav ultrasound c.
    Ahn thrombectomy c.
    Alert c.
    Amplatz left coronary c.
    Amplatz maceration-aspiration
      thrombectomy c. (AMATC)
    Amplatz right coronary c.
    Amplatz Super Stiff c.
    Angiocath Autoguard Shielded IV c.
    Angiocath PRN c.
    angiographic c.
    c. angiography
    AngioJet Xpeedior c.
    angled-tip c.
    angulated c.
    Anthron heparinized c.
    c. aortography
    apheresis c.
    arrhythmia mapping system c.
    arrhythmogenic myocardial tissue
      ablation c.
    Arrow c.
    ARROWgard Blue Line c.
    Arrow-Howes multilumen c.
    c. arteriography
    Ascent guiding c.
    ATB PTA ablation c.
    AtheroCath Bantam coronary
      atherectomy c.
    AtheroTrack c.
    Atlantis SR IVUS c.
    Auth Rotablator atherectomy c.

    balloon biliary c.
    balloon embolectomy c.
    balloon PTA c.
    balloon-tipped angiographic c.
    Bardex Lubricath c.
    Bard Safety Excalibur c.
    B-D Insyte Autoguard shielded
      intravenous c.
    Berenstein c.
    Berman angiographic c.
    Bernstein c.
    Beta-Cath system c.
    biliary drainage c.
    Blue Max high-pressure reinforced
      polyethylene balloon c.
    braided diagnostic c.
    Brevi-Kath epidural c.
    Brite Tip guiding c.
    Bronchitrac L c.
    Broviac long-term c.
    c. bursting pressure
    c. calibration
    Calypso Rely c.
    Camino intracranial c.
    Camino microventricular bolt c.
    Cardiac Assist intraaortic balloon c.
    Cardiomed Bodysoft epidural c.
    Cardiomed endotracheal ventilation
      c.
    Caud-A-Kath c.
    central venous c. (CVC)
    Centurion PTA balloon dilation c.
    Cheetah angioplasty c.
    Chemo-Port c.
    c. cholangiogram
    cholangiography c.
    CliniCath peripherally inserted c.
    coaxillary directed c.
    Cobra 1, 2 c.
    Cobra diagnostic c.
    cobra-shaped c.
    c. coiling sign
    Comfort Cath I, II c.
    condom c.
    conductance c.
    conoventricular defect PTA balloon
      dilation c.
    Conquest PTA balloon dilation c.
    contrast-filled c.
    Cook-Cope-type loop c.
    Cope locking-loop c.
    Cope loop c.
    Cordis Brite Tip guiding c.
    Cordis Predator PTCA balloon c.
    c. coronary angiography
    coudé c.
    Cragg-McNamara multiple-sidehole
      infusion c.
    cutting balloon c.

Datascope c.
Dawson-Mueller drainage c.
decompression c.
Derek Harwood-Nash c.
dilation c.
directional atherectomy c.
double-J indwelling c.
double-J ureteral c.
double-lumen central venous c.
drainage c.
dual-lumen silicone
 hemodialysis/apheresis c.
Du Pen long-term epidural c.
EchoMark c.
electrothermal c.
Endosound endoscopic ultrasound c.
Envoy guiding c.
Epimed spring guide c.
EPT-Dx steerable diagnostic c.
Equinox occlusion balloon c.
ERCP c.
c. exit site
Explorer rotational diagnostic c.
Explorer ST fixed-curve diagnostic
 c.
Export c.
Express PTCA c.
external biliary drainage c.
Fast-Cath introducer c.
FasTracker c.
c. fixation
Flexima biliary drainage c.
Flexi-Tip ureteral c.
fluid-filled c.
Fogarty adherent clot c.
Fogarty balloon embolectomy c.
Fogarty Thru-Lumen c.
8-, 9-French guiding c.
French-tip c.
gastrojejunostomy c.
gastrostomy c.
Glide Cobra c.
Greenfield c.
Grollman pigtail c.
Groshong distal valve c.
Grüntzig balloon dilation c.
guide c.
H1 c.
Headhunter c.
helium-filled balloon c.
hemodialysis c.
Hickman long-term c.
Hickman tunneled indwelling c.
hockey-stick c.
Hopkins hook-guiding c.
H/S Elliptosphere balloon c.
HSG c.
Hydrolyser hydrodynamic
 thrombectomy c.

hydrophilic coated guiding c.
hysterosalpingography c.
ILUS c.
Imager II c.
c. impact artifact
impeller basket c.
implantable access c.
indwelling Foley c.
Infuse-a-Port c.
infusion c.
c. insertion
Insyte Autoguard shielded IV c.
internal/external c.
intraarterial chemotherapy c.
IntraCardiac echocardiography IVUS
 c.
Intracath c.
intraluminal ultrasound c.
intravascular ultrasound c.
IVUS c.
JB1 c.
jejunostomy c.
Jography angiographic c.
Judkins 4 diagnostic c.
Judkins left coronary c.
Judkins right coronary c.
jugular c.
c. kinking
Kumpe c.
large-bore c.
LifeJet c.
8-lumen manometric c.
Maglinte c.
Malecot nephrostomy c.
MammoSite radiation therapy system
 c.
c. mapping
MediPort c.
Medi-tech c.
Medtronic c.
Mercator atrial high-density array c.
Mewissen infusion c.
micromanometer-tipped c.
MicroMewi multiple-sidehole infusion
 c.
c. migration
Motarjeme c.
MR-trackable intramyocardial
 injection c.
multiaccess c.
multielectrode c.
multiple-sidehole infusion c.
multipurpose c.
multisideport infusion c.
multislit c.
Navarre drainage c.
Navi-Star ablation c.
Nd:YAG laser c.
NephroMax balloon c.

catheter (*continued*)

nephrostomy c.
nondetachable balloon c.
nontunneled c.
nylon c.
Oasis thrombectomy c.
Oasis triple-lumen c.
c. obstruction
Omni Flush 3F, 4F, 5F c.
Omni Selective 0-3 c.
OneStep paracentesis drainage c.
Opticath c.
Opti-Flow dialysis c.
Optiplast balloon dilation c.
OptiQue c.
Oracle MegaSonics c.
Oracle Micro Plus c.
Oracle PTCA c.
PASV c.
PE c.
percutaneous cavity drainage c.
percutaneous cholecystotomy c.
peripherally inserted central c.
 (PICC)
peritoneal dialysis c.
pigtail c.
c. placement
Polaris Dx steerable diagnostic c.
Polaris X steerable diagnostic c.
polyethylene c.
polypropylene c.
Possis AngioJet Xpeedior c.
Proforma c.
PU c.
Pulse-Spray/PRO infusion c.
PVC c.
quantum Monorail balloon c.
RadPICC c.
Ranfac cholangiographic c.
Rapid Transit c.
Reddick cystic duct cholangiogram
 c.
Resolution ultrasonic c.
Resolve nonlocking draining c.
retrieval c.
Ring biliary drainage c.
Rosch hepatic c.
rotatable pigtail c.
Royal Flush pigtail c.
Rusch c.
Saf-T-Intima integrated IV c.
Schneider Guider c.
SCOOP model polyurethane
 intratracheal c.
self-retaining Cope loop pigtail c.
c. sheath
Sidewinder diagnostic c.
Silverhawk c.
Simmons c.

Simpson directional atherectomy c.
single-curved Cobra c.
Softouch c.
Soft-Tip c.
Soft Torque uterine c.
Soft-Vu angiographic c.
solid-state manometry c.
Sonicath Ultra imaging c.
Spyglass angiography c.
Steerocath-Dx octapolar valve
 mapping c.
Stimucath continuous nerve block c.
straight endhole c.
straight sidehole c.
sump drainage c.
Swan-Ganz balloon c.
Tamp c.
Teflon c.
temporary pacing c.
Temp Tip drainage c.
Tenckhoff c.
thermodilution c.
thin-walled c.
c. tip
c. tip hockey-stick appearance
c. tip motion
c. tip motion artifact
c. tip position
c. tip position artifact
Torcon blue c.
Tracker 10 c.
Tracker Excel c.
transducer-tipped c.
transhepatic c.
Trax c.
tunneled c.
Ultra ICE c.
Uni-Fuse infusion c.
Van Aman pulmonary pigtail c.
Van Sonnenberg sump c.
Vaxcel peripherally inserted c.
ventriculography c.
visceral c.
water-infusion c.
c. whip artifact
c. with preformed curve
Z-Med balloon c.

catheter-based
 c.-b. inducible enhancer of gene
  expression
 c.-b. interventional MRI
 c.-b. intervention technique
catheter-borne sector transducer
catheter-delivered platinum coil
catheter-directed
 c.-d. approach
 c.-d. extremity thrombolysis
 c.-d. fenestration
 c.-d. interventional procedure

c.-d. thrombolytic therapy
c.-d. urokinase
catheter-induced
c.-i. coronary artery spasm
c.-i. embolus
c.-i. pulmonary artery hemorrhage
c.-i. subclavian vein thrombosis
c.-i. thromboembolization
c.-i. vasospasm
catheterization
antegrade femoral artery c.
balloon c.
cardiac c.
high brachial artery c.
interventional c.
left axillary artery c.
left heart c.
retrograde femoral artery c.
right heart c.
Seldinger c.
superior petrous sinus c.
superselective mesenteric artery
c.
therapeutic cardiac c.
catheter-securing technique
catheter-skin interface
catheter-tissue contact
Cathflo Activase
cathode
c. glow
c. ray
c. ray oscilloscope (CRO)
c. ray tube (CRT)
CathScanner ultrasound imaging system
CathTrack catheter locator system
cation
paramagnetic c.
CAT-MIBI
computed axial
tomography-methoxyisobutyl isonitrile
CAT-MIBI image fusion
cat phantom
cat's
c. cry syndrome
c. tail configuration
catscratch fever
cat's-eye
c.-e. calculus
c.-e. reflex
cauda, *pl.* **caudae**
c. equina
c. equina compression
c. equina syndrome (CES)
caudad
c. direction
c. projection
c. view
caudae (*pl. of* cauda)
Caud-A-Kath catheter

caudal
c. branch
c. canal
c. flexure
c. ligament
c. pharyngeal complex
c. pons
c. regression
c. regression syndrome
c. sheath
c. tilt
c. vertebra
caudal-cranial (*var. of* caudocranial)
caudalward
caudate
c. body
c. lobe
c. lobe of liver
c. nucleus
c. process
c. vein
c. volume
caudocranial, caudal-cranial
c. angulation
c. projection
c. tangential view
caudolateral orbitofrontal cortex
caudothalamic groove
cauliflower appearance
cauliflower-shaped filling
defect
cause-specific survival
caustic
c. esophagitis
c. stricture
cava
azygos continuation of inferior vena
c.
bilateral superior vena c.
collapsed inferior vena c.
duplicated inferior vena c.
inferior vena c. (IVC)
infrahepatic vena c.
juxtarenal c.
membranous obstruction of inferior
vena c.
paired inferior vena c.
persistent left inferior vena c.
persistent left superior vena c.
redirection of inferior vena c.
retrohepatic vena c.
sinus of vena c.
superior bilateral vena c.
superior vena c. (SVC)
suprahepatic vena c.
thrombosed filter-bearing inferior
vena c.
transposition of inferior vena c.
vena c.

C

cavagram (*var. of* cavogram)
caval
  c. filter
  c. fold
  c. lymph node
  c. opening
  c. tourniquet
  c. valve
cavalry bone
CAVATAS
  carotid and vertebral artery
  transluminal angioplasty study
    CAVATAS trial
CAVB
  complete atrioventricular block
cavernoma
  brain c.
  portal vein c.
cavernosogram
cavernosography
  corpus c.
cavernosometry
cavernous
  c. angioma
  c. angiosarcoma
  c. brain angiography
  c. brain hemangioma
  c. groove
  c. lymphangioma
  c. malformation
  c. plexus
  c. portal vein transformation
  c. portion
  c. segment of internal carotid artery
  c. sinus
  c. sinus aneurysm
  c. sinus fistula
  c. sinus lesion
  c. sinus meningioma
  c. sinus syndrome
  c. sinus thrombosis
  c. tissue
  c. transfer of portal vein
  c. transformation of portal vein
  c. tumor
  c. urethra
caviar lesion
cavitary
  c. consolidation
  c. dilation
  c. fluid
  c. infiltrate
  c. lung lesion
  c. mass
  c. metastasis
  c. prostatitis
  c. pulmonary lesion
  c. small bowel lesion
  c. space

  c. squamous cell carcinoma
  c. tuberculosis
cavitate
cavitating
  c. carcinoma
  c. lung metastasis
  c. lung nodule
  c. neoplasia
  c. pattern
  c. pneumonia
cavitation
  collapse c.
  crescent of c.
  lobar c.
  pulmonary c.
  stable c.
  transient c.
Cavitron ultrasonic surgical aspirator (CUSA)
cavity
  abdominal c.
  abdominopelvic c.
  absorption c.
  acetabular c.
  air c.
  amnionic c.
  ancyroid c.
  aneurysmal c.
  axillary c.
  banana-shaped uterine c.
  body c.
  Bragg-Gray c.
  buccal c.
  chest c.
  cleavage c.
  closed c.
  coexistent c.
  cotyloid c.
  cranial c.
  crown c.
  dome-shaped roof of pleural c.
  embryonic abdominal c.
  endometrial c.
  epidural c.
  funnel-shaped c.
  glenoid c.
  grape-skin lung c.
  greater sac of peritoneal c.
  intraperitoneal c.
  joint c.
  c. lavage
  lesser sac of peritoneal c.
  lung c.
  marrow c.
  Meckel c.
  medullary c.
  midcarpal joint c.
  miniature uterine c.
  multiple thin-walled lung c.'s

nasal c.
c. of aneurysm
orbital c.
pericardial c.
peritoneal c.
pleural c.
popliteal c.
pulmonary c.
resection c.
retroperitoneal c.
saclike c.
septum pellucidum c.
sigmoid c.
sinonasal c.
sinus c.
Stafne idiopathic bone c.
subarachnoid c.
subchondral cystic c.
subdural c.
surgically created resection c.
synovial c.
syringohydromyelic c.
syrinx c.
thin-walled lung c.
thoracic c.
trigeminal c.
tubular c.
tympanic c.
uterine c.
ventricular c.
vertebral marrow c.
c. volume
c. wall
cavoatrial junction
cavogram, cavagram
cavography
cavoportal collateral
cavopulmonary connection
cavovalgus
pes c.
talipes c.
cavovarus
c. deformity
pes c.
cavum
c. septum pellucidum
c. veli interpositi
cavus
c. deformity
global c.
local c.
pes c.
posttraumatic c.
talipes c.
Cayler syndrome
CBCL
cutaneous B-cell lymphoma
CBD
common bile duct

CBDE
common bile duct exploration
CBF
cerebral blood flow
CBF index
CBFV
coronary blood flow velocity
CBI
convergent beam irradiation
CBT
corticobulbar tract
CBV
cerebral blood volume
CBV/CBF
cerebral blood volume to cerebral
blood flow ratio
cc
cubic centimeter
CCA
common carotid artery
CCAM
congenital cystic adenomatoid
malformation
CCD
central collodiaphysial
charge-coupled device
crossed cerebellar diaschisis
CCD angle
CCD detector
CCD photodetector
CCDS
color-coded duplex sonography
CCE
capacitative calcium entry
CCF
carotid-cavernous fistula
C-C
convexo-concave
C-C heart valve
CCJ
calcaneocuboid joint
CCK
cholecystokinin
CCL
calcaneocuboid ligament
CCRT
computer-controlled conformal radiation
therapy
C1-C5 segment of internal carotid artery
CCT
cranial computed tomography
CCTA
coronal computed tomographic
arthrography
CD
cluster of differentiation
color Doppler
Cd
cadmium

C

CDFI
color-coded Doppler flow
imaging
CDH
congenital dislocation of hip
CDI
color Doppler imaging
CDR
computed dental radiography
CDRPan digital x-ray system
CDS
color Doppler sonography
CDUS
color Doppler ultrasonography
microbubble-enhanced CDUS
CE
cardioesophageal
CE angle of Wiberg
CE junction
CEA
carotid endarterectomy
CEA-Scan
CEA-S. diagnostic imaging
CEA-S. imaging agent
cebocephaly
ceca (*pl. of* cecum)
cecal
c. appendage
c. appendix
c. bar
c. bascule
c. carcinoma
c. deformity
c. filling defect
c. fold
c. foramen
c. hernia
c. ileus
c. recess
c. serosa
c. sphincter
c. thickening
c. volvulus
**cecitis, typhlitis, typhlenteritis,
caecitis**
cecocutaneous fistula
cecostomy
percutaneous c.
CECT
contrast-enhanced computed tomography
cecum, *pl.* **ceca**
antimesocolic side of c.
caput c.
coned c.
conical c.
c. diameter
kidney-shaped distended c.
c. mobile
subhepatic c.

Cedell
C. fracture
C. fracture of talus
Cedell-Magnusson
C.-M. arthritis classification
C.-M. classification of arthritis
Ceelen-Gellerstedt syndrome
CE-FAST
contrast-enhanced Fourier-acquired
steady-state technique
CE-FAST scan
Celestin tube
celiac
c. angiography
c. arteriography
c. artery aneurysm
c. artery compression syndrome
c. artery dissection
c. axis
c. axis occlusion
c. axis syndrome
c. branch artery
c. disease
c. ganglion
c. ganglion block
c. lymph node
c. lymph node metastasis
c. plexus
c. plexus block
c. plexus blockade
c. plexus neurolysis, endoscopic
ultrasound-guided
c. trunk
celiacography
celioma
celiomesenteric trunk
celioscopy
celiotomy
cell
ABMMN c.
absorption c.
basket c.
cerebellar granule c.
chromium-heated red blood c.
contaminating tumor c.
encroaching endothelial c.
c. engraftment
enterochromaffin c.
epithelial c.
ethmoid air c.
glomerular mesangial c.
homophilic Purkinje c.
human aortic smooth muscle c.
^{111In}-labeled white blood c.
Kulchitsky c.
c. labeling
mast c.
morula-like epithelial c.
Onodi c.

perivascular epithelioid c. (PEC)
photo c.
pluripotential bronchial epithelial
    stem c.
c. polarization
polygonal elongate c.
polymorphonuclear c.
c. preparation bone marrow uptake
protein-nucleic acid synthesis in
    tumor c.
Rael c.
red blood c. (RBC)
Rieder c.
Schwann c.
small c.
stem c.
T4 c.
tagged red c.
tanned red c. (TRC)
technetium-99m-labeled damaged red
    blood c.
technetium 99m red blood c.
    (^{99m}Tc-RBC)
technetium-99m-tagged red blood c.
technetium-tagged red blood c.
T-helper c. (type 1)
totipotential stem c.
c. tumor
white blood c. (WBC)
Zimmerman c.
cella media index
cell-dose threshold
cell-mediated immune response
celloidin section
CellSeek technology
cellular
c. binding site
c. bronchiolitis
c. embolus
c. fibroadenoma
c. tumor
cellularity
cellule formation
cellulitis
iodine-131-induced c.
orbital c.
celomic
c. metaphysis
c. pouch
CEM
central extensor mechanism
Cemax/Icon PACS system
cement
bone c.
c. embolus
c. line
c. mantle
radiopaque bone c.
residual c.

cemental
c. dysplasia
c. fracture
cementation
cementifying fibroma
cementoblastoma
cementoma
gigantiform c.
cementoosseous dysplasia
cementoossifying fibroma
cementoplasty
percutaneous c.
cementosis
cementum
CEMRA
contrast-enhanced magnetic resonance
    angiography
3D CEMRA
Cencit surface scanner
**Centauri Er:YAG dental laser
    system**
center
accessory ossification c.
anechoic c.
bone c.
cortical c.
diaphysial c.
elbow bone c.
emetic c.
enlargement with low-density lymph
    node c.
epileptogenic c.
epiphysial fetal bone c.
epiphysial ossification c.
femoral ossification c.
fetal epiphysial bone c.
c. line artifact
lucent c.
c. of gravity
C. of Metabolic and Experimental
    Imaging
c. of rotation (COR)
ossification c.
ovoid ossification c.
swallowing c.
tibial tubercle ossification c.
vertebral body ossification c.
window c.
center-compression
Houston Advanced Research C.-C.
    (HARC-C)
center-edge
c.-e. angle of Lequesne
c.-e. angle of Wiberg
center-to-center distance
centigray (cGy)
centimeter (cm)
cubic c. (cc)
centra (*pl. of* centrum)

central
   c. airway disease
   c. amaurosis
   c. aorta
   c. aortic pressure
   c. artery
   c. axis depth dose
   c. beaking
   c. blood volume
   c. bone
   c. bronchiectasis
   c. bronchovascular bundle
   c. caged ball occluder valve
   c. caged disc occluder valve
   c. callus
   c. canal stenosis
   c. caseous necrosis
   c. cavity of cerebrum
   c. cementifying fibroma
   c. cerebellar fissure
   c. cervical cord syndrome
   c. channel
   c. chondrosarcoma
   c. collodiaphysial (CCD)
   c. collodiaphysial angle
   c. diabetes insipidus
   c. dislocation
   c. extensor mechanism (CEM)
   c. fat signal intensity
   c. fatty hilum
   c. fibrosarcoma
   c. fracture
   c. groove
   c. gyrus
   c. hemorrhagic component
   c. herniation
   c. high signal intensity stripe
   c. hilar structure
   c. horn
   c. indentation
   c. intraluminal saturation stripe
   c. intrasubstance signal intensity
   c. lung distance (CLD)
   c. lymph node
   c. medullary bone lesion
   c. nervous system (CNS)
   c. nervous system infection
   c. nervous system tumor
   c. neurocytoma
   c. neurofibromatosis
   c. nidus
   c. nidus of high-intensity marrow
   c. ossifying fibroma
   c. osteosarcoma
   c. pancreatic lesion scar
   c. perineal tendon
   c. pit
   c. placenta previa
   c. pneumonia
   c. point artifact
   c. pontile
   c. pontile myelinolysis
   c. ray
   c. rhomboid attachment
   c. sacral line (CSL)
   c. sinus lipomatosis
   c. skeleton
   c. solitary papilloma breast
   c. spinal canal
   c. spinal cord syrinx
   c. spinal stenosis
   c. splanchnic venous thrombosis (CSVT)
   c. sulcus
   c. tegmental tract (CTT)
   c. tendon diaphragm
   c. vein
   c. venous access
   c. venous catheter (CVC)
   c. venous drainage
   c. venous line position
   c. venous obstruction
   c. venous pressure (CVP)
   c. venous pressure line
   c. vertebral osteomyelitis

centralis
   ala lobuli c.
   fovea c.

centrally
   c. ordered phase encoding
   c. uninhibited bladder

centriacinar emphysema

centriciput

centrifugation
   discontinuous density gradient c.

centrilobar
   c. interstitium
   c. opacity

centrilobular
   c. congestion
   c. distribution
   c. emphysema
   c. lesion
   c. micronodule
   c. necrosis
   c. nodule
   c. region of liver
   c. shadow

centroblast

centroblastic lymphoma

centrocyte-like type

centrocytic lymphoma

centrocytoid

centroid
   endocardial c.
   epicardial c.

floating endocardial c.
floating epicardial c.
myocardial c.
centroid-based maximum-intensity projection
centromere
centrum, *pl.* **centra**
    c. commune
    c. ovale
    c. semiovale
    c. semiovale pattern
Centurion PTA balloon dilation catheter
cephalad direction
cephalic
    c. angle
    c. angulation
    c. arch stenosis
    c. flexure
    c. index
    c. pole
    c. presentation
    c. presentation of fetus
    c. tilt view
    c. triangle
    c. vein
    c. ventricle
cephalization of blood flow
cephalized vessel
cephalocaudad direction
cephalocele
    atretic c.
    congenital c.
    occipital c.
    oral c.
    sincipital c.
cephalofacial proportionality
cephalogram imaging
cephalohematocele
cephalohematoma
    parietal c.
cephalomedullary nail fracture
cephalometer
    Bertillon c.
cephalometric
    c. analysis
    c. angle
    c. radiograph
cephalometry
    radiographic c.
    ultrasonic c.
cephalopelvic
    c. disproportion (CPD)
    c. disproportion index
cephalopelvimetry, pelvicephalography, pelvocephalography
cephalosporin
cephalostat

cephalosyndactyly
    Vogt c.
CEqual quantitative analysis
CerASPECT
    C. camera
    C. system
ceratocricoid ligament
cerebella (*pl. of* cerebellum)
cerebellar
    c. anaplasia
    c. aplasia
    c. apoplexy
    c. artery
    c. astrocytoma
    c. atrophy
    c. attachment
    c. cortex
    c. cystic mass
    c. degeneration
    c. diaschisis
    c. ectopia
    c. epidermoid
    c. fiber
    c. folium
    c. gliosarcoma
    c. granule cell
    c. hemangioblastoma
    c. hemisphere
    c. hemorrhage
    c. heterotopia
    c. hypoperfusion
    c. hypoplasia
    c. infarct
    c. notch
    c. pathway
    c. peduncle
    c. peg
    c. sarcoma
    c. syndrome
    c. tonsil
    c. tract
    c. uvula
    c. vermis
    c. vermis hypoplasia, oligophrenia, congenital ataxia, ocular coloboma, hepatic fibrosis (COACH)
    c. view
    c. volume
cerebelli
    falx c.
    tentorium c.
    vallecula c.
    vermis c.
cerebellitis
cerebellolabyrinthine artery
cerebellomedullary cistern
cerebelloolivary degeneration
cerebellopontile (*var. of* cerebellopontine)

C

cerebellopontine, cerebellopontile
    c. angle (CPA)
    c. angle meningioma
    c. angle tumor
    c. cistern
    c. cisternography
    c. recess
cerebelloretinal
    c. hemangioblastoma
    c. hemangioblastomatosis
cerebellum, *pl.* **cerebella,** *pl.* **cerebellums**
    amygdala of c.
    basal ganglion of c.
    dentate nucleus of c.
    fetal c.
    flocculonodular lobe of c.
    Gowers bundle in c.
    inverse c.
    midline c.
    petrosal c.
    towering c.
cerebellums (*pl. of* cerebellum)
cerebra (*pl. of* cerebrum)
cerebral
    c. abscess
    c. amaurosis
    c. amyloid angiopathy
    c. aneurysm
    c. angiography
    c. anoxia
    c. apotentiality
    c. aqueduct
    c. arterial circle
    c. arteriography
    c. arteriosclerosis
    c. arteriovenous fistula
    c. arteriovenous malformation
    c. artery
    c. artery infarct
    c. artery stenosis
    c. astrocytoma
    c. blood flow (CBF)
    c. blood flow study
    c. blood vessel
    c. blood volume (CBV)
    c. blood volume map
    c. blood volume to cerebral blood
    flow ratio (CBV/CBF)
    c. calcification
    c. circulation
    c. circulation time
    c. commissure
    c. congestion
    c. contrast medium
    c. contusion
    c. convexity
    c. convolution
    c. cortex
    c. cortical gyral pattern

    c. CT venography
    c. cyst
    c. death
    c. dominance
    c. dysfunction
    c. edema
    c. embolism
    c. fat embolus
    c. fissure
    c. flexure
    c. flow image technique
    c. gammography
    c. gigantism
    c. glioma
    c. gyri interdigitation
    c. hemiatrophy
    c. hemidecortication
    c. hemisphere
    c. hemorrhage
    c. herniation
    c. hypoperfusion
    c. hypotension
    c. infarct
    c. inflammatory disease
    c. infundibulum
    c. ischemia
    c. ischemic event
    c. lesion
    c. lymphoma
    c. malformation classification
    c. mantle
    c. metabolic oxygen consumption
    c. metabolic rate of glucose
    c. metabolic rate of oxygen
    (CMRO$_2$)
    c. metabolism
    c. metastasis
    c. microembolism
    c. neuroblastoma
    c. nodule
    c. operculum
    c. palsy pathologic fracture
    c. parenchyma
    c. peduncle
    c. perfusion pressure (CPP)
    c. perfusion SPECT imaging
    c. perfusion SPECT scan
    c. perfusion study
    c. pneumoencephalography
    c. pneumography
    c. pneumonia
    c. porosis
    c. radionecrosis
    c. revascularization
    c. ridge
    c. salt wasting
    c. scintigraphy
    c. shunt
    c. sinovenous occlusion

c. sinusography
c. sparganosis
c. SPECT
c. steal syndrome
c. sulcus
c. surface
c. surface atrophy
c. thrombophlebitis
c. toxoplasmosis
c. tuberculoma
c. vascular microlattice
c. vasculature
c. vasoreactivity
c. vasospasm
c. vein
c. venous sinus
c. venous sinus thrombosis (CVST)
c. ventricle
c. ventricular shunt connector
c. ventriculography
c. vesicle
c. Whipple disease
c. white matter hypoplasia

cerebri
choana c.
commotio c.
contusio c.
falx c.
fornix c.
gliomatosis c.
gyri c.
hypophysis c.
pseudotumor c.

cerebriform carcinoma
cerebritis
lupus c.
sinusitis c.

cerebrohepatorenal syndrome (CHRS)
cerebromacular degeneration (CMD)
cerebromeningeal intracerebral
  hemorrhage
cerebropontocerebellar pathway
cerebroside lipidosis
cerebrospinal
c. canal
c. fluid (CSF)
c. fluid circulation
c. fluid-containing lesion
c. fluid diversion
c. fluid fistula
c. fluid flow measurement
c. fluid flow waveform
c. fluid hypovolemia
c. fluid leak
c. fluid obstruction
c. fluid pathway
c. fluid pressure
c. fluid shunt function
c. fluid volume

cerebrotendinous xanthomatosis
cerebrovascular
c. accident (CVA)
c. aneurysmal clip
c. insufficiency
c. insult
c. malformation
c. occlusive disease
c. stroke

cerebrum, *pl.* **cerebra**
central cavity of c.
cistern of lateral fossa of c.
cortex of c.
degenerative disease in c.
c. demyelination
great vein of c.
lateral ventricle of c.
1st ventricle of c.
2nd ventricle of c.
3rd ventricle of c.

Cerefy neuroradiology atlas
Cerenkov
C. calculation
C. count
C. counter
C. measurement
C. radiation
C. radiation production
C. scintillation analysis

Ceretec
C. brain imaging
^{99m}Tc C.
C. radioisotope imaging agent
technetium 99m C.

CereTom portable CT scanner
cerium silicate imaging agent
ceroid gallbladder granuloma
Cerrobend block
cervical
c. adenocarcinoma
c. adenopathy
c. aorta
c. aortic arch
c. canal
c. cancer
c. cord
c. cord injury
c. cord lesion
c. CSF systole
c. CT
c. disc
c. disc disease
c. disc herniation
c. disc syndrome
c. dysplasia
c. enlargement
c. esophagostomy
c. esophagus
c. eversion

cervical (*continued*)
   c. facet
   c. facet dislocation
   c. fascia
   c. flexure
   c. flush
   c. fusion of spine
   c. ganglion
   c. heart
   c. interbody fusion
   c. intraepithelial neoplasia
   c. length
   c. loop
   c. lordosis
   c. lordotic curvature
   c. lymphadenopathy
   c. lymph node tuberculous adenitis
   c. magnetic resonance phlebography
     (CMRP)
   c. meningocele
   c. mover ligament
   c. mucus arborization
   c. muscle
   c. musculature
   c. myelogram
   c. myelography
   c. nerve root
   c. neural foramen
   c. neuroblastoma
   c. osteophyte
   c. outlet
   c. pain syndrome
   c. paraganglioma
   c. paratracheal lymph node
   c. pleura
   c. plexus
   c. polyp
   c. pregnancy
   c. rest
   c. rib
   c. rib anomaly
   c. rib syndrome
   c. sarcoma
   c. segment of internal carotid
     artery
   c. sinus
   c., skull, and shoulder block
   c. skull pillow
   c. spine
   c. spine curve
   c. spine dens view
   c. spine fracture
   c. spine fusion
   c. spine injury
   c. spine spondylosis
   c. spondylotic myelopathy
     (CSM)
   c. spondylotic radiculopathy
   c. stenosis

   c. stroma
   c. structure
   c. synostosis
   c. synspondylism
   c. syringomyelia
   c. thymic cyst
   c. triangle
   c. tuberculosis
   c. tuberculous lymphadenitis
   c. tumor
   c. vein
   c. vertebra
   c. vesicle
cervices (*pl. of* cervix)
cervicitis
cervicoabdominal node
cervicoaxillary canal
cervicocentral compartment
cervicocerebral
cervicocranium
cervicography
cervicomedullary
   c. junction
   c. kink
cervicooccipital fusion
cervicothoracic
   c. ganglion
   c. junction
   c. sagittal scout image
   c. sign
cervicothoracolumbar
cervicotrochanteric fracture
cervigram
cervix, *pl.* **cervices**
   cockscomb appearance of c.
   double c.
   incompetent c.
   c. uteri
   uterine c.
CES
   cauda equina syndrome
cesium
   c. 137 (^{137}Cs, Cs-137)
   c. 139 (^{139}Cs, Cs-139)
   c. chloride imaging agent
   c. implant
   c. iodide input phosphor
   c. iodide scintillator
   c. needle
   c. with barium 137m
Cestan-Chenais syndrome
cestodic tuberculosis
^{252}Cf, Cf-252
   californium 252
Cf
   californium
CFA
   cut-film angiography
   CFA digital camera

CFD
 color-flow Doppler
CFI
 color-flow imaging
CFL
 calcaneofibular ligament
C-flex stent
CFR
 coronary flow reserve
CF-UM3 echocolonoscope
CGI
 common gateway interface
cGy
 centigray
Chaddock sign
chain
 branched c.
 c. cystogram
 c. cystourethrography
 heavy c.
 image c.
 internal mammary lymphatic c.
 J c.
 jugulodigastric c.
 Markov c.
 obturator nodal c.
 sympathetic c.
chain-of-lakes
 c.-o.-l. anatomy
 c.-o.-l. deformity
chalasia, chalasis
chalasis (*var. of* chalasia)
chalky bone
challenge
 ergotamine c.
 solid bolus c.
chamber
 abnormal dimension of cardiac
  c.
 alpha c.
 cardiac c.
 cloud c.
 c. compression
 defective communication between
  cardiac c.'s
 c. dilation
 c. enlargement
 false aneurysmal c.
 hydraulic c.
 infundibular c.
 ion c.
 ionization c.
 irradiation c.
 left atrial c.
 left ventricular c.
 multiwire proportional c.
 c. of heart
 personal ionization c.
 pocket c.

 reduced compliance of c.
 reentrant well c.
 right atrial c.
 right ventricular c.
 rudimentary outlet c.
 rudimentary ventricular c.
 spark c.
 c. volume
 well-type ionization c.
 Wilson cloud c.
2-chamber echocardiography
3-chamber heart
4-chamber
 4-c. apical view
 4-c. echocardiography
 4-c. hypertrophy
 4-c. plane
Chamberlain
 C. line
 C. procedure
Chamberlain-Towne view
champagne
 c. glass iliac wing
 c. glass pelvis
 c. glass ureter
champagne-bottle legs
chance
 c. equivalent
 C. spinal fracture
change
 age-related c.
 arthritic talonavicular c.
 asymmetric signal c.
 atherosclerotic c.
 attritional pattern c.
 basal ganglionic c.
 BOLD time course c.
 bony c.
 consolidative c.
 cystic c.
 deep gray matter nucleus c.
 degenerative osseous c.
 drug-induced brain c.
 dynamic cervical c.
 dystrophic c.
 E-A c.
 edemalike c.
 epithelial degenerative c.
 fatty marrow c.
 fibrocystic c.
 fibrotic c.
 fMRI signal c.
 focal degenerative c.
 high signal intensity ischemic c.
 hydropic c.
 interstitial c.
 interval c.
 ischemic c.
 lytic c.

C

change (*continued*)
  marrow signal c.
  microstructural c.
  mural c.
  myxoid degenerative c.
  nonspecific c.
  osteoarthritic c.
  papillary apocrine c.
  parenchymatous c.
  paroxysmal c.
  pathophysiologic c.
  pelvicalyceal c.
  pleural c.
  polyneuropathy, organomegaly, endocrinopathy, monoclonal gammopathy, skin c.'s (POEMS)
  postbiopsy c.
  postsurgical c.
  posttherapy c.
  postthoracotomy c.
  precancerous c.
  prediverticular c.
  preslip c.
  proliferative c.
  pulmonary parenchymatous c.
  radiation-induced c.
  radiation-related ischemic c.
  radiographic c.
  reciprocal c.
  residual interstitial c.
  residual limb-shaped c.
  senescent c.
  senile c.
  serial c.
  signal c.
  spinal endplate c.
  spondylitic c.
  spongiform c.
  stenotic c.
  vasomotor c.
change-of-angle view
changer
  Elema roll-film c.
  film c.
  Franklin c.
  Puck film c.
  rapid film c.
  Sanchez-Perez cassette c.
  Schonander film c.
  serial film c.
channel
  aberrant vascular c.
  blood c.
  central c.
  collateral venous c.
  deep venous c.
  dentate output c.
  engorged collateral venous c.

  enlarged vascular c.
  false c.
  gastric c.
  haversian c.
  Lambert c.
  lymphatic c.
  pancreaticobiliary common c.
  pyloric c.
  c. pyloric ulcer
  threads-and-streaks vascular c.
  true c.
  vascular c.
2-channel phased-array RF receiver coil system
6-channel posterior coil
chaotic heart
Chaoul
  C. therapy
  C. voltage x-ray tube
Chaput
  C. fracture
  C. tubercle
characteristic
  alternative free-response receiver operating c. (AFROC)
  associated imaging c.
  contrast transfer c.
  c. curve
  echo c.
  c. emission
  excitatory pulse c.
  c. finding
  generator c.
  pathognomonic imaging c.
  c. radiation
  receiver operating c. (ROC)
  signal c.
  suspension c.
  tip dispersion c.
  c. x-ray
characterization
  physicochemical c.
  tissue c.
charcoal
  dextran-coated c.
Charcot
  C. arthropathy
  C. chondroma
  C. cirrhosis
  C. deformity
  C. foot
  C. fracture
  C. joint
  C. spine
  C. triad
Charcot-Bouchard intracerebral microaneurysm
Charcot-Marie-Tooth (CMT)
  C.-M.-T. disease

charge
homogeneous positive c.
c. injection device (CID)
charge-coupled
c.-c. device (CCD)
c.-c. device scanner
c.-c. device TV camera
charged particle
charged-particle radiosurgery
CHARM
chunk acquisition and reconstruction
method
chart
Segre c.
x-ray tube rating c.
chase
bolus c.
c. bolus imaging technique
peripheral bolus c.
chaser
saline c.
Chassaignac muscle
Chassard-Lapiné
C.-L. position
C.-L. projection
C.-L. view
chastity ring artifact
Chauffard point
Chausse
C. III projection
3rd projection of C.
C. view
Chaussier
C. line
C. projection
C. view
CHB
complete heart block
CHD
common hepatic duct
congenital heart defect
congenital heart disease
arachnodactyly CHD
oligemia-related cyanotic CHD
plethora-related cyanotic CHD
check
design rule c.
Check-Flo sheath
Checkmate system
checkrein
c. deformity
c. ligament
check-valve
c.-v. mechanism
c.-v. sheath
Chédiak-Steinbrinck-Higashi syndrome
cheek bone
cheese
c. handler's lung

c. washer's lung
c. wiring
cheesy pneumonia
cheetah
C. angioplasty catheter
C. radiopaque contrast agent
cheirolumbar
cheiromegaly, chiromegaly
cheirospasm, chirospasm
chelate
Cr-HIDA c.
gadolinium c.
Gd-HIDA c.
chelating agent
chelonian pneumonia
chemical
c. dosimeter
c. peritonitis
c. pleurodesis
c. pneumonia
c. pneumonitis
c. potential energy
c. pulmonary edema
c. ray
c. shift
chemically
c. induced
c. induced dynamic nuclear
depolarization
c. induced dynamic nuclear
polarization
c. modified protein
chemical-selective
c.-s. fat-saturation imaging
c.-s. fat-saturation MR
chemical-shift
c.-s. artifact
c.-s. imaging (CSI)
c.-s. imaging technique
c.-s. magnetic resonance imaging
c.-s. misregistration
c.-s. ratio
c.-s. reference
c.-s. selective suppression technique
c.-s. spatial offset
chemiluminescence, chemoluminescence
chemisorb
chemisorption
chemistry
nuclear c.
radiation c.
radiopharmaceutical c.
chemodectoma
chest c.
chemoembolization
HCC c.
hepatic c.
segmental transcatheter arterial c.
c. solution

C

chemoembolization (*continued*)
    therapeutic c.
    transarterial c. (TACE)
    transcatheter arterial c. (TACE)
    transcatheter hepatic arterial c.
    transcatheter oily c.
chemohyperthermia
chemoinductive support
chemokine receptor (2, 3, 5)
chemokine-related receptor
chemoluminescence (*var. of*
  chemiluminescence)
Chemo-Port
    C.-P. catheter
    C.-P. vascular access system
chemoradiotherapy
    concurrent c.
chemotherapy
    antiangiogenic c.
    CT-guided intraarterial c.
    high-dose c.
    intraarterial c.
    intralesional c.
    intraperitoneal hyperthermic c.
    magnetic c.
    neoadjuvant c.
    primary c.
chemotherapy-induced
    c.-i. inflammation
    c.-i. necrosis
    c.-i. neutropenia
    c.-i. pneumonia
chemotoxic reaction
ChemSat fat suppression
chenodeoxycholic acid
Chen-Smith
    C.-S. image coder
    improved C.-S. (ICS)
Cherenkov effect
cherubism
CHESS
    Cornell high-energy synchrotron
    source
    CHESS method
chest
    alar c.
    barrel c.
    blast c.
    c. Bucky
    buffalo c.
    c. cavity
    c. chemodectoma
    cobbler's c.
    cylindrical c.
    dirty c.
    c. empyema
    expiratory c.
    c. film
    flail c.

    c. fluke lung
    c. fluoroscopy
    foveated c.
    funnel c.
    globular c.
    hollow c.
    hourglass c.
    jail-bar c.
    keeled c.
    c. lead
    narrow c.
    paralytic c.
    c. phantom
    phthinoid c.
    pigeon c.
    pneumonectomy c.
    pterygoid c.
    c. radiology
    symmetric c.
    tetrahedron c.
    c. tube
    c. view
    c. wall
    c. wall hamartoma
    c. wall lateral xeromammogram
    c. wall lesion
    c. wall mesenchymoma
    c. wall neuroblastoma
    c. wall paradoxic motion
    c. wall retraction
    c. wall rhabdomyosarcoma
    c. wall trauma
    c. x-ray (CXR)
chevron
    c. bone
    c. fracture
    c. fusion
CHF
    congenital hepatic fibrosis
    congestive heart failure
CHI
    closed head injury
Chiari
    C. formation
    C. I-II malformation
    C. I-IV lesion
Chiari-associated syringomyelia
chiasm, chiasma
    Camper c.
    cistern of c.
    c. of digit of hand
    optic c.
chiasmal
    c. compression
    c. lesion
chiasmatic
    c. cistern
    c. defect
    c. groove

chiasmatic-hypothalamic pilocytic astrocytoma
chiasmaticus
    sulcus c.
Chiba
    C. needle
    C. percutaneous cholangiogram
chickenpox
chicken-wire calcification
Chilaiditi
    C. sign
    C. syndrome
CIIILD
    congenital hemidysplasia with ichthyosiform erythroderma and limb defects
        CHILD syndrome
childhood
    c. discitis
    c. fracture
    c. osteomyelitis
    c. rhabdomyosarcoma
Child-Pugh
    C.-P. liver disease classification
    C.-P. liver function classification (A, B, C)
chimera
    radiation c.
chimney-shaped high aortic arch
Chinese fluke liver
chin-occiput piece
chip
    bone c.
    cancellous bone c.
    corticocancellous bone c.
    c. fracture
chiromegaly (*var. of* cheiromegaly)
chirospasm (*var. of* cheirospasm)
chisel fracture
chisellike truncated appearance
CH20 Kernal and slim 2 profile
Chlamydia
    C. pneumonitis
    C. trachomatis
chloride
    ^{111}In c.
    magnesium c.
    manganese c.
    polyvinyl c. (PVC)
    ^{89}Sr c.
    stannous c.
    strontium-89 c.
    thallium-201 c.
    Tl-201 c.
    triphenyltetrazolium c. (TTC)
    xenon c. (XeCl)
chloriodized oil
chlormerodrin accumulation test
chlormerodrin-cysteine complex

chloroleukemia (*var. of* chloroma)
chloroma, chloroleukemia
    bone c.
    gastric c.
    kidney c.
choana cerebri
choanal
    c. atresia
    c. polyp
chocolate
    c. cyst
    c. joint effusion
choked marrow
cholangeitis (*var. of* cholangitis)
cholangiectasis
    extrahepatic c.
cholangiitis (*var. of* cholangitis)
cholangiocarcinoma
    extrahepatic c.
    hilar c.
    intrahepatic c.
    peripheral c. (PCC)
Cholangiocath
cholangiocatheter
cholangiocellular carcinoma
cholangiodrainage
cholangiodysplastic pseudocirrhosis
cholangiofibromatosis
cholangiogram
    balloon c.
    catheter c.
    Chiba percutaneous c.
    common duct c.
    contrast selective c.
    cystic duct c.
    drip infusion c. (DIC)
    endoscopic retrograde c. (ERC)
    fine-needle transhepatic c. (FNTC)
    intraoperative c.
    intravenous c. (IVC)
    magnetic resonance c. (MRC)
    operative c.
    percutaneous transhepatic c. (PTC, PTCA, PTHC)
    retrograde c.
    serial c.'s
    single-shot MR c.
    transhepatic c. (THC)
    transjugular c.
    T-tube c. (TTC)
cholangiogram:yttrium-aluminum-garnet
    transhepatic c.:y.-a.-g. (THC:YAG)
cholangiography
    breath-hold MR c.
    c. catheter
    computed tomographic c.
    cystic duct c.
    delayed operative c.
    direct percutaneous transhepatic c.

C

cholangiography (*continued*)
    drip infusion c. (DIC)
    endoscopic retrograde c. (ERC)
    c. imaging
    intraoperative c.
    intravenous c.
    percutaneous hepatobiliary c.
    percutaneous transhepatic c. (PTC, PTCA)
    postoperative c.
    transabdominal c.
    T-tube c.
cholangiohepatitis
    Oriental c.
cholangiolithiasis
cholangiopancreatography
    endoscopic percutaneous c.
    endoscopic retrograde c. (ERCP)
    kinematic MR c.
    magnetic resonance c. (MRCP)
cholangioscopy
    contrast-enhanced virtual MR c.
cholangiotomogram
cholangiovenous communication
cholangitic biliary cirrhosis
cholangitis, cholangeitis, cholangiitis
    acute nonsuppurative ascending c.
    acute obstructive c.
    acute suppurative ascending c.
    AIDS c.
    ascending c.
    bacterial c.
    chronic nonsuppurative destructive c.
    fibrous obliterative c.
    intrahepatic sclerosing c.
    nonsuppurative ascending c.
    nonsuppurative destructive c.
    primary sclerosing c.
    progressive suppurative c.
    pyogenic c.
    recurrent pyogenic c.
    sclerosing c.
    secondary sclerosing c.
    septic c.
    suppurative ascending c.
Cholebrine imaging agent
cholecystectomy
    endoscopic laser c.
cholecystenteric anastomosis
cholecystitis
    acalculous c.
    acute c.
    calculous c.
    chronic c.
    emphysematous c.
    gangrenous acalculous c.
    gaseous c.
    c. glandularis proliferans
    lipid c.

    nongangrenous c.
    perforated c.
    c. with cholelithiasis
    xanthogranulomatous c.
cholecystocholangiography
cholecystocholangitis
cholecystocholedochal fistula
cholecystocholedochostomy
    percutaneous c.
cholecystocolic fistula
cholecystocutaneous fistula
cholecystoduodenal
    c. fistula
    c. ligament
cholecystoduodenocolic
    c. fistula
    c. fold
cholecystogram
    Graham-Cole c.
    oral c. (OCG)
cholecystography
    intravenous c.
    oral c.
    post fatty meal c.
cholecystokinetic food
cholecystokinin (CCK)
    c. cholescintigraphy
cholecystolithiasis
cholecystomegaly
cholecystopaque
cholecystopathy
cholecystoptosis
cholecystosis
    hyperplastic c.
cholecystosonography
cholecystostomy
    percutaneous transhepatic c.
    ultrasound-guided percutaneous c.
choledochal
    c. cyst
    c. sphincter
choledochal-colonic fistula
choledochocele
choledochocholedochostomy
choledochoduodenal
    c. fistula
    c. junctional stenosis
choledochofiberscope
    Olympus CHF-BP30 transduodenal c.
choledochogram
choledochograph
choledochography
choledochojejunostomy stricture
choledocholithiasis
choledochopancreatic ductal junction
choledochoscope
choledochoscopy
    percutaneous c.

choledochostomy
choledochous duct
cholegraphy
cholelith, chololith
cholelithiasis, chololithiasis
    cholecystitis with c.
cholelithoptysis
cholescintigraphy, cholescintography
    cholecystokinin c.
    radionuclide c.
    sincalide c.
cholescintography (*var. of*
 cholescintigraphy)
cholestasis
    intrahepatic c.
    progressive familial intrahepatic c.
    (PFIC)
cholestatic liver disease
cholesteatoma
    attic c.
    congenital c.
    c. cyst
    ear c.
    GU tract c.
    inflammatory c.
    pars flaccida c.
    pars tensa c.
    primary acquired c.
    primary CNS c.
    primary temporal bone c.
    secondary acquired c.
cholesterinosis
cholesterol
    c. debris
    c. ear cyst
    c. ear granuloma
    c. embolus
    c. gallbladder polyp
    c. gallstone
    I-labeled c.
cholesterol-based scintigraphy
cholesterol-containing brain lesion
Choletec radionuclide imaging agent
choline tumor
Cholografin
    C. meglumine
    C. meglumine imaging agent
chololith (*var. of* cholelith)
chololithiasis (*var. of* cholelithiasis)
chondral
    c. defect
    c. fracture
    c. fragment
chondrification
chondritis
chondroblastic osteosarcoma
chondroblastoma
    benign c.
    c. straddling

chondrocalcinosis
    familial c.
chondrocyte
    atypical c.
    c. degeneration
    epiphysial c.
    regenerative c.
chondrodiastasis
chondrodysplasia
    c. calcificans
    Jansen-type metaphysial c.
    McKusick-type metaphysial c.
    metaphysial c.
    c. punctata
    Schmid-like metaphysial c.
chondrodystrophia (*var. of*
 chondrodystrophy)
    c. calcificans congenita
    c. fetalis
chondrodystrophy, chondrodystrophia
chondroectodermal dysplasia
chondrofibroma
chondrogenic tumor
chondrogladiolar
chondroid
    c. matrix
    c. syringoma
    c. tissue
chondroid-origin tumor
chondroitin
    c. sulfate iron colloid-enhanced MRI
    c. sulfate proteoglycan 3
chondrolipoma
chondrolysis
    posttraumatic c.
chondroma
    Charcot c.
    extraskeletal c.
    joint c.
    juxtacortical c.
    soft tissue c.
chondromalacia
    c. patéllae
    patellar c.
    ulnar c.
    c. with fibrillation
    c. with surface fraying
chondromanubrial
chondromatosis
    Henderson-Jones c.
    secondary c.
    synovial c.
chondromatous hamartoma
chondromyofibroma
chondromyxoid fibroma (CMF),
 chondromyxoma
chondromyxoma (*var. of* chondromyxoid
 fibroma)
chondromyxosarcoma

C

chondronecrosis
chondroosteodystrophy
chondrophyte
chondroplasia calcificans
chondroporosis
chondrosarcoma
  central c.
  endosteal c.
  exostotic c.
  extraskeletal mesenchymal c.
  extraskeletal myxoid c.
  juxtacortical c.
  malignant c.
  mesenchymal c.
  myxoid extraskeletal c.
  parosteal c.
  peripheral c.
  skeletal myxoid c.
chondrosarcomatosis
chondrosteoma
chondrosternal junction
chondroxiphoid ligament
chop amputation
Chopart
  C. fracture
  C. fracture-dislocation
  C. hindfoot amputation
  C. joint
chopper
  McIlwain tissue c.
Chopper-Dixon fat-suppression
  imaging
Choquet fuzzy integral
choracobrachialis
chord
  contiguous parallel c.'s
  multiple c.'s
chorda, *pl.* chordae
  basal c.
  cleft c.
  commissural c.
  c. magna
  1st-order c.
  2nd-order c.
  3rd-order c.
  strut c.
  chordae tendineae cordis
  chordae tendineae rupture
  c. tympani
  chordae willisii
chordae (*pl. of* chorda)
chordal rupture
chordate
chordocarcinoma
chordoepithelioma
chordoma
  clivus c.
  sacral c.
  sacrococcygeal c.

sphenooccipital c.
spinal c.
vertebral c.
chordosarcoma
chorea
  Huntington c.
choreiform movement
chorioallantoic placenta
chorioamnionic, chorioamniotic
  c. elevation
  c. separation
chorioamniotic (*var. of* chorioamnionic)
chorioangioma
choriocarcinoma
  esophageal c.
  gestational c.
  ovarian c.
  primary ovarian c.
  testicular c.
choriodecidua
choriodecidual reaction
chorionic
  c. carcinoma
  c. disc
  c. gonadotropin
  c. sac
  c. tissue
chorionicity
chorioretinitis
choristoma
  middle ear c.
  renal c.
choroid
  c. glomus
  c. plexus
  c. plexus blush
  c. plexus calcification
  c. plexus carcinoma
  c. plexus cyst
  c. plexus hemorrhage
  c. plexus neoplasia
  c. plexus papilloma
  c. point
  c. vein
choroidal
  c. fissure
  c. hemangioma
  medial posterior c. (MPCh)
  c. metastasis
  c. neovascularization (CNV)
  c. osteoma
  c. pericallosal artery
choroidal-hippocampal fissure complex
choroidea
  tela c.
choroideum
  glomus c.
Christian brachydactyly
Christmas tree appearance

chromaffin
c. paraganglioma
c. tumor
chromated Cr-51 serum albumin imaging agent
chromatic spectrum
chromatid-type aberration
chromatogram
chromatographic-fluorometric technique
chromatographic separation
chromatography
absorption c.
antiidiotypic affinity c.
DEAE-Sephadex A-25 c.
gas-liquid phase c. (GLPC)
high-performance liquid c.
high-performance size-exclusion c.
high-pressure liquid c.
ion-exchange c.
ChromaVision digital analyzer
chromic phosphate suspension
Chromitope sodium
chromium (Cr)
c. CR-51 serum albumin
c. imaging agent
c. phosphate
chromium-heated red blood cell
chromium-hepatic dimethyl iminodiacetic acid (Cr-HIDA)
chromium-thulium-erbium:yttrium-aluminum-garnet (CTE:YAG)
chromium:yttrium-aluminum-garnet
erbium c.:y.-a.-g. (ErCr:YAG)
chromophobe
kidney carcinoma c.
pituitary adenoma c.
chromoscopy time
chromosome
bacterial artificial c. (BAC)
normal male sex c. (type XY)
Philadelphia c.
chronic
c. abdominal inflammation
c. airway obstruction (CAO)
c. alveolar infiltrate
c. atrophic duodenitis
c. atrophic pyelonephritis
c. berylliosis
c. beryllium disease
c. breast abscess
c. bronchitis
c. calcifying pancreatitis
c. cerebral ischemia
c. cholecystitis
c. communicating hydrocephalus
c. constrictive state
c. diffuse confluent lung opacity
c. diffuse reticulation
c. diffuse sclerosing alveolitis

c. diverticulitis
c. duodenal ileus
c. edema
c. esophagitis
c. expanding hematoma
c. extrinsic allergic alveolitis
c. fibrosing alveolitis
c. fibrosing mesenteritis
c. fissure
c. friction and impingement
c. functional instability
c. gastric atony
c. gastritis
c. glomerulonephritis
c. heart failure
c. hemodynamic overload
c. hepatitis
c. hereditary nephritis
c. hydronephrosis
c. hypertrophic emphysema
c. idiopathic intestinal pseudoobstruction (CIIP)
c. ileus duodenum
c. infantile hyperostosis
c. insufficiency of vein
c. intermittent atelectasis
c. interstitial pneumonia
c. interstitial salpingitis
c. interstitial simulating airspace lung disease
c. irritation
c. ischemic brain infarct
c. ligament complex laxity
c. ligamentous injury
c. lung thromboembolism
c. lymphedematous limb
c. lymphocytic leukemia
c. lymphocytic thyroiditis
c. mesenteric ischemia (CMI)
c. multifocal ill-defined lung opacity
c. myeloid leukemia
c. myelomonocytic leukemia (CMML)
c. necrotizing aspergillosis
c. nonsuppurative destructive cholangitis
c. obstructive emphysema
c. obstructive lung disease (COLD)
c. obstructive pancreatitis
c. obstructive pulmonary disease (COPD)
c. obstructive uropathy
c. outward force
c. overuse syndrome
c. parenchymal hemorrhage
c. partial epilepsy
c. passive congestion
c. peptic ulcer
c. periaortitis

C

chronic (*continued*)
    c. peripheral arterial disease (CPAD)
    c. phase
    c. phase chronic myelogenous leukemia
    c. pleurisy
    c. pneumonitis
    c. posttraumatic aortic pseudoaneurysm
    c. pulmonary emphysema (CPE)
    c. recurrent dislocation
    c. recurrent multifocal osteomyelitis (CRMO)
    c. recurrent sialadenitis
    c. renal failure (CRF)
    c. renal failure amyloidosis
    c. renal infarct
    c. renal vein thrombosis
    c. reserve flow
    c. respiratory decompensation
    c. retrocalcaneal bursitis
    c. sclerosing osteomyelitis
    c. simple silicosis
    c. sinusitis
    c. sprain
    c. subdural hematoma (CSDH)
    c. subperitoneal sclerosis
    c. tamponade
    c. testicular torsion
    c. thromboembolic pulmonary hypertension
    c. tuberculous emphysema
    c. ulcerative colitis (CUC)
    c. venous insufficiency
    c. venous stasis
chronologic age
chronology
    imaging c.
chronotherapy
    adjuvant c.
chronotropic incompetence
chronotropy
CHRS
    cerebrohepatorenal syndrome
Chrys CO$_2$ laser
chrysotile asbestos
chunk acquisition and reconstruction method (CHARM)
Churg-Strauss syndrome
chyle
    c. cistern
    effused c.
    c. fistula
    c. leak
    c. vessel
chyli
    ampulla c.
    cisterna c.
chyliferous vessel

chylocele
    nonfilarial c.
chyloma
chylomediastinum
chylopericardium
chylosus
chylothorax
    postoperative c.
chylous
    c. ascites
    c. effusion
    c. fistula
    c. leakage
    c. reflux
chyluria
CI
    cardiac index
Ci
    curie
CIA
    calcaneal inclination angle
cicatrices (*pl. of* cicatrix)
cicatricial
    c. atelectasis
    c. kidney
    c. stricture
cicatrix, *pl.* **cicatrices**
cicatrization atelectasis
CID
    charge injection device
    CID camera
Cidtech camera
cigarroa formula
CIIP
    chronic idiopathic intestinal pseudoobstruction
ciliaris
    zonula c.
ciliary
    c. canal
    c. cartilage
    c. ganglionic plexus
    c. ligament
    c. ring
    c. vein
ciliated border
ciliospinal center of Budge
Cimino
    C. AV shunt
    C. dialysis shunt
CIN
    contrast-induced nephropathy
cine
    c. acquisition
    c. camera
    c. coronary arteriography
    c. CT imaging
    c. film
    c. fistulogram

c. gradient-echo MR imaging
c. gradient-echo sequence
c. gradient magnetic resonance
   imaging
c. left ventriculogram
c. loop
C. Memory with color-flow Doppler
   imaging
c. mode
parallel c.
c. phase-contrast imaging
c. projector
c. raw data
segmented c.
c. study
velocity-encoded c. (VEC)
c. view
c. view imaging
c. view in MUGA scan
cineangiocardiogram (CACG)
cineangiocardiography
cineangiogram
   ventricular c.
cineangiography
   aortic root c.
   axial c.
   biplane c.
   coronary c.
   radionuclide c.
   selective coronary c.
cinearteriography
   Judkins selective left coronary c.
cine-based viewing
cinebronchogram
cinecardioangiography
cine-CT
   c.-CT scan
   c.-CT scanner
cinedefecogram
cinedensigraphy
cine-encoded image
cineesophagogram
cine-FFE breath-hold sequence
cinefluorography
   biplane c.
cinefluoroscopy
   valve c.
cine-gated imaging
cine-magnetic
   c.-m. resonance function image
   c.-m. resonance imaging
   c.-m. resonance tagging
cinematographic
cinematography
cinematoradiography
cinemicrography
cine-mode display
cine-MR
   breath-hold c.-MR

cinepharyngoesophagogram
cinephlebography
cineportography
cineradiofluorography,
   cineroentgenofluorography
cineradiographic view
cineradiography, cineroentgenography
   c. imaging
cinereum
   tuber c.
cineroentgenofluorography (*var. of*
   cineradiofluorography)
cineroentgenography (*var. of*
   cineradiography)
cineurography
cineventriculogram
cineventriculography
   biplanar c.
cingula (*pl. of* cingulum)
cingulate
   c. cortex
   c. gyrus
   c. herniation
   c. sulcus
cingulum, *pl.* **cingula**
cipher
   transposition c.
ciprofloxacin
   ^{99m}Tc c.
   technetium 99m c.
circadian
   c. continuous infusion
   c. pattern
   c. periodicity
   c. variation
circle
   anastomotic arterial c.
   arterial c.
   articular vascular c.
   cerebral arterial c.
   c. loop biliary drainage
   c. of confusion
   c. of Vieussens
   c. of Willis
   c. wire nephrostomy
Circon videocamera
circuit
   anticoincidence c.
   application-specific integrated c.
      (ASIC)
   arrhythmia c.
   bridge c.
   bypass c.
   coincidence c.
   double-broadband triple-resonance
      NMR probe c.
   macroreentrant c.
   magnetic c.
   magnetoresistive sensor c.

C

circuit (*continued*)
    microreentrant c.
    phototube output c.
    quad-resonance NMR probe c.
    reentry c.
    shunting c.
    triple-resonance NMR probe c.
circular
    c. dichroism spectroscopy
    c. fold
    c. lesion
    c. muscle
    c. plane
    c. polarization wave
    c. polarized volume head coil
    c. sinus
    c. supracondylar amputation
    c. syncytium
    c. tomosynthesis
circulares
    plicae c.
circularly polarized coil
circulating blood volume
circulation
    allantoic c.
    anterior carotid c.
    arrested c.
    balanced c.
    bronchial collateral c.
    cardiac c.
    carotid c.
    cerebral c.
    cerebrospinal fluid c.
    codominant c.
    c. collapse
    collateral mesenteric c.
    compensatory c.
    cutaneous collateral c.
    derivative c.
    devoid of c.
    c. disturbance
    extracardiac collateral c.
    extracorporeal c.
    extracranial carotid c.
    extracranial cerebral c.
    c. failure
    fetal c.
    greater c.
    high-impedance c.
    intervillous c.
    intraaneurysmal flow c.
    intracranial c.
    Korotkoff test for collateral c.
    microvascular c.
    peripheral c.
    persistent fetal c.
    placental c.
    portosystemic collateral c.
    posterior fossa c.

    pulmonary arterial c.
    reduced c.
    c. shock
    spiderweb c.
    c. stasis
    systemic arterial c.
    thebesian c.
    thoracoabdominal venous collateral c.
    c. time
    uteroplacental c.
    venous c.
    vertebrobasilar c.
    c. volume
circulator
    sequential c.
circulatory
    c. arrest
    c. compromise
    c. embarrassment
    c. impairment
circumaortic left renal vein
circumaxillary
circumcaval ureter
circumduction
circumduction-adduction shoulder maneuver
circumference
    abdominal c.
    femur length to abdominal c.
    fetal abdominal c.
    fetal head c.
    fetal thoracic c.
    head c.
    head circumference to abdominal c. (HC/AC)
    c. of fetal head
    thoracic c.
circumferential
    c. cartilage
    c. echodense layer
    c. extremity coil
    c. fibrocartilage
    c. fracture
    c. lamella
    c. narrowing
    c. shortening
    c. thickening
    c. venous stenosis
circumflex
    c. branch
    c. coronary artery
    c. groove artery
    humeral c.
    left c.
    c. retroesophageal arch
    c. system
    c. vein
    c. vessel

circummarginate placenta
circummesencephalic cistern
circumscribed
    c. edema
    c. infiltrate
    c. lesion
    c. margin
    c. mass
    c. nodule
    c. pleurisy
    well c.
circumscripta
    calcinosis c.
    myositis ossificans c.
    osteitis fibrosa c.
    osteoporosis c.
circumscript aneurysm
circumvallate papilla
circumventricular organ
cirrhosis
    acholangic biliary c.
    acute juvenile c.
    alcoholic c.
    atrophic c.
    biliary c.
    Budd c.
    calculous c.
    cardiac c.
    Charcot c.
    cholangitic biliary c.
    congestive c.
    Cruveilhier-Baumgarten c.
    cryptogenic c.
    decompensated alcoholic
     c.
    diffuse c.
    endstage c.
    fatty c.
    focal biliary c.
    frank c.
    glabrous c.
    Hanot c.
    hepatic c.
    hypertrophic c.
    Indian childhood c.
    juvenile c.
    liver c.
    macrolobular c.
    medionodular c.
    metabolic c.
    microlobular c.
    micronodular c.
    multilobular c.
    nutritional c.
    obstructive biliary c.
    periportal c.
    pipestem c.
    porta c.
    posthepatitic c.

    postnecrotic c.
    primary biliary c.
    progressive familial c.
    pulmonary c.
    secondary biliary c.
    septal c.
    stasis c.
    Todd c.
    toxic c.
    unilobular c.
    vascular c.
cirrhosis-related fibrosis
cirrhotic
    c. gastritis
    c. inflammation
    c. liver
    c. nodule
cirsoid
    c. aneurysm
    c. placenta
cistern
    ambient wing of quadrigeminal
     c.
    anterior interhemispheric c.
    basal arachnoid c.
    basilar c.
    carotid c.
    cerebellomedullary c.
    cerebellopontine c.
    chiasmatic c.
    chyle c.
    circummesencephalic c.
    crural c.
    c. effacement
    great c.
    increased basilar c.
    c. indium
    interpeduncular c. (IPC)
    c. isotope
    mesencephalic c.
    c. of chiasm
    c. of lamina terminalis
    c. of lateral fossa of cerebrum
    c. of Pecquet
    c. of Sylvius
    opticochiasmatic c.
    c. oxygen
    parasellar c.
    perimesencephalic c.
    pontile c.
    posterior c.
    prepontine c.
    quadrigeminal plate c.
    c. radioisotope
    subarachnoid c.
    suprasellar subarachnoid c.
    sylvian c.
    terminal c.
    trigeminal c.

C

cisterna, *pl.* **cisternae**
 c. chyli
 c. magna
 c. magna effacement
cisternae (*pl. of* cisterna)
cisternal
 c. herniation
 c. puncture
 c. space
cisternogram
 CT c.
 metrizamide CT c.
cisternography
 air c.
 cerebellopontine c.
 computed tomography c.
 CT c.
 gas CT c.
 c. imaging
 isotopic c.
 Katzman infusion of radionuclide c.
 metrizamide computed tomography
 c. (MCTC)
 oxygen c.
 Pantopaque c.
 radioisotope c.
 radionuclide c.
cisternomyelography
citrate
 clomiphene c.
 fentanyl c.
 ferrous c.
 gallium-67 c.
 manganese c.
Citscope disposable arthroscope
CIVI
 continuous intravenous
 infusion
Civinini
 C. canal
 C. ligament
CJD
 Creutzfeldt-Jakob disease
C/kg
 coulombs per kilogram
CKG
 cardiokymography
 CKG imaging
C-labeled
^{11}C-labeled
 ^{11}C.-l. cocaine
 ^{11}C.-l. cocaine imaging agent
 ^{11}C.-l. fatty acid imaging agent
Clado
 C. band
 C. ligament
 C. point
clamshell double umbrella occluder
Clariscan imaging agent

Clarke
 C. arch angle
 C. column
Clarke-Hadefield syndrome
Clark malignant melanoma classification
Clarus spinescope
classic
 c. carpal tunnel view
 c. nephroblastoma
 c. osteosarcoma
 c. scattering
classification
 AAOS acetabular abnormality c.
 acromioclavicular injury c.
 Aitken acromioclavicular injury c.
 AJCC-UICC mediastinal lymph node
 c.
 Allman c.
 Altman c.
 American Spinal Cord Injury
 Association c.
 Amstutz c.
 anatomic brain c.
 Ann Arbor Hodgkin disease c.
 anular tear c.
 AO and Danis-Weber ankle fracture
 c.
 AO ankle fracture c.
 Arco osteonecrosis c.
 Ashhurst transcondylar humeral
 fracture c. (I, II)
 Bayne c.
 Berndt-Hardy talar dome c.
 Bigliani c.
 Bleck metatarsus adductus c.
 Bosniak renal cystic disease c.
 Boyd and Griffin subtrochanteric
 proximal femur fracture c. (I-IV)
 brain anatomy c.
 brain tumor c.
 Breslow melanoma thickness c.
 Broders tumor index c.
 Brooker periarticular heterotopic
 ossification c.
 Butcher staging c.
 Caldwell-Moloy c.
 Canale-Kelly talar neck fracture c.
 Carnesale-Stewart-Barnes hip
 dislocation c.
 Cedell-Magnusson arthritis c.
 cerebral malformation c.
 Child-Pugh liver disease c.
 Child-Pugh liver function
 classification (A, B, C)
 Clark malignant melanoma c.
 CNS anomaly c.
 CNS tumor c.
 Colonna hip fracture c.
 congenital heart disease c.

Copeland-Kavat metatarsophalangeal dislocation c.
Couinaud liver anatomy c.
Danis-Weber ankle fracture c.
D'Antonio acetabular c.
DeBakey aortic c.
Delbet hip fracture c.
Denis c.
Dickhaut-DeLee discoid meniscus c.
distance-based block c.
Essex-Lopresti calcaneal fracture c.
Evans intertrochanteric fracture c.
FAB c.
Fielding-Magliato subtrochanteric fracture c.
fracture c.
Fränkel spinal cord injury c.
Freeman calcaneal fracture c.
Fries rheumatoid arthritis c.
Frykman distal radius fracture c.
Galassi arachnoid cyst c.
Garden femoral neck fracture c.
Gertzbein seatbelt injury c.
Glasscock-Jackson c.
Goldsmith and Woodburne c.
Graf hip dysplasia c.
Grantham femur fracture c.
Gumley seatbelt injury c.
Gustilo-Anderson tibial plafond fracture c.
Hahn-Steinthal capitellum fracture c.
Hansen fracture c.
Hardy-Clapham sesamoid c.
Hawkins talar neck fracture c.
Herbert-Fisher fracture c.
Hinchey c.
Hohl tibial condylar fracture c.
Holdsworth spinal fracture c.
Hughston Clinic injury c.
Hunt-Kosnik c.
Hyams grading of esthesioneuroblastoma c.
Jahss dislocation c.
Jones c.
Judet epiphysial fracture c.
Kalamchi-Dawe congenital tibial deficiency c.
Kazangia and Converse facial fracture c.
Kernohan brain tumor c.
Key-Conwell pelvic fracture c.
Kiel non-Hodgkin lymphoma c.
Kilfoyle condylar fracture c.
Kimura c.
King-Moe c.
Kistler subarachnoid hemorrhage c.
Klatskin tumor c.
Kocher-Lorenz capitellum fracture c. (I-II)

Kostuik-Errico spinal stability c.
Kyle fracture c.
Lauge-Hansen ankle fracture c.
Lie c.
Mason radial fracture c.
Mazur ankle evaluation c.
McCabe-Fletcher c.
McLain-Weinstein spinal tumor c.
Melone distal radius fracture c.
Merland perimedullary arteriovenous fistula c.
Meyer-McKeever tibial fracture c.
Michels c.
Milch elbow fracture c. (I, II)
Mink-Deutsch c.
Mitchell c.
Modic disc abnormality c.
mulberry-type c.
Müller humerus fracture c.
multiaxial c.
Neer-Horowitz humerus fracture c.
Neviaser frozen shoulder c.
Newman radial fracture c.
Nurick spondylosis c.
NYHA congestive heart failure c.
O'Brien radial fracture c.
Ogden epiphysial fracture c.
Olerud and Molander fracture c.
osteoarthritis grading c.
Ovadia-Beals tibial plafond fracture c.
Papile c.
Pauwel femoral neck fracture c.
percentage c.
pineal gland tumor c.
Pipkin femoral fracture c.
pneumoconiosis c.
Poland epiphysial fracture c.
Potter polycystic kidney c.
primary CNS tumor c.
Rappaport c.
Ratliff avascular necrosis c.
REAL c.
rickets c.
Riemann c.
Riordan clubhand c.
Riseborough-Radin intercondylar fracture c.
Robson staging c.
Rockwood acromioclavicular injury c.
Rowe calcaneal fracture c. (type 1a, 1b, 1c, 2a, 2b, 3-5)
Rowe-Lowell fracture-dislocation c.
Ruedi-Allgower tibial plafond fracture c.
Runyon c.
Russell-Rubinstein cerebrovascular malformation c.

C

classification (*continued*)
 Salter-Harris growth plate injury
  c.
 Salter-Harris-Rang epiphysial fracture
  c. (1a, b, c, 2a, b, c, 3a, b, 4a,
  b, 5-9)
 Schatzker fracture c.
 Severin radiographic residual hip
  dysplasia c.
 Shelton femur fracture c.
 Smith sesamoid position c.
 Snyder SLAP lesion c.
 soft tissue lesion c.
 Sorbie calcaneal fracture c.
 Stanford aortic dissection c.
 Steinberg c.
 Steinbrocker rheumatoid arthritis
  c.
 Steinert epiphysial fracture c.
 Stewart-Milford traumatic pediatric
  hip dislocation c. (I-IV)
 talocalcaneal index c.
 Thompson-Epstein femoral fracture
  c.
 Todani c.
 Tronzo intertrochanteric fracture c.
  (1-3)
 Trunkey pelvic fracture c. (I-III)
 Vostal radial fracture c.
 Watanabe discoid meniscus c.
 Watson-Jones tibial tubercle avulsion
  fracture c.
 Werner c.
 Wiberg patellar-type c.
 Wilkins radial fracture c.
 Winquist-Hansen femoral fracture
  (0-IV) c.
 Wiseman c.
 Wolfe mammogram c.
 Working Formulation c.
clasticus
 conus c.
Claude syndrome
claudication
 intermittent c.
 lifestyle-limiting c.
 c. of jaw
Clauss
 C. assay
 C. method
claustra (*pl. of* claustrum)
claustrum, *pl.* **claustra**
clavi (*pl. of* clavus)
clavicle
 absence of outer end of c.
 penciling of distal c.
clavicular
 c. birth fracture
 c. facet

 c. head of sternocleidomastoid
 c. notch
 c. osteitis condensans
clavipectoral
 c. fascia
 c. triangle
clavus, *pl.* **clavi**
 interdigital c.
claw
clawfoot, claw foot
clawhand, claw hand
clawtoe, claw toe
clay
 c. pipe carcinoma
 c. shoveler's fracture
Claybrook sign
CLD
 central lung distance
CLE
 congenital lobar emphysema
clean shadow
cleansing
 electronic c.
 c. enema
clear
 c. cell carcinoma
 c. cell neoplasm of ovary
 c. cell sarcoma
 c. endpoint
 enemas until c.
 C. technique
 c. zone
clearance
 c. curve
 c. half-time
 isotope c.
 multicompartment c.
 multiple-sample c.
 c. phase ventilation scan
 radioactive xenon c.
 radioaerosol c.
 renal c.
 single-sample c.
Clearview CO$_2$ laser
cleavage
 c. cavity
 c. fracture
 plane of c.
 c. tear
cleaved
 c. cell lymphoma
 c. polyprotein precursor molecule
 c. polyprotein precursor molecule
  product
Cleaves
 C. method
 C. position
cleaving
 plaque c.

cleft
    anal c.
    c. chorda
    coronal c.
    c. face syndrome
    facial c.
    full-thickness c.
    gill c.
    Hahn c.
    intergluteal c.
    interinnominoabdominal c.
    intranuclear c.
    intravertebral body vacuum c.
    laryngotracheoesophageal c.
    lateral facial c.
    c. lip
    median facial c.
    median lip c.
    meniscal c.
    midline longitudinal pontile c.
    c. mitral valve
    natal c.
    neural arch c.
    pudendal c.
    radiolucent c.
    retrosomatic c.
    spinal cord c.
    c. spine
    splenic c.
    1st visceral c.
    synaptic c.
    vacuum c.
    ventricular c.
    c. vertebra
cleidocranial
    c. dysostosis
    c. dysplasia
Cleland ligament
Clements-Nakayama position
clenched fist view
Cleopatra view
Clerc-Levy-Cristico syndrome
clidocranial
climbing fiber
clinical
    c. complete response
    c. correlation
    c. dementia rating
    c. estimation of survival
    c. feature
    C. Outcomes Research Initiative
      (CORI)
    c. parameter
    c. partial response
    c. target volume (CTV)
    c. tumor volume
clinically isolated syndrome
CliniCath peripherally inserted catheter
clinicopathologic analysis

clinicoradiologic entity
clinodactyly
    factitious c.
    traumatic c.
clinoid
    c. aneurysm
    c. ligament
    c. process
clinoparietal line
clip
    aneurysmal c.
    cerebrovascular aneurysmal c.
    Lapra-Ty c.
    c. ligation of aneurysm
    sternal c.
    Weck Hem-o-lock c.
clip-editing plane
clipping
    c. of aneurysm
    ureteral c.
clival meningioma
clivi (*pl. of* clivus)
clivus, *pl.* **clivi**
    Blumenbach c.
    c. chordoma
    c. meningioma tumor
    c. metastasis
clivus-canal angle
CLM
    capillary-lymphatic malformation
cloaca, *pl.* **cloacae**
    bone formation c.
cloacae (*pl. of* cloaca)
cloacal
    c. anomaly
    c. exstrophy
    c. formation
    c. malformation
    c. plate
cloaking
    periosteal c.
    perivascular c.
clock cycle
clockwise whirlpool sign
clomiphene citrate
cloning
    subtraction c.
clonogen number
cloppidogrel
Cloquet
    C. canal
    C. fascia
    hyaloid canal of C.
    C. inguinal lymph node
    C. ligament
close apposition
closed
    c. cavity
    c. conducting loop

C

closed (*continued*)
    c. dislocation
    c. exstrophy
    c. flap amputation
    c. fontanelle
    c. fracture
    c. head injury (CHI)
    c. pneumothorax
    c. reduction
    c. spinal dysraphism
closed-break fracture
closed-core transformer
closed-fist configuration
closed-loop intestinal obstruction
closed-mouth view
closer
    Perclose c.
    C. percutaneous suture-mediated
        closure device
close-space thin-section scanning
close-up view
closing
    c. capacity
    c. slope
    c. velocity
    c. volume
closure
    abrupt vessel c.
    aortic c.
    c. device
    growth center c.
    incomplete c.
    native aortic valve c.
    physial c.
    premature valve c.
    sandwich patch c.
    Stanford type B dissection c.
    threatened vessel c.
    tricuspid valve c.
    valve c.
    VasoSeal Elite vascular c.
    velopharyngeal c.
    VHD c.
Clo-Sur PAD closure device
clot
    agonal c.
    autologous blood c.
    blood c.
    internal c.
    intramural c.
    isoechoic c.
    c. lysis
    c. maceration
    marantic c.
    mural c.
    passive c.
    plastic c.
    preformed c.
    c. removal by laser thrombolysis

    c. retraction
    saddle c.
    subarachnoid c.
    subdural c.
clot-filled lumen
clothesline injury
clothing artifact
cloud
    c. chamber
    electron c.
clouding
    alveolar c.
cloudy
    c. sinus
    c. swelling of heart
cloverleaf
    c. deformity
    c. plate
    c. skull
cloverleaf-shaped lumen
Cloward bone graft
clubbed
    c. finger
    c. penis
clubbing
    calyceal c.
    digital c.
clubfoot deformity
clubhand deformity
club-shaped conus
cluneal nerve
cluster
    activated voxel c.
    grapelike c.
    K-means c.
    microcalcification c.
    c. of differentiation (CD)
    c. of radiolucent areas
        (CORLA)
clustered
    c. calcification
    c. data
cluster-of-grapes lung
Clutton painful joint
clysis
Clysodrast
CM
    contrast medium
        iodinated intravascular CM
cm
    centimeter
CMC
    carpometacarpal
        CMC joint
CMD
    cerebromacular degeneration
    corticomedullary differentiation
¹¹C-methionine
    ¹¹C-m. PET scan

^{11}C-m. positron emission
tomography (MET-PET)
CMF
chondromyxoid fibroma
CMI
chronic mesenteric ischemia
CMJ
corticomedullary junction
CMJ imaging
CMML
chronic myelomonocytic
leukemia
CMOS
complementary metal oxide
semiconductor
CMR
congenital mitral regurgitation
CMRO$_2$
cerebral metabolic rate of
oxygen
CMRP
cervical magnetic resonance
phlebography
CMS
compliance matching stent
CMT
Charcot-Marie-Tooth
CMV
cytomegalovirus
CMV encephalitis
CMV enteritis
C/N, CNR
contrast-to-noise ratio
CNS
central nervous system
CNS amyloidosis
CNS anomaly classification
CNS cortical hamartoma
CNS empyema
CNS fibromuscular dysplasia
CNS ghost tumor
CNS juvenile pilocytic
astrocytoma
CNS lymphoma
CNS multifocal tumor
CNS teratoma
CNS toxoplasmosis
CNS tumor classification
CNV
choroidal neovascularization
Co
cobalt
cyanocobalamin Co 57, 58, 60
^{57}Co, Co-57
cobalt 57
^{58}Co, Co-58
cobalt 58
^{60}Co, Co-60
cobalt 60

CO$_2$
carbon dioxide
CO$_2$ angiography
CO$_2$ cylinder
CO$_2$ generator
CO$_2$ insufflation
CO$_2$ laser
CO$_2$ retention
COACH
cerebellar vermis hypoplasia,
oligophrenia, congenital ataxia, ocular
coloboma, hepatic fibrosis
COACH syndrome
coadaptation
coagulation
disseminated intravascular c.
(DIC)
laser c.
microwave tumor c.
c. necrosis
coagulator
argon beam c. (ABC)
coagulography
coagulopathy
intravascular consumption c.
coal
c. macule
c. miner's lung
c. tar
c. worker's lung
c. worker's pneumoconiosis
(CWP)
coalesce
coalescence
coalescent
c. granuloma
c. nodule
coalition
bony c.
calcaneonavicular c.
carpal c.
fibrous c.
intercarpal c.
lunate-triquetral c.
Minaar classification of c.
osseous c.
talocalcaneal c.
talonavicular c.
target c.
tarsal c.
c. view
coanalgesic
coaptation point
coapted leaflet
coarctation
abdominal aortic c.
adult c.
aortic c.
asymptomatic c.

coarctation (*continued*)
    atypical subisthmic c.
    congenital isthmic c.
    infantile c.
    isthmic c.
    juxtaductal aortic c.
    localized c.
    c. of anomalous venous
      connection
    c. of aorta
    postductal aortic c.
    preductal aortic c.
    reversed c.
    c. syndrome
    thoracic aortic c.

coarcted segment

coarse
    c. bronchovascular marking
    c. calcification
    c. injection
    c. linear opacity
    c. lung reticulation
    c. microcalcification
    c. nodularity
    c. pattern
    c. reticular opacity

coarsening

coated
    enteric c. (EC)

coat hanger osteochondroma

coating
    antireflection c.
    Hydro-Sil c.
    c. of aneurysm

Coats disease

coaxial
    c. micropuncture needle
      set
    c. sheath cut-biopsy needle
    c. sheath technique
    c. steering
    c. Temno needle

coaxially
    pass c.

coaxillary directed catheter

cobalt (Co)
    c. 57 (^{57}Co, Co-57)
    c. 58 (^{58}Co, Co-58)
    c. 60 (^{60}Co, Co-60)
    c. alloy stent
    c. megavoltage machine
    c. pneumopathy
    radioactive c.
    c. radioactive source

cobalt-60
    c.-60 beam
    c.-60 beam therapy unit
    c.-60 Gamma knife radiosurgical
      treatment

**cobalt-chromium-molybdenum
(Co-Cr-Mo)**
    c.-c.-m. alloy metal implant

**cobalt-chromium-tungsten-nickel
(Co-Cr-W-Ni)**
    c.-c.-t.-n. alloy metal implant

Cobatope-57

Cobb
    C. measurement
    C. measurement of scoliosis
    C. method
    C. method of measuring
      kyphosis
    C. scoliosis angle
    C. syndrome

cobbler's chest

cobblestone
    c. appearance
    c. appearance of bile duct
    c. appearance of colon
    c. appearance of duodenum
    c. appearance of eosinophilic
      gastroenteritis
    c. appearance of esophagus
    c. appearance of lymphoma
    c. appearance of stomach
    c. degeneration
    c. ileum
    c. lissencephaly
    c. mucosa
    c. pattern
    c. sign

cobblestoning

Coblation

cobra
    C. 1, 2 catheter
    C. diagnostic catheter

cobra-eye sign

cobra-head
    c.-h. anastomosis
    c.-h. appearance
    c.-h. effect
    c.-h. ureter

cobra-shaped catheter

cobweb
    c. appearance
    c. pattern

cocaine
    ^{11}C-labeled c.

Coccidioides
    C. immitis
    C. infection

coccidioidoma

coccidioidomycosis
    bone c.
    disseminated c.
    latent c.
    lung c.
    c. meningitis

Posadas-Wernicke c.
primary c.
progressive c.
secondary c.
coccygeal
c. appendage
c. body
c. bone
c. ganglion
c. gland
c. ligament
c. plexus
c. sinus
c. spine
c. vertebra
c. vestige
c. whorl
coccygeopubic diameter
coccyges (*pl. of* coccyx)
coccygeus
vortex c.
coccyx, *pl.* coccyges
c. bone
c. fracture
cochlea, *pl.* cochleae
apertura externa canaliculi cochleae
c. aplasia
single-cavity c.
cochleae (*pl. of* cochlea)
cochlear
c. anatomy
c. aqueduct
c. canal
c. canaliculus
c. duct
c. implant
c. labyrinth
c. lesion
c. nerve
c. otosclerosis
c. recess
c. root
cochleariform process
cochlearis
stria vascularis ductus c.
cochleate uterus
cochleitis
calcific c.
ossifying c.
cockade image sign
Cockayne syndrome
cocking injury
cock-robin position
cockscomb
c. appearance
c. appearance of cervix
c. papilloma
cocktail
renal c.

cock-up deformity
Co-Cr-Mo
cobalt-chromium-molybdenum
Co-Cr-Mo alloy metal implant
Co-Cr-W-Ni
cobalt-chromium-tungsten-nickel
Co-Cr-W-Ni alloy implant metal
cocurrent flow-related enhancement
COD
computerized optical densitometry
Code and Carlson radiograph
coded-aperture imaging
coded-image aperture
coder
Chen-Smith image c.
ICS c.
improved Chen-Smith c.
codfish
c. deformity
c. vertebra
Codivilla extension
Codman
C. angle
C. cranioplastic type 1 slow set
C. Medos programmable valve
C. sign
C. triangle
C. tumor
codominant
c. circulation
c. vessel
coefficient
absorption c.
apparent diffusion c. (ADC)
attenuation c.
attenuation-correction c.
binary similarity c.
c. conversion
correlation c.
curve-fit c.
diffusion c.
effective mass attenuation c.
Fourier c.
intraclass correlation c.
linear absorption c.
linear attenuation c.
mass absorption c.
mass attenuation c.
c. of variation
Ostwald solubility c.
partition c.
Pearson correlation c.
reflection c.
Spearman correlation c.
stiffness c.
uniform attenuation c.
viscosity c.
coeur en sabot

C

coexistent
>   c. cavity
>   c. intravoxel fat and water

coffee-bean appearance
coffee-grounds material
coffee worker's lung
coffin bone
Cogan lid twitch sign
cognitive
>   c. fMRI
>   c. functional MR imaging

cogwheel sign
coherence
>   multiple quantum c.
>   phase c.
>   steady-state c.

coherent
>   C. CO_2 surgical laser
>   c. scattering
>   C. UltraPulse 5000C laser
>   C. VersaPulse device

coil
>   aneurysmal c.
>   c. array
>   3-axis gradient c.
>   balloon c.
>   bilateral breast c.'s
>   birdcage head c.
>   body c.
>   breast c.
>   butterfly c.
>   catheter-delivered platinum c.
>   6-channel posterior c.
>   circularly polarized c.
>   circular polarized volume head c.
>   circumferential extremity c.
>   c. closure of coronary artery fistula
>   collagen-filled interlocking detachable c.
>   conventional head c.
>   coupled array c.
>   crossed c.
>   custom-curved c.
>   DCS-10, DCS-18 mechanically
>   detachable platinum c.
>   dedicated phased-array c.
>   dedicated shoulder c.
>   c. delivery
>   c. deposition
>   detachable platinum c.
>   detector c.
>   double breast c.
>   electrically detachable c.
>   2-element phased-array c.
>   4-element phased-array c.
>   embedding of stent c.
>   c. embolization
>   endoanal c.
>   endocavitary c.
>   endoesophageal MRI c.

endorectal c.
endoscopic quadrature radiofrequency
    c.
endovaginal c.
endovascular c.
extremity c.
fat-suppressed body c.
fibered Guglielmi detachable c.
field-profiling c.
flexible anterior 6-channel
    phased-array abdominal imaging c.
flexible radiofrequency c.
flexible surface c.
free fibered c.
GDC-10 soft c.
c. geometry
Gianturco occlusion c.
Gianturco-Wallace-Anderson c.
Gianturco-Wallace-Chuang c.
Gianturco wool-tufted wire c.
Golay c.
gonion gradient c.
Gore 1.5T torso array MRI surface
    c.
gradient sheet c.
Guglielmi detachable c. (GDC)
head c.
Helmholtz c.
high-speed gradient c.
Hipper twist-release c.
immediately detachable c.
Intercept vascular internal MR c.
interlocking detachable c. (IDC)
intrarectal c.
intravascular c.
in vitro evaluation of c.
Jackson c.
linearly polarized c.
liver c.
c. loading
local gradient c.
Maxwell c.
MDS c.
mechanically detachable platinum c.
Medrad MRInnervu endorectal colon
    probe c.
micronester platinum embolization c.
c. migration
modified bird-cage c.
MRCP using HASTE with
    phased-array c.
multichannel pelvic phased-array c.
multiply tuned c.
neck c.
nester c.
c. of intestine
opposed loop-pair quadrature NMR
    c.
orthogonal radiofrequency c.

parallel data acquisition c.'s
pelvic phased-array c.
phased-array surface c.
phased-array torso c.
planar circular c.
platinum c.
posterior neck surface c.
c. protrusion
proximal c.
pushable c.
quadrature adult head c.
quadrature body c.
quadrature cervical spine c.
quadrature radiofrequency receiver c.
quadrature terminal latency surface c.
quadrature transmit-receive head c.
radiofrequency transmitter-receiver c.
receive-only circular surface c.
receiver c.
RF c.
right ventricular c.
saddle c.
c. selection
send-receive phased-array extremity
  c.
sensing c.
shielded gradient c.
shim c.
shoulder surface c.
solenoid surface c.
stainless steel c.
steel c.
Stylet esophageal MRI c.
surface c.
Surgi-Vision MRI c.
switchable c.
thrombogenic c.
Tornado c.
torso phased-array c. (TPAC)
transmit-receive c.
transmitter c.
TriSpan detachable c.
twist-release c.
c. vascular stent
volume c.
VortXX c.
whole-volume c.
wool c.
wrist quadrature phased-array surface
  c.

coiled
  c. spring appearance
  c. spring pattern
  c. spring sign
coiling
  c. of anastomosis
  c. of aneurysm
coil-sensitive encoding
coil-to-vessel diameter

coin
  c. artifact
  fracture en c.
  c. lesion
  c. lesion of lung
  c. test
coincidence
  c. circuit
  counting c.
  c. detection
  c. detection mode
  c. detection positron emission
    tomography
  c. detection scan
  c. event
  c. gamma camera
  c. imaging
  c. imaging scanner
  loss c.
  positron c.
  sum-peak c.
coincidence-resolving window
coincidence-summing correction
coin-on-edge vertebra
Colter muscle
Colapinto
  C. needle
  C. sheath
Colbert method
COLD
  chronic obstructive lung disease
cold
  c. breast abscess
  c. defect
  c. defect renal scintigraphy
  c. lesion
  c. nodule of thyroid
  c. quartz germicidal lamp
  c. spine abscess
  c. spot
  c. spot myocardial imaging
  c. vertebra
colectasia
coli
  elastin deposition in taenia c.
  Escherichia c.
  familial polyposis c.
  haustra c.
  pneumatosis c.
colic
  c. artery
  biliary c.
  c. impression
  c. omentum
  c. plexus
  renal c.
  c. sphincter
  c. surface
  c. vein

C

colitis
  chronic ulcerative c. (CUC)
  Crohn c.
  c. cystica profunda
  focal c.
  fulminant c.
  fulminating ulcerative c.
  granulomatous transmural c.
  ischemic c.
  myxomembranous c.
  c. polypoid
  c. polyposa
  pseudomembranous c.
  radiation c.
  radiation-induced c.
  regional c.
  single-stripe c. (SSC)
  transmural c.
  ulcerative c. (UC)
  c. ulcerosa gravis
collagen
  c. brain abscess
  c. defect (type I, II)
  c. fiber separation
  c. fibril
  c. fragmentation
  c. mediated closure device
  microfibrillar c.
  c. plug
  c. plug device
  c. tissue proliferation
collagen-filled interlocking detachable coil
collagenosis
  mediastinal c.
collagenous
  c. perivascular ala
  c. structure
  c. tissue
collagen-vascular disease
collapse
  absorption c.
  acinar c.
  acute vertebral c.
  alveolar c.
  c. cavitation
  circulation c.
  jugular venous pressure c.
  lingular c.
  massive c.
  pressure c.
  pulmonary c.
  scapholunate advanced c. (SLAC)
  scapholunate arthritic c.
  subchondral c.
  vertebral body c.
collapsed
  c. distal ileum
  c. inferior vena cava
  c. lobe

  c. lung
  c. lung field
  c. subpectoral implant
collapsing cord sign
collar
  Cowboy C.
  implant c.
  periosteal bone c.
  periportal c.
  c. sign
  tension c.
collarbone
collar-button
  c.-b. abscess
  c.-b. appearance
  c.-b. chest lesion
  c.-b. ulcer
collateral
  c. arcade
  arterial c.
  c. blood flow
  c. blood supply
  c. branch
  cavoportal c.
  c. circulation in compression of
    artery
  cross-scrotal c.
  developed c.
  c. edema
  c. eminence
  c. fissure
  gastroesophageal c.
  c. hyperemia
  c. ligament
  c. ligament of knee
  c. mesenteric circulation
  parasitized c.
  portosystemic c.
  c. sulcus
  c. system
  tributary c.
  c. trigone
  venous c.
  c. venous channel
  c. vessel
collateral-dependent myocardium
collateralization
collecting
  c. system
  c. system atony
  c. system filling defect
  c. system opacification
  c. tube
  c. tubule
  c. venous pouch
  c. vessel
collection
  abdominal air c.
  air c.

anechoic fluid c.
complex abdominal fluid c.
crescentic c.
EAA c.
extraalveolar air c.
extraaxial fluid c.
extracerebral fluid c.
fluid c.
gas c.
hypoechoic fluid c.
intratendinous fluid c.
list mode data c.
mottled gas c.
c. of contrast material
pancreatic fluid c.
periarticular fluid c.
pericholecystic fluid c.
perifascial fluidlike c.
perinephric fluid c.
peripancreatic fluid c.
pleural fluid c.
posttraumatic subcapsular hepatic
  fluid c.
retrocerebellar CSF c.
retromammary fluid c.
saccular c.
collective paramagnetism
Colles
C. fascia
C. fracture
C. ligament
Collet-Edwards type IV truncus
  arteriosus
Collet-Sicard syndrome
colli
fibromatosis c.
pterygium c.
collicular fracture
colliculi (*pl. of* colliculus)
colliculus, *pl.* **colliculi**
anterior c.
brachium of c.
facial c.
fused c.
inferior c.
posterior c.
seminal c.
superior c.
Collier sign
collimated slice width
collimating system
collimation
asymmetric c.
c. CT
detector c.
dynamic multileaf c.
electronic c.
c. imaging
lead c.

narrow c.
parallel-hole c.
c. scanning
c. scintillation detector
secondary c.
submillimeter c.
tertiary c.
thin c.
c. width
collimator
APC-3, APC-4 c.
automatic c.
c. contamination
converging c.
converging-hole c.
diverging c.
dual shaped c.
Eureka c.
c. exchange effect
fan-beam c.
focusing c.
heart-shaped c.
c. helmet
high-resolution c.
high-resolution fan-beam c.
high-resolution multileaf c.
LEAP c.
LEUHR fan-beam c.
LEUHR parallel-hole c.
Leur-par c.
long-bore c.
low-energy c.
medium-energy c.
MEHR c.
Micro-Cast c.
multihole c.
multileaf c. (MLC)
multirod c.
parallel-hole medium-sensitivity c.
pinhole c.
c. plugging pattern
c. scattering
single-hole c.
slant-hole c.
slat c.
slit c.
thick-septa c.
thin-septa c.
triple-leaf c.
ultrahigh-energy parallel-hole c.
ultrahigh-resolution parallel-hole
  c.
colliquative necrosis
collision
c. detecting
elastic c.
c. tumor
collodiaphysial
central c. (CCD)

C

colloid
c. adenocarcinoma
c. adenoma
^{198}Au c.
c. brain cyst
c. calculus
c. carcinoma
c. cystadenoma
c. cystic tumor
c. cyst of 3rd ventricle
c. degeneration
c. goiter
minimicroaggregated albumin c.
^{99m}Tc sulfur c. (^{99m}Tc SC)
c. nodule
c. oncotic pressure (COP)
radioactive c.
radiogold c.
c. shift
c. shift on scan
sulfur c.
TechneScan sulfur c.
technetium 99m antimony sulfur c.
technetium 99m antimony trisulfide c.
technetium 99m filtered sulfur c.
technetium 99m minimicroaggregated albumin c.
technetium 99m stannous c.
technetium 99m tin c.
technetium sulfur c.

colloidal
c. chromic phosphorus
c. gold nanoparticle
c. sulfur
c. suspension

colobomatous cyst

colocolic
c. anastomosis
c. fistula
c. intussusception

colocutaneous fistula

colography

Colombo count

colon
angiodysplasia of c.
anterior band of c.
ascending c.
barium-filled c.
burned-out c.
c. carcinoma
carpet lesion of c.
cathartic c.
cobblestone appearance of c.
coned-down appearance of c.
Crohn disease of c.
c. cutoff sign
c. cyst duplication
descending c.

distal c.
double-tracking c.
epithelial c.
feces-filled c.
free band of c.
giant c.
hepatodiaphragmatic interposition of c. (HDIC)
hypoganglionosis of c.
iliac c.
inflammation of c.
intramural air in c.
irritable c.
jejunization of c.
c. kinking
knuckle of c.
lateral reflection of c.
left c.
c. margin
mesosigmoid c.
midsigmoid c.
pelvic c.
perisigmoid c.
proximal c.
c. pseudostricture
right c.
sigmoid c.
spastic c.
c. stenting
thumbprinting appearance of c.
transverse c.

colonic
c. activity
c. adenoma
c. adenomatous polyp
c. air
c. angiodysplasia
c. apple-core lesion
c. atresia
c. carpet lesion
c. dilation
c. distention
c. diverticular hemorrhage
c. diverticulitis
c. diverticulosis
c. diverticulum
c. duplication cyst
c. evacuation
c. filling defect
c. fistula
c. flexure
c. gas composition
c. hamartomatous polyp
c. haustrum
c. ileus
c. interposition
c. involvement of endometriosis
c. lead-pipe appearance
c. loop

c. motility
c. mucosal excretion
c. myenteric plexus
c. narrowing
c. necrosis
c. neoplasia
c. obstruction
c. perforation
c. pit
c. pseudoobstruction
c. saddle lesion
c. spasm
c. stricture
c. transit time
c. ulcer
c. urticaria pattern
c. varix
c. volvulus

colonization
saprophytic c.

Colonna hip fracture classification

colonography, colography
bile-tagged 3D magnetic resonance c.
computed tomographic c. (CTC)
CT c.
MR c.
virtual CT c.
volume-rendered CT c.

colonopathy, colopathy
fibrosing c.

colonoscope, coloscope
Olympus CF-1T100L c.
Olympus CF-200Z c.

colonoscopy, coloscopy
endocervical canal c.
virtual c.

ColonoSight system

colony-forming unit

colopathy (*var. of* colonopathy)

coloproctitis

coloptosia (*var. of* coloptosis)

coloptosis, coloptosia

color
c. amplitude imaging
c. Doppler (CD)
c. Doppler imaging (CDI)
c. Doppler recording
c. Doppler signal
c. Doppler sonography (CDS)
c. Doppler twinkling artifact
c. Doppler ultrasonography (CDUS)
c. Doppler ultrasound
c. duplex interrogation
c. duplex ultrasound
c. gain
c. kinesis
c. power angiography

c. power transcranial Doppler sonography
c. power transcranial Doppler ultrasound
c. space conversion
c. space interpolation
c. space interpolator
c. spectrum
c. velocity imaging
c. void

color-coded
c.-c. Doppler flow imaging (CDFI)
c.-c. duplex sonography (CCDS)
c.-c. duplex ultrasound
c.-c. guidewire
c.-c. pulmonary blood flow imaging
c.-c. real-time sonography
c.-c. real-time ultrasound

colorectal
c. adenocarcinoma
c. adenoma
c. anastomosis
c. cancer endoscopy
c. carcinoid
c. carcinoma
c. duplication
c. hemorrhage
c. lymphoma
c. mucosa
c. polyp

colorectal/ovarian (CR/OV)

color-encoded brain MR imaging

color-flame scale

color-flow
c.-f. Doppler (CFD)
c.-f. Doppler real-time 2D blood flow imaging
c.-f. Doppler sonography
c.-f. duplex imaging
c.-f. duplex scan
c.-f. imaging (CFI)
c.-f. imaging Doppler echocardiography
c.-f. mapping

colorimetric
c. color reproduction
c. test

color-scale image

coloscope (*var. of* colonoscope)

coloscopy (*var. of* colonoscopy)

colosigmoid resection

colostogram
augmented pressure c.

colostomy
barium enema through c.
barium injection through c.
fecal diversion c.

colovaginal fistula

colovesical fistula

C

colpocele
colpocephaly
colpoptosia (*var. of* colpoptosis)
colpoptosis, colpoptosia
colposcopy
colpostat applicator
column
>anal c.
>anterior gray c.
>branchial efferent c.
>Clarke c.
>contrast medium c.
>corrugated air c.
>dye c.
>extraction c.
>c. extraction method
>Gowers c.
>head of barium c.
>intermediolateral gray c.
>Lissauer c.
>c. of Bertin
>c. of Burdach
>c. of Morgagni
>Quick Spin Sephadex G-50 c.
>renal c.
>thoracolumbar spine c.
>variceal c.
>vertebral c.
>weighted spin-echo c.
columnar-lined esophagus
columnar metaphysis
2-column injury
3-column injury
columnization of contrast material
column-mode
>c.-m. sinogram image
>c.-m. sinogram imaging
Colyte bowel preparation
coma
>nonketotic hyperosmolar c.
Combidex MRI contrast agent
combination
>c. flow and pressure load
>molybdenum-molybdenum target-filter c.
>molybdenum-rhodium target-filter c.
>rhodium-rhodium target-filter c.
>target-filter c.
combined
>c. anatomic registration
>c. androgen blockade
>c. antiretroviral therapy
>c. CT-fluoroscopy scanner
>c. CT-PET
>c. dynamic 2D and bolus-chase 3D acquisition

>c. flexion-distraction injury and burst fracture
>c. germ cell tumor
>c. leukocyte-marrow imaging
>c. lineonodular radiographic lung pattern
>c. middle and right lower lobe atelectasis
>c. modality therapy
>c. ^{99m}Tc-DMSA and ^{99m}Tc-DTPA scanning
>c. multisection diffuse-weighted and hemodynamically weighted echo-planar MR
>c. Myoscint/thallium imaging
>c. pregnancy
>c. radial-ulnar-humeral fractures
>c. thallium-Tc-HMPAO imaging
>c. transmission-emission scintiphotograph
>c. ventilation-perfusion scintigraphy
comb sign
comedo, *pl.* comedones
>c. necrosis
>c. pattern
comedo-basal cell carcinoma
comedomastitis
comedones (*pl. of* comedo)
comedo-type DCIS
comet sign
comet-tail
>c.-t. artifact
>c.-t. artifact gallbladder
>c.-t. sign
Comfort Cath I, II catheter
comitans, *pl.* comitantes
>vena c.
comitantes (*pl. of* comitans)
comma-shaped
>c.-s. crus
>c.-s. duodenum
commemorative sign
commencement of vessel
comminuted
>c. burst fracture
>c. intraarticular fracture
>c. teardrop fracture
commission
>Atomic Energy C. (AEC)
>International Electrotechnical C. (IEC)
>Nuclear Regulatory C.
commissural
>c. attachment
>c. chorda
>c. function
>c. leaflet
>c. point

commissure
  anterior c. (AC)
  anterior commissure-posterior c.
    (AC-PC)
  anteroseptal c.
  cerebral c.
  fused c.
  gray c.
  mitral valve c.
  posterior c. (PC)
  scalloped c.
  tectum c.
  temporal limb of anterior c.
  valve c.
  vestigial c.
  white matter c.
committee
  Administration of Radioactive
    Substances Advisory C. (ARSAC)
common
  c. atrioventricular canal
  c. atrium
  c. basal vein
  c. bile duct (CBD)
  c. bile duct bifurcation
  c. bile duct diverticulum
  c. bile duct exploration (CBDE)
  c. bile duct obstruction
  c. bile duct spontaneous perforation
  c. bile duct stone
  c. bile duct stricture
  c. bundle
  c. cardinal vein
  c. carotid artery (CCA)
  c. carotid artery bifurcation
  c. carotid plexus
  c. cavity phenomenon
  c. duct cholangiogram
  c. duct dilation
  c. dural sac
  c. extensor tendinosis
  c. facial vein
  c. femoral artery
  c. femoral vein
  c. gall duct
  c. gateway interface (CGI)
  c. hepatic artery
  c. hepatic duct (CHD)
  c. iliac artery
  c. iliac artery thrombosis
  c. iliac lymph node
  c. peroneal artery
  c. pulmonary vein stenosis
  c. synovial flexor sheath
  c. tendinous ring
  c. tendon
commotio cerebri
commune
  centrum c.

  crus c.
  mesenterium c.
  persistent ostium atrioventriculare c.
communicating
  c. artery
  c. artery aneurysm
  c. cavernous ectasia
  c. cyst
  c. fistula
  c. hydrocephalus
  internal carotid-posterior c. (IC-PC)
  c. syringomyelia
  c. vein
  c. vein incompetence
communication
  biliopleural c.
  cholangiovenous c.
  fistulous gas c.
  interatrial c.
  macrofistulous arteriovenous c.
  medical ultrasound 3-dimensional
    portable with advanced c.
    (MUSTPAC)
  peritoneopleural c.
  pleuroperitoneal c.
communis
  extensor digitorum c. (EDC)
community-acquired pneumonia
Comolli sign
compact
  c. bone
  c. fibrillar echotexture
  c. island
  c. osteoma
companion
  c. lymph node
  c. shadow
  c. vein
comparative
  c. genomic hybridization
  c. value
comparison
  beam quality c.
  c. film
  histopathologic c.
  c. view
  yield c.
compartment
  anterior mediastinal c.
  anterior tibial c.
  cervicocentral c.
  deep posterior c.
  distal radioulnar joint c.
  extensor c.
  extracellular c.
  extradural c.
  extravascular c.
  iliopsoas c.
  infracolic c.

C

compartment (*continued*)
    infratentorial c.
    lateral c.
    medial c.
    midcarpal c.
    occluded c.
    patellofemoral c.
    peribronchovascular interstitial c.
    perirenal c.
    plantar c.
    posterior c.
    posterolateral c.
    posteromedial c.
    radiocarpal c.
    superficial posterior c.
    supracolic c.
    supramesocolic c.
    c. syndrome
    4th c.
    5th c.
    6th c.
    vascular c.
    wrist extensor c.
2-, 3-compartment system
3-compartment
    3-c. arthrography
    3-c. wrist angiography
compartmental
    c. analysis
    c. modeling
    c. radioimmunoglobulin therapy
compartmentalization
Compass stereotactic system
compensated
    c. composite spin-lock pulse
    c. congestive heart failure
    c. hydrocephalus
compensating filter
compensation
    attenuation c.
    cardiac gating c.
    depth c.
    flow c.
    free-breathing motion c.
    gradient c.
    2nd-order c.
    respiratory c.
    scatter c.
    section-select flow c.
    supratentorial flow c.
    time-gain c. (TGC)
    velocity c.
compensator
    multivane intensity modulation c.
      (MIMIC)
    scattering foil c.
    tissue deficit c.
compensatory
    c. atrophy

    c. capillary filling
    c. circulation
    c. cortical activation
    c. deformity
    c. emphysema
    c. enlargement
    c. enlargement of ventricle
    c. hyperplasia
    c. lobe hyperexpansion
    c. mechanism
    c. nodular kidney hypertrophy
    c. pause
competence of ureterovesical junction
competent ileocecal valve
competitive
    c. adsorption
    c. inhibition
    c. iron administration
complementary
    c. and alternative medicine (CAM)
    c. hypertrophy
    c. metal oxide semiconductor
      (CMOS)
    c. spatial modulation of
      magnetization (CSPAMM)
complete
    c. anatomic cure
    c. atrioventricular block (CAVB)
    c. atrioventricular dissociation
    c. bladder emptying
    c. bowel obstruction
    c. congenital heart block
    c. dislocation
    c. duplication
    c. fetal heart block
    c. fracture
    c. heart block (CHB)
    c. lymph node dissection
    c. myelography
    c. nerve lesion
    c. occlusion
    c. placenta previa
    c. situs inversus
    c. small bowel malrotation
    c. stent expansion
    c. stress/rest study
    c. tear
    c. transposition of great arteries
    c. vascular stasis
completed stroke
completion
    c. arteriography
    c. thyroidectomy
complex
    c. abdominal fluid collection
    agyria-pachygria c.
    amygdaloid nuclear c.
    c. anatomic relationship
    ankle joint c.

c. anorectal fistula
anterior communicating artery c.
aperiodic c.
apical c.
arcuate c.
atrial c.
c. atrioventricular canal
auricular c.
azygos-hemiazygos c.
basivertebral venous c.
biceps-labral c.
c. block
c. breast cyst
Buford c.
capsulolabral c.
caudal pharyngeal c.
chlormerodrin-cysteine c.
choroidal-hippocampal fissure c.
compound dislocation c.
c. conjugate
Dandy-Walker c.
discoligamentous c.
Eisenmenger c.
epispadias exstrophy c.
c. extraperitoneal rupture
fabellofibular and arcuate ligament c.
fibrocartilage c.
foot-ankle c.
frontonasal dysplasia malformation c.
gadolinium c.
gallium-transferrin c.
gastrocnemius-soleus c.
gastroduodenal artery c.
Ghon c.
Ghon-Sachs c.
growth plate c.
hallux sesamoid c.
hallux valgus-metatarsus primus
  varus c.
hindfoot joint c.
hippocampal-amygdaloid c.
hypoperfusion c.
hypovolemic c.
inferior glenohumeral ligament-labral
  c. (IGLLC)
inverted-Y c.
Kirklin meniscal c.
labral capsular c.
labral-ligamentous c.
labrum-ligament c.
lateral collateral ligament c.
ligamentous c.
limb-body wall c.
Lutembacher c.
mantle c.
mastoid c.
medial collateral ligament c. (MCLC)
mesenteric adenitis-ileitis c.
metal chelate c.

Michaelis c.
multiform ventricular c.
myocardial perfusion imaging Q c.
c. myxoma
nipple-areola c.
c. of vessels
ostiomeatal c.
outer anular/posterior longitudinal
  ligament c.
oxidized c.
pelvic mass c.
c. periosteal reaction
c. platinum microcoil
preintegration c.
primary c.
pulmonary sling c.
Q c.
Ranke c.
c. regional pain syndrome
renal sinus c.
respiratory chain c. (I-VI)
c. sclerosing lesion (CSL)
sesamoid c.
shoulder labral capsular c.
c. simple fracture
sling ring c.
c. solid and cystic mass
subluxation c.
c. subtraction
superior olivary c.
syndesmotic ligament c.
8th cranial nerve c.
tibiocalcaneal joint c.
transluminal coronary artery
  angioplasty c.
transposition c.
triangular fibrocartilaginous c.
  (TFCC)
VATER c.
ventricular premature c. (VPC)
vertebrobasilar c.
VIII nerve c.
von Meyenburg c.
zygomatic c.
zygomaticomaxillary c. (ZMC)

compliance
craniospinal c.
lung c.
c. matching stent (CMS)
reduced pulmonary c.

complicated
c. dislocation
c. fracture
c. hydatid cyst
c. myoma
c. pneumoconiosis
c. renal cyst
c. scleroderma
c. silicosis

complication
    air leak c.
    graft-related c.
    ischemic c.
    nonfetal c.
component
    anatomically graduated c. (AGC)
    central hemorrhagic c.
    cystic c.
    dispersive c.
    extensive intraductal c. (EIC)
    extracellular matrix c.
    frequency c.
    irregularly layered astrocytic c.
    irregularly layered neuronal c.
    markedly accentuated pulmonic c.
    mitral c.
    obstructive c.
    secretory c.
    solid c.
composite
    c. aortic valve
    c. fracture
    C. laryngeal recurrence staging
      system
    c. pulse
    c. signal
composition
    colonic gas c.
    hydropic c.
    renal stone mineral c.
compound
    c. aneurysm
    c. comminuted fracture
    c. complex fracture
    c. dislocation
    c. dislocation complex
    lipophilic c.
    PET c.
    c. pregnancy
    c. presentation
    radiolabeled c.
    reference c.
    c. skull fracture
    thorium c.
    titanium c.
    unsaturated c.
compressed body
compressibility and phasicity study
compression
    aqueduct c.
    c. atrophy
    biliary tree c.
    brachial artery c.
    brachial plexus c.
    brainstem c.
    cardiac c.
    cauda equina c.
    chamber c.

chiasmal c.
coned-down spot c.
contrecoup c.
cord c.
c. device
double-spot c.
external pneumatic calf c.
extrinsic bladder c.
fenestrated alphanumeric c.
fingerprint image c.
c. fracture
image c.
interfragmental c.
intrinsic c.
irreversible c.
lossless image data c.
lossy image data c.
magnification and spot c.
manual c.
medullary c.
multiplanar c.
nerve root c.
c. neuropathy
neurovascular c.
c. of breast
optic nerve c.
orbital mass c.
c. paddle
pancake c.
plaque c.
c. plate
c. plate and screw
radicular c.
c. ratio
real-time c.
root c.
c. sonography
spinal cord c.
spot c.
subchondral trabecular c.
symptomatic metastatic spinal cord
  c.
c. syndrome
thermal c.
c. ultrasonography
ultrasound-guided pseudoaneurysm c.
vascular esophageal c.
vascular tracheal c.
wavelet c.
compression-flexion injury
compressive
    c. atelectasis
    c. edema
    c. hyperextension injury
compromise
    circulatory c.
    Okuda hepatic c. (stage I-III)
    respiratory c.
    vascular c.

compromised
- c. flow
- c. pregnancy
- c. ventricular function

Compton
- C. coherent scattering densitometry
- C. edge
- C. effect
- C. electron
- C. interaction
- C. scatter
- C. scattering
- C. scattering cross-section
- C. scattering photon
- C. suppression spectrometer
- C. suppression system
- C. wavelength

Compuscan
- C. Hittman computerized electrocardioscanner
- C. Hittman computerized imaging

computation
- analogue c.

computational anatomy

computed
- c. axial tomography (CAT)
- c. axial tomography-methoxyisobutyl isonitrile (CAT-MIBI)
- c. dental radiography (CDR)
- c. ejection fraction
- c. myelography
- c. perfusion map
- c. radiography
- c. radiology
- c. tomographic angiography (CTA)
- c. tomographic angiography of pulmonary artery
- c. tomographic cholangiography
- c. tomographic colonography (CTC)
- c. tomographic cystography
- c. tomographic dacryocystography
- c. tomographic enteroclysis
- c. tomographic lymphography
- c. tomographic metrizamide myelography (CTMM)
- c. tomographic pulmonary angiography
- c. tomography (CT)
- c. tomography angiogram
- c. tomography arterial portography
- c. tomography cisternography
- c. tomography dose index (CTDI)
- c. tomography during arterial portography
- c. tomography fluoroscopy (CTF)
- c. tomography-guided percutaneous radiofrequency denervation of sacroiliac joint
- c. tomography laser mammography (CTLM)
- c. tomography-positron emission tomography (CT-PET)
- c. tomography pulmonary venography (CTPV)
- c. tomography scan
- c. tomography/single-photon emission computed tomography (CT/SPECT)
- c. tomography truncation artifact
- c. tomography venography (CTV)
- c. tomography with arterioportography (CTAP)
- c. transmission tomography
- c. transmission tomography imaging

computer
- c. automated scan technology (CAST)
- c. fusion imaging
- image reconstruction c.
- c. information system
- c. method
- c. strain-gauge plethysmography (CSGP)
- c. subtraction technique
- C. Technology and Imaging (CTI)

computer-aided
- c.-a. diagnosis (CAD)
- c.-a. diagnosis scheme
- c.-a. image analysis
- c.-a. joint space analysis (CAJSA)
- c.-a. polyp detection

computer-assisted
- c.-a. blood background subtraction (CABBS)
- c.-a. intracranial navigation
- c.-a. joint motion analysis
- c.-a. myelography (CAM)
- c.-a. resection of cerebral arteriovenous malformation
- c.-a. stereotactic resection
- c.-a. volumetric stereotaxis

computer-controlled
- c.-c. conformal radiation therapy (CCRT)
- c.-c. radiotherapy

computer-generated
- c.-g. artifact
- c.-g. image

computerized
- c. axial tomography (CAT)
- c. cranial tomography
- c. fluoroscopy
- c. optical densitometry (COD)
- c. radiography
- c. radiotherapy
- c. texture analysis of lung nodules and lung parenchyma
- c. thermal imaging system
- c. tomographic hepatic angiography (CTHA)

C

197

computerized (*continued*)
    c. tomographic holography (CTH)
    c. tomography guidance
    c. tomography-guided needle biopsy
    c. tomography/magnetic resonance (CT/MR)
    c. transverse axial image
    c. transverse axial tomography (CTAT)
computer-simulated phantom
conal
    c. cyst
    c. papillary muscle
    c. septum
    c. ventricular septal defect
concatenation of shadows
Concato disease
concave skull disc
concavity
    posterior c.
concavoconvex
concealed
    c. hemorrhage
    c. penis
concentrated bile
concentration
    deoxyhemoglobin c.
    directional gradient c. (DGC)
    hypertensive contrast c.
    maximum permissible c.
    methylene diphosphonate c.
    minimal inhibitory c. (MIC)
    NAWM metabolite c.
    c. of radionuclide
    organ-specific c.
    Poisson distributed activity c.
    synaptic dopamine c.
    time-dependent xenon c.
    c. times time (C × T)
concentration-time curve
concentric
    c. anular tear
    c. atherosclerotic plaque
    c. calcification
    c. circle technique
    c. contraction
    c. fibroma
    c. heart hypertrophy
    c. hernia
    c. herniation
    c. hourglass stenosis
    c. hypertrophic cardiomyopathy
    c. lamella
    c. lesion
    c. narrowing
    c. pantomography
    c. reduction

concentrica
    encephalitis periaxialis c.
concept
    gooseneck c.
    line integral c.
    no-threshold c.
    ring-of-bone c.
conception
    retained products of c. (RPOC)
concertina pattern
concha, *pl.* **conchae**
    c. bullosa
    nasal c.
conchae (*pl. of* concha)
conchal
    c. cartilage
    c. crest
concomitant
    c. boost radiation therapy
    c. defect
    c. finding
    c. infarct
    c. infection
    c. pneumonia
    c. tracheal injury
concordance
    c. of MR finding
    radiologic-pathologic c.
    situs c.
concordant result
concretion
    bile c.
    fecal c.
concurrent chemoradiotherapy
concussion
    brain c.
    spinal c.
condensans
    clavicular osteitis c.
condition
    adnexal c.
    insonation c.
    nonfetal uterine c.
    nonthromboembolic c.
conditioned reflex
condom catheter
conductance catheter
conducting bronchiole
conduction
    c. band
    c. block
    interval intraatrial c.
    nodal c.
    c. ratio
    reciprocating c.
    retrograde ventriculoatrial c.
    c. system
    ventriculoatrial c.
    zone of slow c.

conductive
    c. development
    c. loop
conductivity
    thermal c.
    tissue c.
    vascular hydraulic c.
conductor
    fiberoptic c.
    c. resistivity
conduit
    detour c.
    ileal c.
    intestinal c.
    nonvalved c.
    right ventricle-pulmonary artery c.
    urinary c.
    c. valve
    ventriculoarterial c.
condylar
    c. angle
    c. articulation
    c. axis
    c. canal
    c. emissary vein
    c. flare
    c. fossa
    c. part of occipital bone
    c. plate
    c. skull hypoplasia
    c. split fracture
    c. translation
condyle
    c. cord
    external c.
    femoral c.
    lateral c.
    mandibular c.
    medial c.
    occipital c.
    tibial c.
condyloid
    c. canal
    c. joint
    c. process
condyloma, *pl.* **condylomata**
condylomata (*pl. of* condyloma)
condylomatous atypia lesion
condylus tertius
cone
    arterial c.
    c. beam
    beveled electron beam c.
    c. disc
    c. down
    c. epiphysis
    medullary c.
    c. of extraocular muscle
    parenchymatous c.

    c. spot compression view
    transvaginal c.
cone-beam image
coned
    c. cecum
    c. down
    c. panoramic tomogram
coned-down
    c.-d. appearance of colon
    c.-d. compression view
    c.-d. radiograph
    c.-d. spot compression
CO_2-negative imaging agent
confidence interval
configuration
    adaptic detector c.
    anatomic c.
    back-to-back c.
    batwing c.
    beaklike c.
    bilobate c.
    biventricular c.
    bulbous c.
    bull's-eye c.
    butterfly c.
    cat's tail c.
    closed-fist c.
    Cupid's bow c.
    cylindrical c.
    discoid c.
    dome-and-dart c.
    double-halo c.
    expansile c.
    fishmouth mitral valve c.
    geriatric c.
    globular c.
    Helmholtz c.
    hexagonal c.
    horizontal dipole c.
    horseshoe c.
    hourglass c.
    hybrid detector c.
    inverted-Y c.
    isosceles triangular c.
    left ventricular c.
    lock-washer c.
    masslike c.
    molar tooth c.
    mosaic detector c.
    multilobular c.
    nonplanar c.
    octagonal c.
    planar c.
    reversed-3 c.
    ringlike c.
    rosary bead c.
    sandwich c.
    sawtooth c.
    scalloped luminal c.

C

configuration (*continued*)
    shepherd's crook c.
    sigmoid-shaped c.
    snowman c.
    stellate c.
    streaklike c.
    surface c.
    swallowtail c.
    T c.
    tentorium keyhole c.
    thoracic cage c.
    tombstone pelvis c.
    triangle c.
    triple-peak cerebellum c.
    unidirectional lead c.
    water-bottle c.
    winged c.
    wooden-shoe c.
    Y c.
configurational formula
confinement
    regional tumor c.
confluence
    c. of vascular markings
    pulmonary c.
    stellate c.
confluens sinuum
confluent
    c. areas of atelectasis
    c. consolidation
    c. fibrosis
    c. infiltrate
confocal image
conformal
    c. neutron and photon radiation
      therapy
    c. radiation therapy (CRT)
Conformexx biliary stent
confusion
    circle of c.
congenita
    amyotonia c.
    arthrogryposis multiplex c.
    chondrodystrophia calcificans c.
congenital
    c. abnormality
    c. absence of kidney
    c. absence of pulmonary artery
    c. absence of pulmonary valve
    c. absence of thymus
    c. adrenal hyperplasia (CAH)
    c. adrenocortical hyperplasia
    c. adrenogenital syndrome
    c. amputation
    c. aneurysm of pulmonary artery
    c. anomaly of mitral valve
      (CAMV)
    c. aortic regurgitation
    c. aortic sinus aneurysm

c. arteriosclerotic aneurysm
c. atelectasis
c. bar
c. biliary atresia
c. bipartite scaphoid
c. bronchiectasis
c. bronchogenic cyst
c. cardiac tumor
c. cardiac valve stenosis
c. cephalocele
c. cerebral aneurysm
c. cholesteatoma
c. cystic adenomatoid malformation
  (CCAM)
c. cystic dilation
c. cystic neck lesion
c. deformity
c. diaphragmatic hernia
c. diffuse fibromatosis
c. dilated cardiomyopathy
c. dislocation of hip (CDH)
c. disorder
c. duodenal obstruction
c. dysplasia of hip
c. esophageal stenosis
c. Finnish nephrosis
c. fracture
c. generalized fibromatosis
c. goiter
c. heart block
c. heart defect (CHD)
c. heart disease (CHD)
c. heart disease classification
c. heart malformation
c. hemidysplasia with ichthyosiform
  erythroderma and limb defects
  (CHILD)
c. hemiplegia
c. hepatic cyst
c. hepatic fibrosis (CHF)
c. hip dislocation
c. hip dysplasia
c. hippocampal sclerosis
c. holoprosencephaly
c. hydrocele
c. hydrocephalus
c. hydronephrosis
c. infiltrating lipomatosis of face
c. interruption of aortic arch
c. intestinal atresia
c. intracranial aneurysm
c. isthmic coarctation
c. kidney fibrosarcoma
c. laryngeal atresia
c. laxity of ligament
c. left-sided outflow obstruction
c. left ventricular aneurysm
c. leukodystrophy
c. liver fibrosis

c. lobar emphysema (CLE)
c. lobar hyperinflation
c. lung cyst
c. lymphangiectasis
c. lymphangiectasis of intestine
c. mediastinal arterial variant
c. megacalyx
c. megacolon
c. mesoblastic nephroma
c. mitral regurgitation (CMR)
c. muscular dystrophy
c. nasal mass
c. pelviureteric junction obstruction
c. pericardial absence
c. pneumothorax
c. polyvalvular dysplasia
c. pulmonary arteriovenous fistula
c. pulmonary artery aneurysm
c. pulmonary hypoplasia
c. pulmonary valve insufficiency
c. pulmonary venolobar syndrome
c. radioulnar synostosis
c. renal aneurysm
c. renal hypoplasia
c. renal osteodystrophy
c. ring
c. scoliosis
c. septooptic dysplasia
c. splenomegaly
c. stenosis of pulmonary vein
c. stippled epiphysis
c. subpulmonic obstruction
c. symptomatic AV block
c. tibia vara
c. tracheobiliary fistula
c. tracheobronchomegaly
c. tracheomalacia
c. ureteric obstruction
c. urethral diverticulum
c. urethral stricture
c. valvular insufficiency
c. vascular-bone syndrome (CVBS)
c. vascular malformation (CVM)
c. vertical talus
c. vesicoureteral reflux
congenitally
c. absent pericardium
c. corrected transposition
c. corrected transposition of great arteries
c. short esophagus
congenitum
congential megaureter
congested
c. kidney
c. pleura
congestion
active c.
asymmetric pulmonary c.

capillary c.
cardiac c.
centrilobular c.
cerebral c.
chronic passive c.
hepatic c.
hypostatic c.
c. index
intravascular c.
passive hepatic c.
passive vascular c.
pulmonary vascular c.
pulmonary venous c. (PVC)
splenic c.
symmetric pulmonary c.
vascular c.
venous heart c.
congestive
c. asymmetry
c. atelectasis
c. brain swelling
c. cardiomyopathy
c. cirrhosis
c. heart failure (CHF)
c. splenomegaly
conglomerate
c. calcification
c. mass
nonspecific c.
c. opacity
c. pulmonary nodule
conglutinating complement absorption test
congophilic angiopathy
Congo red stain
congruence
c. angle
patellofemoral c.
congruent
c. articulation
c. point
c. reduction
c. signal intensity abnormality
coni (*pl. of* conus)
conical
c. cecum
c. heart
c. mass
conjoined
c. cusps
c. nerve roots anomaly
c. root sleeves
c. tendons
c. twins
conjugal carcinoma
conjugate
complex c.
c. diameter
c. foramen

conjugate (*continued*)
    c. gradient
    c. ligament
conjugated hyperbilirubinemia
conjunctiva, *pl.* **conjunctivae**
conjunctivae (*pl. of* conjunctiva)
conjunctival vein
conjunctivum
    brachium c.
connate tooth
connectedness
    theory of fuzzy c.
connecting
    c. canal
    c. cartilage
    c. plate
    c. tubule
connection
    anomalous pulmonary venous c.
    atrioventricular c.
    cavopulmonary c.
    coarctation of anomalous venous c.
    corticocerebellar c.
    partial anomalous pulmonary venous c.
    rostral c.
    slip-in c.
    total anomalous pulmonary venous c.
    ventriculoarterial c.
    wispy c.
connective
    c. tissue
    c. tissue disease
    c. tissue fibrous tumor
    c. tissue neoplasia
    c. tissue proliferation
    c. tissue septum
connector
    cerebral ventricular shunt c.
conniventes
    valvulae c.
Conn syndrome
conoid
    c. ligament
    c. process
    c. tubercle
conotruncal congenital anomaly
conoventricular
    c. defect
    c. defect PTA balloon dilation
      catheter
Conquest PTA balloon dilation catheter
Conrad-Bugg trapping of soft tissue in ankle fracture
Conrad-Crosby bone marrow biopsy needle
Conradi-Hünermann syndrome
Conradi line
Conray 30, 43, 400 imaging agent
conscious sedation

consecutive dislocations
consistency
    cake-glaze c.
    glaze c.
console
    Bruker c.
    direct display c. (DDC)
    Siemens Satellite CT evaluation c.
consolidated
    c. infiltrate
    c. lung
consolidation
    airspace c.
    alveolar c.
    batwing lung c.
    bilateral c.
    cavitary c.
    confluent c.
    dense c.
    discrete area of c.
    exudative c.
    focal alveolar c.
    fracture line of c.
    hemorrhage c.
    ill-defined c.
    lobar c.
    lung parenchyma c.
    nonhomogeneous c.
    parenchymatous c.
    patchy area of c.
    peripheral c.
    pulmonary c.
    segmental bronchus c.
    solid c.
    symmetric c.
    unilateral c.
consolidative
    c. change
    c. pneumonia
    c. process
consortium
    Lung Tissue Resource C. (LTRC)
conspicuity
    lesion c.
    tumor c.
constant
    air Kerma rate c.
    Avogadro c.
    coupling c.
    decay c.
    disintegration c.
    equilibrium dissociation c.
    equilibrium dose c.
    c. level appearance
    maximum amplitude c.
    permeability c.
    c. permeability
    Planck c.
    radioactive c.

c. tilt wave
time c.
transformation c.
T1, T2 time c.
constant-infusion excretory urogram
constant-load treadmill testing
constellation
c. of findings
c. of symptoms
constituent
plaque c.
constitutional
c. osteosclerosis
c. symptom
constrained Wallgraft endoprosthesis
constricting esophageal lesion
constriction
airway c.
c. band
c. band syndrome
ductal c.
hourglass c.
occult pericardial c.
postglomerular arteriolar c.
c. ring
supraanular c.
tangential c.
waistlike c.
constrictive
c. bronchiolitis
c. cardiomyopathy
c. pericarditis
construction artifact
consultation
curbstone c.
consumption
cerebral metabolic oxygen c.
myocardial oxygen c.
oxygen c. (QO_2)
contact
bone-on-bone c.
c. B-scan ultrasound
c. carcinoma
catheter-tissue c.
c. effect
c. image
c. lateral view
c. precaution
c. radiation therapy
c. radiograph
c. radiotherapy
screen-film c.
stent-vessel wall c.
c. transscleral laser
cytophotocoagulation (CTLC)
contained
c. aneurysmal rupture
c. aortic rupture
c. disc

c. leak
c. leak of aortic aneurysm
contaminating tumor cell
contamination
collimator c.
radionuclide c.
surface c.
venous c.
content
abdominal c.'s
bone mineral c. (BMC)
bowel c.'s
brain water c.
digestive tract c.'s
disc water c.
fat-suppressing c.
femoral triangular c.
gastric c.'s
herniated abdominal c.'s
homogeneous echogenic uterine c.'s
intestinal c.'s
intravascular c.'s
macromolecular c.
overlying bowel c.'s
retrograde flow of gastric c.'s
small bowel c.'s
tissue water c.
venous oxygen c.
contention
adequate c.
contiguous
c. articular surfaces
c. images
c. interleaved axial sections
c. loops
c. organ involvement
c. parallel chords
c. scans
c. segments
c. slice MEMP
c. slices
c. supramarginal gyri
c. ventricular septal defects
continent urinary diversion
continua (*pl. of* continuum)
continuation
azygos c.
continuity
aortoseptal c.
bowel c.
c. equation
c. of bone
pancreatic-enteric c.
continuous
c. ambulatory peritoneal dialysis
(CAPD)
c. arterial spin-labeling perfusion
MR
c. capillary

continuous (*continued*)
 c. diaphragm sign
 c. hyperfractionated accelerated
  radiation therapy
 c. hyperfractionated accelerated
  radiotherapy
 c. hyperthermic peritoneal perfusion
 c. imaging
 c. intravenous infusion (CIVI)
 c. mode
 c. moving bed MR imaging
 c. psoas compartment block (CPCB)
 c. scanning
 c. suture graft inclusion technique
  (CSGIT)
 c. volumetric acquisition
 c. wave
 c. x-ray spectrum
continuous-loop exercise
 echocardiography
continuous-scan thermograph
continuous-wave
 c.-w. Doppler echocardiography
 c.-w. Doppler imaging
 c.-w. Doppler recording
 c.-w. Doppler ultrasound system
 c.-w. laser system
 c.-w. NMR
continuum, *pl.* **continua**
 Dandy-Walker c.
 epilepsia partialis continua
contortus
 pes c.
contour
 altered aortic c.
 altered mediastinal c.
 convex outward c.
 Cupid's bow c.
 diaphragmatic c.
 double diaphragm c.
 c. extraction
 irregular hazy luminal c.
 isodose c.
 lobulated c.
 local bulge of kidney c.
 local bulge of renal c.
 c. mapping
 mediastinal c.
 patellar c.
 reniform c.
 S c.
 sawtooth irregularity of bowel c.
 scalloping c.
 C. SE microsphere
 smooth c.
 undulating c.
 vascular c.
contoured tilting compression
 mammography

contracted
 c. bladder
 c. bronchus
 c. gallbladder
 c. kidney
 c. pelvis
contractile
 c. function
 c. pattern
 c. reserve
 c. ring dysphagia
 c. stricture
 c. work index
contractility
 cardiac c.
 c. index
 myocardial c.
contraction
 c. band necrosis
 concentric c.
 esophageal c.
 focal myometrial c.
 kissing c.
 myometrial c.
 nodal premature c.
 peristaltic c.
 phasic c.
 premature nodal c. (PNC)
 premature ventricular c. (PVC)
 ringlike c.
 c. stress test (CST)
 uterine c.
 ventricular premature c. (VPC)
 ventricular segmental c.
contracture
 bladder neck c.
 capsular c.
 c. deformity
 Dupuytren c.
 elbow c.
 fixed flexion c.
 flexion c.
 flexion-adduction c.
 gastrocnemius-soleus c.
 hip flexion c.
 ischemic c.
 joint c.
 knee flexion c.
 muscle c.
 myocardial c.
 myostatic c.
 scar c.
 secondary c.
 soft tissue c.
 Volkmann ischemic c.
 web c.
contralateral
 c. artery
 c. hypertrophy

c. kidney
c. lung
c. sign
c. subtraction technique
c. vessel

contrast

c. absorption barrier
c. administration
c. agent
c. angiography
c. aortography
c. arteriography
barium enema with air c.
c. bolus
c. computed arthrotomography
CT scan with c.
c. data
c. ductography
dynamic susceptibility c. (DSC)
echo c.
c. echocardiography
c. enema
c. enhancement
c. enhancement of computed
  tomographic imaging
c. enhancement pattern
c. esophagram
c. extravasation
glioma-to-white-matter c.
image c.
c. improvement factor
c. infiltration
c. inhomogeneity
c. injection
intraarticular c.
iron-dependent c.
c. laryngography
c. left atriography
lesion-to-white-matter c.
c. loading
long-scale c.
c. lymphangiography
magnetization transfer c. (MTC)
c. material
c. material-enhanced intravenous
  lymphography
c. material-enhanced scanning
c. material instillation
c. medium (CM)
c. medium adverse effect
c. medium column
c. medium excretion
c. medium-induced cytotoxicity
c. medium-induced nephropathy
c. medium-induced pulmonary
  vascular hyperpermeability
c. medium leakage
c. medium nephrotoxicity
c. medium washout

near-resonance spin-lock c.
c. opacification
phase c.
c. precipitation
puddling of c.
radiographic c.
c. radiography
Readi-Cat oral c.
c. resolution
c. selective cholangiogram
c. sensitivity
short-scale c.
small-particle iron oxide c.
soft tissue c.
spontaneous echo c.
subject c.
c. subtraction mammography
time to peak c. (TPC)
tissue c.
c. transesophageal
  echocardiography:yttrium-aluminum-
  garnet
c. transfer characteristic
triple c.
unsharp mask-type c.
c. uptake
c. venography
c. ventriculogram
vessel-to-background c.
c. window level
c. window width
c. x-ray angiography

contrast-enhanced

c.-e. color Doppler
c.-e. computed tomography (CECT)
c.-e. CT
c.-e. CT with saline flush technique
c.-e. dynamic snapshot
c.-e. echocardiography
c.-e. FAST
c.-e. Fourier acquired steady-state
  technique (CE-FAST)
c.-e. fundamental imaging
c.-e. magnetic resonance angiography
  (CEMRA)
c.-e. magnetic resonance imaging
c.-e. MR
c.-e. MRA
c.-e. MR angiography
c.-e. MRI
c.-e. MR image
c.-e. near-infrared laser
  mammography
c.-e. power Doppler
c.-e. radiographic examination
c.-e. retrospective
  electrocardiogram-gated spiral
  technique
c.-e. T1-GRE imaging

C

contrast-enhanced (*continued*)
  c.-e. transrectal sonography
  c.-e. T1-weighted fat-suppressed image
  c.-e. T1-weighted spin-echo high field-strength MR imaging
  c.-e. ultrasound
  c.-e. virtual MR cholangioscopy
contrast-enhancing parametric imaging
contrast-filled
  c.-f. catheter
  c.-f. stomach
contrast-induced
  c.-i. nephropathy (CIN)
  c.-i. renal failure
contrast-to-noise
  c.-t.-n. calculation
  c.-t.-n. ratio (C/N, CNR)
contrecoup
  c. compression
  c. fracture
  c. injury
  c. mechanism
control
  c. angiogram
  automatic brightness c. (ABC)
  automatic exposure c. (AEC)
  automatic gain c. (AGC)
  C-arm fluoroscopic c.
  dynamic range c. (DRC)
  fluoroscopic c.
  image c.
  intravenous accurate c. (IVAC)
  locoregional c.
  radiofrequency radiographic c.
  c. radiograph
  radiographic c.
  radiopharmaceutical quality c.
  scintigraphy quality c.
  SPECT quality c.
  Spli-Prest negative c.
  Spli-Prest positive c.
  time-varied gain c.
controlled ventricular response
controller
  Imed Gemini PC-2 volumetric c.
contusio cerebri
contusion
  bone c.
  bony c.
  brain c.
  cerebral c.
  cortical c.
  frontal lobe c.
  lung c.
  myocardial c.
  osseous bone c.
  c. pneumonia

  pontile c.
  pulmonary c.
  rib c.
  soft tissue c.
  spinal c.
  urinary bladder c.
conus, *pl.* **coni**
  c. arteriosus medullaris
  c. artery
  c. branch ostium
  c. clasticus
  club-shaped c.
  c. elasticus
  c. eye
  c. hypoplasia
  c. ligament
  c. medullaris lesion
  c. medullaris position
  c. septum
  c. tip
conventional
  c. angiography
  c. head coil
  c. hysterography
  c. osteosarcoma
  c. planar imaging (CPI)
  c. processor
  c. pulse sequence
  c. radiograph
  c. spin-echo imaging
  c. study
  c. tomography
  c. transverse cross-sectional image
  c. ultrashort echo time
  c. venography
conventionally fractionated stereotactic radiation therapy
convergence zone
convergent
  c. beam irradiation (CBI)
  c. color Doppler
  c. color Doppler imaging
converging collimator
converging-hole collimator
conversion
  bone marrow c.
  coefficient c.
  color space c.
  c. defect
  c. efficiency
  c. electron
  internal c.
  c. ratio
  spontaneous c.
  thoracofemoral c.
converter
  analogue-to-digital c. (ADC)
  digital-to-analogue c. (DAC)
  image c.

motion-compensating format c.
multiplying digital-to-analogue c.
 (MDAC)
real-time format c.
scan c.

convex
c. border of stomach
c. linear array
c. outward contour
c. posterior margin

convexity
brain c.
cerebral c.
frontocentral c.
c. lesion
c. meningioma
c. of lung
paratracheal c.
parietal c.
soft tissue c.

convexobasia
convexoconcave heart valve
convoluted
c. bone
c. T-cell lymphoma
c. tubule

convolution
Arnold c.
ascending frontal c.
ascending parietal c.
Broca c.
cerebral c.
Gratiolet c.
Heschl c.
c. mask
occipitotemporal c.
Zuckerkandl c.

convolutional
c. differencing
c. impression
c. marking
c. pattern

Cook-Cope-type loop catheter
Cook enforcer
cookie
c. bite lesion
c. cutter lesion

coolant
Cooley-Tukey alignment
CoolGlide laser
Coolidge
C. transformer
C. x-ray tube

cooling
tissue c.

Coopernail sign
Cooper suspensory ligament
coordinate
c. axis

c.'s for target lesion
Talairach c.

coordination
meniscocondylar c.

COP
colloid oncotic pressure

COPD
chronic obstructive pulmonary disease
emphysematous COPD

cope
C. biopsy needle
C. locking-loop catheter
C. loop
C. loop catheter
C. loop nephrostomy
C. mandril guidewire
C. method bronchogram
C. point

Copeland-Kavat metatarsophalangeal dislocation classification
Cope-method bronchography
coplanar
c. beam
c. contour point

copper (Cu)
c. 62 (^{62}Cu, Cu-62)
c. 64 (^{64}Cu, Cu-64)
c. 67 (^{67}Cu, Cu-67)
c. filtration
c. imaging agent
c. 7, T intrauterine device
c. wire effect

copper-vapor pulsed laser
copper-zinc
c.-z. superoxide dismutase
 (Cu/Zn-SOD)
c.-z. superoxide dismutase imaging
 agent

coprecipitation
coprolith
coprostasis
copy
magnification hard c.

COR
center of rotation

cor
c. adiposum
c. arteriosum
c. biloculare
c. bovinum
c. dextrum
c. en cuirasse
c. mobile
c. pendulum
c. pulmonale
c. triatriatum
c. triatriatum dexter

coracoacromial
c. arch

C

coracoacromial (*continued*)
    c. ligament
    c. process
coracobrachialis
coracoclavicular
    c. bar
    c. joint
    c. ligament
    c. space
coracohumeral ligament
coracoid
    c. bursa
    c. fracture
    c. notch
    c. process
    c. tip avulsion
    c. tuberosity
coral
    c. calculus
    c. reef atheroma
    c. thrombus
coralline hydroxyapatite ocular implant
cord
    c. angioblastoma
    anterior gray column of c.
    anterior horn of spinal c.
    anterolateral white matter of c.
    astrocytoma c.
    c. atrophy
    cervical c.
    c. compression
    condyle c.
    c. deformation
    dura mater of spinal c.
    c. edema
    c. embarrassment
    ependymoma c.
    c. epidural extramedullary lesion
    false vocal c.
    fibrous c.
    hepatic c.
    c. intradural extramedullary mass
    c. intramedullary lesion
    medullary c.
    meninx of spinal c.
    mucoid degeneration of umbilical c.
    multiple focal lesions of spinal c.
    noncoiled umbilical c.
    nuchal c.
    posterior gray column of c.
    c. presentation
    pretendinous c.
    c. prolapse
    prolapse of umbilical c.
    reactive cyst c.
    c. remodeling
    ropelike c.
    rostral spinal c.
    c. sign

    size of spinal c.
    spermatic c.
    spinal c.
    split spinal c.
    straight c.
    c. structure
    tethered spinal c.
    thoracic spinal c.
    transection of spinal c.
    true vocal c.
    umbilical c.
    velamentous insertion of c.
    2-vessel umbilical c.
    3-vessel umbilical c.
    vocal c.
    Weitbrecht c.
    white commissure of spinal c.
cordate (*var. of* cordiform)
cordiform, cordate
    c. pelvis
cordis
    apex c.
    atrium dextrum c.
    atrium sinistrum c.
    C. Brite Tip guiding catheter
    bulbus c.
    chordae tendineae c.
    ectopia c.
    C. endovascular system
    fetal ectopia c.
    fossa ovalis c.
    C. injector
    C. multipurpose access port
    C. Palmaz Corinthian stent
    C. Palmaz Schatz long medium
      stent
    C. Predator PTCA balloon catheter
    C. sheath
    C. Smart nitinol stent
    ventriculus c.
    vortex c.
cordlike
    c. mass
    c. trunk
cordocentesis
    therapeutic c.
Cordonnier ureteroileal loop
cordotomy
    percutaneous cervical c.
cord-subarachnoid space ratio
corduroy
    c. artery
    c. artifact
    c. cloth pattern
core
    bone c.
    c. bone biopsy needle
    fibrovascular c.
    ischemic c.

c. needle biopsy
nitinol wire c.
coregistered
c. MRI
c. scan
coregistration
image c.
morphologic and physiologic image c.
c. paradigm
voxel-based c.
core-warming maneuver
CORI
Clinical Outcomes Research Initiative
CORI computerized endoscopic
report generator
Corinthian stainless steel
balloon-expandable stent
corked tracheostomy tube
corkscrew
c. appearance
c. appearance of esophagus
c. appearance of hepatic
artery
c. appearance of small bowel
c. pattern
c. ureter
c. vessel
corkscrew-type flow pattern
CORLA
cluster of radiolucent areas
corn
apical c.
corneae
vertex c.
corneal
c. facet
c. tube
Cornell
C. high-energy synchrotron source
(CHESS)
C. protocol
corner
c. film
c. fracture
c. of knee
cornflake
c. esophageal motility study
c., milk, and sugar meal
corniculate
c. cartilage
c. tubercle
corniculopharyngeal ligament
cornu, *pl.* **cornua**
c. of sacrum
c. of uterus
cornua (*pl. of* cornu)
cornual
c. ectopic pregnancy
c. implantation

corona, *pl.* **coronae**
c. radiata
coronae (*pl. of* corona)
coronal
c. angulation
c. bending view
c. cleft
c. cleft vertebra
c. computed tomographic
arthrography (CCTA)
c. ECD brain SPECT image
c. FLAIR MRI
c. GRE MR image
c. maximum-intensity projection
c. oblique technique
c. orientation
c. planar image
c. plane
c. proton density-weighted fast
spin-echo image
c. reconstruction
c. reconstruction view
c. reformation
c. scan
c. section
c. slab
c. slice
c. STIR image
c. suture
c. suture synostosis
c. tomographic reconstruction
c. T1-weighted image
coronary
c. angiography
c. arterial territory
c. arteriography
c. arteriosclerosis
c. arteriosystemic fistula
c. arteriovenous fistula
c. artery
c. artery anatomy
c. artery aneurysm
c. artery bypass graft (CABG)
c. artery bypass graft patency
c. artery bypass surgery (CABS)
c. artery calcification (CAC)
c. artery calcium score (CACS)
c. artery cameral fistula
c. artery disease
c. artery dominance
c. artery ectasia
c. artery embolus
c. artery lesion
c. artery malformation
c. artery of heart
c. artery of stomach
c. artery ostium
c. artery-pulmonary artery fistula
c. artery scan (CAS)

C

coronary (*continued*)
 c. artery scan imaging
 c. artery spasm (CAS)
 c. artery steal syndrome
 c. artery stenosis
 c. artery to right ventricle fistula
 c. artery tree
 c. atherosclerosis
 c. blood flow
 c. blood flow velocity (CBFV)
 c. cineangiography
 c. cusp
 c. electron beam angiography
 c. embolism
 c. flow reserve (CFR)
 c. groove
 c. insufficiency
 c. ischemia
 c. ligament
 c. luminal stenosis
 c. node
 c. occlusion
 c. orifice
 c. ostial revascularization
 c. ostial stenosis
 c. pathology
 c. perfusion gradient
 c. perfusion pressure
 c. plaque burden
 c. plexus
 c. radiation therapy (CRT)
 RDX c.
 c. remodeling
 c. reserve flow (CRF)
 c. sclerosis
 c. sinus
 c. sinus CT
 c. sinus electrogram
 c. sinus of Valsalva
 c. sinus os
 c. sinus ostium
 c. sinus retroperfusion
 c. sinus root
 c. sinus valve
 c. stenosis index (CSI)
 c. sulcus
 c. tendon
 c. thrombosis
 c. vascular resistance
 c. vascular resistance index (CVRI)
 c. vein
 c. vessel aneurysm
 c. vessel geometry
 c. wedge pressure
coronary-subclavian steal syndrome
coronoid
 c. fossa
 c. of mandible
 c. of ulna

 c. process
 c. process fracture
Coroskop Plus cardiac angiography system
corpora (*pl. of* corpus)
corpulence, corpulency
corpulency (*var. of* corpulence)
corpulent
corpus, *pl.* **corpora**
 c. albicans cyst
 c. amylaceum
 anterior c.
 c. callosum
 c. callosum agenesis
 c. callosum dysgenesis
 c. callosum hypoplasia, retardation, adducted thumbs, spastic paraparesis, and hydrocephalus (CRASH)
 c. callosum lipoma
 c. callosum ring-enhancing lesion
 c. carcinoma
 c. cavernosography
 c. cavernosonography imaging
 c. cavernosum penis
 corpora amylacea
 c. fornicis
 c. hemorrhagicum
 c. luteum cyst
 c. luteum hematoma
 c. medullare
 c. restiforme
 c. spongiosum
 c. spongiosum penis
 c. sterni
 c. striatum
 c. uteri
corpuscular radiation
corrected
 c. gradient-echo phase imaging
 c. sinus node recovery time
 c. TIMI frame count (CTFC)
 c. transposition of great arteries
correction
 accidental c.
 adaptive c.
 attenuation c.
 automatic motion c.
 baseline c.
 coincidence-summing c.
 degree of c.
 3D motion c.
 echo phase c. (EPC)
 fuzzy logic contrast c.
 inhomogeneity c.
 multi-illuminant color c.
 navigator-guided motion c.
 2nd-order c.
 on-the-fly random c.
 phase c.

Picker SPECT attenuation c.
prospective acquisition c. (PACE)
scatter c.
section timing c.
1st-order attenuation c.
summing c.
surface variable-attenuation c.
ultrasound aberration c.
correlated spectroscopy (COSY)
correlation
c. analysis
clinical c.
c. coefficient
echocardiograph c.
false-negative c.
functional c.
histologic c.
histopathologic CT c.
imaging-anatomy c.
imaging-pathology c.
in vivo c.
mammographic-histopathologic c.
morphologic c.
neuropathologic c.
neuroradiologic c.
pathologic c.
radiologic-anatomic c.
radiologic-pathologic c.
side-by-side c.
c. time
correlative
c. diagnostic imaging
c. Doppler study
c. multimodality imaging
c. pertechnetate thyroid imaging
Correra line
corresponding ray
Corrigan sign
corrosive
c. esophagitis
c. gastritis
corrugated
c. air column
c. fat-pad surface
Cortenema retention enema
cortex, *pl.* **cortices**
adrenal c.
articular c.
auditory c.
bilateral orbitofrontal cortices
bone c.
calcarine c.
caudolateral orbitofrontal c.
cerebellar c.
cerebral c.
cingulate c.
eloquent c.
entorhinal c.
femoral c.

frontal c.
frontoparietal parasagittal c.
increased renal echogenicity c.
inner adrenal c.
lymphatic c.
mesial frontal c.
motor c.
nonolfactory c.
c. of cerebrum
opercular c.
orbitofrontal c.
ovarian c.
parastriate c.
parietal c.
patchy atrophy of renal c.
perirolandic parietal c.
peristriate c.
perisylvian c.
piriform c.
postfrontal c.
postrolandic parietal c.
prefrontal c.
premotor c.
prepiriform c.
primary auditory c.
primary motor c. (PMC)
primary visual c.
pyramidal layer of cerebral c.
rarefaction of c.
renal c.
renin-angiotensin-dependent outer c.
rolandic c.
sensorimotor c.
somatosensory c.
striate c.
ventral occipitotemporal visual c.
visual c.
Corti
C. canal
C. organ
cortical
c. abrasion
c. activity
c. adenoma
c. artery
c. atrophy
c. blush
c. bone
c. bone infarct
c. bone lesion
c. bone resorption
c. branch
c. center
c. cerebellar degeneration
c. contusion
c. defect
c. deficit
c. desmoid
c. destruction

cortical (*continued*)
    c. diffusion restriction
    c. disruption
    c. dysfunction
    c. dysplasia
    c. flattening
    c. fracture
    c. fragment
    c. gray matter
    c. hamartoma
    c. hinge axis
    c. hyperintensity
    c. hyperostosis
    c. hypointensity
    c. intracerebral hemorrhage
    c. ischemia
    c. kidney arch
    c. kidney arteriography
    c. kidney necrosis
    c. liquor space
    c. mapping
    c. margin
    c. motor area
    c. nephrocalcinosis
    c. nodular hyperplasia
    c. nodule
    c. notching
    c. osteoid osteoma
    c. plate
    c. renal cyst
    c. rim nephrogram
    c. rim sign
    c. ring
    c. ring sign
    c. roughening
    c. scalloping
    c. scarring of kidney
    c. scintigraphy
    c. signet ring shadow
    c. sulcus
    c. thinning
    c. thumb
    c. tissue
    c. transgression
    c. tuber
    c. vein
    c. vein sign
    c. vein thrombosis
    c. venous reflux
    c. white matter
    c. window
corticale
    cryptostroma c.
corticated border
cortices (*pl. of* cortex)
corticobasal ganglionic degeneration
corticobulbar
    c. pathway
    c. tract (CBT)

corticocallosal dysgenesis
corticocancellous
    c. bone
    c. bone chip
    c. strut
corticocerebellar connection
corticogram
corticography
corticomedullary
    c. differentiation (CMD)
    c. junction (CMJ)
    c. phase
corticopontine tract
corticopontocerebellar pathway
corticorubral tract
corticospinal
    c. motor pathway
    c. pathway lesion
    c. tract (CST)
corticosteroid-induced osteoporosis
corticostriatospinal degeneration
cortisol-producing carcinoma
corundum smelter's lung
Corvita endoluminal graft
Corynebacterium brain abscess
cosine
    c. curve
    c. transform
Cosman-Roberts-Wells guided stereotactic aspiration
cosmic radiation
costa, *pl.* costae
    c. fluctuans decima
    c. retraction
    costae spuriae
    costae verae
costae (*pl. of* costa)
costal
    c. angle
    c. bone
    c. cartilage calcification
    c. facet
    c. groove
    c. intraarticular cartilage
    c. margin
    c. notch
    c. osteoma
    c. osteosarcoma
    c. part of diaphragm
    c. pit
    c. pleura
    c. pleurisy
    c. process
    c. sulcus
    c. surface
    c. tubercle
    c. tuberosity
costimulatory molecule
costoaxillary vein

costocervical
    c. artery
    c. trunk
costochondral
    c. joint
    c. junction
    c. junction separation
costochondritis
costoclavicular
    c. ligament
    c. line
    c. maneuver
    c. syndrome
    c. test
costocolic
    c. fold
    c. ligament
costodiaphragmatic
    c. margin
    c. recess
    c. recess of pleura
costolateral
costolumbar angle
costomediastinal
    c. recess
    c. sinus
costophrenic
    c. angle
    c. angle blunting
    c. recess
    c. septal line
    c. sinus
    c. sulcus
costopleural
costosternal angle
costotransverse
    c. foramen
    c. joint
    c. ligament
costovertebral
    c. angle (CVA)
    c. articulation
    c. joint
costoxiphoid ligament
COSY
    correlated spectroscopy
    COSY H-1 MR
      spectroscopy
Cotrel-Dubousset system
co-trimoxazole
cottage loaf appearance
cotton
    C. ankle fracture
    c. ball appearance
    c. fiber embolus
cotton-wool
    c.-w. appearance
    c.-w. sign
    c.-w. spot (CWS)

Cotunnius canal
cotyloid
    c. cavity
    c. ligament
couch view
coudé catheter
cough
    c. fracture of rib
    nonproductive c.
    c. resonance
Couinaud
    C. liver anatomy classification
    C. liver segment (1-8)
coulomb (C)
    c. force
    C. law
    c.'s per kilogram (C/kg)
Coulter counter
coumarin pulsed dye laser
count
    absolute granulocyte c.
    background c.
    Cerenkov c.
    Colombo c.
    corrected TIMI frame c. (CTFC)
    c. density
    direct liquid scintillation c.
    filament-nonfilament c.
    noise effective c. (NEC)
    out-of-field c.
    c.'s per plane
    random c.
    c. rate
    scattered c.
    white blood c. (WBC)
count-density threshold
counter
    automated gamma c.
    boron c.
    Cerenkov c.
    Coulter c.
    event c.
    gamma ray c.
    gamma well c.
    Geiger c.
    Geiger-Müller c.
    G-M c.
    ionization c.
    proportional c.
    radiation c.
    scaler c.
    scintillation c.
    well c.
    whole-body c.
countercurrent
    c. aortography
    c. flow
    c. flow-related enhancement
counteroccluder

C

counterpulsation
    balloon c.
    diastolic c.
    intraaortic balloon c.
    mechanical c.
    percutaneous intraaortic balloon c.
counterstimulation
counting
    c. coincidence
    double-label c.
    c. rate meter
    single-photon c. (SPC)
    whole-body c.
coupled array coil
couplet
    ventricular premature contraction c.
coupling
    c. constant
    dipole c.
    dipole-dipole c.
    dynamic c.
    electric quadrupole c.
    c. exchange
    c. gel
    hyperfine c.
    magnetic dipole-dipole c.
    scalar c.
    spin c.
    spin-spin c.
    static c.
Cournand arteriography needle
Cournand-Grino angiography needle
course
    extracranial c.
    midlateral c.
    c. of artery
    relapsing c.
    remitting c.
    signal time c.
    undulating c.
coursing
    c. of gas
    c. vessel
Courvoisier
    C. gallbladder
    C. law
    C. sign
Courvoisier-Terrier syndrome
Couvelaire uterus
coverage
    interleaved k-space c.
    spiral k-space c.
covered stent
Cowboy Collar
Cowden
    C. disease
    C. syndrome
cow horn deformity

Cowper
    C. gland lesion
    C. ligament
COX
    cyclooxygenase
    cytochrome oxidase
    COX deficiency
coxa, *pl.* **coxae**
    c. adducta
    c. brevis
    c. flexa
    c. magna
    os coxae
    c. plana
    c. saltans
    c. senilis
    c. valga
    c. valga deformity
    c. vara
    c. vara deformity
coxae (*pl. of* coxa)
coxal bone
coxarthrosis
    Postel destructive c.
coxitis fugax
Cox sterilizer and incinerator unit
CP
    Carr-Purcell
    CP angle
    CP sequence
CPA
    cerebellopontine angle
CPAD
    chronic peripheral arterial disease
CPCB
    continuous psoas compartment block
CPD
    cephalopelvic disproportion
CPE
    chronic pulmonary emphysema
CPET
    cardiopulmonary exercise test
    CPET scanner
CPI
    conventional planar imaging
cpm
    cycles per minute
CPMG
    Carr-Purcell-Meiboom-Gill
    CPMG sequence
CPP
    cerebral perfusion pressure
CPPD
    calcium pyrophosphate dihydrate
    CPPD arthritis of hand
    CPPD crystal
cps
    cycles per second

Cr
    chromium
CR103
    OncoScint CR103
crabmeatlike appearance
crack
    c. fracture
    hairline c.
cracked-pot resonance
cracker
    LeVeen plaque c.
    plaque c.
cradle
    alpha c.
    CT scan c.
    Spectrum DG-P pediatric c.
Cragg
    C. EndoPro stent-graft
    C. Endopro System I covered
      stent
    C. FX-wire
    C. thrombolytic brush
Cragg-Castaneda thrombolytic brush
Cragg-McNamara multiple-sidehole
  infusion catheter
Cramer-Rao minimum variance bound
  (CR-MVB)
Crampton
    C. line
    C. muscle
crania (*pl. of* cranium)
cranial, cranialis
    c. aneurysm
    c. angled view
    c. angulation
    c. anomaly
    c. base
    c. bone
    c. capacity
    c. cavity
    c. computed tomography
      (CCT)
    c. diameter
    c. fixation plate
    c. flexure
    c. fontanelle
    c. foramen
    c. fossa
    c. granulomatous arteritis
    c. irradiation
    c. meningocele
    c. nerve
    c. nerve involvement
    c. nerve neoplasia
    c. nerve sheath tumor
    c. nerve sign
    c. nucleus
    c. osteopetrosis
    c. ridge

    c. root
    c. sinus
    c. suture
    c. synchondroses
    c. synostosis
    c. ultrasound
    c. vault
    c. vertebra
    c. vessel
craniales
cranialis (*var. of* cranial)
cranii
    osteoporosis circumscripta c.
    pneumatocele c.
    synchondroses c.
    vertex c.
craniocaudal
    c. axis
    c. needle angulation
    c. projection
    c. view
craniocervical junction
craniofacial
    c. angle
    c. anomaly
    c. bone
    c. dysjunction
    c. dysjunction fracture
    c. dysostosis
    c. notch
    c. pain syndrome
    c. plexiform neurofibroma
    c. remodeling
    c. synostosis
    c. trauma
craniography
craniolacunia
craniomandibular syndrome
craniometric
    c. diameter
    c. point
cranioorbital deformity
craniopagus twin
craniopharyngeal
    c. canal
    c. duct
craniopharyngioma
    adamantinomatous c.
    ectopic c.
    nasopharyngeal c.
cranioschisis
craniosclerosis
cranioskeletal dysplasia
craniospinal
    c. axis
    c. axis radiation therapy
    c. compliance
    c. hemangioblastoma
    c. irradiation (CSI)

C

craniostenosis
craniosynostosis syndrome
craniotabes
craniotelencephalic dysplasia
craniotomy defect
craniotrypesis
craniovertebral
    c. angle
    c. anomaly
    c. junction
    c. junction anatomy
cranium, *pl.* **crania**
    c. bifidum
    c. bifidum occultum
    fetal c.
    split c.
    vertex of bony c.
crankshaft phenomenon
CRASH
    corpus callosum hypoplasia, retardation,
    adducted thumbs, spastic paraparesis,
    and hydrocephalus
    CRASH syndrome
crater
    ulcer c.
craterlike ulcer
crazy
    c. paving
    c. paving appearance
    c. paving pattern
    c. paving pattern on chest CT
      scan
Cr-chromate-labeled red cell technique
CRE
    cumulative radiation effect
C-reactive protein level
crease
    back c.
    infragluteal c.
    inframammary c.
    inguinal c.
    stellate c.
creation
    percutaneous peritoneovenous shunt
    c.
Cree leukoencephalopathy
creep
    cardiac c.
    diaphragmatic c.
    periosteal c.
creeping epithelialization
cremaster
cremasteric
    c. artery
    c. fascia
Cremin M line
crescendo TIA
crescent
    air c.

    c. artifact
    high-attenuation c.
    c. hip line
    c. of cardia
    c. of cavitation
    c. of gas
    c. sign
crescentic
    c. border
    c. collection
    c. lumen
    c. submucosal fold
crescent-in-doughnut sign
crescent-shaped
    c.-s. fibrocartilaginous disc
    c.-s. glomerulonephritis
CREST
    calcinosis cutis, Raynaud phenomenon,
    esophageal motility disorder,
    sclerodactyly, and telangiectasis
    CREST syndrome
crest
    acoustic c.
    acousticofacial c.
    alveolar c.
    ampullary c.
    anterior iliac c.
    arched c.
    arcuate c.
    articular c.
    basilar c.
    bilateral iliac c.'s
    buccinator c.
    conchal c.
    deltoid c.
    dental c.
    ethmoidal c.
    falciform c.
    frontal c.
    ganglionic c.
    gingival c.
    gyral c.
    iliac c.
    infundibuloventricular c.
    intertrochanteric c.
    posterior iliac c.
    pubic c.
    sacral c.
    supraventricular c. (SVC)
    terminal c.
    tibial c.
    urethral c.
Creutzfeldt-Jakob disease
 (CJD)
crevice
    nonpolar c.
CRF
    chronic renal failure
    coronary reserve flow

Cr-HIDA
  chromium-hepatic dimethyl
    iminodiacetic acid
  Cr-HIDA chelate
cribrate
cribration
cribriform
  c. bone
  c. carcinoma
  c. DCIS
  c. fascia
  c. pattern
  c. plate
  c. process
cricket bat shape
cricoarytenoid articular capsule
cricoesophageal tendon
cricoid cartilage
cricopharyngeal
  c. achalasia
  c. bar
  c. diameter
  c. diverticulum
  c. ligament
  c. spasm
  c. sphincter
cricopharyngeus muscle
cricothyreotomy
cricothyroid
  c. articular capsule
  c. cartilage
  c. junction
  c. ligament
  c. membrane
cricotracheal ligament
cri du chat syndrome (*var. of* cri-du-chat
  syndrome)
cri-du-chat syndrome, cri du chat
  syndrome
crimp stop
crinkle artifact
crinkling
  mucosal c.
  patch c.
crisis
  bone c.
  transient aplastic c. (TAC)
  vasoocclusive c.
crisscross heart
crista, *pl.* **cristae**
  c. galli
  c. pulmonis
  c. supraventricularis
  c. terminalis
cristae (*pl. of* crista)
criteria (*pl. of* criterion)
criterion, *pl.* **criteria**
  American College of Rheumatology
  c.

  Biello c.
  Durie-Salmon clinical staging c.
  dynamic c.
  EORTC c.
  error-sum c.
  interpretive c.
  Jones c.
  morphologic c.
  Mourits c.
  Nyquist c.
  PIOPED c.
  radiographic c.
  response c.
  Rose c.
  Schumacher c.
  Schwartz c.
  c. standards
critical
  c. coronary stenosis
  c. dose table
  c. lesion
  c. limb ischemia
  c. mass
  c. organ
  c. valvular stenosis
CRL
  crown-rump length
Cr-labeled red blood cell technique
CRMO
  chronic recurrent multifocal
    osteomyelitis
CR-MVB
  Cramer-Rao minimum variance bound
CR-39 nuclear tract detector
CRO
  cathode ray oscilloscope
crocidolite asbestos
Crohn
  C. colitis
  C. disease
  C. disease of colon
  C. duodenitis
  C. granulomatous enteritis
  C. ileitis
  C. ileocolitis
  C. jejunitis
  C. regional enteritis
Crohn-like lymphoid reaction
Crone-Renkin index of permeability
Cronkhite-Canada syndrome
Cronqvist cranial index
Crookes
  C. space
  C. tube
Crookes-Hittorf tube
cross-aortic
crossbar symptom of Fränkel
cross-calibration
cross-collateralization

cross-correlation technique
cross-ectopic kidney
crossed
    c. cerebellar diaschisis (CCD)
    c. coil
    c. embolus
    c. upstream and downstream
crossed-coil design
crossed-loop resonator
cross-excitation
cross-filling
crossfire
    c. radiation therapy
    c. treatment
cross-fogging
cross-fused renal ectopia
cross-hatch grid
cross-ligament
crosslinked silicone gel
cross-organ and self-absorbed dose
crossover
    femorofemoral c.
    c. of activity
cross-pelvic collateral vessel
cross-polarization
cross-scrotal collateral
cross-section
    bronchovascular anatomy c.-s.
    c.-s. capture
    Compton scattering c.-s.
    distal leg c.-s.
    elastic c.-s.
    hip muscle c.-s.
    normalized c.-s.
    pharynx c.-s.
    thigh muscle c.-s.
    vertebral c.-s.
cross-sectional
    c.-s. area (CSA)
    c.-s. area stenosis
    c.-s. echocardiography (CSE)
    c.-s. enterography
    c.-s. imaging
    c.-s. lung segment anatomy
    c.-s. modality
    c.-s. pattern
    c.-s. plane
    c.-s. transverse projection
    c.-s. ultrasonographic image
    c.-s. zone
cross-table
    c.-t. lateral film
    c.-t. lateral position
    c.-t. lateral projection
    c.-t. lateral view (CTLV)
    c.-t. leg immobilizer
crosstalk effect artifact
cross-trigonal tunnel
cross-union

Crouzon syndrome
CR/OV
    colorectal/ovarian
crowded
    c. carpal sign
    c. dentition
crowding of bronchovascular markings
Crowe pilot point
Crow-Fukase syndrome
crown
    c. cavity
    halo c.
    c. indemnity
    c. tubercle
crowned dens syndrome
crown-heel length
crown-rump length (CRL)
CRT
    cathode ray tube
    conformal radiation therapy
    coronary radiation therapy
    3D CRT
crucial angle of Gissane
cruciate
    c. eminence
    c. ligament
    c. orientation
cruciatum cruris ligament
cruciform
    c. eminence
    c. ligament
crunch
    mediastinal c.
crural
    c. canal
    c. cistern
    c. cistern widening
    c. fascia
    c. fossa
    c. septum
    c. sheath
    c. triangle
crus
    comma-shaped c.
    c. commune
    c. cupula
    diaphragmatic c.
    displaced c.
    c. dome
    c. hiatus
    lateral c.
    left c.
    medial c.
    muscular c.
    c. of diaphragm
    c. of penis
    c. pericardium
    c. pleura
    right c.

crush
  c. artifact
  c. fracture
  c. injury
  c. kidney
  c. preparation
  c. syndrome
  thoracic c.
crushed
  c. eggshell fracture
  c. tissue
Cruveilhier
  C. fascia
  C. joint
  C. ligament
  C. nodule
  C. ulcer
Cruveilhier-Baumgarten
  C.-B. anomaly
  C. B. cirrhosis
cryogen
CRYOguide ultrasound guidance system
CryoHit tumor ablation system
cryomagnet
cryoplasty balloon
cryoprobe
cryosection
cryostable magnet
cryotherapy
crypt
  c. abscess
  anal c.
  enamel c.
  epithelium c.
  ileal c.
  Lieberkühn c.
  Luschka c.
  Morgagni c.
cryptic vascular malformation (CVM)
cryptococcal
  c. lymphadenitis
  c. meningitis
  c. pneumonia
  c. spondylitis
cryptococcoma
  focal parenchymal c.
cryptococcosis
  disseminated c.
  intracranial c.
Cryptococcus
  pulmonary C.
cryptogenic
  c. cirrhosis
  c. fibrosing alveolitis
  c. organizing pneumonia
cryptorchidism, cryptorchism
cryptorchism (*var. of* cryptorchidism)

cryptoscope
cryptostroma corticale
crystal
  BGO c.
  CPPD c.
  c. deposition arthropathy
  c. deposition disease
  c. field theory
  c. gamma camera
  hydroxyapatite c.
  pyrophosphate c.
  scintillation c.
CrystalEyes endoscopic video system
crystal-induced
  c.-i. arthritis
  c.-i. arthrosis
crystalline phosphor detector
crystallogram
crystallography
  x-ray c.
^{137}Cs, Cs-137
  cesium 137
  ^{137}Cs point source
^{139}Cs, Cs-139
  cesium 139
CSA
  cross-sectional area
C300 scanner
CSD
  cardiac support device
CSDH
  chronic subdural hematoma
CSE
  cross-sectional echocardiography
CSF
  cerebrospinal fluid
    CSF 14-3-3 isoform
    CSF oscillatory motion
    CSF 14-3-3 protein
    CSF pulsation artifact
    CSF systole length
    CSF ventricular systole
CSF-suppressed T2-weighted 3D MP-RAGE MR imaging
CSGIT
  continuous suture graft inclusion technique
CSGP
  computer strain-gauge plethysmography
CSI
  chemical-shift imaging
  coronary stenosis index
  craniospinal irradiation
    risk-adapted CSI
    CSI spectroscopy
CsI
  casium iodide

C-sign sensitivity
CSL
    central sacral line
    complex sclerosing lesion
CSM
    cervical spondylotic myelopathy
CSPAMM
    complementary spatial modulation of
      magnetization
C-spine pseudosubluxation
CSS
    carotid sinus syndrome
CST
    contraction stress test
    corticospinal tract
CSVT
    central splanchnic venous thrombosis
CSWT
    cardiac shock wave therapy
CT
    computed tomography
    indirect CT
    intravascular contrast-enhanced CT
      CT angiography
      CT arteriography
      CT arthrography
      CT attenuation value
      biphasic contrast-enhanced helical
        CT
      bit CT
      CT body scanner
      bone quantitative CT (BQCT)
      CT bone window
      CT bone window photography
      cervical CT
      CT cisternogram
      CT cisternography
      collimation CT
      CT colonography
      contrast-enhanced CT
      coronary sinus CT
      CT correction attenuation
      3D drip infusion cholangiography
        CT
      CT densitometer
      CT densitometry
      3D portography using multislice
        helical CT
      3D processed ultrafast CT
      dual-energy CT
      dual-isotope single-photon emission
        CT
      dual-phase CT
      dynamic contrast-enhanced CT
      electrocardiogram-gated multislice
        spiral CT
      enhanced CT
      CT enteroclysis
      expiratory CT

fast dynamic volumetric x-ray
  CT
gestalt impression on CT
HeartView CT
helical thin-section CT
high spatial-resolution cine CT
CT imaging error
indirect CT (CT)
intravascular contrast-enhanced CT
  (CT)
Marconi/Elscint MxTwin CT
CT Max 640 scanner
multidetector CT (MDCT)
multidetector helical CT
multidetector-row CT
multiphasic helical CT
multislice CT
multislice spiral CT (MSCT)
CT myelography
noncontrast head CT (NCCT)
non-ECG-assisted multidetector row
  CT
nonenhanced CT
CT number
perfusion CT
CT Perfusion 2 software
2-phase helical CT
postmyelography CT
Proceed vascular interventional CT
quantitative spirometrically controlled
  CT
CT ratio
CT reconstruction image
renal helical CT
CT scan
CT scan cradle
CT scan gantry
CT scanner beam
CT scan with contrast
CT scan with renal stone protocol
CT sialography
single-detector helical CT
single-photon emission CT
single-slice helical CT
single-slice spiral CT
slip-ring CT
Somatom Plus 4 CT
spiral multidetector CT
spiral volumetric CT
stable Xenon CT
CT stereotactic guide
surgical simulation CT
thallium-201 single-photon emission
  CT
thin-section CT
thin-slice CT
CT tracheobronchography
triphasic spiral CT
twin-beam CT

ultrafast CT
CT unit
W3000 helical CT
xenon-enhanced CT (XeCT)
Z-dependent CT

CTA
computed tomographic angiography
helical CTA
CTA image
multidetector CTA
single-detector CTA
single-slice CTA

CT-aided volumetry

CTAP
computed tomography with
arterioportography

CTAT
computerized transverse axial
tomography
CTAT imaging

CT-based
CT-b. virtual cystoscopy
CT-b. virtual tracheobronchoscopy

CTC
computed tomographic colonography

CTCL
cutaneous T-cell lymphoma

CTDI
computed tomography dose index

CT-directed
CT-d. biopsy
CT-d. hook-wire localization
CT-d. puncture

C-60 teletherapy

C-telopeptide
type II collagen C-t.

CT-estimated superimposed hydrostatic pressure

CTE:YAG
chromium-thulium-erbium:yttrium-
aluminum garnet
CTE:YAG laser

CTF
computed tomography fluoroscopy

CTFC
corrected TIMI frame count

CT-guided
CT-g. intraarterial chemotherapy
CT-g. needle aspiration
CT-g. needle biopsy
CT-g. percutaneous biopsy
CT-g. percutaneous endoscopic
gastrostomy
CT-g. percutaneous excision
CT-g. percutaneous screw placement
for sacroiliac joint
CT-g. stereotactic surgery
CT-g. superior hypogastric plexus
block

CT-g. transsternal core biopsy
CT-g. ultrasound

CTH
computerized tomographic
holography

CTHA
computerized tomographic hepatic
angiography

CTI
Computer Technology and Imaging
CTI 933/04 ECAT scanner
CTI 931 PET scanner

CTLC
contact transscleral laser
cytophotocoagulation
Nd:YAG CTLC

CTLM
computed tomography laser
mammography

CTLV
cross-table lateral view

CTMM
computed tomographic metrizamide
myelography

CT/MR
computerized tomography/magnetic
resonance
CT/MR peritoneography

CT/MRI-compatible stereotactic head frame

CT/MRI-defined
CT/MRI-d. tumor slice image
CT/MRI-d. tumor volume image

CT-PET
computed tomography-positron emission
tomography
combined CT-PET

CTPV
computed tomography pulmonary
venography

CTR
cardiothoracic ratio

C-Trak handheld gamma detector

CT9000, 9800 scanner

CT/SPECT
computed tomography/single-photon
emission computed tomography
CT/SPECT fusion imaging

CTT
central tegmental tract

CTV
clinical target volume
computed tomography venography

⁶²Cu, Cu-62
copper 62
⁶²Cu PTSM imaging agent

⁶⁴Cu, Cu-64
copper 64
⁶⁴Cu imaging agent

^{67}Cu, Cu-67
copper 67
^{67}Cu imaging agent
Cu
copper
cube vertex
cubic
c. centimeter (cc)
c. convolution interpolation
c. voxel
cubital
c. bone
c. bursitis
c. fossa
c. lymph node
c. tunnel
c. tunnel retinaculum
c. tunnel syndrome
cubiti (*pl. of* cubitus)
cubitocarpal
cubitoradial
cubitus, *pl.* **cubiti**
c. valgus
c. valgus deformity
c. varus
c. varus deformity
cuboid, cuboidal
c. articular surface
c. bone
c. fracture
cuboidal (*var. of* cuboid)
**cuboideonavicular
ligament**
cubonavicular joint
CUC
chronic ulcerative
colitis
cue-based image analysis
cuff
c. abscess
aortic c.
atrial c.
bladder c.
inflow c.
musculotendinous c.
pressure c.
rectal muscle c.
right atrial c.
rotator c.
suprahepatic caval c.
urinary bladder c.
vaginal c.
**cuffed endotracheal
tube**
cuffing
peribronchial c.
perivascular c.
CUG
cystourethrogram

cuirasse
carcinoma en c.
cor en c.
cul-de-sac, *pl.* **culs-de-sac**
Douglas c.-d.-s.
dural c.-d.-s.
Culiner theory
Cullen sign
culpocephaly
culprit
c. lesion
c. stenosis
c. vessel
culs-de-sac (*pl. of* cul-de-sac)
cumulative
c. dose
c. microtrauma
c. radiation effect (CRE)
cumulus oophorus
cuneatus
funiculus c.
cunei (*pl. of* cuneus)
cuneiform
c. bone
c. bone of carpus
c. cartilage
c. fracture
c. fracture-dislocation
c. joint
c. lobe
c. mortise
c. tubercle
cuneocerebellar tract
cuneocuboid ligament
cuneonavicular ligament
cuneus, *pl.* **cunei**
CUP
cancer of unknown primary
carcinoma of unknown primary
cup
acetabular c.
Diogenes c.
migration of acetabular c.
prosthetic c.
retroversion of acetabular c.
cup-and-spill stomach
cupboard
RF-shielded c.
Cupid's
C. bow configuration
C. bow contour
C. bow sign
cupola (*var. of* cupula)
cupping
c. of acromion
c. of calyx
cupula, cupola, *pl.* **cupulae**
crus c.
diaphragmatic c.

gas c.
pleural c.
c. sign
cupulae (*pl. of* cupula)
curative irradiation
curbstone consultation
cure
 complete anatomic c.
curie (Ci)
Curie
 C. effect
 C. law
curie-hour
curietherapy
curium
Curix
 C. Capacity Plus film processing
  system
 C. film-screen cassette
 C. Ultra UV-L film
curlicue ureter
curling
 c. esophagus
 C. ulcer
curly toe deformity
currant jelly stool
Currarino triad
current
 alternating c. (AC)
 attenuation-based online modulation
  of tube c.
 beam c.
 direct c. (DC)
 eddy c.
 gradient drive c.
 ionization c.
 c. leak
 c. line distortion
 3-phase c.
 pulsating c.
 pulsing c.
 saturation c.
 single-phase c.
 tube c.
 unidirectional c.
 unmodulated radiofrequency c.
 variable tube c.
**Curry intravascular retriever
 set**
curtain
 subaortic c.
curvatura (*var. of* curvature), *pl.*
 curvaturae
curvaturae (*pl. of* curvatura)
curvature, curvatura
 angular c.
 c. anisotropy
 anterior c.
 backward c.

cervical lordotic c.
dorsal kyphotic c.
fibroid c.
flattening of normal lordotic c.
gingival c.
kyphotic c.
lumbar c.
radius of c.
stomach c.
curve
 area under c. (AUC)
 biexponential fitting of left
  ventricular c.
 biphasic c.
 blood activity-time c.
 Bragg c.
 brightness-time c.
 catheter with preformed c.
 cervical spine c.
 characteristic c.
 clearance c.
 concentration-time c.
 cosine c.
 depth-dose c.
 dye dilution c.
 elimination c.
 flattening of normal lumbar c.
 flow-time c.
 fractionated dose-survival c.
 Frank-Starling c.
 free induction delay c.
 full width at half-maximum of
  lorentzian c.
 gaussian c.
 glow c.
 H and D c.
 Harrison c.
 Hunter and Driffield c.
 indicator dilution c.
 indocyanine dilution c.
 isoclosed c.
 isodose c.
 kinetic c.
 lordotic c.
 lorentzian c.
 loss of sigmoid c.
 lumbar lordotic c.
 lung count c.
 normal lordotic c.
 c. of duodenum
 pulmonary time-activity c.
 receiver operating characteristic
  c.
 renal flow c.
 renogram c.
 ROC c.
 sensitometric c.
 sigmoid density c.
 signal intensity-time c.

C

curve (*continued*)
    spline c.
    Starling c.
    stress-strain c.
    superincumbent spinal c.
    thoracic spine c.
    time-activity c.
    time-attenuation c.
    time-density c.
    time-intensity c. (TIC)
    ventricular function c.
    videodensity c.
    washout c.

curved
    c. multiplanar reformation
    c. planar reformation
    c. radiolucent line
    c. reconstruction
    c. vessel

curved-array transducer
curved-needle biopsy
curve-fit coefficient
curvilinear
    c. calcification
    c. defect
    c. density
    c. reconstruction
    c. subpleural line
    c. threshold of shoulder

CUSA
    Cavitron ultrasonic surgical aspirator
Cushing
    C. disease
    C. paraneoplastic syndrome
    C. phenomenon
    C. triad
    C. ulcer

Cushing-Rokitansky ulcer
cushion
    c. defect
    endocardial c.
    foam c.

cusp
    accessory c.
    anterior c.
    aortic c.
    asymmetric closure of c.
    ballooning mitral c.
    conjoined c.'s
    coronary c.
    c. degeneration
    dysplastic c.
    c. fenestration
    fibrocalcific c.
    fishmouth c.
    fusion of c.
    intact valve c.
    left coronary c.
    left pulmonary c.

    mitral valve c.
    c. motion
    noncoronary c.
    perforated aortic c.
    posterior c.
    prolapse of right aortic valve c.
    pulmonary valve c.
    right coronary c.
    ruptured aortic c.
    semilunar valve c.
    septal c.
    c. shot
    tricuspid valve c.
    valve c.

custom-curved coil
custom-fabricated graft
custom shielding block
cut
    c. and cine film
    high-resolution coronal c.
    off-center c.
    scalpel c.
    tangential c.
    tomographic c.

cutaneous
    c. adenoma
    c. angioma
    c. angiosarcoma
    c. B-cell lymphoma (CBCL)
    c. chylous vesicle
    c. collateral circulation
    c. fissure
    c. lateral branch
    c. lymphoscintigraphy
    c. metastasis
    c. necrotizing venulitis
    c. nodule
    c. pit
    c. pneumocystosis
    c. ridge
    c. T-cell lymphoma (CTCL)
    c. twig
    c. vascular anomaly
    c. vein

[64]Cu-TETA-octreotide imaging agent
cut-film
    c.-f. angiography (CFA)
    c.-f. technique
cuticular overgrowth
Cutie Pie detector
cutis
    atrophia c.
    c. calcinosis
    osteoma c.
    retinaculum c.
    tuberculosis verrucosa c.
cutoff
    arterial c.
    c. sign

cutting
> c. balloon
> c. balloon catheter

Cuvier
> C. canal
> C. duct

Cu/Zn-SOD
> copper-zinc superoxide dismutase
> Cu/Zn-SOD imaging agent

CVA
> cardiovascular accident
> cerebrovascular accident
> costovertebral angle

CVBS
> congenital vascular-bone syndrome

CVC
> central venous catheter

CVD
> cardiovascular disease

CVIS
> cardiovascular information system

CVM
> congenital vascular malformation
> cryptic vascular malformation

CVP
> central venous pressure

CVRI
> coronary vascular resistance index

CVST
> cerebral venous sinus thrombosis

C-wave pressure

CWP
> coal worker's pneumoconiosis

CWS
> cotton-wool spot

CXR
> chest x-ray

CY
> cyanogen
> CY color space

cyanoacrylate
> N-butyl c. (NBCA)
> c. tissue adhesive

cyanocobalamin
> c. Co 57, 58, 60
> c. imaging agent
> radioactive c.

cyanogen (CY)

cyanosis
> peroral c.

cyanotic
> c. congenital heart disease
> c. kidney

Cyber 170/720

CyberKnife
> C. Express device
> C. stereotactic radiosurgery system

Cyberware 3D scanning system

Cybex ergometer

cycle
> breath-hold c.
> clock c.
> Krebs c.
> pentose c.
> c.'s per minute (cpm)
> c.'s per second (cps)
> c. time
> tricarboxylic acid c.

cycle-length window

cyclic, cyclical
> c. adenosine monophosphate
> c. guanosine monophosphate
> c. guanosine triphosphate
> c. idiopathic edema
> c. voiding cystourethrogram

cyclical (*var. of* cyclic)

cycling
> phase c.

cyclooxygenase (COX)
> c. deficiency

cyclopea (*var. of* cyclopia)

cyclophosphamide therapy

cyclopia, cyclopea

cyclops lesion

cyclosporin nephrotoxicity

cyclotron
> medical c.
> multiparticle c.
> negative-ion c.
> positive-ion c.
> c. radiation

cylinder
> abdominal compression c.
> axonal c.
> Burnett c.
> CO_2 c.
> dome c.
> Fletcher-Delclos dome c.
> sum of c.
> vaginal c.

cylindrical
> c. ablation scheme
> c. bronchiectasis
> c. carcinoma
> c. chest
> c. configuration
> c. format
> c. map projection
> c. papilloma
> c. projection map
> c. thorax

cylindroid aneurysm

cylindroma
> lung c.
> c. parotitis

cylindromatous carcinoma

cylindrosarcoma

cyllosis

C

Cyma line
Cypher stent
Cyriax syndrome
cyst

acoustic c.
acquired hepatic c.
adnexal c.
adrenal c.
air c.
air-filled c.
allantoic c.
amnionic inclusion c.
anechoic c.
aneurysmal bone c. (ABC)
apocrine c.
arachnoid brain c.
arachnoid spine c.
aryepiglottic c.
atypical renal c.
Baker c.
benign conal c.
benign hepatic c.
bilateral arachnoid c.'s
bilateral choroid plexus c.'s
Blessig c.
bone aneurysmal c.
bone implantation c.
brain c.
branchial cleft c.
breast c.
bronchial cleft c.
bronchiectatic c.
bronchogenic duplication c.
brown cell c.
calcified pericardial c.
capping c.
cerebral c.
cervical thymic c.
chocolate c.
choledochal c.
cholesteatoma c.
cholesterol ear c.
choroid plexus c.
colloid brain c.
colobomatous c.
colonic duplication c.
communicating c.
complex breast c.
complicated hydatid c.
complicated renal c.
conal c.
congenital bronchogenic c.
congenital hepatic c.
congenital lung c.
corpus albicans c.
corpus luteum c.
cortical renal c.
cysticercus c.
Dandy-Walker c.

daughter c.
decidual c.
dental c.
dentigerous c.
dermoid ovarian c.
dorsal enterogenous c.
duplication c.
echinococcal c.
echinococcus c.
endodermal c.
endometrial c.
endometriotic c.
enteric duplication c.
enterogenous c.
entrapped ovarian c.
ependymal c.
epidermal inclusion c.
epidermoid c.
epididymal c.
epidural arachnoid c.
epithelial inclusion c.
esophageal duplication c.
expansile aneurysmal bone c.
extradural arachnoid c.
extraparenchymal c.
false splenic c.
fluid-filled c.
follicular ovarian c.
foregut c.
functional ovarian c.
functioning parathyroid c.
ganglion c.
Gartner duct c.
gastric duplication c.
gastrogenic c.
gastrointestinal c.
giant cholesterol c.
gurgling c.
hemorrhagic corpus luteum c.
hemorrhagic ovarian c.
hepatic c.
honeycomb c.
hydatid heart c.
hydatid lung c.
hydatid mediastinum c.
implantation c.
inclusion c.
interhemispheric c.
interosseous c.
intestinal duplication c.
intracranial dermoid c.
intraduodenal choledochal c.
intradural arachnoid c.
intramedullary epidermoid c.
intrameniscal c.
intraneural ganglion c.
intraosseous keratin c.
intraparenchymal c.
intrapulmonary bronchogenic c.

intrasellar Rathke cleft c.
intraspinal dermoid c.
intraspinal enteric c.
intraspinal epidermoid c.
intraspinal neurenteric c.
intratesticular c.
intrathoracic c.
intratumoral c.
intraventricular cryptococcal c.
joint c.
keratin testicular c.
kidney c.
Kimura-type choledochal c.
leptomeningeal arachnoid c.
lipid c.
liver c.
lumbar synovial c.
lung c.
luteal c.
lymphoepithelial c.
mammary c.
mediastinal bronchogenic c.
mediastinal dorsal enteric c.
mediastinal duplication c.
meibomian c.
meniscal c.
mesenteric c.
mesothelial c.
midline of brain c.
milk-of-calcium urinary tract c.
morgagnian c.
mucinous c.
mucous retention c.
müllerian duct c.
multilocular renal c.
multiple pulmonary c.'s
multiple thyroid c.'s
myxoid c.
nabothian c.
nasolabial c.
nasopharyngeal mucous retention c.
2nd branchial cleft c.
neoplastic c.
neurenteric c.
neuroenteric c.
noncommunicating c.
nonfunctioning parathyroid c.
nonneoplastic c.
nonteratomatous ovarian c.
nuchal c.
odontogenic c.
oil c.
omental c.
omphalomesenteric duct c.
orbital blood c.
orbital chocolate c.
orbital dermoid c.
c. or polyp
ovarian dermoid c.

ovarian follicular c.
ovarian image signature c.
ovarian retention c.
pancreatic c.
paraglenoid c.
paralabral c.
parameniscal c.
paramesonephric duct c.
parapelvic c.
parapharyngeal space c.
parathyroid c.
paratubal serous c.
paraurethral c.
parotid c.
parovarian c.
pelvic chocolate c.
peribiliary c.
pericalyceal c.
pericardial c.
pericardial duplication c.
perineural arachnoid c.
perineural sacral c.
peripelvic c.
peritoneal inclusion c.
peritumoral c.
physiologic ovarian c.
pilonidal c.
pineal c.
pituitary c.
placental septal c.
pleural c.
pleuropericardial c.
pontile hydatid c.
popliteal c.
porencephalic c.
posterior fossa c.
postmenopausal adnexal c.
posttraumatic oil c.
posttraumatic spinal cord c.
primordial tooth c.
prostatic c.
pulmonary c.
pyelogenic c.
racemose c.
radicular c.
Rathke cleft c.
reactive spinal c.
rectal duplication c.
regressed c.
renal sinus c.
retention c.
retrocerebellar arachnoid c.
retroperitoneal c.
sacral c.
c. sclerosis
sebaceous c.
secondary archnoid c.
seminal vesicle c.
septal placenta c.

C

cyst (*continued*)

serous intraparenchymatous c.
simple bone c.
simple breast c.
simple cortical renal c.
small bowel duplication c.
solitary bone c.
spinal hydatid c.
splenic epidermoid c.
1st branchial cleft c.
subarachnoid c.
subarticular c.
subchondral c.
subcortical c.
subependymal c.
subpleural air c.
syndrome with multiple cortical renal c.'s
synovial c.
synovium-filled degenerative c.
tailgut c.
talar dome c.
Tarlov c.
tarsal c.
tectal c.
tension c.
testicular c.
theca-lutein ovarian c.
thick-walled c.
thin-walled c.
thoracic duct c.
thymic c.
thyroglossal duct c.
thyroid c.
Todani-type c.
Tornwaldt c.
traumatic bone c.
traumatic lipid c.
traumatic lung c.
tunica albuginea c.
umbilical cord c.
unicameral bone c.
unilocular c.
urachal c.
vallecular c.
wolffian c.

cystadenocarcinoma

mucinous ovarian c.
ovarian serous c.
pancreatic c.
pseudomucinous c.
serous c.

cystadenofibroma

ovarian c.

cystadenoma

bile duct c.
biliary c.
colloid c.

endometrioid c.
glycogen-rich pancreatic c.
c. lymphomatosum
macrocystic serous c.
mucinous c.
ovarian c.
pancreatic c.
papillary epididymal c.
serous c.
thyroid c.

cystic

c. abdominal mass
c. adenocarcinoma
c. adenoma
c. adenomatoid malformation
c. airspace HRCT
c. appearance
c. arachnoiditis
c. area thyroid
c. artery
c. blastoma
c. bone angiomatosis
c. breast disease
c. breast mass
c. bronchiectasis
c. calculus
c. change
c. component
c. degeneration
c. dilation
c. disease of breast
c. duct angiography
c. duct cholangiogram
c. duct cholangiography
c. duct lumen
c. duct obstruction
c. duct perforation
c. duct remnant
c. duct remnant stone
c. duct sign
c. duct stump
c. echinococcosis
c. endometrial hyperplasia
c. epididymis lesion
c. fibrosis
c. fibrous dysplasia
c. fistula
c. fluid
c. gall duct
c. ganglioglioma
c. glandular hyperplasia
c. glioma
c. goiter
c. hemangioblastoma
c. hygroma
c. hyperplasia photomicrograph
c. intracranial fetal lesion
c. intraparenchymal meningioma
c. kidney

c. kidney disease
c. liver lesion
c. lung
c. lymph node
c. lysis
c. mastoplasia
c. medionecrosis
c. mesothelioma
c. metastatic node
c. myelomalacia
c. myelopathy
c. neck hygroma
c. nephroma
c. nodal metastasis
c. orbital hygroma
c. osteofibromatosis
c. ovarian disease
c. ovary
c. partially differentiated
  nephroblastoma
c. pattern
c. pilocytic astrocytoma
c. plexus
c. pneumatosis
c. polyp
c. process
c. pulmonary emphysema
c. renal cell carcinoma
c. rheumatoid arthritis
c. sac
c. splenic lesion
c. splenic neoplasia
c. structure
c. teratoma
c. teratomatous mass
c. tuberculosis
c. tuberculous osteomyelitis
c. tumor
c. vein
c. wall

cystica
cystitis c.
mastitis fibrosa c.
osteitis fibrosa c.
pyelitis c.
pyeloureteritis c.
ureteritis c.

cystic-choledochal junction
cysticerci (*pl. of* cysticercus)
cysticercosis
racemose c.
cysticercus, *pl.* **cysticerci**
c. cyst
c. granuloma
cystic malacic area
cysticohepatic triangle
cystine
c. calculus
c. stone

cystinosis
nephropathic c.
cystitis
c. cystica
emphysematous c.
hemorrhagic c.
interstitial c.
radiation c.
tuberculous c.
cystoatrial shunt
cystocarcinoma
cystocele
protrusion of c.
cystocolpoproctography
Cysto-Conray
C.-C. contrast agent
C.-C. II imaging agent
cystoduodenal ligament
cystofiberscope, cystofibroscope
cystofibroma
cystofibroscope (*var. of* cystofiberscope)
Cystografin
Cystografin-Dilute imaging agent
cystogram
air c.
bead-chain c.
chain c.
delayed c.
double-voiding c.
excretory c.
postdrainage c.
radioisotope voiding c.
radionuclide c.
radiopharmaceutical voiding c.
retrograde c.
stress c.
triple-voiding c.
voiding c.
cystography
antegrade c.
bead-chain c.
computed tomographic c.
c. imaging
radionuclide c.
retrograde c.
triple-voiding c.
cystoid
cystojejunostomy
Roux-en-Y c.
cystoma
cystomatous
cystometrography
cystomorphous
cystoplasty
ileocecal c.
cystopyelography
cystoradiogram
cystoradiography
cystosarcoma phyllodes

C

cystoscope
cystoscopic urography
cystoscopy
    CT-based virtual c.
    3D US-based virtual c.
    virtual c.
    virtual reality flexible c.
cystosonography
    echo-enhanced c.
cystostomy
cystoureterogram
cystoureterography
cystourethrogram (CUG)
    cyclic voiding c.
    lateral c.
    micturating c. (MCU)
    voiding c. (VCU, VCUG)
cystourethrography
    chain c.
    expression c.
    isotope voiding c. (IVCU)
    micturating c.
    micturition c.
    radionuclide voiding c.
    retrograde c.
    voiding c. (VCU)
cystourethroscopy imaging
cytoarchitecture
cytochrome
    c. c oxidase
    c. oxidase (COX)

cytomegalovirus (CMV)
    c. encephalitis
    c. esophagitis
    c. immune globulin
    C. infection
Cytomel suppression
cytometer
    FACScan flow c.
cytometry
    DNA flow c.
    flow c.
    image c.
    laser scanning c. (LSC)
    multicolor flow c.
cytophotocoagulation
    contact transscleral laser c.
    (CTLC)
cytophotometry
    DNA c.
cytoreductive surgery
cytosine arabinoside
cytoskeletal
    c. misalignment
    c. perturbation
cytotoxic
    c. drug
    c. edema
    c. edema of gray
    matter
cytotoxicity
    contrast medium-induced c.

D

D point
D signal

d

d, l-HMPAO imaging agent

1D

1-dimensional
1D ultrasound

2D

2-dimensional
2D B-mode ultrasound
2D B-mode ultrasound machine
2D color-coded imaging of blood flow
2D fast spin-echo acquisition
2D filtering process
2D format
2D Fourier transform
2D Fourier transformation imaging
2D gradient-encoded image
2D GRE dynamic protocol
2D IVUS
2D J-resolved 1H MR spectroscopy
2D KWE direct Fourier imaging
2D mapping
2D modified KWE direct Fourier imaging
2D MRDSA
2D multiplanar reformatted technique
2D multislice
multislice FLASH 2D
2D multislice imaging
2D NMR
2D portal image
2D portal image registration
2D pulsatility index mapping
2D resistance index mapping
2D sector scan
2D sequential slice
2D spatially selective radiofrequency pulse
2D technique
2D time-of-flight technique
2D TOF pulse sequencing

3D

3-dimensional
3D acquired/2D reconstructed
3D anatomic dataset
3D CEMRA
3D conformal radiation therapy
3D connect operation
3D contrast-enhanced MR angiography

3D coronary magnetic resonance angiography
3D CRT
3D deformation field
3D dose profile
3D drip infusion cholangiography CT
3D DSA image
3D echo-planar imaging
3D endoluminal view
3D endosonography
3D Faster
3D fast low-angle shot acquisition
3D fast low-angle shot imaging
3D fast spin-echo acquisition
3D fast spin-echo magnetic resonance imaging
3D field echo acquisition with short repetition time and echo reduction
3D FLASH acquisition
3D format
3D Fourier transform gradient-echo sequence with spoiler gradient
3D freehand ultrasound
3D gadolinium-enhanced magnetic resonance angiography
gadolinium-enhanced subtracted MR angiography, 3D
3D gadolinium sequence
3D GDC
3D gradient-echo
3D gradient-echo acquisition technique
3D GRE
3D helical CT angiography
3D hepatic arteriography
3D image reconstruction
3D inflow MR angiography
3D IVUS
3D KWE direct Fourier imaging
3D laparoscope
3D low-pass filtering
3D magnetic resonance microscopy
3D magnetic source imaging
3D magnetization-prepared rapid gradient echo
3D modeling
3D motion correction
3D MRA
3D MRA slab
3D MRI data set
3D MSI
3D neuroimaging
3D phase-contrast magnetic resonance angiography
3D physiologic flow pattern

D

3D (*continued*)
    3D plate
    3D portography using multislice helical CT
    3D postfiltering
    3D postprocessing technique
    3D prefiltering
    3D processed ultrafast computerized imaging
    3D processed ultrafast CT
    3D projection reconstruction imaging
    3D proton MR spectroscopy
    3D pulse design
    3D radiation treatment planning
    3D reconstructed target
    3D reconstruction
    3D reconstruction algorithm
    3D reformatting
    3D RODEO
    3D rotating delivery of excitation off-resonance
    3D rotational angiography
    3D RTP
    3D shape of neuroanatomic structure
    3D spatial encoding
    3D stereotactic surface projection
    3D superficial liposculpture
    3D surface anthropometry
    3D surface detection algorithm
    3D surface digitizer
    3D surface digitizer scanner
    3D surface rendering
    3D technique
    3D time-of-flight magnetic resonance angiographic sequence
    3D transesophageal echocardiographic sequence
    3D transesophageal echocardiography
    3D turbo fluid-attentuated inversion recovery
    3D turbo SE imaging
    3D T1-weighted gradient-echo imaging
    3D ultrasound reconstruction imaging
    3D ultrasound volumetry
    3D US-based virtual cystoscopy
    3D Viewnix software system
    3D volume
    3D volume-rendered helical CT angiography
    3D volume-rendering CT angiography
    3D volume-rendering reconstruction image
    3D volume-rendering technique
    3D volume technique
4D
    4-dimensional
    4D US image

Da
    dalton
DAC
    digital-to-analogue converter
Dacron-coated microcoil
Dacron-covered stent-graft
Dacron stent
dacryoadenitis
dacryocystitis
dacryocystocele
dacryocystogram
dacryocystography
    computed tomographic d.
    d. imaging
    magnetic resonance d.
    radiopharmaceutical d.
dacryocystorhinostomy
    endoscopic laser d.
dacryoscintigraphy
dactylitis
    tuberculous d.
dagger sign
Dagradi classification of esophageal varix
DAI
    diffuse axonal injury
    DAI in vivo
Dalen-Fuchs nodule
DALM
    dysplasia with associated lesion or mass
dalton (Da)
damage
    anthracycline-induced myocardial d.
    diffuse alveolar d.
    drug-induced pulmonary d.
    endothelial d.
    fatigue d.
    focal d.
    hemisphere d.
    hypoxic brain d.
    ischemic brain d.
    physial d.
    projection fiber d.
    renal vascular d.
    renovascular d.
    seminiferous tubule d.
    U-fiber d.
    valvular d.
    vascular cord d.
dammed-up cerebrospinal fluid
dampened
    d. obstructive pulse
    d. pulsatile flow
    d. waveform
dampening
    Doppler waveform d.
damping of catheter tip pressure
Damus-Kaye-Stansel (DKS)

dance
> hilar d.
> D. sign

dancer's
> d. bone
> d. foot malformation
> d. 5th metatarsal fracture

Dandy-Walker
> D.-W. complex
> D.-W. continuum
> D.-W. cyst
> D.-W. deformity
> D.-W. malformation
> D.-W. spectrum
> D.-W. syndrome
> D.-W. variant

Dandy-Walker-Blake spectrum
dangling choroid plexus
Danis-Weber
> D.-W. ankle fracture classification
> D.-W. fracture

DANTE
> delay alternating with nutation for tailored excitation
> DANTE sequence

DANTE-selective pulse
D'Antonio acetabular classification
DAP
> dose area product

dark
> d. lung
> d. Mach band
> d. pixel value
> d. region
> d. signal intensity
> d. signal-intensity rim

darkfield
> d. imaging
> d. microscopy

darkroom error
Darkschewitsch
> nucleus of D.

Darrach-Hughston-Milch fracture
dartoic tissue
dartos muscle
darwinian tubercle
DAS
> data acquisition system

DASA
> distal articular set angle

Daseler-Anson classification of plantaris muscle anatomy
dashboard fracture
DAT
> digital axial tomography
> dopamine transporter
> DAT binding
> symmetric loss of DAT

data (*pl. of* datum)

database
> Talairach Daemon d.

data-clipping detection error artifact
Datascope catheter
dataset
> 3D anatomic d.
> foreshortened image d.
> isotropic d.
> volumetric d.

dating
> 2nd-trimester gestational d.
> 3rd-trimester gestational d.

DaTSCAN
> D. imager
> D. imaging agent

datum, *pl.* **data**
Daubenton
> D. line
> D. plane

daughter
> d. abscess
> d. cyst
> d. element
> d. isotope
> d. nuclide

DAVF
> dural arteriovenous fistula

David Letterman sign
Davidson shunt
Davies
> D. endocardial fibrosis
> D. endomyocardial fibrosis

Davies-Colley syndrome
da Vinci surgical system
Davis intubated pyelotomy
Dawbarn sign
Dawson finger
Dawson-Mueller drainage catheter
daylight processor
d'Azyr
> bundle of Vicq d.

DBA
> duodenal bulb apex

DBC
> dye-binding capacity

DBDC
> distal bile duct carcinoma

DBM
> demineralized bone matrix

DC
> direct current
> DC offset artifact

DCA
> directional color angiography
> directional coronary atherectomy

DCBE
> double-contrast barium enema

D

DCCF
    dural carotid cavernous fistula
DCE-MRI
    dynamic contrast-enhanced magnetic
      resonance imaging
DCIS
    ductal carcinoma in situ
      comedo-type DCIS
      cribriform DCIS
      micropapillary DCIS
      papillary DCIS
      solid DCIS
      Van Nuys prognostic index for
        DCIS
DCM
    dilated cardiomyopathy
DCO
    distal clavicle osteolysis
      nontraumatic DCO
DCS
    distal coronary sinus
DCS-10, DCS-18 mechanically detachable platinum coil
DCT
    dynamic computed tomography
DDC
    direct display console
DDD
    double-dose delay
    dual-mode, dual-pacing, dual-sensing
dD/dt
    derived value on apexcardiogram
DDFP
    dodecafluoropentane
DDH
    developmental dysplasia of hip
DDR
    direct digital radiography
DDREF
    dose/dose-rate effective factor
DDS
    Denys-Drash syndrome
DDSA
    duplex Doppler signal analysis
      Integris V3000 DDSA
DDSS
    double decidual sac sign
2DE
    2-dimensional echocardiography
de
    d. Broglie wavelength
    d. Lange syndrome
    d. Morsier syndrome
    d. Musset sign
    d. novo aneurysm
    d. novo lesion
    d. Quervain disease
    d. Quervain fracture
    d. Quervain tenosynovitis

    d. Quervain thyroiditis
    d. Seze angle
deactivation
dead
    d. bone
    d. bowel
    d. space
    d. time
    d. time loss
    d. tissue
DEAE-Sephadex A-25 chromatography
death
    brain d.
    cerebral d.
    early fetal d.
    fetal d.
    imminent d.
    intermediate fetal d.
    late fetal d.
    quadrant of d.
    sudden cardiac d.
DeBakey aortic classification
deblurring
    histogram-based selective d.
    d. technique
debris
    atheromatous d.
    atherosclerotic d.
    bone d.
    calcium d.
    cholesterol d.
    echogenic d.
    embolic d.
    extraarticular d.
    foreign d.
    gelatinous d.
    grumous d.
    intimal d.
    intraarticular d.
    intraluminal d.
    joint d.
    layering d.
    metallic d.
    necrotic d.
    particulate d.
    thallium d.
debris-fluid level
debulking
    palliative d.
    d. surgery
decade scaler
decalcification
decalcified dorsum sellae
decannulation
decarboxylation
    amine precursor uptake and d. (APUD)
decay
    alpha d.
    beta d.

beta-minus d.
beta-plus d.
branch d.
branching d.
d. constant
energy d.
d. equation
exponential d.
free induction d. (FID)
isomeric d.
isotope d.
d. mode
nuclear d.
positron d.
d. product
radioactive d.
repeated free induction d.
d. scheme
d. series
d. time
decay-activating factor
deceleration-dependent block
deceleration time
decelerative injury
dechondrification
decidua
decidual
d. cyst
d. fissure
d. sac
decidualized endometrium
deciduate placenta
deciduous
decima
costa fluctuans d.
decimalized variance map
decision matrix
decline
ADC d.
declotting
decoding
document image d. (DID)
Viterbi d.
decompensated
d. alcoholic cirrhosis
d. congestive heart failure
decompensation
cardiac d.
chronic respiratory d.
endstage adult cardiac d.
endstage fetal cardiac d.
hemodynamic d.
ischemic d.
respiratory d.
ventricular d.
decomposition
3-level Haar wavelet d.

linear prediction with singular value d.
singular valve d. (SVD)
decompression
arthroscopic d.
biliary d.
bony d.
canal d.
cardiac d.
d. catheter
endoscopic d.
foramen magnum d.
gastric d.
hydrostatic d.
intestinal d.
microvascular d.
d. of fracture
percutaneous transhepatic d.
peripheral nerve d.
portal d.
d. sickness
spinal cord d.
surgical d.
transduodenal endoscopic d.
transpedicular d.
tube d.
d. tube
variceal d.
venous d.
deconditioned exercise response
deconditioning
deconvolution
d. analysis
d. method
d. technique
decortication
cardiac d.
heart d.
lung d.
decoupling
bilinear rotation d. (BIRD)
decrease
intraluminal attenuation d.
split renal function d.
decreased
d. activity
d. attenuation
d. cerebral blood flow
d. closing velocity
d. diffusion anisotropy
d. distal perfusion
d. E-to-F slope
d. intensity
d. peripheral vascular resistance
d. peristalsis
d. placenta size
d. pulmonary vascularity
d. stroke volume
d. systemic resistance
d. thyroid radiotracer uptake

D

decreased (*continued*)
    d. tidal volume
    d. uptake of radiotracer
    d. vital capacity
decrement
    scan d.
DecThreads software
decubitus
    d. calculus
    d. film
    d. pad
    d. position
    d. projection
    d. radiograph
    d. ulcer
    d. view
decussate
decussation
dedicated
    d. head scanner
    d. linear accelerator
    d. mammography system
    d. PET scanner
    d. phased-array coil
    d. shoulder coil
    d. viewer
dedifferentiated
    d. liposarcoma
    d. parosteal osteosarcoma
dedifferentiation
deep
    d. arch
    d. artery
    d. cardiac plexus
    d. collateral ligament
    d. Doppler velocity interrogation
    d. fascia
    d. fascia of penis
    d. gray matter nucleus change
    d. inspiratory breath-hold (DIBrH)
    d. interloop abscess
    d. lateral femoral notch sign
    d. lymphatic vessel
    d. muscle
    d. myometrial invasion
    d. pelvic abscess
    d. perineal pouch
    d. posterior compartment
    d. roentgen ray therapy
    d. sedation
    d. sulcus sign
    d. to nipple
    d. tumor
    d. vein
    d. vein system of leg
    d. venous aplasia
    d. venous channel
    d. venous incompetence
    d. venous insufficiency (DVI)

    d. venous occlusion
    d. venous thromboembolization
    d. venous thrombosis (DVT)
    d. white matter ischemia
    d. white matter track
deep-seated
    d.-s. infection
    d.-s. lesion
    d.-s. tumor
deep-shelled acetabulum
deexcitation
default display protocol
defecating proctogram
defecogram
defecography
    dynamic open magnetic resonance d.
    open magnetic resonance d.
defect
    abdominal wall d.
    anteroapical d.
    aortic septal d.
    aortopulmonary septal d.
    apical d.
    atrial ostium primum d.
    atrial septal d. (ASD)
    atrioventricular canal d.
    atrioventricular nodal septal d.
    atrioventricular septal d. (AVSD)
    bar d.
    beneficial atrial septal d.
    benign cortical d.
    bile duct filling d.
    bony d.
    bridging d.
    calcified medullary d.
    cauliflower-shaped filling d.
    cecal filling d.
    chiasmatic d.
    chondral d.
    cold d.
    collagen d. (type I, II)
    collecting system filling d.
    colonic filling d.
    conal ventricular septal d.
    concomitant d.
    congenital heart d. (CHD)
    congenital hemidysplasia with
      ichthyosiform erythroderma and
      limb d.'s (CHILD)
    conoventricular d.
    contiguous ventricular septal d.'s
    conversion d.
    cortical d.
    craniotomy d.
    curvilinear d.
    cushion d.
    developmental d.
    discoid filling d.
    duodenal filling d.

Eisenmenger d.
endocardial cushion d. (ECD)
endocardial cushion ventricular
  septal d.
esophageal filling d.
extradural d.
extrinsic filling d.
extrinsic ureteral d.
fetal abdominal wall d.
fibrous cortical d.
fibrous medullary d.
fibrous metaphysial-diaphysial d.
field d.
filling d.
fixed intracavitary filling d.
fixed perfusion d.
fixed radiotracer d.
flap-valve ventricular septal d.
focal liver scintigraphic d.
focal plaquelike d.
frondlike filling d.
frontal d.
fusiform d.
fusion d.
gallbladder filling d.
gastric remnant filling d.
global cortical d.
gouge d.
hatchet d.
hernia d.
high d.
Hill-Sachs d. (HSD)
hot d.
incisura d.
inferoapical d.
infracristal ventricular septal d.
infundibular ventricular septal d.
interatrial septal d.
intercalary d.
interventricular septal d. (IVSD)
intraarterial filling d.
intraatrial filling d.
intracavitary filling d.
intraductal breast filling d.
intraluminal filling d.
intramural filling d.
intravascular filling d.
intrinsic filling d.
inverted umbrella d.
ischemic d.
joint capsule d.
junctional cortical d.
junctional parenchymal kidney d.
juxtaarterial ventricular septal d.
juxtatricuspid ventricular septal d.
linear d.
lingular mandibular bony d.
  (LMBD)
lobulated filling d.

lucent d.
luminal d.
lung perfusion d.
luteal phase d.
malaligned atrioventricular septal d.
mapping of d.
mass d.
membranous ventricular septal d.
metaphysial fibrous d.
mismatched d.
monoradicular filling d.
multiple colon filling d.'s
multiple small bowel filling d.'s
mural d.
muscular ventricular septal d.
neural tube d. (NTD)
nonexpansile well-demarcated
  multilocular bone d.
nonexpansile well-demarcated
  unilocular bone d.
nonsubperiosteal cortical d.
nonuniform rotational d. (NURD)
obstructive ventilatory d.
open neural tube d.
organification d.
osseous d.
osteocartilaginous d.
osteochondral d. (OCD)
osteophytic d.
ostium primum atrial septal d.
ostium secundum atrial septal d.
pars interarticularis d.
partial atrioventricular canal d.
pear-shaped d.
pericardial d.
periinfarction conduction d.
perimembranous ventricular septal d.
photopenic d.
plaquelike linear d.
plication d.
pneumatoenteric d.
polypoid filling d.
porta hepatis d.
postcricoid d.
posteroapical d.
postinfarction ventricular septal d.
postoperative skull d.
punched-out bony d.
radial ray d.
radiolucent linear filling d.
resolving ischemic neurologic d.
restrictive ventilatory d.
reversible ischemic d.
right ventricular conduction d.
Roger ventricular septal d.
scan d.
scintigraphic perfusion d.
secundum atrial septal d.
segmental bone d.

D

defect (*continued*)
    segmental bronchus d.
    septal d.
    septation septal d.
    septum transversum d.
    serpiginous luminal filling d.
    sessile filling d.
    single colonic filling d.
    sinus venosus atrial septal d.
    small bowel filling d.
    soft tissue d.
    solitary small bowel filling d.
    spontaneous closure of d.
    stellate d.
    stomach filling d.
    subcortical d.
    subperiosteal cortical d.
    subsegmental perfusion d.
    superior caval d.
    superior marginal d.
    supracristal ventricular septal d.
    Swiss cheese ventricular septal d.
    thyroid organification d.
    thyroid trapping d.
    transient perfusion d.
    trapping thyroid d.
    triangular d.
    triple match d.
    trochlear d.
    tumor d.
    ureteral filling d.
    valvular cardiac d.
    venous d.
    ventilation d.
    ventilation-perfusion d.
    ventral hernia d.
    ventricular septal d.
    wedge-shaped d.
    wire-related d.
defective
    d. communication between cardiac
      chambers
    d. volume regulation delay
deferens, *pl.* **deferentia**
    ductus d.
    vas d.
    vasa deferentia
deferent
    d. canal
    d. duct
deferentia (*pl. of* deferens)
deferential
    d. artery
    d. plexus
deferentis
    ampulla ductus d.
defibrillation
    rectilinear biphasic waveform for
      external d.

defibrillator
    automatic external d. (AED)
defibrination syndrome
deficiency
    acyl CoA oxidase d.
    Aitken femoral d.
    alpha-1-antitrypsin d.
    COX d.
    cyclooxygenase d.
    photon d.
    proximal focal femoral d.
      (PFFD)
    RDS-like d.
    sphingomyelinase d.
    surfactant d.
    zinc d.
deficit
    base d.
    cortical d.
    focal d.
    hand motor d.
    lateralization d.
    neurogenic d.
    posterior column d.
    presynaptic dopaminergic d.
    reversible ischemic neurologic d.
    significant residual d.
    space d.
defined homogeneous calcification
definition
    ground-glass d.
    loss of d.
definitive
    d. abnormality
    d. callus
Definity
    D. contrast agent
    D. injectable suspension
    D. suspension for IV
      injection
deflation
deflection
    full-scale d. (FSD)
    intrinsic d.
deflector
    tip d.
deflexion
defluorescence
defluxion
deformability
deformable
    d. manipulation
    d. template
deformans
    arthritis syphilitica d. (ASD)
    arthrosis d.
    osteitis d.
    osteochondrodystrophia d.
    Paget osteitis d.

spondylitis d.
spondylosis d.

deformation

d. amplitude
cord d.
d. posterior plagiocephaly
shear-strain d.

deformation-based

d.-b. hippocampal segmentation and
shape analysis
d.-b. surface-rendered image

deformity

Åkerlund d.
alpine hunter's cap d.
angular d.
aortic valve d.
Arnold-Chiari d.
back-knee d.
Bankart d.
bayonet d.
bell-and-clapper d.
biconcave d.
bifid thumb d.
bony d.
boutonnière d.
bowing d.
bull's-eye d.
burn boutonnière d.
buttonhole d.
calcaneovarus d.
calcaneus d.
cavovarus d.
cavus d.
cecal d.
chain-of-lakes d.
Charcot d.
checkrein d.
cloverleaf d.
clubfoot d.
clubhand d.
cock-up d.
codfish d.
compensatory d.
congenital d.
contracture d.
cow horn d.
coxa valga d.
coxa vara d.
cranioorbital d.
cubitus valgus d.
cubitus varus d.
curly toe d.
Dandy-Walker d.
digital d.
digitus flexus d.
dinner-fork d.
duodenal bulb d.
endometrial surface d.
equinovalgus d.

equinovarus hindfoot d.
equinus d.
Erlenmeyer flask-like d.
eversion-external rotation d.
femoral head d.
flatfoot d.
flexible spastic equinovarus d.
flexion d.
foot d.
forefoot abduction d.
fracture d.
funnel chest d.
garden spade d.
gastric wall d.
genu valgum d.
genu varum d.
gibbous d.
gooseneck outflow tract d.
gunstock d.
Haglund d.
hallux flexus d.
hallux malleus d.
hallux rigidus d.
hallux valgus d.
hallux varus d.
hammertoe d.
hatchet-head d.
Hill-Sachs d.
hindbrain d.
hindfoot d.
hockey-stick tricuspid valve d.
hourglass d.
humpback d.
Ilfeld-Holder d.
internal rotation d.
intrinsic minus d.
intrinsic plus d.
J-hook d.
joint d.
J-sella d.
keyhole d.
Kirner d.
kleeblatschädel d.
Klippel-Feil d.
knock-knee d.
lanceolate d.
lobster-claw d.
Madelung d.
mallet-finger d.
mermaid d.
metatarsus adductocavus d.
metatarsus adductovarus d.
metatarsus adductus d.
metatarsus atavicus d.
metatarsus latus d.
metatarsus primus varus d.
Michel d.
mitral valve d.
nasal tip d.

D

deformity (*continued*)
neuropathic midfoot d.
pannus d.
parachute mitral valve d.
pectus carinatum d.
pectus excavatum d.
pencil-in-cup d.
penciling d.
pencil-like d.
pencil-point metatarsal d.
perigastric d.
pes arcuatus clawfoot d.
pes cavus clawfoot d.
pes planovalgus d.
pes planus d.
phrygian cap d.
pigeon-breast d.
ping-pong ball d.
pistol-grip femur d.
planovalgus foot d.
plantar flexion-inversion d.
postoperative thoracic d.
procurvature d.
pseudo-Hurler d.
pulmonary valve d.
recurvatum d.
reduction d.
rocker d.
rockerbottom foot d.
rolled-edge d.
rotational d.
rotoscoliotic d.
roundback d.
round shoulder d.
saber-shin d.
sandal-gap d.
scimitar d.
seal-fin d.
shepherd's crook d.
snowman d.
spastic equinovarus d.
spastic hindfoot valgus d.
splayfoot d.
split foot d.
spondylitic d.
Sprengel d.
static foot d.
subtrochanteric varus d.
supination d.
supratip nasal tip d.
swan-neck finger d.
talus foot d.
thoracic d.
thumb-in-palm d.
torsion d.
trefoil d.
tricuspid valve d.
trigger finger d.
triphalangeal thumb d.

turned-up pulp d.
ulnar drift d.
valgus heel d.
varus d.
Velpeau d.
vertical talus foot d.
VISI d.
Volkmann d.
wasp-tail d.
wedging d.
whistling d.
Whitehead d.
windblown d.
windswept d.

degenerated
d. fibroadenoma
d. tissue
d. uterine leiomyoma

degeneration
acquired hepatocerebral d.
angiolithic d.
articular cartilage d.
atheromatous d.
atrophic d.
ballooning d.
bony d.
brain d.
breast d.
calcareous d.
carcinomatous subacute cerebellar d.
cardiac valve mucoid d.
cardiomyopathic d.
cartilaginous d.
cerebellar d.
cerebelloolivary d.
cerebromacular d. (CMD)
chondrocyte d.
cobblestone d.
colloid d.
cortical cerebellar d.
corticobasal ganglionic d.
corticostriatospinal d.
cusp d.
cystic d.
disc d.
Doyne honeycomb d.
dystrophic d.
esophageal d.
facet d.
fatty d.
fibroid d.
frontotemporal lobe d.
gliosis-induced microcystic d.
granulovacuolar d.
gray matter d.
heart d.
hepatic d.
hepatocerebral d.
hepatolenticular d.

Holmes cortical cerebellar d.
honeycomb d.
hyaline d.
hydropic d.
hypertensive vascular d.
hypertrophic olivary d.
internal d.
intimal d.
intrameniscal mucoid d.
liquefaction d.
malignant d.
meniscal d.
Menzel olivopontocerebellar d.
microcystic d.
mitral valve myxomatous d.
Mönckeberg d.
mucinous d.
mucoid umbilical cord d.
mucous d.
mural d.
muscular d.
myocardial cellular d.
myocardial fibrous d.
d. of pancreas
olivary d.
olivopontocerebellar d. (OPCD)
pancreatic d.
paraneoplastic cerebellar d.
parenchymatous cerebellar d.
paving-stone d.
primary progressive cerebellar d.
progressive d.
Regnauld great toe d.
renal tubular d.
retinal d.
retrograde d.
rim d.
sclerotic d.
secondary d.
senile d.
spinal d.
spinocerebellar d.
spongiform d.
spongy white matter d.
striatonigral d.
subacute combined spinal cord d.
testicular d.
thyroid d.
trabecular d.
traumatic d.
wallerian d.
wear-and-tear d.
Zenker d.

degenerative
d. aortic aneurysm
d. arthritis
d. arthrosis
d. atrioventricular node disease
d. atrophy

d. brain disease
d. cardiomyopathy
d. dementia
d. disc
d. disc disease
d. disease in cerebrum
d. horizontal cleavage tear
d. joint disease (DJD)
d. liver
d. microcystic formation
d. narrowing
d. nuclear pattern
d. osseous change
d. osteoarthritis
d. spinal instability
d. spondylolisthesis
d. spondylosis
d. spur
d. spurring

deglutition
d. disorder
d. mechanism
muscle of d.
d. pneumonia

Degos syndrome
degradable starch microsphere
degradation
fibrinogen d.
image quality d.
motion d.
d. of image

degraded
d. liver
d. photon

degranulation
degree
noncircularity d.
d. of correction
d. of head rotation
d. of inspiration
d. of neck obliquity

360-degree rotation
45-degree spinal wedge
55-degree tomography wedge
dehalogenation
dehiscence
anastomotic d.
aortic intimal d.
bronchial d.
Killian d.
valve d.
wound d.

dehiscent jugular bulb
dehydration-induced renal dysfunction
dehydrogenase
succinate d. (SDH)

DEI
diffraction-enhanced imaging
Dejerine-Klumpke syndrome

D

Dejerine-Roussy
  thalamic syndrome of D.-R.
Dejerine sign
Delarnette scanner
delay
  d. alternating with nutation for tailored excitation (DANTE)
  defective volume regulation d.
  double-dose d. (DDD)
  interscan d.
  intraventricular conduction d.
  phase d.
  postinjection scan d.
  readout d.
  regrowth d.
  regular wedge d.
  regurgitant flow d.
  regurgitant lesion d.
  temporal phase d.
  d. time selection
  transition d.
  trigger d.
  upfront d.
delayed
  d. bone age
  d. bone imaging
  d. closure of suture
  d. cystogram
  d. development
  d. eclampsia
  d. excretion of contrast medium
  d. film
  d. fracture union
  d. gadolinium-enhanced magnetic resonance imaging of cartilage (dGEMRIC)
  d. gadolinium-enhanced MRI of cartilage
  d. gastric emptying
  d. hydrocephalus
  d. myelination
  d. operative cholangiography
  d. phase
  d. phase of arteriography
  d. pineal apoplexy
  d. posttraumatic myelopathy
  d. resolution of pneumonia
  d. rupture of spleen
  d. small bowel transit
  d. splenic rupture
  d. transit time
  d. transport of tracer
  d. traumatic intracerebral hematoma (DTICH)
  d. traumatic intracerebral hemorrhage
  d. unilateral nephrogram
  d. visualization
  d. washout

delayed-phase
  d.-p. image
  d.-p. scan
  d.-p. scanning
Delbet
  D. hip fracture classification
  D. sign
deleterious effect
delimitation
delineation
  lumen d.
delivered
  d. by balloon inflation
  d. total dose (DTD)
delivery
  angiogenesis gene d.
  coil d.
  intracavitary d.
  intravascular angiogenesis gene d.
  percutaneous endometrial drug d.
  timed bolus d.
  transcutaneous angiogenesis gene d.
  viral vector d.
Delmege sign of tuberculosis
delphian lymph node
delta
  D. 32 digital stereotactic system
  d. heavy-chain disease
  d. ray
  d. sign
  D. 32 TACT 3-dimensional breast imaging system
DELTAmanager MedImage system
deltoid
  d. branch of posterior tibial artery
  d. bursa
  d. crest
  d. eminence
  d. fascia
  d. ligament
  d. tuberosity
deltoideopectoral
  d. triangle
  d. trigone
deltopectoral
  d. groove
  d. lymph node
demagnetization
  adiabatic d.
  d. field effect
demarcate
demarcation
  d. line
  nidus d.
  shell-like d.
dementia
  degenerative d.
  diffuse Lewy body d. (DLBD)
  frontotemporal lobe d.

multiinfarct d.
subcortical ischemic vascular
d.
vascular d.
Demianoff sign
demifacet
demineralization
bone d.
demineralized
d. bone matrix (DBM)
d. bony structure
demise
embryo d.
imminent d.
intrauterine d.
d. of fetus
demodulator
Demons-Meigs syndrome
Demons method
demyelinating disease
demyelination, demyelinization
age-related d.
brainstem d.
cerebrum d.
infection-related d.
intramedullary d.
ischemic d.
large-fiber d.
leopard skin d.
metabolic d.
posterior column d.
postinfectious d.
primary d.
segmental d.
tigroid d.
toxic d.
white matter d.
demyelinative disorder
demyelinization (*var. of* demyelination)
**DeMyer system of cerebral
malformation**
denatured
d. ^{99m}Tc-RBC
d. ^{99m}Tc-RBC imaging
agent
dendritic
d. calculus
d. carcinoma
d. gynecomastia
d. lesion
d. spine
d. vegetation
dendrocytoma
denervated area
denervation
d. atrophy
autonomic d.
cardiac d.
sympathetic d.

Denis
D. classification
D. classification of spinal fracture
Denker procedure
Dennis tube
Denonvilliers
D. fascia
D. ligament
dens
d. fracture
hypoplasia of d.
d. in dente
d. view
d. view of cervical spine
dense
d. abdominal veins
d. body
d. brain mass
d. breast
d. capillary staining
d. cerebral mass
d. connective tissue
d. consolidation
d. echo
d. enhancing brain lesion
d. lung lesion
d. MCA sign
d. metaphysial band
d. rib
d. scar
d. structure of bone
densitometer
accuDEXA bone d.
Achilles d.
bone d.
CT d.
DEXA scan bone d.
DPX-IQ d.
dual-energy x-ray absorptiometry d.
dual-photon d.
dynamic spiral CT lung d.
Expert-XL d.
Hologic 2000 d.
Lunar DPX d.
Lunar Expert d.
Norland XR26 bone d.
OsteoView digital bone d.
pDEXA peripheral bone d.
Prodigy bone d.
QDR-1500, -2000 bone d.
Sahara portable bone d.
single-photon d.
densitometric measurement
densitometry
bone d.
cardiac output video d.
Compton coherent scattering d.
computerized optical d. (COD)
CT d.

D

densitometry (*continued*)
  dual-photon d.
  dynamic spiral CT lung d.
  Norland bone d.
  photon d.
  pulmonary d.
  QCT 3000 system for bone d.
  quantitative CT d.
  single-photon bone d.
  spirometrically controlled CT lung d.
  d. z score
density
  air d.
  area of abnormal d.
  arterial linear d.
  asymmetric breast d.
  axial spin d.
  background d.
  band of d.
  base d.
  bone mineral d. (BMD)
  calcific d.
  capillary d.
  count d.
  curvilinear d.
  diffuse increase in breast d.
  diffuse reticular d.
  diffuse reticulogranular lung d.
  discrete perihilar d.
  d. discrimination
  double d.
  echo-spin d.
  endoluminal d.
  energy flux d.
  d. equalization filter
  falx increased d.
  fat d.
  fibroglandular d.
  fluid d.
  focal asymmetric d.
  ground-glass d.
  hazy d.
  homogeneous soft tissue d.
  hydrogen spin d.
  ill-defined breast d.
  ill-defined multifocal lung d.
  increased bone d.
  increased splenic d.
  inherent d.
  integrated optical d. (IOD)
  ionization d.
  lamellar body d. (LBD)
  linear d.
  low d.
  lung d.
  magnetic flux d.
  d. matrix theory
  maximum d. (D_{max})

  mean optical d.
  metallic d.
  microvessel d.
  minimum pixel d.
  mixed fat-water lesion d.
  mottled d.
  multiple pleural d.'s
  near-water d.
  nodular d.
  optic d.
  paratracheal d.
  patchy area of d.
  peak count d.
  perihilar d.
  photon d.
  pleural d.
  prostate-specific antigen d.
  PSA d.
  pulmonary d.
  radiographic d.
  radiolucent d.
  radiopaque d.
  reticulogranular pulmonary d.
  retroareolar d.
  retrocardiac d.
  segmental lung d.
  soft tissue d.
  spicular d.
  spin d.
  spleen d.
  strand of increased d.
  streak of increased d.
  subareolar breast d.
  tissue d.
  T-score measurement of bone mineral d.
  tubular lung d.
  urographic d.
  variation in d.
  water d.
  wedge-shaped d.
dental
  d. bulb
  d. contrast material
  d. crest
  d. cyst
  d. granuloma
  d. groove
  d. infection
  d. neck
  d. polyp
  d. radiography
  d. radiology
  d. ridge
  d. root
  d. sac
  d. scan
  d. shelf
  d. tubercle

Dentalaser
    Multi-Operatory D. (MOD)
DentaScan
    D. imaging
    D. multiplanar reformation
dentata
    vertebra d.
dentate
    d. fascia
    d. fissure
    d. fracture
    d. gyrus
    d. ligament
    d. line
    d. nucleus
    d. nucleus calcification
    d. nucleus of cerebellum
    d. output channel
    d. suture
    d. suture of skull
dentatoolivary pathway
dentatorubral pallidoluysian atrophy
dentatothalamic tract
DentCAM
dente
    dens in d.
denticulate, denticulated
    d. ligament
    d. suture
denticulated (*var. of* denticulate)
dentiform
dentigerous cyst
dentin
dentinal
    d. sheath
    d. tubule
dentine
dentinogenesis imperfecta
dentition
    crowded d.
dentoskeletal relationship
denture-supporting structure
Dent-X intraoral x-ray unit
denudation
    area of d.
denutrition
Denver shunt
Denys-Drash
    D.-D. syndrome (DDS)
    D.-D. tumor
Denys syndrome
deossification
    band of d.
6-deoxy-1-galactose
deoxygenated blood
2-deoxyglucose
    2-fluoro 2-d. (FDG)
deoxyglucose
    ^{11}C d.

deoxyguanosine triphosphate
deoxyhemoglobin concentration
deoxyribonucleic acid (DNA)
dependence, dependency
    quadratic d.
    relaxation rate frequency d.
    solvent water TI frequency d.
dependency (*var. of* dependence)
    d. reaction
dependent
    d. atelectasis
    d. edema fluid resorption
    d. extracellular fluid accumulation
    d. lung
    d. opacity
    d. pouch of Douglas
    d. space
dephase-rephase magnitude subtraction
  technique
dephasing
    d. gradient
    intraluminal d.
    intravoxel d.
    odd-echo d.
    rapid d.
    signal d.
    spin d.
depicted Hounsfield unit
depiction
    magnetic resonance d.
    d. of vasculature
depilatory agent
depletion
    intravascular volume d.
deployed stent
deployment
    stent d.
depolarization
    chemically induced dynamic nuclear
    d.
    ventricular premature d. (VPD)
deposit
    amyloid d.
    arteriosclerotic d.
    bony d.
    calcareous d.
    calcium salt d.
    callus d.
    endochondral bone d.
    hemosiderin d.
    intramuscular hemosiderin d.
    pericardial calcareous d.
    rough calcific d.
    smooth calcific d.
deposition
    calcium pyrophosphate dihydrate
      crystal d.
    coil d.
    iron d.

D

245

deposition (*continued*)
    d. of tracer
    radiotracer d.
depreotide
    ^{99m}Tc d.
    d. scan
    technetium 99m d.
depressed
    d. diaphragm
    d. ejection fraction
    fracture simple and d. (FSD)
    d. right ventricular contractile
      function
    d. skull fracture
depression
    biconcave d.
    bone marrow d.
    fragment d.
    hemidiaphragm d.
    iodinated CM-induced cardiac d.
    iodinated contrast material-induced
      cardiac d.
    marginal kidney d.
    myocardial d.
    d. of left mainstem bronchus
    d. of nasal bone
    d. of renal margin
    pacchionian d.
    parasagittal d.
    reciprocal d.
    sinus node d.
    spinal cord d.
    tibial plateau d.
    translucent d.
    ventricular d.
depression-type intraarticular fracture
deprivation dwarfism
depth
    acetabular d.
    d. compensation
    d. dose
    lumbosacral spine d.
    maximum d.
    midplane d.
    d. of tumor invasion assessed by
      EUS
    photon interaction d.
    d. pulse
    d. resolution
    scatterer d.
    signal d.
    skin d.
    target d.
depth-dose
    d.-d. curve
    d.-d. distribution
depth-pulse technique
depth-resolved surface spectroscopy
  (DRESS)

DER
    dual-energy radiograph
deranged tissue development
derangement
    articular d.
    disc d.
    internal d.
    longitudinal transarticular d.
    painful disc d.
    soft tissue d.
derby hat fracture
Derek Harwood-Nash catheter
Derenzo
    D. equation
    D. phantom
derivative
    d. circulation
    hematoporphyrin d. (HpD)
    pyridone d.
    technetium 99m iminodiacetic acid
      d.
derived value on apexcardiogram (dD/dt)
Derma
    D. K laser
    D. 20 laser
dermal
    d. bone
    d. breast calcification
    d. duct tumor
    d. sinus tract
DermaLase laser
dermal-subcutaneous fat interface
dermatoarthritis
    lipoid d.
dermatofibrosarcoma protuberans
dermatomyositis
dermatosis
    radiation d.
dermoid
    mediastinal d.
    monodermal d.
    ovarian d.
    d. ovarian cyst
    d. plug
    spinal d.
    d. tumor
derotate
derotation
DES
    diffuse esophageal spasm
    DES exposure
Desault
    D. dislocation
    D. fracture
descended superior parathyroid adenoma
descending
    d. aorta dissection
    d. colon
    d. duodenum

left anterior d. (LAD)
d. septal artery
d. thoracic aorta
d. tract
d. urography
d. venography

descent
basal d.
epididymal d.
perineal d.

desert rheumatism
desferrioxamine toxicity
desiccated
desiccation
disc d.

design
crossed-coil d.
3D pulse d.
factorial d.
Hanafy piano-concave transducer d.
over-the-wire d.
PORT radiofrequency electrode d.
pulse d.
d. rule check

Desilets-Hoffman introducer
desmectasis
desmocytoma
desmofibromatosis
desmoid
cortical d.
extraabdominal d.
d. lesion
periosteal d.
d. reaction
subperiosteal d.
d. tumor

desmoma
desmoplasia
desmoplastic
d. cerebral astrocytoma of infancy
d. effort
d. fibroma
d. infantile astrocytoma
d. infantile ganglioglioma
d. medulloblastoma
d. reaction
d. response
d. small round-cell tumor (DSRCT)

desmosis
desmosome
d'Espine sign
desquamated epithelial breast hyperplasia
desquamative
d. fibrosing alveolitis
d. interstitial pneumonia (DIP)

destroy and replace method
destruction
bony d.
cortical d.

geographic bone d.
moth-eaten bone d.
mucosal d.
d. of tissue
pattern of d.
permeative bone d.
sellar d.
temporomandibular joint d.
trabecular d.

destructive
d. bone lesion
d. brucellar arthritis
d. discovertebral lesion
d. interference technique
d. process
d. spondyloarthropathy
d. tumor

detachable
d. balloon-modified reducing stent
d. platinum coil

detail
d. burnout
exquisite d.
fetal d.
fine d.
intraluminal d.
low-contrast d. (LCD)
recorded d.
rib d.
suboptimal d.
trabecular bone d.

detectability
lesion d.
low-contrast d.
threshold contrast detail d. (TCDD)

detecting
collision d.
d. Down syndrome by ultrasound
of nose bone
d. module

detection
annihilation coincidence d.
(ACD)
automated polyp d.
beta d.
cardiac shunt d.
coincidence d.
computer-aided polyp d.
d. echocardiography
edge d.
focus d.
ICP-AES d.
magnetic resonance d.
molecular coincidence d. (MCD)
occult d.
photooptical d.
quadrature d.
radioactivity d.
radwaste radioactivity d.

D

detection (*continued*)
>   sonographic d.
>   d. threshold
>   turbidimetric d.
>   d. zone

detective quantum efficiency (DQE)

detector
>   Add-On Bucky direct x-ray d.
>   anular d.
>   d. array
>   bismuth germanate d.
>   block d.
>   cadmium iodide d.
>   CCD d.
>   d. coil
>   d. collimation
>   collimation scintillation d.
>   CR-39 nuclear tract d.
>   crystalline phosphor d.
>   C-Trak handheld gamma d.
>   Cutie Pie d.
>   dielectric track d.
>   digital amorphous silicon flat-panel d.
>   digital x-ray d.
>   diode d.
>   Doppler ultrasonic blood flow d.
>   Doppler ultrasonic velocity d.
>   element-specific d.
>   flame ionization d.
>   flat-panel d.
>   flat-plate d.
>   gamma probe radiation d.
>   gas-filled d.
>   GE d.
>   Geiger-Müller d.
>   glass tract d.
>   HPGe d.
>   ionization d.
>   kinestatic charge d. (KCD)
>   NaI d.
>   Neoprobe 1000, 1500 portable radioisotope d.
>   Neoprobe radioactivity d.
>   passive track d.
>   Pediatric Ingesta Scan metal d.
>   phase-sensitive d.
>   planar d.
>   quadrature phase d. (QPD)
>   radiation d.
>   ring d.
>   scintillation d.
>   semiconductor d.
>   Si(Li) d.
>   slot-scanning d.
>   sodium iodide d.
>   solid-state nuclear track d.
>   d. system
>   thallium-activated sodium iodine d.

>   Thoravision selenium x-ray d.
>   tissue-equivalent d.
>   Wang-Binford edge d.
>   x-ray d.

16-detector PET system

determinant
>   sequential d.

determination
>   Budin-Chandler anteversion d.
>   d. of lung volume
>   particle size d.
>   void d.

deterministic effect

detorsion
>   spontaneous d.

detour conduit

detritus

detrusor
>   d. hyperreflexia
>   d. instability
>   d. muscle

detrusor-sphincter dyssynergia

Detsky modified cardiac risk index

detunable elliptic transmission line resonator

deuterium
>   d. imaging agent
>   d. oxide

deuterium-tritium generator

deuteron, deuton

deuton (*var. of* deuteron)

Deutschländer disease

devascularization
>   paraesophagogastric d.

developed collateral

developer artifact

development
>   anomalous d.
>   branchial cleft d.
>   conductive d.
>   delayed d.
>   deranged tissue d.
>   distal bone marrow d.
>   endocardial cushion d.
>   interval d.
>   lymphatic d.
>   metacarpophalangeal bone marrow d.
>   metatarsophalangeal bone marrow d.
>   tibial bone marrow d.

developmental
>   d. defect
>   d. dysplasia of hip (DDH)
>   d. groove

Deventer
>   D. diameter
>   D. pelvis

deviated mediastinum

deviation
>   angular d.

aortic d.
carpal d.
fracture d.
left axis d. (LAD)
mean d.
mediastinal d.
needle d.
radial d.
right axis d. (RAD)
rotary d.
septal d.
significant axis d.
standard d.
tracheal d.
ulnar d.
ureteral d.
valgus d.
varus d.

device

abdominal left ventricular assist d. (ALVAD)
Accunet distal protection d.
amorphous silicon filmless digital x-ray detection technology d.
Amplatzer septal occluder d.
Amplatz thrombectomy d.
AngioGuard-EX distal protection d.
AngioJet thrombectomy d.
Angiolink EVS closure d.
Angio-Seal closure d.
Angio-Seal diagnostic d.
Angio-Seal therapeutic d.
antisiphon d.
Arrow-Trerotola percutaneous thrombectomy d.
Arrow-Trerotola percutaneous thrombolytic d.
arterial puncture site closure d.
automated gun-needle d.
automatic spring-loaded biopsy d.
BabyFace 3D surface rendering accessory d.
Bard rotary atherectomy d.
Baxter PMT d.
beam-indicating d.
beam-modifying d.
bioabsorbable sheath-delivered vascular d.
biventricular assist d. (biVAD)
BladderManager ultrasound d.
bone fixation d.
Bruker minispec measuring d.
Bucky digital x-ray d.
Burnett BiDirectional TMJ d.
buttoned d.
cardiac support d. (CSD)
charge-coupled d. (CCD)
charge injection d. (CID)

Closer percutaneous suture-mediated closure d.
closure d.
Clo-Sur PAD closure d.
Coherent VersaPulse d.
collagen mediated closure d.
collagen plug d.
compression d.
copper 7, T intrauterine d.
CyberKnife Express d.
directional atherectomy d.
DirectRay direct-to-digital image capture d.
Duett arterial puncture site closure d.
Duett diagnostic d.
Duett therapeutic d.
DynaWell medical compression d.
Electro-Acuscope d.
electrooptical d.
Endostaple d.
EVS mechanical closure d.
expandable foam immobilization d.
external fixation d.
FemoStop compression d.
Filter Wire distal protection d.
FloWire ultrasound d.
gating d.
Gelbfish-Endovasc d.
Glucoband electronic scanning d.
halo d.
hemostatic puncture closure d.
HiSonic ultrasonic bone conduction hearing d.
H2 Score office-based diagnostic d.
Hysterocath hysterosalpingography d.
Ilizarov d.
implantable vascular access d.
internal fixation d.
intramedullary fixation d.
intraoperative d.
intrauterine d. (IUD)
Kendall sequential compression d.
kinematic wrist d.
Laser Lancet laser d.
left ventricular assist d. (LVAD)
lost intrauterine d.
magnetic induction d.
MammoReader mammogram d.
Mobin-Uddin umbrella endoluminal d.
Molteno double-plate drainage d.
Molteno single-plate drainage d.
MultiDop P, T, X transcranial Doppler d.
nail plate d.
NB200 vascular access d.
Neuroshield distal protection d.
nonferromagnetic positioning d.
nuclear magnetic LipoProfile d.

D

device (*continued*)
 Omnisense multisite QUS d.
 Optical Path Difference-Scan optical
  d.
 OsteoAnalyzer bone densitometry d.
 Palpagraph breast mapping d.
 Perclose arterial closure d.
 Perclose diagnostic d.
 Perclose therapeutic d.
 Percusurg distal protection d.
 percutaneous arterial closure d.
 percutaneous suture-mediated
  arteriotomy closure d.
 percutaneous vascular surgical d.
 Pigg-O-Stat pediatric positioning d.
 Prostar-Techstar suture-mediated
  closure d.
 Prostar XL 8, 10 suture-mediated
  closure d.
 RadStat hemostasis d.
 Rashkind double umbrella d.
 rheolytic mechanical thrombectomy d.
 right ventricular assist d. (RVAD)
 scaling d.
 ScopeGuide magnetic resonance
  imaging d.
 ScopeGuide MRI d.
 Second Look breast imaging d.
 Sideris buttoned double-disc d.
 Siemens Magnetom Vision
  whole-body MR d.
 Sonoline Sierra ultrasound imaging d.
 SonoSite 180 hand-carried ultrasound
  d.
 Sonotron electronic therapeutic d.
 spinal fixation d.
 spot film d.
 stereotactic d.
 superconducting quantum interference
  d. (SQUID)
 SuperStitch closure d.
 synchronization d.
 Syvek Patch closure d.
 Telos radiographic stress d.
 T-fastener d.
 The Closer arterial puncture site
  closure d.
 thrombectomy d.
 Trak Back pullback d.
 Trerotola thrombectomy d.
 TriSpan aneurysm neck bridge d.
 tube d.
 vascular access d.
 vascular hemostatic d. (VHD)
 VasoSeal diagnostic d.
 VasoSeal ES, VHD arterial puncture
  site closure d.
 VasoSeal therapeutic d.
 venous access d.

 ventricular assist d.
 woggle d.
 X-Press suture-mediated closure d.
devitalized
 d. allogeneic bone
 d. portion of bone
 d. tissue
devoid of circulation
DEXA
 dual-energy x-ray absorptiometry
  DEXA bone density scan imaging
  DEXA scan
  DEXA scan bone densitometer
dexamethasone suppression test imaging
dexiocardia (*var. of* dextrocardia)
dexter
 cor triatriatum d.
Dexter-Grossman classification of mitral
 regurgitation
dextrad
dextral
dextran
 Gd-DTPA-labeled d.
 iron d.
 technetium 99m d.
dextran-coated
 d.-c. charcoal
 d.-c. particle
dextrocardia, dexiocardia
 mirror-image d.
dextroconcave
dextrogastria
dextro loop
dextroposition
dextropositioned aorta
dextropropoxyphene-IQ (DPX-IQ)
dextrorotary scoliosis (*var. of*
 dextrortoscoliosis)
dextrorotoscoliosis, dextrorotary scoliosis
dextroscoliosis
dextrose 5% in water imaging agent
dextrosinistral
dextrotransposition of great arteries
dextrotropic
dextroversion of heart
dextrum
 cor d.
DFA
 dorsiflexion angle
DFI
 dye fluorescence index
DFP
 diastolic filling pressure
DFS
 distraction-flexion staging
2DFT
 2-dimensional Fourier transform
  2DFT method
  2DFT time-of-flight MR angiography

3DFT
    3-dimensional Fourier transform
      3DFT gradient-echo MR imaging
      3DFT magnetic resonance angiography
      3DFT volume imaging
DFT
    discrete Fourier transform
3DFT-CISS
    3-dimensional Fourier
    transform-constructive interference in
    steady state
      3DFT-CISS sequence
DGC
    directional gradient concentration
dGEMRIC
    delayed gadolinium-enhanced magnetic
    resonance imaging of cartilage
DGHAL
    Doppler-guided hemorrhoid artery
    ligation
DGR
    duodenogastric reflux
DHCT
    dual-phase helical computed
    tomography
DHS
    dynamic hip screw
DI
    diagnostic imaging
Di
    D. Guglielmo disease
    D. Guglielmo syndrome
diabetes
    gestational d.
    d. mellitus (type 1, 2)
diabetic
    d. angiopathy
    d. cardiomyopathy
    d. gastroparesis
    d. ketoacidosis
    d. mastopathy
    d. microangiopathy
    d. nephropathy
    d. neuropathy
diacondylar fracture
DIAGNOdent laser
diagnosis
    computer-aided d. (CAD)
    prenatal d.
    prospective investigation of
    pulmonary embolus d. (PIOPED)
    radiographic d.
    radiologic d.
    sonographic d.
    ultrasound d.
Diagnost 120
diagnostic
    d. and therapeutic technology
    assessment

    d. angiography
    d. arteriography
    d. cascade
    d. efficacy analysis
    d. imaging (DI)
    d. mammography
    d. modality
    d. pneumoperitoneum
    d. pneumothorax
    d. procedure
    d. puncture
    d. radiation
    d. radioiodine scanning
    d. radiology
    d. radiopharmaceutical
    d. range ultrasound
    d. reconstruction
    d. skull series
    d. teleradiology
    d. x-ray camera and imaging source
    d. yield
diagonal
    d. branch
    d. branch of artery
    d. conjugate diameter
diagonalis
    stria d.
diagonalization
diagram
    energy level d. (ELD)
    Ladder d.
    marker-channel d.
    Zurich growth centile d.
diagrammatic radiography
dialysis
    d. arthropathy
    continuous ambulatory peritoneal d.
    (CAPD)
    d. fistula
    d. shunt
    d. tube
diamagnetic
    d. shift
    d. substance
    d. susceptibility
    d. tissue
diamagnetism
    Landau d.
diametaphysial
diametaphysis
diameter
    acetabular depth to femoral head d.
    (AD/FHD)
    anterior sagittal d. (ASD)
    anterior-to-posterior sagittal canal d.
    anteroposterior d.
    aortic root d.
    artery d.
    Baudelocque d.

D

diameter (*continued*)
    bicristal d.
    biischial d.
    biparietal d. (BPD)
    bisacromial d.
    bispinous d.
    bitemporal d.
    bituberous d.
    bronchial d.
    cardiac d.
    cecum d.
    coccygeopubic d.
    coil-to-vessel d.
    conjugate d.
    cranial d.
    craniometric d.
    cricopharyngeal d.
    Deventer d.
    diagonal conjugate d.
    end-diastolic d.
    end-systolic d.
    film d.
    frontomental d.
    frontooccipital d.
    gestational sac d.
    increased anteroposterior d.
    increment in luminal d.
    inferior longitudinal d.
    in-stent d.
    intercristal d.
    internal conjugate d.
    intertubercular d.
    left anterior internal d. (LAID)
    left ventricular internal d. (LVID)
    Löhlein d.
    lumen d.
    maximum anteroposterior d.
    maximum short-axis d. (MSAD)
    mean sac d. (MSD)
    mentooccipital d.
    mentoparietal d.
    midsagittal d. (MSD)
    minimal luminal d. (MLD)
    minimal port d. (MPD)
    narrow anteroposterior d.
    d. obliqua pelvis
    oblique d.
    occipitofrontal d. (OFD)
    occipitomental d.
    orthonormal d.
    parietal d.
    pelvic d.
    posterotransverse d.
    pyloric d.
    right ventricular internal d. (RVID)
    sacropubic d.
    sagittal canal d. (SCD)
    spinal cord d.

spleen d.
stenosis d.
suboccipitobregmatic d.
temporal d.
torsional attenuated d. (TAD)
d. transversa pelvis
transverse cerebellar d. (TCD)
transverse pelvic d.
ureter d.
valve d.
vertebromammary d.
vertical d.
vessel d.
yolk sac d.
diametric pelvic fracture
diamniotic pregnancy
Diamond-Blackfan syndrome
Diamox
diapedesis
diaphanography
diaphanoscope
diaphragm
    above d.
    accessory d.
    antral mucosal d.
    aperture d.
    aponeurotic portion of d.
    below d.
    bilateral elevation of d.
    Bucky d.
    central tendon d.
    costal part of d.
    crus of d.
    depressed d.
    dome of d.
    duodenal d.
    d. duplication
    elevated d.
    d. embryology
    eventration of d.
    excursion of d.
    flattening of d.
    free air under d.
    gastric d.
    inferior vena cava d.
    leaf of d.
    lumbar part of d.
    median arcuate ligament of d.
    muscular crus of d.
    paralysis of d.
    pelvic d.
    polyarcuate d.
    Potter-Bucky d.
    respiratory d.
    sella turcica d.
    sternal part of d.
    sternocostal part of d.
    tenting of d.

thoracoabdominal d.
traumatic rupture of d.
(TRD)
urogenital d.
vertebral part of d.
diaphragma sellae
diaphragmatic
d. attenuation
d. border
d. contour
d. creep
d. crus
d. cupula
d. dome
d. echo
d. elevation
d. esophageal hiatus
d. eventration
d. fascia
d. hernia
d. hump
d. ligament
d. lymph node
d. myocardial infarct (DMI)
d. paralysis
d. pericardium
d. pleura
d. pleurisy
d. rupture
d. sarcoma
d. segment
d. slip
d. surface
d. surface of heart
d. surface of liver
diaphyseal (*var. of* diaphysial)
diaphyses (*pl. of* diaphysis)
diaphysial, diaphyseal
d. aclasis
d. bone length ratio
d. center
d. cortical mortise
d. dysplasia
d. fracture
d. lesion
d. ossification
d. sclerosis
diaphysial-epiphysial fusion
diaphysis, *pl.* **diaphyses**
diaphysitis
luetic d.
diaplasis
diapositive
diarthrodial intervertebral joint
diarthroses (*pl. of* diarthrosis)
diarthrosis, *pl.* **diarthroses**
diaschisis
cerebellar d.

crossed cerebellar d. (CCD)
ipsilateral cortical d.
diascope
diascopy
Diasonics
D. ultrasound
D. ultrasound scanner
diastasis
fracture d.
d. heart period
d. of cranial bone
d. of suture
syndesmotic d.
tibiofibular d.
diastatic
d. fracture
d. lambdoid suture
diastematomyelia
spinal d.
diastole
gastric d.
diastolic
d. atrial volume
d. counterpulsation
d. depolarization phase
d. depolarization pulse
d. doming
d. filling period
d. filling pressure (DFP)
d. function
d. gating
d. gradient
d. heart failure
d. left ventricular index
d. notch impedance
d. overload
d. perfusion pressure
d. perfusion time
d. pressure-time index (DPTI)
d. pseudogating
d. regurgitant velocity
d. reserve
d. velocity ratio
d. zero flow
diastrophic
d. dwarfism
d. dysplasia
diathermic
d. loop
d. vascular occlusion
diathermy ultrasound
diatheses (*pl. of* diathesis)
diathesis, *pl.* **diatheses**
hypertensive d.
diatrizoate
meglumine d.
methylglucamine d.
diatrizoic acid contrast medium

D

DIBrH
    deep inspiratory breath-hold
DIC
    disseminated intravascular
     coagulation
    drip infusion cholangiogram
    drip infusion cholangiography
dicephalus
dichorionic-diamniotic
    d.-d. twin
    d.-d. twin pregnancy
dichromate
    d. dosimeter
    d. dosimetry
**Dickhaut-DeLee discoid meniscus
classification**
DICOM
    Digital Imaging and Communications
     in Medicine
     DICOM format
**DICOM-3-compatible digital computer
format**
dicondylar fracture
Dicopac test
dicrotic notch
DID
    document image decoding
DIDA
    dimethyl iminodiacetic acid
didactylism
didelphia
    uterine d.
didelphic uterus
didelphys
    uterus d.
dielectric
    d. artifact
    d. resonance
    d. track detector
diencephala (*pl. of* diencephalon)
diencephalic herniation
diencephalon, *pl.* **diencephala**
die-punch fracture
DIET
    dual-interval echo train
     DIET fast SE imaging
     DIET method of fat suppression
diet
    d. cola and metoclopramide syrup
    low-iodine d. (LID)
diethylenetriamine
    d. pentaacetic acid (DTPA)
    d. pentaacetic acid imaging
     agent
Dieulafoy
    D. disease
    D. lesion
    D. vascular malformation
DiFerrante syndrome

difference
    field-echo d.
    hemispheric regional lateralization d.
    operator-related d.
    potential d.
    rib-vertebral angle d.
    transient hepatic attenuation d.
     (THAD)
    transient hepatic intensity d. (THID)
differencing
    convolutional d.
    d. fiber
    d. filter
differential
    d. diagnosis bone lesion
    d. diagnostic lung mass feature
    d. interference contrast microscopy
    renal function d.
    scintillation camera linearity d.
    scintillation camera uniformity d.
    d. signal
    d. uniformity
    d. uptake ratio
    d. washout
differentiated
    d. carcinoma
    d. thyroid carcinoma (DTC)
differentiation
    cluster of d. (CD)
    corticomedullary d. (CMD)
    echocardiographic d.
    gray matter-white matter d.
    gray-white d.
    liposarcomatous d.
    nuclear anular d.
difficult-to-treat vascular lesion
diffracting Doppler transducer
diffraction
    beam d.
    high-resolution d.
    high-temperature d.
    low-temperature d.
    d. pattern
    d. peak
    x-ray d.
diffraction-enhanced imaging (DEI)
diffuse
    d. abdominal calcification
    d. adenomyosis
    d. adrenal enlargement
    d. aggressive lymphoma
    d. aggressive polymorphous infiltrate
    d. airspace disease
    d. airspace opacity
    d. alveolar damage
    d. alveolar interstitial infiltrate
    d. aortic atresia
    d. aortic dilation
    d. aortomegaly

d. arterial ectasia
d. arteriolar spasm
d. aspiration bronchiolitis
d. atelectasis
d. axonal injury (DAI)
d. bacterial nephritis
d. bilateral alveolar infiltrates
d. cerebral histiocytosis
d. cerebral swelling
d. cirrhosis
d. CNS sclerosis
d. contrast agent distribution pattern
d. dilation of esophagus
d. edema
d. emphysema
d. enlargement of thymus
d. esophageal spasm (DES)
d. fatty liver infiltrate
d. fibrosis type
d. fine lung reticulation
d. gallbladder wall thickening
d. ganglion
d. haziness
d. hepatic enlargement
d. hyperemia
d. idiopathic skeletal hyperostosis (DISH)
d. increase in breast density
d. infection
d. inflammation
d. intermediate lymphocytic lymphoma
d. interstitial pulmonary fibrosis (DIPF)
d. intimal thickening
d. irregularity
d. large cell lymphoma (DLCL)
d. leiomyomatosis
d. Lewy body dementia (DLBD)
d. liver enlargement
d. low attenuation
d. low-signal replacement of vertebral body
d. lung uptake
d. lymphangioma
d. malformation
d. malignant peritoneal mesothelioma
d. mediastinal widening
d. mixed small and large cell lymphoma
d. mottling
d. mucosal polyposis
d. multinodular infarct
d. myelinoclastic sclerosis
d. narrowing
d. necrosis
d. necrotizing leukoencephalopathy
d. neuroendocrine system
d. osteosclerosis

d. panbronchiolitis
d. pancreatitis
d. parenchymal lung disease
d. parenchymal renal disease
d. periapical sclerosing osteitis
d. pericarditis
d. perivascular infiltrate
d. pleural thickening
d. pleurisy
d. pneumonia
d. pneumonitis
d. pulmonary alveolar hemorrhage
d. pulmonary hemorrhage (DPH)
d. pulmonary neuroendocrine cell hyperplasia
d. pulmonary ossification
d. pulmonary uptake
d. reflector
d. reticular density
d. reticulogranular lung density
d. reticulonodular infiltrate
d. sarcomatosis
d. scleroderma
d. sclerosing alveolitis
d. signal hyperintensity
d. skeletal angiomatosis
d. skeletal metastasis
d. small cell lymphocytic lymphoma
d. spasm of esophagus
d. spatial distribution
d. spondylosis
d. stenosis
d. stippled calcification
d. subarachnoid hemorrhage
d. symmetric hypertrophied cardiomyopathy
d. synovial lipoma
d. thymic enlargement
d. toxic goiter
d. ulcerative lesion
d. uterine enlargement
d. ventricular hypokinesis
d. white matter injury
diffusible tracer
diffusing capacity
diffusion
anisotropic d.
anisotropically rotational d. (ARD)
d. anisotropy
d. anisotropy thresholding
d. characteristic of water
d. coefficient
directional d.
d. encoding strength
d. factor
Fick 1st law of d.

diffusion (*continued*)
- d. gradient
- d. magnetic resonance imaging
- molecular d.
- d. MRI
- d. pulse sequence
- restricted water d.
- d. scan
- spectral d.
- d. spectroscopy
- spin d.
- d. tension
- thermal d.
- d. time
- translational d.

diffusion-perfusion
- d.-p. mismatch
- d.-p. snapshot FLASH

diffusion-sensitive sequence
diffusion-sensitizing gradient
diffusion-tensor (DT)
- d.-t. imaging (DTI)
- d.-t. magnetic resonance imaging
- d.-t. MRI
- d.-t. MR imaging
- d.-t. tractography (DTT)

diffusion-weighted
- d.-w. echo-planar imaging
- d.-w. image
- d.-w. imaging (DWI)
- d.-w. magnetic resonance imaging
- d.-w. MR imaging
- d.-w. pulse sequence
- d.-w. scanning

diffusivity
- mean d.
- preferential d.
- white matter d.

diffusum
- papilloma d.

digastric
- d. fossa
- d. groove
- d. impression
- d. line
- d. muscle
- d. notch
- d. triangle

DiGeorge syndrome
digestive
- d. system
- d. tract
- d. tract contents
- d. tube

digestive-respiratory fistula
DIGGEST
- direct imaging of local gradients by group echo selection tomography

Digibar 190 contrast agent

Digirad
- D. gamma camera
- D. 2020tc imager

Digiscope
- Direx D.

digit
- accessory d.
- arthrodesed d.
- binary d.
- fibroosseous pseudotumor of d.
- flail d.
- photoplethysmographic d.
- replanted d.
- sausage d.
- supernumerary d.
- syndactylization of d.

digital
- d. abdominal radiograph
- D. Add-On Bucky radiographic detector image acquisition system
- d. amorphous silicon flat-panel detector
- d. amputation
- d. aponeurosis
- d. artery of foot
- d. artery of hand
- d. autofluoroscope
- d. autopsy
- d. axial tomography (DAT)
- d. beam attenuation
- d. branch
- d. celiac trunk angiography
- d. chest imaging
- d. chest imaging system
- d. chest radiograph
- d. clubbing
- d. deformity
- d. ejection fraction
- d. equipment system
- d. extensor tendon
- d. flat-panel amorphous silicon detector-radiography system
- d. flexor tendon
- d. fluorography
- d. fluoroscopy
- d. fossa
- d. free hepatic venography
- d. frequency analysis
- d. fundus imager
- d. gray scale
- d. high-speed endoscopy
- d. holography system
- D. Imaging and Communications in Medicine (DICOM)
- d. imaging processing (DIP)
- d. isotope calibrator
- d. livedo reticularis infarct
- d. mammographic system
- d. marking

d. medical system
d. neuroma
D. OsteoView 2000
d. parabola
d. plethysmography
d. process of fat
d. pulsed fluoroscopy (DPF)
d. radiography imaging
d. ray
d. rectal evacuation
d. reformatting knee MRI
d. road mapping
d. rotational angiography (DRA)
d. runoff
d. sampling rate
d. selenium-based chest imaging
  system
d. storage
d. subtraction
d. subtraction angiography (DSA)
d. subtraction aortography
d. subtraction arteriography (DSA)
d. subtraction film
d. subtraction imaging (DSI)
d. subtraction mammography (DSM)
d. subtraction rotational angiography
d. subtraction technique
d. subtraction ventriculogram
d. tomosynthesis
D. Traumex system
d. unraveling
d. vascular imaging (DVI)
d. vein
d. videoangiography
d. video gastrointestinal radiography
d. x-ray detector
digitalis therapy
digitalization noise
digitally
  d. fused CT and radiolabeled
    imaging
  d. fused CT and radiolabeled
    monoclonal antibody SPECT
    image
  d. reconstructed radiograph (DRR)
digital-to-analogue converter (DAC)
digitate ectasia
digiti (*pl. of* digitus)
digitization
digitized
  d. contact mammogram
  d. CT slice
  d. film image
  d. spinography
digitizer
  backlit d.
  3D surface d.
  laser d.
  multiple-jointed d.

multisensor structured light-range d.
Polhemus 3D d.
digitorum
  extensor d.
Digitron
  D. digital subtraction imaging
    system
  D. Koordinat angiography equipment
digitus, *pl.* **digiti**
  d. annularis
  d. flexus deformity
  d. manus
  d. medius
  d. pedis
  d. pedis minimus
  d. primus
  d. secundus
  d. valgus
  d. varus
dihydrate
  calcium pyrophosphate d. (CPPD)
**dihydropyrimidine dehydrogenase
  activity**
dihydroxyphenylalanine (DOPA)
  d. imaging agent
diiodotyrosine
diisopropyl iminodiacetic acid (DISIDA)
dilacerated tooth root
dilatation (*var. of* dilation)
dilatator (*var. of* dilator)
dilated
  d. aortic root
  d. bile duct
  d. bowel loop
  d. bronchus
  d. cardiomyopathy (DCM)
  d. collateral vein
  d. descending aorta
  d. dry small bowel
  d. duodenum
  d. esophagus
  d. fetal bowel
  d. gallbladder
  d. intercavernous sinus
  d. intrahepatic duct
  d. loop of bowel
  d. lymphatics
  d. mammary duct
  d. myocardium
  d. pulmonary artery
  d. pulmonary trunk
  d. rete testis
  d. small airway
  d. small bowel lumen
  d. spinal vein
  d. subareolar duct
  d. ureter
  d. ventricle
  d. wet small bowel

D

dilation, dilatation
 alveolar d.
 d. and hypertrophy
 aneurysmal d.
 antegrade transluminal balloon d.
 anular d.
 aortic root d.
 arterial d.
 ascending aorta d.
 balloon d.
 beaded ductal d.
 bile duct d.
 biliary d.
 bowel loop d.
 bronchial d.
 bronchiolar d.
 calyceal d.
 cardiac d.
 d. catheter
 cavitary d.
 chamber d.
 colonic d.
 common duct d.
 congenital cystic d.
 cystic d.
 diffuse aortic d.
 distal ureteral d.
 ductal d.
 Eder-Puestow d.
 esophageal d.
 extrahepatic biliary cystic d.
 fusiform d.
 gaseous d.
 gastric d.
 hepatic web d.
 idiopathic pulmonary artery d.
 idiopathic right atrial d.
 intestinal d.
 intrahepatic biliary cystic d.
 intrahepatic biliary ductal d.
 intrahepatic biliary tract d.
 intraluminal d.
 junctional d.
 left ventricular d.
 megacolon d.
 multiple mural d.'s
 mural d.
 myocardial d.
 d. of aneurysm
 d. of sulcus
 d. of ureter
 d. of ventricle
 pancreatic duct d.
 paradoxic colon d.
 pelvicalyceal d.
 percutaneous transluminal balloon
  d.
 periportal sinusoidal d.
 pharmacologic d.

 poststenotic d.
 prestenotic d.
 probe d.
 prognathic d.
 proximal d.
 proximal esophagitis d.
 pulmonary artery d.
 pulmonary trunk idiopathic d.
 pulmonary valve stenosis d.
 rectal d.
 respiratory bronchiolar d.
 right ventricular d.
 saccular d.
 stress-induced left ventricular d.
 sulcal d.
 sulcus d.
 thickened irregular small bowel fold
  d.
 thickened smooth small bowel fold
  d.
 tortuous vein d.
 track d.
 transient left ventricular d.
 transluminal d.
 tubular d.
 ureteral d.
 vein d.
 ventricular wall d.
 Virchow-Robin space d.
 Wirsung d.
dilator, dilatator
 angiographic Teflon d.
 balloon d.
 Teflon fascial d.
 telescopic aerial d.
dilution
 isotopic d.
 ultrasound d.
DILV
 double-inlet left ventricle
**Dimaq integrated ultrasound
 workstation**
dimeglumine
 gadobenate d.
 gadolinium d.
 Magnevist gadopentate d.
dimension
 abnormal heart chamber d.
 absolute artery d.
 anteroposterior d.
 aortic root d.
 arterial d.
 axial d.
 fractal d.
 intraluminal d.
 intrathoracic d.
 left ventricular diastolic d. (LVdd)
 left ventricular end-diastolic d.
  (LVEDD)

left ventricular end-systolic d.
(LVESD)
left ventricular internal diastolic d.
(LVIDd)
lumbar spine d.
luminal d.
right ventricular d. (RVD)
spleen d.

1-dimensional (1D)
1-d. chemical-shift imaging
1-d. phase encoding

2-dimensional (2D)
2-d. cine gradient echo-based
tagging
2-d. cine phase-contrast flow
measurement
2-d. cross-sectional echocardiography
2-d. echocardiography (2DE)
2-d. Fourier transform (2DFT)
2-d. magnetic resonance digital
subtraction angiography
2-d. nonlinear filter

3-dimensional (3D)
3-d. analysis
3-d. conformal radiotherapy
3-d. conformation radiotherapy
3-d. contrast-enhanced MR
angiography
3-d. digital subtraction angiography
3-d. driven equilibrium sequence
3-d. Fourier transform (3DFT)
3-d. Fourier transform-constructive
interference in steady state
(3DFT-CISS)
3-d. Fourier transform volume
image
3-d. gradient-echo volumetric
sequence
3-d. magnetic resonance
angiography
3-d. multiple gradient-recalled echo
sequence
3-d. perfusion/motion map software
3-d. stereotactic surface projection
(3D SSP)
3-d. trabecular bone microstructure
3-d. tractography

4-dimensional (4D)
4-d. image
4-d. imaging

dimer
ethyl cysteinate d. (ECD)
ionic hexaiodinated d.
^{99m}Tc ethyl cysteinate d.
^{99m}Tc L-ethyl cysteinate d.
technetium 99m ethyl cysteinate d.
(^{99m}Tc-ECD, Tc99m-ECD)

dimercaptosuccinic acid (DMSA)
dimerization

3,4-dimethoxyphenyl-ethylamine
(DMPE)
dimethyl iminodiacetic acid (DIDA)
dimethylsuccinic acid
diminished
d. airway perfusion
d. lung volume
d. marrow signal intensity
d. systemic perfusion

diminutive
d. interlobar right pulmonary
artery
d. vessel

dimple
blind d.
d. of bone
pretibial d.

dinner-fork deformity
diode
d. detector
infrared light-emitting d.
d. laser
d. measurement
Palomar SLP1000 d.
PIN d.
positive-intrinsic-negative d.
silicone d.
Zener d.

diodone
Diodrast
Diogenes cup
Diomed
D. EVLT laser
D. 630 PDT laser model

Dionosil imaging agent
dioxide
carbon d. (CO_2)
titanium d.

DIP
desquamative interstitial pneumonia
digital imaging processing
distal interphalangeal
DIP joint

dip
apical d.
D. articulation
d. phenomenon
septal d.

DIPF
diffuse interstitial pulmonary fibrosis

diphenhydramine
diphosphate
dipyridoxal d.
manganese dipyridoxyl d.

diphosphine
lipophilic cationic d.

diphosphonate
hydroxymethylene d. (HMDP)
methylene d. (MDP)

D

diphosphonate (*continued*)
 technetium 99m hydroxymethylene
  d. (Tc-99m HMDP)
 technetium 99m methylene d.
  (Tc-99m MDP)
1-diphosphonic acid
diplegia spinalis brachialis traumatica
diploë
diplogram
diploic
 d. canal
 d. vein
diplomyelia
diplopia
dipolar
 d. broadening
 d. interaction
dipole
 d. coupling
 electric d.
 d. field
 magnetic d.
dipole-dipole
 d.-d. coupling
 d.-d. interaction
 proton electron d.-d.
 d.-d. relaxation rate
diprosopus
DIPS
 direct intrahepatic portacaval shunt
dipygus
dipyridamole
 d. echocardiography
 d. echocardiography imaging
 d. handgrip imaging
 d. handgrip test
 d. infusion imaging
 d. technetium-99m-2-methoxyisobutyl
 d. technetium-99m-2-methoxyisobutyl
  isonitrile
 d. thallium-201 imaging
 d. thallium-201 scintigraphy
 d. thallium stress imaging
 d. thallium ventriculogram
dipyridoxal diphosphate
direct
 d. caval cannulation
 d. current (DC)
 d. current generator
 d. current offset artifact
 d. digital radiography (DDR)
 d. display console (DDC)
 d. embolus
 d. Fourier transformation imaging
 d. fracture
 d. fulguration
 d. imaging of local gradients by
  group echo selection tomography
  (DIGGEST)

 d. immunofluorescence analysis
 d. inguinal hernia
 d. intrahepatic portacaval shunt
  (DIPS)
 d. liquid scintillation count
 d. needle puncture
 d. percutaneous transhepatic
  cholangiography
 d. puncture MR phlebogram
 d. puncture phlebography
 d. radiation
 d. radioiodination
 d. ray
 d. saturation effect
 d. slice
 d. spiral computed tomography
  venography
 d. splenoportography
 d. transtorcular approach
 d. visualization
direct-contact transmission
direction
 aborad d.
 anteroposterior flow d.
 caudad d.
 cephalad d.
 cephalocaudad d.
 mediolateral flow d.
 noncollinear d.
 phase-encoding d.
 superoinferior flow d.
 white matter tract d.
directional
 d. atherectomy catheter
 d. atherectomy device
 d. color angiography (DCA)
 d. coronary atherectomy
  (DCA)
 d. diffusion
 d. gradient concentration (DGC)
direction-encoded color mapping
directive
 advance d.
 medical device d. (MDD)
director
 grooved d.
DirectRay direct-to-digital image capture
 device
Directview
 D. CR 900 imaging system
 D. CR mammography system
direct-vision spectroscope
Direx
 D. Digiscope
 D. Thermex
 D. Tripter
dirty
 d. acoustic shadowing
 d. chest

d. fat
d. film artifact
d. mass
d. necrosis
disappearance
d. frequency
d. slope
disappearing
d. bone disease
d. fetus
disarray
myocardial d.
disarticulation
hip d.
disassociation (*var. of* dissociation)
disc, disk
acromioclavicular joint d.
anal d.
anterior intervertebral d.
articular d.
atrial d.
d. ballooning
biconcave d.
bilocular d.
Bowman d.
d. bulge
d. calcification
candle drip d.
cartilaginous d.
cervical d.
chorionic d.
concave skull d.
cone d.
contained d.
crescent-shaped fibrocartilaginous
d.
d. degeneration
degenerative d.
d. derangement
d. desiccation
d. disease
d. displacement
distal radioulnar d.
embryonic d.
Engelmann d.
epiphysial d.
extruded d.
d. extrusion
fibrocartilaginous d.
fibrous ring of d.
fixation d.
d. fragment
frayed d.
growth d.
H d.
herniated intervertebral d. (HID)
d. herniation
hydrodynamic potential of d.
interarticular d.

d. interspace
intervertebral d.
isotropic d.
kidney d.
d. lesion
locking d.
lumbar d.
lumbosacral d.
magnetic d.
magnetooptical d. (MOD)
mandibular d.
d. margin
massive herniated d.
d. maturation
midline herniation of d.
Molnar d.
d. morphology
occult residual herniated d.
d. of ankle
d. of endocardium
d. ossification
d. oxygenator
placental d.
d. plication
d. poppet
protruded d.
d. protrusion
rectangular d.
ruptured d.
sequestered d.
d. sequestration
d. space
d. space height
d. space infection
d. space narrowing
spheric d.
sternoclavicular joint d.
tactile d.
temporomandibular joint d.
thoracic d.
thoracolumbar vertebral d.
d. tissue
d. to magnetic field
d. to magnetic field orientation
triangular d.
unilocular d.
vertebral d.
d. water content
Winchester d.
discectomy, diskectomy
automated percutaneous lumbar d.
(APLD)
percutaneous automated d.
same-day microsurgical arthroscopic
lateral-approach laser-assisted
fluoroscopic d.
stereotactic percutaneous lumbar
d.
discernible venous motion

discharge
    periodic synchronous d. (PSD)
    sympathetic d.
    d. tube
discharging tubule
disci (*pl. of* discus)
discitis, diskitis
    calcific d.
    childhood d.
    infective d.
    juvenile calcific d.
    septic d.
disclike atelectasis
discogenic, diskogenic
    d. disease
    d. osteophyte
    d. vertebral sclerosis
discogram, diskogram
    intervertebral d.
    intranuclear d.
discographer, diskographer
discographic technique
discography, diskography
    functional anesthetic d. (FAD)
discoid
    d. atelectasis
    d. chest mass
    d. configuration
    d. filling defect
    d. kidney
    d. lateral meniscus
    d. shadow
discoligamentous complex
disconnected pancreatic duct syndrome
discontinuous
    d. density gradient
    d. density gradient centrifugation
    d. imaging
    d. scanning
discordance
    radiologic-pathologic d.
discordant
    d. finding
    d. thyroid nodule
    d. twin
discovertebral
    d. infection
    d. osteomyelitis
    d. spondylitis
discovery
    D. LS imaging system
    D. LS, ST^4 PET/CT scanner
discrepancy
    biomechanics of limb-length d.
    leg-length d. (LLD)
    limb-length d. (LLD)
discreta
    porokeratosis plantaris d.

discrete
    d. area of consolidation
    d. area of effusion
    d. bleeding source
    d. cosine transform
    d. focal stenosis
    d. Fourier transform (DFT)
    d. hyperintense focus
    d. hyperintense signal intensity
    d. lesion
    d. mass
    d. narrowing
    d. perihilar density
    d. plaque
    d. pulmonary nodule
    d. segment of normal esophagus
    d. subaortic stenosis
    d. subvalvular aortic stenosis (DSAS)
    d. tumor
discriminant analysis
discriminate
discrimination
    density d.
discriminator setting
disc-shaped bone graft
disc-thecal sac interface
disc-type valve
discus, *pl.* **disci**
disease
    acalculous biliary d.
    acinar airspace d.
    acquired cystic kidney d.
    acquired occupational lung d.
    acquired renal cystic d.
    acquired uremic cystic kidney d.
    active parenchymal d.
    acute d.
    acyanotic congenital heart d.
    Addison d.
    adrenal medullary d.
    adult polycystic kidney d.
    airflow obstruction d. (AOD)
    airspace d.
    airway d.
    Albers-Schönberg d.
    alcoholic liver d. (ALD)
    Alexander d.
    alloimmune d.
    Alpers d.
    alpha heavy-chain d.
    alveolar lung d. (ALD)
    Alzheimer d.
    aneurysmal d.
    angiomatous d.
    anterior horn cell d.
    aortic valvular d. (AVD)
    aortoiliac occlusive d. (AIOD)
    arterial degenerative d.

arteriosclerotic cardiovascular d.
  (ASCVD)
arteriosclerotic heart d. (ASHD)
arteriosclerotic occlusive d.
arteriosclerotic peripheral vascular d.
asbestos-related pleural d.
atheroembolic renal d.
atherosclerotic cardiovascular d.
  (ASCVD)
atherosclerotic carotid artery d.
  (ACAD)
atherosclerotic heart d. (ASHD)
atherosclerotic peripheral vascular d.
  (ASPVD)
atherosclerotic pulmonary vascular d.
atherosclerotic renal occlusive d.
autosomal dominant polycystic
  kidney d. (ADPKD)
autosomal recessive polycystic
  kidney d. (ARPKD)
Baastrup d.
Bamberger-Marie d.
Behçet d.
benign asbestos-related pleural d.
benign breast d. (BBD)
benign ovarian cystic d.
biliary tract d.
Binswanger d.
black lung d.
Blount d.
Bouchard d.
Bouillaud d.
Bourneville d.
Bourneville-Pringle d.
brittle bone d. (BBD)
Brodie d.
Bruck d.
Buerger d.
bullous lung d. (BLD)
Byler d.
caisson d.
calcium hydroxyapatite deposition d.
calcium pyrophosphate dihydrate
  deposition d.
Calvé-Legg-Perthes d.
Calvé-Perthes d.
Camurati-Engelmann d.
Canavan d.
Canavan-van Bogaert-Bertrand d.
cardiopulmonary d.
cardiorenal d.
cardiovascular d. (CVD)
cardiovascular renal d.
Caroli d.
carotid artery d.
carotid atherosclerotic d.
carotid occlusive d.
Carrington d.
Castleman d.

celiac d.
central airway d.
cerebral inflammatory d.
cerebral Whipple d.
cerebrovascular occlusive d.
cervical disc d.
Charcot-Marie-Tooth d.
cholestatic liver d.
chronic beryllium d.
chronic interstitial simulating
  airspace lung d.
chronic obstructive lung d. (COLD)
chronic obstructive pulmonary d.
  (COPD)
chronic peripheral arterial d.
  (CPAD)
Coats d.
collagen-vascular d.
Concato d.
congenital heart d. (CHD)
connective tissue d.
coronary artery d.
Cowden d.
Creutzfeldt-Jakob d. (CJD)
Crohn d.
crystal deposition d.
Cushing d.
cyanotic congenital heart d.
cystic breast d.
cystic kidney d.
cystic ovarian d.
degenerative atrioventricular node d.
degenerative brain d.
degenerative disc d.
degenerative joint d. (DJD)
delta heavy-chain d.
demyelinating d.
de Quervain d.
Deutschländer d.
Dieulafoy d.
diffuse airspace d.
diffuse parenchymal lung d.
diffuse parenchymal renal d.
Di Guglielmo d.
disappearing bone d.
disc d.
discogenic d.
disseminated metastatic d.
disseminated xanthogranulomatous
  infiltrative d.
diverticular colon d.
drug-induced chest d.
drug-induced eosinophilic pulmonary
  d.
drug-induced lung d.
Duroziez mitral stenosis d.
Ekman-Lobstein d.
endstage liver d.
endstage lung d.

D

disease (*continued*)

endstage renal d.
Engelmann d.
eosinophilic lung d.
Erb d.
Erdheim-Chester d.
extracolonic d.
extracranial carotid artery occlusive
   d.
extragenital Bowen d.
extramammary Paget d.
extranodal systemic d.
extrapancreatic autoimmune d.
extrathoracic d.
facet d.
Fahr d.
Fairbank d.
Favre d.
fibrocystic breast d.
fibrocystic lung d.
fibromuscular d. (FMD)
Flatau-Schilder d.
flax-dresser d.
focal lung d.
focal small bowel d.
Fong d.
Forestier d.
Freiberg d.
Friedreich d.
Fukuyama congenital muscular d.
   (FCMD)
gamma heavy-chain d.
Gandy-Nanta d.
Garré d.
gastroesophageal reflux d. (GERD)
Gaucher d.
Gee-Herter d.
Gee-Thaysen d.
Gerstmann-Sträussler-Scheinker d.
gestational trophoblastic d. (GTD)
Gilchrist d.
Glénard d.
Global Initiative for chronic
   obstructive lung d.
glycogen storage d.
Gorham d.
Graves d.
GSS d.
Hallervorden-Spatz d.
heart d.
heavy-chain d.
Heberden d.
hepatic vein d.
hepatic venoocclusive d.
hepatobiliary d.
hepatocerebral d.
higher stage d.
Hirschsprung d.
Hodgkin d.

Hodgson d.
Hoffa d.
Horton d.
Hunter d.
Huntington d.
Huppert d.
hyaline membrane d. (HMD)
hydatid d.
hydroxyapatite deposition d.
   (HADD)
hypertensive cardiovascular d.
hypertensive renal d.
hypertensive vascular d.
idiopathic mural endomyocardial d.
idiopathic Parkinson d. (IPD)
ileocolic d.
iliocaval d.
immature lung d.
immunoproliferative small intestine
   d. (IPSID)
infantile polycystic kidney d.
infectious heart d.
inflammatory bowel d.
infrapopliteal arterial d.
inhalation d.
interfollicular Hodgkin d.
interstitial fibrotic lung d.
interstitial lung d. (ILD)
intracranial stenoocclusive d.
intrasynovial d.
iron storage d.
ischemic bowel d.
Jaffe-Lichtenstein d.
Jansen d.
Jansky-Bielschowsky d.
juvenile autosomal recessive
   polycystic d.
juvenile Paget d.
Kahler d.
Kawasaki d.
Kienböck d.
Keshan d.
Kikuchi d.
Kikuchi-Fujimoto d.
Kinnier-Wilson d.
Köhler d.
Krabbe d.
Kugelberg-Welander d.
Kummel d.
Kussmaul-Maier d.
kyphoscoliotic heart d.
LCP d.
Legg-Calvé-Perthes d. (LCP)
Legionnaires d.
Leigh d.
leptomeningeal d.
Lewy body d.
Lhermitte-Duclos d.
Libman-Sacks endocarditis d.

Lichtenstein-Jaffe d.
light-chain deposition d. (LCDD)
liver hydatid d.
local nodal d.
locoregional d.
maple bark d.
maple syrup urine d.
marble bone d.
Marchiafava-Bignami d.
Marie-Bamberger d.
Marie-Strümpell d.
Martin d.
medullary cystic d.
Ménétrier d.
Ménière d.
Menkes kinky hair d.
mesenteric Weber-Christian d.
metabolic bone d.
metastatic d.
microvascular d.
Mikulicz d.
miliary lung d.
miliary parenchymal d.
Milroy d.
mixed connective tissue d. (MCTD)
mixed tissue d.
Mondor d.
monostotic Paget d.
moyamoya d.
mu heavy-chain d.
multicentric Castleman d. (MCD)
multiple-gland d.
multisegment d.
muscle-eye-brain d.
mushroom picker's d.
necrotizing granulomatous d.
neonatal wet lung d.
neurodegenerative d.
Niemann-Pick d.
Nievergelt d.
nodal d.
nodular lung d.
nodular sclerosis Hodgkin d.
nodular thyroid d.
no evidence of d. (NED)
no evidence of recurrent d. (NERD)
nonatherosclerotic d.
nonthromboembolic pulmonary d.
Norrie d.
obstructive airway d.
obstructive arterial d.
obstructive lung d.
obstructive pulmonary d. (OPD)
occlusive carotid d.
occlusive cerebrovascular d.
occupational lung d.
Ollier d.
optic chiasm d.
Ormond d.

Osgood-Schlatter d.
Osler d.
osseous metastatic d.
Otto d.
Paas d.
Paget jaw d.
pancreatic d.
pancreaticobiliary d.
Panner d.
parenchymatous lung d.
parenchymatous renal d.
Parenti-Fraccaro d.
Parkinson d.
Pelizaeus-Merzbacher d.
Pellegrini-Stieda d.
pelvic inflammatory d.
peptic ulcer d. (PUD)
pericardial d.
perihilar lung d.
perineural d.
periodontal d.
peripheral airspace d.
peripheral arterial occlusive d.
  (PAOD)
peripheral lung d.
peripheral vascular d. (PVD)
peripheral vascular occlusive d.
  (PVOD)
Perthes d.
Peyronie d.
Pfaundler-Hurler d.
Pfeiffer d.
Pick d.
pleural d.
Plummer d.
polycystic kidney d.
polycystic liver d.
polycystic ovarian d. (PCOD, POD)
Pompe d.
popliteal artery occlusive d.
posttransplant coronary artery d.
Pott d.
prediverticular d.
Preiser d.
primary pigmented nodular
  adrenocortical d.
pseudo-Whipple d.
pulmonary collagen vascular d.
pulmonary embolic septic d.
pulmonary interstitial d.
pulmonary thromboembolic d.
pulmonary vascular d.
pulmonary venoocclusive d. (PVOD)
Pyle d.
radiation-induced liver d. (RILD)
ragpicker's d.
reactive airway d. (RAD)
renal cystic d.
renovascular d.

D

disease (*continued*)

respiratory bronchiolitis-associated interstitial lung d. (RB-ILD)
restrictive lung d.
restrictive myocardial d.
reticulonodular lung d.
reversible airway d.
rheumatic heart d.
rheumatic valvular d.
rheumatoid lung d.
Ribbing d.
Roger d.
Rosai-Dorfman d.
Rutherford clinical stage of peripheral vascular d.
Ruysch d.
sacroiliac d.
Salla d.
Santavuori-Haltia d.
Scheuermann d.
Schilder d.
Schmid d.
Schmorl nucleus pulposus d.
Sever d.
Shaver d.
sickle cell d.
silo-filler's d.
Simmond d.
Sinding-Larsen-Johansson patellar tendinitis d.
single-vessel d.
small bowel d.
Spielmeyer-Vogt d.
Still d.
1st-trimester gestational trophoblastic d.
subarachnoid metastatic d.
subarachnoid space d.
synchronous d.
systemic granulomatous d.
Takayasu d.
thromboembolic d. (TED)
thromboembolic lung d.
thyrocardiac d.
thyroid d.
tibial artery d.
tibioperoneal occlusive d.
toxic lung d.
transspatial d.
Trevor d.
tubercular bone d.
Uhl d.
ulcer d.
undercalling d.
upper lung d.
upper respiratory tract d.
urachal remnant d.
uremic medullary cystic d.
valvular d.

valvular heart d.
van Buchem d.
vanishing bone d.
Van Neck d.
Vaquez d.
variant Creutzfeldt-Jakob d. (vCJD)
vascular occlusive d.
venous occlusive d.
venous thromboembolic d. (VTED)
venous thrombotic d.
vertebrobasilar d.
3-vessel coronary d.
von Recklinghausen d.
von Willebrand d.
Voorhoeve d.
Vrolik d.
Warburg d.
warfarin-aspirin symptomatic intracranial d. (WASID)
Werdnig-Hoffmann d.
Werner classification of thyroid eye d.
Westphal-Strümpell d.
wet lung d.
Whipple d.
white matter d.
Wilson d.
Winiwarter-Buerger d.
Zuska d.

disease-free vessel
DISH

diffuse idiopathic skeletal hyperostosis

dishpan fracture
DISI

dorsal intercalated segmental instability

DISIDA

diisopropyl iminodiacetic acid

disintegration

d. constant
myofibrillar d.
nuclear d.
radioactive d.
d. rate
spontaneous d.

disintegrator

electrohydraulic d.

disjointing
disk (*var. of* disc)
Disk-Criminator
diskectomy (*var. of* discectomy)
diskitis (*var. of* discitis)
diskogenic (*var. of* discogenic)
diskogram (*var. of* discogram)
diskographer (*var. of* discographer)
diskography (*var. of* discography)
dislocated

d. hip
d. knee

dislocation
> anterior d.
> anteroinferior d.
> atlantooccipital d.
> axial carpal d.
> Bankart d.
> bayonet d.
> Bennett d.
> bilateral intrafacetal d.
> boutonnière d.
> bursting d.
> central d.
> cervical facet d.
> chronic recurrent d.
> closed d.
> complete d.
> complicated d.
> compound d.
> congenital hip d.
> consecutive d.'s
> Desault d.
> divergent d.
> dysplasia d.
> facet d.
> frank d.
> glenohumeral d.
> Hill-Sachs d.
> hip d.
> hyperextension d.
> incomplete d.
> interfacetal d.
> interphalangeal d.
> irreducible dorsal d.
> isolated d.
> joint d.
> Kienböck d.
> Lisfranc d.
> lunate d.
> midcarpal d.
> milkmaid's elbow d.
> Monteggia d.
> Nélaton d.
> d. of patella
> open d.
> partial d.
> patellar d.
> pathologic d.
> primitive d.
> radiocarpal d.
> recent d.
> recurrent d.
> rotational d.
> scapholunate d.
> shoulder d.
> simple d.
> Smith d.
> sternoclavicular d.
> subastragalar d.
> subspinous d.

> tibiofemoral joint d.
> tibiotarsal d.
> transradial styloid perilunate d.
> transscaphoid perilunate d.
> traumatic d.
> triquetrolunate d.
> unilateral facet d.
> unilateral interfacetal d.
> unilateral intrafacetal d.
> upward and backward d.
> upward lens d.
> volar d.
> wrist d.

dislodgement
> partial d.

dismutase
> copper-zinc superoxide d.
>   (Cu/Zn-SOD)
> superoxide d.

disobliteration
> carotid d.

disodium
> pamidronate d.

disofenin
> technetium 99m d.

disorder
> angiitis-granulomatosis d.
> angiocentric immunoproliferative d.
> articular hand d.
> articular wrist d.
> atypical parkinsonian d.
> autoimmune d.
> bullous d.
> cartilaginous growth plate d.
> congenital d.
> deglutition d.
> demyelinative d.
> drug-induced bullous d.
> dysmyelination d.
> esophageal functional d.
> esophageal morphologic d.
> esophageal motility d.
> evacuation d.
> functional d.
> gastric motor d.
> granular lymphoproliferative d.
> infectious pulmonary d.
> intractable bleeding d.
> lymphoproliferative d.
> lysosomal storage d.
> metabolic bone d.
> migration d.
> mitochondrial respiratory
>   chain d.
> motility d.
> myeloproliferative d.
> National Institute of Neurological
>   and Communicative D.'s
> neurogenic d.

D

disorder (*continued*)
    nonspecific esophageal motility d. (NEMD)
    organic acid d.
    patellofemoral d.
    posttransplant lymphoproliferative d.
    pulmonary lymphoid d.
    surfactant deficiency d. (SDD)
    systemic d.
    underlying d.

disorganized
    d. architecture
    d. folium

dispenser
    film d.

dispersing agent

dispersion
    gradient-induced phase d.
    intravoxel phase d.
    d. mode

dispersive component

disphenoid extraction

displaced
    d. crus
    d. fracture
    d. fracture fragment
    d. fragment of bone
    d. gallbladder
    d. intimal calcification
    d. left paraspinal line
    d. left ventricular apex
    d. osteochondral fragment
    d. vertebra

displacement
    anterior tracheal d.
    arterial brain d.
    atlantoaxial rotary d.
    brainstem d.
    breast tissue d.
    disc d.
    Ellis Jones peroneal d.
    esophageal d.
    d. field-fitting MR imaging
    hilar d.
    inferior d.
    left apexcardiogram, calibrated d. (LACD)
    mediastinal d.
    d. of bowel gas
    d. of brain vessel
    d. of interhemispheric fissure
    palmar d.
    d. placentogram (DPG)
    radial epiphysial d.
    retroperitoneal fat stripe d.
    rotational d.
    superolateral d.
    tracheal d.

display
    A-mode d.
    B-mode d.
    cine-mode d.
    d. coordinate system
    dynamic volume-rendered d.
    image d.
    liquid crystal d. (LCD)
    M-mode d.
    multiparametric color composite d.
    multiplanar d. (MPD)
    real-time d.
    segmentation method for real-time d.
    shaded surface d. (SSD)
    stack mode d.
    static image d.
    tile mode d.

disposable thermometer

disproportion
    cephalopelvic d. (CPD)
    fetal-pelvic d.
    fetal ventricular heart d.
    fiber-type d.
    ventricular d.

disproportionate upper septal thickening

disrupted plaque

disruption
    anastomotic d.
    anterior labral d.
    anular d.
    blood-brain barrier d.
    bony d.
    cortical d.
    epiglottic d.
    facet capsule d.
    glenoid articular rim d. (GARD)
    glenolabral articular cartilage d. (GLAD)
    ligamentous d.
    lymphatic needle d.
    myofascial d.
    d. of cartilaginous synchondrosis
    d. of duct
    retinacular d.
    skeletal d.
    superior peroneal retinaculum d.
    supraspinous ligament d.
    trabecular d.
    traumatic aortic d.
    volar radiocarpal ligament d.

dissecans
    osteochondritis d.
    osteochondrosis d.

dissecting
    d. abdominal aneurysm
    d. aortic aneurysm
    d. aortic hematoma
    d. basilar artery aneurysm

d. intracranial aneurysm
d. intramural hematoma

dissection
abdominal aortic d.
aneurysmal d.
aortic d.
arterial wall d.
axial joint d.
axillary lymph node d. (ALND)
celiac artery d.
complete lymph node d.
descending aorta d.
esophageal d.
extensive d.
extracapsular d.
extrapericardial d.
familial aortic d.
groin d.
intimal medial d.
lymph node d.
medial d.
d. of artery
renal artery d.
selective complete lymph node d.
sentinel node d.
sharp d.
spiral d.
spontaneous carotid d.
spontaneous coronary artery d.
(SCAD)
Stanford type B aortic d.
subintimal d.
therapeutic lymph node d.
thoracic aortic d.
d. tubercle
type B aortic d.
vertebral arterial d.

dissector
balloon d.

disseminata
osteitis fibrosa d.
osteopathia condensans d.
tuberculosis cutis miliaris d.
tuberculosis miliaris d.

disseminated
d. aspergillosis
d. CNS histoplasmosis
d. coccidioidomycosis
d. cryptococcosis
d. inflammation
d. intravascular coagulation (DIC)
d. intravascular coagulation
syndrome
d. lipogranulomatosis
d. metastasis
d. metastatic disease
d. necrotizing leukoencephalopathy
d. sclerosis
d. tuberculosis

d. tumor
d. xanthogranulomatous infiltrative
disease

dissemination
hematogenous d.
lymphogenous d.
lymphohematogenous d.
d. pattern

Disse space

dissociation, disassociation
complete atrioventricular d.
electromechanical d. (EMD)
interference d.
scapholunate d.

dissociative instability
dissolution of gallstone
distal
d. acinar emphysema
d. aorta
d. aortic arch
d. aortic arch aneurysm
d. articular set angle (DASA)
d. bile duct
d. bile duct carcinoma (DBDC)
d. blind stomach
d. bone marrow development
d. branch
d. bronchiectasis
d. bulbar septum
d. carpal row
d. circumflex marginal artery
d. clavicle osteolysis (DCO)
d. colon
d. common bile duct obstruction
d. convoluted tubule
d. coronary perfusion pressure
d. coronary sinus (DCS)
d. duodenum
d. embolization
d. esophageal ring
d. femoral epiphysial fracture
d. femur
d. humoral fracture
d. ileitis
d. interphalangeal (DIP)
d. interphalangeal joint
d. intestinal obstruction syndrome
d. leak (type I)
d. leg cross-section
d. line of reference (DLR)
d. lobular emphysema
d. metatarsal articular angle
(DMAA)
d. occlusal distention
d. radial fracture
d. radioulnar disc
d. radioulnar joint (DRUJ)
d. radioulnar joint compartment
d. radioulnar subluxation

D

distal (*continued*)
    d. rectal adenocarcinoma (DRA)
    d. reference axis (DRA)
    d. runoff
    d. runoff vessel
    d. segment
    d. shift
    d. small bowel
    d. splenorenal shunt
    d. surface
    d. tibial physis
    d. tibiofibular syndesmosis
    d. tissue bed
    d. ureteral dilation
distalward
distance
    acromiohumeral d.
    anterior capsular d. (ACD)
    atlas odontoid d.
    center-to-center d.
    central lung d. (CLD)
    Doppler-derived stroke d.
    fanning of interspinous d.
    film-focus d.
    film-tube d.
    flexion interspinous d.
    focal film d. (FFD)
    focal spot-to-object d.
    focus-film d. (FFD)
    focus-object d. (FOD)
    focus-skin d. (FSD)
    focus-to-detector d.
    focus-to-isocentre d.
    interarch d.
    intercaudate d.
    interlaminar d.
    internuclear d.
    interopercular d.
    interorbital d.
    interpediculate d.
    interridge d.
    interslice d.
    interspinal d.
    interuncal d.
    object-film d. (OFD)
    pisoscaphoid d.
    posterior capsular d.
    probe-surface d.
    source-film d. (SFD)
    source-skin d. (SSD)
    source-surface d. (SSD)
    source-to-image receptor d. (SID)
    source-to-skin d. (SSD)
    source-tray d. (STD)
    surface d.
    target-film d. (TFD)
    target-skin d. (TSD)
    target-trocar d.
    teardrop d.

    ulnotriquetral d.
    widened teardrop d.
distance-based block classification
distant
    d. metastasis
    d. spread
distended
    d. abdomen
    d. central bronchus
    d. gallbladder
    d. kidney
    d. scapulothoracic bursitis
    d. stomach
    d. vein
distensibility
    aortic d.
distensible
distension (*var. of* distention)
distention, distension
    abdominal d.
    alveolar d.
    azygos vein d.
    bladder d.
    bowel d.
    colonic d.
    distal occlusal d.
    gaseous d.
    gastric d.
    hydraulic d.
    intestinal d.
    jugular venous d.
    luminal d.
    maximum radiographic d.
    d. of esophagogastric region
    passive venous d.
    pelvicalyceal d.
    postvagotomy small bowel d.
    radiographic d.
    d. ratio
    rectal d.
    ureteral d.
    venous d.
    vesical d.
distinction
    loss of d.
distorted
    d. anatomy
    d. mucosal fold
distortion
    architectural d.
    barreling d.
    bronchial d.
    current line d.
    focal d.
    geometric d.
    image d.
    pincushion d.
    pituitary stalk d.
    radiographic pincushion d.

radiologic d.
S d.
spicular d.
Y-shaped d.
distraction
bifocal manipulation with d.
d. gap
d. hyperflexion injury
joint d.
d. of fracture
d. osteogenesis
physial d.
segment d.
small-step d.
soft tissue d.
distraction-flexion staging (DFS)
distractor
intramedullary skeletal kinetic d.
(ISKD)
distribution
anatomic d.
anomalous d.
apparent volume of d.
batwing d.
Boltzmann d.
butterfly d.
centrilobular d.
depth-dose d.
diffuse spatial d.
dose d.
gaussian d.
geometric d.
harness-shaped d.
homogeneous susceptibility d.
homogeneous thallium d.
inhomogeneous tracer d.
interstitial lung disease d.
loop d.
lung infiltrate d.
maxwellian d.
mottled d.
normal variant fluorodeoxyglucose
uptake d.
normal whole-body
fluorodeoxyglucose d.
peribronchial d.
perivascular d.
Poisson d.
radioactivity d.
rapid d.
regional myocardial mass d.
reverse d.
rimlike calcium d.
spatial dose d.
spectral noise d.
stem cell d.
symmetric d.
thallium-201 uptake and d.
trace element d.

d. transformer
uniform d.
unusual marrow d.
d. volume ratio (DVR)
distributive shock
disturbance
architectural d.
circulation d.
neurovegetative d.
d. of articulation
disturbed orientation
disuse osteoporosis
diuresis
d. renogram
d. urogram
diuretic
d. radionuclide urography
d. renal imaging
d. renal scan
d. renography
Diva laparoscopic morcellator
divergent
d. dislocation
d. ray projection
d. spiculated pattern
diverging
d. collimator
d. meniscus
diversion
biliopancreatic d.
cerebrospinal fluid d.
continent urinary d.
partial external biliary d.
d. pouch
urinary d.
ventriculoperitoneal d.
diversity segment
diverticula (*pl. of* diverticulum)
diverticular
d. abscess
d. colon disease
d. prostatitis
diverticulitis
acute d.
bladder d.
chronic d.
colonic d.
Meckel d.
sigmoid d.
diverticulogram
diverticulosis
colonic d.
intramural esophageal d.
jejunal d.
tracheal d.
diverticulum, *pl.* **diverticula**
acquired urethral d.
arachnoid d.
bladder d.

D

diverticulum (*continued*)
    calyceal d.
    colonic d.
    common bile duct d.
    congenital urethral d.
    cricopharyngeal d.
    divisional block d.
    dorsal d.
    ductus d.
    duodenal intraluminal d.
    epiphrenic d.
    esophageal d.
    fallopian tube d.
    false d.
    functional d.
    gallbladder d.
    Ganser d.
    gastric d.
    giant sigmoid d.
    Graser d.
    hepatic d.
    Hutch d.
    hypopharyngeal d.
    interaorticobronchial d.
    interbronchial d.
    intestinal d.
    intraluminal duodenal d. (IDD)
    intramural d.
    inverted Meckel d.
    jejunal d.
    jejunoileal d.
    juxtapapillary d.
    Kirchner d.
    Kommerell d.
    Kumeral d.
    Meckel d.
    meningeal d.
    metanephric d.
    midesophageal d.
    Nuck d.
    paraureteral d.
    perforated d.
    periampullary d.
    pharyngoesophageal d.
    pulsion d.
    pyelocalyceal d.
    renal d.
    Rokitansky d.
    roofless 4th ventricle d.
    sigmoid d.
    small bowel d.
    stomach d.
    thoracic pulsion d.
    thoracic root sleeve d.
    4th ventricle d.
    traction d.
    urachal d.
    ureteral d.
    urethral d.
    urinary bladder d.
    Vater d.
    vesical d.
    vesical-urachal d.
    windsock d.
    Zenker d.
diverting stoma
divided dose
diving goiter
division
    mandibular d.
    maxillary d.
    ureteral d.
divisional
    d. block
    d. block diverticulum
divisionary line
divisum
    pancreas d.
divopontocerebellar atrophy
Dixon
    D. fat fraction measurement
    D. method of phase unwrapping
    D. quantitative chemical-shift
      image
dizygotic twin
DJD
    degenerative joint disease
DJF
    duodenojejunal flexure
DJJ
    duodenojejunal junction
DKS
    Damus-Kaye-Stansel
      DKS pulmonary artery to ascending
      aorta anastomosis procedure
DLBD
    diffuse Lewy body dementia
DLCL
    diffuse large cell lymphoma
      limited-stage DLCL
D-loop
    ventricular D-l.
    D-l. ventricular situs
DLR
    distal line of reference
DMAA
    distal metatarsal articular angle
D-malposition of aorta
D_{max}
    maximum density
DMI
    diaphragmatic myocardial
    infarct
DMPE
    3,4-dimethoxyphenyl-ethylamine
dMRI
    dynamic magnetic resonance
    imaging

DMSA
dimercaptosuccinic acid
^{99m}Tc DMSA
technetium 99m DMSA
DNA
deoxyribonucleic acid
DNA cytophotometry
DNA flow cytometry
DNA microinjection technique
DNET
dysembryoplastic neuroepithelial tumor
DNP
dynamic nuclear polarization
DNR
dose nonuniformity ratio
DOBI
dynamic optical breast imaging
DOBI system
dobutamine
low-dose d. (LDD)
d. stress echocardiography (DSE)
d. thallium angiography
DOBV
double-outlet both ventricles
doctrine
Monroe-Kellie d.
documentary arteriography
document image decoding (DID)
Dodd perforating vein group
dodecafluoropentane (DDFP)
d. imaging agent
Dodge
D. area-length method for
ventricular volume
D. method for ejection fraction
D. principle
Dodick laser photolysis system
Doerner-Hoskins distribution law
dog
scotty d.
dolens
phlegmasia cerulea d.
dolichocephalic, dolichocephalous
dolichocephalism (*var. of* dolichocephaly)
dolichocephalous (*var. of* dolichocephalic)
dolichocephaly, dolichocephalism
dolichocolon
dolichoectasia
vertebrobasilar d.
dolichoesophagus
dolichopellic pelvis
dolichosigmoid
dolichostenomelia
DoLi S extracorporeal shock wave lithotriptor
DOLV
double-outlet left ventricle
domain
dose rate d.

extracellular d.
Fourier d.
frequency d.
magnetic d.
scene d.
spatial frequency d.
time d.
dome
anterior talar d.
atrial d.
bladder d.
crus d.
d. cylinder
diaphragmatic d.
d. fracture
lateral talar d.
liver d.
d. of aneurysm
d. of diaphragm
shoulder d.
talar d.
weightbearing acetabular d.
dome-and-dart configuration
dome-shaped
d.-s. heart
d.-s. roof of pleural
cavity
dome-to-neck ratio
dominance
cerebral d.
coronary artery d.
orbitofrontal d.
dominant
anatomically d.
d. follicle
d. hemisphere
d. hemisphere infarct
d. hemisphere lesion
d. left coronary artery
d. right coronary artery
d. vessel
doming
diastolic d.
d. of leaflet
d. of valve
donor
adult-to-adult living related liver
transplant d.
d. graft
d. heart
d. heart-lung block
d. site
d. twin
donor-recipient anatomy
don't-touch lesion
donut (*var. of* doughnut)
DOPA
dihydroxyphenylalanine
DOPA imaging agent

D

dopaminergic
    d. dysfunction
    d. neurotransmission
dopamine transporter (DAT)
dopa-responsive dystonia
Dopascan radiopharmaceutical imaging agent
doped water
Doppler
    D. angle
    D. ankle systolic pressure
    D. artifact
    D. assessment
    ATL HDI 5000 color D.
    D. blood flow monitor
    D. blood flow velocity signal
    D. blood pressure
    color D. (CD)
    color-flow D. (CFD)
    D. color flow
    D. color-flow imaging
    D. color-flow mapping
    D. continuous-wave echocardiography
    contrast-enhanced color D.
    contrast-enhanced power D.
    convergent color D.
    duplex B-mode D.
    D. effect
    D. equation
    D. flow echocardiographic probe
    D. flow index
    D. flowmeter
    D. flowmetry
    D. flow probe study
    D. flow signal enhancement
    D. frequency shift
    D. frequency spectrum
    D. gain
    gray-scale D.
    high-frequency D. (HFD)
    high pulse-repetition frequency D.
    D. insonation
    D. interrogation
    intraoperative D.
    multigated D.
    D. operation
    D. ovary signal
    periorbital bidirectional D.
    pocket D.
    power D.
    D. pulse
    pulsed-wave D.
    D. pulsed-wave echocardiography
    range-gated pulsed D.
    real-time D.
    renal D.
    D. resistive index (DRI)
    D. shift frequency
    D. shift principle
    D. sonography (DS)
    D. sonography of SMA
    SonoSite pulsed-wave D.
    spectral D.
    D. spectral analysis
    D. spectral waveform
    D. study of blood flow
    D. System 97
    D. tissue imaging (DTI)
    transcranial D. (TCD)
    transcranial color-coded D.
    D. tricuspid regurgitation
    D. ultrasonic blood flow detector
    D. ultrasonic fetal heart monitor
    D. ultrasonic velocity detector
    D. ultrasonic velocity detector segmental plethysmography
    D. ultrasonography
    D. ultrasonography imaging
    D. ultrasound
    D. ultrasound segmental blood pressure testing
    D. venous examination
    D. venous imaging
    D. VWF
    D. waveform analysis
    D. waveform dampening
Doppler-derived stroke distance
Doppler-guided hemorrhoid artery ligation (DGHAL)
Dorello canal
Dorendorf
    D. sign
    D. sign of aortic arch aneurysm
dormancy
    tumor d.
Dornier
    D. compact lithotriptor
    D. HM3, HM4 lithotriptor
    D. scanner
Dor reconstruction
dorsa (*pl. of* dorsum)
dorsad
dorsal
    d. abdominal wall
    d. artery
    d. artery of penis
    d. aspect
    d. bend
    d. branch
    d. capsule
    d. decubitus position
    d. dermal sinus
    d. diverticulum
    d. enteric fistula
    d. enteric sinus
    d. enterogenous cyst
    d. induction
    d. induction error

d. intercalated segmental instability (DISI)
d. interosseus
d. kyphotic curvature
d. meningocele
d. metacarpal ligament
d. muscle
d. nerve of penis
d. pancreas
d. pancreatic bud
d. penile vein
d. plate
d. point
d. primary ramus
d. ramus of spinal nerve
d. recumbent position
d. ridge
d. rim
d. rim distal radial fracture
d. root entry zone (DREZ)
d. root entry zone lesion
d. root ganglion (DRG)
d. spinal cord horn
d. spine
d. spinocerebellar tract
d. subaponeurotic space
d. subcutaneous space
d. talar beak
d. talonavicular bone
d. tubercle
d. vertebra
d. view
d. wing fracture
d. wrist ligament

dorsale
os supratrochleare d.
dorsalis
funiculus d.
d. pedis
d. pedis pulse
tabes d.
dorsalward
dorsi (*gen. of* dorsum)
dorsiflexion
d. angle (DFA)
d. view
dorsiflexor
dorsispinal vein
dorsoanterior
dorsocephalad
dorsolateral
d. aspect
d. tract
dorsomedial
d. nucleus
d. thalamotomy
dorsoplantar
d. aspect
d. projection

d. talometatarsal angle
d. talonavicular angle
d. view
dorsoposterior
dorsoradial
dorsorostral
dorsosacral position
dorsum, *pl.* **dorsa**, *gen.* **dorsi**
d. of penis
d. pedis
d. sellae
d. sellae atrophy
DORV
double-outlet right ventricle
dosage
dose
absorbed d.
adult d.
air d.
ALARA radiation d.
d. area product (DAP)
d. area product meter
average radiation d.
bioeffect d. (BED)
biologically equivalent d. (BED)
biologic effective d. (BED)
bolus d.
bone marrow d.
boost d.
d. calibrator
central axis depth d.
cross-organ and self-absorbed d.
cumulative d.
delivered total d. (DTD)
depth d.
d. distribution
divided d.
doubling d.
effective d.
epilation d.
d. equivalent
d. equivalent radiation
erythema d.
exit d.
exposure d.
fractionated d.
fractionation of radiation d.
^{67}Ga higher d.
genetically significant d.
glandular d.
gonadal d.
gray radiation absorbed d.
Haut-Einheits-Dosis unit skin d.
incremental d.
d. infiltration
integral d.
iodine d.
isoeffect d.
joule radiation-absorbed d.

D

dose (*continued*)
    d. kernel
    lethal d.
    matched peripheral d. (MPD)
    maximum permissible d. (MPD)
    maximum tolerated d. (MTD)
    mean central d. (MCD)
    mean gonad d.
    median lethal d.
    medical internal radiation d.
     (MIRD)
    minimal peripheral d.
    minimum tolerance d.
    multiple-scan average d. (MSAD)
    nominal single d.
    nominal standard d.
    d. nonuniformity ratio (DNR)
    normalized average glandular d.
    optimal d.
    optimum d.
    organ tolerance d. (OTD)
    peak skin radiation d.
    percentage depth d. (PDD)
    radiation absorbed d. (rad)
    radiation tolerance d.
    radiopharmaceutical d.
    d. rate
    d. rate domain
    reciprocity theorem d.
    reference d.
    scatter d.
    shielded/unshielded breast d.
    skin d.
    table of radiation d.'s
    tapering d.
    threshold erythema d.
    tissue tolerance d. (TTD)
    total radiation d.
    tracer d.
    tumor lethal d. (TLD)
dose/dose-rate effective factor (DDREF)
dose-length product
dose-limiting toxicity
dose-surface histogram
dose-time relationship
dose-volume
    d.-v. histogram (DVH)
    d.-v. relationship
dosimeter
    chemical d.
    dichromate d.
    electronic d.
    Gardray d.
    high-dose film d.
    LiF thermoluminescence d.
    pencil d.
    pocket d.
    POSL d.
    silicon diode d.

    sucrose d.
    thermoluminescent d. (TLD)
    ultraviolet fluorescent d.
    Victoreen d.
dosimetric penumbra
dosimetrist
dosimetry
    adjacent field x-ray d.
    beam's-eye view d.
    dichromate d.
    electron d.
    4-field x-ray d.
    free-radical d.
    Fricke d.
    high-dose film d.
    large-field x-ray d.
    LiF thermoluminescence d.
    marrow d.
    medical internal radiation d.
     (MIRD)
    phantom d.
    pion d.
    polymer d.
    radiation d.
    radiopharmaceutical d.
    single x-ray d.
    thermoluminescence d.
    transmission d.
    x-ray d.
Dos Santos aortography needle
dot
    quantum d.
    d. scan
    subpleural d.
DOTA
    tetraazacyclododecanetetraacetic acid
dot-and-dash pattern
Dotter
    D. effect
    D. tube
dottering effect
double
    d. aortic arch
    d. aortic arch of Edwards
    d. appendix
    d. autograft
    d. basket
    d. bleb sign
    d. breast coil
    d. bubble
    d. bubble sign
    d. camelback sign of knee
    d. cervix
    d. coronary orifice
    d. decidual ring appearance
    d. decidual sac
    d. decidual sac sign (DDSS)
    d. density
    d. diaphragm contour

d. diaphragm sign
d. duct sign
d. ectopia
d. emission
d. fracture
d. gallbladder
d. halo sign
d. helical CT imaging
d. helical CT scan
d. injection
d. inversion recovery sequence
d. kidney
d. label
d. lesion sign
d. line sign
d. lumen
d. outflow
d. outline
d. PCL sign
d. penis
d. pleurisy
d. pneumonia
d. reverse alpha sigmoid loop
d. ring esophageal sign
d. spin-echo proton spectroscopy
d. systolic apical impulses
d. tracking of barium
d. uterus
d. vagina
double-arc gallbladder shadow
double-arch aorta
double-barrel
d.-b. aorta
d.-b. esophagus
d.-b. lumen
double-bonded carbon
double-broadband triple-resonance NMR probe circuit
double-bubble
d.-b. appearance
d.-b. shadow
double-bulb appearance
double-channel endoscope
double-condom sign
double-contrast
d.-c. arthrography
d.-c. arthrotomography of shoulder
d.-c. barium enema (DCBE)
d.-c. barium meal
d.-c. barium study
d.-c. esophagography
d.-c. eversion examination
d.-c. GI examination
d.-c. laryngography
d.-c. radiograph
d.-c. radiography
d.-c. technique
d.-c. visualization

double-density
d.-d. heart
d.-d. sign
double-dose
d.-d. delay (DDD)
d.-d. delayed-contrast MRI
d.-d. gadolinium imaging
double-echo
d.-e. echo-planar imaging
d.-e. method
double-exposed rib
double-exposure drift artifact
double-freeze technique
double-halo
d.-h. appearance
d.-h. configuration
double-helix
d.-h. acquisition
d.-h. prostatic stent
double-inlet
d.-i. left ventricle (DILV)
d.-i. single ventricle
d.-i. ventricle anomaly
double-J
d.-J indwelling catheter
d.-J stent placement
d.-J ureteral catheter
d.-J ureteral stent
double-label counting
double-lumen
d.-l. breast implant
d.-l. central venous catheter
d.-l. endoprosthesis
double-mode steady state
double-mouthed uterus
double-outlet
d.-o. both ventricles (DOBV)
d.-o. left ventricle (DOLV)
d.-o. right ventricle (DORV)
double-phase technetium-99m sestamibi imaging
double-pigtail endoprosthesis
double-populated detector ring
double-power injector
double-probe pH study
double-pulse interlaced echo imaging
double-ring esophagus
double-spiral CT arterial portography
double-spot compression
double-stem silicone lesser MP implant
double-stick technique
double-strand scission
double-throw
single-pole d.-t. (SPDT)
double-tracking colon
double-track sign
double-umbrella technique
double-voiding cystogram

D

double-wall sign
double-wire atherectomy technique
doubling
    d. dose
    d. time
doughnut, donut
    GE Signa double d.
    d. kidney
    d. lesion
    d. magnet
    d. sign
    sonolucent d.
    d. transformer
doughy mass
Douglas
    D. cul-de-sac
    dependent pouch of D.
    D. fold
    D. ligament
    D. rectouterine pouch
Dow
    D. hollow-fiber analyzer
    D. method for measuring cardiac
     output
dowager's hump
dowel
    iliac d.
dowel-shaped bone graft
down
    cone d.
    coned d.
    ramp d.
    D. syndrome
downhill varix
downscatter
downsloping
downstaging
    axillary tumor d.
    d. effect
downstream
    crossed upstream and d.
    d. sampling method
downward
    d. displacement of apical impulse
    d. slope
    d. vergence
Dox-Spheres
Doyne honeycomb degeneration
DPA
    dual-photon absorptiometry
dP/dt
    upstroke pattern on apexcardiogram
     peak dP/dt
DPF
    digital pulsed fluoroscopy
DPG
    displacement placentogram
DPH
    diffuse pulmonary hemorrhage

DPR
    dynamic planar reconstructor
DPTI
    diastolic pressure-time index
DPX-IQ
    dextropropoxyphene-IQ
     DPX-IQ densitometer
DQE
    detective quantum efficiency
DRA
    digital rotational angiography
    distal rectal adenocarcinoma
    distal reference axis
dragon pyelogram
drain
    external ventricular d. (EVD)
    occlusive d.
    radiopaque d.
    retroperitoneal d.
    rubber d.
    sump d.
drainage
    aberrant venous d.
    biliary d.
    d. catheter
    central venous d.
    circle loop biliary d.
    enteric exocrine d.
    external-internal d.
    extrapleural d.
    gaseous d.
    guided d.
    imaging-guided catheter d.
    infradiaphragmatic totally
     anomalous pulmonary venous
     d.
    internal biliary d.
    intrathoracic catheter d.
    pancreatic pseudocyst d.
    percutaneous abscess d.
    percutaneous antegrade biliary
     d.
    percutaneous biliary d. (PBD)
    percutaneous catheter d. (PCD)
    percutaneous transhepatic biliary d.
     (PTBD)
    percutaneous transhepatic cholangial
     d. (PTCD)
    pulmonary venous d.
    spondylodiscitis d.
    spontaneous d.
    total anomalous pulmonary venous
     d. (TAPVD)
    transhepatic d.
    transvaginal ultrasound-guided d.
    tube d.
    venous d.
    ventricular d.
    water-sealed d.

draining
    d. lymphatic bed
    d. sinus
    d. with venous pressure
drain-out film
draped aorta
Drash syndrome
DRC
    dynamic range control
Drennan metaphysial-epiphysial angle
DRESS
    depth-resolved surface spectroscopy
dressing
    occlusive d.
Dressler syndrome
DREZ
    dorsal root entry zone
    DREZ lesion
DRG
    dorsal root ganglion
DRI
    Doppler resistive index
d-ribose
Driffield
    Hunter and D. (H and D)
drift
    field d.
    radial d.
drifting wedge pressure
drill
    lithoclast miniature pneumatic d.
    magnetic resonance
      imaging-compatible piezoelectric
      power d.
drinking esophagram
drip
    d. infusion cholangiogram
      (DIC)
    d. infusion cholangiography
      (DIC)
    d. infusion pyelography
    d. infusion technique
    d. infusion urography
dripping
    brain candle d.
    candle-wax d.
    d. candle-wax appearance
driven
    d. equilibrium Fourier transform
    d. equilibrium Fourier transform
      technique
    d. inversion spin echo
dromedary hump
drooping
    d. gallbladder
    d. lily appearance
    d. lily sign
    d. shoulder
    d. shoulder sign

drop
    d. finger
    d. heart
    d. metastasis
    d. shoulder
    d. test for pneumoperitoneum
drop-lock ring
dropped stone
drowned lung
DRR
    digitally reconstructed
    radiograph
drug
    adjuvant analgesic d.
    d. administration
    adrenergic d.
    anesthetic d.
    antiadrenergic d.
    anticonvulsant d.
    antidepressant d.
    antimuscarinic d.
    antineoplastic d.
    antipsychotic d.
    cytotoxic d.
    d. dose intensity
    d. efflux
    d. fraction
    macromolecular d.
    noncytotoxic d.
    psychotherapeutic d.
    slow channel-blocking d.
    d. tolerance
drug-associated hemorrhage
drug-delivery system
drug-eluting stent
drug-induced
    d.-i. bone marrow suppression
    d.-i. brain abnormality
    d.-i. brain change
    d.-i. bullous disorder
    d.-i. chest disease
    d.-i. drug resistance
    d.-i. eosinophilic pulmonary
      disease
    d.-i. erythematous lupus
    d.-i. esophagitis
    d.-i. lung disease
    d.-i. nephrotoxicity
    d.-i. pneumonitis
    d.-i. pulmonary damage
drug-resistant
    d.-r. extratemporal epilepsy
    d.-r. tumor
DRUJ
    distal radioulnar joint
Drummond
    D. marginal artery
    D. sign
    D. sign of aortic aneurysm

D

drum spur
drumstick
    d. appearance
    d. phalanx
drusen
    optic nerve d.
dry
    d. bowel preparation
    d. bronchiectasis
    d. heat sterilizer and incinerator unit
    d. laser imaging
    d. pleurisy
    d. swallow
dryer system
Drystar dry imager
DryView laser imaging system
DS
    Doppler sonography
DSA
    digital subtraction angiography
    digital subtraction arteriography
        DSA image
        infrainguinal DSA
DSAS
    discrete subvalvular aortic stenosis
DSC
    dynamic susceptibility contrast
        DSC MR imaging
DSC-MRI
    dynamic susceptibility contrast magnetic resonance imaging
3-Dscope laparoscope
DSCT
    dual-source computed tomography
        DSCT system
DSE
    dobutamine stress echocardiography
D-shaped vessel lumen
DSI
    digital subtraction imaging
        DSI camera
DSM
    digital subtraction mammography
3D-spoiled gradient-recalled echo sequence
DSR
    dynamic spatial reconstructor
        DSR scanner
DSRCT
    desmoplastic small round-cell tumor
DT
    diffusion-tensor
        DT MR imaging
DTC
    differentiated thyroid carcinoma
DTD
    delivered total dose

DTI
    diffusion-tensor imaging
    Doppler tissue imaging
DTICH
    delayed traumatic intracerebral hematoma
D-to-E slope
DTPA
    diethylenetriamine pentaacetic acid
        DTPA CSF flow study
        dysprosium DTPA
        DTPA imaging agent
        ^{111}In DTPA
        iron ascorbate DTPA
        DTPA renography
        technetium 99m DTPA
        technetium 99m iron ascorbate DTPA
        ytterbium-169 DTPA
DTPA-bismethylamide
    dysprosium DTPA-b.
DTPA-Lys(40)-Exendin 4
D-transportation
DTT
    diffusion-tensor tractography
DTU-215 cardiac digital stimulator
DTU-One UltraSure imaging system
dual
    d. atrioventricular node pathways
    d. blood supply
    d. ectopic thyroids
    d. gradient-recalled echo pulse sequence
    d. intracoronary scintigraphy
    d. lateral hand positioner
    d. lateral skull block
    d. leg immobilizer
    d. oblique hand positioner
    d. parathyroid gland hyperplasia
    d. photon
    d. plate
    d. popliteal veins
    d. shaped collimator
    d. single-crystal gamma camera
    d. transverse linear-array sonogram
    d. ventricles
dual-agent imaging
dual-balloon method
dual-B206 isotope myocardial scan
dual-coil imaging
dual-contrast study
dual-demand pacing mode
dual-detector helical CT angiography
dual-echo
    d.-e. and DT MR imaging
    d.-e. chemical shift gradient-echo MRI
    d.-e. DIET fast spin-echo imaging
    d.-e. interleaved spiral out-in imaging

d.-e. sequence
d.-e. turbo spin-echo
dual-emulsion mammography film
dual-energy
  d.-e. contrast-enhanced computed
    tomography
  d.-e. CT
  d.-e. imaging
  d.-e. linear accelerator
  d.-e. mammography
  d.-e. radiograph (DER)
  d.-e. subtraction
  d.-e. x-ray absorptiometry (DEXA,
    DXA)
  d.-e. x-ray absorptiometry
    densitometer
dual-head
  d. h. coincidence camera
  d.-h. coincidence detection system
  d.-h. SPECT
dual-interval echo train (DIET)
dual-isotope
  d.-i. myocardial perfusion imaging
  d.-i. osteomyelitis scan
  d.-i. scanning
  d.-i. single-photon emission CT
  d.-i. SPECT
  d.-i. subtraction technique
  d.-i. TI 201
dual-labeled solid and liquid meal
dual-lookup table algorithm
**dual-lumen silicone hemodialysis/apheresis
  catheter**
**dual-mode, dual-pacing, dual-sensing
  (DDD)**
dual-phase
  d.-p. CT
  d.-p. gastric emptying
  d.-p. helical computed tomography
    (DHCT)
  d.-p. ^{99m}Tc-sestamibi imaging
  d.-p. scan
dual-photon
  d.-p. absorptiometry (DPA)
  d.-p. densitometer
  d.-p. densitometry
dual-probe rectilinear scanner
dual-segment reconstruction
dual-sensing
  dual-mode, dual-pacing, d.-s.
    (DDD)
**dual-source computed tomography
  (DSCT)**
dual-time point imaging
dual-tracer imaging
Dubin-Johnson syndrome
Duchenne
  D. muscular dystrophy
  D. sign

duct
  aberrant intrahepatic bile d.
  accessory bile d.
  accessory hepatic d.
  accessory pancreatic d.
  alveolar d.
  amnionic d.
  arborization of d.
  arterial d.
  asymmetric bile d.
  Bartholin d.
  beaded bile d.
  beaded hepatic d.
  beaded pancreatic d.
  bile d.
  biliary d.
  Botallo d.
  branch d.
  branchial d.
  bucconeural d.
  canalicular d.
  carotid d.
  d. cell adenocarcinoma
  d. cell carcinoma
  choledochous d.
  cobblestone appearance of
    bile d.
  cochlear d.
  common bile d. (CBD)
  common gall d.
  common hepatic d. (CHD)
  craniopharyngeal d.
  Cuvier d.
  cystic gall d.
  deferent d.
  dilated bile d.
  dilated intrahepatic d.
  dilated mammary d.
  dilated subareolar d.
  disruption of d.
  distal bile d.
  duodenal end of dorsal d.
  duodenal end of main d.
  efferent d.
  ejaculatory d.
  endolymphatic d.
  excretory d.
  extrahepatic bile d.
  extralobular terminal d.
  focally dilated d.
  frontonasal d.
  fusiform widening of d.
  galactophorous d.
  gall d.
  Gartner d.
  genital d.
  hepatic d.
  hypophysial Rathke d.
  infundibulum of bile d.

D

duct (*continued*)
interlobular bile d.
intrahepatic bile d.
intralobular terminal d.
involution of d.
lacrimal d.
lactiferous d.
d. lumen
lymph d.
lymphatic d.
main pancreatic d. (MPD)
main papillary d. (MPD)
mammary d.
middle extrahepatic bile d.
müllerian d.
nasofrontal d.
nasolacrimal d.
nipplelike common bile d.
normal-caliber d.
d. obstruction
d. of Bellini
omphalomesenteric d.
pancreatic d.
paramesonephric d.
paraurethral d.
parotid d.
percutaneous dilation of biliary d.
perilobular d.
preampullary portion of bile d.
prepapillary bile d.
prostatic d.
proximal part of dorsal d.
pruned-tree appearance of bile d.
pseudocalculus bile d.
Rathke d.
rat-tail common bile d.
recanalized d.
right hepatic d.
Rivinus d.
ruptured thoracic d.
Santorini d.
solitary dilated d.
sphincter of bile d.
spontaneous perforation of biliary d.
(SPBD)
spontaneous perforation of common
bile d.
Stensen d.
subareolar d.
submandibular d.
subvesical d.
terminal bile d.
thoracic d.
thyroglossal d.
transabdominal catheterization of
thoracic d.
Vater d.
vitelline d.
Wharton d.

window d.
Wirsung d.
wolffian d.
ductal
d. adenoma
d. aneurysm
d. arch
d. architecture
d. breast microcalcification
d. carcinoma in situ (DCIS)
d. constriction
d. dilation
d. ectasia
d. epithelial hyperplasia
d. epithelium
d. in situ breast carcinoma
d. pancreatic adenocarcinoma
d. papillary carcinoma
d. papilloma
d. pattern
d. remnant
ductectatic
d. mucinous cystic neoplasia
d. mucinous tumor
ductogram
mammary d.
ductography
contrast d.
d. of breast
peroral retrograde pancreaticobiliary
d.
duct-penetrating sign
ductular
ductule
ductus *pl.* **ductus**
d. arteriosus
d. arteriosus aneurysm
d. arteriosus occlusion
d. arteriosus patency
d. bump
d. deferens
d. deferens artery
d. diverticulum
d. infundibulum
d. of Kommerell
d. venosus
d. venosus patency
Duett
D. arterial puncture site closure
device
D. diagnostic device
D. therapeutic device
Dulcolax bowel preparation
dullness, dulness
left border of cardiac d. (LBCD)
triangular area of d.
dulness (*var. of* dullness)
dumbbell
d. appearance

d. brain mass
d. lesion
d. loculation
d. needle
d. neurofibroma
d. schwannoma
d. shape
d. tumor
dumbbell-shaped shadow
dumbbell-type neuroblastoma
dummy source
dumping
d. stomach
d. syndrome
Duncan placenta
Dunlop-Shands view
duodena (*pl. of* duodenum)
duodenal
d. adenocarcinoma
d. ampulla
d. artery
d. atresia
d. bulb
d. bulb apex (DBA)
d. bulb deformity
d. button
d. cap
d. C loop
d. diaphragm
d. duplication
d. end of dorsal duct
d. end of main duct
d. erosion
d. extrinsic pressure effect
d. filling defect
d. fossa
d. gastrinoma
d. hematoma
d. hernia
d. hourglass stenosis
d. impression
d. injury
d. intraluminal diverticulum
d. leiomyosarcoma
d. ligament
d. loop
d. lumen
d. malignant tumor
d. narrowing
d. obstruction
d. papilla
d. polyp
d. segment
d. sphincter
d. stricture
d. stump
d. sweep
d. teardrop appearance
d. terminus

d. ulcer
d. ulcer perforation
d. varix
d. vein
d. villus
d. wall hamartoma
d. web
duodeni (*gen. of* duodenum)
duodenal-gastric outlet obstruction
duodenitis
chronic atrophic d.
Crohn d.
erosive d.
hemorrhagic d.
duodenobiliary
d. pressure gradient
d. reflux
duodenocolic fistula
duodenogastric reflux (DGR)
duodenogastroesophageal reflux
duodenogastroscopy
duodenogram
duodenography
hypotonic d.
d. imaging
duodenojejunal
d. angle
d. flexure (DJF)
d. fold
d. fossa
d. junction (DJJ)
d. recess
d. sphincter
duodenojejunitis
duodenomesocolic fold
duodenopancreatic
d. fistula
d. reflux
duodenorenal ligament
duodenoscope
Olympus JF1T10 fiberoptic d.
duodenum, *pl.* **duodena,** *gen.* **duodeni**
ampulla duodeni
chronic ileus d.
C loop of d.
cobblestone appearance
of d.
comma-shaped d.
curve of d.
descending d.
dilated d.
distal d.
d. inversum
d. megabulbus
mobile d.
2nd portion of d.
onion-shaped dilation of d.
postbulbar d.
3rd portion of d.

D

duodenum (*continued*)
    scarified d.
    scarred d.
    1st portion of d.
    supravaterian d.
    suspensory muscle of d.
    d. water trap
    windsock appearance of d.
duografin
Du Pen long-term epidural catheter
duplex
    d. B-mode Doppler
    d. B-mode ultrasound
    d. carotid imaging
    d. carotid ultrasound
    d. Doppler imaging
    d. Doppler scan
    d. Doppler signal analysis (DDSA)
    d. echocardiography
    d. pulsed Doppler sonography
    d. pulsed Doppler ultrasound
    d. scanner
    d. screening test
    d. sonography
    d. ultrasonography (DUS)
    d. ultrasound analysis
    d. ultrasound error
    d. ultrasound of carotid artery
    d. uterus
duplicated
    d. inferior vena cava
    d. renal collecting system
duplication
    d. anomaly
    colon cyst d.
    colorectal d.
    complete d.
    d. cyst
    diaphragm d.
    duodenal d.
    esophageal d.
    foregut d.
    gallbladder d.
    gastrogenic d.
    hindgut d.
    incomplete ureteral d.
    inferior vena cava d.
    intestinal d.
    jejunal d.
    d. of left kidney
    d. of right kidney
    partial ureter d.
    renal d.
    thoracoabdominal d.
    ureteral d.
duplicator
    cardiac pulse d.

DuPont
    D. Cronex x-ray film
    D. scanner
Dupré muscle
Dupuytren
    D. canal
    D. contracture
    D. fracture
    D. sign
dura
    attenuated d.
    bulging d.
    effacement of d.
    lamina d.
    d. mater
    d. mater of brain
    d. mater of spinal cord
    d. mater venous sinus
dural
    d. arachnoid lymphoma
    d. arteriovenous fistula (DAVF)
    d. arteriovenous malformation
    d. artery
    d. attachment
    d. calcification
    d. carotid cavernous fistula (DCCF)
    d. cul-de-sac
    d. ectasia
    d. enhancement
    d. fold
    d. hematoma
    d. impingement
    d. metastasis
    d. ossification
    d. puncture
    d. root pouch
    d. sac
    d. sac effacement
    d. sheath
    d. sinus occlusion
    d. sinus thrombosis infarct
    d. tail
    d. tear
    d. venous sinus
    d. venous sinus thrombosis
Duralyn balloon
Duran ring
Dürck node
Duret
    D. hemorrhage
    D. lesion
Durham flatfoot
Durie-Salmon
    D.-S. clinical staging criterion
    D.-S. PLUS staging system
durocutaneous fistula
Duroliopaque

Duroziez
    D. mitral stenosis disease
    D. sign
durum
    heloma d.
    osteoma d.
    papilloma d.
DUS
    duplex ultrasonography
    dynamic ultrasound of shoulder
dusty lung
Duverney
    D. foramen
    D. fracture
    D. gland
    D. muscle
DVH
    dose-volume histogram
DVI
    deep venous insufficiency
    digital vascular imaging
    DVI Simpson AtheroCath
DVR
    distribution volume ratio
DVT
    deep venous thrombosis
dwarfism
    achondroplastic d.
    acromelic d.
    Amsterdam d.
    bird-headed d.
    deprivation d.
    diastrophic d.
    late-onset d.
    lethal d.
    Lorain-Lévi d.
    mesomelic d.
    metatrophic d.
    micromelic d.
    nonlethal d.
    pituitary d.
    renal d.
    Russell-Silver d.
    thanatophoric d.
    Walt Disney d.
dwarf pelvis
dwell position
DWI
    diffusion-weighted imaging
Dwyer anterior endoscopic correction of scoliosis
DXA, DEXA
    dual-energy x-ray absorptiometry
Dy
    dysprosium
^{166}Dy, Dy-166
    dysprosium 166
Dycal base
dyclonine

Dy-DTPA-BMA imaging agent
dye
    blue d.
    d. column
    d. dilution curve
    d. extravasation
    fill and spill of d.
    d. fluorescence index (DFI)
    halogenated phenolphthalein d.
    indentation of myelography d.
    indocyanine green d.
    d. injection technique
    d. laser
    d. laser system
    lipophilic d.
    d. reduction spot test
    rose bengal d.
    d. uptake
dye-binding capacity (DBC)
2-dye method
^{166}Dy generator
Dyggve-Melchior-Clausen dysplasia
Dyke-Davidoff-Masson syndrome
Dynabead
Dynalink self-expanding stent
dynamic
    d. acquisition
    d. antral scintigraphy
    d. aorta
    d. axial fixator
    d. beat filtration
    d. bolus
    d. bolus tracking technique
    d. cervical change
    d. cervical magnetic resonance imaging
    d. computed tomography (DCT)
    d. computed tomography mammography
    d. computerized tomography
    d. condenser electrometer
    d. conformal therapy
    d. contrast-enhanced CT
    d. contrast-enhanced magnetic resonance imaging (DCE-MRI)
    d. contrast-enhanced MRI
    d. contrast-enhanced subtraction MR imaging
    d. contrast-enhanced subtraction study
    d. contrast MRI
    d. coupling
    d. criterion
    d. CT scan
    d. emission scan
    d. enhancement
    d. entrapment of vertebral artery
    d. filtering
    d. focusing

D

dynamic (*continued*)
  d. hip screw (DHS)
  d. ileus
  d. image
  d. lineshape effect
  d. liver imaging
  d. lung
  d. magnetic resonance imaging (dMRI)
  d. multileaf collimation
  d. nuclear imaging study
  d. nuclear polarization (DNP)
  d. open magnetic resonance defecography
  d. optical breast imaging (DOBI)
  d. pedobarography
  d. planar reconstructor (DPR)
  d. pulmonary hyperinflation
  d. radiation therapy
  d. radionuclide renal scintigraphy
  d. radiotherapy
  d. range
  d. range control (DRC)
  d. renal imaging
  d. scintigraphy imaging
  d. series
  d. snapshot
  d. sonography
  d. spatial reconstructor (DSR)
  d. spiral CT lung densitometer
  d. spiral CT lung densitometry
  d. stabilizer
  d. stereotactic radiosurgery
  d. subaortic stenosis
  d. subtraction magnetic resonance angiogram
  d. supine study
  d. susceptibility contrast (DSC)
  d. susceptibility contrast magnetic resonance imaging (DSC-MRI)
  d. tagging magnetic resonance angiography
  d. ultrasound of shoulder (DUS)
  d. ventilation He-MRI
  d. volume imaging
  d. volume-rendered display
  d. volumetric SPECT
  d. wedge
  d. weightbearing cervical magnetic resonance imaging
dynamite heart
Dynapix
DynaRad portable x-ray system
DynaWell medical compression device
dyne
dynode
dynography
dysarthria-clumsy hand syndrome

dysautonomia
  familial d.
dyschezia
dyschondroplasia
dyschondrosteosis
dyschromia
dyscinesia (*var. of* dyskinesia)
dyscollagenosis
dyscrasic fracture
dysdiadochocinesia (*var. of* dysdiadochokinesia)
dysdiadochokinesia, dysdiadochocinesia
dysembryoplastic neuroepithelial tumor (DNET)
dysfunction
  bladder d.
  bowel and bladder d.
  brain d.
  cerebral d.
  cortical d.
  dehydration-induced renal d.
  dopaminergic d.
  frontal lobe d.
  hepatocellular d.
  left ventricular d. (LVD)
  lower esophageal sphincter d.
  oropharyngeal d.
  positional d.
  regional myocardial d.
  renal d.
  renal proximal tubular d.
  reversible temporary myocardial d.
  right ventricular d. (RVD)
  salivary gland d.
  sinuatrial node d.
  sinus node d.
  small airway d.
  sphincter d.
  swallowing d.
  testis d.
  valvular d.
  ventilatory d.
  ventricular d.
dysfunctional
  d. autogenous hemodialysis fistula
  d. kidney
dysgenesia (*var. of* dysgenesis)
dysgenesis, dysgenesia
  alar d.
  anorectal d.
  callosal d.
  corpus callosum d.
  corticocallosal d.
  epiphysial d.
  gonadal d.
  hindbrain d.
  mixed gonadal d.
  ovarian d.
  renal tubular d.

sacral d.
sacrolumbar d.
segmental spinal d. (SSD)
thyroid d.
tubular d.
dysgenetic kidney
dysgerminoma
brain d.
mediastinal d.
ovarian d.
pineal d.
dysjunction
craniofacial d.
dyskeratosis
kidney d.
dyskinesia, dyskinesis, dyscinesia
bile duct d.
biliary d.
gallbladder d.
regional d.
tardive d.
dyskinesis (*var. of* dyskinesia)
dyskinetic
d. cerebral palsy
d. segmental wall motion
d. segmental wall motion
abnormality
d. septum
dysmaturity
pulmonary d.
dysmorphia (*var. of* dysmorphism)
dysmorphism, dysmorphia
lobar d.
dysmorphology
facial d.
dysmotile
d. cilia syndrome
d. esophagus
dysmotility
esophageal d.
dysmyelination disorder
dysosteogenesis, dysostosis
dysostosis (*var. of* dysosteogenesis)
cleidocranial d.
craniofacial d.
epiphysial d.
mandibulofacial d.
metaphysial d.
d. multiplex
mutational d.
dysphagia, dysphagy
contractile ring d.
esophageal d.
d. inflammatoria
liquid food d.
d. lusoria
oropharyngeal d.
d. paralytica
postvagotomy d.

preesophageal d.
progressive d.
sideropenic d.
soft food d.
solid food d.
d. spastica
vallecular d.
d. valsalviana
dysphagy (*var. of* dysphagia)
dysplasia
acetabular residual d.
acromelic d.
acromesomelic d.
acropectorovertebral d.
arrhythmogenic right ventricular d.
(ARVD)
arteriohepatic d.
asphyxiating thoracic d.
bone d.
bronchopulmonary d. (BPD)
Burke-type metaphysial d.
camptomelic d.
cemental d.
cementoosseous d.
cervical d.
chondroectodermal d.
cleidocranial d.
CNS fibromuscular d.
congenital hip d.
congenital polyvalvular d.
congenital septooptic d.
cortical d.
cranioskeletal d.
craniotelencephalic d.
cystic fibrous d.
diaphysial d.
diastrophic d.
d. dislocation
Dyggve-Melchior-Clausen d.
endocardial d.
epiarticular osteochondromatous d.
epiphysial d.
d. epiphysialis hemimelia
d. epiphysialis multiplex
d. epiphysialis punctata
external auditory canal d.
familial arterial fibromuscular d.
fetal musculoskeletal d.
fibromuscular d.
fibrous temporal bone d.
focal cerebellar d.
focal cortical d.
foot d.
frontonasal d.
hip d.
idiopathic diffuse cerebellar d.
isolated focal cerebellar cortical d.
Jansen metaphysial d.
Joubert focal cerebellar d.

D

dysplasia (*continued*)
 Kniest d.
 lethal bone d.
 lethal musculoskeletal d.
 lymphatic d.
 mammary d.
 McKusick-type metaphysial d.
 mesodermal d.
 mesomelic d.
 metaphysial d.
 metatrophic d.
 Meyer d.
 micromelic d.
 microscopic cortical d.
 Mondini d.
 monostotic fibrous d.
 multicystic d.
 multiple epiphysial d.
 Namaqualand spondyloepiphysial d.
  (NSED)
 neuroectodermal d.
 nonlethal d.
 nonsyndromic focal cerebellar d.
 obstructive renal d.
 odontoid d.
 osseous d.
 osteofibrous d.
 periapical cemental d.
 perimedial d.
 periosteal d.
 polyostotic fibrous d.
 polypoid d.
 Potter d.
 progressive diaphysial d. (PDD)
 pulmonary valve d.
 Pyle d.
 renal artery fibromuscular d.
 retinal d.
 retroareolar d.
 rhizomelic d.
 rib d.
 right ventricular d.
 Scheibe d.
 Schmid-type metaphysial d.
 septooptic d.
 sheetlike d.
 short limb d.
 skeletal d.
 sphenoid d.
 spondylocostal d.
 spondyloepiphysial d.
 spondylothoracic d.
 Streeter d.
 tapetoretinal d.
 Taylor-type d.
 tectal d.
 testis d.
 thanatophoric d.
 thoracic d.

 thymic d.
 transmantle d.
 tricuspid valve d.
 variable cerebral d.
 ventricular d.
 ventriculoradial d.
 d. with associated lesion or mass
  (DALM)
dysplasia-associated lesion
dysplasia-carcinoma sequence
dysplasia-clefting
 ectrodactyly-ectodermal d.-c.
dysplastic
 d. breast
 d. cerebellar gangliocytoma
 d. cusp
 d. kidney
 d. liver nodule
 d. meniscus
 d. pulmonary valve
dysprosium (Dy)
 d. 166 (^{166}Dy, Dy-166)
 d. analogue
 d. DTPA
 d. DTPA-bismethylamide
 d. HP-DO3A imaging agent
dysprosium-diethylenetriamine pentaacetic acid-bismethylamide
dysprosium-holmium in vivo generator
dysproteinemia
dysraphia (*var. of* dysraphism)
dysraphic spine
dysraphism, dysraphia
 closed spinal d.
 occult spinal d.
 spinal d.
 tectocerebellar d.
dysregulation
 vertigo/orthostatic d.
dysrhythmia of fetal heart
dyssynchronous primary tumor
dyssynergia, dyssynergy
 biliary d.
 detrusor-sphincter d.
 Ramsay Hunt cerebellar myoclonic
  d.
 regional d.
 segmental d.
dyssynergy (*var. of* dyssynergia)
dystocia
 fetal d.
 labor d.
 shoulder d.
dystonia
 dopa-responsive d.
dystonic reaction
dystopia
dystrophia (*var. of* dystrophy)

dystrophic
  d. change
  d. degeneration
  d. soft tissue
    calcification
dystrophinopathic cardiomyopathy
dystrophy, dystrophia
  adiposogenital d.
  asphyxiating thoracic d.
  bone d.
  congenital muscular d.
  Duchenne muscular d.

Fukuyama congenital muscular d.
infantile thoracic d.
limb-girdle muscular d.
merosin-deficient congenital muscular
  d.
muscular d.
neuraxonal d.
oculocerebrorenal d.
oculopharyngeal d.
reflex sympathetic d.
Sudeck d.
sympathetic d.

D

E
- E plane
- E point of cardiac apex pulse
- E point on echocardiography
- E point to septal separation (EPSS)
- E sign on x-ray

E₁
- estrone
- prostaglandin E₁

E-A
- E-A change
- E-A wave ratio

EAA
- extraalveolar air
- EAA collection

Eagle-Barrett syndrome

ear
- e. cholesteatoma
- frontal horn Mickey Mouse e.
- inner e.
- middle e.

early
- e. advanced hepatocellular carcinoma
- e. bladder activity
- e. bone scintigraphy
- e. echo
- e. endovascular treatment
- e. fetal death
- e. opening of valve
- e. osteoarthritis
- e. osteomyelitis
- e. pneumonitis
- e. repolarization pattern
- e. satiety
- e. segmental opacification
- e. stromal invasion
- e. systolic peak (ESP)
- e. venous filling

early-phase termination
Eastern Cooperative Oncology Group (ECOG)
Eastman Kodak scanner
Easy Wallstent stent
Eaton agent pneumonia
EBA
- electron beam angiography
- extrahepatic biliary atresia

EBCT
- electron beam computed tomography
- EBCT IV angiography
- volume-mode EBCT

EBDA
- effective balloon-dilated area

EBER
- electron beam electroreflectance

EBIORT
- electron beam intraoperative radiotherapy

EBRT
- external beam radiation therapy

Ebstein
- E. angle
- E. anomaly
- E. lesion
- E. malformation
- E. sign

EBT
- electron beam tomography
- EBT scanner

eburnated bone
eburnation
- bony e.
- trapezium-metacarpal e. (TME)

eburneum
- osteoma e.

EBV
- Epstein-Barr virus

EC
- enteric coated

ECA
- external carotid artery

E-CABG
- endoscopic coronary artery bypass graft

E.CAM dual-head emission imaging system
ECAT
- emission computerized axial tomography
- ECAT Reveal PET/CT imaging system

eccentric
- e. atherosclerotic plaque
- e. atrophy
- e. axis of rotation of ankle
- e. coronary artery
- e. enhancing nodule
- e. epicenter
- e. ledge
- e. left ventricular hypertrophy
- e. medullary bone lesion
- e. monocuspid disc valve
- e. narrowing
- e. pantomography
- e. restenosis lesion
- e. stenosis
- e. vessel

eccentrically placed lumen
eccentricity index
ecchondroma, ecchondrosis

ecchondrosis (*var. of* ecchondroma)
Eccocee CS ultrasound system
eccrine
> e. angiomatous hamartoma
> e. sweat gland

ECD
> endocardial cushion defect
> ethyl cysteinate dimer
> ^{99m}Tc ECD

ECE
> extracapsular extension

EC-folate
ECG, EKG
> electrocardiogram
> ECG trigger

ECG-gated
> ECG-g. multislice
> ECG-g. multislice MR imaging
> ECG-g. spin-echo
> ECG-g. spin-echo MR imaging

ECG-gated
ECG-synchronized digital subtraction angiography
ECG-triggered
> ECG-t. flow-compensated gradient-echo image
> ECG-t. phase contrast cine gradient-echo sequence

ECG-triggered
echinococcal
> e. abscess
> e. cyst

echinococciasis (*var. of* echinococcosis)
echinococcosis, echinococciasis
> alveolar e.
> bone e.
> cystic e.
> liver e.
> lung e.
> pericardial cystic e.

echinococcus cyst
echo
> amphoric e.
> asymmetric e.
> atrial e.
> breath-hold turbo spin e.
> bright e.
> e. characteristic
> e. contrast
> e. contrast agent
> e. delay time
> dense e.
> diaphragmatic e.
> 3D magnetization-prepared rapid gradient e.
> driven inversion spin e.
> early e.
> endometrial e.
> enhanced fast gradient e.

> e. enhancement
> e. enhancer
> even distribution of e.'s
> fast-field e. (FFE)
> fast spin e. (FSE)
> fast spoiled gradient-recalled e. (FSPGR)
> fat-suppressed spin e.
> FID-acquired e.
> field e.
> e. FLASH MR
> fuzzy e.
> generalized interferography using spin echoes and stimulated e.'s
> generation e.
> gradient e. (GE)
> gradient-recalled e. (GRE)
> gradient-refocused e. (GRE)
> gradient spin e.
> hepatic pattern e.
> high-amplitude e.
> highly mobile e.
> highly reflective e.
> homogeneous e.
> e. image
> e. imaging
> inhomogeneous e.
> internal e.
> inversion recovery spin e. (IRSE)
> linear e.
> low-amplitude internal e.
> low-level e.
> magnetization-prepared rapid acquisition gradient e. (MP-RAGE)
> median level e.
> metallic e.
> mirrorlike e.
> multiplanar gradient-recalled e.
> multiple spin e.'s
> navigator e.
> offset radiofrequency spin e.
> out-of-phase gradient e.
> partial saturation spin e.
> particulate e.
> e. pattern
> pencil-beam navigator e.
> e. phase correction (EPC)
> pulsed-gradient spin e. (PGSE)
> radiofrequency spin e.
> e. ranging
> rapid-acquisition spin e. (RASE)
> rapid-acquisition with gradient e.
> rapid gradient e. (RAGE)
> e. reflectivity
> renal sinus e.
> e. rephasing
> reverberation e.
> RF spin e.
> ring-down e.
> salvo of e.'s

SENSE with half-Fourier single-shot turbo spin e. (SShTSE)
shower of e.'s
e. signature
simulated e.
single-shot fast spin e. (SSFSE)
sludgelike intraluminal e.
smokelike e.
solid e.
sonographic e.
e. space
specular e.
spin e.
spin echo using repeated gradient e.'s
spoiled gradient e.
standard single e.
stimulated e.
supraventricular venous e.
swirling smokelike e.
symmetric e.
thick e.
e. time chemical-shift imaging
E. Tip trocar needle
e. train
turbo gradient-refocused e. (turboGRE)
turbo-spin e. (TSE)
T1-weighted conventional spin e.
ultrasonographic e.
ventricular e.

echoaortography
echocardiogram
adenosine e.
e. planar imaging
echocardiograph correlation
echocardiographic
e. automated border
e. differentiation
e. gating
echocardiography
adenosine e.
ambulatory Holter e.
American Society of E.
A-mode e.
aortic root e.
aortic valve e. (AVE)
apical 2-chamber view e.
apical 5-chamber view e.
automated border detection by e.
biplane transesophageal e.
blood pool radionuclide e.
B-mode e.
cardiac output e.
2-chamber e.
4-chamber e.
color-flow imaging Doppler e.
continuous-loop exercise e.
continuous-wave Doppler e.

contrast e.
contrast-enhanced e.
cross-sectional e. (CSE)
detection e.
2-dimensional e. (2DE)
2-dimensional cross-sectional e.
dipyridamole e.
dobutamine stress e. (DSE)
Doppler continuous-wave e.
Doppler pulsed-wave e.
3D transesophageal e.
duplex e.
epicardial Doppler e.
E point on e.
exercise e.
Feigenbaum e.
fetal e.
high pulse-repetition frequency Doppler e.
H-mode e.
hypokinesis on e.
e. imaging
intracardiac e. (ICE)
intracoronary contrast e.
intraoperative cardioplegic contrast e.
Levovist myocardial contrast e.
Meridian e.
mitral valve e.
M-mode e.
multiplanar transesophageal e.
myocardial contrast e. (MCE)
myocardial perfusion e.
parasternal long-axis view e.
parasternal short-axis view e.
pharmacologic stress e.
postcontrast e.
postexercise e.
postinjection e.
postmyocardial infarction e.
precontrast e.
preinjection e.
premyocardial infarction e.
pulsed Doppler transesophageal e.
pulsed-wave Doppler e.
quantitative Levovist myocardial contrast e.
real-time e.
resting myocardial e.
sector e.
short-axis view e.
stress e.
subcostal short-axis view e.
supine bicycle stress e.
THI e.
transesophageal e. (TEE)
transthoracic 3-dimensional e.
ultrasound e.
ventricular wall motion e.

E

echocardiography:yttrium-aluminum-garnet
    contrast transesophageal
      e.:y.-a.-g.
Echo-Coat ultrasound biopsy needle
echocolonoscope
    CF-UM3 e.
echodense
    e. layer
    e. pattern
    e. valve
echodensity
echoencephalogram (EEG)
echoencephalograph (EEG)
    midline e.
echoencephalography
  (EEG)
echoendoscope
    FG-36UX scanning e.
    linear-array e.
    Olympus GF-UM2,
      GF-UM3 e.
    Olympus GIF-1T10 e.
    Olympus JF-UM20 e.
    Olympus VU-M2 e.
    Olympus XIF-UM3 e.
echo-enhanced cystosonography
echo-enhancing agent
echoeSystem digital x-ray
EchoEye 3D ultrasound imaging
  system
echo-free
    e.-f. area
    e.-f. central zone
    e.-f. layer
    e.-f. space
echogastroscope
EchoGen-enhanced ultrasound
echogenic
    e. appearance
    e. band
    e. bile
    e. calculus
    e. debris
    e. fetal bowel
    e. focus
    e. intraluminal thrombus
    e. liver
    e. liver metastasis
    e. mass
    e. nodule
    e. noise
    e. periphery
    e. plaque
    e. plug
    e. renal pyramid
    e. ring
    e. solid lesion
    e. starburst sign
    e. tumor

echogenicity
    brightly increased renal parenchymal e.
    calvarial e.
    focally increased renal e.
    generalized increased liver e.
    increased e.
    internal e.
    normal e.
    parenchymatous e.
    periventricular e. (PVE)
    e. scatterer
    ultrasound e.
EchoGen ultrasound imaging agent
echogram
    mitral valve e.
echographer
echographia
echography
    B-mode e.
    hepatic e.
    ophthalmic biometry by ultrasound
      e.
    transrectal e.
    transvaginal e.
echoic
echoicity
echoing
echolaminography
echolocation
echolucent
    e. pattern
    e. plaque
EchoMark catheter
echophonocardiography
    M-mode e.
echo-planar
    e.-p. diffusion-weighted imaging
    e.-p. FLAIR imaging
    e.-p. GRE T2-weighted imaging
    e.-p. image
    e.-p. imaging (EPI)
    e.-p. imaging method
    e.-p. pulse sequence
    e.-p. readout
echo-poor
    e.-p. area
    e.-p. area of environment
    e.-p. testis
Echospeed
    E. Signa LX 1.5T scanner
    E. 1.5T MR machine
echo-speed gradient
echo-spin density
echo-tagging technique
echotexture
    compact fibrillar e.
    inhomogeneous e.
    internal e.
    mottled e.

echo-train
    e.-t. echo time
    e.-t. length (ETL)
    e.-t. value
Echovist imaging agent
ECI
    ensemble contrast imaging
Eck fistula
eclampsia
    delayed e.
eclipse
    e. effect lung
    E. MR system
    E. TENS unit
    E. TMR laser
ECOG
    Eastern Cooperative Oncology Group
    ECOG scale
ECRB
    extensor carpi radialis brevis
    ECRB muscle
ECRL
    extensor carpi radialis longus
    ECRL muscle
ECS
    electrocerebral silence
ECT
    emission computed
    tomography
ectasia, ectasis
    alveolar e.
    anuloaortic e.
    basilar artery e.
    benign duct e.
    bilateral ductal e.
    communicating cavernous e.
    coronary artery e.
    diffuse arterial e.
    digitate e.
    ductal e.
    dural e.
    gonadal venous e.
    mammary duct e.
    moniliform e.
    e. of aorta
    renal tubular e.
    saccular e.
    seminiferous tubule e.
    tubular e.
    vascular colon e.
ectasis (*var. of* ectasia)
ectatic
    e. aneurysm
    e. aortic valve
    e. bronchus
    e. carotid artery
    e. emphysema
ectocardia
ectodermal groove

ectomesenchyme
ectopia, ectopy
    benign cerebellar e.
    cerebellar e.
    e. cordis
    cross-fused renal e.
    double e.
    familial thyroid e.
    longitudinal renal e.
    posterior pituitary gland e.
    renal e.
    testicular e.
    tonsillar e.
    transverse testicular e.
ectopic
    e. ACTH syndrome
    e. anus
    e. beat
    e. bone growth
    e. craniopharyngioma
    e. endometrial tissue
    e. firing nociceptor
    e. focus
    e. gallbladder
    e. gastric mucosa
    e. gland
    e. impulse
    e. intracavernous pituitary
    microadenoma
    e. intraluminal gallstone
    e. kidney
    e. meningioma
    e. ossification
    e. pancreas
    e. parathyroid
    e. parathyroid adenoma
    e. pinealoma
    e. pregnancy
    e. spleen
    e. testis
    e. thymus
    e. thyroid tissue
    e. ureter
    e. ureterocele
    e. varix
ectopy (*var. of* ectopia)
ectrodactyly-ectodermal dysplasia-clefting
ECTS
    extended computed tomography scale
ECU
    extensor carpi ulnaris
    ECU muscle
EDAMS
    encephaloduroarteriomyosynangiosis
EDAS
    encephaloduroarteriosynangiosis
EDB
    extensor digitorum brevis
    EDB muscle

E

EDC
extensor digitorum communis
EDC muscle

eddy
e. current
e. current artifact
e. current mapping
e. formation
e. ringing artifact

edema
acute interstitial lung e.
acute pulmonary e.
adjacent e.
airspace e.
alveolar pulmonary e.
angioneurotic e.
antral e.
batwing e.
bone marrow e.
brain e.
brainstem e.
breast e.
bronchiolar e.
brown e.
bullous e.
cardiogenic pulmonary e.
cardiopulmonary e.
cerebral e.
chemical pulmonary e.
chronic e.
circumscribed e.
collateral e.
compressive e.
cord e.
cyclic idiopathic e.
cytotoxic e.
diffuse e.
fetal scalp e.
fingerprint e.
e. fluid
focal e.
follicular e.
frank pulmonary e.
fulminant pulmonary e.
generalized pulmonary e.
gravitational e.
gut e.
hemorrhagic pulmonary e.
high-altitude pulmonary e.
  (HAPE)
high-permeability pulmonary e.
hydrostatic e.
hypervolemic pulmonary e.
idiopathic e.
ileocecal e.
immunologic pulmonary e.
increased capillary permeability e.
inflammatory e.
intercellular e.

interstitial pulmonary e.
intracompartmental e.
intraosseous e.
laryngeal e.
leg e.
liver e.
local e.
localized e.
lung e.
lymphatic e.
lymphaticovenous secondary e.
malignant brain e.
massive ovarian e.
massive pulmonary hemorrhagic e.
mediastinal fat e.
mild e.
myelin e.
negative image pulmonary e.
e. neonatorum
nephrotic e.
nerve root e.
neurogenic pulmonary e.
neuronal cytotoxic e.
noncardiac pulmonary e.
noncardiogenic pulmonary e.
e. of epididymis
orbital e.
osmotic e.
ovarian e.
paroxysmal pulmonary e.
passive e.
patchy e.
e. pattern
pericholecystic e.
pericystic e.
perifocal e.
perihilar pulmonary e.
perilesional e.
perineoplastic e.
periorbital e.
peripheral vasogenic e.
peritumoral e.
perivascular e.
placental e.
preosteonecrosis marrow e.
pulmonary e. (PE)
reactive marrow e.
reexpansion pulmonary e.
renal e.
reperfusion lung e.
reversible vasogenic e.
solid e.
stasis e.
stomal e.
subchondral marrow e.
subcutaneous e.
subglottic e.
supraglottic e.
terminal e.

testicular posttraumatic e.
thalamic e.
trace e.
transient bone marrow e.
umbilical cord e.
unilateral pulmonary e.
vasogenic e.
venous e.
vernal e.
visceral e.
white matter e.

edemalike change
edematous
e. brain
e. bronchus
e. gallbladder
e. kidney
e. pancreatitis
e. pleura
e. tissue
Eder-Puestow dilation
edge
boundary e.
Compton e.
e. detection
e. effect
e. enhancement
leading e.
ligament reflecting e.
ligament shelving e.
liver e.
e. misalignment artifact
e. packing
patellar e.
e. response function (ERF)
e. ringing
c. ringing artifact
sawtooth e.
e. shadow
e. stenosis
sternal e.
tentorial e.
ulcer with heaped-up e.'s
edge-boundary artifact
edge-detection
e.-d. angiography
e.-d. procedure
edge-region pixel
E-dial calibration
Edison
E. effect
E. fluoroscope
editing
spectral e.
EDL
extensor digitorum longus
EDL muscle
Edmonton Symptom Assessment Scale

EDQ
extensor digiti quinti
EDQ muscle
EDR
exposure data recognizer
EDTMP
ethylenediamine tetramethylene
phosphoric acid
EDTMP imaging agent
Edwards
double aortic arch of E.
E. Fogarty
E. syndrome
E. Thrombex PMT system
EDXRF
energy-dispersive x-ray fluorescence
EDXRF spectrometer
EEG
echoencephalogram
echoencephalograph
echoencephalography
electroencephalogram
electroencephalograph
electroencephalography
efaproxiral
EFF
electromagnetic focusing field
effaced mucosal fold
effacement
architectural e.
cistern e.
cisterna magna e.
dural sac e.
mesencephalic cistern e.
nerve root sheath e.
e. of dura
pelvicalyceal e.
sulcus e.
ventricle e.
effect
abscopal e.
adverse e.
Anrep e.
arterial sump e.
artifact e.
attenuation e.
Auger e.
Bayliss e.
beam-hardening e.
Bernoulli e.
bilateral vagotomy e.
black blood e.
blood oxygenation level-dependent
e.
Bohr e.
BOLD e.
Bowditch e.
bronchodilator e.
bronchomotor e.

E

effect (*continued*)
bronchospastic e.
butterfly e.
bystander e.
candy-wrapper e.
Cherenkov e.
cobra-head e.
collimator exchange e.
Compton e.
contact e.
contrast medium adverse e.
copper wire e.
cumulative radiation e. (CRE)
Curie e.
deleterious e.
demagnetization field e.
deterministic e.
direct saturation e.
Doppler e.
Dotter e.
dottering e.
downstaging e.
duodenal extrinsic pressure e.
dynamic lineshape e.
edge e.
Edison e.
Faraday e.
flare e.
flow-related enhancement e.
flow void e.
fogging e.
gastrointestinal adverse e.
genitourinary adverse e.
halo e.
heel e.
hematocrit e.
hemispheric mass e.
hemodynamic e.
inhomogeneity e.
isotope e.
lag e.
Laplace e.
localized mass e.
Mach band e.
Macklin e.
macromolecular hydration e.
magic angle e.
magnetization transfer e.
magnetohydrodynamic e.
masquerading e.
mass e.
methemoglobin e.
milking e.
missile e.
multilog e.
near-field e.
negative-contrast e.
neurotoxic e.
nozzle e.

nuclear Overhauser e.
osmotic e.
outflow e.
Overhauser e.
oxygen e.
pacemaker e.
pad e.
paramagnetic e.
passive loss of correlation e.
phase e.
phase-shift e.
photechic e.
photoechoic e.
photoelectric e.
photographic e.
photonuclear e.
piezoelectric e.
pinchcock e.
postvagotomy e.
priming e.
pursestringing e.
radiation e.
radiographic e.
reservoir e.
Russell e.
sausage segment e.
scalar e.
shine-through e.
side e.
silver wire e.
sink e.
skin e.
skin-sparing e.
snowplow e.
sonic e.
star e.
steal e.
stochastic e.
1st-pass e.
streaming e.
stunning e.
susceptibility e.
systematic relaxation e.
teratogenic e.
thermal e.
time-of-flight e.
tracheal mass e.
transient 1st-pass e.
T1, T2 dephasing e.
vacuum cleaner e.
vagatomy e.
vasodilatory e.
Venturi e.
Volta e.
Warburg e.
washboard e.
wash-in e.
washout e.
Wolff-Chaikoff e.

effective
- e. atomic number
- e. balloon-dilated area (EBDA)
- e. dose
- e. focal spot size
- e. half-life
- e. mass attenuation coefficient
- e. path length (EPL)
- e. pulmonary blood flow (EPBF)
- e. pulmonic index
- e. refractory period (ERP)
- e. renal plasma flow (ERPF)
- e. section thickness
- e. transverse relation time

effectiveness
- relative biologic e. (RBE)

effector-target cell interaction

efferent
- e. arteriolar resistance
- e. digital nerve
- e. duct
- e. ductule of testis
- e. loop
- e. loop obstruction
- e. lymph vessel
- e. nipple valve
- e. view

effervescent agent

efficacy study

efficiency
- absolute e.
- conversion e.
- detective quantum e. (DQE)
- full-energy peak e.
- geometric e.
- intrinsic e.
- kidney extraction e.
- quantum detection e. (QDE)
- slice e.
- valvular e.
- window e.

efficient relaxation time

effluent
- radioactive e.

efflux
- drug e.
- e. inhibitor
- e. pump

effort
- desmoplastic e.
- inspiratory e.
- respiratory e.
- shallow inspiratory e.
- suboptimal e.
- e. thrombosis
- ventilatory e.
- voluntary e.

effort-dependent

effused chyle

effusion
- e. artifact
- asbestos-related pleural e.
- Baccelli sign of pleural e.
- benign subdural e.
- bilateral pleural e.'s
- bilateral serous pleural e.'s
- cardiac e.
- chocolate joint e.
- chylous e.
- discrete area of e.
- epidural e.
- exudative pleural e.
- fetal pleural e.
- free pleural e.
- hemorrhagic pleural e.
- inflammatory joint e.
- ipsilateral pleural e.
- joint e.
- Karplus sign of pleural e.
- Kellock sign of pleural e.
- knee joint e.
- large-volume joint e.
- layering e.
- left-sided pleural e.
- liquid pleural e.
- loculated pleural e.
- malignant pleural e.
- massive pleural e.
- milky e.
- moderate-sized-volume joint e.
- noninflammatory joint e.
- parapneumonic e.
- pericardial e. (PE)
- peritoneal e.
- pleural e.
- pleuropericardial e.
- pseudochylous e.
- serofibrinous pericardial e.
- serous e.
- e. shadow
- subdeltoid bursa e.
- subdural e.
- subpleural e.
- subpulmonic e.
- taut pericardial e.
- transient pleural e.
- transudative pleural e.
- tuberculous e.
- unilateral pleural e.

EFOV
- extended field-of-view
- EFOV technique

EFW
- estimated fetal weight

Egan mammography

EGG
- electrogastrogram

egg-on-its-side heart

egg-shaped orbit
eggshell
    e. border of aneurysm
    e. breast calcification
    e. calcification of lymph node
    e. nodal calcification
egress of blood
Egyptian splenomegaly
EHL
    electrohydraulic lithotripsy
    extensor hallucis longus
Ehlers-Danlos syndrome
EHM
    extrahepatic metastasis
EHT
    electrohydrothermal
        EHT electrode
EIC
    extensive intraductal carcinoma
    extensive intraductal component
eigenvalue
eigenvector
    e. analysis
    principal e.
Eindhoven magnet
einsteinium (Es)
    e. 255 (^{255}Es)
Einthoven triangle
EIP
    extensor indicis proprius
        EIP muscle
EIS
    electrical impedance scanning
        EIS spot
        targeted EIS
Eisenmenger
    E. complex
    E. defect
    E. group
    E. reaction
    E. syndrome
EIT
    electrical impedance tomography
ejaculatory
    e. duct
    e. duct obstruction
ejection
    e. fraction
    e. fraction by 1st-pass technique
    e. phase index
    e. time
EJV
    external jugular vein
EKG, ECG
    electrocardiogram
Eklund
    E. technique
    E. view
Ekman-Lobstein disease

EKY
    electrokymogram
El-Ahwany classification of humeral supracondylar fracture
elastance
    maximum ventricular e.
elastic
    e. cartilage
    e. collision
    e. cross-section
    e. imaging
    e. recoil of artery
    e. scattering spectroscopy
    e. stable intramedullary nailing (ESIN)
    e. subtraction spiral CT angiography
elasticity
elasticum
    pseudoxanthoma e.
elasticus
    conus e.
elastin deposition in taenia coli
elastofibroma
elastography
    magnetic resonance e. (MRE)
elastomyofibrosis
elastosis
elbow
    above e. (AE)
    baseball pitcher's e.
    e. bone center
    boxer's e.
    e. contracture
    e. coronal scan
    e. extensor tendon
    e. fat-pad
    e. fat-pad sign
    floating e.
    e. fracture
    golfer's e.
    javelin thrower's e.
    e. joint
    milkmaid's e.
    nursemaid's e.
    reverse tennis e.
    tennis e.
    thrower's e. *Student's*
    wrestler's e.
ELCA
    excimer laser coronary angioplasty
        ELCA laser
ELD
    energy level diagram
elderly onset rheumatoid arthritis
elective TIPS
electric
    e. dipole
    e. field gradient
    General E. (GE)

e. generator
e. induction
e. interaction
e. joint fluoroscopy
e. joint fluoroscopy imaging
e. quadrupole coupling
e. stimulation
e. syringe

electrical
e. activity
e. circulatory arrest
e. grounding pad
e. impedance scanning (EIS)
e. impedance tomography (EIT)
e. potential energy

electrically
e. activated implant
e. detachable coil

Electro-Acuscope device
electrocardiogram (ECG, EKG)
resting e.
signal-averaged e. (SAECG, SaECG)
e. tracing
e. trigger

electrocardiogram-gated
e.-g. high-speed x-ray computed
  tomography
e.-g. MRI
e.-g. MRI imaging
e.-g. multislice spiral CT
e.-g. multislice spiral CT of heart
e.-g. SPECT

electrocardiogram-synchronized digital
  subtraction angiography
electrocardiographic
e. angle between QRS and T
  vectors (QRS-T)
e. gating
e. trigger method
e. variant
e. wave (QRS)

electrocardiograph triggering
electrocardiography
electrocardiography-gated echo-planar
  imaging
electrocardiophonogram
electrocardioscanner
Compuscan Hittman computerized e.

electrocautery
endoluminal radiofrequency e.
monopolar radiofrequency e.

electrocerebral silence (ECS)
electrocoagulation
intraluminal e.

electroconvulsive therapy
electrode
e. array
EHT e.
esophageal pill e.

Medelec DMG 50 Teflon-coated
  monopolar e.
e. monitoring
monopolar e.
MRI-compatible e.
patch e.
polarographic needle e.
subcutaneous array e.

electrodesiccation
electrodiagnosis
electrodiagnostic imaging
electroencephalogram (EEG)
flat e.
isoelectric e.

electroencephalograph (EEG)
Nihon Kohden Neurofax e.

electroencephalography (EEG)
intracranial e.
quantitative e. (QEEG)

electrogastrogram (EGG)
electrogastrograph
electrogram
atrial e.
coronary sinus e.
esophageal e.
high right atrial e.
His bundle e. (HBE)
intraatrial e.
intracardiac e.
right ventricular apical e.
RVA e.
sinus node e.

electrography
electrohydraulic
e. disintegrator
e. fragmentation
e. lithotripsy (EHL)
e. probe
e. shock wave lithotripsy (ESWL)

electrohydrothermal (EHT)
electrohysterogram
electrohysterography
electrokymogram (EKY)
electrokymograph
electroluminescent sensitometer
electrolytic reduction
electromagnet
structured coil e.

electromagnetic
e. absorption
e. articulography (EMA)
e. blood flow imaging
e. blood flow study
e. energy
e. flow probe
e. focusing field (EFF)
e. induction
e. interference (EMI)
e. interference scan

E

electromagnetic (*continued*)
  e. modeling
  e. navigation
  e. position sensor
  e. radiation
  e. radiation exposure
  e. unit (emu, EMU)
  e. wave
electromagnetism
electromechanical dissociation (EMD)
electrometer
  dynamic condenser e.
  vibrating-reed e.
electromotive force
electromyogram (EMG)
electromyography (EMG)
electron
  e. arc therapy
  Auger e.
  backscatter e.
  e. beam
  e. beam angiography (EBA)
  e. beam boost
  e. beam computed tomography (EBCT)
  e. beam CT-derived CAC score
  e. beam CT scanner
  e. beam electroreflectance (EBER)
  e. beam intraoperative radiation
    therapy
  e. beam intraoperative radiotherapy
    (EBIORT)
  e. beam tomography (EBT)
  e. binding energy
  e. bolus
  bound e.
  e. capture
  e. cloud
  Compton e.
  conversion e.
  e. diffraction camera
  e. dosimetry
  emission e.
  e. equilibrium loss
  excited e.
  e. flow
  e. flux
  free e.
  e. gun
  internal conversion e.
  K e.
  L e.
  e. linear accelerator
  e. magneton
  e. microscopy
  e. multiplier tube
  e. neutrino
  e. orbit
  orbital e.
  oscillating e.

  e. paramagnetic resonance (EPR)
  e. paramagnetic resonance spatial
    imaging
  positive e.
  e. radiography
  e. radiography imaging
  recoil e.
  secondary e.
  e. spin
  e. spin resonance (ESR)
  e. stream
  e. theory
  e. time-of-flight (E-TOF)
  transition e.
  valence e.
  e. valence
  e. volt (eV)
electron-beam
electron-capture decay mode
electron-dense
electroneuromyography
electroneuronography (ENoG)
electronic
  e. atlas of hippocampus
  e. cleansing
  e. collimation
  e. dosimeter
  e. focusing field
  e. independent beam steering
  e. linear-array transducer
  e. magnification
  e. microanalyzer (EMA)
  e. picture acquisition
  e. portal imaging
  e. stabilization
electron-photon field matching
electron-positron pair
electron-volt
electrooculogram apparatus
electrooculographic analysis
electrooptical device
electropherogram
electrophilic radioiodination
electrophysiologic mapping
electrophysiology (EP)
electropolished stent
electroradiology
electroradiometer
electroreflectance
  electron beam e. (EBER)
electroretinogram (ERG)
  flicker e.
electroscope
electrospray ionization mass spectroscopy
electrostatic
  e. generator
  e. imaging
  e. imaging system
  e. potential

electrothermal catheter
electrovectorcardiogram
electrovectorcardiography
Elema roll-film changer
element
    blowout lesion of posterior vertebral e.
    daughter e.
    estrogen-response e. (ERE)
    fibroglandular e.
    infiltrative hemorrhagic e.
    inflammatory e.
    neoplastic destruction of spinal e.
    paramagnetic trace e.
    parent e.
    picture e. (pixel)
    radioactive e.
    resolution e.
    e. subluxation
    volume e. (voxel)
elementary
    e. body
    e. fracture
2-element phased-array coil
4-element phased-array coil
element-specific detector
elephant
    e. ears pelvis
    e. trunk aortic graft technique
    e. trunk graft
elephantiasis neuromatosa
elevated
    e. diaphragm
    e. gradient
    e. leg support
    e. lower esophageal sphincter resting
      pressure
    e. retinal hamartoma
elevation
    bilateral diaphragmatic e.
    chorioamnionic e.
    diaphragmatic e.
    periosteal e.
    unilateral diaphragmatic e.
elevatus
    hallux e.
ELF
    extremely low frequency
elimination
    e. curve
    e. half-life
    e. kinetics
    pyelography by e.
elite
    VasoSeal E.
Ellestad protocol
ellipsoid, ellipsoidal
    e. joint
    e. lesion
    e. method

ellipsoidal (*var. of* ellipsoid)
elliptic, elliptical
    e. centric acquisition
    e. centric time-resolved imaging of
      contrast kinetics
    e. lumen
elliptical (*var. of* elliptic)
ellipticity index
Ellis
    E. Jones peroneal displacement
    E. line
    E. technique for Barton fracture
Ellis-Garland line
Ellis-van Creveld syndrome
EL2-LS2 flexible videolaparoscope
Eloesser procedure
elongated
    e. aorta
    e. heart
    e. mass
    e. structure
elongation
    e. and tortuosity
    aortic e.
    e. of ventricle
eloquent
    e. area of brain
    e. cortex
ELPS
    excessive lateral pressure
    syndrome
Elscint
    E. Apex 409-AG ECT camera
    E. Apex 009 Precursor camera
    E. dual-detector cardiac camera
    E. Dual-Head Helix camera
    E. Excel 905 scanner
    E. MR scanner
    E. Prestige MRI system
    E. Twin CT scanner
EL2-TF410 laparoscope
elute
elution, elutriation
elutriation (*var. of* elution)
ELVT
    endolaser venous therapy
EMA
    electromagnetic articulography
    electronic microanalyzer
emanation
    actinium e.
    radium e.
    thorium e.
emanatorium
emanon
emanotherapy
embarrassment
    circulatory e.
    cord e.

E

embarrassment (*continued*)
    nerve root e.
    respiratory e.
Embden-Meyerhof glycolytic pathway
embedding of stent coil
Emblocker technology
EmboGold microsphere
embolectomy
    percutaneous e.
emboli (*pl. of* embolus)
embolic
    e. aneurysm
    e. cerebral infarct
    e. debris
    e. event
    e. material
    e. necrosis
    e. obstruction
    e. occlusion
    e. phenomenon
    e. pneumonia
    e. shower
    e. stroke
embolism
    cerebral e.
    coronary e.
    nonthrombotic pulmonary e.
    pulmonary cement e.
    thrombotic pulmonary e.
    venography-related air e.
    venous e.
embolization
    bronchial artery e. (BAE)
    coil e.
    distal e.
    fibroid e.
    Guglielmi detachable coil e.
    Lipiodol e.
    N-butyl-2-cyanoacrylate e.
    nontarget e.
    ovarian vein e.
    paradoxic e.
    particulate arterial e.
    platinum coil e.
    polyvinyl alcohol particle e.
    pulmonary artery e.
    SAP-MS transarterial e.
    spontaneous hemodialysis catheter
      fracture and e.
    testicular vein e.
    transcatheter arterial e.
      (TAE)
    e. transcatheter therapy
    transhepatic variceal e.
    uterine artery e. (UAE)
    uterine fibroid e. (UFE)
embolotherapy
    bronchial e.
    percutaneous e.

embolus, *pl.* **emboli**
    air e.
    amnionic fluid e.
    arterial e.
    atheromatous e.
    bacillary e.
    bile pulmonary e.
    bland e.
    bone marrow e.
    cancer e.
    capillary e.
    cardiogenic e.
    catheter-induced e.
    cellular e.
    cement e.
    cerebral fat e.
    cholesterol e.
    coronary artery e.
    cotton fiber e.
    crossed e.
    direct e.
    fat e.
    fibrin platelet e.
    foam e.
    foreign body e.
    hematogenous e.
    infective e.
    intracranial e.
    intraluminal e.
    lipid e.
    lymphogenous e.
    massive e.
    e. migration
    miliary e.
    multiple emboli
    obturating e.
    occluding spring e.
    oil e.
    pantaloon e.
    paradoxic cerebral e.
    peripheral e.
    plasmodium e.
    platelet fibrin e.
    polyurethane foam e.
    prosthetic valve e.
    pulmonary e. (PE)
    pulmonary tumor e.
    pulmonary venous-systemic air e.
    pyemic e.
    recurrent e.
    renal cholesterol e.
    retinal e.
    retrograde e.
    riding e.
    saddle e.
    septic e.
    septic pulmonary e.
    silent cerebral e.
    straddling e.

submassive pulmonary e.
therapeutic e.
thrombus e.
trichinous e.
tumor e.
venous thrombosis e.
visceral e.

Embosphere
E. microsphere
E. particle

embryo
adnexal e.
e. demise
e. size

embryogenesis
embryoid body
embryology
airway e.
breast e.
diaphragm e.
genital tract e.
reproductive tract e.
urogenital e.

embryonal
e. adenoma
e. carcinosarcoma
e. cell carcinoma
e. liver sarcoma
e. ovary teratoma
e. rhabdomyosarcoma
e. tumor
e. vein

embryonic
e. abdominal cavity
e. anastomosis
e. aortic arch
e. branchial arch
e. disc
e. organizer
e. ovary
e. period
e. sac
e. truncus arteriosus
e. tumor
e. umbilical vein

embryopathy
warfarin e.

embryotoxon
posterior e.

EMD
electromechanical dissociation

eMed scanner
emetic center
EMF
endomyocardial fibrosis

EMG
electromyogram
electromyography
Neuropack 4, 8 EMG

EMI
electromagnetic interference
EMI brain scanner
EMI CT 500 scanner
EMI scan
EMI 7070 scanner
EMI unit

eminence
arcuate e.
articular e.
collateral e.
cruciate e.
cruciform e.
deltoid e.
facial e.
frontal e.
genital e.
hypothenar e.
iliopectineal e.
iliopubic e.
intercondylar e.
malar e.
medial e.
occipital e.
parietal e.
pyramidal e.
thenar e.
thyroid e.
tibial intercondylar e.

emissary
e. sphenoidal foramen
e. vein

emission
e. and transmission data
e. angiography
beta e.
characteristic e.
e. computed tomography (ECT)
e. computer-assisted tomography
e. computerized axial tomography (ECAT)
double e.
e. electron
filament e.
gamma e.
e. hepatogram
induced acoustic e.
negatron e.
photoelectric e.
e. probability
radioactive e.
e. range
e. renography
source of e.
spectral e.
stimulated acoustic e. (SAE)
thermonic e.
e. tomography

E

emitter
- alpha-particle e.
- Auger electron e.
- beta e.
- gamma e.
- e. grid

EMP
- extramedullary plasmacytoma

emphysema
- acquired lobar e.
- alveolar duct e.
- atrophic e.
- bronchiolar e.
- bullous e.
- centriacinar e.
- centrilobular e.
- chronic hypertrophic e.
- chronic obstructive e.
- chronic pulmonary e. (CPE)
- chronic tuberculous e.
- compensatory e.
- congenital lobar e. (CLE)
- cystic pulmonary e.
- diffuse e.
- distal acinar e.
- distal lobular e.
- ectatic e.
- false e.
- focal dust e.
- gangrenous e.
- gastric e.
- generalized e.
- giant bullous e.
- glass blower's e.
- hypoplastic e.
- idiopathic unilobar e.
- increased markings of e.
- infantile lobar e.
- interlobular e.
- interstitial intestinal e.
- interstitial lung e.
- intestinal e.
- intramural gastric e.
- irregular e.
- linear e.
- liquefactive e.
- lobar e.
- localized obstructive e.
- lung e.
- mediastinal e.
- neck e.
- necrotizing e.
- neonatal cystic pulmonary e.
- obstructive e.
- orbital e.
- oxygen-dependent e.
- panacinar e.
- panlobular e.
- paracicatrial e.

- paraseptal e.
- pericicatricial e.
- perifocal e.
- postoperative e.
- postsurgical e.
- proximal acinar e.
- pulmonary interstitial e. (PIE)
- pulmonary subcutaneous encephalitis e.
- restrictive pulmonary e.
- scar e.
- senile e.
- skeletal e.
- small-lunged e.
- subcutaneous e.
- subpleural e.
- surgical e.
- traumatic e.
- unilateral lobar e.
- unilateral obstructive e.
- vesicular e.

emphysematosa
- vaginitis e.

emphysematous
- e. bleb
- e. bulla
- e. cholecystitis
- e. COPD
- e. cystitis
- e. enterocolitis
- e. expansion
- e. gastritis
- e. lung
- e. pyelitis
- e. pyelonephritis (EPN)

empirical method

empty
- e. collapsed lung
- e. delta sign
- e. gestational sac
- e. heart
- e. sella
- e. sella syndrome
- e. uterus
- e. vertebral body

emptying
- complete bladder e.
- delayed gastric e.
- dual-phase gastric e.
- gastric e.
- incomplete bladder e.
- oropharyngeal e.
- rapid gastric e.
- e. time
- tortuous e.

empyema
- brain e.
- chest e.
- CNS e.
- epidural e.

gallbladder e.
Hawkins accordion-type e.
interlobar e.
intracranial e.
latent e.
left-sided e.
loculated e.
metapneumonic e.
paraspinal e.
pericardial e.
pleural e.
pulsating e.
right-sided e.
spinal e.
subdural e.
synpneumonic e.
thoracic e.
tuberculous e.

E-MRI
extremity magnetic resonance imaging
extremity MRI

emu, EMU
electromagnetic unit

emulsion
e. film
nuclear e.

Emulsoil bowel preparation

en
e. bloc excision
e. bloc resection
e. face
e. face view
e. passage feeder artery

enalaprilat

enalaprilat-enhanced renography

enamel
e. crypt
e. lamella

enantiomer

enarthrosis

encapsulated
e. brain abscess
e. fat-containing lesion
e. fat necrosis
e. fluid
e. gas bubble
e. mass
e. neoplasia
e. radioactive seed
e. subdural hematoma

encased heart

encasement
vascular e.
ventricular e.

encephali
arachnoidea mater e.

encephalic
e. angioma
e. vesicle

encephalitides (*pl. of* encephalitis)

encephalitis, *pl.* **encephalitides**
adult herpes e.
brainstem e.
bronzed sclerosing e.
CMV e.
cytomegalovirus e.
herpes simplex virus type 1 e.
HIV-associated e.
HSV1 e.
Japanese e.
Listeria e.
paraneoplastic e.
e. periaxialis concentrica
postinfectious e.
primary HIV e.
Rasmussen e.
Russian spring-summer e.
subacute e.
toxoplasmosis e.

encephaloarteriography

encephalocele
frontoethmoidal e.
frontosphenoidal e.
occipital e.
parietal e.
sphenoethmoidal e.
sphenoid e.
sphenomaxillary e.
sphenoorbital e.
sphenopharyngeal e.
transethmoidal e.

encephaloclastic
e. lesion
e. porencephaly

encephalocystocele

encephaloduroarteriomyosynangiosis (EDAMS)

encephaloduroarteriosynangiosis (EDAS)

encephalodysplasia

encephalogram

encephalograph

encephalography
air e.
A-mode e.
fractional e.
gamma e.
positive contrast e.

encephaloid carcinoma

encephalolith

encephaloma

encephalomalacia
inherited cavernous angioma-related
posthemorrhage e.
macrocystic e.
microcystic e.
multicystic e.
neonate e.

encephalomeningocele

E

encephalometry
encephalomyelitis
    acute disseminated e. (ADEM)
    enteroviral e.
    postinfectious e. (PIE)
encephalomyelopathy
    subacute necrotizing e.
encephalomyopathy
    mitochondrial e.
encephalopathia (*var. of* encephalopathy)
    e. subcorticalis progressiva
encephalopathy, encephalopathia
    AIDS e.
    anoxic e.
    Binswanger e.
    hepatic e.
    HIV-associated e.
    hypertensive e.
    hypoxic ischemic e.
    ischemic e.
    lead e.
    neonatal e.
    nonhypoxic ischemic e.
    prenatal hypoxic
      ischemic e.
    progressive subcortical e.
    subcortical arteriosclerotic e.
    subcortical atherosclerotic e.
    Wernicke e.
encephalotrigeminal
    e. angiomatosis
    e. syndrome
encerclage
enchondral
    e. bone formation
    e. ossification
enchondroma, endochondroma, *pl.*
  enchondromata
enchondromata (*pl. of* enchondroma)
enchondromatosis
    multiple e.
enchondrosarcoma
encoded
    e. Fourier
    sensitivity e. (SENSE)
encoding
    amplitude of phase e.
    centrally ordered phase e.
    coil-sensitive e.
    1-dimensional phase e.
    3D spatial e.
    frequency e.
    gradient e.
    ordered phase e.
    phase e.
    position e.
    reordering of phase e.
    respiratory ordered phase e.
      (ROPE)

    respiratory sorted phase e.
    sensitivity e. (SENSE)
    spatial e.
    wavelet e.
encroaching endothelial cell
encroachment
    bony e.
    foraminal e.
    luminal e.
    soft tissue canal e.
    stenosis e.
encrustation
    bile e.
encysted
    e. calculus
    e. pleurisy
end
    bone e.
    e. bud
    e. bulb
    e. exhalation
    e. expiration
    fimbriated e.
    e. inhalation
    e. of atrial systole
    e. of saturated bombardment
      (EOSB)
    seen on e.
endarterectomy
    carotid e. (CEA)
    extraluminal e.
    femoral e.
    e. graft
    surgical e.
    transluminal e.
endarteritis obliterans
end-diastole
end-diastolic
    e.-d. aortic-left ventricular pressure
      gradient
    e.-d. diameter
    e.-d. imaging
    e.-d. polar map
    e.-d. pressure-volume relation
    e.-d. velocity measurement
    e.-d. volume
    e.-d. volume index
Endeavor drug-eluting stent
end-expiratory lung volume
endfire transducer
endhole introducer
endoanal
    e. coil
    e. MR imaging
    e. sonography
    e. ultrasound
Endobile
endobiliary stenting
EndoBlade

endobrachyesophagus
endobronchial
    e. anaplastic plasmacytoma
    e. carcinoid
    e. carcinoma
    e. hamartoma
    e. Kaposi sarcoma
    e. lesion
    e. mass
    e. metastasis
    e. obstruction
    e. sarcoidosis
    e. tube
    e. tuberculosis
    e. tumor
endocardia (*pl. of* endocardium)
endocardial
    e. activation mapping
    e. biopsy
    e. catheter mapping
    e. centroid
    e. cushion
    e. cushion defect (ECD)
    e. cushion development
    e. cushion malformation
    e. cushion ventricular septal defect
    e. dysplasia
    e. fibroelastosis
    e. fibrosis
    e. plaque
    e. pressure
    e. sclerosis
    e. trabeculation
    e. volume
endocarditis
    aortic valve e.
    atypical verrucous e.
    bacterial e.
    Löffler fibroplastic e.
    marantic e.
    subacute bacterial e.
    thrombotic e.
endocardium, *pl.* **endocardia**
    disc of e.
    wafer of e.
endocatheter ruler
endocavitary coil
endocervical
    e. canal
    e. canal colonoscopy
    e. mucosa
endochondral
    e. bone
    e. bone deposit
endochondroma (*var. of* enchondroma)
endocranium
endocrine
    e. ablative therapy
    e. gland

    e. gland scintigraphy
    e. imaging
    e. tumor
endocyst
endodermal, endodermic
    e. cyst
    e. pouch
    e. sinus
    e. sinus ovarian tumor
    e. sinus testis tumor
endodermic (*var. of* endodermal)
endodiascope
endodiascopy
endoergic reaction
endoesophageal MRI coil
endofluoroscopic technique
endofluoroscopy
    flexible e.
    percutaneous e.
    rigid e.
endogenic (*var. of* endogenous)
endogenous, endogenic
    e. adenosine contrast
      medium
    e. callus formation
    e. contrast agent
    e. lipid pneumonia
Endografin
endograft
    AneuRx e.
endografting
    transluminal e.
**endolaser venous therapy
  (ELVT)**
endoleak
    e. graft
    type I e. (T1EL)
    type II e. (T2EL)
    type III e. (T3EL)
    type IV e. (T4EL)
endoluminal
    e. density
    e. fly-through
    e. MRI
    e. radiofrequency electrocautery
    e. sonography
    e. view
    e. visualization
endolymphatic
    e. duct
    e. hydrops
    e. sac
    e. sac tumor
    e. stromal myosis
endometria (*pl. of* endometrium)
endometrial
    e. adenoacanthoma
    e. anatomy
    e. atrophy

E

endometrial (*continued*)
    e. canal fluid
    e. carcinoma
    e. cavity
    e. cyst
    e. echo
    e. fluid in canal
    e. hyperplasia
    e. implant
    e. island
    e. polyp
    e. secretory adenocarcinoma
    e. stripe
    e. stromal sarcoma
    e. surface deformity
    e. thickness
endometrioid
    e. cystadenoma
    e. ovarian carcinoma
    e. tumor
endometrioma
endometriosis
    bladder e.
    colonic involvement of e.
    GI tract e.
    gynecologic e.
    e. interna
    sciatic e.
    ureteral e.
endometriotic cyst
endometritis
    inflammatory e.
endometrium, *pl.* **endometria**
    decidualized e.
    FIGO staging of adenocarcinoma of
      e.
    inactive e.
    postmenopausal e.
    proliferative-phase e.
    secretory-phase e.
    thickened irregular e.
endometry
endomotorsonde
endomyelography
endomyocardial
    e. biopsy
    e. fibroplasia
    e. fibrosis (EMF)
endoneural
endoneurium
endoneurosonography
end-on vessel
endopelvic fascia
endophlebitis
Endo-P-Probe
endoprobe
    rotating e.
    single-crystal e.
endoprostheses (*pl. of* endoprosthesis)

endoprosthesis, *pl.* **endoprostheses**
    biliary e.
    Carey-Coons soft-stent biliary e.
    constrained Wallgraft e.
    double-lumen e.
    double-pigtail e.
    Hemobahn e.
    IntraCoil e.
    large-bore bile duct e.
    metallic biliary e.
    self-expanding metallic e.
    Viabahn e.
    Viabil biliary e.
    Viatorr e.
    Wallgraft e.
    Wallstent biliary e.
endopyelotomy
    percutaneous e.
endorectal
    e. coil
    e. coil magnetic resonance imaging
      (erMRI)
    e. ileal pouch
    e. surface-coil MR imaging
    e. ultrasonography
    e. ultrasound (ERU, ERUS)
end-organ
    e.-o. resistance
    e.-o. response
endosaccular packing
endosalpingosis
endoscope
    double-channel e.
    light-induced fluorescence e.
    Olympus EVIS Q-200V e.
    Olympus TJF-100 e.
    virtual e.
    Zeiss EndoLive e.
endoscopic
    e. coronary artery bypass graft
      (E-CABG)
    e. decompression
    e. laser
    e. laser cholecystectomy
    e. laser dacryocystorhinostomy
    e. lithotripsy
    e. optical coherence tomography
      (EOCT)
    e. papillotomy
    e. percutaneous
      cholangiopancreatography
    e. procedure
    e. quadrature radiofrequency coil
    e. retrograde cholangiogram (ERC)
    e. retrograde cholangiography (ERC)
    e. retrograde
      cholangiopancreatography (ERCP)
    e. retrograde pancreatic duct
      cannulation

e. retrograde pancreatography
e. retrograde parenchymography
(ERP)
e. sonography
e. surveillance
e. ultrasound (EUS)
e. ultrasound-guided fine-needle
aspiration (EUS-FNA)
e. variceal sclerosis (EVS)
e. washing pipe

endoscopy
capsule e.
colorectal cancer e.
digital high-speed e.
gastrointestinal e.
intraoperative e.
laser-assisted spinal e. (LASE)
M2A imaging capsule e.
percutaneous e.
upper gastrointestinal e.
velolaryngeal e.
virtual e. (VE)
virtual arterial e.
wireless capsule e.

endoskeleton
endosonographic image
endosonography
3D e.
hydrogen peroxide-enhanced
anal e.
rectal e.
transduodenal e.
transgastric e.
vaginal e.

endosonoscopy
**Endosound endoscopic ultrasound
catheter**
endosseous implant
Endostaple device
⌐ **endosteal** ➤
e. callus
e. chondrosarcoma
e. revascularization
e. scalloping
e. surface

endosteoma
endosteum
endothelia (*pl. of* endothelium)
endothelial
e. damage
e. growth factor
e. hypoplasia
e. injury
e. leukocyte
e. myeloma
e. surface

endothelialization
endothelialized vascular graft
endotheliomatous meningioma

endothelium, *pl.* **endothelia**
arterial e.
capillary e.
pulmonary capillary e.

endothoracic fascia
endothorax
tension e.

endotracheal (ET)
e. intubation
e. tube (ETT)

endovaginal
e. coil
e. sonography
e. ultrasonography
e. ultrasound (EVUS)

endovascular
e. aneurysm repair (EVAR)
e. aortic graft
e. brachytherapy
e. coil
e. embolization femoral approach
e. exclusion
e. flow wire study
e. photoacoustic recanalization
(EPAR)
e. stent graft
e. system
e. technique
e. ultrasonography
e. ultrasound

EndoVasix EPAR laser system
**endovenous laser treatment
(EVLT)**
end-plate (*var. of* endplate)
endplate, end-plate
cartilage e.
cartilaginous e.
hyaline cartilage e.
e. sclerosis
vertebral body e.

endpoint
clear e.
exercise e.
measurable e.
stress e.

end-pressure artifact
endstage
e. adult cardiac decompensation
e. cardiomyopathy
e. cirrhosis
e. fetal cardiac decompensation
e. liver disease
e. lung
e. lung disease
e. renal disease
e. renal failure (ESRF)

end-systole
left ventricular internal dimension at
e.-s. (LVIDs)

E

end-systolic
- e.-s. diameter
- e.-s. polar map
- e.-s. pressure (ESP)
- e.-s. pressure to end-systolic volume (ESP/ESV)
- e.-s. pressure-volume relation
- e.-s. residual volume
- e.-s. reversal
- e.-s. volume (ESV)
- e.-s. volume index (ESVI)
- e.-s. wall index
- e.-s. wall index to end-systolic volume ratio

end-to-end anastomosis

end-to-side biliary-enteric anastomosis

endviewing transducer

Enecat CT concentrated rectal suspension

enema
- air-contrast barium e. (ACBE)
- analeptic e.
- barium e. (BE)
- blind e.
- cleansing e.
- contrast e.
- Cortenema retention e.
- double-contrast barium e. (DCBE)
- full-column barium e.
- Gastrografin e.
- Harris flush e.
- hydrocortisone e.
- hydrogen peroxide e.
- Hypaque e.
- hypertonic e.
- mesalamine e.
- methylene blue e.
- nuclear e.
- oil-retention e. (ORE)
- opaque e.
- phosphate e.
- Phospho-Soda e.
- retention e.
- Rowasa e.
- saline e.
- self-administered cleansing e.
- single-contrast barium e.
- small bowel e.
- soapsuds e.
- tap water e.
- therapeutic barium e.
- e.'s until clear
- water-soluble contrast e.

energetic positron

energy
- e. analysis
- atomic e.
- average positron e.
- beam e.
- binding e.
- chemical potential e.
- e. decay
- electrical potential e.
- electromagnetic e.
- electron binding e.
- e. fluence
- e. flux density
- e. frequency
- gravitational potential e.
- kinetic e.
- laser e.
- e. level
- e. level diagram (ELD)
- low-photon e.
- mechanical potential e.
- nuclear e.
- photon e.
- potential e.
- quadrant e.
- quantum e.
- radiant e.
- radiation e.
- radiofrequency e.
- recoil e.
- e. resolution
- e. spectrum
- e. subtraction
- thermal e.
- e. transfer
- e. transfer process
- treatment e.
- variable e.
- e. wave
- e. wavelength
- e. window
- x-ray e.

energy-dispersive x-ray fluorescence (EDXRF)

enforcer
- Cook e.

Engel alkalinity

Engelmann
- E. disc
- E. disease

engine
- Kodak Mammography CAD e.

engorged
- e. collateral venous channel
- e. tissue
- e. vein

engraftment
- cell e.

enhanced
- e. CT
- e. CT scan

e. fast gradient echo
e. glycolysis
e. imaging

enhancement

absolute percentage loss of e. (APLE)
acoustic e.
artery-like pattern of e.
benign postoperative meningeal e.
bolus contrast e.
bright contrast e.
cocurrent flow-related e.
contrast e.
countercurrent flow-related e.
Doppler flow signal e.
dural e.
dynamic e.
echo e.
edge e.
evanescent e.
exercise-induced contrast e.
e. factor
fast low-angle acquisition with
    relaxation e. (FLARE)
flip-flop e.
flow-related e.
focal nodular e.
gadolinium e.
gyral brain e.
heterogeneous isodense e.
homogeneous e.
hybrid rapid acquisition with
    relaxation e. (HRARE)
inhomogeneous contrast e.
inhomogeneous moderate e.
internal e.
isodense e.
meningeal e.
microbubble contrast e.
e. morphology
multislice flow-related e.
nodular e.
nonhomogeneous e.
nuclear magnetic resonance
    relaxation rate e.
paradoxic e.
paramagnetic contrast e.
parenchymatous e.
e. pattern (type I-IV)
peak of maximum e. (PME)
peripheral lesion e.
peritoneal e.
peritumoral e.
portal vein e.
posterior acoustic e.
proton relaxation e. (PRE)
pulmonary nodule e.
punctate e.
radiation e.

rapid acquisition with relaxation e.
    (RARE)
real-time e.
rim e.
ring e.
scan with contrast e.
serpentine e.
signal e.
sulcal e.
temporal peritumoral e.
time-of-flight e.
transient peritumoral e.
vascular MR contrast e.

enhancer

echo e.
pulmonary stable echo e.
vein contrast e. (VCE)

enhancing

e. brain lesion
e. mass
e. nodule
e. septum
e. ventricular margin

enlarged

e. cardiac silhouette
e. frontal horn
e. gallbladder
e. heart
e. kidney
e. liver
e. presacral space
e. pulmonary vessel
e. thyroid gland
e. vascular channel
e. vertebral foramen
e. vestibular vascular aqueduct
    syndrome

enlargement

airspace e.
azygos vein e.
bilateral hilar e.
bilateral pulmonary artery e.
biventricular e.
bony e.
bulbous e.
cardiac silhouette e.
cervical e.
chamber e.
compensatory e.
diffuse adrenal e.
diffuse hepatic e.
diffuse liver e.
diffuse thymic e.
diffuse uterine e.
epiglottic e.
extraocular muscle e.
gastric fold e.
global renal e.

E

enlargement (*continued*)
    iliopsoas compartment e.
    left atrial e. (LAE)
    lymph node e.
    masseteric e.
    mediastinal lymph node e.
    e. of epididymis
    e. of lacrimal gland
    e. of parotid gland
    e. of subarachnoid space
    e. of uterus
    e. of ventricle
    e. of vertebral body
    e. of vertebral foramen
    optic nerve e.
    panchamber e.
    papilla of Vater e.
    pituitary gland e.
    placenta e.
    right atrial e. (RAE)
    right ventricular e. (RVE)
    sella e.
    sulcal e.
    thymic e.
    unilateral hilar e.
    ventricular e.
    e. with low-density lymph node
        center
ENoG
    electroneuronography
enostosis
ensemble contrast imaging (ECI)
ensheathing callus
ensiform
    e. appendix
    e. cartilage
    e. process
ensisternum cartilage
EnSite 3000 imaging system
Entamoeba histolytica
eNTEGRA workstation
enteric
    e. coated (EC)
    e. drained pancreas transplant
    e. duplication cyst
    e. exocrine drainage
    e. fistula
    e. plexus
    e. stricture
enteritis
    Candida e.
    CMV e.
    Crohn granulomatous e.
    Crohn regional e.
    eosinophilic e.
    e. follicularis
    radiation e.
    regional e.
enterobiliary

enterocele sac
enterochromaffin cell
enterocleisis
enteroclysis
    computed tomographic e.
    CT e.
    helical CT e. (HCTE)
enterococci (*pl. of* enterococcus)
enterococcus, *pl.* **enterococci**
enterocolic fistula
enterocolitis
    emphysematous e.
    granulomatous e.
    Hirschsprung-associated e. (HAEC)
    necrotizing e.
    neutropenic e.
    Yersinia e.
enterocutaneous fistula
enterocystoma
enterocytic processing
enteroenteral fistula
enteroesophageal reflux
enterogenous cyst
enterography
    cross-sectional e.
enterohepatic
enteroinsular axis
enterolith
enteropathica
    acrodermatitis e.
enteropathy
    exudative e.
    gluten-sensitive e.
    protein-losing e.
    radiation e.
enteropathy-associated T-cell lymphoma
enteroperitoneal abscess
enteroptosia (*var. of* enteroptosis)
enteroptosis, enteroptosia
enteroscope
    Olympus SIF-100 video e.
    single-balloon e. (SBE)
enteroscopy
    small bowel e. (SBE)
    virtual e.
enterospinal fistula
enterostomal therapist
enterourethral fistula
enterovaginal fistula
enterovesical fistula
enteroviral encephalomyelitis
Entero Vu contrast medium
entertainment ultrasound
enthesis
enthesitis
enthesopathic transformation
enthesophyte
    plantar calcaneal e.
    subacromial e.

entity
    clinicoradiologic e.
    tumor e.
entorhinal cortex
entrance
    e. block
    e. skin exposure
entrapment
    artery e.
    gas e.
    guidewire e.
    lateral e.
    median nerve e.
    nerve e.
    e. neuropathy
    patellar e.
    popliteal e.
    posterior interosseous nerve e.
    scar tissue e.
    soft tissue e.
    suprascapular nerve e.
    ulnar nerve e.
entrapped
    e. ovarian cyst
    e. plantar sesamoid bone
EntroEase oral radiopaque contrast medium
entry
    capacitative calcium e. (CCE)
    e. flap
    e. point
    e. slice phenomenon artifact
    e. tear
    e. zone
enucleation
    globe e.
envelope
    capsuloperiosteal e.
    fascial e.
    soft tissue e.
    synovial e.
environment
    echo-poor area of e.
    high-tech low-touch examination e.
environmental
    e. factor
    e. plutonium
Envision CT power injector
Envoy guiding catheter
enzyme
    angiotensin-converting e.
    (ACE)
    e. replacement therapy
    e. supplementation therapy
enzyme-linked immunoabsorbent assay
enzyme-multiplied immunoassay technique
EOCT
    endoscopic optical coherence tomography

EORTC
    European Organization for Research and Treatment of Cancer
    EORTC criterion
EOSB
    end of saturated bombardment
eosinophilia
    simple pulmonary e.
    tumor-associated tissue e.
eosinophilic
    e. brain adenoma
    e. enteritis
    e. gastroenteritis
    e. granuloma
    e. infiltrate
    e. leukocyte
    e. lung disease
    e. pneumonia
Eovist contrast agent
EP
    electrophysiology
    HearTwave EP
epactal bone
EPAR
    endovascular photoacoustic recanalization
    EPAR laser system
eparterial bronchus
EPB
    extensor pollicis brevis
    EPB muscle
EPBF
    effective pulmonary blood flow
EPC
    echo phase correction
EP2000 electrophysiology imaging system
ependyma
ependymal cyst
ependymitis
    bacterial e.
    e. granularis
ependymoblastoma
ependymoma
    anaplastic e.
    brain e.
    brainstem e.
    e. cord
    intracranial e.
    intramedullary e.
    malignant e.
    myxopapillary e.
    spinal cord e.
    subcutaneous sacrococcygeal myxopapillary e.
ephemeral pneumonia
EPI
    echo-planar imaging
epiarticular osteochondromatous dysplasia
epiblast

E

315

epicardia (*pl. of* epicardium)
epicardial
    e. attachment
    e. centroid
    e. coronary artery
    e. Doppler echocardiography
    e. Doppler flow sector
      transducer
    e. fat-pad
    e. imaging
    e. implantation
    e. mapping
    e. pacemaker
    e. space
    e. surface
    e. tension
    e. volume
epicardium, *pl.* **epicardia**
epicenter
    eccentric e.
epicolic lymph node
epicondylar
    e. fracture
    e. fracture of humerus
    e. ridge
epicondyle
    humeral e.
    medial e.
epicondylitis
    lateral e.
    medial e.
epicondyloolecranon ligament
Epic ophthalmic 3-in-1 laser
epicortical lesion
epicranial aponeurosis
epidemiology
epidermal, epidermatic, epidermic
    e. carcinoma
    e. inclusion cyst
    e. ridge
epidermatic (*var. of* epidermal)
epidermic (*var. of* epidermal)
epidermoid
    acquired e.
    black e.
    cerebellar e.
    e. cyst
    e. lung carcinoma
    e. mass
    e. mediastinum
    e. spine
    e. tumor
    white e.
epidermoidoma
    incisural e.
    intradural e.
    prepontine white e.
epidermolysis
    e. bullosa, dermal type
    e. bullosa, epidermal type
    e. bullosa, junctional type
epididymal
    e. cyst
    e. descent
    e. fibrosarcoma
epididymides (*pl. of* epididymis)
epididymis, *pl.* **epididymides**
    appendix of e.
    body of e.
    edema of e.
    enlargement of e.
    inflammation of e.
    interstitial congestion of e.
    e. lesion
    ligament of e.
    lobule of e.
    postvasectomy change in e.
    sinus of e.
    tail of e.
epididymitis
epididymography imaging
epididymoorchitis
epididymovesiculography
epidural
    e. abscess
    e. angiolipoma
    e. anular fibrosis
    e. arachnoid cyst
    e. blood
    e. blood patch
    e. cavernous hemangioma
    e. cavity
    e. effusion
    e. empyema
    e. extramedullary lesion
    e. fat
    e. hematoma
    e. hemorrhage
    e. implant
    e. infection
    e. lipoma
    e. lipomatosis
    e. lymphoma
    e. mass
    e. pneumatosis
    e. saline infusion
    e. space
    e. steroid injection
    e. tumor
    e. venography
    e. venous plexus
epidurogram
epidurography
    magnetic resonance e.
epigastria (*pl. of* epigastrium)
epigastric
    e. angle
    e. fold

e. fossa
e. hernia
e. lymph node
e. vein
epigastrium, *pl.* **epigastria**
epiglottic, epiglottidean
    e. carcinoma
    e. cartilage
    e. disruption
    e. enlargement
    e. fold
    e. tubercle
epiglottidean (*var. of* epiglottic)
epiglottiditis (*var. of* epiglottitis)
epiglottitis, epiglottiditis
    bacterial e.
epignathus
epihyal
    e. bone
    e. ligament
epihyoid bone
epilarynx
EpiLaser
epilation dose
epilepsia (*var. of* epilepsy)
    e. partialis continua
epilepsy, epilepsia
    chronic partial e.
    drug-resistant extratemporal e.
    extratemporal e.
    grand mal e.
    idiopathic e.
    postcerebral infarction e.
    structural e.
    temporal lobe e. (TLE)
epileptic focus
epilepticus
    status e.
epileptogenic, epileptogenous
    e. center
    e. focus
    e. lesion
    e. zone
epileptogenous (*var. of* epileptogenic)
Epimed spring guide catheter
epipericardial ridge
epiphora
epiphrenic
    e. bulge
    e. diverticulum
epiphyseal (*var. of* epiphysial)
epiphyses (*pl. of* epiphysis)
epiphysial, epiphyseal
    e. arrest
    e. cartilage
    e. cartilage plate
    e. chondroblastic growth
    e. chondrocyte

e. coxa vara
e. disc
e. dysgenesis
e. dysostosis
e. dysplasia
e. exostosis
e. fetal bone center
e. growth plate
e. hemopoietic marrow
e. hyperplasia
e. hypertrophy
e. ischemic necrosis
e. line
e. ossification center
e. osteochondroma
e. overgrowth
e. plate fracture
e. plate injury
e. slip fracture
e. slippage
e. tibial fracture
epiphysiolysis
    femoral head e.
    idiopathic e.
    juvenile e.
epiphysis, *pl.* **epiphyses**
    anular e.
    atavistic e.
    e. avulsion
    ball-and-socket e.
    balloon e.
    e. bone
    bone lesion e.
    capital femoral e.
    capitular e.
    cartilaginous e.
    cone e.
    congenital stippled e.
    familial avascular necrosis of
      phalangeal e.
    femoral capital e.
    humeral e.
    ossifying e.
    osteochondral separation of e.
    Perthes e.
    pressure e.
    ring e.
    slipped capital femoral e.
      (SCFE)
    slipped upper femoral e. (SUFE)
    tibial e.
    traction e.
epiphysitis
    juvenile e.
    vertebral e.
epiploic
    e. appendage
    e. appendix
    e. foramen

epiploica, *pl.* epiploicae
  appendix e.
  appendices epiploicae
epiploicae (*pl. of* epiploica)
epipteric bone
epirenal septum
episcleral
  e. plaque brachytherapy
  e. space
  e. vein
episode
  ischemic e.
  mitochondrial encephalomyopathy
    with lactic acidosis and strokelike
    e. (MELAS)
  silent ischemic e.
epispadias-exstrophy complex
Epistar
  E. diode laser system
  E. perfusion technique
  E. subtraction angiography
epistaxis~ nose bleed
episternal bone
epitendineum, epitenon
epitenon (*var. of* epitendineum)
epithalamus
epithelia (*pl. of* epithelium)
epithelial
  e. cell
  e. colon
  e. colonic polyp
  e. degenerative change
  e. hyperplasia
  e. inclusion cyst
  e. malignancy
  e. neoplasia
  e. ovarian carcinoma
  e. spleen
  e. tumor
epithelialization, epithelization
  creeping e.
epithelial-myoepithelial carcinoma
epithelioid
  e. angiomatosis
  e. granuloma
  e. hemangioendothelioma
  e. hemangioma
  e. leiomyoma
  e. malignant mesothelioma
  e. osteosarcoma
  e. sarcoma
epithelioma
  calcifying Malherbe e.
epitheliosis
  infiltrating breast e.
epitheliotropism
epithelium, *pl.* epithelia
  atypical e.
  Barrett e.

blind sac e.
e. crypt
ductal e.
normal ovarian surface e. (NOSE)
papilla of columnar e.
squamous metaplasia with white e.
surface e.
tumor of surface e.
white e.
epithelization (*var. of* epithelialization)
epithermal neutron
EpiTouch laser
epitrochlear lymph node
epituberculous infiltrate
epitympanic
  e. recess
  e. space
epitympanum
EPL
  effective path length
  extensor pollicis longus
  EPL muscle
EPN
  emphysematous pyelonephritis
epoch
  VNS e.
eponychium
epoophoron
Eppendorf pO$_2$ histograph
EPR
  electron paramagnetic resonance
epsilon
  e. 2D and tissue velocity imaging
  TDE-derived epsilon (p) and e. (m)
EPSS
  E point to septal separation
Epstein-Barr virus (EBV)
EPT-Dx steerable diagnostic catheter
eptifibatide
epulofibroma
EQP
  extensor quinti proprius
equal in intensity
equalization
  histogram e.
  pressure e.
equalized diastolic pressure
equation
  Bernoulli e.
  bioheat e.
  Bloch e.
  Bohr e.
  Boltzmann e.
  Bragg e.
  Carter e.
  continuity e.
  decay e.
  Derenzo e.
  Doppler e.

Fick e.
hamiltonian e.
Kety e.
Larmor e.
modified Bernoulli e.
Nernst e.
Schroedinger e.
Solomon-Bloembergen e.
Stewart-Hamilton e.
Teichholz e.
tracer concentration e.
transformer e.
equilibration
equilibrium
e. dissociation constant
e. dose constant
e. factor
e. magnetization
e. MUGA imaging
e. MUGA scan
e. phase
e. point
radioactive e.
e. radionuclide angiocardiography
c. radionuclide angiocardiography
technique
e. radionuclide angiography
e. radionuclide ventriculography
secular e.
state of e.
thermal e.
transient e.
e. view
equina
cauda e.
nerve root of cauda e.
equinovalgus
e. deformity
pes e.
equinovarus
e. hindfoot deformity
pes e.
talipes e.
Equinox
E. balloon microcatheter
E. occlusion balloon
catheter
equinus
e. deformity
pes e.
equipment
e. artifact
Austin Medical E. (AME)
Digitron Koordinat angiography e.
Polytron DSA e.
RapidScreen RS-2000 x-ray e.
equivalence, equivalency
mass energy e.
equivalency (*var. of* equivalence)

equivalent
chance e.
dose e.
meconium ileus e.
total effective dose e. (TEDE)
total organ dose e. (TODE)
e. treatment
equivocal finding
^{171}Er
erbium 171
ER
estrogen-receptor
ER positive
Er
erbium
Er-171
erbium 171
erase
background e.
Erb
E. disease
E. injury
E. palsy
E. point
Erb-Duchenne-Klumpke injury
erbium (Er)
e. 171 (^{171}Er, Er-171)
e. chromium:yttrium-aluminum-garnet
(ErCr:YAG)
e. SilkLaser
erbium:YAG
erbium:yttrium-aluminum-garnet
erbium:YAG infrared laser
erbium:yttrium-aluminum-garnet
(erbium:YAG)
ERC
endoscopic retrograde cholangiogram
endoscopic retrograde
cholangiography
ERCP
endoscopic retrograde
cholangiopancreatography
ERCP catheter
ERCP imaging
ERCP manometry
ErCr:YAG
erbium
chromium:yttrium-aluminum-garnet
ErCr:YAG laser
Erdheim
E. cystic medial necrosis
E. tumor
Erdheim-Chester disease
ERE
estrogen-response element
external rotation in extension
erect
e. fluoro spot projection
e. lateral flexion-extension radiograph

erect (*continued*)
  e. position
  e. view
erector spinae
ERF
  edge response function
  external rotation in flexion
ERG
  electroretinogram
ergometer
  bicycle e.
  Cybex e.
  magnetic resonance-compatible pedal e.
ergonomics
  hands-up e.
ergotamine challenge
Erichsen sign
Erlenmeyer
  E. flask
  E. flask appearance
  E. flask-like deformity
erMRI
  endorectal coil magnetic resonance
  imaging
Ernst
  E. angle
  Kumar, Welti and E. (KWE)
erosion
  articular e.
  bony e.
  bronchial e.
  duodenal e.
  focal cartilage e.
  gastric antral e.
  graft-enteric e.
  infraspinatus insertion e.
  linear e.
  marginal e.
  mouse-ear e.
  odontoid e.
  e. of articular surface
  e. of epiphysial bone
  osteoclastic e.
  pedicle e.
  plaque e.
  pressure e.
  rat-bite e.
  salt-and-pepper duodenal e.
  stomach varioliform e.
  tumor e.
  varioliform e.
erosive
  e. duodenitis
  e. gastritis
  e. gingivitis
  e. mucocele
  e. osteoarthritis
ERP
  effective refractory period

endoscopic retrograde
  parenchymography
ERPF
  effective renal plasma flow
error
  ADC quantization e.
  analogue-to-digital conversion
    quantization e.
  CT imaging e.
  darkroom e.
  data clipping detection e.
  data spike detection e.
  e. diffusion method
  dorsal induction e.
  duplex ultrasound e.
  flow-related phase e.
  gating e.
  generalized compensation for
    resonance offset and pulse length
    e.'s (GROPE)
  Hausdorff e.
  interobserver e.
  intraobserver e.
  isocenter placement e.
  magnification e.
  measurement e.
  photoreceptor fractional
    velocity e.
  positioning e.
  preparation e.
  quantization e.
  random e.
  raster spacing e.
  relative e.
  sampling e.
  sensing e.
  size estimation e.
  spatial frequency e.
  systematic e.
  truncation e.
error-sum criterion
ERU, ERUS
  endorectal ultrasound
  gray-scale ERU
eruption
  rhythmic paradoxic e.
  violaceous presternal e.
ERUS
  endorectal ultrasound
ERV
  expiratory reserve volume
erythema
  e. dose
  e. of joint
  radiation e.
  e. threshold
erythematosus
  lupus e. (LE)
  systemic lupus e. (SLE)

erythrocyte
  e. iron turnover
  technetium 99m heat-denatured e.
erythropoietin
  e. assay
  e. bioassay
²⁵⁵Es
  einsteinium 255
Es
  einsteinium
Esaote extremity scanner
escalation
escape
  e. beat
  e. interval
  e. of air into lung connective tissue
escape-capture rhythm
escaped beat
escape-peak ratio
Escherichia coli
ESIN
  elastic stable intramedullary nailing
Esmarch bandage
EsophaCoil stent
esophageal
  e. achalasia pattern
  e. adenocarcinoma
  e. aperistalsis
  e. apple-core lesion
  e. atresia
  e. balloon technique
  e. body
  e. carcinoma
  e. carcinosarcoma
  e. choriocarcinoma
  e. contraction
  e. degeneration
  e. dilation
  e. displacement
  e. dissection
  e. diverticulum
  e. duplication
  e. duplication cyst
  e. dysmotility
  e. dysphagia
  e. electrogram
  e. fibroadenoma
  e. filling defect
  e. fold
  e. functional disorder
  e. function imaging
  e. graft
  e. groove
  e. hernia
  e. hiatus
  e. impression
  e. inflammation
  e. inlet
  e. lead

  e. leiomyoma
  e. leiomyomatosis
  e. leiomyosarcoma
  e. lipomatosis
  e. lumen
  e. manometry
  e. margin serration
  e. morphologic disorder
  e. motility
  e. motility disorder
  e. mucosal nodule
  e. mucosal ring
  e. muscular ring
  e. narrowing
  e. neoplasia
  e. obstruction
  e. obturator airway
  e. opening
  e. peptic stricture
  e. perforation
  e. peristalsis
  e. peristaltic pressure
  e. pill electrode
  e. plaque
  e. plexus
  e. pseudosarcoma
  e. reflux
  e. rupture
  e. shiver
  e. shunt
  e. spasm
  e. sphincter relaxation
  e. stenosis
  e. stent
  e. stricture
  e. tear
  e. transition zone
  e. transit time
  e. tumor
  e. ulcer
  e. variceal sclerosis
  e. varix
  e. vein
  e. vestibule
  e. web
  e. window
esophageal-pleural stripe
esophagectomy
  Ivor Lewis e.
  total thoracic e.
  transhiatal e.
  transthoracic e.
esophagi (*pl. of* esophagus)
esophagitis
  acute e.
  AIDS-related e.
  bile e.
  Candida e.
  caustic e.

E

esophagitis (*continued*)
    chronic e.
    corrosive e.
    cytomegalovirus e.
    drug-induced e.
    herpes e.
    HIV e.
    infectious e.
    peptic e.
    pill e.
    radiation e.
    reflux e. (RE)
    Sonnenberg classification of erosive e.
    stasis e.
    viral e.
esophagogastrectomy
esophagogastric
    e. fat-pad
    e. intubation
    e. junction
    e. orifice
    e. region
    e. tamponade
esophagogastroduodenoscopy
esophagogastrostomy
esophagogram (*var. of* esophagram)
esophagography
    double-contrast e.
    e. imaging
esophagojejunostomy
esophagorespiratory fistula
esophagoscopy
esophagospasm
esophagostomy
    cervical e.
    palliative e.
esophagotracheal fistula
esophagram, esophagogram
    air e.
    barium e.
    barium-water e.
    contrast e.
    drinking e.
    pullback e.
    radionuclide e.
esophagus, *pl.* **esophagi**
    abnormal peristaltic e.
    achalasia of e.
    A level of e.
    aperistaltic e.
    A ring of e.
    atonic e.
    Barrett e.
    bird-beak e.
    B level of e.
    B ring of e.
    cervical e.
    cobblestone appearance of e.
    columnar-lined e.

    congenitally short e.
    corkscrew appearance of e.
    curling e.
    diffuse dilation of e.
    diffuse spasm of e.
    dilated e.
    discrete segment of normal e.
    double-barrel e.
    double-ring e.
    dysmotile e.
    extrinsic impression of e.
    foamy e.
    foreign body in e.
    intramural rupture of e.
    long smooth narrowing e.
    middle 3rd of thoracic e.
    muscular ring e.
    nutcracker e.
    polypoid lesion of lower e.
    rat-tail e.
    rosary beading e.
    scleroderma of e.
    shaggy e.
    shish kabob e.
    short-segment Barrett e. (SSBE)
    spastic e.
    submerged segment of e.
    thoracic e.
    tortuous e.
    upper thoracic e.
    Z line of e.
ESP
    early systolic peak
    end-systolic pressure
e-speed EBT scanner
ESP/ESV
    end-systolic pressure to end-systolic volume
    ESP/ESV ratio
ESR
    electron spin resonance
ESRF
    endstage renal failure
essential
    e. osteolysis
    e. thrombocytosis
    e. tumor
Essex-Lopresti
    E.-L. calcaneal fracture classification
    E.-L. joint depression-type calcaneal fracture
    E.-L. lesion
ester
    iodipamide ethyl e.
esthesioneuroblastoma
esthesioneurocytoma
esthesioneuroepithelioma
estimated fetal weight (EFW)

estimation
> bayesian image e. (BIE)
> fractional moving blood volume e.
> frequency e.
> magnetic resonance volume e.
> stereologic method of volume e.
> volume e.

estradiol
> methoxy-17-alpha-iodvinyl e. (Z-MIVE)

estrogen-producing tumor

estrogen-receptor (ER)
> e.-r. positive

estrogen-response element (ERE)

estrone (E₁)

ESV
> end-systolic volume

ESVI
> end-systolic volume index

ESWL
> electrohydraulic shock wave
>   lithotripsy
> extracorporeal shock wave lithotripsy

ET
> endotracheal

etching
> track e.

ETF
> extension teardrop fracture

ethanol (EtOH)
> e. ablation
> e. injection

Ethiodane

ethiodized
> e. oil
> e. oil contrast medium

Ethiodol imaging agent

ethmocephalus (*var. of* ethmocephaly)

ethmocephaly, ethmocephalus

ethmoid
> e. air cell
> e. bone
> e. canal
> e. sinus
> e. sinus carcinoma

ethmoidal
> e. artery
> e. bulla
> e. crest
> e. foramen
> e. groove
> e. labyrinth
> e. meningoencephalocele
> e. notch
> e. process
> e. vein

ethmoidalis
> bulla e.

ethmoidolacrimal suture

ethmoidomaxillary suture

ethmovomerine plate

ethyl
> e. cysteinate dimer (ECD)
> ^{18}F-labeled polyfluorinated e.

ethylenediamine
> e. tetramethylene phosphonate
> e. tetramethylene phosphoric acid
>   (EDTMP)

ethylenedicysteine
> technetium 99m e. (^{99m}Tc EC,
>   Tc-99m EC)

ethylenedicysteine-folate
> technetium 99m e.-f. (^{99m}Tc
>   EC-folate, Tc-99m EC-folate)

ethyliodophenylundecyl contrast
  medium

etidronate
> e. disodium imaging agent
> ^{186}Re e.
> rhenium-186 e.
> technetium 99m e.

etiology
> fever of unknown e. (FUE)
> multifactorial e.

etiopathogenetic

etiopathology

ETL
> echo-train length

E-TOF
> electron time-of-flight
> E-TOF detecting module

E-to-F
> E-t.-F slope
> E-t.-F slope of valve

EtOH
> ethanol

ETT
> endotracheal tube
> exercise tolerance test

euchromatin

eukinesis

Euler number

EUP
> extrauterine pregnancy

Eureka collimator

European
> E. Association for Study of the
>   Liver
> E. Carotid Surgery Trial
> E. Organization for Research and
>   Treatment of Cancer (EORTC)

europium-activated barium fluorohalide

EUS
> endoscopic ultrasound
>   depth of tumor invasion assessed
>   by EUS

EUS-FNA
> endoscopic ultrasound-guided
> fine-needle aspiration

E

eustachian
    e. canal
    e. tonsil
    e. tube
    e. valve
euthyroid ophthalmopathy
eutopic
eV
    electron volt
ev3
    e. premounted balloon-expandable stent
    e. self-expanding stent
    e. unmounted balloon-expandable stent
Evac-Q-Kwik bowel preparation
evacuation
    colonic e.
    digital rectal e.
    e. disorder
    e. pouchography
    precipitate e.
    e. proctography
evaluation
    e. of glucose metabolism
    e. of mass mammography
    plaque e.
    shunt e.
evanescent enhancement
Evans
    E. blue albumin
    E. blue imaging agent
    E. intertrochanteric fracture classification
    E. ratio
Evans-D'Angio staging system
EVAR
    endovascular aneurysm repair
EVD
    external ventricular drain
even
    e. distribution of echoes
    e. distribution pattern
even-echo rephasing
event
    acute atherothrombotic e.
    cardiac e.
    cardinal e.
    cerebral ischemic e.
    coincidence e.
    e. counter
    embolic e.
    inciting e.
    ischemic e.
    main timing e. (MTE)
    major adverse cardiac e. (MACE)
    precipitating e.
    random coincidence e.

    scattered coincidence e.
    true e.
event-free survival
eventration
    diaphragmatic e.
    e. of diaphragm
event-related paradigm
everolimus
eversion
    cervical e.
    e. of ankle
    e. position
    e. sprain
eversion-external rotation deformity
evidence
    scintigraphic e.
EVLT
    endovenous laser treatment
    EVLT laser
evolution
    E. CT scanner
    stroke in e. (SIE)
    E. XP scanner
evolving
    e. hematoma
    e. myocardial infarct
EVS
    endoscopic variceal sclerosis
    EVS mechanical closure device
evulsion
EVUS
    endovaginal ultrasound
Ewald
    E. node
    E. test meal
Ewart sign
Ewing
    E. sarcoma
    E. sarcoma family of tumors
    E. sarcoma-Wilms tumor 1 (EWS-WT1)
EWS-WT1
    Ewing sarcoma-Wilms tumor 1
EX
    examination
    Filterwire EX
ex
    e. vacuo ventriculomegaly
    e. vivo magnetic resonance imaging
ExAblate 2000 ultrasound system
exacerbation
exact framing
exaggerated
    e. craniocaudal lateral (XCCL)
    e. craniocaudal view
exametazime
    e. imaging agent
    technetium 99m e.

examination (EX)
    barium followthrough e.
    contrast-enhanced radiographic e.
    Doppler venous e.
    double-contrast eversion e.
    double-contrast GI e.
    ^{67}Ga e.
    gated exercise e.
    gray-scale e.
    image-acquisition gated e.
    in vivo e.
    limited e.
    neuroradiologic e.
    postglucose loading e.
    proton brain e. (PROBE)
    reinjection thallium stress e.
    resting redistribution e.
    single-contrast GI e.
    single-voxel proton brain e.
    1-stop-shop e.
    1st-pass e.
    stress-gated blood pool cardiac e.
    stress-redistribution e.
    stress-rest reinjection e.
    suboptimal e.
    transcranial e.
    transforaminal e.
    unsuppressed e.
    venous Doppler e.
    volumetric interpolated breath-hold e.
    (VIBE)
    whole-body nuclear physical e.
    whole-body screening e.
excavation
    saucer-shaped e.
excavatum
    pectus e.
Excelart short-bore MRI
Excel-14 microcatheter
Excelsior microcatheter
excessive
    e. callus formation
    e. lateral pressure syndrome (ELPS)
exchange
    air e.
    coupling e.
    e. guidewire
    half-time of e.
    intestinal gas e.
    narrowing e.
    proton-proton magnetization e.
    pulmonary gas e.
    rapid e. (RX)
    spin e.
excimer
    e. laser
    e. laser coronary angioplasty
    e. laser system
    XeCl e.

excision
    CT-guided percutaneous e.
    en bloc e.
    large loop e.
    total mesorectal e.
excisional biopsy
excitation
    delay alternating with nutation for
      tailored e. (DANTE)
    fast acquisition multiple e. (FAME)
    e. function
    e. function measurement
    magnetization-prepared rapid gradient
      echo-water e. (MP-RAGE-WE)
    nonuniform e.
    number of e.'s (NEX)
    e. profile
    quadrature e.
    rebound e.
    selective e.
    slice-selective e.
    spatial and chemical-shift encoded
      e. (SPACE)
    e. spectrum
    supernormal e.
    tailored e.
    tilted optimized nonsaturating e.
      (TONE)
    uniform TR e.
    variable-angle uniform signal e.
      (VUSE)
    variable flip-angle e.
    volume-selective e.
    wave of e.
excitation-spoiled fat-suppressed
T1-weighted SE image
excitatory
    e. lesion
    e. neurotransmitter
    e. pulse characteristic
excited
    e. atom
    e. electron
    e. proton
excitotoxic
    e. cord injury
    e. mechanism
Excluder stent-graft
exclusion
    endovascular e.
    subtotal gastric e.
exclusion-HPLC technique
excrescence
    bony e.
    papillary e.
excrescentic thickening of optic nerve
excretion
    ammonium e.
    colonic mucosal e.

excretion (*continued*)
  contrast medium e.
  ^{67}Ga e.
  e. pyelography
  uptake and e.
  urinary e.
  e. urography
  vicarious contrast e.
excretory
  e. cystogram
  e. duct
  e. intravenous pyelography
  e. phase
  e. phase imaging
  e. urethrogram
  e. urogram
  e. urography imaging
excursion of diaphragm
exencephalia (*var. of* exencephaly)
exencephaly, exencephalia
exenteration
  anterior e.
  orbital e.
  pelvic e.
exercise
  e. echocardiography
  e. endpoint
  flexion and extension e.'s
  e. image
  e. index
  e. load
  e. LV function
  modified stage e.
  e. myocardial perfusion
    scintigraphy
  e. radionuclide angiocardiography
  e. radionuclide ventriculogram
  e. renography
  e. 1st-pass LVEF
  e. strain-gauge venous
    plethysmography
  e. stress redistribution
    scintigraphy
  e. thallium scintigraphy
  e. thallium-201 stress imaging
  e. thallium-201 tomography
  e. tolerance test (ETT)
exercise-induced
  e.-i. bronchoconstriction
  e.-i. contrast enhancement
  e.-i. renal failure
  e.-i. transient myocardial
    ischemia
exertion
  Borg scale of treadmill e.
exertional
  e. hypertension
  e. rhabdomyolysis
exfoliating tumor

exhalation
  end e.
exit
  e. block
  e. dose
  e. wound
Exner plexus
exocardia
**exoccipital part of occipital
  bone**
exoergic reaction
Exogen
  E. 2000+ low-intensity ultrasound
    fracture healing system
  E. 2000+ noninvasive ultrasound
    therapy
  E. 2000 SAFHS
exogenous
  e. glucose rate
  e. imaging
  e. invasion
  e. lipoid pneumonia
exon-specific primer pair
exophthalmic goiter
exophytic
  e. adenocarcinoma
  e. carcinoma
  e. fibroid
  e. mass
  e. neoplasia
  e. papilloma
exoskeleton
exostoses (*pl. of* exostosis)
exostosis, *pl.* **exostoses**
  blocker's e.
  bony e.
  cartilage-capped e.
  epiphysial e.
  hypertrophic e.
  impingement e.
  marginal e.
  osteocartilaginous e.
  pelvic e.
  retrocalcaneal e.
  tackler's e.
  traction e.
  turret e.
exostotica
  bursa e.
exostotic chondrosarcoma
expandable
  e. foam immobilization device
  e. Gianturco metallic stent
expanded
  e. disability status scale
  e. lung
  e. polytetrafluoroethylene-covered
    nitinol TIPS stent-graft
  e. polytetrafluoroethylene graft

expanding
    e. cavernous sinus brain lesion
    e. intracranial mass
expansile
    e. aneurysmal bone cyst
    e. aortic segment
    e. configuration
    e. lytic lesion
    e. mass
    e. multilocular bone lesion
    e. osteoblastoma
    e. osteolysis
    e. rib lesion
    e. unilocular well-demarcated bone
      lesion
expansion
    air e.
    bone marrow e.
    complete stent e.
    emphysematous e.
    fluid e.
    infarct e.
    localized e.
    lung e.
    passive chest e.
    peripheral e.
    rapid fluid e.
    stent e.
    uneven air e.
expectoration
    bilious e.
expenditure
    resting energy e.
experimental protocol
Expert-XL densitometer
expiration
    end e.
    flow-limited e.
    quantitative CT during e.
    e. view
expiratory
    e. attenuation
    e. chest
    e. computed tomography
    e. CT
    e. film
    e. flow
    e. gating
    e. image
    inspiratory to e.
    e. phase
    e. reserve volume (ERV)
    e. resistance
    e. view
explantation
exploration
    common bile duct e. (CBDE)
explorer
    E. rotational diagnostic catheter

    E. ST fixed-curve diagnostic
      catheter
    E. X70 intraoral radiography system
explosion fracture
explosive follicular hyperplasia
exponential
    e. decay
    e. kinetics
    e. shape
    e. weighting
Export catheter
exposure
    e. angle
    anthrax e.
    asbestos e.
    bioterrorism e.
    bone-tendon e.
    e. data recognizer (EDR)
    DES e.
    e. dose
    electromagnetic radiation e.
    entrance skin e.
    high-intensity e.
    index of e.
    intraperitoneal e.
    ionizing radiation e.
    magnetic radiation e.
    e. meter
    operator e.
    overcouch e.
    radiation e.
    uneven e.
    e. variation
    zero e.
express
    E. balloon-expanded stent
    E. biliary LD premounted stent
      system
    E. biliary LD stent
    E. PTCA catheter
expression
    antigen e.
    AQP4 e.
    catheter-based inducible enhancer of
      gene e.
    e. cystourethrography
    receptor e.
    upregulated AQP4 e.
    e. vector
exquisite detail
exsanguinating hemorrhage
exstrophy
    bladder e.
    cloacal e.
    closed e.
    urinary bladder e.
extended
    E. Brilliance Workspace
    e. cardiac reconstruction

E

extended (*continued*)
    e. computed tomography scale (ECTS)
    e. field-of-view (EFOV)
    e. field-of-view technique
    e. pattern
extended-field
    e.-f. irradiation
    e.-f. irradiation therapy
    e.-f. radiotherapy
extension
    angle of greatest e. (AGE)
    basal e.
    Buck e.
    capital e.
    Codivilla e.
    e. corner avulsion fracture
    external rotation in e. (ERE)
    extraaxial e.
    extracapsular e. (ECE)
    extranodal tumor e.
    extrascleral e.
    hilar e.
    e. injury
    e. injury of spine
    internal rotation in e. (IRE)
    intracavitary e.
    medial e.
    metaphysial e.
    parenchymatous e.
    parietal e.
    perineural e.
    e. position
    radiolucent operating room table e.
    subligamentous e.
    supradiaphragmatic e.
    suprasellar e.
    e. teardrop fracture (ETF)
    thrombus e.
    tumor e.
    e. view
extensive
    e. anterior myocardial infarct
    e. bilateral pneumonia
    e. dissection
    e. head injury
    e. intraductal carcinoma (EIC)
    e. intraductal component (EIC)
extensor
    e. apparatus
    e. carpi radialis brevis (ECRB)
    e. carpi radialis brevis muscle
    e. carpi radialis brevis tendon
    e. carpi radialis longus (ECRL)
    e. carpi radialis longus muscle
    e. carpi radialis longus tendon
    e. carpi ulnaris (ECU)
    e. carpi ulnaris muscle
    e. carpi ulnaris sheath

    e. carpi ulnaris tendon
    e. compartment
    e. digiti longus
    e. digiti minimi tendon
    e. digiti quinti (EDQ)
    e. digiti quinti muscle
    e. digiti quinti tendon
    e. digitorum
    e. digitorum brevis (EDB)
    e. digitorum brevis muscle
    e. digitorum brevis tendon
    e. digitorum communis (EDC)
    e. digitorum communis muscle
    e. digitorum communis tendon
    e. digitorum longus (EDL)
    e. digitorum longus muscle
    e. digitorum longus tendon
    e. hallucis longus (EHL)
    e. hallucis longus muscle
    e. hallucis longus tendon
    e. indicis
    e. indicis muscle
    e. indicis proprius (EIP)
    e. indicis proprius tendon
    e. mechanism
    e. pollicis brevis (EPB)
    e. pollicis brevis muscle
    e. pollicis brevis tendon
    e. pollicis longus (EPL)
    e. pollicis longus muscle
    e. pollicis longus tendon
    e. quinti proprius (EQP)
    e. quinti tendon
    e. retinaculum
    ulnar e.
extensor-supinator group
extensus
    hallux e.
extent
    anular tear e.
exteriorization
externa
    theca e.
externae
    stria laminae granularis e.
external
    e. absorption
    e. acoustic foramen
    e. anal sphincter
    e. artifact
    e. auditory canal atresia
    e. auditory canal dysplasia
    e. auditory meatus
    e. band
    e. beam irradiation
    e. beam radiation
    e. beam radiation therapy (EBRT)
    e. beam radiotherapy
    e. beam with tandem

e. biliary drainage catheter
e. biliary fistula
e. callus
e. capsule
e. carotid
e. carotid artery (ECA)
e. condyle
e. ear mass
e. ear neoplasia
e. elastic lamina
e. fiducial marker
e. fixation device
e. gamma dose reconstruction
e. heat-generating source
e. hemorrhage
e. hernia
e. iliac artery
e. iliac lymph node
e. iliac stenosis
e. inguinal ring
e. jugular vein (EJV)
e. looping technique
e. nose
e. oblique aponeurosis
e. oblique muscle
e. orthovoltage irradiation
e. os
e. pneumatic calf compression
e. pudendal vein
e. retractor
e. ring apex
e. rotation in extension (ERE)
e. rotation in flexion (ERF)
e. rotation view
e. scanning
e. snapping hip
e. table of calvaria
e. tibial torsion
e. urethral orifice
e. urethral sphincter
e. ventricular drain (EVD)
e. wire fixation
e. x-ray therapy

external-internal drainage
externe
horizontal toit e. (HTE)
externum
os tibiale e.
externus
obturator e.
extinction phenomenon
extirpation
e. of saphenous vein
tumor e.
extraabdominal desmoid
extraadrenal
e. chromaffin tissue
e. myelolipoma
e. paraganglioma

e. pheochromocytoma
e. site
extraalveolar
e. air (EAA)
e. air collection
extraarachnoid
e. injection
e. myelography
e. space
extraarticular
e. debris
e. fracture
e. hip fusion
e. posterior ossification
e. resection
extraaxial
e. cavernous hemangioma
e. CNS lesion
e. extension
e. fluid collection
e. infection
e. low-attenuation lesion
e. space
e. tumor
extracapsular
e. ankylosis
e. dissection
e. extension (ECE)
e. fracture
e. invasion
e. ligament
e. metastasis
e. spread
extracardiac
e. anomaly
e. collateral circulation
e. focal uptake
e. mass
extracavitary prosthetic arterial graft
extracellular
c. compartment
e. contrast agent
e. domain
e. fluid
e. fluid volume
e. matrix
e. matrix component
e. space
extracerebral
e. aneurysm
e. cavernous angioma
e. fluid collection
e. hematoma
e. intracranial glioneural hamartoma
e. soft tissue uptake
extrachorial placenta
extracolonic
e. disease
e. structure

E

extracompartmental tumor
extracorporeal
  e. circulation
  e. irradiation
  e. liver
  e. membrane oxygenation
  e. membrane oxygenator
  e. photochemotherapy
  e. shock wave
  e. shock wave lithotripsy (ESWL)
extracranial
  e. aneurysm
  e. carotid artery atherosclerosis
  e. carotid artery occlusive disease
  e. carotid circulation
  e. carotid system
  e. cerebral circulation
  e. cerebral vasculature
  e. course
  e. mass lesion
  e. meningioma
  e. pneumatocele
  e. vertebral artery
  e. vessel
extracranial-intracranial bypass
extraction
  anatomy-based e.
  automatic e.
  e. catheter atherectomy
  e. column
  contour e.
  disphenoid e.
  fringe skeleton e.
  e. generator
  e. method
  stone e.
  1st-pass thallium e.
  vacuum e.
  vascular segmentation and e.
extradural
  e. abscess
  e. anastomosis
  e. arachnoid cyst
  e. artery
  e. brain hematoma
  e. compartment
  e. defect
  e. hemorrhage
  e. mass
  e. space
  e. tumor
  e. venography
  e. vertebral plexus
  e. vertebral plexus of vein
extraembryonic mesoderm
extrafascial hysterectomy
extragastric placement
extragenital Bowen disease
extragonadal seminoma

extrahepatic
  e. bile duct
  e. bile duct carcinoma
  e. biliary atresia (EBA)
  e. biliary cystic dilation
  e. biliary obstruction
  e. cholangiectasis
  e. cholangiocarcinoma
  e. lesion
  e. metastasis (EHM)
  e. portal hypertension
  e. portal vein tributary
  e. primary malignant tumor
  e. pseudoaneurysm
  e. stone
extraintestinal
extralobar sequestration
extralobular
  e. connective tissue
  e. stroma
  e. terminal duct
extraluminal
  e. air
  e. contrast medium
  e. endarterectomy
  e. gas
  e. hemorrhage
extramammary Paget disease
extramedullary
  e. compressive lesion
  e. hemangioma
  e. hemopoiesis
  e. involvement
  e. mass
  e. myeloid tumor
  e. plasma cell tumor
  e. plasmacytoma (EMP)
extramural hemorrhage
extraneous material
extranodal
  e. follicular lymphoma
  e. non-Hodgkin lymphoma
  e. proliferation
  e. site
  e. systemic disease
  e. tumor extension
extraoctave fracture
extraocular
  e. muscle
  e. muscle enlargement
  e. muscle metastasis
extraoral radiograph
extraosseous
  e. angioma
  e. Ewing sarcoma
  e. mass
  e. osteosarcoma
  e. uptake
extraovarian mass

extrapancreatic
    e. autoimmune disease
    e. lesion
extraparenchymal cyst
extrapelvic malignancy
extrapericardial dissection
extraperitoneal
    e. bladder rupture
    c. fascia
    e. fat
    e. implant
    e. organ
extrapleural
    e. drainage
    e. hemorrhage
    e. lesion
    e. mass
    e. pneumothorax
    e. sign
    e. space
extrapolate
extrapolation
    half scan with e.
extrapontine myelinolysis
extrapulmonary
    e. activity
    e. bronchus
    e. sequestration
    e. small cell carcinoma
    e. tuberculosis
    e. uptake
extrapyramidal
    e. reaction
    e. symptom
    e. system
    e. tract
extrarenal renal pelvis
extrascleral extension
extraskeletal
    e. chondroma
    e. mesenchymal
      chondrosarcoma
    e. metastasis
    e. myxoid chondrosarcoma
    e. osteosarcoma
    e. tuberculosis
    e. uptake
extrasphincteric anal fistula
extraspinal neurofibroma
extra-stiff guidewire
extrasynovial
extratemporal
    e. epilepsy
    e. structural lesion
extratesticular
    e. lesion
    e. mass
    e. tumor
extrathecal nerve root

extrathoracic
    e. disease
    e. lesion
    e. metastasis
    e. obstruction
extrathymic malignancy
extrauterine
    e. gestation
    e. pelvic mass
    e. pregnancy (EUP)
extravaginal testicular torsion
extravasated
    e. blood
    e. contrast agent
    e. tracer
extravasation
    bile e.
    contrast e.
    e. detection accessory
    dye e.
    fluid e.
    high-volume e.
    intravascular contents e.
    joint fluid e.
    e. of contrast agent
    radiopaque fluid e.
    renal transplant urine e.
    secondary e.
    spontaneous urinary e.
    urinary e.
extravascular
    e. compartment
    e. fluid
    e. granuloma
    e. mass
    e. pressure
extraventricular obstructive hydrocephalus
extravesical
    e. infrasphincteric ectopic ureter
    e. opacification
extravital ultraviolet
extremely
    e. low frequency (ELF)
    e. low-frequency field
extreme micromelia
extremity
    e. coil
    e. CT angiography
    e. gigantism
    e. hemangioma
    left lower e. (LLE)
    lower e.
    e. magnetic resonance imaging
      (E-MRI)
    e. malformation
    e. MRI (E-MRI)
    e. osteosarcoma
    e. rhabdomyosarcoma
    upper e.

E

331

extrinsic
- e. allergic alveolitis
- e. bladder compression
- e. cellular parameter
- e. esophageal impression
- e. field uniformity
- e. filling defect
- e. foot muscle
- e. impression of esophagus
- e. intraabdominal inflammation
- e. lesion
- e. ligament
- e. malignant obstruction
- e. neoplasia
- e. sphincter
- e. stomach impression
- e. ureteral defect

extrophia vesicalis
extrude
extruded
- e. disc
- e. disc fragment

extrusion
- disc e.
- joint fluid e.

extubate
extubation
exuberant
- e. atheroma formation
- e. callus
- e. granulation tissue
- e. periostitis
- e. synovium
- e. tumor

exudative
- e. bronchiolitis
- e. consolidation
- e. enteropathy
- e. pleural effusion
- e. pleurisy
- e. tuberculosis

eye
- artificial e.
- conus e.
- E. Cubed ultrasound
- e. exposure limit
- fetal e.
- hamartoma of e.
- intraconal portion of e.
- e. myositis
- e. trauma

eyebrow ring artifact
eye-ear plane
eyelet
- rod e.

eyepiece
- Huygens e.

eye-view 3D conformal radiation therapy
E-Z-CAT
- E-Z-CAT Dry barium sulfate
- E-Z-CAT Dry contrast agent

E-Z-CAT
E-Z-EM
- E-Z-EM barium powder
- E-Z-EM cut-biopsy needle

E-Z-EM
E-zero offset
E-Z-Guar mouthpiece
E-Z-Paque barium suspension

F
frequency
F microcatheter
F point of cardiac apex
F T line
^{18}F, F-18
fluorine 18
^{18}F 2-deoxyglucose uptake
^{18}F estradiol imaging agent
^{18}F FDG-negative imaging
^{18}F fludeoxyglucose imaging agent
^{18}F fluorodeoxyglucose imaging agent
^{18}F fluoro-DOPA imaging agent
^{18}F fluoroisonidazole imaging agent
^{18}F fluorotamoxifen imaging agent
^{18}Fl-DOPA imaging agent
^{18}FN-methylspiperone imaging agent
^{18}F sodium fluoride imaging agent
^{18}F spiperone imaging agent
^{19}F, F-19
fluorine 19
FAA
flavone acetic acid
FAB
French-American-British
FAB classification
FAB fragment
Fab
fragment antigen binding
^{131}I-labeled monoclonal Fab
fabella
os f.
fabellofibular
f. and arcuate ligament complex
f. ligament
Fabian stent
Fabricius
bursa of F.
face
congenital infiltrating lipomatosis of f.
en f.
f. presentation
faceless kidney
facet, facette
articular f.
atlas f.
bilateral locked f.'s
capitate f.
f. capsule disruption
f. cartilage
cervical f.
clavicular f.
corneal f.
costal f.

f. degeneration
f. degenerative arthropathy
f. disease
f. dislocation
flat f.
f. fusion
hamate f.
f. hypertrophy
inferior medial f.
f. joint
f. joint arthritis
f. joint capsule
f. joint incongruity
f. joint injection
f. joint vacuum
jumped f.
Lenoir f.
locked f.
lunate f.
occlusal f.
f. osteoarthritis
f. osteoarthritis sign (FOS)
scaphoid f.
squatting f.
superior articular f.
superior costal f.
f. surface of vertebra
f. syndrome
transverse costal f.
f. tropism
facetal imbrication
facetectomy
faceted gallstone
faceting
facette (*var. of* facet)
facial, facialis
f. abnormality
f. artery
f. asymmetry
f. bipartition
f. bone
f. cleft
f. colliculus
f. dysmorphology
f. eminence
f. fracture
f. hemangioma
f. nerve
f. nerve anatomy
f. nerve canal
f. plane
f. plexus
f. root
f. schwannoma
f. thickening

F

facial (*continued*)
    f. trauma
    f. triangle
    f. vein
facialis (*var. of* facial)
facies, *pl.* **facies**
    f. ossea
    Potter f.
facioauriculovertebral syndrome
faciostenosis
FACScan
    fluorescence-activated cell sorter
    FACScan flow cytometer
FACSVantage cell sorter
FACT
    focused appendix computed
    tomography
factitious
    f. clinodactyly
    f. regurgitation
factor
    accelerator f.
    activation f.
    adherence f.
    f. analysis of dynamic series
    (FADS)
    f. analysis of dynamic study
    angiogenic f.
    anisotropy f.
    automotility f.
    backscatter f. (BSF)
    blocking f.
    breast cancer risk f.
    calibration f.
    contrast improvement f.
    decay-activating f.
    diffusion f.
    dose/dose-rate effective f. (DDREF)
    endothelial growth f.
    enhancement f.
    environmental f.
    equilibrium f.
    filling f.
    Fletcher f.
    gamma f.
    geometry f.
    granulocyte colony-stimulating f.
    (GCSF, G-CSF)
    granulocyte
    macophage-colony-stimulating f.
    (GM-CSF)
    grid conversion f. (GCF)
    growth f.
    Hageman f.
    HIV-inducing f.
    human macrophage-monocyte
    chemotactic and activating f.
    inciting f.
    incremental risk f.

    intensification f.
    interferon regulatory f.
    intrinsic f.
    Kerma-to-dose conversion f.
    magnification f.
    Mayneord F f.
    monocyte colony-stimulating f.
    negative f.
    net magnetization f.
    off-axis f. (OAF)
    overrelaxation f.
    pathogenic f.
    peak scatter f.
    platelet f. 3, 4 (PF3, PF4)
    platelet-derived endothelial cell
    growth f.
    protection f.
    quality f.
    radiation weighting f.
    relative conversion f.
    releasing f.
    rheumatoid f.
    scatter degradation f.
    screen-intensifying f.
    therapeutic gain f.
    tissue inhomogeneity f.
    tissue weighting f.
    trefoil f. 3 (TFF3)
    tumor angiogenesis f.
    f. VIII
    wedge f.
factorial design
FAD
    functional anesthetic discography
FADS
    factor analysis of dynamic series
Fahr disease
FAI
    femoroacetabular impingement
    functional aerobic impairment
    FAI syndrome
failed
    f. back surgery syndrome
    (FBSS)
    f. back syndrome (FBS)
    f. pregnancy
    f. valve
failure
    acute heart f.
    acute renal f. (ARF)
    acute respiratory f. (ARF)
    adrenal f.
    backward heart f.
    bypass f.
    cardiac f.
    chronic heart f.
    chronic renal f. (CRF)
    circulation f.
    compensated congestive heart f.

congestive heart f. (CHF)
contrast-induced renal f.
decompensated congestive heart f.
diastolic heart f.
endstage renal f. (ESRF)
exercise-induced renal f.
fetal heart f.
forward heart f.
frank congestive heart f.
fulminant hepatic f. (FHF)
functional classification of congestive
  heart f.
graft f.
heart f.
hepatic f.
high-output heart f.
intractable heart f.
intrauterine cardiac f.
intrauterine heart f.
irreversible organ f.
kidney f.
left-sided heart f.
left ventricular f.
liver f.
low-output heart f.
Mamm-Aire heart f.
multiple-organ f.
neonatal cardiac f.
neonatal heart f.
ovulatory f.
pituitary f.
posttransplant acute renal f.
prerenal f.
pulmonary f.
refractory congestive heart f.
renal f.
respiratory f.
right-sided heart f.
right ventricular f.
systolic heart f.
time-to-distant f.
time to local f.
time-to-treatment f. (TTF)
TIPS f.
ventilatory f.
ventricular f.

failure-free survival
FAIR
  flow-sensitive alternating inversion
  recovery
Fairbank disease
falces (*pl. of* falx)
falciform
  f. cartilage
  f. crest
  f. fold
  f. ligament
  f. ligament sign
  f. process

falcine meningioma
falcotentorial meningioma
falcula
falcular
fallen
  f. fragment sign
  f. lung sign
fallopian
  f. canal
  f. ligament
  f. pregnancy
  f. tube
  f. tube carcinoma
  f. tube diverticulum
  f. tube mass
  f. tube occlusion
  f. tube recanalization
falloposcopy system
Fallot
  pentalogy of F.
  F. syndrome
  F. tetrad
  tetralogy of F.
  (TOF)
  trilogy of F.
fallout
  radioactive f.
  signal f.
false
  f. aneurysm
  f. aneurysmal chamber
  f. ankylosis
  f. bundle-branch block
  f. channel
  f. colonic obstruction
  f. color scale
  f. cord carcinoma
  f. diverticulum
  f. emphysema
  f. frequency
  f. hypocchogenicity
  f. knot
  f. localizing sign
  f. lumen
  f. pelvis
  f. pregnancy
  f. rib
  f. sac
  f. splenic cyst
  f. steal
  f. suture
  f. vertebra
  f. vocal cord
false-negative
  f.-n. correlation
  f.-n. mammogram
  f.-n. ratio
  f.-n. result
  f.-n. test

F

false-positive
    f.-p. ratio
    f.-p. result
    f.-p. test
falx, *pl.* **falces**
    f. artery
    f. calcification
    f. cerebelli
    f. cerebri
    f. cerebri lesion
    f. fenestration
    f. increased density
FAME
    fast acquisition multiple excitation
familial
    f. adenomatous polyposis (FAP)
    f. adenomatous polyposis syndrome
    f. aortic dissection
    f. arterial fibromuscular dysplasia
    f. atresia
    f. avascular necrosis of phalangeal
      epiphysis
    f. cavernous malformation
    f. cerebral ferrocalcinosis
    f. chondrocalcinosis
    f. colorectal polyposis
    f. dysautonomia
    f. fibromuscular dysplasia of artery
    f. gastrointestinal polyposis
    f. goiter
    f. hypertrophic cardiomyopathy (FHC)
    f. hypertrophy
    f. idiopathic hyperphosphatasia
    f. intestinal polyposis
    f. intestinal pseudoobstruction
    f. juvenile polyposis
    f. lymphohistiocytosis
    f. multiple polyposis
    f. myxoma
    f. onychoosteodysplasia
    f. polyposis coli
    f. retinoblastoma
    f. thyroid ectopia
    f. varicose vein
fan
    f. angle
    f. sign
fan-beam
    f.-b. collimator
    f.-b. formula
    f.-b. projection
    f.-b. reconstruction
Fanconi
    F. anemia
    F. syndrome
Fanconi-Hegglin syndrome
fanning
    f. of interspinous distance
    f. of spinous process

fanolesomab
    technetium 99m f.
fan-shaped
    f.-s. mesentery
    f.-s. view
FAP
    familial adenomatous polyposis
farad
Faraday
    F. cage
    F. effect
    F. law
    F. shield
    F. shielded resonator
far field
farmer's lung
FAS
    fetal alcohol syndrome
    MAS in FAS
fas-associated phosphatase-1
fascia, *pl.* **fasciae**, *pl.* **fascias**
    anal f.
    antebrachial f.
    anterior rectus f.
    axillary f.
    bicipital f.
    brachial f.
    broad f.
    buccopharyngeal f.
    Buck f.
    Camper f.
    cervical f.
    clavipectoral f.
    Cloquet f.
    Colles f.
    cremasteric f.
    cribriform f.
    crural f.
    Cruveilhier f.
    deep f.
    deltoid f.
    Denonvilliers f.
    dentate f.
    diaphragmatic f.
    endopelvic f.
    endothoracic f.
    extraperitoneal f.
    Gerota f.
    iliac f.
    infraspinous f.
    investing f.
    Laimer f.
    f. lata
    lateral conal f.
    lateral oblique f.
    lateroconal f.
    lumbar f.
    medial geniculate f.
    obturator internus f.

f. of breast
palmar f.
parietal pelvic f.
pelvic f.
perineal f.
pharyngobasilar f.
prepectoral f.
prevertebral f.
psoas f.
quadratus femoris f.
rectal f.
renal f.
retromammary f.
rim of f.
Scarpa f.
Sibson f.
spigelian f.
subcutaneous f.
superficial temporalis f.
superficial temporoparietal f.
supraanal f.
thoracolumbar f.
transversalis f.
umbilicovesical f.
vesical f.
visceral pelvic f.
Waldeyer f.
Zuckerkandl f.
fasciae (*pl. of* fascia)
fasciagram
fasciagraphy
fascial
   f. band
   f. connective tissue
   f. envelope
   f. incisor
   f. margin necrosis
   f. plane
   f. rent
   f. sheath
   f. stranding
   f. tract
fascias (*pl. of* fascia)
fascicle
   synovium-lined f.
   tibioligamentous f.
   triquetroscaphoid f.
   triquetrotrapezoid f.
fascicular
   f. block
   f. bundle
   f. sarcoma
fasciculata
   zona f.
fasciculation
   tongue f.
fasciculi (*pl. of* fasciculus)
fasciculus, *pl.* **fasciculi**
   arcuate f.

Gowers f.
lenticular f.
longitudinal f.
longitudinalis medialis f.
mamillothalamic f.
medial longitudinal f. (MLF)
occipitofrontal f.
superior longitudinal f.
superior occipitofrontal f.
fasciitis, fascitis
   fulminant f.
   necrotizing f.
   f. ossificans
   palmar f.
   plantar f.
   pseudosarcomatous f.
   scrotal f.
fasciolar gyrus
fascioliasis
fascitis (*var. of* fasciitis)
fashion
   snapshot f.
fasiculoventricular bypass tract
FAST
   focused assessment by sonography for trauma
   Fourier-acquired steady-state technique
   contrast-enhanced FAST
   FAST PC cine MR sequence with echo-planar gradient
   FAST pulse sequence
   reduced-acquisition matrix FAST
   RF-spoiled FAST
   T1-weighted FAST
fast
   f. acquisition multiple excitation (FAME)
   f. adiabatic trajectory in steady state (FATS)
   f. array processor
   f. breeder reactor
   f. cardiac phase contrast cine imaging
   f. dynamic volumetric x-ray CT
   f. FLAIR sequence
   f. fluid-attenuation inversion recovery image
   f. Fourier flow (FFF)
   f. Fourier imaging
   f. Fourier projection (FFP)
   f. Fourier spectral analysis
   f. Fourier transform (FFT)
   f. Fourier transform image
   f. fractionation
   f. gradient-echo sequence
   f. imaging employing steady-state acquisition (FIESTA)
   f. imaging employing steady-state acquisition technique

F

fast (*continued*)
f. imaging with steady-state free precession
f. imaging with steady-state precession (FISP)
f. inversion-recovery Fourier transform (FIRFT)
f. inversion-recovery motion-insensitive (FIRM)
f. low-angle acquisition with relaxation enhancement (FLARE)
f. low-angle shot (FLASH)
f. multiplanar inversion recovery imaging
f. multiplanar spoiled gradient-recalled imaging
f. multislice phase-sensitive inversion recovery sequence
f. neutron
f. neutron radiotherapy
f. routine production
f. short tau inversion recovery
f. spin echo (FSE)
f. spin-echo acquisition
f. spin-echo and fast inversion recovery imaging
f. spin-echo black blood imaging
f. spin-echo MR imaging
f. spin-echo T2-weighted image
f. spin-echo view
f. spoiled gradient-recalled echo (FSPGR)
f. spoiled gradient-recalled MR imaging
f. STIR
f. Talairach transformation
Fastcard
Fast-Cath introducer catheter
FastCINE
FASTER
field echo acquisition with short repetition time and echo reduction
3D FASTER
fast-exchange
f.-e. cellular suspension
f.-e. soft tissue
fast-field echo (FFE)
fast-FLAIR technique
fast-flow
f.-f. lesion
f.-f. malformation
f.-f. vascular anomaly
fasting blood sugar (FBS)
fast-neutron radiation therapy
FasTracker catheter
fast-scan
f.-s. magnetic resonance
f.-s. magnetic resonance imaging
fast-twitch muscle

fat
abdominal f.
f. absorption test
f. and long T2-suppressed ultrashort echo time (FLUTE)
anterior epidural f.
bony glenoid marrow f.
brown f.
f. density
digital process of f.
dirty f.
f. dissociation syndrome
f. embolism syndrome (FES)
f. embolus
epidural f.
extraperitoneal f.
herniated preperitoneal f.
intraabdominal f. (IAF)
f. island
isointense background f.
lipid content of storage f.
f. lobule
f. lung herniation
mediastinal f.
mesocolon f.
f. metabolism
microvesicular f.
mistiness of pericolonic f.
muckiness of pericolonic f.
f. necrosis
parametrial f.
peribursal f.
pericardiac f.
pericolonic f.
perigastric f.
perihilar f.
perinephric f.
perineural f.
perirectal f.
perirenal f.
f. plane
posterior epidural f.
preperitoneal f.
prerenal f.
properitoneal f.
protruding f.
radiolucent f.
renal sinus f.
retrobulbar f.
retromammary f.
f. saturation
f. signal intensity
f. signal suppression
f. stranding
f. stripe
subcutaneous f.
subdiaphragmatic f.
subepicardial f.
tumoral f.

USA f.
ventral epidural f.
visceral f.

fatal dose of radiation

fat- and water-suppressed T2-weighted image

fat-blood
f.-b. interface (FBI)
f.-b. interface sign

fat-containing
f.-c. breast lesion
f.-c. mass

fat-density
f.-d. area
f.-d. line
f.-d. mass

fat-fluid
f.-f. density interface
f.-f. level

fat-fraction measurement

fatigue
f. damage
f. fracture

fat-pad
antimesenteric f.-p.
elbow f.-p.
epicardial f.-p.
esophagogastric f.-p.
foveal f.-p.
haversian f.-p.
heel f.-p.
Hoffa f.-p.
ileocecal f.-p.
infrapatellar f.-p.
intracapsular f.-p.
intrapatellar f.-p.
ischiorectal f.-p.
patellar f.-p.
pericardial f.-p.
pre-Achilles f.-p.
scalene f.-p.
f.-p. sign

FATS
fast adiabatic trajectory in steady
state

fat-saturated
f.-s. axial image
f.-s. spin-echo proton
density-weighted image
f.-s. T2-weighted fast spin-echo
image

fat-selective presaturation

fat-spared
f.-s. area in fatty liver
f.-s. area in pancreas

fat-suppressed
f.-s. acquisition with TE and TR
times shortened
f.-s. body coil

f.-s. 3D gradient-echo image
f.-s. 3D-spoiled gradient-echo
FLASH MR imaging
f.-s. 3D-spoiled gradient-recall echo
imaging
f.-s. gadolinium-enhanced imaging
f.-s. spin echo
T1-weighted f.-s. (T1FS)
f.-s. T1-weighted 3D-spoiled
gradient-echo image
f.-s. T2-weighted fast spin-echo
sequence
f.-s. T2-weighted FSE technique
f.-s. ultrashort echo time (FUTE)

fat-suppressing content

fat-suppression
f.-s. pulse
f.-s. pulse sequence
f.-s. technique

fatty
f. acid metabolism
f. cirrhosis
f. degeneration
f. filum
f. filum terminale
f. halo
f. heart
f. infiltrate
f. intima streak
f. kidney
f. liver
f. marrow
f. marrow change
f. meal
f. meal sonogram (FMS)
f. meal sonography
f. mesentery
f. metastatic lesion
f. necrosis
f. plaque
f. prostatic tissue
f. renal capsule
f. soft tissue tumor
f. sparing
f. streak atherosclerosis

fat-water
f.-w. chemical-shift imaging
f.-w. interface
f.-w. out of phase
f.-w. signal cancellation
f.-w. signal separation

fauces, *pl.* **fauces**
anterior pillar of f.
arch of f.

faucial
f. pillar
f. tonsil

fault
sagittal plane f.

F

faulty
> f. radiofrequency shielding
> f. radiofrequency shielding artifact
> f. union

faveolate

Favre disease

FBI
> fat-blood interface
> FBI sign

FBM
> fetal breathing movement

FBP
> filtered back projection
> FBP method

FBS
> failed back syndrome
> fasting blood sugar

FBSS
> failed back surgery syndrome

FCMD
> Fukuyama congenital muscular disease

FCPA-2
> fiber chirped pulse amplification
> FCPA-2 laser

FCR
> flexor carpi radialis
> FCR Velocity-U digital imaging
> system

FCS
> full cervical spine
> FCS series
> FCS view

FDA
> Food and Drug Administration

FDDNP
> fluorine-18
> 2-dialkylamino-6-acylmalononitrile
> substituted naphthalene
> FDDNP PET scan contrast medium

FDG
> ^{18}F-fluoro-2-deoxyglucose
> 2-fluoro 2-deoxyglucose
> fluorodeoxyglucose
> FDG myocardial imaging
> FDG positron emission tomography
> FDG SPECT
> FDG uptake

FDG-blood flow mismatch

FDG-labeled positron imaging

^{18}FDG-PET
> ^{18}F-fluorodeoxyglucose positron
> emission tomography
> ^{18}FDG-PET scan

FDG-PET
> fluorodeoxyglucose positron emission
> tomography
> positron emission tomography with
> fluorodeoxyglucose
> FDG-PET scan

FDG-6-phosphate

FDI
> frequency domain imaging
> 1st digital interosseous
> FDI muscle
> FDI ultrasound

FDL
> flexor digitorum longus
> FDL muscle

FDQB
> flexor digiti quinti brevis
> FDQB muscle

FDS
> flexor digitorum sublimis
> flexor digitorum superficialis
> FDS muscle

^{52}Fe, Fe-52
> iron 52

^{55}Fe, Fe-55
> iron 55

^{59}Fe, Fe-59
> iron 59

Fe
> iron

feasibility of image registration

FeatherTouch CO_2 laser

feathery
> f. appearance
> f. pattern

feature
> clinical f.
> differential diagnostic lung mass f.
> geriatric f.
> mammographic f.
> mongoloid f.
> proctographic f.

featureless appearance

fecal
> f. concretion
> f. diversion colostomy
> f. fistula
> f. impaction
> f. incontinence
> f. material
> f. obstruction
> f. residue
> f. stone
> f. tumor

fecalith

fecaloid

fecaloma

fecaluria

feces
> impacted f.
> inspissated f.
> semiliquid f.

feces-filled colon

feculence

feculent

Fédération Internationale de Gynécologie Obstétrique (International Federation of Gynecology) (FIGO)
feedback
    breathing f.
    real-time respiratory f.
feeder
    f. artery
    f. vein
feeding
    f. artery of aneurysm
    f. branch
    f. branch of artery
    f. mean arterial pressure (FMAP)
    f. tube
    f. vessel
    f. vessel sign
FEER
    field-echo sequence with even-echo rephasing
    field even-echo rephasing
feet (*pl. of* foot)
Fe-Ex orogastric tube magnet
Feigenbaum echocardiography
feign tumor
Feiss line
Feist-Mankin position
fellow
    F. of the American College of Nuclear Medicine
    F. of the American College of Nuclear Physicians
Felson
    silhouette sign of F.
Felty syndrome
female
    f. genital tract calcification
    f. genital tract rhabdomyosarcoma
    intersex f.
    f. pelvis
    f. pseudohermaphroditism
    f. urethra
fem-fem
    femorofemoral
feminine aorta
feminization
    testicular f.
feminizing
    f. adrenal tumor
    f. testis syndrome
femora (*pl. of* femur)
femoral
    f. access
    f. antetorsion
    f. anteversion
    f. artery
    f. artery approach
    f. artery pseudoaneurysm
    f. articulation

    f. bone
    f. capital epiphysis
    f. condylar shaving
    f. condyle
    f. cortex
    f. endarterectomy
    f. fossa
    f. head
    f. head amputation
    f. head deformity
    f. head epiphysiolysis
    f. head vascularity
    f. hernia
    f. intertrochanteric fracture
    f. leak
    f. ligament
    f. medullary canal
    f. neck
    f. neck fracture
    f. nerve
    f. ossification center
    f. physial scar
    f. plate
    f. plexus
    f. pulsatility index (FPI)
    f. pulse
    f. retrotorsion
    f. retroversion
    f. ring
    f. runoff angiography
    f. runoff arteriography
    f. septum
    f. shaft
    f. shaft axis
    f. shaft fracture
    f. sheath
    f. stress fracture
    f. supracondylar fracture
    f. torsion V angle
    f. triangle
    f. triangular content
    f. tuberosity
    f. varus derotational osteotomy
    f. vein
    f. vein percutaneous insertion
    f. venous approach
    f. view
femorale
    calcar f.
femoris (*gen. of* femur)
femoroacetabular impingement (FAI)
femorocerebral catheter angiography
femorocrural graft
femorodistal popliteal bypass graft
femorofemoral (fem-fem)
    f. bypass graft
    f. crossover
femorofemoropopliteal
femoropatellar joint

F

femoroperoneal in situ vein bypass graft

femoropopliteal (fem-pop)
    f. artery
    f. atheromatous stenosis
    f. bypass graft
    f. Gore-Tex graft
    f. system
    f. thrombosis
    f. vessel

femorotibial
    f. angle (FTA)
    f. bypass graft

FemoStop compression device

fem-pop
    femoropopliteal

femtocurie

femtoliter

femtosecond
    f. laser keratome
    f. laser system

femur, *pl.* **femora,** *gen.* **femoris**
    apex of f.
    body of f.
    distal f.
    greater trochanter of f.
    head of f.
    isthmus of f.
    f. length
    f. length to abdominal
      circumference
    lesser trochanter of f.
    neck of f.
    NSA of f.
    nutrient artery of f.
    proximal f.
    quadratus femoris
    quadriceps femoris
    rectus femoris
    tensor fasciae femoris

fencer's bone

fender fracture

fenestra, *pl.* **fenestrae**

fenestrae (*pl. of* fenestra)

fenestral otosclerosis

fenestram
    fissula ante f.

fenestrated
    f. alphanumeric compression
    f. compression plate
    f. sheath
    f. tube
    f. vessel

fenestration
    aortopulmonary f.
    apical f.
    arterial f.
    balloon f.
    balloon catheter f.

    catheter-directed f.
    cusp f.
    falx f.
    interchordal space f.
    middle cerebral artery f.
    f. of basilar artery
    f. of dissecting aneurysm
    vertebral artery f.

fenoldopam mesylate

fentanyl citrate

Fe_3O4
    magnetite
    magnetite albumin imaging agent

Ferguson
    F. angle
    F. method
    F. method for measuring scoliosis
    F. sacroiliac view

Feridex IV MRI contrast agent

fermium (Fm)
    f. 255 (^{255}Fm)

fernlike pattern

ferpentetate
    technetium 99m f.

Ferrein
    F. canal
    F. foramen
    F. ligament

ferric ammonium citrate-cellulose paste

ferrite

ferritin-labeled yttrium

ferrocalcinosis
    familial cerebral f.

ferroelectric relaxor

ferrokinetic data

ferromagnetic
    f. artifact
    f. implant
    f. material
    f. microembolization
    f. microembolization treatment
    f. microsphere
    f. particle spill
    f. relaxation
    f. tamponade

ferrous citrate

ferruginous body

Fertinex

ferucarbotran MR imaging agent

feruglose contrast agent

ferumoxide imaging agent

ferumoxsil imaging agent

ferumoxtran-enhanced
    f.-e. echo-planar GRE T2-weighted
      imaging
    f.-e. echo-planar SE T2-weighted
      and echo-planar GRE
    f.-e. echo-planar SE T2-weighted
      imaging

ferumoxtran imaging agent
FES
    fat embolism syndrome
    flame emission spectroscopy
    fluoroestradiol
fetal
    f. abdominal circumference
    f. abdominal cystic mass
    f. abdominal wall
    f. abdominal wall defect
    f. abnormality
    f. adenocarcinoma
    f. adenoma
    f. age
    f. alcohol syndrome (FAS)
    f. amputation
    f. aortic flow volume
    f. ascites
    f. asphyxia
    f. attitude
    f. biometry
    f. biometry of ulna
    f. biophysical profile score
    f. bowel obstruction
    f. BPS
    f. breathing movement (FBM)
    f. cardiac anomaly
    f. cardiosplenic syndrome
    f. cerebellum
    f. chest anomaly
    f. circulation
    f. CNS anomaly
    f. cranium
    f. cystic adenomatoid
      malformation
    f. cystic fibrosis
    f. cystic hygroma
    f. death
    f. death in utero
    f. detail
    f. dystocia
    f. echocardiographic view
    f. echocardiography
    f. echocardiography in utero
    f. ectopia cordis
    f. epiphysial bone center
    f. eye
    f. femoral length
    f. foot length measurement
    f. fracture
    f. gallbladder
    f. gastrointestinal anomaly
    f. goiter
    f. growth acceleration
    f. growth retardation
    f. hand malformation
    f. head circumference
    f. heart
    f. heart anomaly

    f. heart failure
    f. hydrops
    f. hypomineralization
    f. incarceration
    f. intraabdominal calcification
    f. kidney lobation
    f. lie
    f. liver biopsy
    f. liver magnetic resonance
      imaging
    f. lobe
    f. lobulation
    f. long bone measurement
    f. lung hypoplasia
    f. lymphoid tissue
    f. mesenchymal tumor
    f. mesenchymal tumor of kidney
    f. midface
    f. movement
    f. musculoskeletal dysplasia
    f. musculoskeletal system
    f. neck anomaly
    f. neck pseudomembrane
    f. period
    f. placenta
    f. pleural effusion
    f. pole
    f. position
    f. pyelectasis
    f. renal function
    f. renal hamartoma
    f. renal obstruction
    f. scalp edema
    f. skin biopsy
    f. small part
    f. sonography
    f. spine
    f. stress test
    f. swallowing
    f. thoracic circumference
    f. ultrasound
    f. urinary tract anomaly
    f. urogenital tract
    f. uterus
    f. ventricular heart disproportion
    f. ventriculomegaly
    f. weight
fetalis
    chondrodystrophia f.
    nonimmune hydrops f.
fetal-pelvic
    f.-p. disproportion
    f.-p. index
feticide
fetogram
fetography
fetometry
fetu
    fetus in f.

F

fetus
- amorphous f.
- calcified f.
- cephalic presentation of f.
- demise of f.
- disappearing f.
- growth-retarded f.
- impacted f.
- f. in fetu
- intrauterine f.
- malpositioned f.
- maturity of f.
- multiple fetuses
- nonviable f.
- paper-doll f.
- f. papyraceus
- parasitic f.
- postterm f.
- previable f.
- retained dead f.
- small for gestational age f.
- small part of f.
- stunted f.
- syndactyly in f.
- tissue of f.
- trisomic f.
- viable f.

Feuerstein-Mims syndrome

fever
- catscratch f.
- Mediterranean f.
- f. of unknown etiology (FUE)
- f. of unknown origin (FUO)

FFA
- free fatty acid

FFD
- focal film distance
- focus-film distance

FFE
- fast-field echo

FFF
- fast Fourier flow

F-1200,-2000,-4500 fluorescence spectrophotometer

^{18}F-fluorocholine
- radiation dosimetry of ^{18}F-f.

^{18}F-fluoro-2-deoxyglucose (FDG)

^{18}F-fluorodeoxyglucose positron emission tomography (^{18}FDG-PET)

^{18}F-fluoro-6-thia-heptadecanoic acid (FTHA)

FFP
- fast Fourier projection

FFR
- fractional flow reserve

FFT
- fast Fourier transform

FG-36UX scanning echoendoscope

FHC
- familial hypertrophic cardiomyopathy

FHF
- fulminant hepatic failure

FHI
- frontal horn index

FI
- fusion inhibitor
- FI method
- FI projection

fiber, fibre, fibra
- anular f.
- asbestos f.
- association f.
- atrio-His f.
- Bergman f.
- cardiac muscle f.
- cerebellar f.
- climbing f.
- differencing f.
- gastric sling f.
- Herxheimer f.
- long f.
- Mahaim and James f.
- mossy f.
- Müller f.
- muscle f. (type I, II)
- myocardial f.
- myoclonic epilepsy and ragged red f.'s (MERRF)
- nodoventricular bypass f.
- notch from gastric sling f.
- obliquely oriented f.
- onionskin configuration of collagenous f.
- parasympathetic f.
- pontocerebellar f.
- postganglionic gray f.
- postganglionic sympathetic f.
- precharred f.
- Purkinje f.
- radial glial f.
- f. retraction
- Rosenthal f.
- Sharpey f.
- skeletal muscle f.
- sling muscle f.
- f. tracking
- type I, II muscle f.
- unmyelinated nerve f.

fiber-bundle striation
fibered Guglielmi detachable coil
fiberglass pneumoconiosis
Fiberlase laser
fiberoptic
- f. bronchogram
- f. bronchoscopy (FOB)
- f. bundle
- f. conductor

f. light source
f. probe
f. taper
f. video glasses
FiberScan laser
fiberscopic
fiber-shortening velocity
4-fiber therapy
fiber-type disproportion
fibra (*var. of* fiber)
fibrae (*pl. of* fibra)
fibre (*var. of* fiber)
fibril
collagen f.
fibrillary astrocytoma
fibrillation
atrial f.
chondromalacia with f.
Fibrimage diagnostic imaging agent
fibrin
f. mass
f. platelet embolus
f. polymerization
f. sleeve stripping
fibrinogen
f. degradation
f. equivalent unit
iodinated I-125 f.
labeled f.
radiolabeled f.
fibrinoid necrosis
fibrinolytic
f. therapy
f. treatment
fibrinoma
fibrinopeptide (A, B)
fibrinopurulent pleurisy
fibrinous
f. inflammation
f. pleurisy
f. pneumonia
f. polyp
fibrin-specific contrast agent
fibrin-split product
fibroadenolipoma
breast f.
fibroadenoma
breast f.
calcified f.
cellular f.
degenerated f.
esophageal f.
giant breast f.
hyalinized breast f.
involuting f.
juvenile f.
noncalcified f.

fibroadenomatosis
breast f.
fibroadipose tissue
fibroareolar tissue
fibroblastic
f. meningioma
f. osteosarcoma
fibroblastoma
perineural f.
fibroblast radiosensitivity
fibrocalcific
f. cusp
f. residual
fibrocalcification
fibrocartilage
avascular f.
circumferential f.
f. complex
intraarticular plate of f.
labral f.
triangular f. (TFC)
fibrocartilaginous
f. disc
f. labrum
f. meniscus
f. nodule
f. overgrowth
f. pad
f. ridge
f. scar
f. tissue
f. volar plate
fibrocaseous
fibrocavitary infiltrate
fibrochondrogenesis
fibrocollagenous
f. connective tissue
f. stroma
fibrocongestive splenomegaly
fibrocystic
f. breast
f. breast disease
f. breast syndrome
f. change
f. lung disease
f. residual
fibrodysplasia ossificans progressiva
fibroelastic
f. band
f. cartilage
fibroelastoma
f. of heart valve
papillary f.
fibroelastosis
endocardial f.
fibroepithelial
f. papilloma
f. urethral polyp

F

fibroepithelioma
   urinary tract f.
fibrofatty
   f. breast tissue
   f. layer
   f. plaque
fibrogenesis imperfecta ossium
fibrogenic pneumoconiosis
fibroglandular
   f. density
   f. element
   f. tissue
fibrohistiocytic
   f. lesion
   f. tumor
fibrohistiocytoma
fibrohistiocytosis
fibroid
   f. adenoma
   calcified f.
   f. curvature
   f. degeneration
   f. embolization
   exophytic f.
   f. heart
   intramural f.
   f. lung
   f. myocarditis
   pedunculated uterine f.
   f. polyp
   submucosal f.
   subserosal f.
   f. tumor
   uterine f.
   f. uterus
fibroinflammatory tissue
fibrointimal hyperplasia
fibrolamellar
   f. HCC
   f. hepatocarcinoma
   f. hepatocellular carcinoma
fibroleiomyoma
   metastasizing f.
fibrolipoma
   filum terminale f.
   neural f.
fibrolipomatosis
   pelvic f.
   renal pelvic f.
fibrolipomatous nerve hamartoma
fibroma
   ameloblastic f.
   aponeurotic f.
   benign pleural f.
   calcified f.
   cardiac f.
   cementifying f.
   cementoossifying f.
   central cementifying f.

central ossifying f.
chondromyxoid f. (CMF)
concentric f.
desmoplastic f.
giant cell f.
heart f.
irritation f.
juvenile aponeurotic f.
juvenile ossifying f.
meningeal f.
f. molle
f. molle gravidarum
f. molluscum
musculoaponeurotic f.
f. myxomatodes
nonossifying f.
nonosteogenic f.
f. of lung
ossifying bone f.
ossifying skull f.
osteogenic bone f.
ovarian f.
periosteal f.
peripheral ossifying f.
periungual f.
polypoid f.
psammomatoid ossifying f.
recurrent digital f.
scrotal f.
senile f.
Shope f.
sinonasal psammomatoid ossifying f.
soft tissue f.
subcutaneous f.
subungual f.
telangiectatic f.
ungual f.
fibroma-thecoma tumor of ovary
fibromatogenic
fibromatoid
fibromatosis
   abdominal f.
   aggressive infantile f.
   f. colli
   congenital diffuse f.
   congenital generalized f.
   infantile digital f.
   juvenile f.
   mesenteric f.
   multicentric f.
   multiple congenital f.
   musculoaponeurotic f.
   palmar f.
   penile f.
   plantar f.
fibromatous
fibromuscular
   f. band
   f. disease (FMD)

f. dysplasia
f. lesion
f. pelvic floor
f. renal artery stenosis
f. ridge
f. subaortic stenosis
f. tissue
fibromyoma
fibromyositis
fibromyxoid sarcoma
fibromyxoma
kidney f.
odontogenic f.
pleural f.
fibronodular infiltrate
fibronuclear
fibroosscous
f. attachment
f. lesion
f. pseudotumor of digit
f. tunnel
fibroosteoma of tooth
fibroplasia
adventitial f.
endomyocardial f.
intimal f.
medial f.
perimedial renal artery f.
retrolental f.
fibroplastic
f. process
f. proliferation
fibroproductive tuberculosis
fibroretractive
fibrosa, *pl.* **fibrosae**
hepatica f.
osteodystrophia f.
pseudoaneurysm of mitral-aortic f.
fibrosae (*pl. of* fibrosa)
fibrosarcoma
ameloblastic f.
bone f.
cardiac f.
central f.
congenital kidney f.
epididymal f.
infantile f.
inflammatory f.
nonmetastasizing f.
periosteal f.
f. variant
fibrosclerosis
multifocal f.
fibrosclerotic
fibrosed muscle
fibrosing
f. arachnoiditis
f. colonopathy
f. cryptogenic alveolitis

f. inflammation
f. inflammatory pseudotumor
f. mediastinitis
f. mesenteritis
f. mesothelioma
f. piecemeal necrosis
f. tissue
fibrosis
acute diffuse interstitial f.
alcoholic f.
anular f.
arachnoid f.
asbestos-induced pleural f.
basilar f.
benign meningeal f.
bone marrow f.
brachytelephalangic type of cystic f.
breast f.
cerebellar vermis hypoplasia,
  oligophrenia, congenital ataxia,
  ocular coloboma, hepatic f.
  (COACH)
cirrhosis-related f.
confluent f.
congenital hepatic f. (CHF)
congenital liver f.
cystic f.
Davies endocardial f.
Davies endomyocardial f.
diffuse interstitial pulmonary f.
  (DIPF)
endocardial f.
endomyocardial f. (EMF)
epidural anular f.
fetal cystic f.
focal f.
hepatic f.
horseshoe f.
hyalinized fibroadenoma with f.
idiopathic interstitial pulmonary f.
idiopathic pulmonary f. (IPF)
inflammatory f.
interstitial prematurity f.
interstitial pulmonary f. (IPF)
intimal f.
intraalveolar f.
intralobular f.
leptomeningeal f.
massive f.
mediastinal f.
meningeal f.
mesenteric f.
mural endomyocardial f.
nephrogenic systemic f.
nodal f.
nodular subepidermal f.
noncirrhotic portal f. (NCPF)
nonnodular f.
f. of lung

F

fibrosis (*continued*)
    pancreatic cystic f.
    parietal lobe gray matter cytosolic
      choline pathogenetic mechanism of
      myocardial f.
    periadventitial f.
    perialveolar f.
    periaortic f.
    peribronchial f.
    pericentral f.
    periductal f.
    peridural f.
    perihilar f.
    perimuscular f.
    perineural f.
    periportal f.
    periureteral f.
    perivascular f.
    perivenular f.
    pipestem f.
    portal f.
    portal-to-portal f.
    postinflammatory pulmonary f.
    postirradiation f.
    postradiation f.
    posttraumatic f.
    primary retroperitoneal f.
    progressive interstitial pulmonary f.
    progressive massive f. (PMF)
    progressive nodular pulmonary f.
    pulmonary f.
    pulmonary interstitial
      idiopathic f.
    pulmonary vein f.
    radiation-induced f. (RIF)
    reactive f.
    replacement f.
    retroperitoneal f. (RPF)
    secondary retroperitoneal f.
    subadventitial f.
    subintimal f.
    subserosal f.
    Symmers f.
    transmural f.
fibrosum
    molluscum f.
    pericardium f.
fibrosus
    anulus f.
    bulging anulus f.
fibrothorax
fibrotic
    f. cavitating pattern
    f. change
    f. honeycombing
    f. island
    f. kidney
    f. neoplasm
    f. plaque

    f. residual
    f. resolution
    f. scarring
    f. tissue
fibrous, fibrosa
    f. ankylosis
    f. attachment
    f. band
    f. bar
    f. bone lesion
    f. cap
    f. cartilage
    f. coalition
    f. connective tissue
    f. connective tissue tumor
    f. cord
    f. cortical defect
    f. GI tract polypoid lesion
    f. goiter
    f. hamartoma
    f. histiocytoma
    f. hood
    f. intima plaque
    f. mastopathy
    f. medullary defect
    f. meningioma
    f. metaphysial-diaphysial
      defect
    f. nodular pattern
    f. nodule
    f. nonunion
    f. obliterative cholangitis
    f. osteodystrophy
    f. osteoma
    f. pericardium
    f. plaque atherosclerosis
    f. pleural adhesion
    f. pneumonia
    f. pseudocapsule
    f. renal capsule
    f. ring
    f. ring of disc
    f. scar tissue
    f. septum
    f. sheath
    f. skeleton
    f. temporal bone dysplasia
    f. tissue hyperplasia
    f. trigone
    f. tubercle
    f. tumor pleura
    f. union
    f. urinary tract polyp
    f. web
fibrovascular
    f. core
    f. polyp
    f. stalk
    f. tissue

fibroxanthoma
    malignant f.
    multiple f.'s
    pediatric f.
fibroxanthosarcoma
fibula, *pl.* **fibulae,** *pl.* **fibulas**
    apex of f.
    caput fibulae
    inferior tip of f.
    nutrient artery of f.
    proximal f.
fibulae (*pl of* fibula)
fibular
    f. articular surface
    f. collateral ligament
    f. fracture
    f. hallux sesamoid
    f. lymph node
    f. notch
    f. physis
    f. sesamoid bone
    f. vein
fibulas (*pl. of* fibula)
fibulotalar ligament
fibulotalocalcaneal (FTC)
    f. ligament
Ficat
    F. and Axlet staging system
    F. stage of avascular necrosis
    F. staging
Fick
    F. cardiac index
    F. equation
    F. law
    F. method
    F. method for measuring cardiac output
    F. position
    F. principle
    F. 1st law of diffusion
Ficoll gradient
FID
    free induction decay
FID-acquired echo
fiducial
    f. alignment system
    f. movement
    f. skin marker
4-field
    4-f. technique
    4-f. x-ray dosimetry
field
    f. alignment
    blocked vertex f.
    Brodmann cytoarchitectonic f.
    f. cancerization
    collapsed lung f.
    3D deformation f.
    f. defect

    dipole f.
    disc to magnetic f.
    f. drift
    f. echo
    f. echo acquisition with short repetition time and echo reduction (FASTER)
    electromagnetic focusing f. (EFF)
    electronic focusing f.
    f. emission tube
    f. even-echo rephasing (FEER)
    extremely low-frequency f.
    far f.
    fringe f.
    Gibbs random f.
    gonion gradient magnetic f.
    f. gradient
    gradient magnetic f.
    harmonic f.
    helmet f.
    high-powered f.
    f. inhomogeneity
    insonifying wave f.
    involved f.
    large hinge-angle electron f.
    f. lock
    lower lung f.
    lung f.
    magnetic fringe f.
    mantle f.
    Markov random f.
    midlung f.
    near f.
    f. of view (FOV)
    oscillating magnetic f.
    parietal eye f. (PEF)
    perturbing magnetic f.
    radiofrequency electromagnetic f.
    rotational f.
    f. size
    skimming of magnetic f.
    spade f.
    static magnetic f.
    stationary f.
    stippling of lung f.
    stray neutron f.
    f. strength
    tangential breast f.
    Tesla f.
    time-varying magnetic f.
    f. uniformity
    upper lung f.
    f. variation
    Z axis f.
field-echo
    f.-e. difference
    f.-e. imaging
    f.-e. pulse sequence

F

field-echo (*continued*)
    f.-e. sequence with even-echo
      rephasing (FEER)
    f.-e. sum
field-fitting
    f.-f. analysis
    f.-f. technique
**field-focusing nuclear magnetic resonance
(FONAR)**
**Fielding-Magliato subtrochanteric fracture
classification**
field-of-view
    extended f.-o.-v. (EFOV)
    f.-o.-v. imaging
    f.-o.-v. information
field-profiling coil
field-strength
    high f.-s.
Fiessinger-Leroy-Reiter syndrome
Fiessinger-Leroy syndrome
FIESTA
    fast imaging employing steady-state
    acquisition
      micro-MRI with FIESTA
      FIESTA technique
fighter's fracture
FIGO
    Fédération Internationale de
      Gynécologie Obstétrique (International
      Federation of Gynecology)
      FIGO stage carcinoma
      FIGO staging of adenocarcinoma of
      endometrium
FIGURA
    fused imaging-guided
    radiotherapy
FIGURAsystem
figure
    acetabular teardrop f.
    teardrop f.
figure-8 appearance
figure-4 position
figure-3 sign
fila (*pl. of* filum)
filament
    f. emission
    f. transformer
filament-nonfilament count
filarial infection
file
    Indian f.
filiform
    f. appendix
    f. polyp
    f. polyposis
filigree pattern
filipuncture
fill and spill of dye
filler block

filling
    augmented f.
    capillary f.
    compensatory capillary f.
    f. defect
    early venous f.
    f. factor
    late venous f.
    passive f.
    peak f.
    f. pressure
    rapid f.
    reduced f.
    retrograde f.
    subintimal f.
    time to peak f. (TTPF)
    ureteral f.
    ventricular f.
    vessel f.
    zero f.
film
    f. alternator
    anteroposterior f.
    f. badge
    biplane axial f.
    bitewing f.
    Bucky f.
    f. changer
    chest f.
    cine f.
    comparison f.
    corner f.
    cross-table lateral f.
    Curix Ultra UV-L f.
    cut and cine f.
    decubitus f.
    delayed f.
    f. density calibration
    f. diameter
    digital subtraction f.
    f. dispenser
    drain-out f.
    dual-emulsion mammography f.
    DuPont Cronex x-ray f.
    emulsion f.
    expiratory f.
    flat plate f.
    f. fog
    gamma f.
    GLP7 f.
    f. graininess
    grid f.
    f. hanger
    high-contrast f.
    horizontal beam f.
    in-department f.
    intraoperative f.
    kidneys, ureters, and bladder f.
    Knuttsen bending f.

Kodak Min-R f.
Kodak X-OMAT f.
late f.
lateral cervical spine f.
lateral decubitus f.
latitude f.
limited f.
low-contrast f.
low-dose f.
manual subtraction f.
mobility f.
nitrocellulose f.
normal chest f.
oblique f.
occlusal f.
overhead f.
overpenetrated f.
f. oxygenator
PA and lateral f.'s
panoramic x-ray f.
periapical f.
photo plotter f.
plain f.
Polaroid f.
port f.
portable chest f.
posteroanterior chest f.
postevacuation f.
postexercise f.
postreduction f.
postvoiding f.
preliminary f.
prone f.
radiochromic f.
right or left lateral decubitus f.
runoff f.
Scopix Laser f.
scout f.
screenless mammography f.
screen-type f.
semierect f.
sequential f.'s
serial subtraction f.'s
shoot-through lateral x-ray f.
silver halide f.
simulation f.
skull f.
f. slippage
f. speed
spot f.
stress f.
suboptimal f.
subtraction f.
supine f.
survey f.
UP7 f.
upright chest f.
upright compression spot f.
weightbearing f.

wide-latitude f.
working f.
x-ray f.
film-based
f.-b. screening mammogram
f.-b. viewing
FilmFax teleradiology system
film-focus distance
filmless
f. imaging
f. radiography
film-screen
f.-s. cassette
f.-s. contact test
f.-s. magnification
f.-s. mammography
f.-s. radiography
film-tube distance
filter
adaptive noise reduction f.
bandpass f.
bird's-nest f.
Butterworth f.
caval f.
compensating f.
density equalization f.
differencing f.
2-dimensional nonlinear f.
flattening f.
gaussian f.
Greenfield vena cava f.
Günther Tulip vena cava MReye f.
Hamming f.
Hann f.
helix f.
high-pass f.
inferior vena cava f.
inherent f.
inline low-pass f.
Kalman f.
K-edge f.
Keeper vena cava f.
leukoreduction f.
low-pass f.
Metz spatially varying f.
Mobin-Uddin vena cava f.
f. mold
nitinol inferior vena cava f.
OptEase permanent vena cava f.
over-the-wire Greenfield f.
10-pole Butterworth f.
prophylactic IVC f.
ramp f.
Recovery f.
Recovery nitinol f.
retrievable IVC f.
rhodium f.
SafeFlo IVC f.
sigma f.

F

filter (*continued*)
    Simon nitinol IVC f.
    Simon nitinol vena cava f.
    software-controlled internal
        hardware f.
    spatial f.
    stainless steel Greenfield f.
    Tempofilter vena cava f.
    temporal f.
    Thoreau f.
    titanium Greenfield f.
    translation-invariant f.
    TrapEase inferior vena cava f.
    TrapEase permanent IVC f.
    vena cava f.
    Vena Tech LGM vena cava f.
    Vena Tech low-profile f.
    Vena Tech LP vena cava f.
    wall f.
    wedge f.
    Weiner spatially varying f.
    Wiener MRI f.
    F. Wire distal protection
        device
    F. Wire EX
    Wratten 6B f.
filtered
    f. back projection (FBP)
    f. back-projection method
filtering
    3D low-pass f.
    dynamic f.
    low-pass f.
    morphologic f.
    multidimensional adaptive f.
    phase f.
filtration
    beam f.
    copper f.
    dynamic beat f.
    f. fraction
    glomerular f.
    postbeat f.
    supplemental beam f.
filum, *pl.* **fila**
    fatty f.
    f. terminale
    f. terminale fibrolipoma
fimbriated end
finding
    ancillary imaging f.
    angiographic f.
    atypical f.
    auscultatory f.
    cardinal f.
    characteristic f.
    concomitant f.
    concordance of MR f.
    constellation of f.'s

    discordant f.
    equivocal f.
    focal lateralizing f.
    incidental f.
    lateralizing f.
    no discernible f.
    nonspecific f.
    pathognomonic f.
    radiographic f.
    secondary sonographic f.
    specious f.
    spurious f.
    ultrasonographic f.
fine
    f. calcification
    f. detail
    f. injection
    f. peripheral reticular pattern
    f. speckled appearance
fine-needle
    f.-n. aspiration (FNA)
    f.-n. aspiration biopsy
    f.-n. puncture
    f.-n. transhepatic cholangiogram
        (FNTC)
finger
    baseball f.
    base of f.
    bolster f.
    bony tuft of f.
    clubbed f.
    Dawson f.
    drop f.
    football f.
    f. fracture
    hippocratic f.
    index f.
    jammed f.
    jersey f.
    little f.
    long f.
    f. lucent lesion
    mallet f.
    middle f.
    f. of tumor
    overlapping f.
    pedicle f.
    pulley of f.
    pulp of f.
    replantation of f.
    ring f.
    sausage f.
    spade f.
    speck f.
    spider f.
    stoved f.
    f. sweep
    tapered f.
    telescoping f.

trigger f.
f. web
webbed f.
finger-in-glove
f.-i.-g. pattern
f.-i.-g. sign
fingerlike
f. mucous plug
f. projection
f. villus
fingerprint
f. edema
f. image compression
f. mark artifact
f. pattern
fingertip
f. amputation
f. calcification
f. lesion
Finkelstein
F. sign
F. test
fire
side f.
firearm injury
FIRFT
fast inversion-recovery Fourier
transform
firing
f. of ectopic atrial focus
f. temperature
FIRM
fast inversion-recovery
motion-insensitive
firm
f. mass
f. neoplasia
F. sequence
Firooznia
threshold of F.
Fischer sign
Fischgold
F. bimastoid line
F. biventer line
FISH
fluorescence in situ hybridization
fish
f. flesh appearance
f. vertebra sign
Fisher subarachnoid hemorrhage (grade 1-4)
fish-hooking
urethral f.-h.
fishmeal worker's lung
fishmouth
f. amputation
f. configuration of mitral valve
f. cusp
f. fracture

f. mitral stenosis
f. mitral valve configuration
f. vertebra
fishnet appearance
fish-scale gallbladder
fishtail
f. tear
f. vertebra
FISP
fast imaging with steady-state
precession
mirrored FISP
FISP pulse sequence
fission
nuclear f.
f. product
f. track analysis
fissula ante fenestram
fissuration
fissure
abdominal f.
accessory azygos f.
anal f.
anterior interhemispheric f.
anterior median f.
antitragohelicine f.
auricular f.
azygos f.
brain f.
bulging lung f.
calcarine f.
callosomarginal f.
central cerebellar f.
cerebral f.
choroidal f.
chronic f.
collateral f.
cutaneous f.
decidual f.
dentate f.
displacement of interhemispheric
f.
f. fracture
glaserian f.
hepatic f.
hippocampal f.
horizontal f.
f. in ano
incomplete pulmonary f.
inferior accessory f.
inferior orbital f.
interhemispheric f. (IHF)
interlobar f.
lateral f.
ligamentum venosum f.
liver f.
longitudinal f.
lung f.
main f.

F

fissure (*continued*)
    major f.
    minor f.
    nasopalatal f.
    oblique f.
    occipital f.
    f. of anulus
    f. of lung
    f. of Rolando
    oral f.
    orbital f.
    palpebral f.
    portal f.
    rolandic f.
    f. sign
    studded f.
    superior orbital f.
    supraorbital f.
    sylvian f.
    transitional zone f.
    umbilical f.
    widened superior orbital f.
fissured atheromatous plaque
fisting
    rectal f.
fistula, *pl.* **fistulae,** *pl.* **fistulas**
    abdominal f.
    aerodigestive f.
    anal f.
    anorectal f.
    anovaginal f.
    aortic-enteric f.
    aortic-left ventricular f.
    aortic-right ventricular f.
    aortic sinus to right ventricle f.
    aortocaval f.
    aortoduodenal f.
    aortoenteric f.
    aortoesophageal f.
    aortojejunal f.
    aortopulmonary f.
    aortosigmoid f.
    arterial-arterial f.
    arterial-portal f.
    arteriobiliary f.
    arterioportobiliary f.
    arteriosinusoidal penile f.
    arteriovenous f. (AVF)
    autogenous hemodialysis f.
    biliary f.
    biliary-cutaneous f.
    biliary-duodenal f.
    biliary-enteric f.
    biliary-gastric f.
    bilioenteric f.
    bladder f.
    Blom-Singer tracheoesophageal f.
    BP f.
    branchial f.

Brescia-Cimino f.
bronchobiliary f.
bronchocavitary f.
bronchocutaneous f.
bronchoesophageal f.
bronchopleural f.
bronchopulmonary f.
cameral f.
caroticocavernous f.
carotid-cavernous f. (CCF)
carotid-cavernous sinus f.
carotid-dural f.
carotid-jugular f.
cavernous sinus f.
cecocutaneous f.
cerebral arteriovenous f.
cerebrospinal fluid f.
cholecystocholedochal f.
cholecystocolic f.
cholecystocutaneous f.
cholecystoduodenal f.
cholecystoduodenocolic f.
choledochal-colonic f.
choledochoduodenal f.
chyle f.
chylous f.
coil closure of coronary artery f.
colocolic f.
colocutaneous f.
colonic f.
colovaginal f.
colovesical f.
communicating f.
complex anorectal f.
congenital pulmonary arteriovenous f.
congenital tracheobiliary f.
coronary arteriosystemic f.
coronary arteriovenous f.
coronary artery cameral f.
coronary artery-pulmonary artery f.
coronary artery to right ventricle f.
cystic f.
dialysis f.
digestive-respiratory f.
dorsal enteric f.
duodenocolic f.
duodenopancreatic f.
dural arteriovenous f. (DAVF)
dural carotid cavernous f. (DCCF)
durocutaneous f.
dysfunctional autogenous hemodialysis f.
Eck f.
enteric f.
enterocolic f.
enterocutaneous f.
enteroenteral f.
enterospinal f.

enterourethral f.
enterovaginal f.
enterovesical f.
esophagorespiratory f.
esophagotracheal f.
external biliary f.
extrasphincteric anal f.
fecal f.
f. formation
gastric f.
gastroabdominal f.
gastrobiliary f.
gastrocolic f.
gastrocutaneous f.
gastroduodenal f.
gastrointestinal f.
gastrojejunocolic f.
genitourinary f.
graft-enteric f.
hepatic arteriovenous f.
hepatic artery-portal vein f.
hepatopleural f.
hepatoportal biliary f.
high-flow arteriovenous f.
horseshoe f.
H-type tracheoesophageal f.
hyperdynamic AV f.
iatrogenic iliocaval f.
ileosigmoid f.
f. in ano
infralevator f.
intersphincteric anal f.
intracranial arteriovenous f.
intradural retromedullary
  arteriovenous f.
intrahepatic arterial-portal f.
intrahepatic AV f.
intrapulmonary arteriovenous f.
jejunocolic f.
labyrinthine f.
Mann-Bollman f.
mediastinal f.
mesenteric f.
metroperitoneal f.
microvenoarteriolar f.
mucous f.
neurenteric f.
orofacial f.
f. ostium
pancreatic cutaneous f.
pancreaticopleural f.
paraprosthetic-enteric f.
parietal f.
periareolar f.
perineovaginal f.
persistent bronchopleural f.
pilonidal f.
pleural f.
pleurocutaneous f.

postbiopsy renal AV f.
premedullary arteriovenous f.
pulmonary arteriovenous f.
radial artery to cephalic vein f.
radiation f.
radiculomeningeal f.
rectal f.
rectovaginal f.
rectovesical f.
respiratory-esophageal f.
retroperitoneal f.
spinal dural arteriovenous f.
splanchnic AV f.
splenic AV f.
splenobronchial f.
supralevator f.
suprasphincteric f.
TE f.
thoracic duct-cutaneous f.
thoracobiliary f.
tracheobiliary f.
tracheobronchial f.
tracheobronchoesophageal f.
tracheoesophageal f. (TEF)
f. tract study
transdural f.
transsphincteric anal f.
trigeminal cavernous f.
type A carotid cavernous f.
ureteral f.
ureterocutaneous f.
ureterointestinal f.
ureteroperitoneal f.
ureterovaginal f.
urethrovaginal f.
urinary f.
vaginal f.
vein of Galen f.
venobiliary f.
vertebrojugular f.
vertebrovertebral f.
vesical f.
vesicocolic f.
vesicovaginal f.
vitelline f.
fistulae (*pl. of* fistula)
fistulas (*pl. of* fistula)
fistulogram
  cine f.
  venous f.
fistulography
fistulous
  f. gas communication
  f. tract
fit
  smoothed curve f.
fitting
  peak f.
Fitz-Hugh and Curtis syndrome

F

fixation
  f. articulation
  atlantoaxial rotary f.
  bowel loop f.
  catheter f.
  f. disc
  external wire f.
  intramedullary f.
  intrapedicular f.
  metallic rod f.
  f. of scoliosis
  open reduction and internal f.
    (ORIF)
  plate-and-screw f.
  screw f.
  spinal f.
  suprasyndesmotic f.
  transsyndesmotic screw f.
  triangular external ankle f.
  wire f.
fixator
  dynamic axial f.
  f. muscle
fixed
  f. airway obstruction
  f. coronary obstruction
  f. flexion contracture
  f. gantry
  f. intracavitary filling defect
  f. mass
  f. perfusion defect
  f. pulmonary valvular resistance
  f. radiotracer defect
  f. 3rd-degree AV block
  f. segment of bowel
fixed-orifice aortic stenosis
fixed-shaped coplanar or nonplanar
  radiation beam bouquet
fixer
fixing time
flabby heart
^{18}F-labeled
  fluorine-18-labeled
  ^{18}F-labeled fatty acid
  ^{18}F-labeledHFA
  ^{18}F-labeled polyfluorinated
    ethyl
F-labeled levodopa PET scan
Flack sinuatrial node
flag
  Rudick red f.
flail
  f. air
  f. chest
  f. digit
  f. foot
  f. joint
  f. mitral valve
  f. shoulder

FLAIR
  fluid-attenuated inversion recovery
    FLAIR echo-planar imaging
    FLAIR image
FLAIR-FLASH
  fluid-attenuated inversion recovery-fast
    low-angle shot
    FLAIR-FLASH imaging
FLAK
  flow artifact killer
    FLAK technique
flake
  f. fracture
  f. fracture of hamate
flake-shaped injury
flaking of cartilage
flaky calcification
flame
  f. appearance
  f. emission spectroscopy
    (FES)
  f. ionization detector
Flamingo stent
flange
  shaft f.
flank
  f. bone
  f. stripe
flap
  bone f.
  bursal f.
  entry f.
  foramen ovale f.
  intimal f.
  Karapandzic lip reconstruction f.
  liver f.
  localized intimal f.
  lytic area bone f.
  necrotic f.
  osteoplastic f.
  pedicle f.
  pericardial f.
  pleural f.
  f. positioning
  postangioplasty intimal f.
  rotary door f. (RDF)
  scapular f.
  scimitar-shaped f.
  subclavian f.
  f. tear
  TRAM f.
flaplike valve
flap-valve
  f.-v. mechanism
  f.-v. ventricular septal defect
flare
  condylar f.
  f. effect
  metaphysial f.

f. phenomenon
f. reaction
tibial f.
trochanteric f.
FLARE
fast low-angle acquisition with
relaxation enhancement
flared ilium
FLASH
fast low-angle shot
FLASH acquisition
diffusion-perfusion snapshot FLASH
FLASH image
FLASH magnetic resonance imaging
FLASH photolysis
flashlamp-pulsed dye laser
flashlamp-pumped pulsed dye laser
FlashPoint image-guided surgical
instrument
flask
Erlenmeyer f.
vascular f.
flask-shaped
f.-s. heart
f.-s. ulcer
flat
f. adenoma
f. bone
f. colorectal carcinoma
f. diastolic slope
f. electroencephalogram
f. facet
f. neck vein
f. pelvis
f. plate
f. plate film
f. plate of abdomen
f. suture
f. time-intensity profile
f. vertebral body
f. waist sign
Flatau-Schilder disease
flat-field imaging
flatfoot
calcaneovalgus f.
f. deformity
Durham f.
flat-hand test
flat-panel
f.-p. detector
f.-p. detector-based volumetric
computed tomography
f.-p. megavoltage imager
f.-p. volume computed tomography
(FPVCT)
flat-plate detector
flattened
f. arch
f. duodenal fold

f. E-to-F slope
f. longitudinal arch of foot
flattening
cortical f.
f. filter
f. filter beam
f. of diaphragm
f. of gyrus
f. of normal lordotic curvature
f. of normal lumbar curve
f. ratio
flat-top
f.-t. bladder
f.-t. talus
flaval ligament
flavone acetic acid (FAA)
flavum
ligamentum f.
pleating of ligamentum f.
flawed
f. image
f. imaging
flax-dresser disease
Flechsig bundle
Fleckinger view
fleck sign
fleecy mass
fleet
F. Phospho-Soda bowel preparation
F. Prep Kit (1, 2, 3)
fleeting lung infiltrate
Fleischmann bursa
Fleischner
F. line
F. position
F. sign
Fletcher
F. afterloader
F. dyspnea scale
F. factor
F. projection
F. rule of irradiation tolerance
Fletcher-Delclos dome cylinder
Fletcher-Suit-Delclos (FSD)
F.-S.-D. tandem
Fletcher-Suit system for radium therapy
fleur-de-lis pattern
flexa
coxa f.
Flexart MRI scanner
flexible
f. anterior 6-channel phased-array
abdominal imaging coil
f. biopsy needle
f. endofluoroscopy
f. nephroscope
f. over-wire system
f. radiofrequency coil
f. spastic equinovarus deformity

F

flexible (*continued*)
 f. surface coil
 f. surface coil-type resonator
 (FSCR)
flexible-tip guidewire
Flexiflo
Flexima biliary drainage catheter
flexion
 f. and extension exercises
 f. and extension views
 angle of greatest f. (AGF)
 f. burst fracture
 f. contracture
 f. deformity
 external rotation in f. (ERF)
 internal rotation in f. (IRF)
 f. interspinous distance
 f. maneuver
 f. position
 f. teardrop fracture
flexion-adduction contracture
flexion-compression fracture
flexion-distraction
 f.-d. fracture
 f.-d. injury
flexion-extension
 f.-e. injury
 f.-e. plane
 f.-e. projection
 f.-e. radiography
flexion-rotation injury
Flexi-Tip ureteral catheter
Flexlase 600 laser
flexor
 f. bursa
 f. canal
 capital f.
 f. carpi radialis (FCR)
 f. carpi radialis muscle
 f. carpi radialis tendon
 f. carpi ulnaris
 f. carpi ulnaris aponeurosis
 f. carpi ulnaris tendon
 f. digiti minimi
 f. digiti minimi brevis
 f. digiti quinti brevis (FDQB)
 f. digiti quinti brevis muscle
 f. digitorum brevis
 f. digitorum communis tendon
 f. digitorum longus (FDL)
 f. digitorum longus muscle
 f. digitorum longus tendon
 f. digitorum profundus
 f. digitorum profundus muscle
 f. digitorum profundus tendon
 f. digitorum sublimis (FDS)
 f. digitorum sublimis tendon
 f. digitorum superficialis (FDS)
 f. digitorum superficialis muscle

 f. digitorum superficialis tendon
 f. hallucis brevis
 f. hallucis brevis muscle
 f. hallucis brevis tendon
 f. hallucis longus
 f. hallucis longus tendon
 F. introducer
 f. plate
 f. pollicis brevis
 f. pollicis brevis tendon
 f. pollicis longus
 f. pollicis longus tendon
 f. profundus tendon
 f. retinaculum
 f. sublimis tendon
 f. tendon sheath
 f. tenosynovitis
flexor-pronator muscle group
FlexStent
 Gianturco-Roubin F.
FlexStrand cable
Flex-T guidewire
flexural pseudotumor
flexure
 caudal f.
 cephalic f.
 cerebral f.
 cervical f.
 colonic f.
 cranial f.
 duodenojejunal f. (DJF)
 hepatic f.
 inferior duodenal f. (IDF)
 left colonic f.
 right colonic f.
 sigmoid f.
 splenic f.
flicker electroretinogram
Flint colon injury scale
flip
 f. angle
 spin f.
 tristimulus value f.
 value f.
flip-angle image
flip-flop
 f.-f. enhancement
 f.-f. pattern
 f.-f. phenomenon
flipped meniscus sign
floating
 f. arch fracture
 f. cartilage
 f. elbow
 f. endocardial centroid
 f. epicardial centroid
 f. gallbladder
 f. gallstone
 f. image

f. kidney
f. knee
f. leaflet
f. ligament
f. liver
f. organ
f. osteophyte
f. palate fracture
f. patella
f. prostate
f. rib
f. spleen
f. thumb
f. tooth
f. villus
f. viscera sign
floccular fossa
flocculation of barium
flocculent focus of calcification
flocculi (*pl. of* flocculus)
flocculonodular
f. lobe
f. lobe of cerebellum
f. tumor
flocculus, *pl.* **flocculi**
Flocks and Kadesky system
flood
intrinsic f.
F. ligament
f. phantom
f. section
f. source
floor
bladder f.
fibromuscular pelvic f.
inguinal f.
f. of orbit
f. of ventricle
pelvic f.
sellar f.
floppy
f. mitral valve
f. thumb sign
f. valve syndrome
Flo-Rester vessel occluder
florid
f. callus
f. cardiac tamponade
f. duct lesion
f. follicular hyperplasia
f. plaque
f. reactive periostitis
flottant
pouce f.
flow
absolute blood f.
f. acceleration
aliased f.
altered blood f.

anatomic shunt f.
antegrade bile f.
antegrade blood f.
antegrade diastolic f.
aortic f.
f. arrest
f. artifact killer (FLAK)
autoregulation of cerebral blood f.
azygos blood f.
backward f.
bile f.
blood f.
capillary blood f.
cephalization of blood f.
cerebral blood f. (CBF)
chronic reserve f.
collateral blood f.
f. compensation
compromised f.
coronary blood f.
coronary reserve f. (CRF)
countercurrent f.
f. cytometric DNA measurement
f. cytometry
f. cytometry sample preparation
f. cytometry technique
dampened pulsatile f.
2D color-coded imaging of blood f.
decreased cerebral blood f.
diastolic zero f.
Doppler color f.
Doppler study of blood f.
f. effect artifact
effective pulmonary blood f. (EPBF)
effective renal plasma f. (ERPF)
electron f.
expiratory f.
fast Fourier f. (FFF)
fluid f.
flush f.
forward f.
Ganz formula for coronary sinus f.
global cerebral blood f. (gCBF)
global intracranial blood f.
great cardiac vein f. (GCVF)
hepatofugal f.
hepatopetal f.
high-velocity f.
hyperemic f.
f. imaging
inspiratory f.
intercoronary collateral f.
internal carotid systolic peak f. (ICSPF)
intramyocardial coronary blood f.
intrarenal arterial f.
intrasac f.
jet f.
krypton f.

F

flow (*continued*)
laminar f.
left-to-right f.
local bone blood f.
low-velocity f.
lung volume loop f.
maintenance of f.
f. mapping technique
maximum midexpiratory f. (MMEF)
microcirculatory blood f.
midexpiratory tidal f.
mitral valve f.
mixed petal-fugal f.
myocardial blood f. (MBF)
f. of contrast material
peak expiratory f. (PEF)
peak flush f.
peak velocity of blood f.
peripheral blood f.
petal-fugal f.
f. phenomenon
physiologic shunt f.
plug f.
Poiseuille f.
portal f.
f. portion of bone scan
preferential f.
protodiastolic reversal of blood f.
pulmonary blood f. (PBF)
pulmonary output f.
pulmonary versus systemic f.
f. quantification
Quintero umbilical artery blood f.
  (stage 1-4)
f. rate
real-time phase-contrast f.
real-time quantitative f.
f. redistribution
regional cerebral blood f. (rCBF)
regional myocardial blood f.
regurgitant pandiastolic f.
regurgitant systolic f.
relative cerebral blood f.
relative regional blood f. (rrBF)
relative shunt f.
resistance blood f.
f. respiratory artifact obliteration
  with directed orthogonal pulses
  (FRODO)
resting regional myocardial blood f.
restoration of f.
retrograde systolic f.
reversed vertebral blood f.
F. Rider microcatheter
sluggish f.
stasis of blood f.
straight-line f.
f. study
supratentorial cerebral blood f.

systemic blood f. (SBF)
systemic output f.
through-plane f.
time-averaged f.
tissue f.
to-and-fro f.
total cerebral blood f. (TCBF)
f. tract
transmitral f.
tricuspid valve f.
turbulent blood f.
turbulent intraluminal f.
unequal pulmonary blood f.
uterine blood volume f.
f. velocity
f. velocity profile
f. velocity signal
f. velocity waveform
f. void
f. void effect
f. volume
xenon-enhanced cerebral blood f.
  (X-CBF)
zero net f.
flow-compensated
f.-c. gradient-echo sequence
f.-c. image
flow-compromising lesion
flow-controlled valve
flow-dependent obstruction
flow-directed approach
flow-encoded image
flow-encoding gradient
flow-function mismatch
flow-induced artifact
flowing
f. anterior vertebra ossification
f. spin
FloWire
F. Doppler ultrasound
F. ultrasound device
flow-limited expiration
flow-limiting
f.-l. lesion
f.-l. stenosis
flowmeter, flow meter
Doppler f.
Gould electromagnetic f.
Parks bidirectional Doppler f.
pulsed Doppler f.
flowmetry
blood f.
Doppler f.
laser Doppler f. (LDF)
Narcomatic f.
Parks 800 bidirectional Doppler f.
Statham electromagnetic f.
**flow-mode ultrafast computed
tomography**

flow-on gradient-echo image
flow-related
    f.-r. artifact
    f.-r. enhancement
    f.-r. enhancement effect
    f.-r. phase error
    f.-r. phase shift
flow-sensitive
    f.-s. alternating inversion recovery
    (FAIR)
    f.-s. MR imaging
flow-time curve
flow-volume loop
FLT
    fluorodeoxythymidine
flu
    influenza
fluctuant mass
fluctuation
    Poisson noise f.
fluence
    energy f.
    photon f.
    f. profile
fluffy
    f. amorphous calcification
    f. infiltrate
    f. margin
    f. periosteal reaction
    f. pulmonary nodule
    f. rarefaction
fluid
    abdominal collection of f.
    f. accumulation
    amnionic f.
    anechoic f.
    articular f.
    ascitic f.
    bloodless f.
    bursal f.
    cavitary f.
    cerebrospinal f. (CSF)
    f. collection
    cystic f.
    dammed-up cerebrospinal f.
    f. density
    edema f.
    encapsulated f.
    endometrial canal f.
    f. expansion
    extracellular f.
    f. extravasation
    extravascular f.
    f. flow
    free abdominal f.
    free cul-de-sac f.
    free peritoneal f.
    high-signal intratendinous collection
      of f.

    increased interstitial f.
    f. intake
    f. interface
    interstitial f.
    intestinal f.
    intraperitoneal f.
    joint f.
    f. level
    loculated pleural f.
    f. overload
    pelvic f.
    pericardial f.
    pericerebral f.
    pericholecystic f.
    pericolonic f.
    periesophageal f.
    perigraft f.
    peritoneal cavity f.
    pleural f.
    prostatic f.
    proteinaceous f.
    f. resorption
    retained fetal lung f.
    f. retention
    f. sequestration
    serohemorrhagic f.
    serosanguineous f.
    f. signal
    silicone f.
    f. space
    spinal f.
    subgaleal cerebrospinal f.
    subphrenic f.
    subpulmonic f.
    synovial f.
    transudation of f.
    transudative pericardial f.
    f. volume
    f. wave
fluid-attenuated
    f.-a. inversion recovery
    (FLAIR)
    f.-a. inversion recovery-fast
    low-angle shot (FLAIR-
    FLASH)
    f.-a. inversion recovery imaging
fluid-blood layer
fluid-filled
    f.-f. bronchogram
    f.-f. catheter
    f.-f. cyst
    f.-f. kidney mass
    f.-f. loop of bowel
    f.-f. sac
fluid-flow artifact
fluid-fluid
    f.-f. level
    f.-f. level sign
fluid-sensitive sequence

F

fluke
    liver f.
    lung f.
    Oriental lung f.
Fluoratec imaging agent
fluorescein
    f. angiogram
    f. indocyanine green angiography
    f. sodium
    f. uptake
fluorescence
    energy-dispersive x-ray f. (EDXRF)
    f. in situ hybridization (FISH)
    f. resonance energy transfer
    (FRET)
    f. resonance energy transfer
    microscopy
    f. spectroscopy
fluorescence-activated
    f.-a. cell sorter (FACScan)
    f.-a. cell sorting
fluorescent
    f. micelle
    f. phosphor
    f. ray
    f. scan
    f. screen
Fluorescite injection
fluoride
    argon f. (ArF)
    barium f.
    holmium-yttrium lithium f.
    (holmium-YLF)
    f. ion positron emission tomography
    lithium f. (LiF)
    neodymium:yttrium-lithium f.
    (Nd:YLF)
    yttrium lithium f. (YLF)
fluorine
    f. 18 (^{18}F, F-18)
    f. 19 (^{19}F, F-19)
    f. imaging agent
fluorine-18
    f.-18 2-dialkylamino-6-
    acylmalononitrile substituted
    naphthalene (FDDNP)
    f.-18 fluorocholine (F-18 FCH)
    f.-18 fluoro-2-deoxyglucose imaging
    agent (F-18 FDG)
    f.-18 fluorodeoxyglucose-positron
    emission tomography
    f.-18 fluorodeoxythymidine (F-18
    FLT)
    f.-18 fluoroethyltyrosine
    (F-18 FET)
2-[fluorine-18]fluoro-2-deoxy-D-glucose
fluorine-18-labeled (^{18}F-labeled)
fluorine-19 spectroscopy
Fluor-I-Strip

Fluor-I-Strip-AT
fluorocaptopril
fluorocarbon-based ultrasound contrast
  agent
fluorochloride
    barium f.
fluorocholine
    fluorine-18 f. (F-18 FCH)
fluorochrome
fluorodeoxyglucose (FDG)
    f. F-18 injection
    f. imaging agent
    f. positron emission tomography
    (FDG-PET)
    positron emission tomography with
    f. (FDG-PET)
2-fluoro 2-deoxyglucose (FDG)
18-fluoro-deoxyglucose PET scan
fluorodeoxyglucose-6-phosphate
fluorodeoxythymidine (FLT)
    fluorine-18 f. (F-18 FLT)
fluorodeoxyuridine
fluoro-DOPA
fluoroestradiol (FES)
fluoroethyltyrosine
    fluorine-18 f. (F-18 FET)
fluorography
    digital f.
    spot film f.
fluorohalide
    europium-activated barium f.
fluorometer
    96-well scanning f.
fluorometry
    image intensification f.
    2-plane f.
fluoromibolerone
fluoromisonidazole
Fluoroplex
FluoroPlus
    F. angiography
    F. cardiac digital fluoroscopy
    F. cardiac digital imaging system
    F. real-time digital imaging system
fluoropropylepidepride
fluoroptic thermometry system
fluoropyrimidine
fluororoentgenography
FluoroScan C-arm fluoroscopy
fluoroscope
    Edison f.
fluoroscopic
    f. assistance
    f. control
    f. gantry
    f. guidance
    f. image
    f. imaging
    f. localization

fluoroscopy *(continued)*
f. observation
f. programmed radiography (FPR)
f. pushing technique
radiographic and f.
f. road-mapping technique
f. triggering
f. view

fluoroscopy
airway f.
biplane f.
C-arm f.
chest f.
computed tomography f. (CTF)
computerized f.
digital f.
digital pulsed f. (DPF)
electric joint f.
FluoroPlus cardiac digital f.
FluoroScan C-arm f.
high-resolution f.
image-amplified f.
mobile f.
Orca C-arm f.
orthogonal C-arm f.
portable C-arm image
  intensifier f.
radiography and f. (R&F)
real-time CT f.
region-of-interest f.
simultaneous f.
spinal f.
f. time
video f.

fluoroscopy-guided
f.-g. condylar lift-off imaging
f.-g. subarachnoid phenol block
  therapy

fluorosis
osteophytosis in f.

fluorotamoxifen
Fluoro Tip cannula
**FluoroTrak fluoroscopy-based surgical
  navigation system**
fluorotropapride
fluorotyrosine
FluoroVision
flush
f. angiogram
f. aortogram imaging
f. aortography
cervical f.
f. flow
saline solution f.

flush-tank sign
FLUTE
fat and long T2-suppressed ultrashort
  echo time

flutter
atrial fetal f.

flux
electron f.
improved photon f.
magnetic f.
photon f.

fluxionary hyperemia
flying
f. focal spot
f. spot excimer laser
f. spot excimer laser system

fly-swatterlike pad
fly-through
endoluminal f.-t.
f.-t. viewing
virtual f.-t.

^{255}Fm
fermium 255

Fm
fermium

FMAP
feeding mean arterial pressure

FMD
fibromuscular disease

FMH
1st metatarsal head

F-misonidazole
fMR
functional magnetic resonance
  fMR tube

fMRA
functional magnetic resonance
  angiography

fMRI
functional magnetic resonance
  imaging
    cognitive fMRI
    integrated fMRI
    fMRI signal change
    VNS-synchronized BOLD fMRI

FMS
fatty meal sonogram

FNA
fine-needle aspiration

FNH
focal nodular hyperplasia
follicular nodular hyperplasia

FNTC
fine-needle transhepatic
  cholangiogram

foam
f. cushion
f. embolus
minimally attenuating medical-grade
  f.
f. vacuum pillow

foam-padded Velcro restraint
foamy esophagus
FOB
fiberoptic bronchoscopy

F

focal

f. alimentary tract calcification
f. alveolar consolidation
f. alveolar infiltrate
f. and diffuse lung texture analysis
f. area of hemorrhage
f. area of hypometabolism
f. articular cartilage lesion
f. asymmetric density
f. asymmetry
f. atrophy
f. attenuation
f. back pain
f. bacterial nephritis
f. biliary cirrhosis
f. bone sclerosis
f. caliectasis
f. cartilage erosion
f. cecal apical thickening
f. cerebellar dysplasia
f. cerebral ischemia
f. cold liver lesion
f. colitis
f. cortical dysplasia
f. cortical hyperplasia
f. cranial radiation therapy
f. damage
f. decreased radiotracer uptake
f. deficit
f. degenerative change
f. disc herniation
f. distortion
f. dust emphysema
f. eccentric stenosis
f. edema
f. endocardial hemorrhage
f. esophageal narrowing
f. fat necrosis
f. fatty infiltration of liver
f. fibrocartilaginous dysplasia of tibia
f. fibrosis
f. film distance (FFD)
f. gallbladder wall thickening
f. gigantism
f. hemispheric lesion
f. hepatic necrosis
f. high-intensity zone
f. hot liver lesion
f. hydronephrosis
f. hyperinflation
f. hypoechoic lesion
f. indentation
f. inflammation
f. interstitial infiltrate
f. intimal thickening
f. ischemic lesion
f. lateralizing finding
f. length

f. limb abnormality
f. liver hot spot
f. liver scintigraphic defect
f. lobular carcinoma
f. lung disease
f. malformation
f. mass
f. metabolic abnormality
f. myometrial contraction
f. neurologic sign
f. nodular enhancement
f. nodular hyperplasia (FNH)
f. nuclear herniation
f. organizing pneumonia
f. osseous offset
f. pancreatitis
f. parenchymal brain lesion
f. parenchymal cryptococcoma
f. pattern
f. perihepatitis
f. perivascular infiltrate
f. plane tomography
f. plaquelike defect
f. pleural plaque
f. pool
f. pooling of tracer
f. pulmonary hemorrhage
f. pulmonary uptake
f. pyloric hypertrophy
f. renal hypertrophy
f. small bowel disease
f. sparing
f. splenic lesion
f. spot (FS)
f. spot blur
f. spot size
f. spot-to-film angle
f. spot-to-object distance
f. spot tracking
f. subluxation of vertebra
f. tumor
f. ulcer
f. wall motion abnormality
f. white matter signal abnormality
f. zone

focally

f. decreased renal neoplasia
f. dilated duct
f. increased renal echogenicity

foci (*pl. of* focus)
focus, *pl.* **foci**

Assmann f.
atrial f.
basal ganglion echogenic f.
bright cystic f.
brightly echogenic f.
f. detection
discrete hyperintense f.
echogenic f.

ectopic f.
epileptic f.
epileptogenic f.
firing of ectopic atrial f.
Ghon f.
hemorrhagic f.
hot f.
hyperechoic f.
hypermetabolic activity f.
inflammatory f.
junctional f.
linear f.
mesial frontal f.
metastatic f.
midline parasagittal f.
multifocal residual f.
multiple foci
multizone transmit-receive f.
nodular hyperintense f.
occipital f.
f. of calcification
f. of tumor
punctate hyperintense f.
radiolucent f.
residual f.
satellite cartilaginous f.
Simon f.
stationary f.
subependymal/subpial f.

focused
f. appendix computed tomography
(FACT)
f. assessment by sonography for
trauma (FAST)
f. assessment with sonography in
trauma
f. grid
f. nuclear magnetic resonance
f. segmented ultrasound machine
f. ultrasound
focus-film distance (FFD)
focusing
f. collimator
dynamic f.
zone f.
focus-object distance (FOD)
focus-skin distance (FSD)
focus-to-detector distance
focus-to-isocentre distance
FOD
focus-object distance
fog
f. artifact
base f.
film f.
Fogarty
F. adherent clot catheter
F. balloon embolectomy
catheter

Edwards F.
F. maneuver
F. Thru-Lumen catheter
fogging
f. effect
f. phenomenon
foil
scattering f.
Foix-Alajouanine syndrome
Foix-Chavany-Marie syndrome
fold
abnormal esophageal f.
abnormal small bowel f.
accordion f.
adipose f.
alar f.
amnionic f.
aryepiglottic f.
axillary f.
blunted mucosal f.
caval f.
cecal f.
cholecystoduodenocolic f.
circular f.
costocolic f.
crescentic submucosal f.
distorted mucosal f.
Douglas f.
duodenojejunal f.
duodenomesocolic f.
dural f.
effaced mucosal f.
epigastric f.
epiglottic f.
esophageal f.
falciform f.
flattened duodenal f.
fragmented mucosal f.
gastric f.
gastropancreatic f.
genital f.
giant gastric f.
glossoepiglottic f.
glossopalatine f.
gluteal f.
Guérin f.
haustral f.
Hensing f.
hepatopancreatic f.
hidebound small bowel f.
ileocecal f.
ileocolic f.
inferior transverse rectal f.
inframammary f.
inguinal f.
irregular mucosal f.
Kerckring f.
Kohlrausch f.
lateral umbilical f.

F

fold (*continued*)
    longitudinal esophageal f.
    medial umbilical f.
    mucosal f.
    Nélaton f.
    palatopharyngeal f.
    paraduodenal f.
    f. pattern
    pericardial f.
    peritoneal f.
    pleuroperitoneal f.
    prepyloric f.
    rectal f.
    rectouterine f.
    rugal f.
    sacrogenital f.
    semilunar f.
    sentinel f.
    sickle-shaped f.
    sigmoid f.
    skin f.
    smooth thickened mucosal f.
    spiral f.
    stack-of-coins mucosal f.
    submucosal circular f.
    superior duodenal f.
    superior transverse rectal f.
    tethered small bowel f.
    thickened duodenal f.
    thickened esophageal f.
    thickened gastric f.
    thickened nodular irregular small
      bowel f.
    thickened stomach f.
    thickened straight small bowel f.
    transverse esophageal f.
    uteric f.
    Vater f.
    ventriculoinfundibular f.
    vestigial f.
folded
    f. fundus of gallbladder
    f. lung
    f. step ramp
folding potential analysis
foldover
    f. artifact
    image f.
folia (*pl. of* folium)
folial pattern
folium, *pl.* **folia**
    cerebellar f.
    disorganized f.
    shrunken f.
    folia vermis
Folius muscle
follicle
    aggregated lymphatic f.
    anovular ovarian f.

    ascendant f.
    atretic ovarian f.
    dominant f.
    gastric lymphatic f.
    geographic f.
    graafian f.
    intestinal f.
    inverse f.
    luteinized unruptured f.
    lymphoid f.
    f. lysis
    malpighian f.
    nabothian f.
    primordial f.
    ruptured f.
    thyroid f.
    unruptured f.
follicular
    f. B-cell lymphoma
    f. bronchiectasis
    f. bronchiolitis
    f. bronchitis
    f. carcinoma
    f. center cell lymphoma
    f. edema
    f. gastritis
    f. involution
    f. mixed small cleaved lymphoma
    f. nodular hyperplasia (FNH)
    f. ovarian cyst
    f. pattern
    f. phase
    f. predominantly large cell
      lymphoma
    f. predominantly small cell
      lymphoma
    f. salpingitis
    f. thyroid adenoma
    f. thyroid carcinoma
folliculare
    oophoroma f.
follicularis
    enteritis f.
followthrough
    barium meal and f.
    small bowel f. (SBFT)
    upper GI with small bowel f.
    f. view
followup duplex Doppler sonography
fomes, *pl.* **fomites**
fomites (*pl. of* fomes)
FONAR
    field-focusing nuclear magnetic
      resonance
      FONAR Standing Ovation MRI
        system
FONAR-360 MRI scanner
Fong disease
Fontana canal

fontanelle
anterior f.
anterolateral f.
bregmatic f.
bulging f.
closed f.
cranial f.
frontal f.
fused f.
Gerdy f.
mastoid f.
occipital f.
open f.
overriding suture of f.
posterior f.
posterolateral f.
sagittal f.
sphenoid f.
tense f.
triangular f.
Fontan operation
food
F. and Drug Administration (FDA)
f. bolus obstruction
cholecystokinetic f.
retention of f.
foot, *pl.* **feet**
abnormal position of f.
f. architecture
arch of f.
ball of f.
calcaneocavus f.
Charcot f.
Claw f.
f. deformity
digital artery of f.
f. dysplasia
flail f.
flattened longitudinal arch of f.
f. fracture
Friedreich f.
hollow f.
large-vessel disease of diabetic f.
lateral spring ligament of f.
Madura f.
march f.
neuropathic Charcot f.
phalanx of f.
planovalgus f.
f. plate
f. revascularization
rockerbottom f.
valgus f.
varus f.
foot-ankle complex
football
f. finger
f. player's shoulder
f. sign

footling presentation
foot-plate (*var. of* footplate)
footplate, foot-plate, foot plate
intraluminal polymeric f.
footprint analysis
foot-progression angle (FPA)
foramen, *pl.* **foramina**
alveolar f.
anterior condyloid f.
anterior palatine f.
anterior sacral f.
aortic f.
apical f.
arachnoidal f.
base of skull f.
Bichat f.
blind f.
Bochdalek f.
Botallo f.
brain mass in jugular f.
carotid f.
cecal f.
cervical neural f.
conjugate f.
costotransverse f.
cranial f.
Duverney f.
emissary sphenoidal f.
enlarged vertebral f.
enlargement of vertebral f.
epiploic f.
ethmoidal f.
external acoustic f.
Ferrein f.
Froesch f.
frontal f.
greater palatine f.
greater sciatic f.
great sacrosciatic f.
Huschke f.
Hyrtl f.
intertransverse f.
interventricular f.
intervertebral f.
jugular f.
f. lacerum
lesser sciatic f.
Magendie f.
f. magnum
f. magnum decompression
f. magnum herniation
mandibular f.
mastoid f.
mental f.
Morgagni f.
neural f.
nutrient f.
obturator f.
f. of Luschka

F

foramen (*continued*)
 f. of Monro
 f. of Vesalius
 f. of Winslow
 optic f.
 f. ovale
 f. ovale flap
 f. ovale valve
 palatine f.
 parietal f.
 petrosal f.
 restrictive bulboventricular f.
 Retzius f.
 f. rotundum
 sacral f.
 sacrosciatic f.
 skull base f.
 sphenopalatine f.
 f. spinosum
 spinous f.
 Stensen f.
 stylomastoid f.
 sublabral f.
 superior maxillary f.
 supraorbital f.
 thebesian f.
 f. transversarium
 f. venosum
 vertebral f.
 Weitbrecht f.
 zygomaticofacial f.
foramina (*pl. of* foramen)
foraminal
 f. encroachment
 f. node
 f. space
 f. stenosis
force
 chronic outward f.
 coulomb f.
 electromotive f.
 magnetic line of f.
 nuclear f.
 pascal of f.
 radial resistive f.
 reserve f.
 rotational f.
 shearing f.
 Starling f.
 stroke f.
 tensile f.
 torsion impaction f.
 transverse plane f.
forced
 f. expiratory volume
 f. flexion injury
force-frequency relation
forceful parasternal motion
force-length relation

force-velocity relation
forearm
 f. amputation
 f. fracture
forebrain
forefoot
 f. abduction deformity
 f. angulation
 narrowing of f.
foregut
 bronchopulmonary f.
 f. cyst
 f. duplication
foreign
 f. body
 f. body embolus
 f. body granuloma
 f. body in esophagus
 f. body sensation
 f. body upper airway obstruction
 f. debris
 f. material artifact
Forel
 H field of F.
foreshortened image dataset
foreshortening
 anular f.
 f. artifact
Forestier disease
forking
 aqueductal f.
 f. of sylvian aqueduct
form
 ring-shaped f.
Formad kidney
formaldehyde, formic aldehyde
format
 cylindrical f.
 2D f.
 3D f.
 DICOM f.
 DICOM-3-compatible digital
  computer f.
 hemodynamic f.
 slice f.
 tag image file f. (TIFF)
formation
 abscess f.
 batwing f.
 beaklike osteophyte f.
 bone f.
 bony callus f.
 brainstem reticular f.
 bulla f.
 bunion f.
 callosal f.
 callus f.
 cellule f.
 Chiari f.

cloacal f.
degenerative microcystic f.
eddy f.
enchondral bone f.
endogenous callus f.
excessive callus f.
exuberant atheroma f.
fistula f.
gcodc f.
glomeruloid f.
Gothic arch f.
hematoma f.
heterotopic bone f.
hippocampal f.
honeycomb f.
hooklike osteophyte f.
image f.
intracavitary clot f.
lateral reticular f.
marginal osteophyte f.
mesencephalic reticular f.
microcystic f.
midbrain reticular f. (MRF)
mural thrombus f.
mycetoma f.
myelin ball f.
neointima f.
new bone f.
nipplelike osteophyte f.
osteoid f.
osteophyte f.
palisade f.
pannus f.
paramedian pontile reticular f.
  (PPRF)
periosteal new bone f.
pontile parareticular f.
pontile reticular f.
pseudoaneurysm f.
pseudogland f.
pseudointimal f.
pseudopod f.
reticular activating f.
ruffled border f.
saccular f.
scar f.
semilunar bone f.
sparsity of bone f.
spur f.
thrombin f.
thrombus f.
tophus f.
vesical stone f.
formatter
former
  low-risk single-stone f.
formic aldehyde (*var. of* formaldehyde)
formula, *pl.* **formulae,** *pl.* **formulas**
  autotransformer f.

bayesian f.
Boyd f.
cigarroa f.
configurational f.
fan-beam f.
Poisson-Pearson f.
projection f.
rapid dissolution f.
formulae (*pl. of* formula)
formulas (*pl. of* formula)
Forney syndrome
fornicatus
  gyrus f.
forniceal rupture
fornices (*pl. of* fornix)
fornicis (*gen. of* fornix)
fornix, *pl.* **fornices,** *gen.* **fornicis**
  f. cerebri
  corpus fornicis
  vaginal f.
forward
  f. flow
  f. heart failure
  f. positioning of head
  f. stroke volume (FSV)
  f. subluxation
  f. transport
  f. velocity
forward-angle light scattering
FOS
  facet osteoarthritis sign
fossa, *pl.* **fossae**
  acetabular f.
  adipose f.
  amygdaloid f.
  anconal f.
  antecubital f.
  anterior recess of ischiorectal f.
  articular f.
  axillary f.
  biloma in gallbladder f.
  bony f.
  cardiac f.
  condylar f.
  coronoid f.
  cranial f.
  crural f.
  cubital f.
  digastric f.
  digital f.
  duodenal f.
  duodenojejunal f.
  epigastric f.
  femoral f.
  floccular f.
  gallbladder f.
  glenoid f.
  Gruber f.
  hepatorenal f.

F

fossa (*continued*)
    hyaloid f.
    hypoglossal f.
    hypophysial f.
    iliac f.
    infraspinous f.
    infrasternal f.
    infratemporal f.
    interpeduncular f.
    intratemporal f.
    ischiorectal f.
    Jobert f.
    Landzert f.
    malleolar f.
    mandibular f.
    meningioma of posterior f.
    mesentericoparietal f.
    middle cranial f.
    f. navicularis
    olecranon f.
    f. ovalis
    f. ovalis cordis
    ovarian f.
    paraduodenal f.
    pararectal f.
    paravesical f.
    patellar f.
    pituitary f.
    popliteal f.
    posterior cranial f.
    posterior pituitary f.
    pterygoid f.
    pterygopalatine f.
    radial f.
    rectouterine f.
    retroappendiceal f.
    rhomboid f.
    Rosenmüller f.
    sphenoid f.
    stylomastoid f.
    subscapular f.
    supraclavicular f.
    Sylvius f.
    temporal f.
    tonsillar f.
    Treitz f.
    uterovesical f.
    valve of navicular f.
    Waldeyer f.
fossae (*pl. of* fossa)
fourchette
Fourier
    F. analysis
    F. coefficient
    F. 2-dimensional imaging
    F. 2-dimensional projection
     reconstruction
    F. direct transform imaging
    F. discrete transform

    F. domain
    encoded F.
    F. imaging technique
    F. multislice modified KWE direct
     imaging
    F. optical theory
    F. pulsatility index
    F. transfer
    F. transform
    F. transform imaging
    F. transform infrared spectroscopy
    F. transform NMR spectrometry
    F. transform Raman spectroscopy
    F. transform reconstruction
    F. transform zeugmatography
Fourier-acquired
    F.-a. steady state
    F.-a. steady-state technique
    (FAST)
Fourier-encoded
Fourmentin thoracic index
Fournier phase
FOV
    field of view
    FOV imaging
fovea, *pl.* **foveae**
    f. capitis
    f. centralis
    f. inferior
foveae (*pl. of* fovea)
foveal fat-pad
foveated chest
foveola, *pl.* **foveolae**
    gastric f.
foveolae (*pl. of* foveola)
Fowler
    F. position
    F. test
FP
    frontopolar
    FP artery
FPA
    foot-progression angle
FPI
    femoral pulsatility index
FPR
    fluoroscopic programmed
    radiography
FPRNA
    1st-pass radionuclide angiography
FPS
    frames per second
FPVCT
    flat-panel volume computed
    tomography
fractal
    f. analysis
    f. dimension
fractal-based method

fraction
absorbed f.
active emptying f.
area-length method for ejection f.
blood flow extraction f.
blunted ejection f.
branching f.
cardiac scintigraphy ejection f.
computed ejection f.
depressed ejection f.
digital ejection f.
Dodge method for ejection f.
drug f.
ejection f.
filtration f.
gallbladder ejection f.
global ejection f.
globally depressed ejection f.
interval ejection f.
Kennedy method for calculating
  ejection f.
left atrial active emptying f.
left ventricular ejection f. (LVEF)
Maddahi method of calculating right
  ventricular ejection f.
MB f.
myofibril volume f.
oxygen extraction f. (OEF)
packing f.
penetration f.
photopeak f.
radionuclide ejection f.
regional ejection f.
regional oxygen extraction f. (rOEF)
regurgitant f.
resting left ventricular ejection f.
right ventricular ejection f. (RVEF)
scatter f.
shortening f.
shunt f.
S-phase f.
1st-3rd ejection f.
systolic ejection f.
Teichholz ejection f.
thermodilution ejection f.
thickening f.
unattached f.
ventricular ejection f.
well-preserved ejection f.

fractional
f. anisotropy
f. area
f. encephalography
f. flow reserve (FFR)
f. moving blood volume
f. moving blood volume estimation
f. myocardial shortening
f. pneumoencephalography
f. shortening of left ventricle

f. vascular volume
f. volumetric analysis

fractionated
f. dose
f. dose-survival curve
f. external beam irradiation
f. external beam radiation therapy
f. radiation
f. stereotactic radiation therapy
f. stereotactic radiotherapy (FSR)
f. total body irradiation

fractionation
accelerated f.
fast f.
f. of radiation dose
quasiaccelerated f.
S-phase f.

fracture
abduction f.
abduction-external rotation f.
acetabular posterior wall f.
acetabular rim f.
acute avulsion f.
acute on chronic f.
adduction f.
adult type III TIE f.
agenetic f.
Aitken classification of epiphysial f.
alveolar bone f.
anatomic f.
Anderson-Hutchins tibial f.
angulated f.
ankle mortise f.
anterior column f.
anterior wedge compression f.
anterior wedge compression f.
anteroinferior corner f.
anterolateral compression f.
anular f.
AO classification of ankle f.
apophysial f.
arch f.
articular mass separation f.
articular pillar f.
artificial f.
Ashhurst-Bromer classification of
  ankle f.
Atkin epiphysial f.
atlas f.
atrophic f.
avulsion chip f.
avulsion stress f.
axial compression f.
axial load 3-part 2-plane f.
axial load teardrop f.
axis f.
backfire f.
banana f.
Bankart f.

F

fracture (*continued*)

Barton f.
Barton-Smith f.
basal neck f.
basal skull f.
baseball finger f.
basicervical f.
basilar femoral neck f.
basilar skull f.
bayonet f.
beak f.
bedroom f.
bending f.
Bennett f.
bicondylar T-shaped f.
bicondylar Y-shaped f.
bicycle spoke f.
bimalleolar ankle f.'s
bipartite f.
f. blister
blow-in f.
blowout f.
bone f.
boot-top f.
Bosworth f.
both-bone f.
both-column f.
bowing f.
boxer's f.
Boyd type I-IV f.
f. bracing
bronchial f.
bucket-handle pattern of f.
bucket-handle pelvic f.
buckle f.
bumper f.
bunk-bed f.
Burkhalter-Reyes method of
  phalangeal f.
burst f.
butterfly f.
buttonhole f.
calcaneal avulsion f.
calcaneal displaced f.
calcaneal stress f.
f. callus
f. callus loading
calvarial f.
capitate f.
capitellar f.
capitulum humeri f.
carpal bone stress f.
carpal navicular f.
carpal scaphoid bone f.
carpometacarpal joint f.
cartwheel f.
Cedell f.
cemental f.
central f.

cephalomedullary nail f.
cerebral palsy pathologic f.
cervical spine f.
cervicotrochanteric f.
Chance spinal f.
Chaput f.
Charcot f.
chevron f.
childhood f.
chip f.
chisel f.
chondral f.
Chopart f.
circumferential f.
f. classification
clavicular birth f.
clay shoveler's f.
cleavage f.
closed f.
closed-break f.
coccyx f.
Colles f.
collicular f.
combined flexion-distraction injury
  and burst f.
combined radial-ulnar-humeral f.'s
comminuted burst f.
comminuted intraarticular f.
comminuted teardrop f.
complete f.
complex simple f.
complicated f.
composite f.
compound comminuted f.
compound complex f.
compound skull f.
compression f.
condylar split f.
congenital f.
Conrad-Bugg trapping of soft tissue
  in ankle f.
contrecoup f.
coracoid f.
corner f.
coronoid process f.
cortical f.
Cotton ankle f.
crack f.
craniofacial dysjunction f.
crush f.
crushed eggshell f.
cuboid f.
cuneiform f.
dancer's 5th metatarsal f.
Danis-Weber f.
Darrach-Hughston-Milch f.
dashboard f.
decompression of f.
f. deformity

Denis classification of spinal f.
dens f.
dentate f.
depressed skull f.
depression-type intraarticular f.
de Quervain f.
derby hat f.
Desault f.
f. deviation
diacondylar f.
diametric pelvic f.
diaphysial f.
f. diastasis
diastatic f.
dicondylar f.
die-punch f.
direct f.
dishpan f.
displaced f.
distal femoral epiphysial f.
distal humoral f.
distal radial f.
distraction of f.
dome f.
dorsal rim distal radial f.
dorsal wing f.
double f.
Dupuytren f.
Duverney f.
dyscrasic f.
El-Ahwany classification of humeral
  supracondylar f.
elbow f.
elementary f.
Ellis technique for Barton f.
f. en coin
f. en rave
epicondylar f.
epiphysial plate f.
epiphysial slip f.
epiphysial tibial f.
Essex-Lopresti joint depression-type
  calcaneal f.
explosion f.
extension corner avulsion f.
extension teardrop f. (ETF)
extraarticular f.
extracapsular f.
extraoctave f.
facial f.
fatigue f.
femoral intertrochanteric f.
femoral neck f.
femoral shaft f.
femoral stress f.
femoral supracondylar f.
fender f.
fetal f.
fibular f.

fighter's f.
finger f.
fishmouth f.
fissure f.
flake f.
flexion burst f.
flexion-compression f.
flexion-distraction f.
flexion teardrop f.
floating arch f.
floating palate f.
foot f.
forearm f.
f. fragment
f. fragment separation
f. frame
Freiberg f.
frontal f.
Frykman classification of hand f.
Frykman radial f.
fulcrum f.
Gaenslen f.
Galeazzi f.
f. gap
Gartland classification of humeral
  supracondylar f.
glenoid rim f.
Gosselin f.
greater trochanteric femoral f.
greater tuberosity f.
greenstick f.
grenade thrower's f.
gross f.
growing f.
growth plate f.
Guérin f.
gunshot f.
Gustilo-Anderson open clavicular f.
gutter f.
hairline f.
hamate tail f.
hand f.
hangman's f.
Hawkins classification of talar f.
head-splitting humeral f.
healing f.
heat f.
hemicondylar f.
hemitransverse f.
Henderson f.
Herbert scaphoid bone f.
Hermodsson f.
hickory-stick f.
Hill-Sachs posterolateral
  compression f.
hip f.
hockey-stick f.
Hoffa f.
Holstein-Lewis f.

F

fracture (*continued*)
  hook of hamate f.
  hoop stress f.
  horizontal maxillary f.
  humeral condylar f.
  humeral head-splitting f.
  humeral physial f.
  humeral supracondylar f.
  Hutchinson f.
  hyperextension teardrop f.
  hyperflexion teardrop f.
  ice skater's f.
  idiopathic f.
  iliac insufficiency f.
  iliofemoral wing f.
  impacted subcapital f.
  impacted valgus f.
  implant f.
  f. in close apposition
  incomplete f.
  indented f.
  indirect f.
  inflammatory f.
  infraction f.
  insufficiency f.
  intercondylar femoral f.
  intercondylar humeral f.
  intercondylar tibial f.
  internally fixed f.
  interperiosteal f.
  intertrochanteric 4-part f.
  intraarticular calcaneal f.
  intraarticular proximal tibial f.
  intracapsular femoral neck f.
  intraoperative f.
  intraperiosteal f.
  intrauterine f.
  inverted-Y f.
  ipsilateral femoral neck f.
  ipsilateral femoral shaft f.
  irreducible f.
  ischioacetabular f.
  isolated hook f.
  Jefferson burst f.
  Jefferson cervical f.
  Jeffery classification of radial f.
  joint depression f.
  Jones classification of diaphysial f.
  juvenile Tillaux f.
  juxtaarticular f.
  juxtacortical f.
  Kapandji radical f.
  Key-Conwell classification of
    pelvic f.
  Kilfoyle classification of condylar f.
  knee f.
  Kocher f.
  labral and anteroinferior glenoid rim
    f.'s

LaGrange classification of humeral
  supracondylar f.
laryngeal f.
lateral column calcaneal f.
lateral condylar humeral f.
laterally displaced f.
lateral malleolar f.
lateral tibial plateau f.
lateral wedge f.
Laugier f.
lead-pipe f.
Le Fort fibular f.
Le Fort I, II, III f.
Le Fort mandibular f.
Le Fort-Wagstaffe f.
lesser trochanteric f.
f. line
linear skull f.
f. line of consolidation
Lisfranc f.
local compression f.
local decompression f.
long-bone f.
longitudinal tibial fatigue f.
long oblique f.
loose f.
lorry driver's f.
low-energy f.
low-T humerus f.
lumbar spine f.
lunate f.
Maisonneuve fibular f.
malar f.
Malgaigne pelvic f.
malignant vertebral compression f.
malleolar f.
mallet f.
malunited f.
mandibular f.
march f.
marginal f.
Marmor-Lynn f.
Mathews classification of
  olecranon f.
maxillary f.
maxillofacial f.
medial column calcaneal f.
medial epicondyle f.
medial malleolar f.
medial wall f.
metacarpal f.
metaphysial f.
metatarsal f.
midface f.
midfacial f.
midfoot f.
midshaft f.
midwaist scaphoid f.
Milch classification of humeral f.

milkman's f.
minimally displaced f.
Moberg-Gedda f.
molar tooth f.
monomalleolar f.
Monteggia f.
Montercaux f.
Moore f.
Mouchet f.
multangular ridge f.
multipartite f.
multiple f.'s
multiray f.
nasal f.
nasoethmoid f.
nasomaxillary f.
nasoorbital f.
navicular body f.
navicular hand f.
naviculocapitate f.
neck f.
Neer classification of shoulder f.
Neer-Horowitz classification of
  humeral f.
neoplastic f.
neural arch f.
neurogenic f.
neuropathic f.
neurotrophic f.
Newman classification of radial
  neck and head f.'s
nightstick f.
nonarticular radial head f.
noncontiguous f.
nondisplaced f.
nonphysial f.
nonrotational burst f.
f. nonunion
nonunited f.
nutcracker f.
oblique spiral f.
O'Brien classification of radial f.
obturator avulsion f.
occipital condyle f.
occult osseous f.
occult sacral f.
odontoid condyle f.
odontoid f. (type I-III)
f. of astragalus
f. of necessity
Ogden classification of epiphysial f.
olecranon tip f.
open f.
open-book f.
open-break f.
orbital blowout f.
orbital floor f.
osteochondral slice f.
osteoporotic compression f.

overlapping f.
Pais f.
panfacial f.
Papavasiliou classification of
  olecranon f.
paranasal sinus f.
parasymphysial f.
paratrooper's f.
parry f.
pars interarticularis f.
1-, 2-, 3-, 4-part f.
patellar f.
patellar sleeve f.
pathologic f.
pedicle f.
pelvic insufficiency f.
pelvic rim f.
pelvic ring f.
pelvic straddle f.
penetrating f.
perforating f.
periarticular f.
peripheral f.
periprosthetic f.
peritrochanteric f.
phalangeal diaphysial f.
physial plate f.
Piedmont f.
pillar f.
pillion f.
pillow f.
pilon ankle f.
ping-pong f.
pisiform f.
plafond f.
plaque f.
plastic bowing f.
plateau tibial f.
pond f.
Posada f.
posterior arch f.
posterior element f.
posterior ring f.
posterior wall f.
postirradiation f.
Pott ankle f.
pressure f.
pronation-abduction f.
pronation-eversion f.
proximal femoral f.
proximal humeral f.
proximal tibial metaphysial f.
pseudo-Bennett f.
pseudo-Jefferson f.
puncture f.
pyramidal f.
quadruped f.
Quinby classification of pelvic f.
radial head f.

F

fracture (*continued*)

radial neck f.
radial styloid f.
radiographically occult f.
f. reduction
resecting f.
retrodisplaced f.
reverse Barton f.
reverse Colles f.
reverse Monteggia f.
reverse Segond f.
rib f.
ring f.
ring-disrupting f.
Rolando f.
rotational burst f.
Ruedi-Allgower tibial plafond f.
f. running length of bone
sacral insufficiency f. (SIF)
sacroiliac f.
Sakellarides classification of calcaneal f.
Salter-Harris classification of epiphysial f. (group 1-5)
sandbagging f.
scaphoid hand f.
scotty dog f.
seatbelt f.
secondary f.
segmental bronchus f.
Segond f.
Seinsheimer classification of femoral f.
senile subcapital f.
sentinel f.
SER type I-IV f. (SER)
shaft f.
shear f.
Shepherd f.
short oblique f.
sideswipe f.
silver fork f.
f. simple and depressed (FSD)
simple skull f.
sinus f.
f. site
skier's f.
Skillern f.
skull f.
sleeve f.
slice f.
Smith f.
snowboarder's f.
sphenoid bone f.
spinal f.
spinous process f.
spiral oblique f.
splintered f.

split compression f.
split heel f.
splitting f.
spontaneous f.
sprain f.
Springer f.
sprinter's f.
stability of f.
stable f.
stairstep f.
stellate skull f.
stellate undepressed f.
stepoff of f.
Stieda f.
straddle f.
strain f.
stress f.
strut f.
subcapital f.
subchondral f.
subcutaneous f.
subperiosteal f.
subtrochanteric f.
supination-adduction f.
supination-eversion f.
supination-external rotation type IV f.
supracondylar femoral f.
supracondylar humeral f.
supracondylar Y-shaped f.
surgical neck f.
T f.
talar avulsion f.
talar dome f.
talar neck f.
talar osteochondral f.
T condylar f.
teacup f.
teardrop burst f.
teardrop-shaped flexion-compression f.
temporal bone f.
tension f.
testis f.
thoracic spine f.
thoracolumbar burst f.
thoracolumbar junction f.
f. threshold
through-and-through f.
thrower's f.
Thurston Holland f.
tibial bending f.
tibial condyle f.
tibial diaphysial f.
tibial open f.
tibial pilon f.
tibial plafond f.
tibial plateau f.
tibial shaft f.

tibial stress f.
tibial triplane f.
tibial tuberosity f.
tibiofibular f.
Tillaux f.
Tillaux-Chaput anterolateral tibial
  epiphysis f.
Tillaux-Kleiger f.
toddler's f.
tongue-type intraarticular f.
torsion f.
torus f.
total condylar depression f.
trabecular f.
tracheal f.
traction f.
trampoline f.
transcaphoid f.
transcapitate f.
transcervical femoral f.
transchondral talar dome f.
transcondylar f.
transepiphysial f.
transhamate f.
transiliac f.
transsacral f.
transscaphoid dislocation f.
transtriquetral f.
transverse comminuted f.
transversely oriented endplate
  compression f.
transverse maxillary f.
transverse process f.
trapezium f.
traversing the f.
trimalleolar ankle f.
triplane f.
tripod f.
triquetral f.
trophic f.
T-shaped f.
tuft f.
ulnar f.
uncinate process f.
undepressed skull f.
undisplaced f.
unicondylar f.
unilateral f.
unimalleolar f.
unstable f.
ununited f.
upper thoracic spine f.
vertebral body f.
vertebral compression f.
  (VCF)
vertebral plana f.
vertebral wedge compression f.
vertical shear f.
volar rim distal radial f.

Volkmann f.
V-shaped f.
Wagstaffe f.
Walther hip f.
Weber C f.
wedge compression f.
wedge flexion-compression f.
western boot in open f.
willow f.
Wilson f.
wrist f.
Y f.
Y-T f.
ZMC f.
f. zone
zygomaticomaxillary f.

fractured
  f. bronchus
  f. kidney
  f. vertebra
fracture-dislocation
  Chopart f.-d.
  cuneiform f.-d.
  Galeazzi f.-d.
  intermediate cuneiform f.-d.
  Monteggia f.-d.
  pedicolaminar f.-d.
  perilunate f.-d.
  posterior f.-d.
fragilitas ossium
fragility
  acquired f.
fragment
  alignment of fracture f.'s
  anteroinferior triangular f.
  f. antigen binding (Fab)
  apoptic nuclear f.
  articular f.
  avulsed fracture f.
  bayoneting of fracture f.
  bone f.
  butterfly fracture f.
  calcified free f.
  capital f.
  chondral f.
  cortical f.
  f. depression
  disc f.
  displaced fracture f.
  displaced osteochondral f.
  extruded disc f.
  FAB f.
  fracture f.
  free disc f.
  free-floating cartilaginous f.
  iodine-125-labeled f.
  jagged bone f.
  Klenow f.
  loose osteochondral f.

F

fragment (*continued*)
    LymphoScan Tc99m-labeled murine antibody f.
    major fracture f.
    malunion of fracture f.'s
    metallic f.
    nonunion of fracture f.'s
    ^{99m}Tc-labeled anti-E-selectin Fab f.
    osteochondral fracture f.
    overriding of fracture f.
    retropulsed fracture f.
    smear f.
    Spengler f.
    technetium 99m Fab f.
    torsion of fracture f.
    union of fracture f.'s
fragmentation
    collagen f.
    electrohydraulic f.
    meniscal f.
    f. myocarditis
    f. of apophysis
    f. of barium
    f. therapy
    unilateral f.
fragmented
    f. mucosal fold
    f. pattern
fragment-in-notch sign
fragmentocytosis
frame
    adduction f.
    adiabatic demagnetization in rotating f. (ADRF)
    Balkan fracture f.
    Brown-Roberts-Wells f.
    CT/MRI-compatible stereotactic head f.
    fracture f.
    imaging-compatible stereotactic coordinate f.
    ISAH stereotactic immobilization f.
    Komai stereotactic head f.
    Laitinen stereotactic head f.
    Leksell D-shaped stereotactic f.
    Leksell-Elekta stereotactic f.
    Malcolm-Lynn C-RXF cervical retractor f.
    open reading f. (ORF)
    peak arterial f.
    pelvic fracture f.
    f.'s per second (FPS)
    radiolucent spine f.
    Radionics CRW stereotactic head f.
    Reichert-Mundinger-Fischer stereotactic f.
    robotics-controlled stereotactic f.
    rotating f.
    stereotactic head f.
    stereotactic localization f.
    Stryker f.
2-frame gated imaging
frameless
    f. stereotactic digital subtraction angiography
    f. stereotactic guidance
    f. stereotaxis
framing
    exact f.
frank
    f. breech presentation
    f. cerebral gumma
    f. cirrhosis
    f. congestive heart failure
    f. disc herniation
    f. dislocation
    f. hemorrhage
    f. lesion
    f. necrosis
    f. pulmonary edema
    f. rupture
    F. vectorcardiography
Fränkel
    crossbar symptom of F.
    F. spinal cord injury classification
    F. typhus nodule
    F. white line
Frankfort
    F. horizontal plane
    F. line
    F. mandibular incisor angle
    F. mandibular notch
    F. plane
Franklin changer
Frank-Starling
    F.-S. curve
    F.-S. mechanism
    F.-S. relation
Franseen needle
fraternal twin
Fraunhofer zone
frayed
    f. disc
    f. metaphysis
frayed-string appearance
fraying
    chondromalacia with surface f.
Frederick-Miller tube
free
    f. abdominal fluid
    f. air passage
    f. air under diaphragm
    f. band of colon
    f. body
    f. body calcification
    f. breathing
    cancer f.

f. cul-de-sac fluid
f. disc fragment
f. electron
f. fatty acid (FFA)
f. fibered coil
f. flap of cartilage
f. gas bubble
f. hepatic venography
f. induction decay (FID)
f. induction decay signal
f. induction delay curve
f. intraperitoneal air
f. intraperitoneal gas
f. iodine
f. knee joint
f. pericardial space
f. peritoneal air
f. peritoneal fluid
f. pertechnetate
f. pleural effusion
f. precession
f. precession sequence steady state
f. radical
f. reflux
f. subphrenic gas
free-breathing motion compensation
freedom from progression
FreeDop Doppler monitor
FreeFlo
F. proximal nitinol stent
F. stent-graft
free-floating
f.-f. cartilaginous fragment
f.-f. loop of bowel
f.-f. meniscus
f.-f. retinaculum
free-fragment disc herniation
freehand
f. interventional sonography
f. interventional ultrasound
f. probe
freely movable mass
Freeman calcaneal fracture classification
free-radical dosimetry
freestanding workstation
Freiberg
F. disease
F. fracture
F. infarction
F. infraction
French-American-British (FAB)
8-, 9-French guiding catheter
French-tip catheter
French T-tube
F-15 renogram
frenulum of valve
frequency (F)
f. analysis
angular f.

f. component
disappearance f.
f. domain
f. domain image
f. domain imaging (FDI)
Doppler shift f.
f. encoding
energy f.
f. estimation
extremely low f. (ELF)
false f.
halftone f.
high f.
f. intensification
Larmor f.
Nyquist f.
offset f.
peak repetition f.
pelvic mass f.
precessional f.
pulse repetition f.
f. range
raster f.
resonance f.
respiratory f.
rotational f.
f. separation
spatial f.
f. spectrum
f. synthesizer
vibration f.
water proton resonance f.
frequency-encoding gradient
frequency-related peak
frequency-selective
f.-s. fat saturation
f.-s. inversion
f.-s. pulse
Fresnel
F. zone
F. zone plate
FRET
fluorescence resonance energy transfer
Freund anomaly
Frey syndrome
friability
friable
f. anulus
f. artery
f. lesion
f. mass
f. mucosa
f. thickened degenerated intima
f. tumor
f. vegetation
f. wall
Fricke
F. dosimetry
F. gel

F

friction-fit
friction neuritis
Friedländer pneumonia
Friedman
    F. method
    F. position
Friedreich
    F. ataxia
    F. ataxic cardiomyopathy
    F. disease
    F. foot
    F. phenomenon
    F. sign
Fries rheumatoid arthritis classification
fringe
    f. field
    moiré f.
    f. of osteophyte
    f. skeleton extraction
    synovial f.
FRODO
    flow respiratory artifact obliteration
    with directed orthogonal pulses
        FRODO technique
Froesch foramen
frogleg
    f. lateral projection
    f. lateral view
    f. position
    f. view of hips
froglike appearance
Frohse
    arcade of F.
    F. ligamentous arcade
Froment sign
frond
    villous f.
frondlike
    f. appearance
    f. filling defect
frondy lesion
frontal
    f. abscess
    f. arteriovenous malformation
    f. artery
    f. biauricular plane
    f. bone
    f. bossing
    f. bossing of Parrot
    f. cephalometric radiograph
    f. cortex
    f. crest
    f. defect
    f. eminence
    f. fontanelle
    f. foramen
    f. fracture
    f. gyrus
    f. horn

    f. horn asymmetry
    f. horn index (FHI)
    f. horn Mickey Mouse ear
    f. horn of lateral ventricle
    f. hypoperfusion
    f. lobe
    f. lobe contusion
    f. lobe dysfunction
    f. lobe infarct
    f. lobe lesion
    f. lobe sign
    f. lobe tumor
    f. nerve
    f. notch
    f. operculum
    f. plane loop
    f. plane vectorcardiography
    f. plate
    f. pole
    f. process
    f. projection
    f. section
    f. sinus
    f. sinus mucocele
    f. sulcus
    f. suture
    f. vein
    f. view
frontalis
    apertura sinus f.
frontier ulcer
frontocentral convexity
frontoethmoidal
    f. encephalocele
    f. giant cell reparative granuloma
    f. mucocele
    f. suture
frontolacrimal suture
frontomalar suture
frontomaxillary suture
frontomental diameter
frontonasal
    f. duct
    f. dysplasia
    f. dysplasia malformation
      complex
    f. process
    f. suture
frontooccipital diameter
frontoorbital advancement
frontoparallel plane
frontoparietal
    f. arteriovenous malformation
    f. parasagittal cortex
    f. suture
frontopolar (FP)
    f. artery
    f. point
frontopontine tract

frontosphenoidal
- f. encephalocele
- f. process

frontosphenoid suture

frontotemporal
- f. atrophy
- f. lobe degeneration
- f. lobe dementia
- f. muscle
- f. tract

frontozygomatic suture

Frostberg sign

frosted liver

frothy colonic mucosa

Frouin
- quadrangulation of F.

frozen
- f. hemithorax
- f. joint
- f. pelvis
- f. shoulder

FRP
- functional refractory period

Frykman
- F. classification of hand fracture
- F. distal radius fracture classification
- F. radial fracture

FS
- focal spot
- FS burst MR imaging
- FS projection

F-scan

FSCR
- flexible surface coil-type resonator

FSD
- Fletcher-Suit-Delclos
- focus-skin distance
- fracture simple and depressed
- full-scale deflection

FSE
- fast spin echo

FSE-T2 with fat suppression

FSPGR
- fast spoiled gradient echo
- FSPGR technique

FSR
- fractionated stereotactic radiotherapy

FS-069 sterile injectable sonography contrast agent

FSU
- functional subunit

FSV
- forward stroke volume

FTA
- femorotibial angle

FTC
- fibulotalocalcaneal
- FTC ligament

FTHA
- ^{18}F-fluoro-6-thia-heptadecanoic acid

Fuchs
- F. adenoma
- F. odontoid view
- F. position
- F. principle

fucose

fucosidosis

FUE
- fever of unknown etiology

fugax
- amaurosis f.
- coxitis f.

Fuji
- F. AC2 storage phosphor computed radiology system
- F. computed radiography mammography suite
- F. FCR9000 computed radiology system
- F. QA 771 workstation

Fukuyama
- F. congenital muscular disease (FCMD)
- F. congenital muscular dystrophy

fulcra (*pl. of* fulcrum)

fulcrum, *pl.* **fulcra,** *pl.* **fulcrums**
- f. fracture
- joint f.
- f. test

fulcrums (*pl. of* fulcrum)

fulguration
- direct f.
- indirect f.
- nephroscopic f.

full
- f. bladder ultrasound
- f. cervical spine (FCS)
- f. cervical spine series
- f. cervical spine view
- f. column view
- f. 3-dimensional mode
- f. energy peak
- f. lateral position
- f. scan with interpolation
- f. scan with interpolation projection
- f. thickness
- f. width at half-maximum (FWHM)
- f. width at half-maximum of lorentzian curve

full-blown cardiac tamponade

full-body
- f.-b. CT scan
- f.-b. echo-planar system imager

full-column
- f.-c. barium enema
- f.-c. technique

F

full-energy peak efficiency
Fuller earth pneumoconiosis
full-field
    f.-f. digital mammography
    f.-f. digital mammography system
full-intensity needle
full-length view
full-line scanning
full-ring
    f.-r. dedicated BGO PET/CT camera
    f.-r. scanner
full-scale deflection (FSD)
full-scan
    f.-s. method
    f.-s. projection
full-thickness
    f.-t. button of aortic wall
    f.-t. Carrel button
    f.-t. chondral lesion
    f.-t. cleft
    f.-t. infarct
    f.-t. tear
full-to-empty VAD mode
full-volume loop spirometry
full-wave
    f.-w. rectification
    f.-w. rectifier
fulminant
    f. cerebral lymphoma
    f. colitis
    f. fasciitis
    f. hepatic failure (FHF)
    f. hydrocephalus
    f. pulmonary edema
    f. tuberculosis
fulminating ulcerative colitis
function
    abnormal tubular f.
    arterial input f. (AIF)
    atrial-phase volumetric f.
    autocorrelation f.
    brain f.
    bundle f.
    cerebrospinal fluid shunt f.
    commissural f.
    compromised ventricular f.
    contractile f.
    depressed right ventricular
      contractile f.
    diastolic f.
    edge response f. (ERF)
    excitation f.
    exercise LV f.
    fetal renal f.
    gaussian f.
    global ventricular f.
    gonadal f.
    harmonic f.
    impaired renal f.

    Kaiser-Bessel window f.
    leaflet f.
    left atrial f.
    left ventricular systolic/diastolic f.
    left ventricular systolic pump f.
    line spread f. (LSF)
    midbrain f.
    mitochondrial f.
    modulation transfer f. (MTF)
    myocardial contractile f.
    nasal mucociliary clearance f.
    pharyngoesophageal f.
    point-spread f. (PSF)
    rectosigmoid f.
    regional left ventricular f.
    regional myocardial f.
    reserve cardiac f.
    resting left ventricular f.
    resting right ventricular f.
    right and left atrial phasic
      volumetric f.
    right ventricular systolic/diastolic f.
    Shepp-Logan filter f.
    sinusoid reference f.
    stress perfusion and rest f.
    swallowing f.
    systolic f.
    time correlation f.
    tubular f.
    velocity distribution f.
    ventricular contractility f. (VCF)
    volumetric f.
    Zeeman hamiltonian f.
functional
    f. abnormality
    f. aerobic impairment (FAI)
    f. anatomic mapping
    f. anesthetic discography (FAD)
    f. bladder capacity
    f. bowel syndrome
    f. brain imaging
    f. classification of congestive heart
      failure
    f. correlation
    f. data
    f. diffusion anisotropy
    f. disorder
    f. diverticulum
    f. hyperlordosis
    f. hypertrophy
    f. ileus
    f. immaturity of bowel
    f. magnetic resonance (fMR)
    f. magnetic resonance angiography
      (fMRA)
    f. magnetic resonance imaging
      (fMRI)
    f. map
    f. marrow

f. megacolon
f. MRI
f. MR tube
f. neuroimaging
f. obstruction
f. ovarian cyst
f. paraganglioma
f. radioiodine scintigraphy
f. reentry
f. refractory period (FRP)
f. residual capacity
f. scoliosis
f. sphincter
f. spin-echo imaging
f. subunit (FSU)
f. unit of spine
f. ureteral obstruction
functioning
f. neoplasia
f. nodule
f. parathyroid cyst
f. pituitary adenoma
FuncTool software
fundal
f. leiomyoma
f. placenta
fundamental Doppler mode
fundamental-mode ultrasound imaging
fundi (*pl. of* fundus)
fundic-antral junction
fundic metaphysis
fundiform ligament
fundoplication
Nissen f.
fundus, *pl.* **fundi**
aneurysmal f.
bald gastric f.
bladder f.
gallbladder f.
gastric f.
f. of aneurysm
saddle-shaped uterine f.
stomach f.
urinary bladder f.
f. uteri
uterine f.
vaginal f.
Funduscein injection
fungal (*var. of* fungous)
fungating tumor
fungiform papilloma
fungoides
tumeur d'emblée mycosis f.
fungous, fungal
f. hypha
f. infection
f. meningitis
f. plaque
f. pneumonia

fungus ball
funic, funicular
f. souffle
funicular (*var. of* funic)
f. inguinal hernia
funiculi (*pl. of* funiculus)
funiculus, *pl.* **funiculi**
f. cuneatus
f. dorsalis
f. gracilis
f. medullae spinalis
f. ventralis
funnel
f. chest
f. chest deformity
funnellike cardiomegaly
funnel-shaped
f. s. cavity
f.-s. pelvis
FUO
fever of unknown origin
furosemide
f. imaging agent
f. renography
furrier's lung
furrow
fused
f. ankle
f. colliculus
f. commissure
f. fontanelle
f. image technology
f. imaging-guided radiotherapy (FIGURA)
f. kidney
f. papillary muscle
f. pelvic kidney
f. physis
f. rib
f. vertebra
fusiform
f. aneurysm
f. bronchiectasis
f. defect
f. dilation
f. enlargement of optic nerve
f. gyrus
f. high signal intensity
f. malformation
f. mass
f. narrowing of artery
f. shadow
f. swelling
f. syrinx
f. thickening
f. widening of duct
fusion
ankle f.
anterior cervical f. (ACF)

F

fusion (*continued*)
    anterior spine f. (ASF)
    atlantooccipital f.
    bony f.
    calcaneotibial f.
    carpometacarpal f.
    CAT-MIBI image f.
    cervical interbody f.
    cervical spine f.
    cervicooccipital f.
    chevron f.
    f. defect
    diaphysial-epiphysial f.
    extraarticular hip f.
    facet f.
    Hatcher-Smith cervical f.
    image f.
    f. image
    f. imaging
    f. inhibitor (FI)
    interbody f.
    interphalangeal f.
    intersegmental laminar f.
    interspinal process f.
    intraarticular knee f.
    joint f.
    Kellogg-Speed lumbar spinal f.
    metatarsocuneiform joint f.
    metatarsophalangeal joint f.
    multilevel f.
    nuclear f.

    occipitoatlantoaxial f.
    occipitocervical f.
    f. of cusp
    pantalar f.
    PET/MRI f.
    f. plate
    posterior lumbar interbody f. (PLIF)
    posterior spine f. (PSF)
    sacroiliac joint f.
    spinal f.
    splenogonadal f.
    2-stage f.
    talar body f.
    talocrural f.
    tibiocalcaneal f.
    tibiotalocalcaneal f.
    transfibular f.
    vertebral f.
Fusobacterium
FUTE
    fat-suppressed ultrashort echo time
fuzzy
    f. echo
    f. logic contrast correction
    f. set theory
FWHM
    full width at half-maximum
FX-wire
    Cragg FX-w.

G
- gauss
  - immunoglobulin G (IgG)
  - indium-111-labeled human nonspecific immunoglobulin G
  - [111In]-labeled human nonspecific immunoglobulin G

Ga
- gallium

67Ga, Ga-67
- gallium 67
  - 67Ga bone scan
  - 67Ga citrate scintigraphy
  - 67Ga examination
  - 67Ga excretion
  - 67Ga GABA uptake carrier
  - 67Ga higher dose
  - 67Ga uptake

68Ga, Ga-68
- gallium 68

G/A
- globulin/albumin
  - G/A recombinant

GABA
- gamma-aminobutyric acid

gadobenate
- g. dimeglumine
- g. dimeglumine contrast agent

gadobenic acid imaging agent
gadobutrol imaging agent
gadodiamide imaging agent
gadofosveset trisodium
gadolinium (Gd)
- g. 153 ([153Gd], Gd-153)
- g. benzylopropionic tetracetate (Gd-BOPTA)
- g. chelate
- g. complex
- g. dimeglumine
- g. enhancement
- g. ethylenediamine tetraacetic acid
- g. fast multiplanar spoiled gradient (Gd-FMPSPGR)
- intraarticular g.
- g. iron
- g. oxide imaging agent
- g. oxyorthosilicate
- g. oxysulphide
- sandwiched g.
- g. scan
- g. silicate
- g. sucralfate
- g. tetraazacyclododecanetetraacetic acid (Gd-DOTA)
- g. texaphyrin (Gd-Tex)

gadolinium-based contrast agent
gadolinium-diethylenetriamine
- g.-d. pentaacetic acid (Gd-DTPA)
- g.-d. pentaacetic acid
- g.-d. pentaacetic acid-bismethylamide (Gd-DTPA-BMA)

gadolinium-enhanced
- g.-e. elliptically reordered 3-dimensional MR angiography
- g.-e. imaging group
- g.-e. MR imaging
- g.-e. subtracted MR angiography
- g.-e. subtracted MR angiography, 3D
- g.-e. T1-weighted axial image
- g.-e. T1-weighted MRI image
- g.-e. venographic technique

gadolinium-ethoxybenzyl-diethylenetriamine pentaacetic acid (Gd-EOB-DTPA)
gadolinium-hepatoiminodiacetic acid (Gd-HIDA)
gadolinium-159 hydroxycitrate
gadolinium-rich nanoparticle
Gadolite oral suspension contrast agent
Gadomer
gadopentetate
- g. contrast agent
- g. dimeglumine imaging agent

gadopentetic acid
gadopentolate-polylysine
gadoterate-enhanced digital subtraction angiography
gadoterate meglumine
gadoteridol imaging agent
gadoversetamide
- g. contrast agent
- g. imaging agent

Gadovist
gadoxetate
gadoxetic acid
Gaeltec catheter-tip pressure transducer
Gaenslen
- G. fracture
- G. sign

Gaffney joint
gain
- accelerated phase g.
- brightness g.
- color g.
- Doppler g.
- phase g.
- power g.

G

gain (*continued*)
>   quadratic phase g.
>   time-compensated g.
>   time-varied g. (TVG)

Gaisböck syndrome

gait
>   tandem g.

galactocele

galactogram
>   mammary g.

galactography

galactophoritis

galactophorous
>   g. canal
>   g. duct

galactose-based suspension

galactose contrast medium

galactosyl human serum albumin (GSA)

Galassi arachnoid cyst classification

galea aponeurotica

galeal extension of tumor

Galeazzi
>   G. fracture
>   G. fracture-dislocation
>   G. sign

Galen
>   great cerebral vein of G.
>   G. Scan scanner
>   G. teleradiology system
>   G. thrombosis
>   G. vein aneurysm
>   G. ventricle

galenic venous malformation

Galileo intravascular radiotherapy system

gall duct

gallbladder, gall bladder
>   g. adenoma
>   g. agenesis
>   g. bed
>   bilobate g.
>   blunt trauma of g.
>   body of g.
>   calcified g.
>   g. calculus
>   g. carcinoma
>   comet-tail artifact g.
>   contracted g.
>   Courvoisier g.
>   dilated g.
>   displaced g.
>   distended g.
>   g. diverticulum
>   double g.
>   drooping g.
>   g. duplication
>   g. dyskinesia
>   ectopic g.

>   edematous g.
>   g. ejection fraction
>   g. empyema
>   enlarged g.
>   fetal g.
>   g. filling defect
>   fish-scale g.
>   floating g.
>   folded fundus of g.
>   g. fossa
>   g. function test
>   g. fundus
>   gangrene of g.
>   g. gravel
>   hourglass constriction of g.
>   g. hydrops
>   g. hypoplasia
>   g. ileus
>   g. imaging
>   g. infundibulum
>   g. lift
>   g. lithiasis
>   g. metastasis
>   mobile g.
>   multiseptated g.
>   neck of g.
>   nonfunctioning g.
>   nonvisualization of g.
>   pearl necklace g.
>   g. perforation
>   g. polyp
>   porcelain g.
>   porcine g.
>   sagging g.
>   septated g.
>   g. septation
>   g. series (GBS)
>   shrunken g.
>   g. size
>   g. sludge
>   small g.
>   S-shaped g.
>   stasis g.
>   g. stone
>   strawberry g.
>   g. study
>   thick-walled g.
>   thin-walled g.
>   g. torsion
>   g. trauma
>   g. ultrasound
>   g. villus
>   g. wall
>   g. wall abscess
>   wandering g.

gallbladder-gastrointestinal (GB-GI)
>   g.-g. series

gallbladder-vena cava line

galli
>ala cristae g.
>crista g.

Gallie H-graft

gallium (Ga)
>g. 67 (^{67}Ga, Ga-67)
>g. 68 (^{68}Ga, Ga-68)
>g. bone scintigraphy
>g. imaging agent
>g. lung imaging
>g. lung scintigraphy
>radioactive g.
>g. scan
>g. scintigraphy of lymphoma
>g. titrate
>g. tumor scintigraphy
>g. uptake

gallium-arsenide laser
gallium-67-avid lesion
gallium-avid thymic hyperplasia
gallium-67 citrate
gallium-67-labeled leukocyte
gallium-transferrin complex
gallstone
>asymptomatic g.
>cholesterol g.
>dissolution of g.
>g. dissolution therapy
>ectopic intraluminal g.
>faceted g.
>floating g.
>gas-containing g.
>g. ileus
>innocent g.
>intraluminal g.
>laminar g.
>layered g.'s
>layering of g.'s
>g. migration
>mulberry g.
>opacifying g.
>radiolucent g.
>retained g.
>silent g.
>solitary g.
>symptomatic g.

GALT
>gut-associated lymphoid tissue

galvanometer
gamekeeper's thumb
gamma
>g. aminobutyrate
>g. camera
>g. cascade
>g. emission
>g. emitter
>g. encephalography
>g. factor
>g. film
>g. heating
>g. heavy-chain disease
>g. irradiation
>G. Knife-stereotactic radiosurgery (GK-SRS)
>G. nail
>g. photon
>g. probe
>g. probe radiation detector
>g. radiation
>g. radiography
>g. ray
>g. ray attenuation
>g. ray capture
>g. ray counter
>g. ray level indicator
>g. ray scanner
>g. ray spectrometer
>g. ray spectrum
>g. ray therapy
>g. scan
>g. scanning
>g. signal
>g. spectrometric analysis
>g. tocopherol (gamma-T)
>g. transverse colon loop
>g. unit
>g. well counter

gamma-aminobutyric acid (GABA)
gamma-detection probe
gamma-emitting isotope
gamma-irradiated plug
GammaPlan software
gamma-ribbon radiation therapy
gamma-T
>gamma tocopherol

Gammex
>G. RBA-5 radiation beam analyzer
>G. RMI DAP meter
>G. RMI scanner

gammography
>cerebral g.

gammopathy
>monoclonal g.

Gamna-Gandy nodule
Gamna nodule
Gandy-Nanta disease
ganglia (*pl. of* ganglion)
gangliocytic paraganglioma
gangliocytoma
>dysplastic cerebellar g.

ganglioglioma
>cystic g.
>desmoplastic infantile g.
>infantile g.
>intracerebral g.

gangliolysis
>radiofrequency g.

G

ganglioma
    intracerebral g.
ganglion, *pl.* **ganglia,** *pl.* **ganglions**
    aberrant g.
    acousticofacial g.
    Acrel g.
    aorticorenal g.
    auditory g.
    auricular g.
    basal g.
    calcification of basal g.
    cardiac g.
    carotid g.
    celiac g.
    g. cell tumor
    cervical g.
    cervicothoracic g.
    coccygeal g.
    g. cyst
    diffuse g.
    dorsal root g. (DRG)
    gasserian g.
    geniculate g.
    g. impar block
    intraarticular g.
    intraosseous g.
    ipsilateral basal g.
    otic g.
    palmar g.
    paravertebral g.
    periosteal g.
    petrosal g.
    posterior root g.
    prevertebral g.
    pterygopalatine g.
    radiocapitellar joint g.
    g. ridge
    Scarpa g.
    sensory g.
    soft tissue g.
    sphenopalatine g.
    spinal g.
    submandibular g.
    superior cervical g.
    superior mesenteric g.
    sympathetic g.
    trigeminal g.
    uterine cervical g.
    vestibular g.
    Wrisberg cardiac g.
ganglioneuroblastoma
  (GNB)
ganglioneurofibromatosis
    mucosal g.
ganglioneuroma
    adrenal g.
ganglionic
    g. canal
    g. crest

ganglions (*pl. of* ganglion)
gangliosidosis
    GM_1/GM_2 g.
gangrene
    bowel g.
    g. of gallbladder
    g. of lung
gangrenous
    g. acalculous cholecystitis
    g. emphysema
    g. pneumonia
    g. tissue
Gans
    incisura dextra of G.
Ganser diverticulum
gantry
    g. angulation
    CT scan g.
    fixed g.
    fluoroscopic g.
    g. rotation
    g. rotation time
    g. tilt
gantry-free gamma camera
Gantzer muscle
Ganz formula for coronary sinus
  flow
gap
    air g.
    artifactual g.
    Bochdalek g.
    g. calculation
    distraction g.
    fracture g.
    intersection g.
    interslice g.
GARD
    glenoid articular rim disruption
    GARD lesion
garden
    G. femoral neck fracture angle
    G. femoral neck fracture
      classification
    g. spade deformity
Gardner bone syndrome
Gardray dosimeter
garland
    g. sign
    G. triad
    G. triangle
GARP
    globally optimized alternating-phase
      rectangular pulse
Garré
    G. disease
    G. sclerosing osteomyelitis
Garren-Edwards
    G.-E. gastric (GEG)
    G.-E. gastric bubble

Garth shoulder view
Gartland classification of humeral supracondylar fracture
Gartner
    G. canal
    G. duct
    G. duct cyst
Gärtner phenomenon
gas
    abdominal g.
    accumulation of g.
    aneurysmal wall g.
    g. angiocardiography
    bile duct g.
    biliary tree g.
    bowel g.
    g. bubble
    g. collection
    coursing of g.
    crescent of g.
    g. CT cisternography
    g. cupula
    g. density line
    displacement of bowel g.
    g. entrapment
    extraluminal g.
    free intraperitoneal g.
    free subphrenic g.
    g. gangrene of uterus
    genital tract g.
    hyperpolarized ^{129}Xe g.
    g. insufflation
    intestinal g.
    intrahepatic portal
      vein g.
    intramural g.
    intrauterine g. (IUG)
    g. mediastinography
    natural neon g.
    noble g.
    overlying bowel g.
    g. pattern
    paucity of bowel g.
    portal venous g.
    pulmonary g.
    radioactive g.
    radiopaque xenon g.
    scrotal g.
    small bowel g.
    soft tissue g.
    subcutaneous tissue g.
    superimposed bowel g.
    g. target
    g. trapping
    urinary tract g.
    g. ventilation imaging
    g. ventilation study
    g. volume
gas-bloat syndrome

gas-containing
    g.-c. gallstone
    g.-c. stone
gaseous
    g. cholecystitis
    g. dilation
    g. distention
    g. drainage
    g. injection
    g. mediastinography
    g. oxygen artifact
gas-filled detector
gas-fluid level
gasless
    g. abdomen
    g. laparoscopic system
gas-liquid phase chromatography (GLPC)
^{67}GaSPECT
gasserian ganglion
Gasser syndrome
gastric
    g. adenocarcinoma
    g. adenopapillomatosis
    g. air bubble
    g. antral erosion
    g. antrum
    g. artery
    g. atony
    g. atresia
    g. atrophy
    g. bezoar
    g. bypass surgery (GBS)
    g. canal
    g. capacity
    g. cardia
    g. channel
    g. chloroma
    g. contents
    g. decompression
    g. diaphragm
    g. diastole
    g. dilation
    g. distention
    g. diverticulum
    g. duplication cyst
    g. emphysema
    g. emptying
    g. emptying half-time
    g. emptying imaging
    g. emptying rate
    g. emptying scan
    g. fistula
    g. fold
    g. fold enlargement
    g. foveola
    g. fundus
    Garren-Edwards g. (GEG)
    g. groove
    g. hamartomatous polyposis

G

gastric (*continued*)
- g. hemic calculus
- g. hemorrhage
- g. hernia
- g. heterotopia
- g. hypersecretion
- g. impression
- g. insufficiency
- g. interposition
- g. intramural-extramucosal lesion
- g. leiomyoma
- g. leiomyosarcoma
- g. lumen
- g. lymphatic follicle
- g. lymph node
- g. lymphoma
- g. metaplasia
- g. metastasis
- g. motor disorder
- g. mucosa
- g. mucosa imaging
- g. mucosal pattern
- g. narrowing
- g. neuroendocrine carcinoma
- g. omentum
- g. outlet obstruction
- g. outline
- g. parietography
- g. partition
- g. pit
- g. plexus
- g. pneumatosis
- g. polyp
- g. pool
- g. pouch
- g. pseudolymphoma
- g. pullthrough procedure
- g. pull-up
- g. reflux of bile
- g. remnant
- g. remnant carcinoma
- g. remnant filling defect
- g. residual
- g. rugae
- g. sclerosis
- g. secretion
- g. sling fiber
- g. stump
- g. stump carcinoma
- g. surface
- g. thumbprinting
- g. transit time
- g. transposition
- g. tumor
- g. ulcer
- g. varix
- g. vein
- g. volvulus
- g. wall deformity
- g. wall thickening
- g. window
- g. xanthoma

gastrica
- area g.

gastrinoma
- duodenal g.

gastritis
- acute erosive g. (AEG)
- antral g.
- atrophic g.
- bile reflux g.
- bilious g.
- chronic g.
- cirrhotic g.
- corrosive g.
- emphysematous g.
- erosive g.
- follicular g.
- giant hypertrophic g.
- hypertrophic g.
- necrotizing g.
- phlegmonous g.
- pseudomembranous radiation g.
- radiation g.
- reflux g.
- zonal g.

gastroabdominal fistula
gastrobiliary fistula
gastrocardiac syndrome
gastrocnemial ridge
gastrocnemius
- g. bursa
- g. muscle
- g. tendon

gastrocnemius-semimembranosus bursa
gastrocnemius-soleus
- g.-s. complex
- g.-s. contracture
- g.-s. junction
- g.-s. muscle group
- g.-s. tendon

gastrocolic
- g. fistula
- g. ligament
- g. omentum

gastrocutaneous fistula
gastrodiaphragmatic ligament
gastroduodenal
- g. artery
- g. artery complex
- g. fistula
- g. junction
- g. lumen
- g. lymph node
- g. mucosal prolapse
- g. orifice

gastroduodenitis
gastroduodenoscopy

gastroduodenostomy
> Billroth I, II g.

gastroenteric anastomosis

gastroenteritis
> cobblestone appearance of
>   eosinophilic g.
> eosinophilic g.
> viral g.

gastroenterocolitis

gastroenteroptosis

gastroenterostomy
> percutaneous g.
> g. stoma

gastroepiploic
> g. arcade
> g. artery
> g. lymph node
> g. vein
> g. vessel

gastroesophageal (GE)
> g. angle
> g. collateral
> g. incompetence
> g. junction
> g. junction carcinoma
> g. junction stricture
> g. junction tumor
> g. reflux disease (GERD)
> g. variceal plexus

gastrogenic
> g. cyst
> g. duplication

Gastrografin
> G. enema
> G. imaging agent
> G. swallow

gastrohepatic
> g. bare area
> g. ligament
> g. ligament node
> g. omentum

gastrointestinal (GI)
> g. adverse effect
> g. bleeding
> g. bleeding localization nuclear
>   study
> g. carcinoma
> g. cyst
> g. endoscopic ultrasound
> g. endoscopy
> g. fibrous tumor (GIFT)
> g. fistula
> g. glial/schwannoma tumor
> g. leiomyogenic tumor (GILT)
> g. lymphoma
> g. malignancy
> g. motility imaging
> g. plaque
> g. protein loss test

> g. renal transplant hemorrhage
> g. scintigraphy
> g. series
> g. stoma
> g. stromal tumor (GIST)
> g. tract
> g. tract adenocarcinoma
> g. tract obstruction
> g. tuberculosis
> g. ulcer
> upper g. (UGI)

gastrointestinal-associated tissue

gastrojejunal mucosal prolapse

gastrojejunocolic fistula

gastrojejunostomy
> Billroth I, II g.
> g. catheter

gastrolienal ligament

GastroMARK oral imaging agent

gastroomental lymph node

gastropancreatic
> g. fold
> g. ligament

gastroparesis
> diabetic g.

gastropathy
> hyperplastic g.

gastropexy

gastrophrenic ligament

gastroplasty

Gastroport

gastroptosia (*var. of* gastroptosis)

gastroptosis, gastroptosia

gastrorenal shunt

gastroschisis

gastroscope
> Olympus XQ230 g.
> Pentax ELLB 6000, 6500 ultrasound
>   g.

gastroscopy

gastrosphincteric pressure gradient

gastrosplenic
> g. ligament
> g. omentum

gastrostomy
> g. catheter
> CT-guided percutaneous endoscopic
>   g.
> percutaneous endoscopic g. (PEG)
> radiologic percutaneous g. (RPG)
> g. tube

gastrotomy

Gastroview imaging agent

Gastrovist imaging agent

gate
> g. array
> g. signal

G

gated
- g. blood pool angiography
- g. blood pool scan
- g. blood pool scintigraphy
- g. blood pool ventriculogram
- g. cardiac blood pool imaging
- g. cine imaging
- g. CT scanner
- g. 3D reconstruction
- g. equilibrium blood pool scanning
- g. equilibrium cardiac blood pool imaging
- g. equilibrium radionuclide angiography
- g. exercise examination
- g. image
- g. imaging study
- g. inflow magnetic resonance
- g. inflow technique
- g. magnetic resonance imaging
- g. nuclear angiography
- g. nuclear ventriculogram
- g. planar study
- g. radionuclide angiocardiography
- g. radionuclide ventriculogram
- g. RNA
- g. single-photon emission computed tomography (GSPECT)
- g. SPECT myocardial perfusion imaging
- g. stress myocardial perfusion
- g. stress myocardial perfusion slice
- g. system
- g. view

gating
- cardiac g.
- g. device
- diastolic g.
- echocardiographic g.
- electrocardiographic g.
- g. error
- expiratory g.
- heartbeat g.
- inspiratory g.
- motion g.
- peripheral pulse g.
- respiratory g.
- retrospective respiratory g.
- spirometric g.
- systolic g.

Gaucher
- G. disease
- G. nodule
- G. splenomegaly

gauge
- x-ray thickness g.

gauss (G)

gaussian
- g. curve
- g. distribution
- g. dose-volume histogram
- g. filter
- g. function
- g. line
- g. line saturation
- g. line shape
- g. noise
- g. radiofrequency
- g. smoothing

gaussian-mode profile laser beam

Gavard muscle

Gaynor-Hart method

GB-GI
- gallbladder-gastrointestinal
- GB-GI series

GBM
- glioblastoma multiforme
- glomerular basement membrane

GBS
- gallbladder series
- gastric bypass surgery

gCBF
- global cerebral blood flow

GCF
- grid conversion factor

GCH
- giant cavernous hemangioma

GCS
- Glasgow coma scale

G-CSF, GCSF
- granulocyte colony-stimulating factor

GCVF
- great cardiac vein flow

^{153}Gd, Gd-153
- gadolinium 153

Gd
- gadolinium

Gd-153, ^{153}Gd
- gadolinium 153
  - Gd-153 imaging agent

Gd-BOPTA
- gadolinium benzylopropionic tetracetate

Gd-BOPTA/Dimeg imaging agent

GDC
- Guglielmi detachable coil
  - 3D GDC
  - UltraSoft GDC

GDC-10 soft coil

Gd-DOTA
- gadolinium tetraazacyclododecanetetraacetic acid
  - Gd-DOTA contrast medium

Gd-DOTA-enhanced subtraction dynamic study

Gd-DTPA
gadolinium-diethylenetriamine
pentaacetic acid
Gd-DTPA PGTM imaging agent
Gd-DTPA radioisotope
Gd-DTPA with mannitol contrast
agent
Gd-DTPA-BMA
gadolinium-diethylenetriamine
pentaacetic acid-bismethylamide
**Gd-DTPA-enhanced turbo FLASH
MRI**
Gd-DTPA-labeled
Gd-DTPA-l. albumin
Gd-DTPA-l. dextran
Gd-enhanced
Gd-e. imaging agent
Gd-e. MR angiography
Gd-EOB-DTPA
gadolinium-ethoxybenzyl-
diethylenetriamine pentaacetic
acid
Gd-EOB-DTPA imaging agent
Gd-FMPSPGR
gadolinium fast multiplanar spoiled
gradient
Gd-FMPSPGR imaging
Gd-HIDA
gadolinium-hepatoiminodiacetic acid
Gd-HIDA chelate
Gd-HP-DO3A imaging agent
Gd-Tex
gadolinium texaphyrin
GDx
Nerve Fiber Analyzer GDx
GE
gastroesophageal
General Electric
gradient echo
GE 400AC/T STAR II camera
GE Advance PET scanner
GE Advantage 1.5T imager
GE CT Advantage scanner
GE CT HiSpeed Advantage CT
system
GE CTI 9800 scanner
GE CTI single-detector scanner
GE CT Max scanner
GE CT Pace scanner
GE CT/T 8800 scanner
GE CT/T7 scanner
GE detector
GE Discovery LS CT/PET scanner
GE EchoSpeed 1.5T whole-body
MR imager
GE gamma camera
GE Genesis CT scanner
GE GN300 multinuclear
spectrometer

GE GN scanner
GE 9800 high-resolution CT scanner
GE HiSpeed Advantage helical CT
scanner
GE HiSpeed single-detector scanner
GE Lightspeed CT scanner
GE Millennium MG camera
GE MR Max scanner
GE MR Signa scanner
GE MR Vectra scanner
GE Neurocam camera
GE NMR spectrometer
GE OEC Series 9600 cardiac system
GE Omega scanner
GE Pace CT scanner
GE proton head coil probe
GE QE scanner
GE Senographe 2000D digital
mammography system
GE Signa double doughnut
GE Signa 5.4 Genesis MR imager
GE Signa 5.5 Horizon EchoSpeed
MR imager
GE Signa 4.7 MRI scanner
GE Signa 1.5T magnet
GE Signa 1.5T scanner
GE Signa 5.2 with SR-230 3-axis
EPI gradient upgrade scanner
GE single-detector SPECT-capable
camera
GE SPECT
GE Spiral CT scanner
GE Starcam single-crystal
tomographic scintillation camera
GE Vectra MR scanner
GE Viewer software
GE Voluson 730 4D ultrasound
system
GE-Amersham merger signal
Gee-Herter disease
Gee-Thaysen disease
GEG
Garren-Edwards gastric
GEG bubble
Gehan methodology
Geiger counter
Geiger-Müller (G-M)
G.-M. counter
G.-M. detector
G.-M. survey meter
G.-M. tube
gel
acoustic g.
g. bleed
coupling g.
crosslinked silicone g.
Fricke g.
methylcellulose g.
ultrasound g.

G

gelatin
  g. phantom
  g. sponge
  g. sponge particle
  g. sponge pledget
  g. sponge powder
gelatinous
  g. ascites
  g. brain pseudocyst
  g. carcinoma
  g. debris
  g. hematoma
  g. tissue
Gelbfish-Endovasc device
gemellary pregnancy
gemellus
gemistocytic astrocytoma
gemistocytoma
gene
  BRCA1 g.
  BRCA2 g.
  human androgen receptor g.
  retinoblastoma g.
  g. therapy
general
  G. Electric (GE)
  g. pattern matching
generalized
  g. angiofollicular lymph node
    hyperplasia
  g. arteriosclerosis
  g. autocalibrating partial parallel
    acquisition (GRAPPA)
  g. breast hyperplasia
  g. calcinosis
  g. capillary leak
  g. compensation for resonance offset
    and pulse length errors (GROPE)
  g. cortical hyperostosis
  g. cortical hyperstasis
  g. emphysema
  g. hamartomatosis
  g. hazy opacity
  g. increased liver echogenicity
  g. interferography using spin echoes
    and stimulated echoes
  g. lymphadenopathy syndrome
  g. lymphangiectasis
  g. nephrographic (GNG)
  g. osteoarthritis
  g. pulmonary edema
  g. seizure
  g. SENSE
generation
  g. echo
  G. 6 integrated radiotherapy system
  vertical g.
generator
  anterior current g.

carbon dioxide g.
g. characteristic
CO_2 g.
CORI computerized endoscopic
  report g.
deuterium-tritium g.
direct current g.
^{166}Dy g.
dysprosium-holmium in vivo g.
electric g.
electrostatic g.
extraction g.
high-voltage g.
^{166}Ho in vivo g.
molybdenum-99 g.
molybdenum-technetium g.
nuclide g.
3-phase g.
piezoelectric g.
polyphase g.
6-pulse 3-phase g.
12-pulse 3-phase g.
radiofrequency g.
radionuclide g.
resonance g.
spark gap g.
Super 50 CP high-voltage g.
supervoltage g.
g. system
technetium 99m g.
Triphasix g.
Van de Graaf g.
video signal g.
Vnus radiofrequency g.
waveform g.
wet/dry g.
x-ray g.
generator-produced ^{188}Re
Genesis
  G. 2000 carbon dioxide laser
  G. stent
Genesys camera
genetically
  g. engineered oncolytic adenovirus
  g. homogeneous
  g. significant dose
genial, genian
  g. tubercle
  g. tubercle of mandible
genian (*var. of* genial)
genicula (*pl. of* geniculum)
geniculate
  g. body
  g. branch
  g. ganglion
  g. ganglion schwannoma
geniculocalcarine tract
geniculum, *pl.* **genicula**
genioglossus muscle

genital
- g. blood pooling
- g. canal
- g. carcinoma
- g. duct
- g. eminence
- g. fold
- g. groove
- g. ligament
- g. ridge
- g. tract
- g. tract calcification
- g. tract embryology
- g. tract gas
- g. tract outflow obstruction
- g. visualization

genitalia
- ambiguous g.

genitoinguinal ligament

genitourinary (GU)
- g. adverse effect
- g. anomaly
- g. carcinoma
- g. fistula
- g. injury
- g. reflex
- g. rhabdomyosarcoma
- g. system
- g. system scintigraphy
- g. tract
- g. tract trauma
- g. tuberculosis

Gennari
- G. band
- line of G.
- G. stripe

genome
- mitochondrial g.
- nuclear g.

genomic instability

genotype

GentleLASE
- G. Plus laser
- G. Plus laser system

gentle lordosis

genu, *pl.* **genua**
- g. of corpus callosum
- g. recurvatum
- g. valgum
- g. valgum deformity
- g. varum
- g. varum deformity

genua (*pl. of* genu)

geode formation

geographic
- g. bone destruction
- g. follicle
- g. lesion
- g. pattern
- g. skull

geography
- brain g.

geometric
- g. blur
- g. distortion
- g. distribution
- g. efficiency
- g. unsharpness

geometry
- beam g.
- coil g.
- coronary vessel g.
- g. factor
- g. factor map
- Golay g.
- scintillation camera g.
- slice g.

geophagia artifact

GERD
- gastroesophageal reflux disease

Gerdy
- G. fontanelle
- G. interatrial loop
- G. interauricular loop
- G. ligament
- G. tubercle

Gerhardt
- G. sign
- G. triangle

geriatric
- g. configuration
- g. feature

germ
- g. cell neoplasm
- g. cell tumor

germanate
- bismuth g. (BGO)

German horizontal plane

germanium
- high-purity g. (HPGe)

germinal
- g. bleed matrix
- g. matrix-intraventricular hemorrhage
- g. pole

germinolysis
- subependymal g.

germinoma
- intracranial g.
- mediastinal g.
- multicentric g.
- pineal g.
- suprasellar hemorrhagic g.

Gerota
- G. capsule
- G. fascia
- G. method

G

Gerstmann-Sträussler-Scheinker (GSS)
    G.-S.-S. disease
Gerstmann syndrome
Gertzbein seatbelt
  classification
gestalt impression on CT
gestation
      extrauterine g.
      intrauterine g.
      multiple g.'s
      nonviable g.
      normal g.
      triplet g.
gestational
      g. age
      g. choriocarcinoma
      g. diabetes
      g. ring
      g. sac (GS)
      g. sac abnormality
      g. sac diameter
      g. sac measurement
      g. trophoblastic disease (GTD)
      g. trophoblastic neoplasia
      g. trophoblastic tumor
      g. week
geyser sign
GFR
    glomerular filtration rate
GGO
    ground-glass opacification
GHA
    glucoheptanoic acid
GHCH
    giant hepatic cavernous hemangioma
Ghon
      G. complex
      G. focus
      G. node
      G. primary lesion
      G. tubercle
Ghon-Sachs complex
ghost
      g. image
      red cell g.
      g. reduction by equalized acquisition
        triplets (GREAT)
      separation of g.'s
      g. tumor
ghosting artifact
GHz
    gigahertz
GI
    gastrointestinal
      GI bleed
      Imagent GI
      Innerview GI
      GI tract
      GI tract amyloidosis

      GI tract endometriosis
      GI tract lipoma
      GI tract lymphoid hyperplasia
      GI tract mastocytosis
      GI tract scintigraphy
      GI tract trauma
      GI tract tuberculosis
Gianotti-Crosti syndrome
giant
      g. bone island
      g. brain aneurysm
      g. breast fibroadenoma
      g. bullous emphysema
      g. cavernous hemangioma (GCH)
      g. cell adenocarcinoma
      g. cell arteritis
      g. cell astrocytoma
      g. cell carcinoma of thyroid
        gland
      g. cell fibroma
      g. cell interstitial pneumonia (GIP)
      g. cell lung carcinoma
      g. cell pneumonitis
      g. cell reparative granuloma
      g. cell sarcoma
      g. cell tumor
      g. cell tumor of tendon sheath
      g. cell-type MFH
      g. cervical parathyroid adenoma
      g. cholesterol cyst
      g. colon
      g. duodenal ulcer
      g. follicle lymphoma
      g. follicular hyperplasia
      g. gastric fold
      g. hepatic cavernous hemangioma
        (GHCH)
      g. hyperplasia lymph node
      g. hypertrophic gastritis
      g. left atrium (GLA)
      g. myofibroblastoma
      g. osteoid osteoma
      g. parathyroid adenoma
      g. peptic ulcer
      g. saccular aneurysm
      g. serpentine aneurysm
      g. sigmoid diverticulum
      g. villous adenoma
giantism (*var. of* gigantism)
Gianturco
      G. biliary Z-stent
      G. occlusion coil
      G. stent
      G. wool-tufted wire coil
Gianturco-Rosch biliary stent
Gianturco-Roubin FlexStent
Gianturco-Wallace-Anderson coil
Gianturco-Wallace-Chuang coil
giardiasis

gibbous deformity
Gibbs
    G. random field
    G. ringing
    G. sampling
Gibbs-Donnan law
gibbus
    thoracic g.
Gierke respiratory bundle
GIFT
    gastrointestinal fibrous tumor
gigabecquerel
gigahertz (GHz)
gigantiform cementoma
gigantism, giantism
    cerebral g.
    extremity g.
    focal g.
Gilchrist disease
gill
    g. arch skeleton
    g. cleft
    G. lesion
Gillette
    G. joint
    G. suspensory ligament
Gillies suture
GILT
    gastrointestinal leiomyogenic
    tumor
Gimbernat ligament
gingival
    g. carcinoma
    g. crest
    g. curvature
    g. metastasis
    g. septum
    g. space
gingivitis
    erosive g.
    necrotizing ulcerative g.
    (NUG)
gingivobuccal groove
gingivodental ligament
gingivolabial groove
GIP
    giant cell interstitial pneumonia
girdle
    limb g.
    pectoral g.
    pelvic g.
    shoulder g.
girth
    abdominal g.
Gissane
    G. calcaneal x-ray angle
    crucial angle of G.
GIST
    gastrointestinal stromal tumor

given
    G. diagnostic imaging system
    G. imaging capsule/M2A capsule
GK-SRS
    Gamma Knife-stereotactic radiosurgery
    GK-SRS boost
GLA
    giant left atrium
glabella
glabelloalveolar line
glabellomeatal line
glabrous cirrhosis
glacial acetic acid
GLAD
    glenolabral articular cartilage disruption
    GLAD lesion
gladiolus
gladiomanubrial
gland
    absorbent g.
    accessory thyroid g.
    admaxillary g.
    adrenal g.
    Albarran g.
    alveolar g.
    anteprostatic g.
    aortic g.
    apical g.
    apocrine sweat g.
    aporic g.
    arterial g.
    arteriococcygeal g.
    axillary sweat g.
    Bartholin g.
    Bruch g.
    Brunner g.
    bulbocavernous g.
    bulbourethral g.
    calcified pineal g.
    carotid g.
    coccygeal g.
    Duverney g.
    eccrine sweat g.
    ectopic g.
    endocrine g.
    enlarged thyroid g.
    enlargement of lacrimal g.
    enlargement of parotid g.
    giant cell carcinoma of thyroid g.
    globate g.
    glomiform g.
    haversian g.
    hilar g.
    hyperplastic parathyroid g.
    interscapular g.
    lacrimal g.
    Littré g.
    lymph g.
    mammary g.

G

gland (*continued*)
  Montgomery g.
  mucosal g.
  ovarian g.
  pancreas g.
  paramediastinal g.
  parathyroid g.
  paraurethral g.
  parotid g.
  periurethral g.
  pineal g.
  pituitary g.
  prostate g.
  salivary g.
  Stensen g.
  subaortic g.
  sublingual g.
  submandibular g.
  submaxillary g.
  substernal thyroid g.
  supernumerary parathyroid g.
  suprarenal g.
  testicular g.
  thymus g.
  thyroid g.
  urethral g.
  Virchow g.
  g. volume
  Wharton g.
glandes (*pl. of* glans)
glandular
  g. carcinoma
  g. dose
  g. papilloma
  g. proliferation
glans, *pl.* **glandes**
  g. carcinoma
  g. penis
glare
  imaging chain veiling g.
  scatter and veiling g. (SVG)
  veiling g.
glaserian fissure
Glasgow
  G. coma scale (GCS)
  G. outcome scale (GOS)
  G. sign
glass
  g. blower's emphysema
  g. eye artifact
  fiberoptic video g.'s
  ground g.
  hepatic test of G.
  quartz g.
  g. ray
  g. thermometer
  g. tract detector
  vita g.
  wine g.

Glasscock-Jackson classification
glaucoma
  juvenile-onset g.
glaze consistency
Glazunov tumor
Gleason
  G. grade
  G. score
Glénard disease
Glenn
  G. anastomosis
  G. shunt
  G. superior vena cava to right
   pulmonary artery anastomosis
   procedure
glenohumeral
  g. dislocation
  g. instability
  g. joint
  g. ligament
glenoid
  g. articular rim disruption (GARD)
  g. articular rim disruption lesion
  g. cavity
  g. fossa
  g. labral ovoid body
  g. labrum
  g. labrum capsule
  g. labrum injury
  g. ligament
  g. ovoid mass
  g. point
  g. process
  g. rim
  g. rim fracture
  g. surface
glenolabral
  g. articular cartilage disruption
   (GLAD)
  g. articular disruption lesion
  g. ovoid mass (GLOM)
Gliadel wafer
glial
  g. brain tumor
  g. limiting membrane
  g. nodule
  g. rest
  g. scarring
  g. stranding
  g. tumor calcification
GliaSite radiotherapy system
Glidecath
  Radifocus G.
GlideCatheter
Glide Cobra catheter
Glidewire
  angled G.
  long-taper stiff-shaft G.
  Radifocus G.

gliding
    g. joint
    g. sign
glioblast
glioblastoma
    butterfly g.
    multicentric g.
    g. multiforme (GBM)
glioma
    anaplastic cerebral g.
    brainstem g.
    butterfly g.
    cerebral g.
    cystic g.
    high-grade g.
    hypothalamic g.
    intracranial g.
    low-grade g.
    malignant g.
    multicentric malignant g.
    nonanaplastic g.
    optic nerve g.
    pontile g.
    pontocerebellar g.
    recurrent high-grade malignant g.
    rolandoparietal g.
    spinal cord g.
    supratentorial g.
    tectal g.
    temporooccipital g.
    thalamic g.
gliomatosis
    arachnoidal g.
    g. cerebri
    g. peritonei
glioma-to-white-matter contrast
glioneural hamartoma
gliosarcoma
    cerebellar g.
gliosis
    astrocytic g.
    ischemic g.
    g. of sylvian aqueduct
    progressive subcortical g.
    reactive g.
    secondary g.
gliosis-induced microcystic
  degeneration
Glisson capsule
global
    g. cavus
    g. cell leukodystrophy
    g. cerebral blood flow (gCBF)
    g. cerebral hypoperfusion
    g. cerebral ischemia
    g. cortical defect
    g. ejection fraction
    g. hypokinesis
    g. hypometabolism

    G. Initiative for chronic obstructive
      lung disease
    g. intracranial blood flow
    g. myocardial ischemia
    g. phantogeusia
    g. renal enlargement
    g. tissue loss
    g. ventricular function
    g. wall motion abnormality
globally
    g. depressed ejection fraction
    g. optimized alternating-phase
      rectangular pulse (GARP)
globate gland
globe
    g. enucleation
    optic g.
globe-orbit relationship
globi (*pl. of* globus)
globoid heart
globular
    g. cardiomegaly
    g. chest
    g. configuration
    g. meningioma
    g. tumor
    g. valve
globule, globulus
    human milk fat g.
globulin
    cytomegalovirus immune g.
    technetium 99m human
      g.
globuli ossei
globulus (*var. of* globule)
globus, *pl.* **globi**
    g. major
    g. minor
    g. pallidus
    g. sensation
glocoprotein
    P g. (P-gp)
Glofil-125 injection
GLOM
    glenolabral ovoid mass
    GLOM lesion
glomangioma
glomera (*pl. of* glomus)
glomerular, glomerulose
    g. basement membrane (GBM)
    g. filtration
    g. filtration agent
    g. filtration rate (GFR)
    g. lesion
    g. mesangial cell
    g. nephritis
glomeruli (*pl. of* glomerulus)
glomerulocytoma
glomeruloid formation

G

glomerulonephritides (*pl. of* glomerulonephritis)
glomerulonephritis, *pl.*
  glomerulonephritides
    acute g.
    chronic g.
    crescent-shaped g.
    membranous g.
    necrotizing g.
    proliferative g.
    segmental necrotizing g.
glomerulopathy
glomerulosa
    zona g.
glomerulosclerosis
glomerulose (*var. of* glomerular)
glomerulus, *pl.* glomeruli
    renal g.
glomiform gland
glomus, *pl.* glomera
    g. body
    g. body tumor
    g. bone tumor
    choroid g.
    g. choroideum
    g. jugulare
    g. jugulare tumor
    g. jugulotympanicum tumor
    g. neck tumor
    g. of choroid plexus
    g. tympanicum
    g. vagale
glomus-type arteriovenous malformation
glossoepiglottic, glossoepiglottidean
    g. fold
    g. ligament
glossoepiglottidean (*var. of* glossoepiglottic)
glossopalatine fold
glottic
    g. carcinoma
    g. larynx
    g. narrowing
glottides (*pl. of* glottis)
glottis, *pl.* glottides
glove
    optic g.
    g. phenomenon
    g. phenomenon artifact
    radiation-attenuating surgical g.
gloved-finger
    g.-f. shadow
    g.-f. sign
glow
    cathode g.
    g. curve
    g. modular tube
GLPC
    gas-liquid phase chromatography

GLP7 film
glucagon imaging agent
glucagonoma
glucarate imaging agent
glucaric acid-labeled contrast medium
gluceptate
    TechneScan g.
Glucoband electronic scanning device
glucoheptanoate
    ^{99m}Tc g.
    technetium 99m g.
glucoheptanoic acid (GHA)
glucose
    cerebral metabolic rate of g.
    g. water
glucosyl-galactosyl-pyridinoline
    urinary g.-g.-p.
glue
    Technovit 7210 VLC contact g.
    TruFill n-BCA surgical g.
glutamate spectroscopy
glutaric aciduria (type I, II)
gluteal
    g. bonnet
    g. fold
    g. line
    g. lymph node
    g. ridge
    g. tendinitis
gluten-sensitive enteropathy
gluteus
    g. maximus
    g. maximus muscle
    g. medius
    g. minimus
glycerolphosphorylcholine (GPC)
glycogenic acanthosis
glycogen-rich pancreatic cystadenoma
glycogen storage disease
glycol
    isosmotic polyethylene g.
    polyethylene g. (PEG)
glycolysis
    enhanced g.
glycoprotein-secreting adenoma
glycosaminoglycan
glycoside
    cardiac g.
G-M
    Geiger-Müller
      G-M counter
GM
    gray matter
      GM segmentation
GM-CSF
    granulocyte
      macophage-colony-stimulating factor
GM₁/GM₂ gangliosidosis

GMN
    gradient moment nulling
GMR
    gradient moment reduction
    gradient moment rephasing
    gradient motion rephasing
gnathic osteosarcoma
GNB
    ganglioneuroblastoma
GNG
    generalized nephrographic
      GNG phase imaging
goblet cell carcinoid
goblet-shaped pelvis
Godwin tumor
Goethe bone
goggles
    Avotec MR-compatible liquid crystal
      display g.
goiter
    adenomatous g.
    Basedow g.
    colloid g.
    congenital g.
    cystic g.
    diffuse toxic g.
    diving g.
    exophthalmic g.
    familial g.
    fetal g.
    fibrous g.
    intrathoracic g.
    iodide g.
    iodine-deficiency g.
    lingual g.
    multinodular g.
    nodular g.
    nontoxic g.
    parenchymatous g.
    retrotracheal g.
    retrovascular g.
    simple g.
    substernal g.
    suffocative g.
    thyroid g.
    toxic multinodular g.
    toxic nodular g.
    vascular g.
    wandering g.
goitrogen
Golay
    G. coil
    G. geometry
gold (Au)
    g. imaging agent
    g. particle
    g. radioactive source
    g. seed
Goldblatt kidney

golden
    motility of G.
    G. S sign
    S sign of G.
Goldenhar syndrome
gold-195m
    g.-195m radionuclide
    g.-195m tracer
gold-marked stent
Goldsmith and Woodburne
  classification
Goldthwait sign
Gold-tip micro guidewire
golfer's elbow
Golgi tendon
GoLYTELY bowel preparation
gonad
    indifferent g.
gonadal
    g. artery
    g. dose
    g. dysgenesis
    g. function
    g. neoplasia
    g. shielding
    g. steroid-dependent benign smooth
      muscle tumor
    g. stroma
    g. stromal tumor
    g. vein reflux
    g. venography
    g. venous ectasia
gonadoblastoma
gonadotroph cell adenoma
gonadotrophin (*var. of*
  gonadotropin)
gonadotropic hormone
gonadotropin, gonadotrophin
    chorionic g.
gonadotropin-secreting adenoma
gonecystic calculus
gonia (*pl. of* gonion)
gonial angle
goniometer
    Sceratti g.
gonion, *pl.* **gonia**
    g. gradient coil
    g. gradient magnetic field
gonion-gnathion plane
Goodpasture syndrome
Good Samaritan law
goose foot tendon
gooseneck
    g. concept
    g. outflow tract deformity
    g. shape
Gordon-Bröstrom single-contrast
  arthrography
Gordon sign

G

Gore
  G. covered biliary stent-graft
  G. 1.5T torso array MRI surface
    coil
Gorham disease
Gorlin
  G. formula for aortic valve area
  G. formula for mitral valve area
  G. method for measuring cardiac
    output
  G. syndrome
Gorlin-Goltz syndrome
GOS
  Glasgow outcome scale
Gosling pulsatility index
Gosselin fracture
Gosset
  spiral band of G.
gossypiboma
  aseptic g.
Gothic arch formation
Gottron
  G. papule
  G. sign
gouge defect
Gould
  G. electromagnetic flowmeter
  G. Statham pressure transducer
gout
  articular g.
  spinal tophaceous g.
  tophaceous g.
gouty
  g. arthritis
  g. arthropathy
  g. node
  g. tophus
Gowers
  G. bundle
  G. bundle in cerebellum
  G. column
  G. fasciculus
  G. sign
GPC
  glycerolphosphorylcholine
g-probe localization
graafian
  g. follicle
  g. vesicle
**Grace method of metatarsal length
  ratio**
gracile
  g. bone
  g. habitus
gracilis
  funiculus g.
  g. tendon
gradation
  subtle g.

grade
  Gleason g.
  histologic g.
  osteoarthritis g.
  placental g.
  Scharff-Bloom-Richardson g.
  Severin g.
  thrombolysis in brain ischemia flow g.
  tumor regression g.
graded
  g. compression sonography
  g. compression sonography technique
  g. compression ultrasound
  g. infusion
gradient
  g. acquisition
  g. across valve
  g. amplifier
  g. amplitude
  aortic outflow g.
  aortic valve g. (AVG)
  aortic valve peak instantaneous g.
  aortic valve pressure g.
  arteriovenous pressure g.
  atrioventricular g.
  balanced g.
  biliary-duodenal pressure g.
  bipolar g.
  brain-core g.
  g. compensation
  conjugate g.
  coronary perfusion g.
  dephasing g.
  3D Fourier transform gradient-echo
    sequence with spoiler g.
  diastolic g.
  diffusion g.
  diffusion-sensitizing g.
  discontinuous density g.
  g. drive current
  duodenobiliary pressure g.
  g. echo (GE)
  echo-speed g.
  electric field g.
  elevated g.
  g. encoding
  end-diastolic aortic-left ventricular
    pressure g.
  FAST PC cine MR sequence with
    echo-planar g.
  Ficoll g.
  field g.
  flow-encoding g.
  frequency-encoding g.
  gadolinium fast multiplanar spoiled
    g. (Gd-FMPSPGR)
  gastrosphincteric pressure g.
  hepatic venous pressure g.
  holosystolic g.

imaging g.
instantaneous g.
left ventricular outflow pressure g.
linear g.
g. linearity
g. magnetic field
magnetic field g. (MFG)
maximum estimated g.
mean mitral valve g.
mean systolic g.
mitral valve g.
g. moment nulling (GMN)
g. moment reduction (GMR)
g. moment rephasing (GMR)
motion-nulling g.
g. motion rephasing (GMR)
negligible pressure g.
nonisotropic g.
oscillating g.
osmotic g.
outflow tract g.
peak diastolic g.
peak instantaneous g.
peak pressure g.
peak right ventricular-right atrial
  systolic g.
peak systolic g.
peak-to-peak pressure g.
perfusion g.
phase-encoding g.
portosystemic g.
potential g.
Power Trak 6000 g.
pressure-flow g.
pre-TIPS g.
pullback pressure g.
pulmonary artery to right ventricle
  diastolic g.
pulmonary outflow g.
pulmonary valve g.
g. pulse
g. pump
readout g.
rephasing g.
residual g.
g. reversal
right ventricle to main pulmonary
  artery pressure g.
g. scheme
g. selection
sensitizing g.
g. sheet coil
g. slew rate
slice select g.
g. spin echo
Stejskal-Tanner g.
stenotic g.
g. subsystem in MRI
subvalvular g.

g. switching noise
g. system
systolic g.
thoracoabdominal g.
g. timing
transaortic systolic g.
transjugular intrahepatic
  portosystemic shunt g.
translesional pressure g.
transmitral g.
transpulmonic g.
transstenotic g.
transtricuspid valve diastolic g.
transvalvular pressure g.
tricuspid valve g.
twister g.
velocity g.
ventricular g.
voxel g.
washout g.
g. waveform
X g.
Z g.

gradient-echo
  g.-e. axial image
  g.-e. cine technique
  g.-e. coronal image
  3D g.-e.
  g.-e. 3-dimensional Fourier transform
    volume imaging
  g.-e. flow imaging
  g.-e. imaging sequence
  g.-e. method
  g.-e. MR imaging
  g.-e. MR with magnetization transfer
  g.-e. phase imaging
  g.-e. pulse sequence
  g.-e. recall technique
  g.-e. sequence imaging
  g.-e. single-photon
    emission-computed tomography
  spin-lock g.-e. (SL-GRE)
  g.-e. T2-weighted image
gradient-encoded image
gradient-induced phase dispersion
gradient-recalled
  g.-r. acquisition in steady state
    (GRASS)
  g.-r. echo (GRE)
  g.-r. echo image
gradient-refocused echo (GRE)
gradient-to-noise imaging
grading
gradually tapering border
Graf
  G. alpha angle
  G. beta angle
  G. hip dysplasia classification
  G. method

G

graft

Ancure tube g.
aorticorenal g.
aortic tube g.
aortobifemoral g.
aortofemoral bypass g. (AFBG)
aortoiliac bypass g.
aortoplasty with patch g.
arterial bypass g.
autogenous vein bypass g.
autologous patch g.
autologous vein g.
axillary-axillary bypass g.
axillary-brachial bypass g.
axillary-femoral bypass g.
axillary-femorofemoral bypass g.
axillobifemoral bypass g.
bifemoral g.
bifurcation g.
bilateral myocutaneous g.
bone g.
bone-tendon-bone g.
Brescia-Cimino g.
bypass g.
carotid-carotid venous bypass g.
Cloward bone g.
coronary artery bypass g.
  (CABG)
Corvita endoluminal g.
custom-fabricated g.
disc-shaped bone g.
donor g.
dowel-shaped bone g.
elephant trunk g.
endarterectomy g.
endoleak g.
endoscopic coronary artery bypass
  g. (E-CABG)
endothelialized vascular g.
endovascular aortic g.
endovascular stent g.
esophageal g.
expanded polytetrafluoroethylene g.
extracavitary prosthetic arterial g.
g. failure
femorocrural g.
femorodistal popliteal bypass g.
femorofemoral bypass g.
femoroperoneal in situ vein
  bypass g.
femoropopliteal bypass g.
femoropopliteal Gore-Tex g.
femorotibial bypass g.
H g.
hepatorenal saphenous vein
  bypass g.
iliac-renal bypass g.
ilioprofunda bypass g.
infected extracavitary g.

infected thrombosed g.
infrainguinal arterial bypass g.
infrainguinal vein bypass g.
inlay g.
in situ g.
interbody bone g.
internal thoracic artery g.
interposition g.
g. interstitium
intraabdominal arterial bypass g.
ITA g.
jump vein g.
g. kinking
limb of bifurcation g.
loop g.
occluded g.
g. occlusion
onlay g.
osseous g.
g. patency
patency of vein g.
pedicle bone g.
polytetrafluoroethylene g.
prosthetic femoral distal g.
g. revascularization
reversed vein g.
g. roof impingement
saphenous vein bypass g.
Sauvage filamentous velour g.
sequence bypass g.
g. shrinkage
Smith-Robinson bone g.
snake g.
splenorenal arterial bypass g.
g. stenosis
straight interposition g.
subcutaneous arterial bypass g.
suprailiac aortic mesenteric g.
synthetic vascular bypass g.
Varivas loop g.
vascular bypass g.
g. vascularization
vein g.
venous bypass g.
venous interposition g.
Zenith AAA endovascular g.

graft-enteric

g.-e. erosion
g.-e. fistula

grafting

aortoaortic bypass g.
lymphovenous g.

graft-related complication
graft-versus-host disease of liver
graft-versus-tumor response
Graham-Burford-Mayer syndrome
Graham-Cole

G.-C. cholecystogram
G.-C. test

grain handler's lung
graininess
    film g.
gram-negative rod infection
grand
    g. mal epilepsy
    g. mal seizure
Granger
    G. line
    G. projection
    G. view
Grantham femur fracture classification
granular
    g. breast cell myoblastoma
    g. calcification
    g. infiltrate
    g. kidney
    g. leukocyte
    g. lung cell myoblastoma
    g. lymphoproliferative disorder
    g. microcalcification
    g. opacity
    g. sella cell myoblastoma
granularis
    ependymitis g.
granulation
    arachnoid g.
    Bayle g.
    pacchionian g.
    g. stenosis
    g. tissue
granule
    neurosecretory g.
granulocyte
    antibody-labeled circulating g.
    g. colony-stimulating factor (GCSF, G-CSF)
    g. macophage-colony-stimulating factor (GM-CSF)
granulocytic sarcoma
granuloma, *pl.* **granulomas,** *pl.*
  granulomata
    actinic g.
    apical g.
    aspergillotic g.
    beryllium g.
    bilharzial g.
    button sequestrum eosinophilic g.
    calcified cysticercus g.
    caseating g.
    ceroid gallbladder g.
    cholesterol ear g.
    coalescent g.
    cysticercus g.
    dental g.
    eosinophilic g.
    epithelioid g.
    extravascular g.
    foreign body g.

    frontoethmoidal giant cell reparative g.
    giant cell reparative g.
    histoplasmosis g.
    Hodgkin g.
    hyalinizing g.
    inactive g.
    inguinal g.
    lethal midline g.
    liver g.
    lung g.
    malarial g.
    mediastinal g.
    midline g.
    Mignon g.
    miliary g.
    noncaseating g.
    paracoccidioidal g.
    periapical g.
    plasma cell g.
    pseudopyogenic g.
    pulmonary hyalinizing g.
    reparative giant cell g.
    reticulohistiocytic g.
    rheumatic g.
    root end g.
    sarcoid g.
    sea urchin g.
    silicone g.
    sperm g.
    spleen g.
    stellate g.
    swimming pool g.
    thorium dioxide g.
    tracheal g.
    tuberculous g.
    umbilical g.
    xanthomatous g.
    zirconium g.
granulomas (*pl. of* granuloma)
granulomata (*pl. of* granuloma)
granulomatosis
    allergic g.
    bronchocentric g.
    lipoid g.
    lymphomatoid g.
    mainline g.
    Miescher g.
    necrotizing respiratory g.
    organic g.
    pulmonary mainline g.
    Wegener g.
granulomatous
    g. brain abscess
    g. enterocolitis
    g. ileitis
    g. inflammation of bronchus
    g. lesion of sinus
    g. lymphadenitis
    g. lymphoma

G

granulomatous (*continued*)
  g. mediastinitis
  g. myositis
  g. pneumonia
  g. pneumonitis
  g. transmural colitis
  g. uveitis
granulometry
granulomonocyte
granulosa
  g. cell carcinoma
  pyoderma g.
granulosa-theca
  g.-t. cell tumor
  g.-t. neoplasia
granulovacuolar degeneration
grapelike
  g. cluster
  g. multilocular cystic lesion
  g. vesicle
grape-skin lung cavity
graph
  scatter g.
  spin-phase g.
  velocity-time g.
graphics
  Reality Engine g.
graphite fibrosis of lung
GRAPPA
  generalized autocalibrating partial
    parallel acquisition
Graser diverticulum
Grashey
  G. method
  G. position
  G. shoulder view
grasping technique
GRASS
  gradient-recalled acquisition in steady
    state
  GRASS MR imaging
  GRASS pulse sequence
  spoiled GRASS
  GRASS system
Gratiolet
  G. convolution
  radiation of G.
gravel
  gallbladder g.
Graves
  G. disease
  G. hyperthyroidism
  G. ophthalmopathy
gravidarum
  fibroma molle g.
gravid uterus
gravis
  colitis ulcerosa g.
  myasthenia g.

gravitational
  g. edema
  g. potential energy
gravity
  center of g.
gravity-dependent atelectasis
Grawitz tumor
gray (Gy)
  g. box system
  g. commissure
  g. horn in spinal canal
  g. lung
  g. matter (GM)
  g. matter abnormality
  g. matter degeneration
  g. matter heterotopia
  g. matter spectrum
  g. matter-white matter differentiation
  periventricular g. (PVG)
  g. radiation absorbed dose
  g. reticular
  g. scale
  g. unit
gray-level
  g.-l. histogram
  g.-l. spacing
  g.-l. thresholding
gray-scale
  g.-s. baseline imaging
  g.-s. Doppler
  g.-s. endorectal ultrasound
  g.-s. ERU
  g.-s. examination
  g.-s. image
  g.-s. inversion
  g.-s. monitor
  g.-s. range
  g.-s. sonography
  g.-s. ultrasonography
Grayson ligament
gray-to-white
  g.-t.-w. matter activity ratio
  g.-t.-w. matter contrast ratio
  g.-t.-w. matter interface
  g.-t.-w. matter utilization ratio
gray-white
  g.-w. differentiation
  g.-w. matter junction
GRE
  gradient-recalled echo
  gradient-refocused echo
    GRE breath-hold hepatic imaging
    3D GRE
    ferumoxtran-enhanced echo-planar SE
      T2-weighted and echo-planar GRE
    GRE gadolinium chelate-enhanced
      imaging
    GRE magnetic resonance imaging
    GRE technique

great
    g. cardiac plexus
    g. cardiac vein
    g. cardiac vein flow
      (GCVF)
    g. cerebral vein of Galen
    g. cistern
    g. sacrosciatic foramen
    g. terminal vertebra
    g. toe sesamoid bone
    g. vein of cerebrum
    g. vessel
    g. vessel transposition
    g. vessel view
GREAT
    ghost reduction by equalized
    acquisition triplets
greater
    g. arc injury
    g. circulation
    g. curvature of stomach
    g. curvature ulcer
    g. multangular bone
    g. omentum
    g. palatine canal
    g. palatine foramen
    g. pelvis
    g. peritoneal sac
    g. petrosal
    g. sac of peritoneal cavity
    g. saphenous system
    g. saphenous vein
    g. sciatic foramen
    g. sciatic notch
    g. sigmoid notch
    g. sphenoid wing
    g. sphenoid wing lesion
    g. superficial petrosal nerve
    g. trochanter
    g. trochanteric femoral
      fracture
    g. trochanter of femur
    g. tubercle
    g. tuberosity
    g. tuberosity fracture
green
    iodocyanine g. (ICG)
Greene
    G. biopsy set
    G. needle
Greenfield
    G. catheter
    G. vena cava filter
greenstick fracture
GRE-in
    GRE-i. image
    GRE-i. imaging
grenade thrower's fracture
grenz ray

GRE-out
    GRE-o. image
    GRE-o. imaging
Greulich
    G. and Pyle atlas
    G. and Pyle method
Grey Turner sign
grid
    antiscatter g.
    Bucky g.
    g. conversion factor (GCF)
    cross-hatch g.
    emitter g.
    g. film
    focused g.
    localization g.
    Lysholm g.
    megavoltage g.
    oscillating g.
    Potter-Bucky g.
    g. ratio
    scatter g.
    g. technique
    g. therapy
Griesinger sign
griffe
    simian g.
Griffith point
Grisel syndrome
Grocco sign
Grocott methenamine silver
groin
    g. dissection
    g. mass
Grollman pigtail catheter
groove
    alveolingual g.
    alveolobuccal g.
    alveololabial g.
    anal intersphincteric g.
    anterior interventricular g.
    anterolateral g.
    anteromedian g.
    arterial g.
    atrioventricular g.
    basilar g.
    bicipital g.
    bronchial g.
    buccal g.
    carotid g.
    carpal g.
    caudothalamic g.
    cavernous g.
    central g.
    chiasmatic g.
    coronary g.
    costal g.
    deltopectoral g.
    dental g.

G

groove (*continued*)
   developmental g.
   digastric g.
   ectodermal g.
   esophageal g.
   ethmoidal g.
   gastric g.
   genital g.
   gingivobuccal g.
   gingivolabial g.
   Harrison g.
   infraorbital g.
   interatrial g.
   intercollicular g.
   intercondylar g.
   intertubercular g.
   interventricular g.
   labial g.
   lacrimal g.
   Liebermeister g.
   meningeal artery g.
   middle meningeal artery g.
   neural g.
   paravertebral g.
   patellar g.
   posterior coronary g.
   posterior interventricular g.
   proximal trochlear g.
   radial neck g.
   Ranvier g.
   retromalleolar g.
   sagittal g.
   Sibson g.
   spindle colonic g.
   striatothalamic g.
   supraorbital g. (SOG)
   trochlear g.
   trochleocapitellar g.
   ulnar g.
   urethral g.
   vascular g.
   venous g.
   Verga lacrimal g.
   vertebral g.
   Waterston g.
grooved director
grooving of articular surface
GROPE
   generalized compensation for resonance
   offset and pulse length errors
Groshong
   G. distal valve catheter
   G. NXT PICC
gross
   g. fracture
   g. lesion
   g. total resection
   g. tumor
   g. tumor volume (GTV)

Grossman
   G. principle
   G. scale for regurgitation
ground
   g. glass
   g. plate
   g. state
ground-glass
   g.-g. appearance
   g.-g. attenuation
   g.-g. definition
   g.-g. density
   g.-g. infiltrate
   g.-g. lesion
   g.-g. nodule
   g.-g. opacification (GGO)
   g.-g. opacity
   g.-g. osteoporosis
   g.-g. pattern
   g.-g. phenomenon
   g.-g. texture
group
   Dodd perforating vein g.
   Eastern Cooperative Oncology G.
    (ECOG)
   Eisenmenger g.
   extensor-supinator g.
   flexor-pronator muscle g.
   gadolinium-enhanced
    imaging g.
   gastrocnemius-soleus muscle g.
   Imaging Solutions G. (ISG)
   interosseous muscle g.
   iodinated tyrosine g.
   thalamogeniculate g. (TGG)
   g. viewing
growing fracture
growth
   g. acceleration
   g. arrest line
   g. center closure
   g. center of bone
   g. disc
   ectopic bone g.
   epiphysial chondroblastic g.
   g. factor
   g. hormone-producing adenoma
   g. hormone-releasing factor
    tumor
   g. impairment
   lepidic g.
   morphologic g.
   nutrient artery g.
   papillomatous g.
   g. parameter
   g. plate
   g. plate abscess
   g. plate arrest
   g. plate complex

g. plate fracture
g. plate injury
g. plate widening
g. retardation
spinal g.
targetoid g.
twin pregnancy discordant g.
Virchow law of skull g.

growth-retarded fetus

Gruber
G. fossa
petrosphenooccipital suture of G.
G. suture

grumous
g. debris
g. tissue

Grüntzig
G. balloon dilation catheter
G. PTCA technique

Grynfeltt triangle

GS
gestational sac
GS diameter

GSA
galactosyl human serum albumin
GSA imaging agent

Gsell-Erdheim syndrome

GSPECT
gated single-photon emission computed
tomography

GSS
Gerstmann-Sträussler-Scheinker
GSS disease

GSW
gunshot wound

GTD
gestational trophoblastic disease

GTF-A
Olympus Gastrocamera
GTF-A

GTV
gross tumor volume

GU
genitourinary
GU tract cholesteatoma
GU tract tuberculosis

GuardWire
G. distal balloon
G. Plus

gubernacular canal

gubernaculi
pars infravaginalis g.

Gubler
G. line
G. tumor

Guérin
G. fold
G. fracture
G. sinus

Guglielmi
G. detachable coil (GDC)
G. detachable coil embolization

guidance
active biplanar MR imaging g.
angioscopic g.
biplanar MR imaging g.
computerized tomography g.
fluoroscopic g.
frameless stereotactic g.
indirect ultrasound g.
mammographic g.
puncture g.
radiologic g.
sonographic g.
g. system selection
ultrasonic g.

Guidant
G. Ancure endograft procedure
G. Megalink peripheral stent

guide
Brown-Roberts-Wells CT stereotactic
g.
BRW CT stereotactic g.
g. catheter
CT stereotactic g.
side-exiting g.
g. wire

guided
g. biopsy
g. drainage

guideline
American Academy of Pediatrics g.
Mallinckrodt Institute of Radiology
g.'s
MIR g.'s
string g.

guidewire, guide wire
Amplatz Super Stiff g.
angiographic g.
angulated hydrophilic g.
Athlete GT coronary g.
basket g.
color-coded g.
Cope mandril g.
g. entrapment
exchange g.
g. exchange technique
extra-stiff g.
flexible-tip g.
Flex-T g.
Gold-tip micro g.
Headliner g.
Hi-Torque Floppy g.
Hi-Torque Modified J-GW g.
Hi-Torque steerable g.
hydrophilic coated g.
InQwire g.
intracoronary Doppler flow g.

G

guidewire (*continued*)
　　J-tipped g.
　　Katzen infusion g.
　　Lunderquist exchange g.
　　Lunderquist-Ring g.
　　movable core g.
　　Newton g.
　　nitinol g.
　　Nitrex ev3 g.
　　Nitrex nitinol g.
　　open-ended g.
　　Platinum Plus g.
　　platinum-tip g.
　　Radifocus hydrophilic coated g.
　　Ring g.
　　Roadrunner NaviGuide g.
　　Rosen curved g.
　　Silver Speed g.
　　Sniper Elite hydrophilic Ni-Ti
　　　alloy g.
　　standard fixed-core g.
　　stiff g.
　　straight g.
　　super-stiff g.
　　SV-5 g.
　　TAD steerable g.
　　tapered-core g.
　　tapered-tip g.
　　Teflon-coated g.
　　Terumo g.
　　through-and-through g.
　　tip-deflecting g.
　　torqueable g.
　　torque-control g.
　　Transend steerable g.
　　variable-stiffness g.
　　V18 Control Wire g.
　　V18 micro g.
　　WaveWire angioplasty g.
　　Wholey steerable g.
　　x-shaped g.
guiding
　　g. sheath
　　g. shot
Guillain-Barré syndrome
guillotine rib
guilt screen
Gumley seatbelt injury
　classification
gumma, *pl.* **gummata,** *pl.* **gummas**
　　frank cerebral g.
　　g. of rib
gummas (*pl. of* gumma)
gummata (*pl. of* gumma)
gun
　　automated biopsy g.
　　Biopty biopsy g.
　　electron g.
Gunn crossing sign

gunshot
　　g. fracture
　　g. wound (GSW)
gunstock deformity
Günther Tulip vena cava MReye
　filter
Günzberg ligament
gurgling cyst
Gustilo-Anderson
　　G.-A. open clavicular fracture
　　G.-A. tibial plafond fracture
　　　classification
gut
　　aging g.
　　blind g.
　　g. edema
　　large g.
　　primitive g.
　　g. signature
　　small g.
gut-associated lymphoid tissue
　(GALT)
Guthrie muscle
gutter
　　anterolateral g.
　　g. fracture
　　lateral g.
　　left g.
　　paracolic g.
　　parapelvic g.
　　paravertebral g.
　　peritoneal g.
　　right g.
　　sacral g.
　　synovial g.
Guyon
　　G. amputation
　　G. canal
Gy
　　gray
gymnast's wrist
Gynecare Versascope hysteroscope
gynecography
gynecoid pelvis
gynecologic endometriosis
gynecomastia, gynecomasty
　　dendritic g.
gynecomasty (*var. of* gynecomastia)
gynecophoric canal
gynogram
gynography
gyral
　　g. abnormality
　　g. brain enhancement
　　g. crest
　　g. infarct
gyration
Gyratome
gyri (*pl. of* gyrus)

gyriform
> g. calcification
> g. pattern

gyromagnetic ratio

Gyroscan
> G. ACS-NT
> G. ACS-NT MRI scanner
> G. ACS-NT MR unit
> G. ACS-NT 1.5T MR scanner
> G. Interna scanner
> G. NT 10 magnet
> G. S15 scanner
> G. 1.5T superconducting magnet

gyrus, *pl.* **gyri**
> angular g.
> ascending parietal g.
> Broca g.
> callosal g.
> central g.
> gyri cerebri
> cingulate g.
> contiguous supramarginal gyri
> dentate g.
> G. endourology system
> fasciolar g.
> flattening of g.
> g. fornicatus
> frontal g.
> fusiform g.
> Heschl transverse g.
> hippocampal g.
> inferior frontal g.
> inferior temporal g.
> infracalcarine g.
> insular g.
> lamination of g.

lateral occipitotemporal g.
lingual g.
marginal g.
medial occipitotemporal g.
middle frontal g.
middle temporal g.
occipital g.
occipitotemporal g.
olfactory g.
orbital g.
paracentral g.
parahippocampal g.
paraterminal g.
parietal g.
postcentral g.
posterior central g.
posterior cingulate g.
precentral g.
preinsular g.
quadrate g.
g. rectus
sensorimotor g.
short insular g.
1st temporal g.
subcallosal g.
subcollateral g.
superior frontal g.
superior parietal lobule g.
superior temporal g.
supracallosal g.
supramarginal g.
temporal g.
transverse temporal g.
Turner marginal g.
uncal g.
uncinate g.

G

H

H and D curve
H band
H disc
H field of Forel
H graft
H ray
H vertebra sign

H-1

H-1 MR spectroscopic imaging
H-1 MR spectroscopy

HAART

highly active antiretroviral therapy

Haas

H. method
H. position
H. trapezius muscle transfer

habenula, *pl.* **habenulae**
habenulae (*pl. of* habenula)
habenular commissure calcification
habitus

body h.
gracile h.
large h.
twisted body h.

HADD

hydroxyapatite deposition disease

hadron therapy
HAEC

Hirschsprung-associated enterocolitis

haematobium

Schistosoma h.

Haemophilus influenzae
Hageman factor
Hagie pin
HAGL

humeral avulsion of glenohumeral
ligament
HAGL lesion

Haglund

H. deformity
H. syndrome

Hahn

H. cleft
H. spin-echo sequence

**Hahn-Steinthal capitellum fracture
classification**
HAI

hepatic arterial infusion

Haifa camera
**Haines-McDougall medial sesamoid
ligament**
hair

h. artifact
h. shaft

hairbrush pattern
hair-containing sinus
hairline

h. crack
h. fracture

hair-on-end

h.-o.-e. appearance
h.-o.-e. of skull
h.-o.-e. periosteal reaction
h.-o.-e. sign

hairpin vessel
hairy heart
Hajdu-Cheney syndrome
half

h. emptying time (T 1/2)
h. scan with extrapolation
h. scan with extrapolation
projection

half-axial

h.-a. anteroposterior projection
h.-a. view

half-body radiation therapy
**half-dose enhanced MRI with
MT**
half-Fourier

h.-F. acquisition single-shot turbo
spin-echo (HASTE)
h.-F. 3-dimensional technique
h.-F. imaging (HFI)
h.-F. RARE image
h.-F. transformation technique

half-intensity needle
half-life (HL)

antibody h.-l.
biologic h.-l.
effective h.-l.
elimination h.-l.
h.-l. layer
physical h.-l.
positronium h.-l.
radioactive h.-l.
short h.-l.

half-maximum

full width at h.-m. (FWHM)

half-moon

h.-m. artifact
h.-m. patella
h.-m. shape
h.-m. sign

half-Nex imaging
half-ring
half-scan (HS)

h.-s. reconstruction

half-thickness

narrow-beam h.-t.

H

413

half-time
 blood clearance h.-t.
 clearance h.-t.
 gastric emptying h.-t.
 h.-t. of exchange
 pressure h.-t.
halftone
 h. banding
 h. frequency
halftoning
 iterative h.
half-value layer (HVL)
half-wedged field technique
Hallermann-Streiff-François syndrome
Hallervorden-Spatz disease
hallmark
 histopathic h.
 radiofrequency radiographic h.
hallucal pronation
halluces (*pl. of* hallux)
hallucis
 adductor h.
 hyperdynamic abductor h.
hallus (*var. of* hallux)
hallux, hallus, *pl.* **halluces**
 h. abductovalgus
 h. dorsiflexion angle
 h. elevatus
 h. extensus
 h. flexus deformity
 h. interphalangeal joint
 h. interphalangeus angle (HIA)
 intrinsic minus h.
 h. limitus
 h. malleus deformity
 h. migration
 h. rigidus
 h. rigidus deformity
 h. saltans
 h. sesamoid bone
 h. sesamoid complex
 h. valgus (HV)
 h. valgus angle (HVA)
 h. valgus deformity
 h. valgus interphalangeus angle
 h. valgus-metatarsus primus varus
   complex
 h. varus
 h. varus deformity
 halo
 h. crown
 h. device
 h. effect
 fatty h.
 hypoechoic h.
 lucent h.
 nodule h.
 pericardial h.

 perinuclear h.
 periventricular h.
 radiolucent fat h.
 h. ring
 h. sign
 signal h.
 h. sign of hydrops
 sonolucent h.
 subendometrial h.
 h. vest
halofuginone probucol
halogenated
 h. phenolphthalein dye
 h. pyrimidine
 h. thymidine analogue
 h. thymidine analogue radiosensitizer
HAMA
 human antimouse antibody
hamartoma
 angiomatous lymphoid h.
 astrocytic h.
 benign fetal h.
 brain h.
 breast h.
 cardiac h.
 cartilaginous h.
 chest wall h.
 chondromatous h.
 CNS cortical h.
 cortical h.
 duodenal wall h.
 eccrine angiomatous h.
 elevated retinal h.
 endobronchial h.
 extracerebral intracranial
   glioneural h.
 fetal renal h.
 fibrolipomatous nerve h.
 fibrous h.
 glioneural h.
 hypothalamic h.
 leiomyomatous kidney h.
 lung h.
 lymphoid h.
 mesenchymal liver h.
 multiple bile duct h.'s
 myoid h.
 h. of eye
 h. of kidney
 pancreatic h.
 pigmented iris h.
 pulmonary h.
 renal h.
 retrorectal cystic h.
 h. spleen
 splenic h.
 subcortical CNS h.
 subependymal h.

tuber cinereum h.
vascular h.
ventromedial hypothalamic h.
hamartomatosis
generalized h.
hamartomatous
h. gastric polyp
h. lesion
h. polyposis syndrome
hamate
h. bone
h. facet
flake fracture of h.
h. tail fracture
hamiltonian equation
Hamilton-Stewart formula for measuring cardiac output
Hamman-Rich syndrome
Hamman sign
hammer
hypothenar h.
hammered
h. brass appearance
h. silver
h. silver appearance
h. silver skull
hammer-marked skull
hammertoe deformity
Hamming filter
hammocking of mitral valve leaflet
hammock ligament
Hampson unit
Hampton
H. hump
H. hump sign
H. line
H. maneuver
H. technique
H. view
hamstring tendon
hamuli (*pl. of* hamulus)
hamulus, *pl.* **hamuli**
pterygoideus h.
Hanafy piano-concave transducer design
hand
h. and forearm artery scoring (level I-V)
h. angiography
apelike h.
bear's paw h.
bipenniform muscle of h.
Breuerton view of h.
calcium pyrophosphate dihydrate h.
chiasm of digit of h.
claw h.
CPPD arthritis of h.
digital artery of h.
h. fracture

hypothenar muscle group of h.
h. injection
h. injection of contrast medium
h. motor deficit
opera-glass h.
h. osteoarthritis
phalanx of h.
spadelike h.
tangential layer of h.
trident h.
ulnar h.
h. vascularization
windswept h.
hand-agitated imaging agent
hand-carried ultrasound-guided pericardiocentesis
handheld
h. Doppler probe
h. exploring electrode probe
h. focused assessment with sonography for trauma (HHFAST)
h. mapping probe
handle
Amplatz radiolucent h.
hand-shaped bend
hands-up ergonomics
hand/wrist arthritis
hanger
film h.
hanging
h. heart
h. hip
hanging-block technique
hanging-fruit pattern
hangman's fracture
Hann filter
Hannover canal
Hanot cirrhosis
Hansen fracture classification
Hapad metatarsal arch
HAPE
high-altitude pulmonary edema
HAPS
hepatic artery perfusion scintigraphy
HARC-C
Houston Advanced Research Center-Compression
HARC-C wavelet compression technique
hard
h. disc herniation
h. metal pneumoconiosis
h. palate carcinoma
h. papilloma
h. ray
h. x-ray
hard-copy image

H

hardened
    h. lung
    h. pelvis
hardening
    h. artifact
    beam h.
    bone h.
Hardy-Clapham sesamoid classification
Hare syndrome
Harken valve
harlequin sign
harmonic
    h. field
    h. function
    h. imaging
harmonics
    simultaneous acquisition of spatial h. (SMASH)
    spatial h.
Harms cage
harness-shaped distribution
Harrington
    H. rod
    H. rod insertion
Harris
    H. band
    H. flush enema
    H. line
    H. tube
    H. view
Harris-Beath axial hindfoot view
Harrison
    H. curve
    H. groove
    H. sulcus
HART
    hyperfractionated accelerated radiation therapy
Hartmann
    H. closure of rectum
    H. perforated sigmoid diverticulitis resection
    H. point
    H. pouch
    H. solution
Harvard multidetector scanner
harvested vein
harvester's lung
Hashimoto thyroiditis
hashing
    image h.
HASTE
    half-Fourier acquisition single-shot turbo spin-echo
        magnetic resonance cholangiography with HASTE
        HASTE MRI
        HASTE sequence

HAT
    head-arms-trunk
        HAT transformed imaging
Hatcher-Smith cervical fusion
hatchet
    h. defect
    h. sign
hatchet-head deformity
Hatle method to calculate mitral valve area
Haudek niche
Hausdorff
    H. error
    H. measurement
haustra (*pl. of* haustrum)
haustral
    h. blunting
    h. fold
    h. indentation
    h. marking
    h. pattern
    h. pouch
haustration
haustrum, *pl.* **haustra**
    haustra coli
    colonic h.
Haut-Einheits-Dosis (HED)
    H.-E.-D. unit skin dose
haversian
    h. canal
    h. canaliculus
    h. channel
    h. fat-pad
    h. gland
Hawkin hookwire
Hawkins
    H. accordion catheter drainage set
    H. accordion-type empyema
    H. breast lesion localization needle
    H. classification of talar fracture
    H. inside-out nephrostomy set
    H. line
    H. method
    H. sign
    H. 1-stick needle
    H. talar neck fracture classification
Hawkins-Akins needle
hay-fork sign
Haygarth node
hazard
    sandbag h.
haze
    hilar h.
haziness
    diffuse h.
    pericolic h.
    subtle h.

hazy
> h. density
> h. infiltrate
> h. opacity
> h. opaque lung

HBAT
> hypermetabolic brown adipose tissue

HBCT
> helical biphasic computed tomography
>> HBCT imaging

HBE
> His bundle electrogram

HBHC
> hemiballismus-hemichorea

HBI
> hemibody irradiation
> human blood index

HC/AC
> head circumference to abdominal
> circumference
>> HC/AC ratio

H1 catheter

HCC
> hepatocellular carcinoma
>> HCC chemoembolization
>> fibrolamellar HCC

HCCM
> high-concentration contrast medium

HCM
> hypertrophic cardiomyopathy

HCS
> hematocystic spot

HCTA
> helical computed tomographic
> angiography

HCTE
> helical CT enteroclysis

HDI
> high-definition imaging
>> HDI 1000, 3000, 3500, 4000, 5000
>> ultrasound imaging system

HDIC
> hepatodiaphragmatic interposition of
> colon

HDR
> high dose rate

³He
> helium 3

⁴He
> helium 4

head
> h. and neck squamous cell
> carcinoma
> cartilaginous cap of phalangeal h.
> h. circumference
> circumference of fetal h.
> h. circumference to abdominal
> circumference (HC/AC)
> h. coil

> femoral h.
> forward positioning of h.
> h. injury
> ischemic necrosis of femoral h.
> (INFH)
> large fetal h.
> long h.
> metatarsal h.
> h. of barium column
> h. of caudate nucleus
> h. of femur
> h. of humerus
> h. of pancreas
> h. of rib
> pancreatic h.
> radial h.
> radial facing of metacarpal h.
> h. shape
> short h.
> 1st metatarsal h. (FMH)
> strawberry-shaped h.
> terminal h.
> transillumination of h.
> h. trauma
> ulnar h.
> ulnar facing of metacarpal h.

3-head
> 3-h. gamma camera-based SPECT
> system
> 3-h. scan

headache
> orthostatic h.
> paradoxic h.
> postural h.
> sentinel h.
> spontaneous postural h.

head-arms-trunk (HAT)

4-head camera

Headhunter catheter

Headisc

Headliner guidewire

headphones
> Avotec MR-compatible h.

head-splitting humeral fracture

Heaf test

healed gastric ulcer

healing
> bony h.
> h. flare response
> h. fracture
> h. infarct
> resorption phase of h.
> h. ulcer

heart
> abdominal h
> air-driven artificial h.
> alcoholic h.
> h. amyloidosis
> h. and great vessel

H

heart (*continued*)
    angioreticuloendothelioma of h.
    angiosarcoma of h.
    h. anomaly
    anterior border of h.
    aortic opening of h.
    apex of h.
    apical surface of h.
    armored h.
    artificial h.
    athlete's h.
    axis of h.
    balloon-shaped h.
    base of h.
    Baylor total artificial h.
    beer h.
    beriberi h.
    h. block
    boat-shaped h.
    bony h.
    booster h.
    boot-shaped h.
    h. border
    bread-and-butter h.
    h. bulb
    cardiogenic shock h.
    cervical h.
    3-chamber h.
    chamber of h.
    chaotic h.
    cloudy swelling of h.
    conical h.
    coronary artery of h.
    h. count-mediastinum count ratio
      (H/M)
    crisscross h.
    H. CT scan
    h. decortication
    h. degeneration
    dextroversion of h.
    diaphragmatic surface of h.
    h. disease
    dome-shaped h.
    donor h.
    double-density h.
    drop h.
    dynamite h.
    dysrhythmia of fetal h.
    egg-on-its-side h.
    electrocardiogram-gated multislice
     spiral CT of h.
    elongated h.
    empty h.
    encased h.
    enlarged h.
    h. failure
    fatty h.
    fetal h.
    fibroid h.

    h. fibroma
    flabby h.
    flask-shaped h.
    globoid h.
    hairy h.
    hanging h.
    Holmes h.
    horizontal h.
    hyperdynamic h.
    hyperkinetic h.
    hyperthyroid h.
    hypertrophied h.
    hypokinesis of h.
    hypoplastic right h.
    hypothermic h.
    inferior border of h.
    inflammation of h.
    intermediate h.
    irritable h.
    ischemic h.
    H. laser
    left border of h.
    L-loop h.
    malpositioned h.
    massively enlarged h.
    mesoversion of h.
    mildly enlarged h.
    mogul of h.
    movable h.
    h. muscle necrosis
    myxedema of h.
    h. myxoma
    myxoma of h.
    ovoid h.
    ox h.
    paracorporeal h.
    parasternal view of h.
    parchment h.
    pear-shaped h.
    pectoral h.
    pendulous h.
    h. position
    posterior border of h.
    h. pseudoaneurysm
    pulmonary h.
    Quain fatty degeneration of h.
    h. rate reserve mechanism
    h. remnant
    resting h.
    rhabdomyoma of h.
    right border of h.
    right ventricle of h.
    round h.
    sabot h.
    h. sac
    h. scintigraphy
    semihorizontal h.
    semivertical h.
    h. shadow

shift of h.
shoulder of h.
h. silhouette
single-outlet h.
snowman appearance of h.
soldier's h.
h. sounds
spastic h.
squared-off h.
sternocostal surface of h.
stone h.
h. stroke volume
superior border of h.
superoinferior h.
suspended h.
swinging h.
systemic h.
h. tamponade
Taussig-Bing congenital malformation
  of h.
teardrop h.
thrush breast h.
thymoma of h.
tobacco h.
total artificial h.
h. transplant
transverse h.
Traube h.
triatrial h.
trilocular h.
h. tumor
univentricular h.
upstairs-downstairs h.
h. valve
h. valve calcification
h. valve leaflet
h. valve vegetation
venting of h.
1-ventricle h.
vertical h.
wandering h.
water-bottle h.
wooden-shoe h.
heartbeat gating
heart-lung
  h.-l. ratio (HLR)
  h.-l. transplant
heart-shaped
  h.-s. collimator
  h.-s. pelvis
  h.-s. uterus
heart-to-background ratio
heart-to-lung ratio (HLR)
heart-to-thorax volume
HeartView
  H. cardiac reconstruction software
  H. CT
  H. CT cardiac monitor
HearTwave EP

heat
  h. fracture
  h. shape
  h. shaping
  h. unit
heat-damaged ^{99m}Tc-RBC
**heat-denatured autologous RBC SPECT
  imaging**
heater
  resistance wire h.
heat-generating source
heating
  gamma h.
  hot-source h.
  interstitial conductive h.
  nonablative h.
heave
  h. and lift
  sustained left ventricular h.
heavily penetrated view
heaving precordial motion
heavy
  h. chain
  h. charged particle
  h. charged-particle Bragg peak
    radiosurgery
  h. hydrogen
  h. ion imaging
  h. ion irradiation
  h. metal injection
  h. water
heavy-chain disease
heavy-duty standard exchange wire
heavy-particle
  h.-p. irradiation
  h.-p. therapy
Heberden
  H. disease
  H. node
Hecht pneumonia
Hector
  tendon of H.
HED
  Haut-Einheits-Dosis
heel
  black-dot h.
  h. bone
  h. effect
  h. fat-pad
  h. pad sign
  h. pad thickening
  Sorbol h.
  h. spur
  h. tendon
  varus h.
Hegglin syndrome
Heidelberg
  H. protocol
  H. retina tomograph II (HRT-II)

H

Heidenhain
H. pouch
H. variant
height
disc space h.
intervertebral disc space h.
knee joint space h.
radial h.
relative peak h.
vertebral body h.
Heim-Kreysig sign
Heimlich MicroTrach
Heineke-Mikulicz maneuver
Heinig view
Heister
valve of H.
helical
h. biphasic computed tomography
(HBCT)
h. computed tomographic
angiography (HCTA)
h. CTA
h. CT angiography
h. CT enteroclysis (HCTE)
h. CT holography
h. CT scanner
h. CT scanning protocol
h. hydro-CT
h. pattern
h. technique
h. thin-section CT
h. thin-section CT scan
helices (*pl. of* helix)
helicine artery
Helicobacter **infection**
helicoid
Helios
H. diagnostic imaging
H. laser system
Helioseal
heliotropic periorbital rash
helium
h. 3 (^{3}He)
h. 4 (^{4}He)
hyperpolarized h.
h. ion beam
h. magnetic resonance imaging
(He-MRI)
helium-cadmium laser
helium-filled balloon catheter
helium-neon (HeNe)
h.-n. laser
helix, *pl.* **helixes,** *pl.* **helices**
H. camera
h. filter
helixes (*pl. of* helix)
helmet
collimator h.
h. field

Helmholtz
H. axis ligament
H. coil
H. configuration
helminth
helminthic infestation
helminthoma
heloma
h. durum
h. molle
hemal
h. arch
h. canal
h. node
hemangioblastoma
capillary h.
cerebellar h.
cerebelloretinal h.
craniospinal h.
cystic h.
3rd ventricular h.
retinal h.
spinal capillary h.
hemangioblastomatosis
cerebelloretinal h.
hemangioendothelial
h. bone sarcoma
h. liver sarcoma
hemangioendothelioma
capillary h.
epithelioid h.
infantile h.
kaposiform h. (KHE)
malignant h.
osseous h.
hemangioepithelioma
hemangiofibroma
hemangiolymphangioma
hemangioma
arteriovenous h.
bone capillary h.
brain calcification h.
capillary h.
cardiac h.
cavernous brain h.
choroidal h.
epidural cavernous h.
epithelioid h.
extraaxial cavernous h.
extramedullary h.
extremity h.
facial h.
giant cavernous h. (GCH)
giant hepatic cavernous h. (GHCH)
hepatic h.
infantile hepatic h.
intraarticular h.
intramuscular h.
liver capillary h.

lung h.
orbital capillary h.
osseous h.
pediatric h.
pulmonary sclerosing h.
sclerosing h.
small bowel h.
soft tissue h.
splenic h.
subcutaneous h.
subglottic h.
synovial h.
trigeminal h.
umbilical cord h.
urinary bladder h.
vascular h.
venous h.
verrucous h.
vertebral h.
hemangiomatosis
pulmonary capillary h.
hemangiopericytoma
meningeal h.
primary pulmonary h.
renal h.
hemangiosarcoma
liver h.
hemarthrosis
hemathorax (*var. of* hemothorax)
hematobilia
hematocele
scrotal h.
hematochezia
hematocolpos
hematocrit effect
hematocystic spot (HCS)
hematogenous
h. dissemination
h. embolus
h. metastasis
h. osteomalacia
h. route
h. spread
h. tuberculosis
hematologic parameter
hematoma
acute intramural h.
acute subdural h.
adrenal h.
aneurysmal h.
aortic intramural h.
axillary h.
balancing subdural h.
basal ganglion h.
bladder flap h.
bowel wall h.
brain h.
breast h.
carotid plaque h.

chronic expanding h.
chronic subdural h. (CSDH)
corpus luteum h.
delayed traumatic intracerebral h.
  (DTICH)
dissecting aortic h.
dissecting intramural h.
duodenal h.
dural h.
encapsulated subdural h.
epidural h.
evolving h.
extracerebral h.
extradural brain h.
h. formation
gelatinous h.
hemispheric h.
infected pelvic h.
interhemispheric subdural h.
intermuscular h.
interstitial loculated h.
intracerebral h.
intracranial h.
intramural h. (IMH)
intraparenchymal h.
intrarenal h.
intraventricular h.
isodense subdural h.
mediastinal h.
mural h.
nasal septum h.
nasopharyngeal h.
organized h.
parenchymatous h.
perianal h.
periaortic mediastinal h.
pericardial h.
peridiaphragmatic h.
perigraft h.
perinephric h.
perirenal h.
posterior fossa h.
postoperative breast h.
primary intracerebral h.
rectal sheath h.
rectus muscle h.
retromembranous h.
retroperitoneal h.
retropharyngeal h.
retroplacental h.
scalp h.
small bowel h.
spontaneous h.
subacute subdural h.
subcapsular renal h.
subchorionic h.
subdural h.
subdural interhemispheric h.
subfascial h.

H

hematoma (*continued*)
    subgaleal h.
    submembranous placental h.
    subperiosteal h.
    umbilical cord h.
hematometra, hemometra
hematometrocolpos
hematomyelia
hematopoiesis (*var. of* hemopoiesis)
hematopoietic (*var. of* hemopoietic)
hematoporphyrin derivative (HpD)
hematosalpinx, hemosalpinx
hematoxylin and eosin stain
hematoxylin-eosin stain
hematuria
    painless h.
hemiagenesis
hemianopia
    homonymous h.
hemianopsia
    altitudinal h.
hemiarch
hemiatrophy
    cerebral h.
hemiaxial view
hemiazygos vein
hemiballism (*var. of* hemiballismus)
hemiballismus, hemiballism
hemiballismus-hemichorea (HBHC)
    hyperglycemia-induced h.-h.
hemiblock
    left anterior h.
    left anterosuperior h. (LASH)
    left bundle-branch h.
hemibody
    h. irradiation (HBI)
    h. radiotherapy
hemicardium
hemic calculus
hemicolon
hemicondylar fracture
hemicord
hemicranium
hemidecortication
    cerebral h.
hemidesmosome
hemidiaphragm
    accessory h.
    h. attenuation
    h. depression
    h. rupture
    tenting of h.
hemidiaphragmatic paralysis
hemifacial
    h. microsomia
    h. spasm
hemihypertrophy
hemimegalencephaly
    ipsilateral h.

hemimelia
    bilateral dysplasia epiphysialis h.
    dysplasia epiphysialis h.
hemimyelocele
hemiparkinsonism
hemipelvis
hemiplegia
    congenital h.
    infantile h.
    spinal h.
hemiscrotum
hemisection
    spinal cord h.
hemisensory syndrome
hemisphere
    h. atrophy
    cerebellar h.
    cerebral h.
    h. damage
    dominant h.
    left h.
    h. lesion
    mesial h.
    right h.
    h. stroke
    swollen brain h.
hemispheric
    h. demyelinating lesion
    h. hematoma
    h. infarct
    h. mass effect
    h. regional lateralization
    difference
    h. vein
hemithorax
    frozen h.
    h. opacification
hemitransverse fracture
hemitruncus
hemivertebra, *pl.* **hemivertebrae**
    balanced h.
    unbalanced h.
hemivertebrae (*pl. of* hemivertebra)
hemivertebral
hemizygosity
Hemobahn
    H. endoprosthesis
    H. PTFE-covered stent-graft
    H. stent
hemochromatosis
Hemochron
HemoCue photometer
hemodialysis catheter
hemodialysis-related venous stenosis
hemodynamic
    h. alteration
    h. assessment
    h. decompensation
    h. effect

h. format
h. impotence
h. index
h. pattern
h. penumbra
h. reserve impairment
h. response

hemodynamically
  h. relevant stenosis
  h. significant lesion
  h. significant stenosis
  h. weighted echo-planar MR
    imaging

hemoglobin
  sickle h.

hemolymph node

hemolytic
  h. autoimmune anemia
  h. splenomegaly
  h. uremic syndrome

hemomediastinum

hemometra (*var. of* hematometra)

hemoperfusion

hemopericardium

hemoperitoneum

hemophagocytic lymphohistiocytosis
  (HLH)

hemophilic pseudotumor

hemopneumothorax, pneumohemothorax

hemopoiesis, hematopoiesis
  extramedullary h.

hemopoietic, hematopoietic
  h. bone marrow
  h. reticulum
  h. stem cell transplant

hemopoietically active bone marrow

hemoptysis, haemoptysis

hemorrhage, haemorrhage
  abdominal h.
  acute idiopathic h. (AIPII)
  acute subarachnoid h.
  adrenal h.
  alveolar h.
  anastomotic h.
  aneurysmal h.
  antepartum h.
  arterial h.
  8-ball h.
  basilar intracerebral h.
  bladder h.
  brainstem h.
  brain stenosis h.
  bulbar intracerebral h.
  capillary h.
  carotid h.
  catheter-induced artery h.
  cerebellar h.
  cerebral h.
  cerebromeningeal intracerebral h.

choroid plexus h.
chronic parenchymal h.
colonic diverticular h.
colorectal h.
concealed h.
h. consolidation
cortical intracerebral h.
delayed traumatic intracerebral h.
diffuse pulmonary h. (DPH)
diffuse pulmonary alveolar h.
diffuse subarachnoid h.
drug-associated h.
Duret h.
epidural h.
exsanguinating h.
external h.
extradural h.
extraluminal h.
extramural h.
extrapleural h.
Fisher subarachnoid h. (grade 1–4)
focal area of h.
focal endocardial h.
focal pulmonary h.
frank h.
gastric h.
gastrointestinal renal transplant h.
germinal matrix-intraventricular h.
hypertensive brain h.
hypothalamic h.
idiopathic pulmonary h.
infant gastrointestinal h.
interhemispheric extraaxial h.
internal capsule intracerebral h.
interstitial h.
intertrabecular h.
intraabdominal arterial h.
intracerebral h. (ICH)
intracranial subarachnoid h.
intradural h.
intraluminal h.
intramural arterial h.
intramural gastrointestinal tract h.
intraparenchymal h.
intraplaque h. (IPH)
intrapleural h.
intrapontine intracerebral h.
intrapulmonary h.
intrathecal h.
intratumoral h.
intraventricular h. (IVH)
intraventricular neonate h.
labyrinthine h.
life-threatening h.
lobar intracerebral h.
lower gastrointestinal h.
lung h.
massive exsanguinating h.
mediastinal h.

H

hemorrhage (*continued*)
    meningeal h.
    multifocal h.
    neonatal choroid plexus h.
    neonatal intracerebellar h.
    neonatal intracranial h.
    neonatal intraventricular h.
    neonatal subdural h.
    nonaneurysmal perimesencephalic
      subarachnoid h.
    nondominant putaminal h.
    nontraumatic epidural h.
    nontumoral h.
    obstetric h.
    old h.
    ovarian h.
    pancreatic h.
    parenchymatous h.
    periaqueductal h.
    peribronchial h.
    perigestational h.
    perimesencephalic nonaneurysmal
      subarachnoid h.
    perinephric space h.
    perirenal h.
    placental h.
    plaque h.
    pontile h.
    postoperative mediastinal h.
    posttraumatic h.
    preplacental h.
    pulmonary h.
    pulmonary artery h.
    putaminal h.
    retrobulbar h.
    retroperitoneal h.
    retropharyngeal h.
    retroplacental h.
    salmon-patch h.
    sentinel transoral h.
    slit h.
    small bowel h.
    spinal epidural h. (SEH)
    spinal subarachnoid h.
    spinal subdural h. (SSH)
    spontaneous renal h.
    striate h.
    1st-trimester h.
    subacute h.
    subarachnoid h. (SAH)
    subchorionic h.
    subcortical intracerebral h.
    subdural h. (SDH)
    subependymal h.
    subgaleal h.
    submassive h.
    submucosal h.
    subperiosteal h.
    subserosal h.

    thalamic h.
    traumatic meningeal h.
    tumoral h.
    upper gastrointestinal h.
    variceal h.
    venous h.
    ventricular intracerebral h.
    vitreous h.
hemorrhagic
    h. brain infarct
    h. bronchopneumonia
    h. consolidation of lung
    h. corpus luteum cyst
    h. cystitis
    h. duodenitis
    h. focus
    h. hereditary telangiectasia
    h. lesion
    h. leukemia
    h. liver laceration
    h. lung nodule
    h. mediastinal
      adenopathy
    h. metastasis
    h. necrosis
    h. neoplasm
    h. ovarian cyst
    h. pericarditis
    h. pleural effusion
    h. pleurisy
    h. pneumonia
    h. pulmonary edema
    h. salpingitis
    h. stroke
    h. transformation
hemorrhagicum
    corpus h.
hemorrhoidal plexus
hemosalpinx (*var. of* hematosalpinx)
hemosiderin deposit
hemosiderosis
    idiopathic pulmonary h.
    pituitary h.
    pulmonary h.
hemostatic puncture closure device
hemosuccus pancreaticus
hemothoraces (*pl. of* hemothorax)
hemothorax, hemathorax, *pl.*
  hemothoraces
hemp seed calculus
He-MRI
    helium magnetic resonance imaging
    dynamic ventilation He-MRI
Henderson fracture
Henderson-Jones
  chondromatosis
HeNe
    helium-neon
    HeNe laser

Henke
    H. triangle
    H. trigone
Henle
    H. canal
    jejunal loop interposition of H.
    H. ligament
    loop of H.
    H. sheath
    trapezoid bone of H.
Hennekam syndrome
Henoch-Schönlein syndrome
Henry
    master knot of H.
    vertebral artery of H.
Henschke
    H. afterloader
    H. seed applicator
Hensen
    H. canal
    H. node
    H. plane
Hensing
    H. fold
    H. ligament
hen worker's lung
heparin
    low molecular weight h. (LMWH)
hepar lobatum
hepatectomy
    segmental h.
hepatic
    h. abscess
    h. adenoma
    h. anaplastic sarcoma
    h. angiomyolipoma
    h. angiosarcoma
    h. angle
    h. architecture
    h. arterial anastomosis
    h. arterial angiography
    h. arterial infusion (HAI)
    h. arterial perfusion
    h. arterial phase
    h. arteriography
    h. arterioportal shunting
    h. arteriovenous fistula
    h. artery
    h. artery anatomy
    h. artery aneurysm
    h. artery perfusion scintigraphy
      (HAPS)
    h. artery-portal vein fistula
    h. artery pseudoaneurysm
    h. artery stenosis
    h. artery system
    h. artery thrombosis
    h. bed
    h. bleeding

h. calcification
h. calculus
h. capsular rupture
h. capsule
h. carcinoma
h. chemoembolization
h. cirrhosis
h. congestion
h. cord
h. cyst
h. degeneration
h. diverticulum
h. duct
h. ductal system
h. duct bifurcation
h. echography
h. echo pattern
h. encephalopathy
h. failure
h. fibrosis
h. fissure
h. flexure
h. fungal infection
h. hemangioma
h. hilum
h. hydrothorax
h. insufficiency
h. ligament
h. lipoma
h. lobe
h. lymph node
h. metabolism
h. metastasis
h. necrosis
h. neoplasia
h. nerve plexus
h. non-Hodgkin lymphoma
h. outflow tract
h. parenchyma
h. pattern echo
h. resistive artery index
h. sarcoidosis
h. sclerosis
h. sinusoid
h. steatosis
h. stiffness
h. test of Glass
h. transplant
h. trauma
h. tumor
h. vein
h. vein disease
h. vein thrombosis
h. venography
h. venoocclusive disease
h. venous outflow
h. venous outflow obstruction
h. venous pressure gradient
h. venous system

H

hepatic (*continued*)
  h. web
  h. web dilation
  h. wedge pressure (HWP)
hepatica fibrosa
hepaticojejunostomy, hepatojejunostomy
  percutaneous h.
  Roux-en-Y h.
hepatis
  parenchymatous peliosis h.
  phlebectatic peliosis h.
  porta h.
  sagittal porta h.
hepatitis
  h. activity index
  acute h.
  chronic h.
  neonatal h.
  radiation h.
  recurrent pyogenic h.
hepatization
  lung h.
hepatobiliary
  h. carcinoma
  h. contrast agent
  h. disease
  h. ductal system imaging
  h. pathway
  h. scan
  h. scintigraphy
  h. tree
hepatoblastoma
hepatocarcinogenesis
hepatocarcinoma
  fibrolamellar h.
hepatocellular
  h. adenoma
  h. carcinoma (HCC)
  h. dysfunction
hepatocerebral
  h. degeneration
  h. disease
hepatocholescintigraphy
hepatoclavicular view
hepatocolic ligament
hepatocystocolic ligament
hepatocyte tracer uptake
hepatodiaphragmatic
  h. interposition
  h. interposition of colon
  (HDIC)
hepatoduodenal ligament
hepatoesophageal ligament
hepatofugal flow
hepatogastric ligament
hepatogastroduodenal ligament
hepatogram
  emission h.
hepatography

hepatoid adenocarcinoma
hepatoiminodiacetic
  h. acid (HIDA)
  h. acid scan
hepatojejunal anastomosis
hepatojejunostomy (*var. of*
  hepaticojejunostomy)
hepatojugular reflux
hepatolenticular degeneration
hepatolienography
Hepatolite
  H. imaging agent
  technetium 99m H.
hepatolithiasis
hepatoma
hepatomalacia
hepatomegalia (*var. of* hepatomegaly)
hepatomegaly, hepatomegalia
hepatonephric (*var. of* hepatorenal)
hepatopancreatic
  h. ampulla
  h. fold
hepatopancreatica
  ampulla h.
hepatopathy
hepatopetal flow
hepatophlebography
hepatophrenic ligament
hepatopleural fistula
hepatoportal
  h. biliary fistula
  h. sclerosis
hepatoportoenterostomy
hepatoptosis
hepatopulmonary
  h. shunt
  h. syndrome
hepatorenal, hepatonephric
  h. angle
  h. fossa
  h. ligament
  h. pouch
  h. recess
  h. saphenous vein bypass
  graft
  h. syndrome (HRS)
hepatoscan
hepatosplenic
hepatosplenography
hepatosplenomegaly (HSM)
hepatoumbilical ligament
herald
  h. bleed
  h. patch lesion
Herbert-Fisher fracture classification
Herbert scaphoid bone fracture
Hercules
  H. 7000 mobile x-ray unit
  H. power injector

hereditary
- h. amyloidosis
- h. clear cell renal carcinoma
- h. diffuse leukoencephalopathy
- h. flat adenoma syndrome
- h. hemorrhagic telangiectasia (HHT)
- h. nonpolyposis colorectal cancer (HNPCC)
- h. nonpolyposis colorectal carcinoma (HNPCC)
- h. papillary renal carcinoma
- h. predisposition
- h. right heart syndrome (HRHS)
- h. stenosis of aqueduct of Sylvius (HSAS)

Hering canal
Hermansky-Pudlak syndrome
hermaphrodism (*var. of* hermaphroditism)
hermaphroditism, hermaphrodism
- true h.

HERMES
heterogeneous reasoning and mediator system

Hermodsson
- H. fracture
- H. tangential projection

Herndon hump
hernia, *pl.* **hernias,** *pl.* **herniae**
- abdominal wall h.
- axial hiatal h.
- Barth h.
- Béclard h.
- bladder h.
- Bochdalek h.
- broad ligament h.
- h. canal
- cecal h.
- concentric h.
- congenital diaphragmatic h.
- h. defect
- diaphragmatic h.
- direct inguinal h.
- duodenal h.
- epigastric h.
- esophageal h.
- external h.
- femoral h.
- funicular inguinal h.
- gastric h.
- hiatal h.
- Holthouse h.
- incarcerated h.
- incisional h.
- incomplete h.
- indirect inguinal h.
- inguinal h.
- internal h.
- interstitial h.
- intrapericardial diaphragmatic h.

- Lesgaft h.
- lesser sac h.
- Littré h.
- lumbar h.
- mediastinal h.
- mixed h.
- Morgagni h.
- newborn h.
- obturator h.
- ovarian h.
- pantaloon h.
- paraduodenal h.
- paraesophageal hiatal h.
- parahiatal h.
- paraileostomal h.
- h. paralysis
- parastomal h.
- peritoneal h.
- peritoneopericardial diaphragmatic h.
- h. pouch
- properitoneal h.
- Richter h.
- Rieux h.
- rolling hiatal h.
- h. rupture
- h. sac
- scrotal h.
- short esophagus-type hiatal h.
- sliding hiatal h.
- spigelian h.
- strangulated bladder h.
- strangulated inguinal h.
- transient hiatal h.
- traumatic diaphragmatic h.
- Treitz h.
- tubular hiatal h.
- ultrasound-guided reduction of spigelian h.
- umbilical h.
- ventral h.

herniae (*pl. of* hernia)
hernial aneurysm
hernias (*pl. of* hernia)
herniated
- h. abdominal contents
- h. bowel
- h. bowel loop
- h. intervertebral disc (HID)
- h. nucleus pulposus (HNP)
- h. preperitoneal fat

herniation
- acute interosseous disc h.
- brain tissue h.
- central h.
- cerebral h.
- cervical disc h.
- cingulate h.
- cisternal h.
- concentric h.

H

herniation (*continued*)
    diencephalic h.
    disc h.
    fat lung h.
    focal disc h.
    focal nuclear h.
    foramen magnum h.
    frank disc h.
    free-fragment disc h.
    hard disc h.
    hippocampal h.
    impending h.
    inguinal bladder h.
    intercervical disc h.
    internal disc h.
    intradural disc h.
    intraspongy nuclear disc h.
    lateral disc h.
    lumbosacral intervertebral
     disc h.
    nuclear h.
    nucleus pulposus h.
    h. of brain
    phalangeal h.
    physiologic h.
    h. pit
    posterolateral disc h.
    soft disc h.
    subfalcine h.
    subligamentous disc h.
    supraligamentous disc h.
    temporal lobe h.
    tentorial notch h.
    thoracic disc h.
    tonsillar h.
    transtentorial h.
    uncal h.
herniography
heroin vapor leukoencephalopathy
herophili
    torcular h.
herpes
    h. esophagitis
    neonatal h.
    h. simplex virus (HSV)
    h. simplex virus 1 (HSV1)
    h. simplex virus 1 thymidine kinase
     (HSV1-tk, HSV-TK)
    h. simplex virus type 1
     encephalitis
    h. virus
herpesvirus (HV), herpes virus
    human h. (HHV)
    h. pneumonia
herpetic whitlow
herringbone pattern
Herring tube
hertz (Hz)
Herxheimer fiber

Heschl
    H. convolution
    H. transverse gyrus
Hesselbach
    H. ligament
    H. triangle
heterocladic anastomosis
heterocyclic
    h. aromatic amine
    h. free radical
heterodense soft tissue mass
heterogeneity
heterogeneous
    h. appearance
    h. breast mass
    h. carotid plaque
    h. color speckling
    h. hyperattenuation
    h. internal echo pattern
    h. isodense enhancement
    h. microdistribution
    h. perfusion pattern
    h. radiation
    h. reasoning and mediator system
     (HERMES)
    h. signal intensity
    h. uptake
heterophilic leukocyte
heterotaxia, heterotaxy, heterotaxis
    abdominal h.
    h. syndrome
    visceral h.
heterotaxis (*var. of* heterotaxia)
heterotaxy (*var. of* heterotaxia)
heterotopia
    band h.
    cerebellar h.
    gastric h.
    gray matter h.
    subependymal h.
heterotopic
    h. bone
    h. bone formation
    h. gray matter
    h. nodule
    h. pancreas
    h. pregnancy
    h. scar ossification
    h. white matter island
Heubner
    H. artery
    recurrent artery of H.
Hewlett-Packard (HP)
    H.-P. color-flow imager
    H.-P. phased-array ultrasound
     imaging system
    H.-P. scanner
    H.-P. ultrasound
Hexabrix imaging agent

hexadactylism (*var. of* hexadactyly)
hexadactyly, hexadactylism
hexafluoride
    sulfur h.
hexagonal configuration
hexametazime
**hexamethylpropyleneamine oxime
(HMPAO)**
hexokinase reaction
Hey
    H. amputation
    H. ligament
HF
    high-frequency
    HF infrared laser
HFA
    hydrofluoroalkane
    ^{18}F-labeled HFA
HFD
    high-frequency Doppler
HFI
    half-Fourier imaging
H-graft
    Gallie H-g.
H/G recombinant
HGSIL
    high-grade squamous intraepithelial
    lesion
HHFAST
    handheld focused assessment with
    sonography for trauma
HHT
    hereditary hemorrhagic
    telangiectasia
HHV
    human herpesvirus
HIA
    hallux interphalangeus angle
5-HIAA
    5-hydroxyindoleacetic acid
hiatal hernia
hiatus, *pl.* **hiatus**
    adductor h.
    aortic h.
    crus h.
    diaphragmatic esophageal h.
    esophageal h.
    patulous h.
    popliteal h.
    h. semilunaris
**Hibbs metatarsocalcaneal
angle**
hibernating myocardium
hibernation
    myocardial h.
hibernoma
Hickey
    H. method
    H. position

Hickman
    H. line
    H. long-term catheter
    H. tunneled indwelling catheter
hickory-stick fracture
HID
    herniated intervertebral disc
HIDA
    hepatoiminodiacetic acid
    HIDA imaging
    HIDA scan
    TechneScan HIDA
hidebound small bowel fold
hierarchical
    h. information
    h. scanning pattern
Hieshima microcatheter
HIFU
    high-intensity focused ultrasound
high
    h. arch
    h. brachial artery catheterization
    h. cervical spinal cord lesion
    h. defect
    h. dose rate (HDR)
    h. dose-rate brachytherapy
    h. dose-rate intracavitary radiation
    therapy
    h. dose-rate remote afterloading
    h. endothelial venule
    h. field strength
    h. field-strength MR imaging
    h. field-strength scanner
    h. filling pressure
    h. Fowler position
    h. frame rate
    h. frame-rate run
    h. frequency
    h. frequency-induced thermotreatment
    h. heat-capacity x-ray tube
    h. hydrophilicity
    h. interstitial pressure
    h. jugular bulb (HJB)
    h. lateral wall myocardial infarct
    h. left main diagonal artery
    h. linear energy transfer radiation
    h. minute ventilation
    h. normal
    h. pitch
    h. pontile lesion
    h. pulse-repetition frequency Doppler
    h. pulse-repetition frequency Doppler
    echocardiography
    h. reflectivity
    h. right atrial electrogram
    h. right atrium (HRA)
    h. signal intensity
    h. signal intensity
    h. signal intensity ischemic change

H

high (*continued*)
    h. signal intensity yellow marrow
    h. signal intensity zone
    h. small bowel obstruction
    h. spatial resolution cine computed tomography (HSRCCT)
    h. spatial-resolution cine CT
    h. spatial resolution imaging
    h. spatial resolution mode
    h. speech pitch
    h. spin
    h. takeoff
    h. temporal resolution
    h. temporal resolution cine computed tomography (HTRCCT)
    h. temporal resolution mode
    h. tibial osteotomy
    h. torque
    h. velocity
    h. wedge pressure
high-altitude pulmonary edema (HAPE)
high-amplitude
    h.-a. echo
    h.-a. impulse
high-attenuation
    h.-a. blood
    h.-a. crescent
    h.-a. stone
high-caliber low-velocity handgun injury
high-concentration contrast medium (HCCM)
high-contrast film
high-definition
    h.-d. 3-dimensional analysis
    h.-d. imaging (HDI)
high-density
    h.-d. barium
    h.-d. barium imaging agent
    h.-d. lesion
    h.-d. linear array
    h.-d. object
    h.-d. rim
    h.-d. structure
high-dose
    h.-d. chemotherapy
    h.-d. film dosimeter
    h.-d. film dosimetry
    h.-d. radiotherapy
    h.-d. therapy
high-dose-rate
high-energy
    h.-e. bent-beam linear accelerator
    h.-e. image
    h.-e. imaging
    h.-e. laser
    h.-e. proton
    h.-e. trauma
higher stage disease

high-field
    h.-f. magnet
    h.-f. open MRI scanner
    h.-f. system
Highflex large stone retrieval basket
high-flow arteriovenous fistula
high-frequency (HF)
    h.-f. Doppler (HFD)
    h.-f. Doppler ultrasound
    h.-f. Doppler ultrasound imaging
    h.-f. miniature probe
    h.-f. therapeutic ultrasound
    h.-f. transducer
high-grade
    h.-g. AV block
    h.-g. glioma
    h.-g. infiltrative astrocytoma
    h.-g. malignancy
    h.-g. narrowing
    h.-g. obstruction
    h.-g. obstructive lesion
    h.-g. partial tear
    h.-g. proximal stenosis
    h.-g. signal intensity
    h.-g. squamous intraepithelial lesion (HGSIL)
    h.-g. surface osteosarcoma
    h.-g. tumor
high-gradient field strength
high-impedance circulation
high-intensity
    h.-i. exposure
    h.-i. focused ultrasound (HIFU)
    h.-i. lesion
    h.-i. transient signal (HITS)
    h.-i. zone (HIZ)
high-kV technique
highly
    h. active antiretroviral therapy (HAART)
    h. mobile echo
    h. reflective echo
    h. vascular tumor
high-lying patella
Highmore
    H. antrum
    antrum of H.
high-osmolar
    h.-o. contrast agent (HOCA)
    h.-o. contrast medium (HOCM)
high-output
    h.-o. heart failure
    h.-o. state
high-pass filter
high-performance
    h.-p. liquid chromatography
    h.-p. size-exclusion chromatography
high-permeability pulmonary edema
high-pitched signal

high-powered field
high-pressure
    h.-p. Blue Max balloon
    h.-p. liquid chromatography
    h.-p. mercury arc lamp
high-probability lesion
high-purity germanium (HPGe)
high-quality pitch
high-rate
    h.-r. detect interval
    h.-r. ventricular response
high-resolution
    h.-r. B-mode imaging
    h.-r. bone algorithm technique
    h.-r. collimator
    h.-r. computed tomography (HRCT)
    h.-r. coronal cut
    h.-r. CT imaging
    h.-r. CT mammography
    h.-r. 3DFT MR imaging
    h.-r. diffraction
    h.-r. 3D microcomputed tomography
    h.-r. 3D spoiled-GRASS image
    h.-r. fan-beam collimator
    h.-r. fluoroscopy
    h.-r. infrared (HRI)
    h.-r. infrared imaging
    h.-r. linear-array transducer
    low-energy h.-r. (LEHR)
    h.-r. low-speed radiography
    h.-r. magnetic resonance (HR-MR)
    h.-r. magnetic resonance lymphangiography (HR-MRL)
    h.-r. magnification
    medium-energy h.-r. (MEHR)
    h.-r. magnetic resonance imaging (HR-MRI)
    h.-r. multileaf collimator
    h.-r. multisweep (HRMS)
    h.-r. storage phosphor imaging
    h.-r. storage phosphor managing
    h.-r. susceptibility-weighted imaging
    h.-r. transverse view image
    h.-r. ultrasound
    h.-r. ultrasound scanning
    h.-r. volumetric sequence
high-riding
    h.-r. patella
    h.-r. 3rd ventricle
    h.-r. scapula
    h.-r. variant
high-risk primary breast cancer
high-sensitivity measurement
high-signal
    h.-s. abnormality
    h.-s. intratendinous collection of fluid

h.-s. lesion
h.-s. mass
high-speed
    h.-s. gradient coil
    h.-s. imaging
HighSpeed CT scanner
high-tech low-touch examination environment
high-temperature diffraction
high-velocity
    h.-v. flow
    h.-v. gunshot wound
    h.-v. jet
    h.-v. signal loss
high-voltage
    h.-v. generator
    h.-v. pulsed galvanic stimulation (HVPGS)
    h.-v. radiotherapy
    h.-v. roentgen therapy
    h.-v. stimulation (HVS)
    h.-v. transformer
high-volume extravasation
Hilal
    H. embolization apparatus
    H. microcoil
hilar
    h. adenopathy
    h. area
    h. artery
    h. cap
    h. cell tumor of ovary
    h. cholangiocarcinoma
    h. dance
    h. displacement
    h. extension
    h. gland
    h. haze
    h. height ratio
    h. kidney lip
    h. lipoma
    h. lymph node
    h. mass
    h. obstruction
    h. plate
    h. prominence
    h. reaction
    h. shadow
    h. sign
    h. structure
    h. tumor
    h. vessel
Hildreth sign
Hilgenreiner
    H. acetabular index
    H. epiphysial angle
    H. line
HiLight Advantage System CT scanner
Hillock arch

H

Hill-Sachs
> H.-S. defect (HSD)
> H.-S. deformity
> H.-S. dislocation
> H.-S. posterolateral compression
> fracture
> H.-S. shoulder lesion
> H.-S. sign

Hill sign

Hilton
> H. law
> H. muscle

hilum
> central fatty h.
> hepatic h.
> kidney h.
> lip of h.
> lung h.
> h. measurement
> h. of tendon
> pruned h.
> pulmonary h.
> renal h.
> splenic h.
> waterfall h.

Hinchey classification

hindbrain
> h. deformity
> h. dysgenesis
> h. malformation

hindfoot
> h. deformity
> h. instability
> h. joint complex
> h. valgus

hindgut
> h. duplication
> primitive h.

Hine-Duley phantom

hinged implant

hinge joint

hip
> h. bone
> h. bump
> congenital dislocation of h. (CDH)
> congenital dysplasia of h.
> developmental dysplasia of h.
> (DDH)
> h. disarticulation
> dislocated h.
> h. dislocation
> h. dysplasia
> external snapping h.
> h. flexion contracture
> h. fracture
> frogleg view of h.'s
> hanging h.
> h. hump
> h. joint capsule

> h. joint space
> h. muscle cross-section
> h. pinning
> h. pointer
> h. protrusion
> h. replacement
> snapping h.
> transient osteoporosis of h.
> transient synovitis of h.

Hippel-Lindau
> von H.-L.

Hipper twist-release coil

hippocampal
> h. atrophy
> h. fissure
> h. formation
> h. gyrus
> h. head, body, and tail
> h. herniation
> h. infarct
> h. magnetic resonance volumetry
> h. sclerosis
> h. sulcus
> h. volume

hippocampal-amygdaloid complex

hippocampi (*pl. of* hippocampus)

hippocampus, *pl.* **hippocampi**
> electronic atlas of h.

hippocratic finger

hippuran
> I h.
> h. imaging agent

hip-to-ankle view

Hirschberg sign

Hirschfeld canal

Hirschsprung-associated enterocolitis (HAEC)

Hirschsprung disease

His
> H. angle
> H. band
> H. bundle
> H. bundle electrogram (HBE)
> bundle of H.
> H. canal
> H. line
> H. spindle

HiSonic ultrasonic bone conduction hearing device

HiSpeed
> H. Advantage helical scanner
> H. Advantage System CT
> scanner

Hi-Star MRI system

histiocyte
> sinusoidal h.

histiocytic
> h. bone lymphoma
> h. bone tumor origin

h. brain lymphoma
h. chest lymphoma
histiocytoma
angiomatoid malignant fibrous h.
atypical benign fibrous h.
benign fibrous h.
fibrous h.
malignant fibroosseous h.
malignant fibrous h. (MFH)
myxoid malignant fibrous h.
primary pulmonary malignant
fibrous h.
scrotal h.
storiform-pleomorphic malignant
fibrous h.
histiocytosis
diffuse cerebral h.
Langerhans cell h. (LCH)
Langerhans lung cell h.
sinus h.
systemic non-Langerhans cell h.
h. X
Histoacryl embolic agent
histogenesis
histogram
average diffusivity h.
dose-surface h.
dose-volume h. (DVH)
h. equalization
gaussian dose-volume h.
gray-level h.
integrated optical density h.
multisectional dose-volume h.
volume h.
**histogram-based selective
deblurring**
histogram-derived metrics
histograph
Eppendorf pO$_2$ h.
histologic, histological
h. correlation
h. grade
histological (*var. of* histologic)
histology
bone h.
histolytica
Entamoeba h.
histomorphometric
h. image
h. measurement
histomorphometry
bone h.
plaque h.
histopathic hallmark
histopathologic
h. comparison
h. CT correlation
histopathology
ischemic h.

Histoplasma capsulatum
histoplasmoma
histoplasmosis
disseminated CNS h.
h. granuloma
lung h.
pulmonary h.
historadiography
history
problem-focused h.
Hitachi
H. AIRIS II MR system
H. Altaire Open MRI system
H. CT scanner
H. EUB-555 diagnostic ultrasound
system
H. 4-head system
H. MR scanner
H. Open MRI system scanner
H. rotating detector array
system
H. SPECT 2000H-40 camera
H. 0.3T unit scanner
H. ultrasound
hitchhiker's thumb
Hi-Torque
H.-T. Floppy guidewire
H.-T. Modified J-GW guidewire
H.-T. steerable guidewire
HITS
high-intensity transient signal
HIV
human immunodeficiency virus
HIV esophagitis
HIV nephropathy
HIV nucleocapsid protein
HIV pneumonia
HIV pulmonary infection
HIV-associated
HIV-a. encephalitis
HIV-a. encephalopathy
HIV-inducing factor
HIV-related TB
HIZ
high-intensity zone
HJB
high jugular bulb
HL
half-life
HLA
human leukocyte antigen
HLA imaging
HLA-A3 histocompatibility antigen
HLA-B7 histocompatibility antigen
HLA-B14 histocompatibility antigen
HLH
hemophagocytic lymphohistiocytosis
HLHS
hypoplastic left heart syndrome

H

433

HLR
  heart-lung ratio
  heart-to-lung ratio
H/M
  heart count-mediastinum count ratio
HMD
  hyaline membrane disease
HMDP
  hydroxymethylene diphosphonate
H-mode echocardiography
HMPAO
  hexamethylpropyleneamine oxime
  ^{99m}Tc HMPAO
HNP
  herniated nucleus pulposus
HNPCC
  hereditary nonpolyposis colorectal
    cancer
  hereditary nonpolyposis colorectal
    carcinoma
Hobb sternoclavicular joint view
hobnail liver
HOC
  hypertrophic obstructive cardiomyopathy
HOCA
  high-osmolar contrast agent
hockey-stick
  h.-s. appearance of catheter tip
  h.-s. appearance of ureter
  h.-s. catheter
  h.-s. deformity of tricuspid valve
  h.-s. fracture
  h.-s. guiding sheath
  h.-s. tricuspid valve deformity
HOCM
  high-osmolar contrast medium
  hypertrophic obstructive
    cardiomyopathy
Hodge plane
Hodgkin
  H. disease
  H. granuloma
  H. lymphoma
  H. tumor
Hodgson
  H. aneurysmal dilation of aorta
  H. disease
Hodson-type kidney
Hoffa
  H. disease
  H. fat-pad
  H. fracture
Hoffman brain phantom
Hoffmann
  H. atrophy
  H. sign
Hofmeister
  H. anastomosis
  H. gastrectomy procedure

**Hohl tibial condylar fracture
  classification**
^{166}**Ho in vivo generator**
hold
  last image h. (LIH)
Holdaway ratio
holder
  limb h.
  Vogele-Bale-Hohner head h.
Holdsworth spinal fracture classification
holdup in flow of barium
hole
  black h.
  h. pattern
hole-within-hole
  h.-w.-h. appearance
  h.-w.-h. bone lesion
holiday heart syndrome
Holl ligament
hollow
  h. albumin microsphere
  h. bone
  h. chest
  h. foot
  h. organ
  h. ribbon
  h. structure
  h. viscus
  h. viscus injury
hollow-point bullet
holly leaf appearance
Holmes
  H. cortical cerebellar degeneration
  H. heart
  H. syndrome
  H. tremor
holmium
  h. 166
  h. imaging agent
  h. laser
holmium-YLF
  holmium-yttrium lithium fluoride
**holmium:yttrium-aluminum-garnet
  (Ho:YAG)**
  h.:y.-a.-g. laser
**holmium-yttrium lithium fluoride
  (holmium-YLF)**
holoacardius
holocord
  h. hydromyelia
  h. syringohydromyelia
Hologic
  H. 2000 densitometer
  H. QDR 1000W dual-energy x-ray
    absorptiometry scanner
  H. 2000 scanner
holography
  computerized tomographic h. (CTH)
  helical CT h.

h. imaging
medical h.
multiple-exposure volumetric h.
volumetric multiplexed transmission h.
Voxgram multiple-exposure h.

holoprosencephaly
alobar h.
congenital h.
h. lesion
lobar h.
microform of h.
semilobar h.

holosystolic
h. gradient
h. mitral valve prolapse

holoventricle
Holstein-Lewis fracture
Holthouse hernia
Holt-Oram syndrome
Holzknecht
H. space
H. unit

Holz phlegmon
home infusion care
homeostasis
brain h.

Homer
H. Mammalok needle
H. needle/wire localizer

Homerlok needle
homing
h. mechanism
h. molecule
stem cell h.

homogeneity
homogeneous
h. appearance
h. carotid plaque
h. echo
h. echogenic uterine contents
h. echo pattern
h. enhancement
genetically h.
h. intrasellar mass
h. lesion
h. MR pattern
h. opacity
h. perfusion
h. positive charge
h. radiation
h. signal intensity
h. soft tissue density
h. susceptibility distribution
h. thallium distribution

homogeneously
homograft
aortic root h.

homology mapping

homonuclear spin system
homonymous hemianopia
homophilic Purkinje cell
homospoil
homovanillic acid (HVA)
homunculus
Honda sign appearance
honeycomb
h. appearance
h. cyst
h. degeneration
h. formation
h. lung
h. pattern
h. vertebra

honeycombing
fibrotic h.
subpleural h.

hood
fibrous h.

hood-shaped ureter
hooked
h. acromion
h. bone
h. vertebra

hooklike osteophyte formation
hook of hamate fracture
hookwire
Hawkin h.
Kopans spring h.
metallic h.

hoop
h. strength
h. stress
h. stress fracture

hoop-shaped loop of bowel
Hoover sign
Hopkins
H. hook-guiding catheter
H. rod

Hopmann
H. papilloma
H. polyp

hop test
horizon
H. LX scanner
H. LX 1.5T superconducting magnet

horizontal
h. beam film
h. beam radiography
h. beam study
h. boundary
h. dipole configuration
h. fissure
h. fissure of lung
h. heart
h. lie
h. long axis

H

horizontal (*continued*)
    h. long-axis slice
    h. long-axis SPECT image
    h. maxillary fracture
    h. overframing
    h. plane
    h. plane loop
    h. position
    h. segment of middle cerebral
      artery
    h. striping
    h. toit externe (HTE)
    h. toit externe angle
hormesis
    radiation h.
hormone
    adrenocorticotropic h. (ACTH)
    gonadotropic h.
    mediobasal hypothalamus luteinizing
      hormone-releasing h.
    parathyroid h. (PTH)
    h. receptor-negative carcinoma
    recombinant human
      thyroid-stimulating h.
    syndrome of inappropriate
      antidiuretic h. (SIADH)
    thyroid-stimulating h. (TSH)
    thyrotropin-releasing h. (TRH)
hormone-resistant
    h.-r. prostate cancer
    h.-r. prostate carcinoma
horn
    Ammon h.
    anterior h.
    central h.
    dorsal spinal cord h.
    H. endootoprobe laser
    enlarged frontal h.
    frontal h.
    iliac h.
    lateral h.
    meniscal h.
    occipital h.
    h. of uterus
    posterior gray h.
    posterior spinal cord h.
    projectile h.
    spinal dorsal h.
    splaying of frontal h.
    temporal h.
    uterine h.
    ventral h.
    ventricular h.
Horner
    H. muscle
    H. sign
    H. syndrome
horseshoe
    h. abscess

    h. appearance
    h. configuration
    h. configuration of brain
    h. fibrosis
    h. fistula
    h. kidney
    h. lung
    h. osteophyte
    h. placenta
    h. shape
Horsley anastomosis
Horton disease
hose-pipe appearance of terminal ileum
hot
    h. area
    h. cathode x-ray tube
    h. caudate lobe
    h. defect
    h. focus
    h. laser
    h. lesion
    h. light
    h. nose sign
    h. pulmonary nodule
    h. quartz lamp
    h. spot
    h. spur sign
hot-cross
    h.-c. bun appearance
    h.-c. bun skull
hot-source heating
hot-spot
    h.-s. artifact
    h.-s. heart imaging
    h.-s. myocardial imaging
hot-tipped laser probe
Hough
    H. transform (HT)
    H. transform mapping
Hounsfield
    H. calcium density measurement
      unit
    H. number
    H. unit (HU)
4-hour delayed thallium imaging
hourglass
    h. appearance
    h. bladder
    h. chest
    h. configuration
    h. constriction
    h. constriction of gallbladder
    h. constriction of hip capsule
    h. deformity
    h. membrane
    h. pattern
    h. phalanx
    h. shape
    h. stenosis

h. stomach
h. tumor
h. ventricle
h. vertebra
hourglass-shaped lesion
House grading system
housemaid's knee
housing
x ray tube h.
Houston
H. Advanced Research
Center-Compression
(HARC-C)
H. muscle
valve of H.
Howell-Evans syndrome
Howship-Romberg sign
Howtek Scanmaster DX scanner
Ho:YAG
holmium:yttrium-aluminum-garnet
Ho:YAG laser
Hoyeraal-Hreidarsson syndrome
HP
Hewlett-Packard
hypoparathyroidism
Profasi HP
ScleroPLUS HP
HP Sonos 5500 ultrasound
echocardiography system
HP Sonos 5500 ultrasound imaging
system
HPA
hypothalamic-pituitary-adrenal
HpD
hematoporphyrin derivative
HpD photosensitizing agent
HPGe
high-purity germanium
HPGe detector
**H2-150 positron emission
tomography**
HPS
hypertrophic pyloric stenosis
HPV
human papillomavirus
HPV16-associated tumor
HPV18-associated tumor
H&R
hysterectomy and radiation
HRA
high right atrium
HRARE
hybrid rapid acquisition with relaxation
enhancement
HRCT
high-resolution computed tomography
cystic airspace HRCT
inhomogeneous lung attenuation
HRCT

interstitial nodule HRCT
noncontiguous expiratory HRCT
volumetric expiratory HRCT
HRHS
hereditary right heart syndrome
hypoplastic right heart syndrome
HRI
high-resolution infrared
HRI imaging
HR-MR
high-resolution magnetic resonance
sagittal HR-MR
HR-MRI
high-resolution magnetic resonance
imaging
HR-MRL
high-resolution magnetic resonance
lymphangiography
HRMS
high-resolution multisweep
HRS
hepatorenal syndrome
HRT-II
Heidelberg retina tomograph (II)
IIS
half-scan
HSA, HuSA
human serum albumin
^{99m}Tc HSA
HSAS
hereditary stenosis of aqueduct of
Sylvius
H2 Score office-based diagnostic device
HSD
Hill-Sachs defect
H/S Elliptosphere balloon catheter
HSG
hysterosalpingogram
hysterosalpingography
hysterosonography
HSG catheter
H-shaped
H-s. vertebra
H-s. vertebral body
HSM
hepatosplenomegaly
HSRCCT
high spatial resolution cine computed
tomography
HSSG
hysterosalpingosonography
HSV
herpes simplex virus
HSV1
herpes simplex virus 1
HSV1 encephalitis
HSV-TK, HSV1-tk
herpes simplex virus 1 thymidine
kinase

H

HT
    Hough transform
    hypothyroidism
HTE
    horizontal toit externe
    HTE angle
HTRCCT
    high temporal resolution cine
    computed tomography
H-type tracheoesophageal fistula
HU
    Hounsfield unit
Huckman number
Hudson attachment
Hueck ligament
Hughes-Stovin syndrome
Hughston
    H. Clinic injury classification
    H. patella view
Huguier canal
Huisman percutaneous drainage set
Huldshinsky radiation
Hulten variance
human
    h. albumin microsphere
    h. androgen receptor gene
    h. antimouse antibody (HAMA)
    h. aortic smooth muscle cell
    h. blood index (HBI)
    h. herpesvirus (HHV)
    h. immunodeficiency virus (type 1,
    2) (HIV)
    h. immunodeficiency virus-associated
    non-Hodgkin lymphoma
    h. leukocyte antigen (HLA)
    h. macrophage-monocyte chemotactic
    and activating factor
    h. mammary tumor virus
    h. milk fat globule
    h. papillomavirus (HPV)
    h. serum albumin (HSA, HuSA)
    h. serum albumin imaging agent
    h. T-cell leukemia virus
    h. thrombin
    h. visual sensitivity weighting
humanized anti-human IL-2 receptor
  antibody
HumaSPECT imaging agent
humeral
    h. avulsion of glenohumeral
    ligament (HAGL)
    h. bone
    h. capitellum
    h. circumflex
    h. condylar fracture
    h. epicondyle
    h. epiphysis
    h. head-splitting fracture
    h. length

    h. line
    h. mechanism
    h. metaphysis
    h. physial fracture
    h. ridge
    h. supracondylar fracture
humeri (*pl.* and *gen. of* humerus)
humeroradial articulation
humeroulnar articulation
humerus, *pl.* **humeri,** *gen.* **humeri**
    capitulum humeri
    epicondylar fracture of h.
    head of h.
    pseudocyst of h.
    pseudodislocation of h.
    surgical neck of h.
humidifier lung
hump
    buffalo h.
    diaphragmatic h.
    dowager's h.
    dromedary h.
    Hampton h.
    Herndon h.
    hip h.
    Kumpe h.
humpback deformity
Humphry ligament
hunchback
    Kokopelli h.
hunger
    air h.
Hunner ulcer
hunt
    H. and Hess aneurysm (grade I-V)
    H. and Hess aneurysm grading
    system
    H. and Hess subarachnoid
    hemorrhage scale
    H. and Kosnik aneurysm (grade
    O-V)
hunter
    H. and Driffield (H and D)
    H. and Driffield curve
    H. aneurysm ligation
    H. canal
    H. disease
    H. ligament
    H. syndrome
hunterian ligation of aneurysm
Hunter-Schreger band
Hunter-Sessions
Huntington
    H. chorea
    H. disease
Hunt-Kosnik
    H.-K. classification
    H.-K. classification of aneurysm
    (grade 0–4)

Huppert disease
Hurler-Scheie syndrome
Hurler syndrome
Hurst phenomenon
Hurter
Hürthle cell adenoma
HuSA, HSA
    human serum albumin
Huschke
    H. canal
    H. foramen
    H. ligament
Hutch diverticulum
Hutchinson
    H. fracture
    H. plaque
    H. syndrome
    H. teeth
Hutchinson-Gilford syndrome
Hutchinson-type neuroblastoma
Hutinel-Pick syndrome
Hutson loop
Huygens
    H. eyepiece
    H. principle
HV
    hallux valgus
    herpesvirus
HVA
    hallux valgus angle
    homovanillic acid
HVL
    half-value layer
HVPGS
    high-voltage pulsed galvanic
      stimulation
HVS
    high-voltage stimulation
HWP
    hepatic wedge pressure
hyaline
    h. arteriosclerosis
    h. articular cartilage
    h. cartilage endplate
    h. cartilage plate
    h. degeneration
    h. membrane disease (HMD)
    h. necrosis
hyalinized
    h. breast fibroadenoma
    h. fibroadenoma with fibrosis
    h. fibrocollagenous tissue
hyalinizing granuloma
hyalocapsular ligament
hyaloid
    h. artery
    h. canal
    h. canal of Cloquet
    h. fossa

hyaloserositis pleura
Hyams grading of esthesioneuroblastoma
   classification
hybrid
    h. approach
    h. detector configuration
    h. imaging
    h. magnet
    h. MRI imaging agent
    h. PET/SPECT camera
    h. probe
    h. rapid acquisition with relaxation
      enhancement (HRARE)
    h. SPECT/CT system
    h. subtraction technique
hybridization
    comparative genomic h.
    fluorescence in situ h.
     (FISH)
    h. probe
hybridization-subtraction technique
hybrid-RARE imaging
hydatid
    alveolar h.
    h. disease
    h. heart cyst
    h. lung cyst
    h. mediastinum cyst
    Morgagni h.
    h. polyp
    h. pregnancy
    sessile h.
    Virchow h.
hydatidosis
    cardiac h.
    osseous h.
Hydradjust IV table
hydramnion (*var. of* hydramnios)
hydramnios, hydramnion
hydranencephaly
hydrated pyelogram
hydraulic
    h. chamber
    h. distention
hydraulics
    vascular h.
Hydra Vision Plus DR, ES, HP urologic
   imaging system
hydrazinonicotinyl-Tyr3-octreotide
   (HYNIC-TOC)
    technetium 99m h.-T.-o.
hydrocalycosis
hydrocalyx
hydrocarbon aspiration
hydrocele
    bilateral h.'s
    congenital h.
    idiopathic h.
    infantile h.

H

hydrocele (*continued*)
  primary h.
  secondary h.
hydrocephalic obstruction
hydrocephalocele
hydrocephalus, hydrocephaly
  acquired h.
  acute h.
  asymptomatic h.
  bilateral h.
  chronic communicating h.
  communicating h.
  compensated h.
  congenital h.
  corpus callosum hypoplasia,
    retardation, adducted thumbs,
    spastic paraparesis, and h.
    (CRASH)
  delayed h.
  extraventricular obstructive h.
  h. ex vacuo
  fulminant h.
  hyperdynamic h.
  idiopathic h.
  infantile h.
  intraventricular obstructive h.
  low-pressure h.
  mass-effect h.
  noncommunicating h.
  nonobstructive h.
  normal-pressure h.
  normotensive h.
  obstructive h.
  occult h.
  posthemorrhagic h.
  postinfectious h.
  posttraumatic h.
  primary h.
  progressive h.
  secondary h.
  shunted h.
  symptomatic obstructive h.
  unilateral h.
  unshunted h.
hydrocephaly (*var. of* hydrocephalus)
HydroCoil embolic system
hydrocolpocele, hydrocolpos
hydrocolpos (*var. of* hydrocolpocele)
hydrocortisone enema
hydro-CT
  helical hydro-CT
hydrodynamic
  h. potential of disc
  h. thrombectomy
    system
hydroencephalocele
hydroencephalomeningocele
hydrofluoroalkane (HFA)
hydrogel plug

hydrogen
  heavy h.
  h. peroxide enema
  h. peroxide-enhanced anal
    endosonography
  h. peroxide imaging agent
  h. proton imaging
  h. spin density
hydrogen-1, -2, -3 MR spectroscopy
hydrography
  MR h.
**Hydrolyser hydrodynamic thrombectomy
  catheter**
hydrolysis in vivo
hydrolyzed technetium
hydroma (*var. of* hygroma)
hydromer-coated microguidewire
hydrometra
hydrometrocolpos
hydro-MRI
hydromyelia
  holocord h.
hydromyoma
hydronephrosis
  acute h.
  chronic h.
  congenital h.
  focal h.
  in utero h.
hydronephrotic
  h. kidney
  h. sac
hydronephroureter
hydropericardium
hydroperitoneum, hydroperitonia
hydroperitonia (*var. of* hydroperitoneum)
hydrophilic
  h. coated guidewire
  h. coated guiding catheter
  h. contrast agent
  h. nonflocculating barium
  h. polymer-coated
hydrophilicity
  high h.
hydrophone
  needle h.
hydrophthalmos
hydropic
  h. change
  h. composition
  h. degeneration
  h. villus
hydropneumothorax, pneumohydrothorax
  loculated h.
hydrops
  h. canal
  endolymphatic h.
  fetal h.
  gallbladder h.

halo sign of h.
labyrinthine h.
nonimmune fetal h.
semicircular canal h.
transient gallbladder h.
h. tubae profluens
hydropyonephrosis
hydrosalpinx
Hydro-Sil coating
hydrosoluble contrast agent
hydrostatic
h. decompression
h. edema
h. pressure of blood
hydrosyringomyelia
hydrotherapy
hydrothorax
hepatic h.
refractory hepatic h.
hydroureter
hydroureteronephrosis
hydroxide
iron h.
hydroxyapatite, hydroxylapatite
air plasma spray h.
calcium h. (CaHA)
h. crystal
h. deposition disease (HADD)
h. implant
h. rheumatism
hydroxycitrate
gadolinium-159 h.
hydroxyethylidene-1,1-diphosphonic acid,
1-diphosphonic acid
5-hydroxyindoleacetic acid (5-HIAA)
hydroxylapatite (*var. of* hydroxyapatite)
hydroxymethylene diphosphonate (HMDP)
hygroma, hydroma
cystic h.
cystic neck h
cystic orbital h.
fetal cystic h.
pseudocystic h.
subdural h.
hymen
imperforate h.
HYNIC-TOC
hydrazinonicotinyl-Tyr3-octreotide
hyoepiglottic ligament
hyoglossus muscle
hyoid
h. arch
h. bar
h. bone
hyopharyngeal carcinoma
hyoscine butylbromide imaging agent
hypacusis, hypoacusis
Hypaque
H. enema

H. meglumine imaging agent
H. myelography
H. sodium imaging agent
H. swallow
Hypaque-Cysto imaging agent
Hypaque-76 imaging agent
Hypaque-M imaging agent
hyparterial bronchus
hyperabduction
h. maneuver
h. syndrome
hyperactive peristalsis
hyperacute
h. ischemic brain infarct
h. myocardial infarct
h. stroke
hyperaemia
hyperaesthesia (*var. of* hyperesthesia)
hyperalgesia, hyperalgia
hyperalgia (*var. of* hyperalgesia)
hyperattenuated
h. blood
h. intrasellar mass
hyperattenuation
heterogeneous h.
hyperbilirubinemia
conjugated h.
hypercalcemia
malignant h.
hypercalcemic supravalvular aortic
stenosis
hypercapitation
hypercellular reconverted bone marrow
hypercholesteremia (*var. of*
hypercholesterolemia)
hypercholesterinemia (*var. of*
hypercholesterolemia)
hypercholesterolemia, hypercholesteremia,
hypercholesterinemia
hypercinesia (*var. of* hyperkinesis)
hypercinesis (*var. of* hyperkinesis)
hyperconcentration of contrast medium
hypercortisolism
hypercycloidal tomography
hyperdense
h. brain lesion
h. mass
h. middle cerebral artery sign
h. neoplasm
h. sinus secretion
h. spleen
hyperdontia
hyperdynamic
h. abductor hallucis
h. AV fistula
h. heart
h. hydrocephalus
h. right ventricular impulse
h. 4th ventricle

H

hyperechogenicity
hyperechoic
  h. area
  h. breast mass
  h. focus
  h. region
  h. renal medulla
  h. renal nodule
  h. splenic spot
  h. structure with shadowing
  uniformly h.
hyperechoicity
hyperemia
  active h.
  arterial h.
  collateral h.
  diffuse h.
  fluxionary h.
  mucous membrane h.
  passive h.
  reactive h.
  reperfusion h.
  subchondral marrow h.
  venous h.
hyperemic flow
hypereosinophilic syndrome
hyperesthesia
hyperexpanded lobe
hyperexpansion
  compensatory lobe h.
hyperextensibility
  joint h.
hyperextension
  h. dislocation
  h. injury
  h. of neck
  h. teardrop fracture
hyperfine coupling
hyperfixation
  ^{99m}Tc HMPAO h.
hyperflexion
  spine h.
  h. teardrop fracture
hyperflexion-hyperextension cervical injury
hyperflexion-rotation injury
hyperfractionated
  h. accelerated radiation therapy (HART)
  h. radiation
  h. radiotherapy
  h. total body irradiation
hyperfractionation
  accelerated h.
hyperfunction
  adrenocortical h.
hyperfunctioning thyroid nodule
hypergastrinemia

hyperglycemia-induced hemiballismus-hemichorea
hyperglycinemia
hypergonadotropic hypogonadism
hyperhydration
hyperinflation
  bilateral lung h.
  congenital lobar h.
  dynamic pulmonary h.
  focal h.
  lobar h.
  pulmonary h.
hyperintense
  h. marrow space
  h. mass
  h. muscle
  h. periventricular brain lesion
  h. ring sign
  h. signal
hyperintensity
  cortical h.
  diffuse signal h.
  incidental punctate white matter h.
  localized h.
  multifocal area of h.
  muscle h.
  pulvinar h.
  punctate white matter h.
  sacral h.
  senescent periventricular h.
  white matter signal h.
Hyperion
  H. LTK laser
  H. LTK system
hyperkinesia (*var. of* hyperkinesis)
hyperkinesis, hyperkinesia, hypercinesis, hypercinesia
hyperkinetic
  h. heart
  h. segmental wall motion
  h. segmental wall motion abnormality
hyperlordosis
  functional h.
hyperlucency
  unilateral pulmonary h.
hyperlucent
  h. lung
  h. rib
hypermaturation
hypermetabolic
  h. activity focus
  h. adenopathy
  h. brown adipose tissue (HBAT)
  h. lesion
  h. nodule
  h. region
  h. tumor
hypermetabolism

hypermobile
> h. joint
> h. kidney
> h. 1st ray

hypermotility
hypermyelination
hypernephroid carcinoma
hypernephroma
hyperosmolar
hyperosmotic solution
hyperostosis
> ankylosing h.
> bony h.
> Caffey h.
> chronic infantile h.
> cortical h.
> diffuse idiopathic skeletal h. (DISH)
> h. frontalis interna
> generalized cortical h.
> idiopathic cortical h. (ICH)
> infantile cortical h.
> h. of Morgagni
> senile ankylosing h.
> skeletal h.
> skull h.
> sternoclavicular h.
> vertebral h.

HyperPACS teleradiology system
hyperparathyroidism
> brown tumor of h.
> persistent h.
> primary h.
> recurrent h.
> secondary h.
> tertiary h. (tHPT)

hyperperfusion
> h. abnormality of liver
> ictal h.
> mesial h.
> septal h.
> h. therapy

hyperperistalsis
hyperpermeability
> contrast medium-induced pulmonary vascular h.

hyperphenylalaninemia
hyperphosphatasia
> familial idiopathic h.

hyperplasia
> adaptive h.
> adenomatous h.
> adrenal h.
> adrenocortical h.
> alveolar epithelial h.
> angiofibroblastic h.
> angiofollicular lymph node h.
> angiolymphoid h.
> antral G-cell h.
> arachnoid h.

atypical ductal h.
atypical lobular h. (ALH)
atypical lobular breast h.
atypical regenerative h.
benign prostatic h. (BPH)
bone marrow lymphoid h.
breast h.
Brunner gland h.
compensatory h.
congenital adrenal h. (CAH)
congenital adrenocortical h.
cortical nodular h.
cystic endometrial h
cystic glandular h.
desquamated epithelial breast h.
diffuse pulmonary neuroendocrine cell h.
dual parathyroid gland h.
ductal epithelial h.
endometrial h.
epiphysial h.
epithelial h.
explosive follicular h.
fibrointimal h.
fibrous tissue h.
florid follicular h.
focal cortical h.
focal nodular h. (FNH)
follicular nodular h. (FNH)
gallium-avid thymic h.
generalized angiofollicular lymph node h.
generalized breast h.
giant follicular h.
GI tract lymphoid h.
idiopathic adrenocortical h.
intimal h.
intravascular papillary endothelial h.
lipoid adrenal h.
localized angiofollicular lymph node h.
lung lymphoid h.
lymphoid h.
lymphonodular h.
medial h.
mucosal h.
mucous cell h.
myeloid h.
myointimal h.
neointimal h.
neoplastic C-cell h.
nodular adrenal h.
nodular lymphoid h.
nodular regenerative h. (NRH)
paracortical h.
parathyroid h.
physiologic h.
pituitary h.
plantar h.

H

443

hyperplasia (*continued*)
  polypoid lymphoid h.
  prostatic h.
  pseudoangiomatous stromal h.
   (PASH)
  pseudointimal h.
  pulmonary neuroendocrine cell h.
  reactive follicular h.
  reactive lymphoid h.
  sclerosing duct h.
  sinus h.
  smooth h.
  splenic h.
  subadventitial h.
  tenocyte h.
  thymic h.
  thyroid h.
  torus h.
  unicentric angiofollicular lymph
   node h.
hyperplastic
  h. adenomatous polyp
  h. bone
  h. cholecystosis
  h. colon polyp
  h. gastric polyp
  h. gastropathy
  h. inflammation
  h. lesion
  h. parathyroid gland
  h. stomach polyp
  h. synovium
  h. tissue
hyperpolarized
  h. ^{3}He imaging agent
  h. helium
  h. ^{129}Xe gas
  h. ^{129}Xe imaging agent
hyperpressure
hyperreactivity
  airway h. (AHR)
hyperreflexia
  detrusor h.
hyperreninemic hypertension
hyperrugosity
hypersecretion
  gastric h.
  mucous h.
hypersegmentation
  manubrium h.
hypersensitivity
  alveolar h.
  carotid sinus h.
  inflammatory h.
  h. lung
  h. pneumonia
  h. pneumonitis
  h. reaction
  tracheobronchial h.

hypersplenism
hyperstasis
  generalized cortical h.
hyperstereoroentgenography
hyperstimulation of ovary
hypertelorism
hypertension
  acute thromboembolic pulmonary
   arterial h.
  arterial h.
  benign intracranial h.
  chronic thromboembolic pulmonary
   h.
  exertional h.
  extrahepatic portal h.
  hyperreninemic h.
  hypoxic pulmonary h.
  idiopathic intracranial h.
  idiopathic noncirrhotic portal h.
  idiopathic portal h. (IPH)
  idiopathic pulmonary h.
  h. injury
  intracranial h.
  isolated systolic arterial h.
   (ISAH)
  obstructive pulmonary arterial
   h.
  persistent pulmonary h.
  portal h.
  precapillary lung h.
  primary pulmonary h. (PPH)
  pulmonary h.
  pulmonary arterial h. (PAH)
  pulmonary venous h. (PVH)
  refractory h.
  renal artery h.
  renal transplant h.
  renovascular h. (RVH)
  secondary intracranial h.
   (SIH)
  segmental portal h.
  sinistral portal h.
  suprahepatic h.
  systemic arterial h.
  systemic venous h.
  systolic h.
  venous h.
hypertensive
  h. arteriosclerosis
  h. brain hemorrhage
  h. cardiovascular disease
  h. contrast concentration
  h. diathesis
  h. encephalopathy
  h. ischemic ulcer
  h. left ventricular hypertrophy
  h. lower esophageal sphincter
  h. renal disease
  h. stroke

h. vascular degeneration
h. vascular disease

hyperthermia
anular phased-array h.
interstitial h.
locoregional h.
malignant h.
microwave h.
h. probe
radiofrequency h.
radiotherapy with h.
radiotherapy without h.
volumetric interstitial h.

hyperthyroid heart
hyperthyroidism
Graves h.
neonatal h.

hypertonic
h. airway
h. enema
h. solution

hypertransradiancy
hypertrophia (*var. of* hypertrophy)
hypertrophic
h. asymmetry
h. bladder
h. cardiomyopathy (HCM)
h. cirrhosis
h. duct network
h. exostosis
h. gastritis
h. inflammation
h. infundibular subpulmonic
stenosis
h. lingual tonsil
h. marginal spurring
h. nonunion
h. obstructive cardiomyopathy (HOC, HOCM)
h. olivary degeneration
h. pulmonary osteoarthropathy
h. pyloric stenosis (HPS)
h. pyloric string-sign stenosis
h. pyloric target-sign stenosis
h. pylorus
h. subaortic stenosis
h. tissue

hypertrophicans
osteodermopathia h.

hypertrophied
h. heart
h. intima
h. myocardium
h. trigone

hypertrophy, hypertrophia
adaptive h.
adenoid h.
apical h.
asymmetric septal h. (ASH)

asymptomatic h.
benign prostatic h. (BPH)
biatrial h.
biventricular h.
bladder h.
bone h.
Brunner gland h.
cardiac h.
4-chamber h.
compensatory nodular kidney h.
complementary h.
concentric heart h.
contralateral h.
dilation and h.
eccentric left ventricular h.
epiphysial h.
facet h.
familial h.
focal pyloric h.
focal renal h.
functional h.
hypertensive left ventricular h.
interatrial septal h.
left atrial h.
left ventricular h. (LVH)
ligamentous-muscular h.
ligamentum flavum h.
lipomatous h.
muscular h.
myocardial cellular h.
olivary h.
panchamber h.
physiologic h.
prostatic h.
pyloric h.
right atrial h.
right ventricular h. (type A-C) (RVH)
Romhilt-Estes score for left ventricular h.
scalenus anticus muscle h.
septal h.
septate h.
smooth muscle h.
symmetric heart h.
trigeminal trigonal h.
trigonal h.
unilateral h.
ventricular h.
villous h.
Wigle scale for ventricular h.

hypervariable
h. region
h. sequence

hypervascular
h. arterialization
h. granulation tissue
h. hepatocellular carcinoma
h. liver metastasis

H

hypervascular (*continued*)
    h. mediastinal mass
    h. pancreatic tumor
hypervascularity
hypervolemia of pregnancy
hypervolemic pulmonary edema
hypesthesia, hypoesthesia
hypha, *pl.* **hyphae**
    fungous h.
hyphae (*pl. of* hypha)
hypoacusis (*var. of* hypacusis)
hypoaeration
hypoattenuating
    h. lesion
    h. mass
hypoattenuation
hypocellular marrow
hypochordal arch
hypocinesia (*var. of* hypokinesis)
hypocinesis (*var. of* hypokinesis)
hypocycloidal tomography
hypodense
    h. area
    h. basal ganglion brain lesion
    h. mass
    h. mesencephalic low-density brain
      lesion
hypodensity
    periventricular h.
    white matter h.
hypodiploid tumor
hypodiploidy
hypodontia
hypoechogenic
    h. retroplacental myometrial
      zone
    h. tumor
hypoechogenicity
    false h.
hypoechoic
    h. area
    h. area of ultrasound
    h. band
    h. fluid collection
    h. halo
    h. layer
    h. liver
    h. mantle
    h. plaque
    h. renal sinus
    h. rim
    h. solid tumor
    h. structure
    h. testis
    h. tissue
    h. zone
hypoenhanced
    h. area
    h. tissue

hypoesthesia (*var. of* hypesthesia)
hypofractionated
    h. radiation
    h. radiation therapy
hypofrontality
hypogammaglobulinemia
hypoganglionosis of colon
hypogastric
    h. artery
    h. plexus
hypogastrium
hypogenetic
    h. lung
    h. lung syndrome
hypoglossal, hypoglossus
    h. canal
    h. fossa
    h. nerve
    h. trigone
hypoglossus (*var. of*
  hypoglossal)
hypogonadism
    hypergonadotropic h.
    hypogonadotropic h.
hypogonadotropic hypogonadism
hypohidrosis
hypoinflation of lung
hypointense
    h. fibrous capsule
    h. marrow signal
    h. nodule
    h. sella lesion
    h. signal inhomogeneity
    h. signal shadowing
hypointensity
    cortical h.
hypokinesia (*var. of* hypokinesis)
hypokinesis, hypokinesia, hypocinesis,
  hypocinesia
    apical h.
    cardiac h.
    diffuse ventricular h.
    global h.
    inferior wall h.
    h. of heart
    h. on echocardiography
    regional h.
    septal h.
    wall h.
hypokinetic
    h. left ventricle
    h. myocardium
    h. segment
    h. segmental wall motion
    h. segmental wall motion
      abnormality
hypolordosis
hypolucency of lung
hypometabolic area

hypometabolism
  bilateral superior
    parietal h.
  biparietotemporal h.
  focal area of h.
  global h.
  lesion h.
  occipital h.
hypomineralization
  fetal h.
hypoparathyroidism (HP)
  idiopathic h.
  secondary h.
hypoperfused state
hypoperfusion
  acute alveolar h.
  apical h.
  cerebellar h.
  cerebral h.
  h. complex
  frontal h.
  global cerebral h.
  peripheral h.
  pulmonary h.
  resting regional myocardial h.
  septal h.
  systemic h.
hypoperistalsis
hypopharyngeal
  h. carcinoma
  h. diverticulum
  h. tumor
hypopharynx
hypophosphatemic osteomalacia
hypophyseal (*var. of* hypophysial)
hypophysial, hypophyseal
  h. fossa
  h. pouch
  h. Rathke duct
hypophysis
  h. cerebri
  infundibulum of h.
hypophysitis
  lymphocytic h.
  lymphoid h.
hypopituitarism
  hypothalamic h.
hypoplasia
  anular h.
  aortic tract complex h.
  ascending aorta h.
  basiocciput h.
  biliary h.
  bone marrow h.
  cartilage-hair h.
  cerebellar h.
  cerebral white matter h.
  condylar skull h.
  congenital pulmonary h.

congenital renal h.
conus h.
endothelial h.
fetal lung h.
gallbladder h.
isolated cerebellar h.
left ventricular h.
lung h.
lymphatic h.
mandible h.
maxillary sinus h.
medullaris h.
occipital condyle h.
h. of dens
optic nerve h.
pontocerebellar h.
pulmonary h.
radius h.
seminal vesicle h.
sinus h.
skeletal h.
transverse h.
tubular aortic h.
uterine h.
vermian h.
vermian-cerebellar h.
vermis h.
hypoplastic
  h. aortic arch
  h. aortic syndrome
  h. disc interval
  h. emphysema
  h. heart ventricle
  h. horizontal rib
  h. left heart syndrome
    (HLHS)
  h. left parietal syndrome
  h. left ventricle
  h. lung
  h. penis
  h. right heart
  h. right heart syndrome
    (HRHS)
  h. right ventricle
  h. subpulmonic outflow
  h. thumb
  h. tricuspid orifice
  h. valve
hypopnea
  obstructive h.
hyposensitization
hyposmia
hyposplenism
hypostatic
  h. bronchopneumonia
  h. congestion
  h. pneumonia
  h. pulmonary insufficiency
hypotelorism

H

hypotension
  arterial h.
  cerebral h.
  spontaneous intracranial h.
    (SIH)
hypothalamic
  h. glioma
  h. hamartoma
  h. hemorrhage
  h. hypopituitarism
  h. hypothyroidism
  h. infundibulum
  h. lesion
  h. sulcus
hypothalamic-pituitary-adrenal (HPA)
  h.-p.-a. axis
hypothalamic-pituitary axis
hypothalamic-pituitary-gonadal axis
hypothalamohypophysial tract
hypothalamoneurohypophysial axis
hypothalamopituitary axis
hypothalamus
  anterior h.
  rostral h.
  h. tumor
hypothenar
  h. eminence
  h. hammer
  h. muscle group of hand
hypothermia
  scalp h.
hypothermic
  h. heart
  h. perfusion
hypothyroidism (HT)
  hypothalamic h.
  primary h.
  secondary h.
  tertiary h.
hypotonia, hypotonus
hypotonic
  h. bladder
  h. duodenography
  h. duodenography imaging
hypotonus (*var. of* hypotonia)
hypovascular zone
hypoventilation
hypovolemia
  cerebrospinal fluid h.
  h. trauma

hypovolemic
  h. complex
  h. shock
hypoxemia
  arterial h.
hypoxia
  ischemic h.
  relative h.
  tumor h.
hypoxia-ischemia
hypoxic
  h. brain damage
  h. injury
  h. ischemic encephalopathy
  h. pulmonary hypertension
  h. pulmonary vasoconstriction
hypoxic-ischemic insult
Hyrtl foramen
hysterectomy
  abdominal h.
  h. and radiation (H&R)
  h. and radiation therapy
  extrafascial h.
  supracervical h.
  Wertheim h.
hysteresis
Hysterocath hysterosalpingography device
hysterogram
hysterograph
hysterography
  conventional h.
  ultrasonic h.
hysterometry
hysteromyoma
hysterosalpingo-contrast sonography
hysterosalpingogram (HSG)
hysterosalpingography (HSG)
  h. catheter
  h. imaging
  ultrasonic h.
hysterosalpingosonography (HSSG)
hysteroscope
  Gynecare Versascope h.
hysteroscopy
hysterosonography (HSG)
  transvaginal h. (TVHS)
hysterotubogram
hysterotubography
Hz
  hertz

I
iodine
I hippuran
¹¹¹I, I-111
iodine 111
¹²³I, I-123
iodine 123
¹²³I BMIPP imaging
¹²³I brain imaging spectamine
¹²³I heptadecanoic acid
¹²³I isopropyl iodoamphetamine
¹²³I metaiodobenzylguanidine
¹²³I metaiodobenzylguanidine
scintigraphy
¹²⁵I, I-125
iodine 125
¹²⁵I fibrinogen scan
¹²⁵I interstitial radiation implant
¹²⁷I, I-127
iodine 127
¹³¹I, I-131
iodine 131
¹³¹I radioactive iodine
¹³¹I therapy
¹³²I, I-132
iodine 132
¹⁹²I, I-192
iodine 192
IABP
intraaortic balloon pump
IADSA
intraarterial digital subtraction
angiography
IAF
intraabdominal fat
IAR
instantaneous axis of rotation
IAS
interatrial septum
iatrogenic
i. avulsion
i. cardiomegaly
i. dural tear
i. esophageal perforation
i. iliocaval fistula
i. pseudoaneurysm
i. trauma
i. ureteral injury
iatrogenically induced artifact
IAVB
incomplete atrioventricular
block
IBC
inflammatory breast carcinoma

IBM
ideal body mass
IBM field-cycling research
relaxometer
IBM NMR spectrometer
**I-B1 radiolabeled antibody injection
radiation therapy**
ibritumomab
yttrium-90 i.
IBS
irritable bowel syndrome
IBTR
ipsilateral breast tumor recurrence
ICA
internal carotid artery
intracranial aneurysm
juxtasellar ICA
petrous ICA
supraclinoid ICA
ice
i. cream cone shape
i. skater's fracture
ICE
intracardiac echocardiography
iceberg
i. lesion
i. radiotherapy
ice-pick view
ICEUS
intracaval endovascular ultrasonography
intracaval endovascular ultrasound
ice-water swallow
ICG
iodocyanine green
ICH
idiopathic cortical hyperostosis
intracerebral hemorrhage
ichorous pleurisy
ICIS
integrated clinical information system
icon
Siemens I.
ICP
intracranial pressure
ICP-AES
inductively coupled plasma atomic
emission spectrometry
ICP-AES detection
IC-PC
internal carotid-posterior communicating
IC-PC artery
IC-PC artery aneurysm
ICR
intercostal retraction

ICRP
>International Commission on
>Radiological Protection

ICRT
>intracoronary radiation therapy

ICRU
>International Commission on Radiation
>Units
>>ICRU reference point

ICS
>improved Chen-Smith
>>ICS coder

ICSPF
>internal carotid systolic peak flow

ictal
>i. hyperperfusion
>i. ^{99m}Tc HMPAO brain SPECT
>i. PET scan
>i. phase study
>i. SPECT scan

ICUS
>intracoronary ultrasound

ICV
>internal cerebral vein
>intracerebroventricular
>>ICV reservoir

ICW
>intracranial width

IDA
>image display and analysis
>iminodiacetic acid
>>IDA scanning

IDC
>idiopathic dilated cardiomyopathy
>interlocking detachable coil
>intraductal carcinoma

IDD
>intraluminal duodenal diverticulum

ideal body mass (IBM)

identification
>particle i.
>peak i.
>phase i.
>topographic i.

IDET
>intradiscal electrothermal therapy

IDF
>inferior duodenal flexure

idiopathic
>i. adrenocortical hyperplasia
>i. amyloidosis
>i. avascular necrosis
>i. cortical hyperostosis (ICH)
>i. diffuse cerebellar dysplasia
>i. dilated cardiomyopathy (IDC)
>i. dilated pulmonary artery
>i. edema
>i. epilepsy
>i. epiphysiolysis

>i. fibrous mediastinitis
>i. fracture
>i. gastric perforation
>i. hydrocele
>i. hydrocephalus
>i. hypertrophic subaortic sclerosis
>(IHSS)
>i. hypertrophic subaortic stenosis
>i. hypoparathyroidism
>i. interstitial pneumonia (IIP)
>i. interstitial pneumonitis
>i. interstitial pulmonary fibrosis
>i. intestinal pseudoobstruction
>i. intracranial hypertension
>i. megacolon
>i. multicentric osteolysis
>i. mural endomyocardial disease
>i. myelofibrosis
>i. noncirrhotic portal hypertension
>i. obstruction
>i. osteonecrosis
>i. Parkinson disease (IPD)
>i. pleural calcification
>i. portal hypertension (IPH)
>i. pulmonary arteriosclerosis (IPA)
>i. pulmonary artery dilation
>i. pulmonary fibrosis (IPF)
>i. pulmonary hemorrhage
>i. pulmonary hemosiderosis
>i. pulmonary hypertension
>i. restrictive cardiomyopathy
>i. right atrial dilation
>i. scoliosis
>i. thrombocytopenic purpura (ITP)
>i. unilateral hyperlucent lung
>i. unilobar emphysema
>i. varicocele

idiosyncratic anaphylactoid reaction
idioventricular rhythm (IVR)
IDIS
>intraoperative digital subtraction
>>IDIS angiography system

IDK
>internal derangement of knee

IDP
>imidodiphosphonate

IDSA
>intraoperative digital subtraction
>angiography

IDSI
>internodular difference in signal
>intensity
>>IDSI scanner

IDXrad radiology information system
I/E
>inspiratory-to-expiratory ratio

IEC
>International Electrotechnical
>Commission

IES
  inferior esophageal sphincter
IFT
  inverse Fourier transform
IgG
  immunoglobulin G
  ^{111}In IgG
  indium-111-labeled IgG
Iglesias fiberoptic resectoscope
IGLLC
  inferior glenohumeral ligament-labral
  complex
IGRT
  image-guided radiation therapy
IHA
  intrahepatic atresia
IHF
  interhemispheric fissure
IHSA
  iodinated human serum albumin
IHSS
  idiopathic hypertrophic subaortic
  sclerosis
IIP
  idiopathic interstitial pneumonia
^{123}**I-IPPA**
  iodine-123 iodophenyl pentadecanoic
  acid
IJV
  internal jugular vein
I-labeled
  I-l. cholesterol
  I-l. macroaggregated albumin
  I-l. rose bengal
^{131}**I-labeled**
  ^{131}I-l. human MoAb
  ^{131}I-l. monoclonal Fab
^{123}**I-labeled Z-MIVE**
iLab ultrasound imaging system
ILBBB
  incomplete left bundle-branch
  block
ILD
  interstitial lung disease
ileal
  i. atresia
  i. conduit
  i. crypt
  i. inflow tract
  i. jejunization
  i. loop
  i. loopography
  i. motility
  i. neobladder
  i. obstruction
  i. pouch-anal anastomosis
  i. spill
  i. S pouch
  i. stenosis

ileitis
  backwash i.
  Crohn i.
  distal i.
  granulomatous i.
  obstructive dysfunctional i.
  prestomal i.
  reflux i.
  terminal i.
ileoanal pouch
ileocecal
  i. cystoplasty
  i. edema
  i. fat-pad
  i. fold
  i. insufficiency
  i. junction
  i. mass
  i. orifice
  i. pouch
  i. recess
  i. syndrome
  i. valve
  i. valve abnormality
ileococcygeus muscle
ileocolic, ileocolonic
  i. anastomosis
  i. artery
  i. disease
  i. fold
  i. intussusception
  i. lymph node
  i. plexus
  i. vein
  i. vessel
ileocolitis
  Crohn i.
ileocolonic (*var. of* ileocolic)
ileocolostomy
ileoentectropy
ileogram
ileoileal intussusception
ileorectal anastomosis (IRA)
ileosacral (IS)
ileosigmoid
  i. fistula
  i. knot
ileostogram
ileostomy
ileotransverse colon anastomosis
ileum
  antimesenteric border of distal i.
  cobblestone i.
  collapsed distal i.
  hose pipe appearance of
    terminal i.
  jejunization of i.
  neoterminal i.
  terminal i.

ileus
  adhesive i.
  adynamic i.
  adynamic/paralytic i.
  cecal i.
  chronic duodenal i.
  colonic i.
  dynamic i.
  functional i.
  gallbladder i.
  gallstone i.
  localized i.
  mechanical i.
  meconium i.
  nonobstructive i.
  occlusive i.
  paralytic i.
  postoperative i. (POI)
  reflex i.
  spastic i.
Ilfeld-Holder deformity
iliac
  i. apophysitis
  i. artery
  i. artery aneurysm
  i. artery stenosis
  i. artery stenting
  i. artery stent placement
  i. bifurcation
  i. canal
  i. cancellous bone
  i. circumflex lymph node
  i. colon
  i. crest
  i. dowel
  i. fascia
  i. fossa
  i. fossa abscess
  i. horn
  i. index
  i. insufficiency fracture
  i. lesion
  i. plaque
  i. PTA category (1–4)
  i. spine
  i. tubercle
  i. tuberosity
  i. vein
  i. vein compression syndrome
  i. vein obstruction
  i. venography
  i. vessel
  i. wing
iliac-renal bypass graft
iliacus
ilii
  osteitis condensans i.
iliocaval
  i. disease

  i. junction
  i. thrombus
  i. tree
iliocostal muscle
iliofemoral
  i. artery
  i. crossover bypass
  i. ligament
  i. thrombosis
  i. triangle
  i. vein
  i. venous stenosis
  i. wing fracture
ilioinguinal lymph node
ilioischial line
iliolumbar ligament
iliopectineal
  i. eminence
  i. ligament
  i. line
ilioprofunda bypass graft
iliopsoas
  i. abscess
  i. bursa
  i. bursitis
  i. compartment
  i. compartment enlargement
  i. impingement
  i. muscle
  i. muscle shadow
  i. sign
  i. tendon
iliopubic
  i. eminence
  i. ligament
iliotibial (IT)
  i. band
  i. band friction syndrome
  i. ligament
  i. tract
iliotrochanteric ligament
ilium
  flared i.
Ilizarov
  I. device
  I. ring
ill-defined
  i.-d. appearance
  i.-d. breast density
  i.-d. consolidation
  i.-d. margin
  i.-d. mass
  i.-d. multifocal lung
    density
illuminator
  Mammo Mask i.
ILUS
  intraluminal ultrasound
  ILUS catheter

IM
> intramedullary
>> IM joint
>> IM rod
>> IM rodding

IMA
> inferior mesenteric artery
> intermetatarsal angle
> internal mammary artery

image
> acetazolamide dual-isotope i.
> i. acquisition
> i. acquisition time
> Add-On Bucky radiographer detector i.
> i. aliasing
> alignment and registration of 3D i.
> i. amplifier
> amplitude i.
> i. analysis system
> anatomic i.
> anatomometabolic i.
> arm-down i.
> arm-up i.
> arterial flow-phase i.
> artifact i.
> ascending dynamic flow i.
> attenuated i.
> attenuation-corrected i.
> axial fat-suppressed T2-weighted i.
> axial gradient-echo i.
> axial proton density-weighted i.
> axial transabdominal i.
> bead i.
> binarized i.
> binary i.
> black blood cardiac i.
> i. blur
> bolus-chase i.
> bone phase i.
> breath-hold fast spin-echo i.
> bull's-eye i.
> calculated i.
> cervicothoracic sagittal scout i.
> i. chain
> cine-encoded i.
> cine-magnetic resonance function i.
> color-scale i.
> column-mode sinogram i.
> i. compression
> computer-generated i.
> computerized transverse axial i.
> cone-beam i.
> confocal i.
> contact i.
> contiguous i.'s
> i. contrast
> contrast-enhanced MR i.
> contrast-enhanced T1-weighted
>> fat-suppressed i.

> i. control
> conventional transverse
>> cross-sectional i.
> i. converter
> i. coregistration
> coronal ECD brain SPECT i.
> coronal GRE MR i.
> coronal planar i.
> coronal proton density-weighted fast
>> spin-echo i.
> coronal STIR i.
> coronal T1-weighted i.
> cross-sectional ultrasonographic i.
> CTA i.
> CT/MRI-defined tumor slice i.
> CT/MRI-defined tumor volume i.
> CT reconstruction i.
> i. cytometry
> i. data reconstruction
> 3DDSA i.
> deformation-based surface-rendered i.
> degradation of i.
> delayed-phase i.
> 2D gradient-encoded i.
> diffusion-weighted i.
> digitally fused CT and radiolabeled
>> monoclonal antibody SPECT i.
> digitized film i.
> 4-dimensional i.
> 3-dimensional Fourier transform
>> volume i.
> i. display
> i. display and analysis (IDA)
> i. distortion
> Dixon quantitative chemical-shift i.
> 2D portal i.
> DSA i.
> 4D US i.
> 3D volume-rendering reconstruction
>> i.
> dynamic i.
> ECG-triggered flow-compensated
>> gradient-echo i.
> echo i.
> echo-planar i.
> endosonographic i.
> excitation-spoiled fat-suppressed
>> T1-weighted SE i.
> exercise i.
> expiratory i.
> fast fluid-attenuation inversion
>> recovery i.
> fast Fourier transform i.
> fast spin-echo T2-weighted i.
> fat- and water-suppressed
>> T2-weighted i.
> fat-saturated axial i.
> fat-saturated spin-echo proton
>> density-weighted i.

image (*continued*)

fat-saturated T2-weighted fast spin-echo i.
fat-suppressed 3D gradient-echo i.
fat-suppressed T1-weighted 3D-spoiled gradient-echo i.
FLAIR i.
FLASH i.
flawed i.
flip-angle i.
floating i.
flow-compensated i.
flow-encoded i.
flow-on gradient-echo i.
fluoroscopic i.
i. foldover
i. formation
frequency domain i.
i. fusion
fusion i.
gadolinium-enhanced T1-weighted axial i.
gadolinium-enhanced T1-weighted MRI i.
gated i.
ghost i.
gradient-echo axial i.
gradient-echo coronal i.
gradient-echo T2-weighted i.
gradient-encoded i.
gradient-recalled echo i.
gray-scale i.
GRE-in i.
GRE-out i.
half-Fourier RARE i.
hard-copy i.
i. hashing
high-energy i.
high-resolution 3D spoiled-GRASS i.
high-resolution transverse view i.
histomorphometric i.
horizontal long-axis SPECT i.
imaginary i.
immediate postflow i.
inhomogeneous i.
ink-blot i.
in-phase T1-weighted i.
i. intensification
i. intensification fluorometry
i. intensifier
intercondylar sagittal i.
intermediate i.
inversion recovery i.
inversion recovery-weighted i.
IR i.
isotropic thin-section i.
large field-of-view i.
latent i.
late-phase i.

lateral breast-prone i.
lateral sagittal i.
localizing i.
longitudinal i.
lower-energy i.
magnetic resonance multispectral color i.
magnetic susceptibility-weighted i.
magnetization transfer gradient-echo i.
magnitude i.
matrix i.
maximum-intensity projection and source i.
midcoronal oblique i.
midplane sagittal i.
midsagittal MR i.
minimum-intensity projection i.
MIP i.
mirror i.
misleading i.
i. modulation
modulus i.
motion-triggered cine kinematic MR i.
multiecho axial i.
multiecho coronal i.
multiplanar volume-reformatted i.
multiple planar gradient-recalled i.'s
native i.
2nd echo i.
near-isotropic reformatted i.
negative i.
i. noise
nonattenuation-corrected i.
nonmagnetization transfer gradient-refocused echo i.
nonmagnified i.
nonsubtracted i.
nonsubtraction i.
nuclear magnetic resonance i.
opposed GRE i.
opposed-phase T1-weighted i.
overlapping i.
panoramic i.
parallel-tagged MR i.
parametric i.
parasagittal i.
parenchymatous phase i.
phantom i.
phase i.
phase-corrected GRE i.
phase-velocity i.
pinhole i.
plain-paper i.
planar left anterior oblique i.
postchemotherapy i.
postexercise i.
postfire i.
postintraarticular paramagnetic contrast injection T1-weighted i.

postprandial i.
i. postprocessing
i. postprocessing error artifact
poststress i.
prechemotherapy i.
prefire i.
i. processing workstation
projectional i.
proton-density axial i.
proton density-weighted fast
  spin-echo i.
pulse-echo i.
PVP i.
i. quality
i. quality degradation
quasiradiographic i.
radiographic i.
rapid half-Fourier T2-weighted i.
real-time echo-planar i.
reconstructed i.
i. reconstruction
i. reconstruction computer
i. reconstruction time
i. recording system
recovery time i.
reference i.
i. reformation
reformatted T1 magnetic resonance i.
i. registration
registration and alignment of 3D i.
renal i.
respiratory triggered fat-saturated
  axial i.
sagittal fat-suppressed T1-weighted
  3D spoiled gradient-echo i.
sagittal scout i.
sagittal T1-weighted MR i.
saturation recovery i.
scout i.
scrambled i.
see-through i.
SE proton density-weighted i.
sequential postcontrast MR i.
i. set
i. shading
i. sharpness
short-axis i.
short tau inversion recovery i.
single-section 2D i.
single-slice gradient-echo i.
i. slice thickness
sliding thin-slab maximum-intensity
  projection i.
smoked glass i.
spatial modulation of magnetization i.
i. spatial resolution
spectral-spatial i.
spin-echo pilot i.
spin-echo T1-weighted i.

spin-lattice T1 i.
spin-lock-induced T1-rho-weighted i.
SPIR-FLAIR i.
spot compression i.
spot magnification i.
spot planar i.
standard-dose enhanced conventional
  T1-weighted i.
static i.
stop-action i.
1st-pass contrast bolus perfusion i.
stress-and-rest i.
stress thallium i.
striation across i.
stroke count i.
stroke volume i.
subtracted i.
subtraction i.
summed i.
tensor diffusion-weighted MR i.
T1 1st field-echo dynamic perfusion i.
T1FS i.
T2-gradient refocused i.
thick-slab 3D multiplanar
  reformatted i.
thin collimation i.
thin-cut axial CT i.
thin-section axial i.
tomographic emission i.
transaxial fat-saturated 3D i.
transcoronal STIR i.
transient punctate cortical
  hyperintensity on T1-weighted i.
transmission silhouette i.
transverse ECD brain SPECT i.
transverse-plane PET i.
trauma register i.
TSE i.
T1, T2 i.
turboSTIR i.
T1-weighted i. (T1WI)
T2-weighted i. (T2WI)
T1-weighted axial i.
T2-weighted axial i.
T1-weighted coronal i.
T1-weighted fat-suppressed
  gadolinium-enhanced SE i.
T2-weighted sagittal oblique i.
T2-weighted spin-echo i.
T2-weighted turbo SE i.
ultrasonic tomographic i.
underexposed i.
i. uniformity
unopposed i.
variance i.
velocity-encoded i.
ventilation i.
ventricular function equilibrium i.
i. volume

image (*continued*)
    volume-rendered 3D i.
    volumetric i.
    i. wraparound artifact
    x-ray i.
    zebra stripe i.
image-acquisition
    i.-a. gated examination
    i.-a. gated scan imaging
image-amplified fluoroscopy
Imagecast imaging system
ImageChecker CT CAD software system
image-degrading scattering
image-forming system
image-guided
    i.-g. injection technique
    i.-g. radiation therapy (IGRT)
    i.-g. radiofrequency tumor ablation
    i.-g. radiosurgery
    i.-g. surgery
    i.-g. therapeutic intervention
image-intensifier
    i.-i. node
    i.-i. system
    i.-i. tube
ImageMASTER
Imagent
    I. BP
    I. GI
    I. GI US imaging agent
    I. LN
image-processing software
imager
    Acuson 128EP i.
    Agfa LR 3300 laser i.
    DaTSCAN i.
    Digirad 2020tc i.
    digital fundus i.
    Drystar dry i.
    flat-panel megavoltage i.
    full-body echo-planar system i.
    GE Advantage 1.5T i.
    GE EchoSpeed 1.5T whole-body
      MR i.
    GE Signa 5.4 Genesis MR i.
    GE Signa 5.5 Horizon EchoSpeed
      MR i.
    Hewlett-Packard color-flow i.
    I. II catheter
    Integris V3000 i.
    IRIS III i.
    Kodak Digital Science 1200, 3600
      distributed medical i.
    laser i.
    Lorad digital breast i.
    Magnetom SP MRI i.
    NeuroScan 3D i.
    O-arm multidimensional surgical i.
    Sonata i.

    Tesla magnetic resonance i.
    Voxar Plug-n-View 3D i.
imager/spectrometer
    1.5T Signa whole-body i./s.
**image-selected in vivo spectroscopy
(ISIS)**
imaginary
    i. image
    i. mode
    i. number
    i. signal
imaging
    acetazolamide challenge brain
      SPECT i.
    acoustic i.
    AC-PC referenced MR i.
    acute cerebral infarct i.
    adenosine stress i.
    adrenal i.
    A-FAIR i.
    i. agent
    agent detection i.
    air-contrast i.
    air enema fluoroscopic i.
    Aloka i.
    amplitude i.
    AMT-25-enhanced MR i.
    angiography i.
    anisotropically rotational diffusion i.
    anisotropic 3D i.
    annotated i.
    antegrade pyelography i.
    anthropometric i.
    antifibrin antibody i.
    aortography i.
    aperiodic functional MR i.
    AquariusBLUE 3D i.
    arteriovenous shunt i.
    arthrography i.
    Artoscan MRI i.
    A-scan i.
    ascending contrast phlebography i.
    attenuation i.
    axial echo-planar diffusion-weighted i.
    axial gradient-echo i.
    axial plane i.
    axial T1-weighted spin-echo i.
    balloon expulsion i.
    balloon test occlusion i.
    barium enema i.
    barium swallow i.
    bile duct i.
    biliary tract CT scan i.
    binary i.
    birdcage coil designed for wrist i.
    black blood T2-weighted
      inversion-recovery MR i.
    blipped echo-planar i.
    blood flow i.

I

blood oxygenation level-dependent
functional magnetic resonance i.
(BOLD-fMRI)
blood oxygenation level-dependent
magnetic resonance i.
(BOLD-MRI)
blood oxygen level-dependent
contrast i.
blood pool i.
blush on i.
BMIPP SPECT scan i.
B-mode i.
body-coil i.
body section radiography i.
BOLD contrast i.
bolus challenge i.
bone age i.
bone density i.
bone length i.
bone marrow edema pattern on MR i.
bone mineral content i.
bone phase i.
bone scintiscan i.
brain atlas for functional i.
brain scan i.
breath-hold segmented k-space
gradient-echo i.
breath-hold T1-weighted
gradient-echo i.
breath-hold T1-weighted MP-GRE
MR i.
breath-hold ungated i.
breath-hold velocity-encoded cine-MR i.
bright-blood i.
bright-field i.
bronchial provocation i.
bronchogram i.
B-scan i.
bull's-eye i.
captopril-stimulated renal i.
cardiac blood pool i.
cardiac catheterization i.
cardiac positron emission
tomography i.
cardiac radiography i.
cardiac wall motion i.
Cardiolite scan i.
cardiotocography i.
cardiovascular radioisotope scan and
function i.
carotid duplex i.
carotid sinus i.
CAS i.
CEA-Scan diagnostic i.
i. center information system
Center of Metabolic and
Experimental I.
cephalogram i.
cerebral perfusion SPECT i.

Ceretec brain i.
i. chain veiling glare
chemical-selective fat-saturation i.
chemical-shift i. (CSI)
chemical-shift magnetic resonance i.
cholangiography i.
Chopper-Dixon fat-suppression i.
i. chronology
cine CT i.
cine-gated i.
cine gradient-echo MR i.
cine gradient magnetic resonance i.
cine-magnetic resonance i.
Cine Memory with color-flow
Doppler i.
cine phase-contrast i.
cineradiography i.
cine view i.
cisternography i.
CKG i.
CMJ i.
coded-aperture i.
cognitive functional MR i.
coincidence i.
cold spot myocardial i.
collimation i.
color amplitude i.
color-coded Doppler flow i. (CDFI)
color-coded pulmonary blood flow i.
color Doppler i. (CDI)
color-encoded brain MR i.
color-flow i. (CFI)
color-flow Doppler real-time 2D
blood flow i.
color-flow duplex i.
color velocity i.
column-mode sinogram i.
combined leukocyte-marrow i.
combined Myoscint/thallium i.
combined thallium-Tc-HMPAO i.
Compuscan Hittman computerized i.
computed transmission tomography i.
computer fusion i.
Computer Technology and I. (CTI)
continuous i.
continuous moving bed MR i.
continuous-wave Doppler i.
contrast-enhanced fundamental i.
contrast-enhanced magnetic resonance i.
contrast-enhanced T1-GRE i.
contrast-enhanced T1-weighted
spin-echo high field-strength MR i.
contrast enhancement of computed
tomographic i.
contrast-enhancing parametric i
conventional planar i. (CPI)
conventional spin-echo i.
convergent color Doppler i.
coronary artery scan i.

imaging (*continued*)

corpus cavernosonography i.
corrected gradient-echo phase i.
correlative diagnostic i.
correlative multimodality i.
correlative pertechnetate thyroid i.
cross-sectional i.
CSF-suppressed T2-weighted 3D
  MP-RAGE MR i.
CTAT i.
CT/SPECT fusion i.
cystography i.
cystourethroscopy i.
dacryocystography i.
darkfield i.
3D echo-planar i.
delayed bone i.
DentaScan i.
DEXA bone density scan i.
dexamethasone suppression test i.
3D fast low-angle shot i.
3D fast spin-echo magnetic
  resonance i.
2D Fourier transformation i.
3DFT gradient-echo MR i.
3DFT volume i.
diagnostic i. (DI)
DIET fast SE i.
diffraction-enhanced i. (DEI)
diffusion magnetic resonance i.
diffusion-tensor i. (DTI)
diffusion-tensor magnetic resonance i.
diffusion-tensor MR i.
diffusion-weighted i. (DWI)
diffusion-weighted echo-planar i.
diffusion-weighted magnetic
  resonance i.
diffusion-weighted MR i.
digital chest i.
digitally fused CT and radiolabeled i.
digital radiography i.
digital subtraction i. (DSI)
digital vascular i. (DVI)
4-dimensional i.
1-dimensional chemical-shift i.
dipyridamole echocardiography i.
dipyridamole handgrip i.
dipyridamole infusion i.
dipyridamole thallium-201 i.
dipyridamole thallium stress i.
direct Fourier transformation i.
discontinuous i.
displacement field-fitting MR i.
diuretic renal i.
2D KWE direct Fourier i.
3D KWE direct Fourier i.
3D magnetic source i.
2D modified KWE direct Fourier i.
2D multislice i.

Doppler color-flow i.
Doppler tissue i. (DTI)
Doppler ultrasonography i.
Doppler venous i.
double-dose gadolinium i.
double-echo echo-planar i.
double helical CT i.
double-phase technetium-99m
  sestamibi i.
double-pulse interlaced echo i.
3D processed ultrafast computerized i.
3D projection reconstruction i.
dry laser i.
DSC MR i.
DT MR i.
3D turbo SE i.
3D T1-weighted gradient-echo i.
dual-agent i.
dual-coil i.
dual-echo and DT MR i.
dual-echo DIET fast spin-echo i.
dual-echo interleaved spiral out-in i.
dual-energy i.
dual-isotope myocardial perfusion i.
dual-phase ^{99m}Tc-sestamibi i.
dual-time point i.
dual-tracer i.
3D ultrasound reconstruction i.
duodenography i.
duplex carotid i.
duplex Doppler i.
dynamic cervical magnetic resonance i.
dynamic contrast-enhanced magnetic
  resonance i. (DCE-MRI)
dynamic contrast-enhanced
  subtraction MR i.
dynamic liver i.
dynamic magnetic resonance i. (dMRI)
dynamic optical breast i. (DOBI)
dynamic renal i.
dynamic scintigraphy i.
dynamic susceptibility contrast
  magnetic resonance i. (DSC-MRI)
dynamic volume i.
dynamic weightbearing cervical
  magnetic resonance i.
ECG-gated multislice MR i.
ECG-gated spin-echo MR i.
echo i.
echocardiogram planar i.
echocardiography i.
echo-planar i. (EPI)
echo-planar diffusion-weighted i.
echo-planar FLAIR i.
echo-planar GRE T2-weighted i.
echo time chemical-shift i.
elastic i.
electric joint fluoroscopy i.
electrocardiogram-gated MRI i.

electrocardiography-gated echo-planar i.
electrodiagnostic i.
electromagnetic blood flow i.
electronic portal i.
electron paramagnetic resonance spatial i.
electron radiography i.
electrostatic i.
end-diastolic i.
endoanal MR i.
endocrine i.
endorectal coil magnetic resonance i. (erMRI)
endorectal surface-coil MR i.
enhanced i.
ensemble contrast i. (ECI)
epicardial i.
epididymography i.
epsilon 2D and tissue velocity i.
equilibrium MUGA i.
ERCP i.
esophageal function i.
esophagography i.
excretory phase i.
excretory urography i.
exercise thallium-201 stress i.
exogenous i.
extremity magnetic resonance i. (E-MRI)
ex vivo magnetic resonance i.
fast cardiac phase contrast cine i.
fast Fourier i.
fast multiplanar inversion recovery i.
fast multiplanar spoiled gradient-recalled i.
fast-scan magnetic resonance i.
fast spin-echo and fast inversion recovery i.
fast spin-echo black blood i.
fast spin-echo MR i.
fast spoiled gradient-recalled MR i.
fat-suppressed 3D-spoiled gradient-echo FLASH MR i.
fat-suppressed 3D-spoiled gradient-recall echo i.
fat-suppressed gadolinium-enhanced i.
fat-water chemical-shift i.
FDG-labeled positron i.
FDG myocardial i.
ferumoxtran-enhanced echo-planar GRE T2-weighted i.
ferumoxtran-enhanced echo-planar SE T2-weighted i.
fetal liver magnetic resonance i.
^{18}F FDG-negative i.
field-echo i.
field-of-view i.
filmless i.

FLAIR echo-planar i.
FLAIR-FLASH i.
FLASH magnetic resonance i.
flat-field i.
flawed i.
flow i.
flow-sensitive MR i.
fluid-attenuated inversion recovery i.
fluoroscopic i.
fluoroscopy-guided condylar lift-off i.
flush aortogram i.
Fourier 2-dimensional i.
Fourier direct transform i.
Fourier multislice modified KWE direct i.
Fourier transform i.
FOV i.
2-frame gated i.
frequency domain i. (FDI)
FS burst MR i.
functional brain i.
functional magnetic resonance i. (fMRI)
functional spin-echo i.
fundamental-mode ultrasound i.
fusion i.
gadolinium-enhanced MR i.
gallbladder i.
gallium lung i.
gastric emptying i.
gastric mucosa i.
gastrointestinal motility i.
gas ventilation i.
gated cardiac blood pool i.
gated cine i.
gated equilibrium cardiac blood pool i.
gated magnetic resonance i.
gated SPECT myocardial perfusion i.
Gd-FMPSPGR i.
GNG phase i.
i. gradient
gradient-echo 3-dimensional Fourier transform volume i.
gradient-echo flow i.
gradient-echo MR i.
gradient-echo phase i.
gradient-echo sequence i.
gradient-to-noise i.
GRASS MR i.
gray-scale baseline i.
GRE breath-hold hepatic i.
GRE gadolinium chelate-enhanced i.
GRE-in i.
GRE magnetic resonance i.
GRE-out i.
half-Fourier i. (HFI)

imaging (*continued*)

half-Nex i.
harmonic i.
HAT transformed i.
HBCT i.
heat-denatured autologous RBC
   SPECT i.
heavy ion i.
Helios diagnostic i.
helium magnetic resonance i.
   (He-MRI)
hemodynamically weighted
   echo-planar MR i.
hepatobiliary ductal system i.
HIDA i.
high-definition i. (HDI)
high-energy i.
high field-strength MR i.
high-frequency Doppler ultrasound i.
high-resolution B-mode i.
high-resolution CT i.
high-resolution 3DFT MR i.
high-resolution infrared i.
high-resolution magnetic resonance
   imaging (HR-MRI)
high-resolution storage phosphor i.
high-resolution susceptibility-weighted i.
high spatial resolution i.
high-speed i.
HLA i.
H-1 MR spectroscopic i.
holography i.
hot-spot heart i.
hot-spot myocardial i.
4-hour delayed thallium i.
HRI i.
hybrid i.
hybrid-RARE i.
hydrogen proton i.
hypotonic duodenography i.
hysterosalpingography i.
^{123}I BMIPP i.
image-acquisition gated scan i.
infarct-avid i.
infection i.
Infecton i.
infrared i.
initial i.
in-phase GRE i.
integrated functional magnetic
   resonance i.
intermediate i.
interventional magnetic resonance i.
   (I-MRI)
intracoronary i.
intracranial i.
intraoperative i.
intraperitoneal technetium-sulfur
   colloid i.

intrathecal i.
intravascular ultrasound i.
intravenous fluorescein angiography i.
inversion recovery echo-planar i.
   (IR-EPI)
in vivo He-3 MR i.
^{111}In white blood cell i.
iodine fluorescence i.
iodomethyl-norcholesterol scintigraphy
   i.
irreversible compression of MR i.
Isocam scintillation i.
isotope colloid i.
isotope hepatobiliary i.
isotope-labeled fibrinogen i.
isotope shunt i.
isotopic 3D i.
isotropic diffusion-weighted i.
IVFA i.
KCD i.
kidney function i.
kidney radionuclide i.
kidneys, ureters, and bladder i.
kinematic magnetic resonance i.
kinestatic charge detector i.
KUB i.
laser-polarized helium MR i.
laser projection i. (LPI)
limitation of MR i.
limited i.
line i.
linear scan i.
lipid-polarized helium MR i.
lipid-sensitive MR i.
liver-specific contrast ultrasound i.
liver-spleen i.
localizing i.
longitudinal section i.
loopogram i.
lower extremity i.
lower limb venography i.
low field-strength MR i.
low flip-angle gradient-echo i.
low-resolution i.
lung i.
lymphangiography i.
lymphatic i.
lymph node i.
macromolecular contrast-enhanced
   MR i.
magic angle spinning i.
Magnes 2500 whole-head i.
magnetic resonance i. (MRI)
magnetic resonance catheter i.
magnetic resonance diffusion i.
magnetic resonance perfusion i.
magnetic resonance spectroscopic i.
   (MRSI)
magnetic source i. (MSI)

magnetization and spin-lock transfer i.

magnetization-prepared contrast-enhanced breath-hold volume-targeted i.

magnetization transfer weighted i.

magnetoacoustic i.

malignant melanoma gallium i.

mammary ductogram i.

mammary galactogram i.

mangafodipir trisodium-enhanced MR i.

i. manifestation

marker transit i.

mass i.

material spin echocardiogram total volume i.

Matrix LR3300 laser i.

maxillofacial i.

maximum-intensity projection i.

MCD i.

mediastinal cross-sectional i.

micro CT i.

microscopic i.

microwave i.

middle field-strength MR i.

midsagittal MR i.

miniature i.

minimum-intensity projection i.

mirror i.

misleading i.

M-mode echocardiogram i.

i. modality

molecular i.

morphologic i.

motion-free i.

moving tabletop MR i.

MRA i.

MR echo-planar i.

MR enteroclysis i.

MRI-guided laser-induced interstitial i.

^{99m}Tc-HMPAO cerebral perfusion SPECT i.

^{99m}Tc-labeled denatured autologous RBC i.

^{99m}Tc Myoview myocardial perfusion i.

MUGA cardiac blood pool i.

multiecho i.

multiformatted i.

multigated spectral Doppler i. (MSDI)

multimodality i.

multiorgan i.

multiphase-multisection T2-weighted MR i.

multiplanar MR i.

multiplanar reformatted radiographic and digitally reconstructed radiographic i.

multiple-echo i.

multiple gated blood pool i.

multiple line-scan i. (MLSI)

multiple-plane i.

multiple-slice i.

multisection diffusion-weighted magnetic resonance i.

multisection gradient-echo echo-planar i.

multishot echo-planar i. (MS-EPI)

multishot spin-echo/echo-planar i.

multislice modified KWE direct Fourier i.

multislice 1st-pass myocardial perfusion i.

multitime point i.

multitracer i.

multivoxel i.

musculoskeletal i.

MUSTPAC ultrasound i.

myelography i.

myocardial I-123 MIBG i.

myocardial infarct i.

myocardial perfusion i. (MPI)

myocardial thallium i.

Myoscint i.

^{23}Na magnetic resonance i.

native tissue harmonic i. (NTHI)

navigated spin-echo diffusion-weighted MR i.

2nd harmonic i.

neonatal morphologic i.

nephrostogram i.

nephrotomography i.

neurodiagnostic i.

neuroradiologic i.

neurotransmitter i.

nonattenuation-corrected SPECT i.

nonavid infarct i.

noninvasive i.

nonsubtraction i.

nuclear bone i.

nuclear cardiovascular i.

nuclear gated blood pool i.

nuclear hepatobiliary i.

nuclear magnetic resonance i.

nuclear medicine i.

nuclear perfusion i.

oblique axial MR i.

oblique magnetic resonance i.

oblique sagittal EKG-gated spin-echo magnetic resonance i.

OCG i.

octreotide i.

off-resonance saturation pulse i.

online portal i.

opposed-phase GRE MR i.

optic surface i. (OSI)

optimal angle i.

imaging (*continued*)

optoacoustic i.
oral cholecystogram i.
organ-specific scintigraphic i.
orthopantogram i.
out-of-phase GRE i.
oxygenation-sensitive functional
  MR i.
oxygen-enhanced lung MR i.
PACS PathSpeed MR i.
pancreas ultrasonography i.
pancreatography i.
panoramic i.
parallel i.
parallel-hole collimated i.
paramagnetic enhancement
  accentuation by chemical-shift i.
parathyroid ultrasonography i.
partial Fourier i.
PASTA i.
pediatric nuclear medicine i.
percutaneous intracoronary
  angioscopy i.
perfusion and ventilation lung i.
perfusion MR i.
perfusion-weighted i. (PWI)
perineogram i.
peripheral vascular i.
peritoneogram i.
Persantine thallium i.
PET lung i.
PET metabolic i.
PET myocardial fatty acid i.
PET perfusion metabolism i.
PETT i.
3-phase i.
2-phase computed tomographic i.
2-phase CT i.
phased-array body coil MR i.
phased-array multicoil i.
phased-array surface coil MR i.
phase-dependent spectroscopic i.
phase-encoded time-reduced
  acquisition sequence i.
phase-inversion harmonic i.
phase-sensitive gradient-echo
  MR i.
phase-velocity i.
3-phase whole-body bone i.
photostimulable phosphor digital i.
physiologic i.
pinhole collimated i.
PIPIDA hepatobiliary i.
plain film i.
planar radionuclide i.
planar spin i.
planar thallium i.
i. plane
point i.

polarity-altered spectral-selective
  acquisition i.
POMP i.
portal venous phase i.
postcontrast MR i.
postdrainage i.
postexercise i.
postinjection i.
postmetrizamide CT i.
postoperative cholangiography i.
postwash i.
power Doppler i. (PDI)
precontrast i.
preoperative i.
pressure perfusion i.
pretherapy i.
projection-reconstruction i.
projection tract i.
protodensity MR i.
proton chemical-shift i.
proton density-weighted i.
proton-electron double-resonance i.
  (PEDRI)
proton MR spectroscopic i.
pseudodynamic MR i.
pullback i.
pulmonary perfusion i.
pulmonary ventilation i.
pulsed-electron paramagnetic i.
pulsed magnetization transfer MR i.
pulse-echo i.
pulse-inversion contrast harmonic i.
  (PICHI)
pulse-inversion harmonic i. (PIHI)
pulse sequence echo-planar i.
PunctSURE vascular access i.
pyelography i.
PYP i.
pyrophosphate i.
QCT i.
quantitative brain i.
quantitative chemical-shift i.
  (QCSI)
quantitative fluorescence i.
quantitative lung perfusion i.
quantitative magnetic resonance i.
  (qMRI, QMRI)
quantitative spirometrically controlled
  CT i.
radioactive fibrinogen i.
radiographically normal i.
radioisotope cisternography i.
radioisotope gallium i.
radioisotope indium-labeled white
  blood cell i.
radioisotope technetium i.
radiolabeled antibody i.
radionuclide gated blood pool i.
radionuclide milk i.

radionuclide renal i.
radionuclide renography i.
radionuclide thyroid i.
rapid axial MR i.
rapid-excitation MR i.
rapid-sequence i.
^{82}Rb-based cardiac i.
real-time color Doppler i.
real-time 2D blood flow i.
receptor i.
reconstructed radiographic i.
reconstruction from projection i.
reconstructive i.
rectilinear bone scan i.
redistribution thallium-201 i.
regional ejection fraction i.
renal angiography i.
renal CT i.
renal cyst i.
renal duplex i.
renal perfusion i.
renal ultrasonography i.
renogram i.
respiratory gated i.
resting MUGA i.
resting myocardial perfusion i.
resting redistribution i.
resting thallium-201 myocardial i.
reticuloendothelial i.
ring-type i.
rose bengal sodium I-131 biliary i.
rotating delivery of excitation
  off-resonance MR i.
rotating-frame i.
rotationally invariant i.
row-mode sinogram i.
R-to-R i.
sagittal fast spin-echo T2-weighted
  MR i.
sagittal gradient-echo i.
sagittal oblique i.
sagittal transabdominal i.
saline-enhanced MR i.
scanogram i.
3-Scape real-time 3D i.
scintigraphic scan i.
scintillation i.
scout i.
sector-scan echocardiography i.
segmental k-space turbo
  gradient-echo breath-hold sequence
  i.
segmented echo-planar i. (SEPI)
segmenting dual-echo MR i.
selective excitation projection
  reconstruction i.
selenium-labeled bile acid i.
Senographe 2000D digital
  mammography i.

sensitive plane projection
  reconstruction i.
sequential echo-planar i.
sequential line i.
sequential plane i.
sequential point i.
sequential quantitative MR i.
sequential 1st-pass i.
serial contrast MR i.
serial duplex i.
serial dynamic i.
seriography i.
sestamibi stress scan i.
shaded surface display i.
short echo-time chemical-shift i.
short inversion recovery i.
short T1 inversion recovery i.
1-shot echo-planar i.
shuntogram i.
sialography i.
silhouette i.
simultaneous volume i.
single-dose gadolinium i.
single-echo diffusion i.
single-shot gradient echo-planar i.
single-voxel proton brain
  spectroscopy i.
sinus tract i.
slip-ring i.
small field-of-view MR i.
SmartScore CT i.
sodium i.
I. Solutions Group (ISG)
SonoCT real-time compound i.
Sonoline Antares 4D ultrasound i.
source i.
spastic electron paramagnetic
  resonance i.
SPECT i.
spectamine brain i.
SPECT myocardial perfusion i.
spectral Doppler i.
spike-related functional MR i.
spin-echo cardiac i.
spin-echo magnetic resonance i.
spin-echo T1-weighted transaxial
  MR i.
spin-lock and magnetization transfer
  i.
spin-warp i.
SPIO-enhanced MR i.
spiral echo-planar i.
splanchnic vascular i.
spleen ultrasonography i.
splenoportography i.
split-brain i.
SSD i.
stacked-scan i.
static 3D FLASH i.

imaging (*continued*)
    static liver i.
    steady-state free precession i.
    steady-state gradient-echo i.
    STIR i.
    stop-action i.
    storage phosphor i.
    1st-pass myocardial perfusion i.
    strain-rate MR i.
    stress myocardial perfusion i.
    stress-only perfusion i.
    stress-redistribution i.
    stress thallium-201 myocardial i.
    i. study
    subsecond FLASH i.
    subtraction i.
    superparamagnetic iron oxide MR i.
    i. surveillance
    susceptibility-weighted MR i.
    tagged magnetic resonance i.
    target-to-nontarget ratio for myocardial i.
    technetium 99m anti-CEA Fab murine monoclonal antibody i.
    technetium 99m Infecton i.
    technetium 99m pertechnate/thallium-201 radionuclide subtraction i.
    technetium 99m pyrophosphate i.
    technetium 99m tetrofosmin exercise-rest SPECT myocardial perfusion i.
    technetium stannous pyrophosphate i.
    technetium-thallium subtraction i.
    tensor i.
    thallium-201 i.
    thallium myocardial perfusion i.
    thallium myocardial scan with SPECT i.
    thallium rest-redistribution i.
    thallium scintography i.
    thallium stress i.
    thermoacoustic i.
    thick-slice i.
    thin collimation i.
    thin-slice i.
    thoracic duct i.
    ThromboScan i.
    through-transfer i.
    thyroid ultrasonography i.
    i. time
    timed i.
    time-of-flight echo-planar i.
    time-resolved 3D i.
    i. timing artifact
    TIPS i.
    tissue Doppler i.
    tissue harmonic i. (THI)

    TOF i.
    tomographic i.
    Toshiba Aspire continuous i.
    total body scan i.
    transabdominal i.
    transaxial i.
    transcervical catheterization of fallopian tube i.
    transcranial real-time color Doppler i.
    transesophageal Doppler color-flow i.
    transfer i.
    transform i.
    transjugular intrahepatic portosystemic shunt i.
    transthoracic i.
    transverse breath-hold gradient-echo cine-magnetic resonance i.
    transverse section i.
    triple-dose gadolinium i.
    triple-head coincidence i.
    triple inversion recovery-prepared FSE i.
    triple-phase bone scan i.
    true dynamic joint i.
    TSPP i.
    tumor i.
    turboFLAIR i.
    turboFLASH i.
    T1-weighted coronal i.
    T1-weighted sagittal i.
    twofold accelerated parallel i.
    UBM i.
    ultrafast CT i.
    ultrasonic tomographic i.
    ultrasound backscatter microscopy i.
    ultrasound-based strain rate and strain i.
    unaccelerated 2D cine SSFP i.
    unenhanced MR i.
    unsuppressed i.
    urethrocystography i.
    urography i.
    vagus nerve-stimulated functional magnetic resonance i. (VNS-fMRI)
    vascular flow i.
    VEC i.
    vectorcardiography i.
    velocity i.
    velocity-density i.
    velocity-encoded cine-MR i.
    venography i.
    venous i.
    ventilation-perfusion i.
    vesiculography i.
    videofluoroscopic i.
    virtual dissection i.
    virtual reality i.
    Vitrea 3D i.

volume i.
volumetric i.
V/Q i.
VScore with AutoGate cardiac i.
wall motion i.
water-selective spin-echo i.
wavelet-encoded magnetic resonance
  i.
wet laser i.
white blood cell i.
whole-body echo-planar MR i.
whole-body scan i.
whole-body thallium i.
i. workstation
xenon-133 SPECT i.
zoom i.
imaging-anatomy correlation
imaging-based stereotaxis
imaging-compatible stereotactic coordinate frame
imaging-directed 3D volumetric information
imaging-guided catheter drainage
imaging-pathology correlation
Imagopaque contrast medium
Imagyn microlaparoscope
Imatron
  I. C-100 EBT scanner
  I. C-150L EBCT scanner
  I. C-1000 UFCT scanner
  I. C-100 Ultrafast CT scanner
  I. C-150XL CT scanner
  I. C-100XP CT scanner
  I. Fastrac C-100 cine x-ray CT
    scanner
  I. Ultrafast CT scanner
imbalance
  biomechanical i.
  i. of gain artifact
  i. of phase artifact
  ventilatory capacity-demand i.
imbrication
  capsular i.
  facetal i.
Imed Gemini PC-2 volumetric controller
IMH
  intramural hematoma
IMI
  inferior myocardial infarct
imidoacetic acid imaging agent
imidodiphosphonate (IDP)
iminodiacetic acid (IDA)
immature
  i. bone
  i. lung
  i. lung disease
  i. lung syndrome
  i. ovarian teratoma
  skeletally i.

immaturity
  structural pulmonary i.
immediate
  i. postflow image
  i. postictal period
immediately detachable coil
immersion
  i. B-scan ultrasound
  i. technique
imminent
  i. death
  i. demise
immitis
  Coccidioides i.
immobilization
  bone mineral i.
immobilizer
  Angle-Iron skull i.
  AP-PA skull i.
  i. board
  cross-table leg i.
  dual leg i.
  molded i.
  Pigg-O-Stat mechanical i.
  sheet i.
  shoulder i.
  tomographic skull i.
  Velcro strap i.
  waist i.
immobilizing vest
immovable joint
immune
  i. electron microscopy
  i. response
immunity
  acquired i.
  active acquired i.
  artificial active acquired i.
  artificial passive acquired i.
  natural active acquired i.
  passive acquired i.
immunoblastic large cell lymphoma
immunocytic amyloidosis
immunocytochemical staining
immunofluorescence antibody
immunofluorimetric assay
immunoglobulin G (IgG)
immunologic
  i. injury
  i. pulmonary edema
immunolymphoscintigraphy
immunomagnetic
  i. bead
  i. purging
Immuno-mini NJ-2300 microplate reader
immunoprecipitate
immunoproliferative small intestine disease (IPSID)

immunoradioassay
immunoreactivity
immunoscintigraphy
immunoscintimetry
immunostained surface
immunosuppression
ImmuRAID antibody imaging
 agent
IMN
    internal mammary node
impacted
    i. calculus
    i. feces
    i. fetus
    i. subcapital fracture
    i. urethral stone
    i. valgus fracture
impaction
    anteromedial superior humeral
      head i.
    fecal i.
    lateral compartment i.
    i. lesion
    mucoid i.
    stone i.
impact velocity
impaired
    i. renal function
    i. renal perfusion
    i. tubular transit
    i. venous return
    i. ventilation-perfusion
impairment
    axonal transport i.
    circulatory i.
    functional aerobic i. (FAI)
    growth i.
    hemodynamic reserve i.
    inspiratory muscle function i.
    mild cognitive i.
    motor i.
    posterior cingulate functional i.
    renal function i.
    sensory i.
Impax PACS system
impedance
    acoustic i.
    aortic i.
    diastolic notch i.
    i. matching
    i. MR phlebogram
    multichannel intraluminal i. (MII)
    i. phlebography
    i. plethysmography (IPG)
    pulmonary arterial input i.
    pulmonary vascular bed i.
    respiratory modulation of vascular i.
    vascular i.
    i. venography

impeller basket catheter
impending
    i. herniation
    i. myocardial infarct
imperfecta
    amelogenesis i.
    dentinogenesis i.
    osteogenesis i. (OI)
    Sillence classification of osteogenesis
      i.
imperfect regeneration
imperforate
    i. anus
    i. hymen
impingement
    anterolateral i.
    cam i.
    chronic friction and i.
    dural i.
    i. exostosis
    femoroacetabular i. (FAI)
    graft roof i.
    iliopsoas i.
    lateral i.
    ligamentous i.
    nerve root i.
    outlet i.
    pincer i.
    pincer-type i.
    posterior i.
    posterosuperior glenoid i.
    repetitive osseous i.
    rotator cuff i.
    shoulder i.
    sidewall i.
    i. spur
    syndesmotic i.
    i. syndrome
    talar i.
    talofibular i.
    triquetral i.
    ulnolunate i.
impinging osteophyte
implant
    Baerveldt glaucoma drainage i.
    biodegradable i.
    bone i.
    bowel serosal endometrial i.
    BrachySeed PD-103 i.
    carcinomatous i.
    cesium i.
    cobalt-chromium-molybdenum alloy
      metal i.
    cobalt-chromium-tungsten-nickel alloy
      metal i.
    cochlear i.
    Co-Cr-Mo alloy metal i.
    collapsed subpectoral i.
    i. collar

coralline
  ocular i.
double-lumen breast i.
double-stem silicone
  MP i.
electrically activated i.
endometrial i.
endosseous i.
epidural i.
extraperitoneal i.
ferromagnetic i.
i. fracture
hinged i.
hydroxyapatite i.
^{125}I interstitial radiation i.
interstitial low dose-rate iridium-192
  needle i.
intracavitary i.
iridium-192 endobronchial i.
iridium-192 wire i.
i. irradiation
Joseph valve i.
Krupin-Denver eye valve-to-disc i.
malignant pleural i.
mammary i.
mechanically activated i.
metallic otologic i.
methyl methacrylate bead i.
ocular i.
open-cord tendon i.
otologic i.
palladium i.
^{103}Pd prostatic i.
penile i.
peritoneal metastatic i.
permanent interstitial i.
polymethylmethacrylate i.
prostate i.
prosthetic i.
retropectoral mammary i.
saline i.
serosal endometrial i.
silicone elastomer rubber ball i.
silicone wrist i.
single-lumen silicone breast i.
subglandular i.
subpectoral i.
synthetic bone i.
temporary interstitial i.
total knee i.
transperineal i.
transvaginal i.
tumor i.
VDS i.
ventral derotating spinal i.
Volz wrist i.
implantable
  i. access catheter
  i. drug delivery system

i. infusion port
i. infusion pump
i. vascular access device
implantation
  i. bleeding in pregnancy
  cornual i.
  i. cyst
  epicardial i.
  percutaneous transperineal seed i.
  peroral i.
  radon seed i.
  i. site
  2-stage stent i.
  stem cell i.
  subxiphoid i.
  transluminal aortic endograft i.
  transvenous i.
implanted
  i. imaging opaque marker
  i. NCP
  i. pacemaker
  i. port
impotence, impotency
  arteriogenic i.
  hemodynamic i.
  vasogenic i.
impotency (*var. of* impotence)
impression
  basilar i.
  cardiac i.
  colic i.
  convolutional i.
  digastric i.
  duodenal i.
  esophageal i.
  extrinsic esophageal i.
  extrinsic stomach i.
  gastric i.
  liver i.
  renal i.
  suprarenal i.
imprint
  tissue i.
improved
  i. Chen-Smith (ICS)
  i. Chen-Smith coder
  i. photon flux
improvement
  interval i.
impulse
  apical i.
  bifid precordial i.
  double systolic apical i.'s
  downward displacement of apical i.
  ectopic i.
  high-amplitude i.
  hyperdynamic right ventricular i.
  jugular venous i.
  nodal i.

impulse (*continued*)
  prolonged left ventricular i.
  sustained apical i.
  systolic i.
  undulant i.
I-MRI
  interventional magnetic resonance imaging
IMRT
  intensity-modulated radiation therapy
  intensity-modulated radiotherapy treatment
    SmartBeam IMRT
    step-and-shoot IMRT
IMT
  intimal-medial thickness
  iodomethyltyrosine
in
  i. situ
  i. situ graft
  i. situ pinning
  i. toto
  i. utero
  i. utero detection of cardiac anomaly
  i. utero hydronephrosis
  i. utero MRI
  i. utero ultrasound
  i. vitro evaluation of coil
  i. vitro labeling
  i. vivo
  i. vivo balloon pressure
  i. vivo correlation
  i. vivo disposition study
  i. vivo examination
  i. vivo He-3 MR imaging
  i. vivo imaging agent
  i. vivo labeling
  i. vivo method
  i. vivo microscopy
  i. vivo optical spectroscopy (INVOS)
  i. vivo 31P MR spectroscopy
  i. vivo proton MR spectroscopy
  i. vivo stereologic assessment
  i. vivo technique
In
  indium
¹¹¹In, In-111
  Indium 111
    ¹¹¹In antimyosin scintigraphy
    ¹¹¹In chloride
    ¹¹¹In DTPA
    ¹¹¹In IgG
    ¹¹¹In imciromab pentetate
    ¹¹¹In labeling
    ¹¹¹In murine monoclonal antibody Fab to myosin

    ¹¹¹In octreotide
    ¹¹¹In oxine
    ¹¹¹In oxine WBC
    ¹¹¹In pentetreotide
    ¹¹¹In satumomab pendetide
    ¹¹¹In WBC
    ¹¹¹In white blood cell imaging
inactivator
inactive
  i. endometrium
  i. granuloma
  i. mode
inadequate
  i. bowel preparation
  i. calvarial calcification
  i. cardiac output
  i. cranial calcification
  i. runoff
  i. visualization
inadvertent arterial injection
incarcerated
  i. hernia
  i. omentum
  i. placenta
incarceration
  bladder i.
  fetal i.
incessant ovulation
incidence
incident
  i. angle
  i. ray
incidental
  i. finding
  i. lung uptake
  i. punctate white matter hyperintensity
incidentaloma
  adrenal i.
  brain i.
  thyroid i.
incision
  Brödel bloodless line of i.
incisional hernia
incisive
  i. bone
  i. canal
  i. suture
incisor
  fascial i.
  i. tooth
incisura, *pl.* **incisurae**
  i. angularis
  aortic i.
  cardiac i.
  i. defect
  i. dextra of Gans
  i. scapulae
  stomach defect i.

incisurae (*pl. of* incisura)
incisural
    i. epidermoidoma
    i. sclerosis
inciting
    i. event
    i. factor
inclination
    radial i.
    ulnar i.
    urethral i.
    volar i.
inclinometer
inclusion cyst
incoherence
    magnetic resonance spin i.
incoherent
    i. motion
    i. spin
incompetence, incompetency
    aortic valvular i.
    chronotropic i.
    communicating vein i.
    deep venous i.
    gastroesophageal i.
    mitral valve i.
    myocardial i.
    postphlebitic valvular i.
    pulmonary i.
    saphenous vein i.
    sphincter i.
    traumatic tricuspid i.
    tricuspid i.
    valvular i.
incompetency (*var. of* incompetence)
incompetent
    i. blood-brain barrier
    i. cervix
    i. ileocecal valve
    i. lymph valve
    i. perforator
incomplete
    i. atrioventricular block (IAVB)
    i. bladder emptying
    i. closure
    i. dislocation
    i. fracture
    i. fracture of bone
    i. heart block
    i. hernia
    i. left bundle-branch block
    (ILBBB)
    i. lower esophageal sphincter
    relaxation
    i. neurofibromatosis
    i. obstruction
    i. placenta previa
    i. pulmonary fissure
    i. resolution of pneumonia

    i. right bundle-branch block
    (IRBBB)
    i. ring sign
    i. stroke
    i. tumor
    i. unfolding
    i. ureteral duplication
incongruity
    angle of i.
    facet joint i.
    joint i.
    patellofemoral i.
incontinence
    bladder i.
    bowel i.
    fecal i.
    motor urge i.
    stress i.
increased
    i. airway
    i. anteroposterior diameter
    i. attenuation
    i. basilar cistern
    i. bone density
    i. capillary permeability edema
    i. carrying angle
    i. central venous pressure
    i. cerebrovascular resistance
    i. density of spleen
    i. echogenicity
    i. echo signal
    i. extracellular fluid volume
    i. interstitial fluid
    i. interstitial marking
    i. intracranial pressure
    i. intrapericardial pressure
    i. isotope uptake
    i. lateral joint space
    i. left ventricular ejection time
    i. markings of emphysema
    i. myocardial oxygen requirement
    i. outflow resistance
    i. peripheral resistance
    i. peristalsis
    i. prominence of pulmonary vessels
    i. pulmonary arterial pressure
    i. pulmonary obstruction
    i. pulmonary vascularity
    i. pulmonary vascular marking
    i. pulmonary vascular resistance
    i. pulmonary vasculature
    i. renal echogenicity cortex
    i. skull thickness
    i. splenic density
    i. thyroid uptake
    i. tracer activity
    i. tracer uptake
    i. uptake of radiotracer
    i. ventricular afterload

increase in intensity
increasingly dense nephrogram
increment
    i. in luminal diameter
    i. of perfusion
incremental
    i. dose
    i. risk factor
incrementation
    time-proportional phase i.
    (TPPI)
increta
    placenta i.
incubator
    MR-compatible i.
incudes (*pl. of* incus)
incus, *pl.* **incudes**
    i. bone
indemnity
    crown i.
indentation
    anterior central i.
    central i.
    focal i.
    haustral i.
    irregular extrinsic i.
    i. of myelography dye
    posterior central i.
    semilunar i.
indented
    i. fracture
    i. fracture of skull
in-department film
independent jaw
indeterminate age
index, *pl.* **indices,** *pl.* **indexes,**
  gen. **indicis**
    acceleration i. (AI)
    acetabular head i. (AHI)
    amnionic fluid i. (AFI)
    angiographic muscle mass i.
    ankle-arm i. (AAI)
    ankle-brachial i. (ABI)
    apnea-hypopnea i. (AHI)
    arch length i.
    Ashman i.
    axial acetabular i. (AAI)
    Benink tarsal i.
    bicaudate i. (BCI)
    bifrontal i. (BFI)
    biliary saturation i.
    body mass i. (BMI)
    Broca i.
    bromodeoxyuridine labeling i.
    calculated splenic i.
    cardiac i. (CI)
    cardiothoracic i.
    carpal height i.
    CBF i.

    cella media i.
    cephalic i.
    cephalopelvic disproportion i.
    computed tomography dose i.
    (CTDI)
    congestion i.
    contractile work i.
    contractility i.
    coronary stenosis i. (CSI)
    coronary vascular resistance i.
    (CVRI)
    Cronqvist cranial i.
    Detsky modified cardiac risk i.
    diastolic left ventricular i.
    diastolic pressure-time i.
    (DPTI)
    Doppler flow i.
    Doppler resistive i. (DRI)
    dye fluorescence i. (DFI)
    eccentricity i.
    effective pulmonic i.
    ejection phase i.
    ellipticity i.
    end-diastolic volume i.
    end-systolic volume i. (ESVI)
    end-systolic wall i.
    exercise i.
    extensor indicis
    femoral pulsatility i. (FPI)
    fetal-pelvic i.
    Fick cardiac i.
    i. finger
    Fourier pulsatility i.
    Fourmentin thoracic i.
    frontal horn i. (FHI)
    Gosling pulsatility i.
    hemodynamic i.
    hepatic resistive artery i.
    hepatitis activity i.
    Hilgenreiner acetabular i.
    human blood i. (HBI)
    iliac i.
    Insall-Salvati i.
    International Prognostic I. (IPI)
    intervertebral disc i.
    ischemic i.
    lattice i.
    left ventricular end-diastolic volume
    i. (LVEDI)
    left ventricular end-systolic volume
    i. (LVESVI)
    left ventricular fractional shortening
    i.
    left ventricular mass i. (LVMI)
    left ventricular stroke work i.
    (LVSWI)
    lithogenic i.
    lumbar vertebral body i.
    maturation i.

mean ankle-brachial systolic pressure i.
mean wall motion score i.
Mengert i.
metacarpal i.
metastatic efficiency i.
migration i.
Miller i.
mitosis-karyorrhexis i. (MKI)
mitral flow velocity i.
myocardial infarct recovery i.
myocardial jeopardy i.
myocardial O₂ demand i.
Nakata i.
O₂ consumption i.
i. of exposure
i. of runoff resistance
i. of sensitivity
patellofemoral i.
penile-brachial pressure i. (PBPI)
perfusion i.
pipestemming of ankle-brachial i.
ponderal i.
portal vein congestion i.
positive cephalopelvic disproportion i.
postexercise i.
poststress ankle-arm Doppler i.
Pourcelot i.
predicted cardiac i.
profundal popliteal collateral i.
proliferative i.
pulmonary arterial resistance i.
pulmonary blood volume i. (PBVI)
pulmonary output i.
pulmonary vascular resistance i. (PVRI)
pulsatility i.
pyloric i.
qualitative i.
quantitative i.
quantum mottle i.
rectosigmoid i.
renal resistive i.
reproducibility i.
resistive i.
resting ankle-arm pressure i.
resting ankle pressure i. (RAPI)
retention i.
right and left ankle indices
right ventricular stroke work i. (RVSWI)
Ritchie i.
runoff resistance i.
saturation i.
scoliosis i.
short-increment sensitivity i.
Singh osteoporosis i.

stroke volume i. (SVI)
stroke-work i. (SWI)
superomedial acetabular i. (SMAI)
systemic arteriolar resistance i.
systemic output i.
systemic vascular resistance i. (SvO₂, SVRI)
systolic pressure-time i.
systolic toe/brachial i.
talocalcaneal i.
tension-time i. (TTI)
therapeutic i.
thoracic i.
thymic i.
thymidine labeling i. (TLI)
tritiated thymidine labeling i.
truncated arch i.
tubular fertility i.
ulnar styloid process i. (USPI)
valgus i.
venous distensibility i. (VDI)
ventricular i.
vertebral body i.
wall motion score i.
water perfusable tissue i.
weighted computed tomography dose i.
weighted CT dose i.
widened anterior meningeal i.
Wood unit i.
indexes (*pl. of* index)
India ink artifact
Indian
 I. childhood cirrhosis
 I. file
Indiana pouch
indicator
 i. dilution curve
 i. dilution method for cardiac output measurement
 i. dilution method of perfusion assessment
 i. dilution therapy
 i. fractionation principle
 gamma ray level i.
 xylol pulse i.
indices (*pl. of* index)
indicis (*gen. of* index)
Indiclor
indifferent gonad
indigo
 i. calculus
 I. LaserOptic
 I. LaserOptic treatment system
indirect
 i. blood supply
 i. computed tomographic lymphography
 i. computed tomography

indirect (*continued*)
   i. CT (CT)
   i. fracture
   i. fulguration
   i. hernia sac
   i. inguinal hernia
   i. laryngoscopy
   i. MR arthrography
   i. MR arthrography of knee
   i. placentography
   i. ray
   i. ultrasound guidance
indirect-contact transmission
indiscernible
indiscrete
indiscriminate lesion
indistinct
   i. endometrial margin
   i. interface
indium (In)
   i. 111 (^{111}In, In-111)
   cistern i.
   i. imaging agent
   i. oxine
   tin with i. 113m
   i. transferrin
indium-111
   i.-111 capromab pendetide
   i.-111 leukocyte scan
   i.-111 pentetreotide
   i.-111 zevalin antibody scan
indium-111-labeled
   i.-111-l. human nonspecific
     immunoglobulin G
   i.-111-l. IgG
   i.-111-l. leukocyte
   i.-111-l. white blood cell scan
individualized functional status
  assessment
indocyanine
   i. dilution curve
   i. green angiography
   i. green dye
   i. green imaging agent
indoleamine
indolent
   i. lesion
   i. myeloma
   i. radiation-induced rectal ulcer
Indomitable scanner
induced
   i. acoustic emission
   i. biopotential
   chemically i.
   i. pneumothorax
   i. radioactivity
   i. thrombosis of aortic aneurysm
inducible basal state
inductance

inductance-capacitance
induction
   dorsal i.
   electric i.
   electromagnetic i.
   magnetic i.
   neuromuscular system electric i.
   ovulation i.
   i. therapy
inductively coupled plasma atomic
  emission spectrometry (ICP-AES)
inductive reactance
indurated
   i. mass
   i. tissue
indurativa
   tuberculosis cutis i.
indurative
   i. necrosis
   i. pleurisy
   i. pneumonia
indwelling
   i. cannula
   i. Foley catheter
   i. nonvascular shunt
   i. stent
inelastic pericardium
inequality
   limb-length i.
   ventilation-perfusion i.
inert dust pneumoconiosis
inexorable progression
infancy
   desmoplastic cerebral astrocytoma of
     i.
   melanotic neuroectodermal tumor of
     i. (MNTI)
infant
   i. cranial Doppler ultrasonography
   i. gastrointestinal hemorrhage
infantile
   i. arteriosclerosis
   i. cardiomyopathy
   i. coarctation
   i. coarctation of aorta
   i. cortical hyperostosis
   i. digital fibromatosis
   i. embryonal carcinoma
   i. fibrosarcoma
   i. ganglioglioma
   i. hemangioendothelioma
   i. hemangioendothelioma of liver
   i. hemiplegia
   i. hepatic hemangioma
   i. hydrocele
   i. hydrocephalus
   i. lobar emphysema
   i. myofibromatosis
   i. pneumonia

I

i. polycystic kidney disease
i. pylorospasm
i. thoracic dystrophy
i. tibia vara
i. uterus
infantile-onset leukodystrophy
infantilism
intestinal i.
infarct, infarction
acute ischemic brain i.
acute myocardial i.
acute nonhemorrhagic i.
acute renal i.
age-indeterminate i.
anemic i.
anterior communicating artery
  distribution i.
anterior septal myocardial i.
anterior wall myocardial i.
anteroinferior myocardial i.
anterolateral myocardial i.
anteroseptal myocardial i.
apical-lateral wall myocardial i.
apical myocardial i.
arrhythmic myocardial i.
atherothrombotic brain i.
atrial i.
basal ganglion i.
bicerebral i.
bilateral i.'s
bland i.
bone i.
bowel i.
brain i.
brainstem i.
capsular i.
capsulocaudate i.
capsuloputaminal i.
capsuloputaminocaudate i.
cardiac i.
cerebellar i.
cerebral i.
cerebral artery i.
chronic ischemic brain i.
chronic renal i.
concomitant i.
cortical bone i.
diaphragmatic myocardial i. (DMI)
diffuse multinodular i.
digital livedo reticularis i.
dominant hemisphere i.
dural sinus thrombosis i.
embolic cerebral i.
evolving myocardial i.
i. expansion
extensive anterior myocardial i.
frontal lobe i.
full-thickness i.
gyral i.

healing i.
hemispheric i.
hemorrhagic brain i.
high lateral wall myocardial i.
hippocampal i.
hyperacute ischemic brain i.
hyperacute myocardial i.
impending myocardial i.
inferior myocardial i. (IMI)
inferolateral wall myocardial i.
inferoposterior wall myocardial i.
inferoposterolateral myocardial i.
intestinal i.
ischemic brainstem i.
kidney i.
lacunar brain i.
lateral myocardial i.
lobar renal i.
lung i.
marrow i.
medullary bone i.
mesencephalic i.
mesenteric i.
middle cerebral artery i.
multifocal i.
multiple cortical i.'s
muscle i.
myocardial i. (MI)
nonarrhythmic myocardial i.
nonembolic i.
nonhemorrhagic i.
nonseptic embolic brain i.
nontransmural myocardial i.
occipital lobe i.
occipitoparietal i.
occlusive mesenteric i.
i. of pons
old myocardial i.
omental i.
papillary muscle i.
paramedian i.
parenchymatous i.
periventricular hemorrhagic i.
pituitary i.
placental i.
pontile i.
posterior cerebral territory i.
posterior wall myocardial i.
posterobasal wall myocardial i.
posteroinferior myocardial i.
posterolateral wall myocardial i.
postmyocardial i.
postmyocardiotomy i.
pulmonary i.
Q-wave myocardial i.
radiation-induced i.
red i.
renal i.
renal graft i.

infarct (*continued*)
    right ventricular i.
    rule out myocardial i. (ROMI)
    i. scan
    segmental bowel i.
    segmental omental i.
    septal myocardial i.
    septic pulmonary i.
    silent cerebral i.
    silent myocardial i. (SMI)
    sinuatrial node i.
    i. size limitation
    small bowel i.
    small, deep, recent i. (SDRI)
    spinal cord i.
    splenic i.
    subacute cerebral i.
    subacute ischemic brain i.
    subacute myocardial i.
    subcortical i.
    subendocardial i. (SEI)
    subendocardial myocardial i.
    temporal lobe i.
    testicular i.
    thalamic i.
    thromboembolic pontile i.
    thrombolysis in myocardial i.
      (TIMI)
    thrombotic i.
    transmural myocardial i.
    traumatic i.
    uncomplicated myocardial i.
    uninfected i.
    venous i.
    ventral pontile i.
    watershed brain i.
    wedge-shaped i.
    white matter i.
infarct-avid imaging
infarcted
    i. heart muscle
    i. lung segment
    i. myocardium
    i. scar
    i. testis
infarction (*var. of* infarct)
    Freiberg i.
infarct-localized asynergy
infarct-related artery
infected
    i. aneurysm
    i. bone
    i. extracavitary graft
    i. pelvic hematoma
    i. thrombosed graft
infection
    actinomycotic i.
    acute varicella i.
    alveolar i.

    anaerobic bacterial i.
    aortic graft i.
    brain i.
    buccal space i.
    Campylobacter i.
    cardiovascular i.
    central nervous system i.
    Coccidioides i.
    concomitant i.
    Cytomegalovirus i.
    deep-seated i.
    dental i.
    diffuse i.
    discovertebral i.
    disc space i.
    epidural i.
    extraaxial i.
    filarial i.
    fungous i.
    gram-negative rod i.
    Helicobacter i.
    hepatic fungal i.
    HIV pulmonary i.
    i. imaging
    intercurrent i.
    interstitial i.
    intraabdominal i.
    intracranial mycobacterial i.
    intracranial opportunistic i.
    intravascular catheter-related i.
    listerial i.
    masticator space i.
    mycotic lung i.
    nonpyogenic i.
    opportunistic lung cavity i.
    orbital i.
    paracytic i.
    parenchymatous i.
    pelvic i.
    periprosthetic i.
    pneumocystic i.
    postoperative i.
    pulmonary i.
    pulmonary parenchymatous i.
    pyogenic i.
    renal fungal i.
    respiratory tract i.
    retroperitoneal i.
    rickettsial lung i.
    sacroiliac i.
    salivary gland i.
    sinus i.
    skeletal i.
    spinal i.
    spirochete i.
    subdural i.
    subperiosteal i.
    superimposed fungal i.
    temporal space i.

tendon sheath space i.
tubercular bone i.
urinary tract i. (UTI)
vascular graft i.
vessel displacement brain i.

infection-related demyelination

infectious

i. aortitis
i. arthritis
i. bubbly bone lesion
i. cardiomyopathy
i. esophagitis
i. heart disease
i. pulmonary disorder
i. splenomegaly

infective

i. discitis
i. embolus
i. thrombosis

Infecton

I. imaging
I. scintigraphy
I. uptake

inferior

i. accessory fissure
i. alveolar nerve
apertura pelvis i.
apertura thoracis i.
i. aspect
i. beaking
i. border
i. border of heart
i. cardiac branch
i. cerebellar peduncle
i. colliculus
i. dental canal
i. displacement
i. dorsal radioulnar ligament
i. duodenal flexure (IDF)
i. duodenal recess
i. epigastric artery
i. esophageal sphincter (IES)
i. extensor retinaculum
fovea i.
i. frontal gyrus
i. gemellus muscle
i. glenohumeral ligament-labral
    complex (IGLLC)
i. jugular vein bulb
i. lobe
i. lobe bronchus
i. lobe of lung
i. longitudinal diameter
i. margin of superior rib
i. medial facet
i. mediastinum
i. mesenteric artery (IMA)
i. mesenteric plexus
i. mesenteric vein

i. myocardial infarct (IMI)
i. olive
i. ophthalmic vein
i. orbital fissure
i. parathyroid adenoma
i. parietal lobule
i. peroneal retinaculum
i. pole
i. pubic ramus
i. pulmonary ligament
i. pulmonary vein
i. quadriceps retinaculum
i. rectal vein
i. sagittal sinus (ISS)
i. spur
i. syndrome of red nucleus
i. temporal gyrus
i. temporal lobule
i. thyroid vein
i. tip of fibula
i. tip of scapula
i. transverse rectal fold
i. triangle sign
i. turbinate bone
i. vena cava (IVC)
i. vena cava diaphragm
i. vena cava duplication
i. vena cava filter
i. vena cava obstruction
i. vena cava orifice
i. vena cava syndrome
i. vena cava transposition
i. venacavogram (IVCV)
i. venacavography (IVCV)
i. wall
i. wall akinesis
i. wall branch
i. wall hypokinesis
i. wall MI
i. wall motion
zygapophysis i.

inferiormost

inferoanterior count ratio

inferoapical

i. aspect of myocardium
i. defect
i. segment
i. wall

inferobasal segment

inferolateral

i. displacement of apical beat
i. surface of prostate
i. wall myocardial infarct

inferolaterally

inferomedial

inferoposterior

i. segment
i. wall myocardial infarct

inferoposterolateral myocardial infarct

inferred presence
infestation
  helminthic i.
INFH
  ischemic necrosis of femoral head
infiltrate
  active i.
  acute alveolar i.
  aggressive interstitial i.
  aggressive perivascular i.
  alveolar i.
  apical i.
  Assmann tuberculous i.
  basilar zone i.
  benign i.
  bilateral interstitial pulmonary i.'s
  bilateral upper lobe cavitary i.'s
  bone marrow i.
  brachial plexus i.
  bronchocentric inflammatory i.
  butterfly pattern of i.
  calcareous i.
  calcium i.
  cavitary i.
  chronic alveolar i.
  circumscribed i.
  confluent i.
  consolidated i.
  diffuse aggressive polymorphous i.
  diffuse alveolar interstitial i.
  diffuse bilateral alveolar i.'s
  diffuse fatty liver i.
  diffuse perivascular i.
  diffuse reticulonodular i.
  eosinophilic i.
  epituberculous i.
  fatty i.
  fibrocavitary i.
  fibronodular i.
  fleeting lung i.
  fluffy i.
  focal alveolar i.
  focal interstitial i.
  focal perivascular i.
  granular i.
  ground-glass i.
  hazy i.
  interstitial nonlobar i.
  invasive angiomatous interstitial i.
  linear i.
  lingular i.
  lung base i.
  lymphoplasmacytic i.
  marrow i.
  massive i.
  meningeal i.
  micronodular i.
  migratory patchy i.
  mottled i.

  multifocal aggressive i.
  mural i.
  parasitic i.
  patchy migratory i.
  peribronchial i.
  pericapsular fat i.
  perihilar batwing i.
  peripheral i.
  perivascular i.
  pneumonic i.
  pulmonary i.
  pulmonary parenchymatous i.
  punctate i.
  recurrent fleeting i.
  reticular i.
  reticulonodular i.
  retrocardiac i.
  reverse peripheral batwing i.
  soft i.
  subcutaneous i.
  sulfasalazine-induced pulmonary i.
  transient symmetric pulmonary i.
  tuberculous i.
infiltrating
  i. adenocarcinoma
  i. breast epitheliosis
  i. ductal carcinoma
  i. esophageal carcinoma
  i. lesion
  i. lipoma
  i. lobular carcinoma
  i. plaque
infiltration
  blastic i.
  contrast i.
  dose i.
  marrow i.
  myocardial i.
  pathologic marrow i.
  i. pattern
  i. suture
infiltrative
  i. astrocytoma
  i. cardiomyopathy
  i. hemorrhagic element
  i. lymphoma
infinitesimal Z spectrum
inflamed
  i. bronchus
  i. pleura
inflammation
  abdominal i.
  acute phase of i.
  adhesive i.
  alveolar septal i.
  aortic i.
  atrophic i.
  bronchial i.
  bursal i.

calcaneal bursa i.
cardiac muscle i.
chemotherapy-induced i.
chronic abdominal i.
cirrhotic i.
diffuse i.
disseminated i.
esophageal i.
extrinsic intraabdominal i.
fibrinous i.
fibrosing i.
focal i.
hyperplastic i.
hypertrophic i.
interstitial i.
intrinsic intraabdominal i.
lung i.
meningeal i.
mucosal i.
myocardial i.
necrotic i.
obliterative i.
i. of bone
i. of brain
i. of colon
i. of epididymis
i. of heart
parenchymatous i.
pill-induced i.
polyarticular symmetric tophaceous
  joint i.
proliferative i.
pseudomembranous i.
radionuclide i.
renal i.
retrodiscal temporomandibular joint
  pad i.
sclerosing i.
spinal i.
spleen i.
subacute i.
suppurative i.
tendon i.
thyroid gland i.
transmural i.
tumor i.
vein i.
inflammatoria
dysphagia i.
inflammatory
i. adhesion
i. aortic aneurysm
i. bowel disease
i. bowel disease arthritis
i. breast cancer
i. breast carcinoma (IBC)
i. carotid pseudotumor
i. cholesteatoma
i. colonic polyp

i. edema
i. element
i. endometritis
i. esophagogastric polyp
i. fibroid polyp
i. fibrosarcoma
i. fibrosis
i. focus
i. fracture
i. heart block
i. hypersensitivity
i. idiopathic orbital pseudotumor
i. intestinal pseudotumor
i. joint effusion
i. lesion
i. MFH
i. myofibroblastic tumor
i. osteoarthritis
i. polyp in sinus
i. polypoid mass
i. reaction
i. spleen
i. stomach polyp
i. synovial process
inflation
air i.
balloon i.
delivered by balloon i.
sequential balloon i.
simultaneous balloon i.
inflicted injury
inflow
aortic i.
blood i.
i. cuff
i. disease progression
i. MRA
3rd i.
i. tract of left ventricle
inflow/outflow method
influence
paramagnetic i.
influenza (flu)
influenzae
Haemophilus i.
information
field-of-view i.
hierarchical i.
imaging-directed 3D volumetric i.
infraapical
infraaxillary
infracalcaneal bursitis
infracalcarine gyrus
infracardiac-type total anomalous venous return
infraclavicular
i. area
i. node
i. pocket

infraclusion, infraocclusion
infracolic
    i. compartment
    i. midline
infracostal
infracristal ventricular septal defect
infraction
    i. fracture
    Freiberg i.
infradiaphragmatic
    i. adenopathy
    i. application
    i. totally anomalous pulmonary
      venous drainage
    i. vein
**infragastric infragenicular popliteal
  artery**
infragenicular
    i. popliteal artery
    i. position
    i. revascularization
infrageniculate
infraglenoid
    i. recess
    i. tuberosity
infraglottic
    i. larynx
    i. space
infragluteal crease
infrahepatic
    i. arteriography
    i. inferior vena cava anastomosis
    i. vena cava
infrahilar area
infra-His block
infrahyoid lymph node
infrainguinal
    i. arterial bypass graft
    i. bypass stenosis
    i. DSA
    i. percutaneous transluminal
      angioplasty
    i. revascularization
    i. vein bypass graft
infralevator fistula
inframamillary
inframammary
    i. crease
    i. fold
inframesocolic space
infranuclear lesion
infraocclusion (*var. of* infraclusion)
infraorbital
    i. canal
    i. groove
    i. line
    i. margin (IOM)
    i. suture
infraorbitomeatal line (IOML)

infrapatellar
    i. aspect
    i. bursa
    i. contracture syndrome (IPCS)
    i. fat-pad
    i. ligament
    i. plica
    i. tendon
    i. view
infrapopliteal
    i. arterial disease
    i. artery occlusion
    i. vessel
infrapulmonary position
infrared
    i. camera
    high-resolution i. (HRI)
    i. imaging
    i. light
    i. light-emitting diode
    i. navigation system
    near i. (NIR)
    i. radiation
    i. ray
    i. spectrum
    i. thermography
infrarenal
    i. abdominal aorta
    i. abdominal aortic aneurysm
    i. stenosis
infraroentgen ray
infrascapular
infraspinatus
    i. insertion erosion
    i. muscle
    i. tendon
infraspinous
    i. fascia
    i. fossa
infrasternal
    i. angle
    i. fossa
infratemporal fossa
infratentorial
    i. compartment
    i. gray matter
    i. Lindau tumor
infraumbilical
    i. mound
    i. omphalocele
infravesical obstruction
infundibula (*pl. of* infundibulum)
infundibular
    i. atresia
    i. chamber
    i. pulmonary stenosis
    i. septum
    i. stalk
    i. subpulmonic stenosis

i. systolic-diastolic ratio
i. tilt
i. tumor
i. ventricular septal defect
infundibuloovarian ligament
infundibulopelvic ligament
infundibuloventricular crest
infundibulum, *pl.* **infundibula**
    bile duct i.
    cerebral i.
    ductus i.
    gallbladder i.
    hypothalamic i.
    junctional i.
    i. of bile duct
    i. of hypophysis
    i. of kidney
    os i.
    pituitary i.
    right ventricular i.
    tumor of i.
    i. widening
infundibulum-bulb ratio
Infuse-a-Port catheter
infuser
    IVAC P4000 i.
    Ohio i.
infusion
    arterial i.
    balloon-occluded arterial i.
    i. catheter
    circadian continuous i.
    continuous intravenous i. (CIVI)
    epidural saline i.
    graded i.
    hepatic arterial i. (HAI)
    intralymphatic i.
    intraportal i.
    intrathrombus i.
    intravenous i.
    isolated hepatic i.
    isoproterenol i.
    local streptokinase i.
    i. nephrotomography
    pericardial i.
    prostaglandin i.
    protective cold saline i.
    protracted venous i. (PVI)
    Pulse-Spray i.
    i. pyelogram
    i. pyelography
    regional intraarterial i.
    retrograde coronary sinus i.
    stepwise i.
    subcutaneous i.
    superselective i.
    systemic intravenous i.
    i. transcatheter therapy
    viral i.

infusothorax
Ingenor silicone mixture
ingrowth
    bone i.
    peripheral perimeniscal capillary i.
    porous i.
inguinal
    i. bladder herniation
    i. bulge
    i. canal
    i. crease
    i. floor
    i. fold
    i. granuloma
    i. hernia
    i. ligament
    i. ligament syndrome
    i. lymph node
    i. lymph node metastasis
    i. mass
    i. mesh prosthesis
    i. pseudoaneurysm
    i. ring
    i. triangle
    i. trigone
inguinale
    papilloma i.
inhalation
    i. anthrax
    i. bronchopneumonia
    i. disease
    end i.
    i. of krypton 77
    i. pneumonia
    radioactive xenon gas i.
    i. study
    i. technique
    tin oxide i.
    i. tuberculosis
inhaled
    i. oxygen imaging agent
    i. radionuclide
inherent
    i. density
    i. filter
inherited cavernous angioma-related
  posthemorrhage encephalomalacia
inhibition
    competitive i.
inhibitor
    efflux i.
    fusion i. (FI)
    nonnucleoside reverse transcriptase i.
    reverse transcriptase i.
    thrombin activatable fibrinolysis i.
    (TAFI)
inhibitory
    i. neurotransmitter
    i. syndrome

inhomogeneity
    contrast i.
    i. correction
    i. effect
    field i.
    hypointense signal i.
    metaphysial-diaphysial low signal
        intensity red marrow i.
    off-axis dose i.
    shim i.
    signal intensity i.
inhomogeneous
    i. attenuation
    i. contrast enhancement
    i. echo
    i. echo pattern
    i. echotexture
    i. image
    i. lung attenuation HRCT
    i. moderate enhancement
    i. perfusion
    i. tracer distribution
iniencephaly
inion bump
initial
    i. atelectasis
    i. imaging
initiative
    Clinical Outcomes Research I.
        (CORI)
injectable procoagulant mixture
injectate
injection
    accidental intradural i.
    air i.
    barium i.
    bismuth i.
    bolus intravenous i.
    coarse i.
    contrast i.
    Definity suspension for IV i.
    double i.
    epidural steroid i.
    ethanol i.
    extraarachnoid i.
    facet joint i.
    fine i.
    Fluorescite i.
    fluorodeoxyglucose F-18 i.
    Funduscein i.
    gaseous i.
    Glofil-125 i.
    hand i.
    heavy metal i.
    inadvertent arterial i.
    intraamnionic i.
    intraarterial i.
    intracavernosal i.
    intradermal i.

    intradiscal i.
    intramuscular fetal i.
    intraparenchymal i.
    intraperitoneal fetal i.
    intrathecal i.
    intratumoral 90Y glass microsphere
        i.
    intravascular i.
    intravenous bolus i.
    intravenous fetal i.
    iobenguane I-123 i.
    iodinated I-131 aggregated albumin
        i.
    ipsilateral i.
    kit for preparation of technetium
        depreotide i.
    i. leakage
    machine i.
    manual i.
    i. mass
    Miraluma i.
    multiphasic contrast i.
    Omnipaque i.
    opacifying i.
    paratumoral i.
    percutaneous ethanol i. (PEI)
    percutaneous ultrasound-guided
        thrombin i.
    perinephric air i.
    peritumoral i.
    i. port
    power i.
    prostaglandin E_1 i.
    radionuclide i.
    resting i.
    retrograde i.
    i. scan interval (ISI)
    sclerosing i.
    selective arterial i.
    serial i.'s
    silicone i.
    straight AP pelvic i.
    subarachnoid i.
    subareolar i.
    subcutaneous i.
    subdermal i.
    subdural contrast i.
    subureteric Teflon i. (STING)
    test i.
    transduodenal fiberscopic duct i.
    trigger point i.
    ultrasonographically guided i.
    ultrasound-guided methotrexate i.
    venous i.
injector
    Cordis i.
    double-power i.
    Envision CT power i.
    Hercules power i.

Injectron CT2 power i.
Mark V Plus automatic i.
Medrad automated power i.
Medrad contrast medium i.
Medrad power angiographic i.
MR-compatible power i.
Optistat power i.
power i.
pressure i.
Pulse-Spray i.
Renovist II i.
single-power i.
Spectris MR-compatible i.
Spectris power i.
Stellant dual-head i.
Taveras i.

Injectron CT2 power injector

injury

acute radiation i.
acute stretch i.
acute thoracic aortic i.
acute traumatic aortic i. (ATAI)
ankle inversion i.
anterior cruciate ligament i.
anterior urethral i.
aortic-brachiocephalic i.
apophysial i.
avulsion i.
axial compression i.
axial loading i.
ballistic i.
barked i.
bilateral incomplete ureteral i.'s
blunt i.
bony trabecular i.
brachial plexus birth i.
brainstem primary i.
brainstem secondary i.
burst i.
cervical cord i.
cervical spine i.
chronic ligamentous i.
closed head i. (CHI)
clothesline i.
cocking i.
2-column i.
3-column i.
compression-flexion i.
compressive hyperextension i.
concomitant tracheal i.
contrecoup i.
crush i.
decelerative i.
diffuse axonal i. (DAI)
diffuse white matter i.
distraction hyperflexion i.
duodenal i.
endothelial i.
epiphysial plate i.

Erb i.
Erb-Duchenne-Klumpke i.
excitotoxic cord i.
extension i.
extensive head i.
firearm i.
flake-shaped i.
flexion-distraction i.
flexion-extension i.
flexion-rotation i.
forced flexion i.
genitourinary i.
glenoid labrum i.
greater arc i.
growth plate i.
head i.
high-caliber low-velocity handgun i.
hollow viscus i.
hyperextension i.
hyperflexion-hyperextension cervical
  i.
hyperflexion-rotation i.
hypertension i.
hypoxic i.
iatrogenic ureteral i.
immunologic i.
inflicted i.
intercostal nerve i.
intraoperative gastrointestinal i.
intraperitoneal i.
inversion i.
irradiation i.
ischemic reperfusion i.
isolated airway i.
Klumpke brachial plexus i.
Kulkarni i.
labral i.
lateral bending i.
lateral compartment traumatic bony
  i.
lateral talar dome i.
lesser arc i.
lethal myocardial i.
Lisfranc i.
low back i.
Maisonneuve i.
matrix i.
mechanism of i.
medial talar dome i.
medial talar osteochondral i.
meniscal i.
metatarsal i.
midtarsal i.
mild head i.
mild traumatic brain i
motor vehicle i.
multifocal traumatic axonal i.
multiple recurrent inversion i.'s
muscle-crushing i.

injury (*continued*)
    myocardial reperfusion i.
    nerve i.
    nonaccidental i.
    nonlethal myocardial ischemic i.
    occult osseous i.
    osseous cervical spine i.
    osteochondral i.
    overuse i.
    penetrating head i.
    penetrating lung i.
    pericarinal i.
    perinatal i.
    peripheral nerve i.
    peroneal tendon i.
    phrenic nerve i.
    physial i.
    plexus i.
    posterior cruciate ligament i.
    posterior urethral i.
    posterolateral corner i.
    postnatal i.
    prenatal i.
    pronation-abduction i.
    pronation-external rotation i.
    proximity i.
    pulmonary parenchymatous i.
    radial vascular thermal i.
    radiation i.
    radiation-induced skin i.
    radiocontrast-induced i.
    rapid deceleration i.
    rectal radiation i.
    renal i.
    repetitive strain i. (RSI)
    repetitive stress i. (RSI)
    rotation-shearing i.
    Sage-Salvatore classification I-III of acromioclavicular joint i.
    scalp i.
    seatbelt i.
    sesamoid i.
    i. severity scale (ISS)
    i. severity score (ISS)
    shaken impact i.
    shear i.
    shearing white matter i.
    shear-type brain i.
    skier's i.
    softball sliding i.
    soft tissue i.
    solid viscus i.
    spinal cord i. (SCI)
    spinal nerve root i.
    straddle i.
    stress i.
    subendocardial i.
    superior labral anteroposterior i.
    supination-adduction i.
    supination-external rotation i.
    supination-outward rotation i.
    talar dome osteochondral i.
    talofibular ligament i.
    tensile i.
    through-and-through i.
    throwing arm i.
    tracheobronchial i. (TBI)
    transcutaneous crush i.
    traumatic aortic i. (TAI)
    traumatic brain i. (TBI)
    traumatic head i.
    ultrasonic assessment of i.
    unilateral locked facet i.
    urethral straddle i.
    valgus-external rotation i.
    vesical i.
    wafer-shaped i.
    weightbearing rotation i.
    whiplash i.
    white matter shearing i.
    windup i.

ink-blot image
inking the margin
^{111}In-labeled
    ^{111}In-l. human nonspecific immunoglobulin G
    ^{111}In-l. white blood cell
inlay graft
inlet
    esophageal i.
    pelvic i.
    i. position
    thoracic i.
    transaxial thoracic i.
inline low-pass filter
inner
    i. adrenal cortex
    i. bright layer
    i. ear
    i. ear anatomy
    i. ear atresia
    i. ear mass
    i. ear vestibule
    i. isoattenuated appearance
    i. stripe of Baillinger
    i. table
    i. table of frontal bone
    i. table of skull
    i. table thickening
innermost intercostal muscle
InnerVasc vascular access system
innervation
    sympathetic i.
Innerview GI
Innervision MR scanner
innocent gallstone
innocuous

innominate
    i. absence of line
    i. aneurysm
    i. angiography
    i. artery
    i. artery buckling
    i. artery compression syndrome
    i. artery kinking
    i. artery stenosis
    i. artery stenting
    i. bone
    i. canaliculus
    i. vein
inoperable brain tumor
inorganic phosphorus
^{111}In-oxime-labeled leukocyte
^{111}In pentetreotide scan
In-pentetreotide scintigraphy
in-phase
    i.-p. GRE imaging
    i.-p. sequence
    i.-p. T1-weighted image
in-plane
    i.-p. spatial resolution
    i.-p. vessel
InQwire guidewire
Insall ratio
Insall-Salvati
    I.-S. index
    I.-S. ratio
insertion
    anomalous i.
    Bosworth bone peg i.
    capsular i.
    catheter i.
    femoral vein percutaneous i.
    Harrington rod i.
    ligamentous i.
    percutaneous pin i.
    percutaneous tube i.
    sartorius i.
    tendinous i.
    velamentous i.
inside-out x-ray
inside-to-outside segmentation
InSightec
Insight Millennium scan
insipidus
    central diabetes i.
    nephrogenic diabetes i.
InSite Her-2/neu kit
insoluble
insonation
    angle of i.
    i. condition
    Doppler i.
    transforaminal i.
    transtemporal i.
insonifying wave field

Inspec-100
inspection
    surgical i.
    visual i.
inspiration
    i. and expiration views
    degree of i.
    shallow i.
    suspended i.
inspiratory
    i. effort
    i. flow
    i. flow rate
    i. gating
    i. increase in venous pressure
    i. muscle function impairment
    i. phase
    i. reserve volume (IRV)
    i. retraction
    i. spasm
    i. to expiratory
    i. view
inspiratory-to-expiratory ratio (I/E)
inspired air
inspissated
    i. feces
    i. material
    i. secretion
instability
    alveolar i.
    ankle i.
    anterolateral rotary knee i.
    articular i.
    atlantoaxial i. (AAI)
    atraumatic multidirectional bilateral
      radial i. (AMBRI)
    chronic functional i.
    degenerative spinal i.
    detrusor i.
    dissociative i.
    dorsal intercalated segmental i.
      (DISI)
    genomic i.
    glenohumeral i.
    hindfoot i.
    inversion i.
    ischemic i.
    joint i.
    lateral rotatory ankle i.
    ligamentous i.
    microsatellite i. (MSI)
    midcarpal i.
    nondissociative i.
    osseous i.
    phase i.
    posterolateral rotatory i.
    postlaminectomy i.
    rotary ankle i.
    rotational i.

instability (*continued*)
  rotatory i.
  shoulder joint i.
  sonographic measurement of subtalar
    joint i.
  spinal i.
  1st ray i.
  subtalar i.
  sympathetic vascular i.
  truncal i.
  varus-valgus i.
  ventricular electrical i.
  volar-flexed intercalated segment i.
  volar intercalated segment i.
    (VISI)
instantaneous
  i. axis of rotation (IAR)
  i. enhancement rate
  i. gradient
InstaScan scanner
in-stent
  i.-s. diameter
  i.-s. lumen
  i.-s. restenosis
  i.-s. stenosis
instillation
  contrast material i.
  percutaneous ethanol i.
  subarachnoid i.
institute
  National Heart, Lung, and
    Blood I.
instrument
  Bard Monoply reusable core
    biopsy i.
  FlashPoint image-guided
    surgical i.
  ionization i.
  Magnum biopsy i.
  i. output
  Sabourand-Noiré i.
  single-headed i.
  United States Catheter and I.
    (USCI)
instrumentation
  advanced breast biopsy i. (ABBI)
  interspinous segmental spinal i.
    (ISSI)
  long-term venous i.
  RealHand i.
insufficiency
  acute cerebrovascular i.
  adrenal i.
  aortic valvular i.
  arterial i.
  autonomic i.
  basilar artery i.
  brachial-basilar i.
  cardiac i.

  cardiopulmonary i.
  cerebrovascular i.
  chronic venous i.
  congenital pulmonary valve i.
  congenital valvular i.
  coronary i.
  deep venous i. (DVI)
  i. fracture
  gastric i.
  hepatic i.
  hypostatic pulmonary i.
  ileocecal i.
  mesenteric vascular i.
  mitral i. (MIS)
  muscular i.
  myocardial i.
  nonocclusive mesenteric arterial i.
  nonrheumatic aortic i.
  pad sign of aortic i.
  parathyroid i.
  postirradiation vascular i.
  posttraumatic pulmonary i.
  primary adrenal i.
  pulmonary i.
  pulmonary arterial flow i.
  pulmonary valve i.
  pyloric i.
  renal i.
  respiratory i.
  rheumatic aortic i.
  secondary venous i.
  Sternberg myocardial i.
  subchondral i.
  thyroid i.
  transient ischemic carotid i.
  tricuspid i.
  uterine i.
  uteroplacental i.
  valvular aortic i.
  vascular i.
  velopharyngeal i.
  venous i.
  vertebrobasilar i. (VBI)
insufficient
  i. acoustic penetration
  i. cochlear turn
  i. venous opacification
insufflation
  air i.
  CO_2 i.
  gas i.
  mechanical i.
  perirenal i.
  retroperitoneal gas i.
  tubal i.
insufflator
  ProtoCO$_2$l automated CO_2 i.
insula, *pl.* **insulae**
insulae (*pl. of* insula)

insular
- i. gyrus
- i. lobe
- i. region
- i. region of brain
- i. ribbon sign
- i. segment of middle cerebral artery
- i. triangle

insulinase

insulin-iodine

insulinoma

insult
- aortic i.
- bihemispheral i.
- cerebrovascular i.
- hypoxic-ischemic i.
- mechanical i.
- myocardial i.
- notable cerebral i.
- occlusive cerebrovascular i.
- thermal i.
- vascular i.

Insyte Autoguard shielded IV catheter

intact
- i. valve cusp
- i. ventricular septum

intake
- fluid i.

integral
- Choquet fuzzy i.
- i. dose
- systolic velocity-time i.
- time-velocity i.
- i. uniformity scintillation camera

integrated
- i. clinical information system (ICIS)
- i. CT scanner
- i. fMRI
- i. functional magnetic resonance imaging
- i. optical density (IOD)
- i. optical density histogram
- i. parallel acquisition technique (iPAT)
- i. reference air Kerma (IRAK)

integration
- time delay i. (TDI)

Integrilin

Integris
- I. 3D RA
- I. III-V DSA system
- I. 3000 scanner
- I. V3000 DDSA
- I. V3000 digital subtraction system
- I. V3000 imager

integrity
- spinal i.

Intelect Legend Combo stimulator and ultrasound unit

intense uptake

intensification
- i. factor
- frequency i.
- image i.

intensified radiographic imaging system (IRIS)

intensifier
- image i.
- portable C-arm i.

intensifying
- i. screen
- i. screen artifact

intensity
- absolute dose i. (ADI)
- amorphous high signal i.
- beam i.
- bright signal i.
- calcified sequestra of low signal i.
- central fat signal i.
- central intrasubstance signal i.
- dark signal i.
- decreased i.
- diminished marrow signal i.
- discrete hyperintense signal i.
- drug dose i.
- equal in i.
- fat signal i.
- fusiform high signal i.
- heterogeneous signal i.
- high-grade signal i.
- high signal i.
- high signal i.
- homogeneous signal i.
- increase in i.
- intermediate signal i.
- internodular difference in signal i. (IDSI)
- intrameniscal signal i.
- intravascular signal i.
- juxtaarticular low signal i.
- linear degenerative signal i.
- linear high signal i.
- low signal i.
- luminous i.
- marrow fat signal i.
- maximum i.
- nuclear magnetic resonance signal i.
- ovoid high signal i.
- pedicle signal i.
- photostimulable luminescence i.
- radiant i.
- radiation i.
- reduced signal i.
- relative dose i.
- reverse pattern of signal i.
- scene i.
- signal i. (grade 1-3)
- single-photon maximum i.

intensity (*continued*)
site of maximum i.
spatial average-pulse average i.
spatial average-temporal average i.
spatial peak-temporal average i.
symmetric confluent high
 signal i.
temporal average i.
temporal peak i.
time to peak i.
variable i.
vertebral body marrow signal i.
waterlike signal i.
i. windowing
intensity-modulated
i.-m. arc therapy
i.-m. photon beam
i.-m. radiation therapy (IMRT)
i.-m. radiotherapy
i.-m. radiotherapy treatment
 (IMRT)
intentional reversible thrombosis
interaction
capacitive i.
Compton i.
dipolar i.
dipole-dipole i.
effector-target cell i.
electric i.
magnetic i.
mind-body i.
photoelectric i.
proton dipole-dipole i.
interactive
i. electronic scalpel
i. gradient optimization
i. MR-guided biopsy
i. triangulation
interaorticobronchial diverticulum
interapophysial joint
interarch distance
interarticular
i. cartilage
i. disc
i. ridge
interarticularis
pars i.
interatrial
i. baffle leak
i. communication
i. groove
i. septal defect
i. septal hypertrophy
i. septum (IAS)
i. transposition of venous return
interbody
i. bone graft
i. bone plug
i. fusion

interbronchial
i. angle
i. diverticulum
i. mass
intercalary defect
intercalated segment
intercalating agent
intercalation
intercapital ligament
intercarpal
i. angle
i. articulation
i. coalition
i. joint
i. ligament
intercartilaginous rim
intercaudate distance
intercaval band
intercavernous
i. anastomosis
i. sinus
intercellular
i. edema
i. space
intercept
I. esophagus microcoil
I. prostate microcoil
I. urethra microcoil
I. vascular internal MR
 coil
intercervical disc herniation
interchondral joint
interchordal space fenestration
interclavicular
i. ligament
i. notch
interclinoid ligament
intercollicular groove
intercomparison
i. measurement
i. measurement technique
intercondylar, intercondylic,
 intercondyloid
i. eminence
i. femoral fracture
i. groove
i. humeral fracture
i. joint space
i. notch
i. process
i. roof
i. sagittal image
i. tibial fracture
i. tubercle
intercondylic (*var. of* intercondylar)
intercondyloid (*var. of*
 intercondylar)
intercornual ligament
intercoronary collateral flow

intercostal
    i. artery
    i. artery angiography
    i. lymph node
    i. muscle
    i. nerve
    i. nerve block
    i. nerve injury
    i. neuromuscular bundle
    i. retraction (ICR)
    i. space
    i. vein
    i. vessel
intercostobrachial nerve
intercristal diameter
intercuneiform ligament
intercurrent infection
interdigital
    i. clavus
    i. ligament
    i. neoplasia
    i. neuroma
interdigitation
    cerebral gyri i.
    i. of vastus lateralis
interecho
    i. spacing
    i. time
interest
    region of i. (ROI)
    volume of i. (VOI)
interface
    acetabular-prosthetic i.
    acoustic i.
    air i.
    air-soft tissue i.
    bidirectional i.
    body i.
    bone-air i.
    bone-implant i.
    brain-computer i. (BCI)
    catheter-skin i.
    common gateway i. (CGI)
    dermal-subcutaneous fat i.
    disc-thecal sac i.
    fat-blood i. (FBI)
    fat-fluid density i.
    fat-water i.
    fluid i.
    gray-to-white matter i.
    indistinct i.
    joint i.
    lumen-intima i.
    lung-mediastinum i.
    magnetic resonance user i.
      (MRUI)
    media-adventitia i.
    muscle-fat i.
    paraspinal i.

    reactive i.
    shear i.
    i. sign
    socket-stump i.
    tissue-air i.
    transducer-skin i.
interfacetal dislocation
interfacial canal
interference
    i. dissociation
    electromagnetic i. (EMI)
    i. phenomenon
    i. screw
    slice i.
interferential current therapy
interferometric synthetic aperture
  microscopy (ISAM)
interferometry
    phase-shifting i.
interferon regulatory factor
interfibrosis
interfollicular Hodgkin disease
interfoveolar ligament
interfraction interval
interfragmental compression
interfragmentary plate
intergluteal cleft
interhaustral septum
interhemispheric
    i. asymmetry
    i. cyst
    i. extraaxial hemorrhage
    i. fissure (IHF)
    i. pathway
    i. subdural hematoma
    i. transfer
interictal
    i. brain SPECT
    i. normalization
    i. PET FDG study
    i. phase
    i. SPECT scan
    i. SPECT study
    i. spiking
interiliac
    i. lymph node
    i. plane
interinnominoabdominal cleft
interlacing
interlaminar distance
interleaved
    i. axial slab
    i. BOLD-fMRI scanning
    i. GRE sequence
    i. image acquisition
    i. imaging pass
    i. inversion readout segment
    i. k-space coverage
    i. phase-contrast technique

interligamentous bursa
interlobar
    i. artery
    i. empyema
    i. fissure
    i. pleurisy
    i. septal line
    i. septum
    i. space
interlobular
    i. bile duct
    i. emphysema
    i. lung septum
    i. septal thickening
    i. tissue
    i. vasculature
    i. vessel
interlocking detachable coil (IDC)
interloop abscess
intermaxillary
    i. bone
    i. spine
    i. suture
intermedia
    beta-thalassemia i.
intermediate
    i. bronchus
    i. bursa
    i. callus
    i. coronary artery
    i. coronary syndrome
    i. CT slice
    i. cuneiform bone
    i. cuneiform fracture-dislocation
    i. fetal death
    i. heart
    i. image
    i. imaging
    i. nerve of Wrisberg
    i. ray
    i. signal intensity
    i. signal intensity layer
    i. signal-intensity mass
    i. signal striation
intermediolateral
    i. gray column
    i. tract
intermedius
    bronchus i.
    nervus i.
    vastus i.
intermesenteric
    i. abscess
    i. plexus
intermetacarpal articulation
intermetatarsal
    i. angle (IMA)
    i. bursitis
    i. joint

    i. ligament
    i. space
intermetatarsophalangeal
    i. bursa
    i. bursitis
intermittent
    i. claudication
    i. diffuse esophageal spasm
    i. obstruction
    i. occlusion
    i. 3rd-degree AV block
    i. sinus arrest
intermodality image registration
intermuscular
    i. hematoma
    i. septum
interna
    endometriosis i.
    hyperostosis frontalis i.
    theca i.
internae
    stria laminae granularis i.
    stria laminae pyramidalis i.
internal
    i. abdominal ring
    i. aberrant carotid artery
    i. and external rotation views
    i. architecture
    i. auditory canal
    i. auditory canal anatomy
    i. auditory canal enhancing lesion
    i. auditory meatus
    i. band
    i. biliary drainage
    i. biliary stent
    i. caliber
    i. capsule
    i. capsule intracerebral hemorrhage
    i. carotid
    i. carotid angiography
    i. carotid artery (ICA)
    i. carotid artery aneurysm
    i. carotid artery occlusion
    i. carotid balloon test
    i. carotid-posterior communicating (IC-PC)
    i. carotid-posterior communicating artery
    i. carotid system
    i. carotid systolic peak flow (ICSPF)
    i. cerebral vein (ICV)
    i. cervical os
    i. clot
    i. collateral ligament
    i. conjugate diameter
    i. conversion
    i. conversion electron
    i. cyclotron target

I

i. degeneration
i. derangement
i. derangement of knee (IDK)
i. disc herniation
i. echo
i. echogenicity
i. echotexture
i. enhancement
i. femoral rotation
i. fixation device
i. hernia
i. iliac artery
i. inguinal ring
i. intercostal muscle
i. intermuscular septum
i. jugular bulb
i. jugular triangle
i. jugular vein (IJV)
i. mammary artery (IMA)
i. mammary artery pedicle
i. mammary lymphatic chain
i. mammary lymph node
i. mammary lymphoscintigraphy
i. mammary node (IMN)
i. oblique aponeurosis
i. oblique radiograph
i. pudendal artery
i. pudendal vessel
i. radiation therapy
i. retention mechanism
i. rotation deformity
i. rotation in extension (IRE)
i. rotation in flexion (IRF)
i. table of calvaria
i. thoracic artery (ITA)
i. thoracic artery graft
i. thoracic vein
i. tibial torsion (ITT)
i. tibiofibular torsion
i. ureteral stent
i. urethral orifice
i. urethrotomy
internal/external catheter
internally fixed fracture
internasal suture
international
    I. Commission on Radiation Units (ICRU)
    I. Commission on Radiological Protection (ICRP)
    I. Electrotechnical Commission (IEC)
    I. Organization of Standardization (ISO)
    I. Prognostic Index (IPI)
    i. reference preparation
    i. standard
    I. System for staging lung cancer
internervous plane

internodular difference in signal intensity (IDSI)
internuclear distance
internus
    obturator i.
interobserver
    i. error
    i. variation
interopercular distance
interorbital distance
interossei
    plantar i.
interosseous
    i. border
    i. cyst
    i. membrane (IOM)
    i. muscle
    i. muscle group
    i. nerve
    i. ridge
    i. sacroiliac ligament
    i. space
    1st digital i. (FDI)
    i. talocalcaneal ligament
    i. tendon
interosseus
    dorsal i.
    palmar i.
interpalatine suture
interparietal
    i. bone
    i. suture
interpectoral lymph node
interpedicular (*var. of* interpediculate)
interpediculate, interpedicular
    i. distance
    i. distance widening
interpeduncular
    i. cistern (IPC)
    i. fossa
    i. notch
    i. space
interperiosteal fracture
interphalangeal (IP)
    i. articulation
    i. dislocation
    distal i. (DIP)
    i. fusion
    i. joint
    i. osteoarthritis
    proximal i. (PIP)
interpleural space
interpolation
    color space i.
    cubic convolution i.
    full scan with i.
    i. kernel
    linear i.
    object-based i.

interpolation (*continued*)
    prism i.
    scene-based i.
    sinc i.
    trilinear i.
    zero-fill i.
interpolator
    color space i.
    linear i.
Interpore bone replacement material
interposed
    i. colon segment
    i. colon segment obstruction
interpositi
    cavum veli i.
interposition
    colonic i.
    gastric i.
    i. graft
    hepatodiaphragmatic i.
    soft tissue i.
interpretation
    mirror-image i.
    radiographic i.
interpretive
    i. criterion
    i. variability
interpulse
    i. interval
    i. time
interpupillary line
interridge distance
interrogation
    color duplex i.
    deep Doppler velocity i.
    Doppler i.
    pulse Doppler i.
    radiation i.
interrupted
    i. duct sign
    i. periosteal reaction
interruption
    aortic arch i.
    bony cortex i.
    juxtahilar bronchus i.
    pulmonary artery i.
    surgical venous i.
intersacral canal
interscalene approach
interscan delay
interscapular gland
interscapulothoracic amputation
intersection gap
intersegmental
    i. aberration
    i. laminar fusion
    i. tract
intersesamoid ligament

intersex
    i. female
    true i.
intersigmoid recess
interslice
    i. distance
    i. gap
interspace
    ballooning of vertebral i.
    disc i.
    vertebral disc i.
    wedging of vertebral i.
Interspec Apogee RX400 diagnostic ultrasound system
intersperse
interspersed lucency
intersphincteric
    i. abscess
    i. anal fistula
    i. plane
interspinal, interspinous
    i. distance
    i. ligament
    i. muscle
    i. plane
    i. process
    i. process fusion
    i. widening
interspinous (*var. of* interspinal)
    i. segmental spinal instrumentation (ISSI)
interstice (*var. of* interstitium), *pl.* **interstices**
interstices (*pl. of* interstice)
interstitial
    i. abnormality
    i. absorption
    i. afterloading nylon tube
    i. atrophy
    i. boost
    i. brachytherapy
    i. calcinosis
    i. change
    i. conductive heating
    i. congestion of epididymis
    i. cystitis
    i. ectopic pregnancy
    i. fibrotic lung disease
    i. fluid
    i. fluid hydrostatic pressure
    i. fluid space
    i. heat-generating source
    i. hemorrhage
    i. hernia
    i. hyperthermia
    i. hyperthermia treatment
    i. infection
    i. inflammation
    i. intestinal emphysema

i. laser photocoagulation
i. loculated hematoma
i. low dose-rate iridium-192 needle implant
i. lung disease (ILD)
i. lung disease distribution
i. lung disease with increased lung volume
i. lung emphysema
i. lung pattern
i. marking
i. meniscal tear
i. nephritis
i. nodule
i. nodule HRCT
i. nonlobar infiltrate
i. opacity
i. organizing pneumonia
i. plasma cell pneumonia
i. pneumonia air leak
i. pneumonitis
i. prematurity fibrosis
i. probe
i. prominence
i. pulmonary edema
i. pulmonary fibrosis (IPF)
i. radiation
i. radiation source
i. radiation therapy
i. radioactive colloid therapy
i. radioelement application
i. radiosurgery
i. radiotherapy
i. radium therapy
i. salpingitis
i. scarring
i. shadowing
i. tear pattern
i. template irradiation
i. thickening
i. tissue
i. water proton

interstitium, interstice
alveolar i.
axial i.
bone i.
bronchovascular i.
centrilobar i.
graft i.
lung i.
parenchymatous i.
peripheral i.
pulmonary i.
renal i.
subpleural i.

intertarsal
interthalamica
interthalamic bridge

intertrabecular
i. hemorrhage
i. soft tissue

intertransverse
i. foramen
i. ligament
i. muscle

intertrochanteric
i. crest
i. 4-part fracture
i. plate
i. ridge

intertubercular
i. bursitis
i. diameter
i. groove
i. plane

intertumoral variability
intertwin membrane
interuncal distance
interureteric ridge
interval
acromiohumeral i. (AHI)
i. articulation
atlantoaxial i.
atlantodens i. (ADI)
basion axial i. (BAI)
basion dens i. (BDI)
i. change
confidence i.
i. development
i. ejection fraction
escape i.
high-rate detect i.
hypoplastic disc i.
i. improvement
injection scan i. (ISI)
interfraction i.
interpulse i.
i. intraatrial conduction
lucent i.
preejection i.
i. progression
prolonged i.
QRS i.
reconstruction i.
i. resolution
rotator i.
supracricoid i.
upper rate i.
ventriculoatrial i.

intervention
image-guided therapeutic i.
magnetic-assisted i. (MAI)
nonvascular i.
percutaneous nonvascular abdominal i.
percutaneous transluminal therapeutic i.
stage-matched i.

intervention (*continued*)
    i. study
    therapeutic i.
interventional
    i. angiography
    i. catheterization
    i. magnetic resonance imaging (I-MRI)
    i. neuroradiology
    i. procedure
    i. radiography
    i. radiology
    i. reference point (IRP)
    i. vascular angiogram
interventionalist
interventricular
    i. block
    i. foramen
    i. groove
    i. septal defect (IVSD)
    i. septal rupture
    i. septal thickness (IVST)
    i. septum
intervertebral
    i. cartilage calcification
    i. disc
    i. disc calcification
    i. disc index
    i. disc narrowing
    i. discogram
    i. disc space
    i. disc space height
    i. disc space uniformity
    i. foramen
    i. joint
    i. ligament
    i. notch
    i. osteochondrosis
intervertebralis
    symphysis i.
intervillous
    i. circulation
    i. lacuna
    i. placental thrombosis
interzone
intestinal
    i. atony
    i. Behçet syndrome
    i. bypass procedure
    i. calculus
    i. canal
    i. carcinoid tumor
    i. conduit
    i. contents
    i. decompression
    i. dilation
    i. distention
    i. diverticulum
    i. duplication

    i. duplication cyst
    i. emphysema
    i. fluid
    i. follicle
    i. gas
    i. gas exchange
    i. gas pattern
    i. hypoperistalsis syndrome
    i. infantilism
    i. infarct
    i. intussusception
    i. invagination
    i. ischemia
    i. kinking
    i. lipodystrophy
    i. loop
    i. lumen
    i. lymphangiectasis
    i. mesentery
    i. metaphysis
    i. metaplasia
    i. necrosis
    i. obstruction
    i. peptide TFF3
    i. perforation
    i. polyposis
    i. prolapse
    i. tract
    i. tract malrotation
    i. tube
    i. ulcer
    i. ureter
    i. villous architecture
    i. villus
    i. wall
    i. web
intestinalis
    pneumatosis cystoides i.
intestine
    blind i.
    bullous emphysema of i.
    coil of i.
    congenital lymphangiectasis of i.
    kink in i.
    large i.
    malrotation of i.
    papillary adenoma of large i.
    small i.
intima, *pl.* **intimae**
    arterial i.
    friable thickened degenerated i.
    hypertrophied i.
    pulmonary artery i.
    tunica i.
intimae (*pl. of* intima)
intimal
    i. arteriosclerosis
    i. atherosclerosis
    i. attachment of diseased vessel

i. debris
i. degeneration
i. fibroplasia
i. fibrosis
i. flap
i. hyperplasia
i. irregularity
i. medial dissection
i. proliferation
i. remodeling
i. tear
i. thickening
intimal-medial thickness (IMT)
intimate attachment
intraabdominal
i. abscess
i. arterial bypass graft
i. arterial hemorrhage
i. fat (IAF)
i. fetal calcification
i. infection
i. lymphadenopathy
i. mass
i. viscus
intraacetabular
intraacinar pulmonary artery
intraalveolar fibrosis
intraamnionic injection
intraaneurysmal
i. flow circulation
i. inflow pattern
i. outflow pattern
i. thrombus
intraaortic
i. balloon assist
i. balloon counterpulsation
i. balloon pump (IABP)
i. endovascular sonography
intraarterial
i. ABMMN cell transplant
i. chemotherapy
i. chemotherapy catheter
i. chemotherapy pump
i. digital subtraction angiography (IADSA)
i. filling defect
i. injection
i. secretin
i. stereotactic digital subtraction angiography
i. superselective nimodipine
i. therapy
i. thrombosis
i. thrombus
intraarticular
i. adhesion
i. calcaneal fracture
i. contrast
i. debris

i. gadolinium
i. ganglion
i. hemangioma
i. knee fusion
i. ligament
i. localized nodular synovitis
i. loose body
i. plate of fibrocartilage
i. proximal tibial fracture
i. radiopharmaceutical therapy
i. tumor
intraatrial
i. block
i. electrogram
i. filling defect
i. reentry
i. thrombus
intraauricular muscle
intraaxial
i. brain lesion
i. brain tumor
i. varix
Intrabeam intraoperative radiotherapy system
intracanalicular irradiation
intracapsular
i. ankylosis
i. fat-fluid level
i. fat-pad
i. femoral neck fracture
i. osteoid osteoma
intracardiac
i. calcification
i. calcium
i. echocardiography (ICE)
I. echocardiography IVUS catheter
i. electrogram
i. lead
i. mass
i. mixing
i. pressure
i. pressure waveform analysis
i. shunt
i. thrombus
i. tumor
intracartilaginous
i. bone
i. ossification
Intracath catheter
intracaval
i. endovascular ultrasonography (ICEUS)
i. endovascular ultrasound (ICEUS)
i. fat mass
intracavernosal injection
intracavernous internal carotid artery
intracavitary
i. afterloading applicator
i. application brachytherapy
i. clot formation

intracavitary (*continued*)
   i. delivery
   i. extension
   i. extension of tumor
   i. filling defect
   i. hyperthermia treatment
   i. implant
   i. irradiation
   i. radiation source
   i. radiation therapy
   i. radioactive colloid therapy
   i. radioelement application
   i. radiotherapy
   i. radium
intracavity mass
intracellular
   i. adhesion molecule
   i. water
intracerebral
   i. aneurysm
   i. arteriovenous malformation
   i. artery
   i. blood
   i. ganglioglioma
   i. ganglioma
   i. hematoma
   i. hemorrhage (ICH)
   i. lesion
   i. lymphoma
   i. thrombolysis
   i. tumor
   i. vascular malformation
intracerebroventricular (ICV)
intrachondral bone
intraclass correlation coefficient
IntraCoil
   I. endoprosthesis
   I. self-expanding peripheral
     stent
intracompartmental
   i. edema
   i. ischemia
   i. tumor
intraconal
   i. lesion
   i. portion of eye
intracondyloid
intracoronary
   i. artery radiation
   i. contrast echocardiography
   i. Doppler flow guidewire
   i. imaging
   i. radiation therapy (ICRT)
   i. stenting
   i. stent placement
   i. thrombolytic therapy
   i. ultrasound (ICUS)
intracorporeal liver

intracortical
   i. lesion
   i. osteosarcoma
intracranial
   i. air
   i. aneurysm (ICA)
   i. arteriovenous fistula
   i. arteriovenous malformation
   i. berry aneurysm
   i. carotid artery atherosclerosis
   i. cavernous angioma
   i. circulation
   i. cryptococcosis
   i. dermoid cyst
   i. electroencephalography
   i. embolus
   i. empyema
   i. ependymoma
   i. epidural pressure
   i. fat prolapse
   i. germinoma
   i. glioma
   i. hematoma
   i. hypertension
   i. imaging
   i. leptomeningeal vascular anomaly
   i. lipoma
   i. mass
   i. mass lesion
   i. metastasis
   i. MR angiography
   i. mycobacterial infection
   i. neoplasia
   i. neuroblastoma
   i. opportunistic infection
   i. physiologic calcification
   i. pneumatocele
   i. pneumocephalus
   i. pressure (ICP)
   i. pulse pressure
   i. saccular aneurysm
   i. seeding
   i. shift
   i. sinus thrombosis
   i. stenoocclusive disease
   i. structure
   i. subarachnoid hemorrhage
   i. tuberculoma
   i. tumor
   i. vascular abnormality
   i. vascular lesion
   i. vascular occlusion
   i. vertebral artery
   i. vessel
   i. volume
   i. width (ICW)
intractable
   i. bleeding disorder

i. heart failure
i. ulcer
intracystic
   i. bleeding
   i. breast carcinoma
   i. breast papillary carcinoma in situ
   i. solid mass
intracytoplasmic
intradecidual sign
intradermal, intradermic
   i. angioma
   i. injection
   i. neurilemoma
intradermic (*var. of* intradermal)
intradiaphragmatic aortic segment
intradiscal, intradiskal
   i. administration of gadolinium
      followed by MRI
   i. electrothermal therapy (IDET)
   i. injection
intradiskal (*var. of* intradiscal)
intraductal
   i. breast filling defect
   i. breast papillomatosis
   i. bridge
   i. calcification
   i. carcinoma (IDC)
   i. mucin-producing tumor
   i. papillary carcinoma
   i. papillary mucinous neoplasia (IPMN)
   i. papillary mucinous tumor (IPMT)
   i. papillary mucinous tumor of
      pancreas
   i. papilloma
   i. pressure
   i. solid mass
   i. ultrasonography
intraduodenal choledochal cyst
intradural
   i. abscess
   i. arachnoid cyst
   i. disc herniation
   i. epidermoidoma
   i. extramedullary lesion
   i. extramedullary mass
   i. extramedullary tumor
   i. hemorrhage
   i. intramedullary tumor
   i. lipoma
   i. nerve root
   i. retromedullary arteriovenous fistula
   i. rootlet
   i. spinal AVM
   i. vessel
intraforaminal vein
intragastric
   i. bubble
   i. placement

intraglandular calcified lithiasis
intragraft stenosis
intrahepatic
   i. abscess
   i. arterial-portal fistula
   i. atresia (IHA)
   i. AV fistula
   i. bile duct
   i. biliary atresia
   i. biliary calculus
   i. biliary carcinoma
   i. biliary cystic dilation
   i. biliary ductal dilation
   i. biliary neoplasia
   i. biliary stasis
   i. biliary tract
   i. biliary tract dilation
   i. biliary tree
   i. biloma
   i. cholangiocarcinoma
   i. cholestasis
   i. portal vein branch
   i. portal vein gas
   i. sclerosing cholangitis
   i. stone
   i. umbilical vein
intra-His block
intrahisian block
intralabyrinthine
intralaminar thalamus
intralesional chemotherapy
intraligamentary pregnancy
intraligamentous bursa
intralobar sequestration
intralobular
   i. connective tissue
   i. fibrosis
   i. interstitial thickening
   i. line
   i. terminal duct
intraluminal
   i. adenocarcinoma
   i. air
   i. attenuation decrease
   i. brachytherapy
   i. debris
   i. dephasing
   i. detail
   i. dilation
   i. dimension
   i. duodenal diverticulum (IDD)
   i. electrocoagulation
   i. embolus
   i. esophageal pressure
   i. filling defect
   i. foreign body
   i. gallstone
   i. hemorrhage

intraluminal (*continued*)
    i. intubation
    i. membrane
    i. plaque
    i. polymeric footplate
    i. polyp
    i. stomach mass
    i. stone
    i. thrombus
    i. ultrasound (ILUS)
    i. ultrasound catheter
intralymphatic
    i. infusion
    i. radioactivity administration
intramammary
    i. lesion
    i. lymph node
intramedullary (IM)
    i. arteriovenous malformation
    i. canal
    i. compartment neoplasia
    i. cord lesion
    i. demyelination
    i. ependymoma
    i. epidermoid cyst
    i. fixation
    i. fixation device
    i. lipoma
    i. marrow involvement
    i. mass
    i. nail
    i. osteosarcoma
    i. rodding
    i. skeletal kinetic distractor (ISKD)
    i. skeletal kinetic distractor system
    i. space-occupying lesion
    i. spinal cord metastasis
    i. spinal cord tumor
    i. spinal lesion
    i. tumor biopsy
intramembranous
    i. bone
    i. ossification
intrameniscal
    i. cyst
    i. mucoid degeneration
    i. signal intensity
intramesenteric abscess
intramural
    i. air in colon
    i. arterial hemorrhage
    i. clot
    i. colonic air
    i. coronary artery aneurysm
    i. diverticulum
    i. esophageal diverticulosis
    i. esophageal pseudodiverticulosis
    i. esophageal rupture
    i. fibroid

    i. filling defect
    i. gas
    i. gastric emphysema
    i. gastrointestinal tract hemorrhage
    i. hematoma (IMH)
    i. hematoma of aorta
    i. leiomyosarcoma
    i. mapping
    i. mechanics
    i. myoma
    i. portion of distal ureter
    i. rupture of esophagus
    i. thrombus
    i. tumor
    i. tunnel
intramural-extramucosal stomach lesion
intramuscular
    i. aortic segment
    i. fetal injection
    i. fluid pressure
    i. hemangioma
    i. hemosiderin deposit
    i. metastasis
    i. myxoma
    i. venous malformation
intramyocardial coronary blood flow
intranasal microbubble
intraneural ganglion cyst
intraneuronal neurofibrillary tangle
intranodal
    i. architecture
    i. block
    i. myofibroblastoma
in-transit
    i.-t. metastasis
    i.-t. node
intranuclear
    i. cleft
    i. discogram
intraobserver
    i. error
    i. variation
intraocular
    i. calcification
    i. foreign body
    i. lesion
    i. pressure
    i. spread
Intra-Op autotransfusion system
intraoperative
    i. arteriography
    i. cardioplegic contrast echocardiography
    i. cholangiogram
    i. cholangiography
    i. device
    i. digital subtraction (IDIS)
    i. digital subtraction angiography (IDSA)
    i. Doppler

i. electrocortical stimulation
i. electrocortical stimulation mapping
i. endoscopy
i. film
i. fracture
i. gamma probe
i. gastrointestinal injury
i. high dose rate (IOHDR)
i. imaging
i. laser photocoagulation
i. lymphatic mapping
i. MIBG scanning
i. pancreatography
i. radiation therapy
i. radiograph
i. radiography
i. radiolymphoscintigraphy
i. radiotherapy
i. red light therapy (IRLT)
i. scanning technique
i. sonography (IOS)
i. ultrasonography
i. ultrasound (IOUS)
i. ventriculogram
i. view
i. x-ray visualization

intraoral
i. cone irradiation
i. periapical radiography
i. projection
i. radiograph
i. radiology
i. radiotherapy

intraorbital air
intraosseous
i. abscess
i. arteriovenous malformation
i. bone lesion
i. desmoid tumor
i. edema
i. ganglion
i. hemophilic pseudotumor
i. keratin cyst
i. lipoma
i. loculation
i. low-grade osteosarcoma
i. meningioma
i. vascular malformation
i. venography
i. vessel
i. wiring

intrapancreatic obstruction
intrapapillary terminus
Intraparenchymal
i. bleed
i. blood
i. cyst
i. hematoma
i. hemorrhage

i. injection
i. lung tumor
i. lymph node
i. meningioma
i. metastasis
i. microvessel
i. tuberculoma

intrapatellar fat-pad
intrapedicular fixation
intrapericardial
i. bleeding
i. diaphragmatic hernia
i. patch lead placement
i. portion
i. pressure

intraperiosteal fracture
intraperitoneal
i. abscess
i. air
i. bladder rupture
i. cavity
i. drug administration
i. exposure
i. fetal injection
i. fluid
i. hyperthermic chemotherapy
i. hyperthermic perfusion (IPHP)
i. injury
i. lesion
i. pregnancy
i. rupture of bladder
i. technetium-sulfur colloid imaging
i. tumor
i. viscus

intrapixel sequential processing (IPSP)
intraplacental venous lake
intraplaque hemorrhage (IPH)
intrapleural
i. hemorrhage
i. pressure

intrapontine intracerebral hemorrhage
intraportal
i. endovascular ultrasonography
   (IPEUS)
i. infusion

intrapulmonary
i. arteriovenous fistula
i. baffle
i. barotrauma
i. bronchogenic cyst
i. bronchus
i. hemorrhage
i. lymph node (IPLN)
i. nodule
i. pressure
i. shunt

intrarectal
i. coil
i. ultrasound

intrarenal
- i. arterial flow
- i. collecting system
- i. hematoma
- i. pelvis
- i. reflux
- i. stenosis

intrarun realignment
intrasac
- i. flow
- i. spectral Doppler flow velocity

intrascapular ligament
intrascrotal
- i. abscess
- i. lesion

intrasellar
- i. brain mass
- i. lesion
- i. Rathke cleft cyst
- i. tumor

intrasinus air-fluid level
Intrasound
  Medtronic Pulsor I.
intraspinal
- i. adenoma
- i. dermoid cyst
- i. enteric cyst
- i. epidermoid cyst
- i. lesion
- i. neurenteric cyst
- i. tumor

intrasplenic
- i. nodule
- i. tissue

intraspongy nuclear disc herniation
IntraStent
- I. DoubleStrut biliary stent
- I. DoubleStrut ParaMount XS premounted stent biliary system
- I. DS, LD, LP balloon-expanded stent

intrasubstance cleavage tear
intraswallowing aspiration
intrasynaptic space
intrasynovial disease
intratemporal fossa
intratendinous
- i. bursa
- i. fluid collection
- i. rupture

intratendon sheath
intratentorial lipoma
intratesticular
- i. band
- i. cyst

intrathecal (IT)
- i. drop metastasis
- i. hemorrhage
- i. imaging

- i. injection
- i. lipoma
- i. root
- i. space

intrathoracic
- i. catheter drainage
- i. cyst
- i. dimension
- i. dislocation of shoulder
- i. fetal mass
- i. goiter
- i. Kaposi sarcoma
- i. low-attenuation mass
- i. pressure
- i. stomach
- i. thyroid
- i. trachea
- i. upper airway obstruction

intrathrombus infusion
intrathymic parathyroid adenoma
intrathyroid superior parathyroid adenoma
intratracheal
intratumoral
- i. accumulation
- i. agent
- i. calcification
- i. cyst
- i. hemorrhage
- i. necrosis
- i. structure
- i. variability
- i. 90Y glass microsphere injection

intrauterine
- i. cardiac failure
- i. demise
- i. device (IUD)
- i. fetus
- i. fracture
- i. gas (IUG)
- i. gestation
- i. growth restriction
- i. growth retardation (IUGR)
- i. heart failure
- i. membrane
- i. pregnancy (IUP)
- i. sac

intravaginal
- i. radiotherapy
- i. torsion

intravasation
  venous i.
intravascular
- i. angiogenesis gene delivery
- i. catheter-related infection
- i. clotting process
- i. coil
- i. congestion
- i. consumption coagulopathy

I

i. contents
i. contents extravasation
i. contrast-enhanced computed tomography
i. contrast-enhanced CT (CT)
i. contrast medium
i. filling defect
i. foreign body
i. injection
i. leiomyosarcoma
i. mass
i. MRI
i. MRI catheter-based technique
i. pacemaker
i. papillary endothelial hyperplasia
i. radiopharmaceutical therapy
i. sickling
i. signal intensity
i. space
i. stent
i. stent artifact
i. stenting
i. thrombosis
i. tumor thrombus
i. ultrasound (IVUS)
i. ultrasound catheter
i. ultrasound imaging
i. volume depletion

intravenous (IV)
i. access
i. accurate control (IVAC)
i. administration of contrast material
i. angiocardiography
i. aortography
i. block
i. bolus
i. bolus injection
i. cholangiogram (IVC)
i. cholangiography
i. cholecystography
i. contrast medium
i. digital subtraction angiography (IVDSA)
i. fetal injection
i. fluorescein angiography (IVFA)
i. fluorescein angiography imaging
i. infusion
i. infusion line
i. injection of isotope
i. microbubble contrast agent
i. pyelogram (IVP)
i. pyelography (IVP)
i. renal angiography
i. stereotactic digital subtraction angiography
i. urography (IVU)

intravenously
i. enhanced CT scan
i. enhanced MRI

intraventricular
i. aberration
i. blood
i. brain tumor
i. conduction block
i. conduction delay
i. cryptococcal cyst
i. heart block
i. hematoma
i. hemorrhage (IVH)
i. mass
i. meningioma
i. neonate hemorrhage
i. neoplasm
i. neuroblastoma
i. neurocytoma
i. obstruction
i. obstructive hydrocephalus
i. systolic tension
i. thrombus

intravertebral
i. body vacuum cleft
i. vacuum cleft sign

intravesical
i. obstruction
i. stone
i. ureter

intravital ultraviolet
intravoxel
i. coherent motion
i. dephasing
i. incoherent motion (IVIM)
i. phase dispersion

intrinsic
i. cellular parameter
i. compression
i. deflection
i. efficiency
i. energy resolution
i. factor
i. field uniformity
i. field uniformity test
i. filling defect
i. flood
i. foot muscle
i. intraabdominal inflammation
i. ligament
i. minus deformity
i. minus hallux
i. plus deformity
i. spatial linearity
i. stenotic lesion
i. stomach wall lesion
i. vein graft stenosis

introducer
Desilets-Hoffman i.
endhole i.
Flexor i.
Tuohy-Borst i.

introduction
single-stick catheter i.
Intropaque
intubated small bowel series
intubation
endotracheal i.
esophagogastric i.
intraluminal i.
nasal i.
nasogastric i.
nasotracheal i.
oral i.
orotracheal i.
intussusception
appendiceal i.
bowel i.
colocolic i.
ileocolic i.
ileoileal i.
intestinal i.
jejunoduodenogastric i.
jejunogastric i.
pneumatic reduction of i.
rectal i.
rectorectal i.
retrograde jejunoduodenogastric i.
stomal i.
transient i.
vein i.
venous i.
intussusceptum
intussuscipiens
Inutest
invagination
basilar i.
intestinal i.
i. of skull base
transient i.
invasion
arterial i.
blood vessel i.
capillary lymphatic space i.
capsular i.
deep myometrial i.
early stromal i.
exogenous i.
extracapsular i.
lymphatic vessel i.
mediastinal i.
neoplastic i.
occipital condyle i.
perineural i.
seminal vesicle i. (SVI)
transmural i.
tumoral i.
vascular i.
invasive
i. angiomatous interstitial infiltrate
i. assessment

i. breast carcinoma
i. ductal carcinoma
i. lesion
i. lobular carcinoma
i. malignant sheath tumor
i. papillomatosis
i. pulmonary aspergillosis (IPA)
i. radiologic vascular procedure
i. surgical staging
i. thermometry
inverse
i. cerebellum
i. comma appearance
i. follicle
i. follicle pattern
i. Fourier transform (IFT)
i. inspiratory-expiratory time ratio
i. radiotherapy technique
i. symmetry
inversion
i. ankle stress view
cardiac i.
frequency-selective i.
gray-scale i.
i. injury
i. injury of ankle
i. instability
isolated ventricular i.
magnetic i.
i. position
i. pulse
i. recovery (IR)
i. recovery echo-planar imaging
(IR-EPI)
i. recovery image
i. recovery spin echo (IRSE)
i. recovery spin-echo sequence
i. recovery technique
i. recovery-weighted image
selective population i. (SPI)
i. sprain
terminal i.
i. time (TI)
torcular-lambdoid i.
i. transfer
ventricular i.
inversion-eversion
inversum
duodenum i.
inversus
abdominal situs i.
cardiac situs i.
complete situs i.
situs i.
inverted
i. left atrial appendage
i. Meckel diverticulum
i. Napoleon hat sign
i. papilloma

I

i. pelvis
i. teardrop sign
i. umbrella defect
inverted-T
    i.-T appearance
    i.-T appearance of mainstem
    bronchus
inverted-V sign
inverted-Y
    i.-Y block
    i.-Y complex
    i.-Y configuration
    i.-Y field irradiation
    i.-Y field radiotherapy
    i.-Y fracture
investing fascia
invisible
    i. light
    i. main pulmonary artery
    i. spectrum
involucra (*pl. of* involucrum)
involucre (*var. of* involucrum)
involucrum, involucre, *pl.* **involucra**
involuting fibroadenoma
involution
    follicular i.
    i. of duct
    spontaneous i.
involutional breast calcification
involved field
involved-field irradiation
involved-region irradiation
involvement
    arcuate fiber i.
    axillary node i.
    contiguous organ i.
    cranial nerve i.
    extramedullary i.
    intramedullary marrow i.
    lymph node i.
    metastatic axillary i.
    pagetoid epidermal i.
    supraclavicular node i.
    thalamotegmental i.
INVOS
    in vivo optical spectroscopy
    INVOS 3100, 3100A cerebral
      oximeter monitoring system
    INVOS 2100 optical
      spectroscopy
inwardly displaced calcification
iobenguane I-123 injection
iobenzamic acid
iobitridol imaging agent
iocarmate meglumine
iocarmic acid
iocetamic
    i. acid
    i. acid imaging agent

IOCM
    isosmolar contrast medium
IOD
    integrated optical density
iodamine imaging agent
iodide
    casium i. (CsI)
    i. contrast medium
    i. goiter
    potassium i.
    propidium i.
    silver i.
    sodium i. (NaI)
    thallium-activated sodium i.
    i. transport
iodinated
    i. CM-induced cardiac depression
    i. contrast material
    i. contrast material-induced cardiac
    depression
    i. human serum albumin
    (IHSA)
    i. I-131 aggregated albumin
    i. I-131 aggregated albumin
    injection
    i. I-125 fibrinogen
    i. imaging agent
    i. intravascular CM
    i. intravascular contrast
    medium
    i. I-125 serum albumin
    i. I-131 serum albumin
    i. nanoparticle
    i. radiologic contrast medium
    (IRCM)
    i. tyrosine group
iodination
iodine (I)
    i. 111 (^{111}I, I-111)
    i. 123 (^{123}I, I-123)
    i. 125 (^{125}I, I-125)
    i. 127 (^{127}I, I-127)
    i. 131 (^{131}I, I-131)
    i. 132 (^{132}I, I-132)
    i. 192 (^{192}I, I-192)
    i. allergy
    butanol-extractable i. (BEI)
    i. dose
    i. fluorescence imaging
    free i.
    ^{131}I radioactive i.
    ^{132}I radioactive i.
    i. load
    protein-bound i. (PBI)
    radioactive i.
    i. radioactive source
    i. scintigraphy
    thyroxine i. (TI)
    i. uptake

iodine-123
    i.-123 iodomethyltyrosine (I-123 IMT)
    i.-123 iodophenyl pentadecanoic acid (^{123}I-IPPA, I-123 IPPA)
    i.-123 metaiodobenzylguanidine (I-123 MIBG)
    i.-123 MIBG radioactive imaging agent
    i.-123 orthoiodohippurate
    i.-123 thyroid
iodine-131
    i.-131 antiferritin treatment
    i.-131 isotope
    i.-131 metaiodobenzylguanidine
    i.-131 MIBG radioactive imaging agent
    i.-131OIH
    i.-131 orthoiodohippurate
    i.-131 outcome analysis
    sodium iodide i.-131
    i.-131 triolein
    i.-131 whole-body scan
    i.-131 whole-body scintigraphy
iodine-containing contrast medium
iodine-deficiency goiter
iodine-131-induced cellulitis
iodine-125-labeled fragment
iodine-labeled product
iodine-particle ratio
iodipamide
    i. ethyl ester
    i. meglumine
    i. meglumine imaging agent
    i. methylglucamine
iodixanol contrast medium
iodized
    i. oil imaging agent
    i. oil study
    i. poppy seed oil
iodoalphionic acid
iodoamphetamine
    ^{123}I isopropyl i.
iodobenzamide
iodocholesterol
iodocyanine green (ICG)
iododeoxyuridine (IUdR)
    i. labeling
5-iodo-2-deoxyuridine imaging agent
Iodo-gen imaging agent
iodohippurate
    i. sodium
    i. sodium imaging agent
iodomethamate
iodomethyl-norcholesterol-59 scintigraphy
iodomethyl-norcholesterol scintigraphy imaging
iodomethyltyrosine (IMT)
    iodine-123 i. (I-123 IMT)

iodopanoic acid
iodophendylate contrast medium
iodophenyl pentadecanoic acid
Iodotope imaging agent
iodovinylestradiol
iodoxamate meglumine
ioglunide contrast medium
ioglycamic
    i. acid
    i. acid contrast medium
ioglycamide
IOHDR
    intraoperative high dose rate
    IOHDR brachytherapy
iohexol
    i. CT ventriculogram
    i. imaging agent
IOM
    infraorbital margin
    interosseous membrane
iomeprol
Iomeron 150, 250, 300, 350 contrast medium
IOML
    infraorbitomeatal line
ion
    amphoteric dipolar i.
    calcium i.
    i. chamber
    i. IntraOperative navigation system
    i. pump
ion-bound water
ion-exchange chromatography
ionic
    i. binding
    i. contrast agent
    i. dimer contrast medium
    i. hexaiodinated dimer
    i. monomer
    i. monomeric contrast medium
    i. paramagnetic contrast medium
    i. paramagnetic imaging agent
    i. polar valence
    i. potassium
ionization
    i. chamber
    i. counter
    i. current
    i. density
    i. detector
    i. instrument
    i. potential
    i. radiation
    i. track
ionized atom
ionizing
    i. radiation
    i. radiation exposure
ionograph

ionography
iopamidol imaging agent
Iopamiron 310, 370 imaging agent
iopanoic
    i. acid
    i. acid imaging agent
iopentol nonionic imaging agent
iophendylate
    i. imaging agent
    i. oil
iophenoxic acid
iopromide
    i. contrast medium
    i. nonionic imaging agent
iopydol
IOS
    intraoperative sonography
iosefamic acid imaging agent
iothalamate
    i. meglumine imaging agent
    i. sodium
    i. sodium imaging agent
iothalamic acid
iotrol (*var. of* iotrolan)
iotrolan, iotrol
iotroxamide contrast medium
iotroxic acid imaging agent
IOUS
    intraoperative ultrasound
ioversol imaging agent
ioxaglate
    i. meglumine
    i. meglumine imaging agent
    i. sodium
    i. sodium imaging agent
ioxaglic
    i. acid
    i. acid contrast medium
ioxilan imaging agent
ioxithalamate contrast medium
ioxithalamic acid contrast agent
IP
    interphalangeal
        IP joint
        IP Plus image-processing software
IPA
    idiopathic pulmonary arteriosclerosis
    invasive pulmonary aspergillosis
iPAT
    integrated parallel acquisition
       technique
IPC
    interpeduncular cistern
IPCS
    infrapatellar contracture syndrome
IPD
    idiopathic Parkinson disease
IPEUS
    intraportal endovascular ultrasonography

IPF
    idiopathic pulmonary fibrosis
    interstitial pulmonary fibrosis
IPG
    impedance plethysmography
IPH
    idiopathic portal hypertension
    intraplaque hemorrhage
IPHP
    intraperitoneal hyperthermic perfusion
IPI
    International Prognostic Index
iPlan BOLD MRI
I-Plant brachytherapy seed
IPLN
    intrapulmonary lymph node
IPMN
    intraductal papillary mucinous
       neoplasia
IPMT
    intraductal papillary mucinous
       tumor
       IPMT of branch duct type
ipodate
    i. calcium imaging agent
    i. sodium
    i. sodium imaging agent
ipodic acid contrast agent
ipomeanol
IPSID
    immunoproliferative small intestine
       disease
ipsilateral
    i. antegrade arteriography
    i. antegrade site
    i. basal ganglion
    i. breast tumor recurrence
      (IBTR)
    i. bundle-branch block
    i. cortical diaschisis
    i. downstream artery
    i. femoral neck fracture
    i. femoral shaft fracture
    i. hemimegalencephaly
    i. hemispheric carotid TIA
    i. injection
    i. jugular lymphatic bed
    i. lateral ventricle
    i. lung volume
    i. margin
    i. pleural effusion
IPSP
    intrapixel sequential processing
       IPSP neuron evaluation method
IR
    inversion recovery
    arrhythmia-insensitive flow-sensitive
       alternating IR
    IR image

Ir
iridium
^{192}Ir, Ir-192
iridium 192
^{192}Ir ribbon
^{192}Ir seed therapy
^{192}Ir wire
^{194}Ir, Ir-194
iridium 194
IRA
ileorectal anastomosis
^{132}I radioactive iodine
IRAK
integrated reference air Kerma
IRA-400 resin
IRBBB
incomplete right bundle-branch
block
IRCM
iodinated radiologic contrast
medium
IRE
internal rotation in extension
IR-EPI
inversion recovery echo-planar
imaging
Irex
I. Exemplar ultrasound
I. Exemplar ultrasound scanner
IRF
internal rotation in flexion
Iriditope
iridium (Ir)
i. 192 (^{192}Ir, Ir-192)
i. 194 (^{194}Ir, Ir-194)
i. imaging agent
i. needle
i. wire
iridium-192
i.-192 endobronchial implant
i.-192 wire implant
IRIS
intensified radiographic imaging
system
IRIS III imager
IRIS scanner
irislike stenosis
^{192}Ir-loaded stent
IRLT
intraoperative red light therapy
iron (Fe)
i. 52 (^{52}Fe, Fe-52)
i. 55 (^{55}Fe, Fe-55)
i. 59 (^{59}Fe, Fe-59)
i. accumulation in kidney
i. ascorbate DTPA
brain i.
i. chelation therapy
i. deposition

i. dextran
gadolinium i.
i. hydroxide
i. overload artifact
radioactive i.
i. storage disease
iron-dependent contrast
iron-sensitive imaging technique
iron-transporting protein mechanism
IRP
interventional reference point
irradiate
irradiated zinc
irradiating
irradiation
abdominal i.
adjuvant i.
axillary i.
breast i.
cardiac i.
i. chamber
convergent beam i. (CBI)
cranial i.
craniospinal i. (CSI)
curative i.
extended-field i.
external beam i.
external orthovoltage i.
extracorporeal i.
fractionated external beam i.
fractionated total body i.
gamma i.
heavy ion i.
heavy-particle i.
hemibody i. (HBI)
hyperfractionated total body i.
implant i.
i. injury
interstitial template i.
intracanalicular i.
intracavitary i.
intraoral cone i.
inverted-Y field i.
involved-field i.
involved-region i.
local i.
low-intensity laser i. (LILI)
mantle field i.
neutron i.
palliative i.
partial brain i.
i. phenomenon
phosphorus-32 intracavitary i.
i. pneumonia
proton i.
radical i.
selective i.
stereotactic external beam i. (SEBI)
stereotactic proton i.

subtotal lymphoid i.
subtotal nodal i.
template i.
i. tolerance
total body i.
total lymphoid i.
ultraviolet i.
vaginal code i.
whole-body i.
whole-brain i.

irradiator
MDS-2000 microwave i.

irreducible
i. dorsal dislocation
i. fracture

irregular
i. block
i. bone
i. border
i. calcification
i. emphysema
i. enchondral ossification
i. extrinsic indentation
i. gallbladder wall thickening
i. hazy luminal contour
i. kidney
i. mass
i. mucosal fold
i. shape
i. tapered appearance

irregularity
avulsive cortical i.
diffuse i.
intimal i.
luminal i.
margin i.
nodular i.
sinus i.
tendon i.

irregularly
i. layered astrocytic component
i. layered neuronal component
i. shaped lesion

irreversible
i. airway obstruction
i. compression
i. compression of MR imaging
i. ischemia
i. narrowing of bronchiole
i. organ failure

irrigoradioscopy
irrigoscopy
irritability
atrial i.
cardiac i.
muscle i.
myocardial i.
nerve root i.
ventricular i.

irritable
i. bowel syndrome (IBS)
i. colon
i. heart
i. stricture

irritant
i. bronchitis
primary i.

irritation
chronic i.
i. fibroma

IRSE
inversion recovery spin echo
IRSE sequence

IRV
inspiratory reserve volume

IS
ileosacral

ISAH
isolated systolic arterial hypertension
ISAH stereotactic immobilization
frame
ISAH stereotactic immobilizing
mask

ISAM
interferometric synthetic aperture
microscopy

ischemia
acute leg i.
acute mesenteric i. (AMI)
anoxic i.
balanced i.
brachiocephalic i.
brain i.
brainstem i.
cardiac i.
carotid artery i.
cerebral i.
chronic cerebral i.
chronic mesenteric i.
(CMI)
coronary i.
cortical i.
critical limb i.
deep white matter i.
exercise-induced transient myocardial
i.
focal cerebral i.
global cerebral i.
global myocardial i.
intestinal i.
intracompartmental i.
irreversible i.
limb-threatening i.
mesenteric i.
myocardial i.
neonatal intracranial i.
nonhemorrhagic i.
nonlocalized i.

ischemia (*continued*)
    nonocclusive mesenteric i.
      (NOMI)
    organ i.
    periinfarction i.
    provocable i.
    radiation-induced i.
    radiation-related i.
    regional myocardial i.
    regional transmural i.
    remote i.
    reversible myocardial i.
    rostral brainstem i.
    segmental bronchus i.
    silent myocardial i.
    stress-induced i.
    subendocardial i.
    talar dome i.
    testicular i.
    transient cerebral i.
    transient myocardial i.
    vertebrobasilar i.

ischemic
    i. area
    i. bowel
    i. bowel disease
    i. brain damage
    i. brainstem infarct
    i. change
    i. colitis
    i. complication
    i. congestive cardiomyopathy
    i. contracture
    i. core
    i. decompensation
    i. defect
    i. demyelination
    i. encephalopathy
    i. episode
    i. event
    i. gliosis
    i. heart
    i. histopathology
    i. hypoxia
    i. index
    i. instability
    i. lesion
    i. mesentery
    i. necrosis
    i. necrosis of femoral head
      (INFH)
    i. nephropathy
    i. penumbra
    i. reperfused myocardium
    i. reperfusion injury
    i. segment
    i. sinus tachycardia
    i. stroke
    i. time
    i. ulcer
    i. viable myocardium
    i. zone

ischemically mediated mitral
** regurgitation**

ischia (*pl. of* ischium)

ischial
    i. bone
    i. bursitis
    i. spine
    i. tuberosity

ischioacetabular fracture

ischiocapsular ligament

ischiocavernosus muscle

ischiofemoral ligament

ischiogluteal
    i. bursa
    i. bursitis

ischiopagus twin

ischiopubic
    i. junction
    i. ramus
    i. synchondrosis

ischiorectal
    i. abscess
    i. fat-pad
    i. fossa
    i. fossa lesion
    i. fossa plane

ischiospongiosus muscle of penis

ischium, *pl.* **ischia**
    ascending ramus of i.
    ramus of i.
    transverse diameter between ischia

ISG
    Imaging Solutions Group
    ISG medical imaging workstation

ISI
    injection scan interval

ISIS
    image-selected in vivo spectroscopy

ISKD
    intramedullary skeletal kinetic distractor
    ISKD system

island
    bone i.
    bony i.
    cartilage i.
    compact i.
    endometrial i.
    fat i.
    fibrotic i.
    giant bone i.
    heterotopic white matter i.
    mucosal i.
    i. of red marrow
    i. of tissue
    Pander i.
    Reil i.

sclerotic calvarial bone i.
tissue i.
islet cell tumor
ISO
International Organization of
Standardization
isoattenuating
isoattenuation
isobaric transition
isobar nuclide
isobutyl
Isocam
I. scintillation imaging
I. scintillation imaging system
I. SPECT imaging system
isocapnic hyperventilation-induced
bronchoconstriction
isocenter
i. placement error
i. shift method
shoulder i.
single i.
isochromatic
isoclosed curve
Isocon camera
isodense
i. appearance
i. enhancement
i. mass
i. subdural hematoma
isodose
i. contour
i. curve
i. line
i. plan
i. shift method
i. width
isoechoic
i. breast mass
i. clot
isoefamate contrast medium
isoeffect dose
isoeffective bronchial mucosa
isoelectric
i. electroencephalogram
i. line
i. period
isoflurane
isoform
CSF 14-3-3 i.
isoimmunization
rhodium i.
isointense
i. background fat
i. lesion
i. signal
i. soft tissue
isointensity
Isolar rod

isolated
i. airway injury
i. cerebellar hypoplasia
i. clustered calcifications
i. dislocation
i. focal cerebellar cortical dysplasia
i. hepatic infusion
i. hepatic perfusion
i. hepatic portal and arterial
perfusion
i. hook fracture
i. systolic arterial hypertension
(ISAH)
i. ventricular inversion
isolation
i. perfusion
protective i.
strict i.
isoleucine
isomer
i. nuclide
optic i.
isomeric
i. decay
i. transition
isomerism
atrial i.
isonitrile
computed axial
tomography-methoxyisobutyl i.
(CAT-MIBI)
dipyridamole
technetium-99m-2-methoxyisobutyl i.
isoosmotic (*var. of* isosmotic)
Isopaque contrast medium
isophil
isoporosis
isopotential line
isoproterenol infusion
isosceles triangular configuration
isosexual precocity
isosmolar contrast medium (IOCM)
isosmotic, isoosmotic
i. polyethylene glycol
i. water solution
isotone nuclide
isotonicity
isotope
beta-emitting i.
i. bone scan
i. calibrator
carrier-free i.
cistern i.
i. clearance
i. colloid imaging
daughter i.
i. decay
i. dilution analysis
i. effect

isotope (*continued*)
    gamma-emitting i.
    i. hepatobiliary imaging
    intravenous injection of i.
    iodine-131 i.
    labeling of i.
    i. lung scan
    i. meal
    i. nephrography
    neutron-deficient short-lived
     i.
    i. nuclide
    parent i.
    ^{103}Pd i.
    phosphorus i.
    poorly concentrated i.
    radioactive i.
    i. renogram
    rhenium i.
    i. scintigraphy
    short-range i.
    i. shunt imaging
    stable i.
    strontium i.
    i. uptake
    i. venography
    i. ventriculography
    i. voiding cystourethrography
     (IVCU)
isotope-labeled fibrinogen imaging
isotope-tagged marker
isotopic
    i. cisternography
    i. dilution
    i. 3D imaging
    i. 3D study
    i. ratio
    i. skeletal survey
    i. volume study
isotretinoin
isotropic, isotropous
    i. dataset
    i. diffusion-weighted imaging
    i. disc
    i. motion
    i. resolution
    i. thin-section image
    i. tissue
    i. voxel
isotropous (*var. of* isotropic)
isotropy
isotype
isovolumetric (*var. of* isovolumic)
isovolumic, isovolumetric
    i. contraction time
    i. period
    i. relaxation
    i. relaxation time (IVRT)

Isovue
    I. nonionic imaging agent
    I. prefilled syringe
Isovue-200, -250, -300, -370 imaging agent
Isovue-M 200, 300 imaging agent
Isovue-370 prefilled syringe
Israel camera
israelii
    Actinomyces i.
ISS
    inferior sagittal sinus
    injury severity scale
    injury severity score
ISSI
    interspinous segmental spinal
    instrumentation
isthmian (*var. of* isthmic)
isthmic, isthmian
    i. coarctation
    i. organizer
    i. region
    i. spondylolisthesis
isthmi, isthmuses
isthmus, *pl.* **isthmi, isthmuses,**
 pl. **isthmuses**
    aortic i.
    i. of corpus callosum
    i. of femur
    i. of uterus
    i. of Vieussens
    pontile i.
    renal i.
    stenotic i.
    temporal i.
    thyroid i.
    uterine i.
isthmuses (*pl. of* isthmus)
IT
    iliotibial
    intrathecal
    IT band
ITA
    internal thoracic artery
    ITA graft
iterative
    i. algorithm
    i. halftoning
    i. reconstruction
    i. sweep
ITP
    idiopathic thrombocytopenic purpura
ITT
    internal tibial torsion
IUD
    intrauterine device
IUdR
    iododeoxyuridine

IUG
    intrauterine gas
IUGR
    intrauterine growth retardation
        asymmetric IUGR
        late flattening IUGR
        low-profile IUGR
        mixed IUGR
        symmetric IUGR
IUP
    intrauterine pregnancy
IV
    intravenous
IVAC
    intravenous accurate control
        IVAC P4000 infuser
Ivalon
        I. particle
        I. plug
        I. sponge
IVC
    inferior vena cava
    intravenous cholangiogram
        solitary left IVC
IVC-to-portal vein shunt
IVCU
    isotope voiding cystourethrography
IVCV
    inferior venacavogram
    inferior venacavography
IVDSA
    intravenous digital subtraction
    angiography

Ivemark CHD syndrome
IVFA
    intravenous fluorescein angiography
        IVFA imaging
IVH
    intraventricular hemorrhage
IVIM
    intravoxel incoherent motion
Ivor Lewis esophagectomy
ivory
        i. osteoma
        i. phalanx
        i. phalanx sign
        i. vertebra
IVP
    intravenous pyelogram
    intravenous pyelography
        rapid-sequence IVP
IVR
    idioventricular rhythm
IVRT
    isovolumic relaxation time
IVSD
    interventricular septal defect
IVST
    interventricular septal thickness
IVU
    intravenous urography
IVUS
    intravascular ultrasound
        IVUS catheter
        2D IVUS
        3D IVUS

J

joule
    J chain
    J junction
    J loop
    J point
Jaboulay amputation
Jaccoud
    J. arthritis
    J. arthropathy
    J. sign
JACE-Stim electrotherapy unit
jackknife position
Jackson
    J. and Huber classification of
      bronchial segments
    J. coil
    J. sign
    J. staging system
Jacobson canal
Jadassohn-Lewandowsky syndrome
Jaffe-Campanacci syndrome
Jaffe-Lichtenstein disease
jagged
    j. bone fragment
    j. osteophyte
Jahss dislocation classification
jail-bar
    j.-b. appearance
    j.-b. chest
    j.-b. rib
James bundle
jammed finger
Janeway lesion
Jansen
    J. disease
    J. metaphysial dysplasia
Jansen-type metaphysial chondrodysplasia
Jansky-Bielschowsky disease
Japanese
    J. classification of gastric carcinoma
    J. encephalitis
    J. Gastric Cancer Association
japonicum
    Schistosoma j.
Jaquet apparatus
Jarcho-Levin syndrome
Jarjavay ligament
Jaszczak phantom
Jatene transposition
jaundice
    painless j.
javelin thrower's elbow
jaw
    ameloblastoma of j.

    j. bone
    claudication of j.
    independent j.
    osteosarcoma of j.
JB1 catheter
Jefferson
    J. burst fracture
    J. cervical fracture
Jeffery classification of radial fracture
jejunal
    j. atresia
    j. diverticulosis
    j. diverticulum
    j. duplication
    j. leiomyosarcoma
    j. loop
    j. loop interposition of Henle
    j. motility
    j. obstruction
    j. pouch
    j. ulcer
jejuni
    Campylobacter j.
jejunitis
    Crohn j.
    ulcerative j.
jejunization
    ileal j.
    j. of colon
    j. of ileum
    vascular j.
jejunocolic fistula
jejunoduodenogastric intussusception
jejunogastric intussusception
jejunoileal (JI)
    j. bypass (JIB)
    j. diverticulum
    j. shunt
jejunoileitis
    ulcerative j.
jejunostomy catheter
jejunum
    proximal j.
jelly-belly appearance
jeopardized myocardium
jersey finger
jet
    aqueductal j.
    j. area
    j. flow
    high-velocity j.
    j. length
    j. lesion
    j. phenomenon
    pressurized fluid j.

J

jet (*continued*)
  regurgitant j.
  ureteral j.
Jeune syndrome
Jewett nail
JGA
  juxtaglomerular apparatus
J-hook
  J-h. deformity
  J-h. deformity of distal ureter
JI
  jejunoileal
  JI shunt
JIB
  jejunoileal bypass
J-modulation
JNPA
  juvenile nasopharyngeal angiofibroma
Jobert fossa
Jod-Basedow phenomenon
Jography angiographic catheter
Johnson-Jahss classification of posterior tibial tendon tear
Johnson position
joint
  acromioclavicular j. (ACJ)
  ankle j.
  j. ankylosis
  apophysial j.
  j. arthrography
  j. articular surface
  j. articulation
  atlantoaxial j.
  atlantooccipital j.
  bail-lock knee j.
  ball-and-socket j.
  basal j.
  Budin j.
  calcaneocuboid j. (CCJ)
  j. calculus
  capitate hamate j.
  capitolunate j.
  j. capsule
  j. capsule defect
  j. capsule thickening
  carpophalangeal j.
  j. cavity
  Charcot j.
  j. chondroma
  Chopart j.
  Clutton painful j.
  CMC j.
  computed tomography-guided percutaneous radiofrequency denervation of sacroiliac j.
  condyloid j.
  j. contracture
  coracoclavicular j.
  costochondral j.

costotransverse j.
costovertebral j.
Cruveilhier j.
CT-guided percutaneous screw placement for sacroiliac j.
cubonavicular j.
cuneiform j.
j. cyst
j. debris
j. deformity
j. depression fracture
diarthrodial intervertebral j.
DIP j.
j. dislocation
distal interphalangeal j.
distal radioulnar j. (DRUJ)
j. distraction
j. effusion
elbow j.
ellipsoid j.
erythema of j.
facet j.
femoropatellar j.
flail j.
j. fluid
j. fluid extravasation
j. fluid extrusion
free knee j.
frozen j.
j. fulcrum
j. fusion
Gaffney j.
Gillette j.
glenohumeral j.
gliding j.
hallux interphalangeal j.
hinge j.
j. hyperextensibility
hypermobile j.
IM j.
immovable j.
j. incongruity
j. instability
interapophysial j.
intercarpal j.
interchondral j.
j. interface
intermetatarsal j.
interphalangeal j.
intervertebral j.
IP j.
j. kinematics
knee j.
j. laxity
lesser metatarsophalangeal j.
j. line
Lisfranc Charcot j.
loss of parallelism of facet j.
lunotriquetral j.

Luschka j.
manubriosternal j.
MCP j.
metacarpophalangeal j. (MCPJ)
metatarsal j.
metatarsocuneiform j.
metatarsophalangeal j.
midcarpal j.
middle facet of subtalar j.
midtarsal j. (MTJ)
j. morphology
mortise j.
MTP j.
naviculocuneiform j.
near-anatomic position of j.
neuropathic tarsometatarsal j.
neurotrophic j.
occipitoaxial j.
j. of trunk
osteolysis on both sides of j.
parallelism of facet j.
patellofemoral j.
perched facet j.
PIP j.
pisotriquetral j.
pivot j.
j. play
primary cartilage j.
proximal interphalangeal j. (PIPJ)
proximal radioulnar j.
pseudo-Charcot j.
pseudoneuropathic j.
pulvinar hip j.
radiocapitellar j.
radiocarpal j.
radioscaphoid j.
radioulnar j.
Regnauld degeneration of MTP j.
J. Review Committee on Education
   in Radiologic Technology (JRCERT)
sacrococcygeal j.
sacroiliac j.
saddle j.
scaphocapitate j.
scapholunate j.
scaphotrapeziotrapezoid j.
scapulothoracic j.
seagull j.
secondary cartilaginous j.
j. segment
sesamoidometatarsal j.
shoulder j.
SI j.
signal j.
silastic finger j.
SL j.
j. space
j. space narrowing
j. space pseudowidening

sternal j.
sternoclavicular j.
sternocostal j.
sternomanubrial j.
STT j.
subluxed facet j.
subtalar j.
j. survey
Swanson finger j.
j. swelling
symphysis cartilage j.
synovial diarthrodial j.
talocalcaneal j
talocalcaneonavicular j.
talocrural j.
talofibular j.
talonavicular j.
tarsal j.
tarsometatarsal j.
temporomandibular j. (TMJ)
thoracic j.
tibiofibular j.
tibiotalar j.
j. tissue
transverse tarsal j.
trapeziometacarpal j.
trapezioscaphoid j.
trapeziotrapezoid j.
triquetrohamate j.
uncovertebral j.
unstable j.
weightbearing j.
widened sacroiliac j.
j. widening
wrist j.
xiphisternal j.
zygapophysial j.

joint-restricting ossification
Joliot method
Jomed
   J. Flexmaster stent
   J. peripheral stent
   J. peripheral stent-graft
Jones
   J. classification
   J. classification of diaphysial
      fracture
   J. criterion
   J. view
Jones-Mote reaction
Joseph valve implant
Jostent
   J. covered stent
   J. peripheral stent-graft
   J. SelfX nitinol stent
Joubert
   J. focal cerebellar dysplasia
   J. malformation
   J. syndrome

joule (J)
    j. radiation-absorbed dose
    J. shock
JPA
    juvenile pilocytic astrocytoma
J-pouch
    small colonic J-p.
JPS
    juvenile polyposis syndrome
JRA
    juvenile rheumatoid arthritis
JRCERT
    Joint Review Committee on Education in Radiologic Technology
J-sella deformity
J-shaped
    J-s. anastomosis
    J-s. sella
    J-s. stomach
    J-s. tube
    J-s. ureter
J-tipped
    J-t. guidewire
    J-t. wire
Jude
    J. pelvic view
    J. pelvic x-ray
Judet
    J. epiphysial fracture classification
    J. view
Judkins
    J. coronary arteriography
    J. 4 diagnostic catheter
    J. left coronary catheter
    J. right coronary catheter
    J. selective left coronary cinearteriography
    J. technique
jugal
    j. ligament
    j. suture
jugular
    j. bulb anomaly
    j. bulb tumor
    j. catheter
    j. chain adenopathy
    j. compression maneuver
    j. foramen
    j. foramen schwannoma
    j. foramen syndrome
    j. foraminal mass
    j. lymph node
    j. megabulb
    j. node metastatic carcinoma
    j. process
    j. technique
    j. tubercle
    j. vein
    j. vein thrombosis

    j. venous access
    j. venous distention
    j. venous impulse
    j. venous oxygen saturation
    j. venous pressure
    j. venous pressure collapse
jugulare
    glomus j.
jugulodigastric
    j. chain
    j. node
juguloomohyoid lymph node
jumped facet
jumper's knee
jumping
    bite j.
jump vein graft
junction
    abnormal pancreatobiliary j. (APBJ)
    anomalous craniovertebral j.
    anorectal j. (ARJ)
    aortic sinotubular j.
    arch-isthmic j.
    atlantooccipital j.
    atriocaval j.
    atrioventricular j.
    beaked cervicomedullary j.
    bird-beak taper at esophagogastric j.
    bulbous costochondral j.
    caniocervical j.
    cardioesophageal j.
    cardiophrenic j.
    cavoatrial j.
    CE j.
    cervicomedullary j.
    cervicothoracic j.
    choledochopancreatic ductal j.
    chondrosternal j.
    competence of ureterovesical j.
    corticomedullary j. (CMJ)
    costochondral j.
    craniocervical j.
    craniovertebral j.
    cricothyroid j.
    cystic-choledochal j.
    duodenojejunal j. (DJJ)
    esophagogastric j.
    fundic-antral j.
    gastrocnemius-soleus j.
    gastroduodenal j.
    gastroesophageal j.
    gray-white matter j.
    ileocecal j.
    iliocaval j.
    ischiopubic j.
    J j.
    lateral margin of esophagogastric j.
    j. line
    meniscocapsular j.

J

meniscosynovial j.
metaphysial-diaphysial j.
midbrain-hindbrain j.
mucocutaneous j.
musculotendinous j.
myoneural j.
myotendinous j.
neuromuscular j.
occipitocervical j.
pancreaticobiliary ductal j.
pelviureteric j. (PUJ)
phrenovertebral j.
pontomedullary j.
pontomesencephalic j.
prostaticovesical j.
pyloroduodenal j.
rectosigmoid j.
saphenofemoral j.
sinotubular j.
splenoportal j.
sternochondral j.
supraspinatus-musculotendinous j.
sylvian-rolandic j.
temporooccipital j.
temporoparietooccipital j.
tracheoesophageal j.
ureteropelvic j. (UPJ)
ureterorenal j.
ureterovesical j.
uterovesical j.
venous j.

junctional
j. cortical defect
j. dilation
j. epidermolysis bullosa
j. focus
j. infundibulum
j. nest
j. parenchymal kidney defect
j. zone

Junghans pseudospondylolisthesis
juvenile
j. ankylosing spondylitis
j. aponeurotic fibroma
j. autosomal recessive polycystic disease
j. breast papillomatosis
j. calcific discitis
j. chronic polyarthritis
j. cirrhosis
j. embryonal carcinoma
j. epiphysiolysis
j. epiphysitis
j. fibroadenoma
j. fibromatosis
j. idiopathic scoliosis
j. laryngeal papillomatosis
j. nasopharyngeal angiofibroma (JNPA)
j. nephrophthisis

j. orbital pilocytic astrocytoma
j. ossifying fibroma
j. osteoporosis
j. Paget disease
j. pelvis
j. pilocytic astrocytoma (JPA)
j. polyp
j. polyposis
j. polyposis syndrome (JPS)
j. rheumatoid arthritis (JRA)
j. spondyloarthropathy
j. Tillaux fracture
j. T-wave pattern
j. xanthogranuloma

juvenile-onset glaucoma
juvenilis
kyphosis dorsalis j.
osteochondrosis deformans j.

juxtaanastomotic stenosis
juxtaarterial ventricular septal defect
juxtaarticular
j. fracture
j. low signal intensity
j. osteoid osteoma

juxtaarticulation
juxtacortical
j. bone lesion
j. chondroma
j. chondrosarcoma
j. fracture
j. osteosarcoma

juxtacrural
juxtadiaphragmatic location
juxtaductal
j. aortic coarctation
j. coarctation of aorta

juxtaepiphysial
juxtaglomerular
j. apparatus (JGA)
j. tumor

juxtahilar bronchus interruption
juxtaintestinal node
juxtapapillary diverticulum
juxtaphrenic
j. peak
j. peak sign

juxtaposition
atrial appendage j.

juxtapyloric ulcer
juxtarenal
j. aortic aneurysm
j. aortic atherosclerosis
j. cava

juxtarestiform body
juxtasellar ICA
juxtaspinal
juxtatricuspid ventricular septal defect
juxtavesical
J-Vision workstation

K

potassium
K capture
K electron
K radiation
K shell

^{38}**K, K-38**
potassium 38

^{39}**K, K-39**
potassium 39

^{40}**K, K-40**
potassium 40

^{42}**K, K-42**
potassium 42

^{43}**K, K-43**
potassium 43

Kadish
K. staging
K. staging system

Kager Achilles tendon triangle
Kahler disease
Kaiser-Bessel window function
Kalamchi-Dawe congenital tibial deficiency classification
Kallmann syndrome
Kalman filter
Kanavel sign
Kantor string sign
kaolin
k. lung nodule
k. pneumoconiosis

Kapandji radical fracture
Kaplan
K. PenduLaser 115
K. PenduLaser 115 laser system

kaposiform hemangioendothelioma (KHE)
Kaposi sarcoma (KS)
Karapandzic lip reconstruction flap
Karplus
K. relationship
K. sign
K. sign of pleural effusion

Kartagener
K. syndrome
K. triad

Kasabach-Merritt syndrome
Kasai portoenterostomy procedure
Kast syndrome
Katayama syndrome
Katzen infusion guidewire
Katzman infusion of radionuclide cisternography

Katz-Wachtel phenomenon
Kauppi method
Kawasaki disease
Kayser-Fleischer ring
Kazangia and Converse facial fracture classification
KBR
kidney length to body height ratio
KCC
Kulchitsky cell carcinoma
KCD
kinestatic charge detector
KCD imaging
kCi
kilocurie
Kearns-Sayre syndrome
K-edge filter
keel
laryngeal k.
keeled chest
Keeper vena cava filter
Kehr sign
Keith
K. node
K. sinuatrial bundle
Keith-Flack sinuatrial node
Kellgren arthritis
Kellock
K. sign
K. sign of pleural effusion
Kellogg-Speed lumbar spinal fusion
Kelly-Goerss Compass system
Kempe series
Kendall sequential compression device
Kennedy method for calculating ejection fraction
Kensey-Nash lithotrite
Kent
bundle of K.
Kent-His bundle
keratectomy
phototherapeutic k. (PTK)
keratin
k. pearl
k. plug
k. testicular cyst
k. urinary tract ball
keratinizing squamous metaplasia
keratocyst
odontogenic k.
keratoma
keratome, keratotome
femtosecond laser k.

K

keratoplasty
    laser thermal k. (LTK)
keratoses (*pl. of* keratosis)
keratosis, *pl.* **keratoses**
    k. pilaris
keratotome (*var. of* keratome)
Kerckring
    K. fold
    K. nodule
    K. ossicle
Kerley A, B, C line
Kerma
    kinetic energy released per unit mass air K.
    integrated reference air K. (IRAK)
    total reference air K. (TRAK)
Kerma-to-dose conversion factor
kernel
    dose k.
    interpolation k.
    large k.
    noise reconstruction k.
    k. size
    soft tissue k.
    spheric k.
kernel-of-corn appearance
Kernig sign
Kernohan brain tumor classification
Keshan disease
ketamine
ketanserin
ketene
ketoacidosis
    diabetic k.
ketone body
Kety equation
Kety-Schmidt method
keV
    kiloelectron volt
    keV gamma ray
Key-Conwell
    K.-C. classification of pelvic fracture
    K.-C. pelvic fracture classification
keyhole
    k. deformity
    k. method
keystone
    k. of calcar arch
    k. wedging
kg
    kilogram
KHE
    kaposiform hemangioendothelioma
kHz
    kilohertz
kick
    atrial k.

Kidner lesion
kidney
    abdominal k.
    k. abscess
    absent k.
    k. adenocarcinoma
    k. adenoma
    k. amyloidosis
    k. anatomy
    k. aneurysm
    k. angiomyolipoma
    k. anomaly
    k. arteriosclerosis
    arteriosclerotic k.
    Ask-Upmark k.
    atrophic k.
    k. atrophy
    atypical angiomyolipoma of k.
    bilateral large k.'s
    bilateral small k.'s
    blunt trauma of k.
    cake k.
    k. calcification
    k. calculus
    k. carcinoma chromophobe
    k. chloroma
    cicatricial k.
    congenital absence of k.
    congested k.
    contracted k.
    contralateral k.
    cortical scarring of k.
    cross-ectopic k.
    crush k.
    cyanotic k.
    k. cyst
    cystic k.
    k. disc
    discoid k.
    distended k.
    double k.
    doughnut k.
    duplication of left k.
    duplication of right k.
    dysfunctional k.
    dysgenetic k.
    k. dyskeratosis
    dysplastic k.
    ectopic k.
    edematous k.
    enlarged k.
    k. extraction efficiency
    faceless k.
    k. failure
    fatty k.
    fetal mesenchymal tumor of k.
    k. fibromyxoma
    fibrotic k.

floating k.
Formad k.
fractured k.
k. function imaging
k. function study
k. fungus ball
fused k.
fused pelvic k.
Goldblatt k.
granular k.
hamartoma of k.
k. hilum
Hodson-type k.
horseshoe k.
hydronephrotic k.
hypermobile k.
k. infarct
infundibulum of k.
iron accumulation in k.
irregular k.
k. leiomyoma
k. length to body height ratio
  (KBR)
lobe of k.
lobulated k.
long axis of k.
lower pole of k.
lumbar k.
lump k.
k. lymphoma
k. malrotation
k. mass growth pattern
medullary sponge k.
mesonephric k.
k. metastasis
movable k.
multicystic k. (MCK)
multicystic dysgenetic k.
multicystic dysplastic k. (MCDK)
mural k.
k. mycetoma
native k.
k. neurofibromatosis
nonfunctioning k.
k. oxalosis
Page k.
pancake k.
k. papillary blush
partially polycystic k.
pelvic k.
pelvis of k.
k. pole
pole-to-pole length of k.
polycystic k.
porous k.
Potter type IV k.
k. pseudotumor
ptotic k.

putty k.
k. radionuclide imaging
Rose-Bradford k.
sacciform k.
k. scan
scarred k.
sclerotic k.
k. shadow
shattered k.
shriveled k.
sigmoid k.
single functioning k.
k. sinus mass
k. size
sponge k.
k. stone
supernumerary k.
suspension of k.
thoracic k.
k. tomography
k. transplant
k. trauma
tree-barking k.
unicalyceal k.
unilateral large smooth k.
unilateral small k.
unipapillary k.
upsloping curve of k.
k.'s, ureters, and bladder film
k.'s, ureters, and bladder imaging
k.'s, ureters, bladder (KUB)
k. vessel
wandering k.
k. washout
kidney-pancreas transplant
kidney-shaped
  k.-s. distended cecum
  k.-s. placenta
kidney-to-background ratio
Kiel non-Hodgkin lymphoma classification
Kienböck
  K. disease
  K. dislocation
  K. unit
Kienböck-Adamson point
Kikuchi disease
Kikuchi-Fujimoto disease
Kilfoyle
  K. classification of condylar fracture
  K. condylar fracture classification
Kilian
  K. line
  K. pelvis
killer
  flow artifact k. (FLAK)
  natural k. (NK)
Killian dehiscence
kilocurie (kCi)

K

kiloelectron volt (keV)
kilogram (kg)
    coulombs per k. (C/kg)
kilohertz (kHz)
kilomegacycle
kilovolt (kV)
    k. peak (kVp)
kilovoltage
Kimmelstiel-Wilson syndrome
Kimura classification
Kimura-type choledochal cyst
kinase
    k. C antiglioma monoclonal
      antibody imaging agent
    herpes simplex virus 1 thymidine k.
      (HSV1-tk, HSV-TK)
    nucleoside diphosphate k.
      (NDP-K)
kindling phenomenon
kinematic
    k. magnetic resonance imaging
    k. MR cholangiopancreatography
    k. MRCP
    k. MRI study
    k. MR technique
    k. wrist device
kinematics
    joint k.
kineradiography
kinesis
    color k.
kinestatic
    k. charge detector (KCD)
    k. charge detector imaging
kinetic
    k. cervical spine
    k. curve
    k. energy
    k. energy released per unit mass
      (Kerma)
    k. parameter analysis
    k. perfusion parameter
kinetics
    elimination k.
    elliptic centric time-resolved imaging
      of contrast k.
    exponential k.
    sorption k.
    time-resolved imaging of contrast k.
      (TRICKS)
    washout k.
kinetocardiogram
kinetoscopy
Kinevac imaging agent
King classification of thoracic
  scoliosis
King-Moe
    K.-M. classification
    K.-M. classification of scoliosis

kinin
kininogen
kininogenase
kink
    k. artifact
    cervicomedullary k.
    k. in intestine
    Lane k.
kinked
    k. aorta
    k. bowel
    k. ureter
kinking
    aortic k.
    arterial k.
    blood vessel k.
    bronchial k.
    carotid artery k.
    catheter k.
    colon k.
    graft k.
    innominate artery k.
    intestinal k.
    limb k.
    patch k.
    ureteral k.
Kinnier-Wilson disease
Kinsbourne syndrome
Kirchner diverticulum
Kirk distal thigh amputation
Kirklin meniscal complex
Kirner deformity
Kirsch laser
Kirschner wire (K-wire, K wire)
kissing
    k. artifacts
    k. atherectomy technique
    k. balloons
    k. balloons technique
    k. contraction
    k. lesions
    k. sequestra
    k. spines
    k. stents
    k. ulcers
Kistler subarachnoid hemorrhage
  classification
Kistner tracheal button
kit
    ARROWgard Blue Plus multilumen
      central venous catheter k.
    A·S·KMerit safety access k.
    Banyan emergency k.
    Fleet Prep K. (1, 2, 3)
    k. for preparation of technetium
      depreotide injection
    InSite Her-2/neu k.
    k. ligand
    k. preparation

Pyrolite k.
Ultra Tag k.
vascular access safety k.
kite angle
Klatskin
K. tumor
K. tumor classification
Klebsiella
kleeblatschädel deformity
Kleffner-Landau syndrome
Klein
K. muscle
K. technique
Klemm sign
Klenow fragment
Klinefelter syndrome
Klippel-Feil
K.-F. deformity
K.-F. sequence
K.-F. syndrome
Klippel-Trenaunay syndrome (KTS)
Klippel-Trenaunay-Weber syndrome
Klumpke
K. brachial plexus injury
K. paralysis
klystron
K-means cluster
knee
anterior cruciate deficit of k.
k. arthrography bolster
breaststroker's k.
Brodie k.
collateral ligament of k.
corner of k.
dislocated k.
double camelback sign of k.
k. flexion contracture
floating k.
k. fracture
housemaid's k.
indirect MR arthrography of k.
internal derangement of k. (IDK)
k. joint
k. joint effusion
k. joint space height
jumper's k.
k. knob
locked k.
medial and lateral support structures of k.
medial plica of k.
motorcyclist's k.
reefing of medial retinaculum of k.
k. rest
runner's k.
spontaneous osteonecrosis of k. (SONK)

surfer's k.
tricompartmental chondromalacia of k.
k. view
wrenched k.
kneecap
kneelike bend
Kniest dysplasia
knife, *pl.* **knives**
Leksell cobalt-60 Gamma k.
roentgen k.
UltraCision ultrasonic k.
knives (*pl. of* knife)
knob
absent aortic k.
aortic k.
blurring of aortic k.
knee k.
notched aortic k.
knobby process
knocked-down shoulder
knock knee
knock-knee deformity
knot
false k.
ileosigmoid k.
lovers' k.
surfer's k.
true umbilical cord k.
known primary carcinoma
knuckle
aortic k.
k. bone
boxer's k.
k. of colon
k. sign
knuckle-shaped
Knuttsen bending film
Koch
K. sinuatrial node
K. triangle
K. triangle apex
Kocher
K. anastomosis
K. dilation ulcer
K. fracture
K. maneuver
Kocher-Lorenz capitellum fracture classification (I-II)
Kock pouch
Kodak
K. Digital Science 1200, 3600 distributed medical imager
K. Mammography CAD engine
K. Min-R film
K. Min-R screen
K. RP X-OMAT processor
K. software
K. X-OMAT film

K

Kodros radiolucent awl
Koeppe nodule
Köhler
    K. disease
    K. line
Kohlrausch fold
Kokopelli hunchback
Köllicker nucleus
Komai stereotactic head
  frame
Kommerell
    K. aneurysm
    K. diverticulum
    ductus of K.
Konica scanner
Konstram angle
Kopans
    K. needle
    K. spring hookwire
Korányi-Grocco triangle
Kore
    pore of K.
Kormed liver biopsy needle
Korotkoff test for collateral
  circulation
Korsakoff syndrome
Kostuik-Errico spinal stability
  classification
Kovalevsky canal
Kozhevnikov syndrome
Kr
  krypton
Krabbe
    K. diffuse sclerosis
    K. disease
Krause
    K. ligament
    transverse suture of K.
Krebs cycle
Kretztechnik ultrasound system
Krigel staging system
kringle
Kromayer lamp
Krönlein orbitotomy
Krukenberg tumor
Krupin-Denver eye valve-to-disc
  implant
Kruskal-Wallis test
krypton (Kr)
    k. 77
    k. flow
    inhalation of k. 77
    k. laser
    k. laser photocoagulation
    k. 81, 81m
    k. scan
KS
    Kaposi sarcoma

k-space
    k-s. matrix
    k-s. trajectory
    k-s. traversal
    k-s. velocity mapping
k-t BLAST
KTP
    potassium titanyl phosphate
KTS
    Klippel-Trenaunay syndrome
KUB
    kidneys, ureters, bladder
    KUB imaging
    KUB view
Kubelka-Munk theory
Kugel
    K. anastomosis
    K. artery
Kugelberg-Welander disease
Kulchitsky
    K. cell
    K. cell carcinoma (KCC)
Kulkarni injury
Kumar
    K., Welti and (KWE)
    K., Welti and Ernst method
Kumeral diverticulum
Kummel disease
Kumpe
    K. catheter
    K. hump
Kupffer cell sarcoma
Kürner septum
kurtosis
Kuslich
    Bagby and K. (BAK)
Kussmaul-Maier disease
Kussmaul sign
kV
    kilovolt
kVp
    kilovolt peak
    kVp meter
kwashiorkor
KWE
    Kumar, Welti and Ernst
    KWE method
K-wire
    Kirschner wire
kx-ky plane
kY
    sliding interleaved kY (SLINKY)
Kyle fracture classification
kyllosis
kymograph
kymography
    rocntgen k.
kymoscopy

kyphoplasty
kyphoscoliosis
kyphoscoliotic
    k. heart disease
    k. pelvis
kyphosis
    Cobb method of measuring k.
    k. dorsalis juvenilis
    loss of thoracic k.
    lumbar k.

    lumbosacral k.
    postlaminectomy k.
    Scheuermann juvenile k.
    thoracic k.
    thoracolumbar k.
kyphotic
    k. angulation
    k. curvature
    k. pelvis
    k. view

K

L
   amyloid L
   L electron
   L shell
L-159
   ^{11}C L-159
L/A
   liver-aorta
   L/A peak ratio
LA
   leukoaraiosis
LAA
   left atrial appendage
LA/AR
   left atrium-aortic root ratio
LABA
   laser-assisted balloon angioplasty
Labbé
   L. triangle
   L. vein
label
   double l.
   long wavelength
     photo l.
   radioactive l.
   radionuclide l.
   single l.
   triple l.
labeled
   l. atom
   l. fibrinogen
   l. free fatty acid scintigraphy
   l. leukocyte scan
   l. phosphorus
   l. positron
   l. RBC
   l. red blood cell sequestration
   l. thyroxine
labeling
   l. abnormality
   antibody l.
   cell l.
   ^{111}In l.
   in vitro l.
   in vivo l.
   iododeoxyuridine l.
   microglobulin l.
   l. of isotope
   pulse l.
   pulsed arterial spin l.
   radioactive l.
   radioisotope l.
   site-specific l.
   technetium 99m antibody l.
   technetium-tagged RBC l.

labial
   l. groove
   l. vein
labile blood pressure
laboratory
   nickel-titanium naval ordnance l.
     (nitinol)
labor dystocia
labra (*pl. of* labrum)
labral
   l. and anteroinferior glenoid rim
     fractures
   l. capsular complex
   l. fibrocartilage
   l. injury
   l. variant
labral-ligamentous complex
labrum, *pl.* **labra**
   acetabular l.
   anterior glenoid l. (AGL)
   articular l.
   fibrocartilaginous l.
   glenoid l.
   osseous l.
labrum-ligament complex
labyrinth
   artery of l.
   bony l.
   cochlear l.
   ethmoidal l.
   membranous l.
   osseous l.
   renal l.
   vestibular l.
labyrinthine
   l. artery
   l. fistula
   l. hemorrhage
   l. hydrops
   l. structure
labyrinthitis ossificans
LACD
   left apexcardiogram, calibrated
     displacement
lacelike
   l. appearance
   l. trabecular pattern
laceration
   bladder l.
   brain l.
   hemorrhagic liver l.
   liver l.
   lung l.
   parenchymatous l.
   spinal cord l.

L

laceration (*continued*)
 spleen l.
 tendon l.
 traumatic spleen l.
lacerum
 foramen l.
Lachman sign
lachrymal (*var. of* lacrimal)
laciniate
 l. ligament
 l. ligament of ankle
lack of acoustic penetration
lacrimal, lachrymal
 l. artery
 l. bone
 l. canal
 l. duct
 l. gland
 l. gland lesion
 l. groove
 l. mass
 l. nerve
 l. recess
 l. sac
 l. scan
 l. scintigraphy
lacrimalis
 ampulla canaliculi l.
lacrimoconchal suture
lacrimoethmoidal suture
lacrimomaxillary suture
lacrimoturbinal suture
lactate
 l. proton
 l. resonance
lactating adenoma
lacteal
 l. calculus
 l. vessel
lactiferous
 l. duct
 l. sinus
lactobezoar
lactoferrin production
lacuna, *pl.* **lacunae**
 bone l.
 cartilage l.
 intervillous l.
 Morgagni l.
 osseous l.
 resorption l.
lacunae (*pl. of* lacuna)
lacunar
 l. abscess
 l. brain infarct
 l. ligament
 l. node
 l. skull
 l. stroke

LAD
 left anterior descending
 left axis deviation
LADARVision excimer laser
Ladd band
Ladder diagram
ladderlike pattern
Lady Windermere syndrome
LAE
 left atrial enlargement
LAFB
 left anterior fascicular block
lag
 l. effect
 l. screw
LAG
 lymphangiogram
Lagios classification system
LaGrange classification of humeral supracondylar fracture
LAID
 left anterior internal diameter
Laimer
 L. fascia
 triangle of L.
LAIS
 Litvack Advanced Interventional Systems
 LAIS excimer laser
Laitinen
 L. CT guidance system
 L. stereotactic head frame
lake
 bile l.
 capillary l.
 intraplacental venous l.
 lipid l.
 maternal l.
 mucous l.
 venous intraplacental l.
 venous skull l.
LAM
 lymphangioleiomyomatosis
lambda
 L. Plus PDL1, PDL2 laser
 white matter l.
lambdoid
 l. cranial suture
 l. synostosis
Lambert
 L. canal
 L. channel
 L. projection
Lambert-Eaton myasthenic syndrome
lamella, *pl.* **lamellae**
 anular l.
 articular l.
 basal l.
 circumferential l.

concentric l.
enamel l.

lamellae (*pl. of* lamella)
lamellar
l. body
l. body density (LBD)
l. bone
l. periosteal reaction

lamina, *pl.* **laminae**
l. dura
external elastic l.
medullary l.
osseous spiral l.
l. papyracea
l. propria
vertebral l.

laminae (*pl. of* lamina)
laminagram, laminogram
laminagraph, laminograph
laminagraphy, laminography
cardiac l.

laminaplasty (*var. of* laminoplasty)
laminar, laminated
l. brain necrosis
l. calcification
l. flow
l. gallstone
l. intraluminal thrombus

laminated (*var. of* laminar)
lamination of gyrus
laminectomy
laminogram (*var. of* laminagram)
laminograph (*var. of* laminagraph)
laminography (*var. of* laminagraphy)
laminoplasty, laminaplasty
laminotomy
lamp
cold quartz germicidal l.
high-pressure mercury arc l.
hot quartz l.
Kromayer l.
mercury arc l.
mercury vapor l.
quartz l.
sun l.
ultraviolet l.
Wood l.
xenon arc l.

lanceolate deformity
lancet
Laser L.

Lancisi
L. muscle
L. sign

Landau diamagnetism
Landau-Kleffner syndrome
landmark
anatomic l.
bony skull l.

l. registration
Talairach l.

Landolfi sign
Landry vein light Venoscope
landscape
anatomic l.

Landsmeer ligament
Landzert fossa
lane
L. band
L. kink

Lanex medium screen
Langenbeck triangle
Langer-Giedion syndrome
Langerhans
L. cell histiocytosis (LCH)
L. lung cell histiocytosis

Langer line
Lannelongue ligament
lanthanide
l. metal
paramagnetic l.
l. shift reagent (LSR)

lanthanide-induced shift
lanthanum
Lanz
L. line
L. point

LAO
left anterior oblique
LAO position
LAO projection

LAP
left atrial pressure

laparoscope
3D l.
3-Dscope l.
EL2-TF410 l.
Surgiview l.

laparoscopic
l. contact ultrasonography (LCU)
l. intracorporeal ultrasound (LICU)
l. laser
l. port-site metastasis (LPSM)
l. ultrasound (LUS)
l. ultrasound probe
l. uterosacral nerve ablation (LUNA)

laparoscopy
laparotomy
radioguided l.

L-A peak ratio
Laplace
L. effect
L. mechanism

Lapra-Ty clip
large
l. airway
l. airway narrowing
l. B-cell lymphoma

L

large (*continued*)
l. bowel
l. bowel obstruction (LBO)
l. cell neuroendocrine carcinoma (LCNEC)
l. cell thyroid lymphoma
l. cell undifferentiated carcinoma
l. cleaved cell lymphoma
l. clothing artifact
l. colloidal particle
l. duct papilloma
l. fetal head
l. field of view (LFOV)
l. field-of-view gamma camera
l. field-of-view image
l. for gestational age
l. gut
l. habitus
l. hinge-angle electron field
l. intestine
l. kernel
l. loop excision
l. obtuse marginal branch
l. solid adrenal mass
l. spleen
l. susceptibility artifact
l. thymus shadow
l. utricle
l. venous tributary
l. vestibule
large-bore
l.-b. bile duct endoprosthesis
l.-b. catheter
l.-b. magnet
l.-b. 0.6T, 1.5T imaging system scanner
large-caliber tube
large-core
l.-c. technique
l.-c. ultrasound-guided biopsy
large-droplet fatty liver
large-fiber demyelination
large-field
l.-f. radiation therapy
l.-f. radiotherapy
l.-f. x-ray dosimetry
large-for-dates uterus
larger-caliber cutting needle
large-vessel
l.-v. disease of diabetic foot
l.-v. thrombosis
l.-v. vasculitis
large-volume joint effusion
Larkin position
Larmor
L. equation
L. frequency
L. precession

Larsen
method of L.
L. syndrome
laryngeal
l. atresia
l. carcinoma
l. cartilage
l. drop procedure
l. edema
l. fracture
l. giant cell tumor
l. keel
l. musculature fluorodeoxyglucose uptake
l. nerve
l. nodule
l. papilloma
l. papillomatosis
l. part of pharynx
l. polyp
l. skeleton
l. tuberculosis
l. ventricle
l. vestibule
l. web
laryngectomy
supraglottic l.
vertical partial l.
larynges (*pl. of* larynx)
laryngitis
laryngocele
laryngogram
laryngography
contrast l.
double-contrast l.
laryngomalacia
laryngopharyngography
laryngopyocele
laryngoscope
Benjamin binocular slimline l.
Benjamin pediatric l.
Bullard l.
Olympus ENF-P2 l.
laryngoscopy
indirect l.
laryngotracheoesophageal cleft
larynx, *pl.* **larynges**
appendix of ventricle of l.
glottic l.
infraglottic l.
supraglottic l.
ventricle of l.
vestibule of l.
larynx-sparing surgery
LASE
laser-assisted spinal endoscopy
Lasègue sign
laser
AccuLase excimer l.

acupuncture l.
alexandrite l.
AlexLAZR l.
Apex Plus excimer l.
ArF excimer l.
argon l.
argon/krypton l.
argon pumped-dye l.
Aura desktop l.
Aurora diode soft tissue l.
l. beam
l. biliary lithotripsy
biocavity l.
BriteSmile l.
Candela pulsed dye l.
carbon dioxide l.
Chrys CO_2 l.
Clearview CO_2 l.
CO_2 l.
l. coagulation
Coherent CO_2 surgical l.
Coherent UltraPulse 5000C l.
CoolGlide l.
copper-vapor pulsed l.
l. correlational spectroscopy (LCS)
coumarin pulsed dye l.
CTE:YAG l.
Derma 20 l.
Derma K l.
DermaLase l.
l. desiccation of thrombus
DIAGNOdent l.
l. diffraction scanning
l. digitizer
diode l.
Diomed EVLT l.
l. Doppler flowmetry (LDF)
l. Doppler flowmetry probe
l. Doppler velocimetry
dye l.
Eclipse TMR l.
ELCA l.
endoscopic l.
l. energy
l. energy absorption
Epic ophthalmic 3-in-1 l.
EpiTouch l.
erbium:YAG infrared l.
ErCr:YAG l.
EVLT l.
excimer l.
FCPA2 l.
FeatherTouch CO_2 l.
Fiberlase l.
FiberScan l.
flashlamp-pulsed dye l.
flashlamp-pumped pulsed dye l.
Flexlase 600 l.
flying spot excimer l.

gallium-arsenide l.
Genesis 2000 carbon dioxide l.
GentleLASE Plus l.
Heart l.
helium-cadmium l.
helium-neon l.
HeNe l.
HF infrared l.
high-energy l.
holmium l.
holmium:yttrium-aluminum-garnet
   l.
Horn endootoprobe l.
hot l.
Ho:YAG l.
Hyperion LTK l.
l. imager
Kirsch l.
krypton l.
LADARVision excimer l.
LAIS excimer l.
Lambda Plus PDL1, PDL2 l.
L. Lancet
L. Lancet laser device
laparoscopic l.
Laserscope l.
LaserSonics EndoBlade l.
LaserSonics Nd:YAG Laserblade l.
LaserSonics Surgiblade l.
Laserthermia l.
LaserTripter MDL 3000 l.
Lasertrolysis l.
Lastec System angioplasty l.
LightSheer SC diode l.
Lightstic 180, 360 fiberoptic l.
low-energy l. (LEL)
LX 20 l.
Lyra l.
Mainster retina l.
Maloney endootoprobe l.
Microlase transpupillary diode l.
Microlight 830 l.
Microprobe l.
microsecond pulsed
   flashlamp-pumped dye l.
midinfrared l.
Nd:YLF l.
neodymium:yttrium-aluminum-garnet
   l.
Nidek EC-5000 excimer l.
NovaLine Litho-S DUV excimer l.
NovaPulse CO_2 l.
Nuvolase 660 l.
OcuLight SL diode l.
OmniPulse-MAX holmium l.
Opmilas CO_2 multipurpose l.
Optical Biopsy System l.
OptiVision l.
OtoLAM l.

L

laser (*continued*)
Pegasus PIV l.
PhotoGenica V-Star l.
PhotoPoint l.
Polaris Nd:YAG l.
Prima l.
l. projection imaging (LPI)
pulsed-dye l.
pulsed infrared l.
pulsed metal vapor l.
PulseMaster l.
Pulsion FS l.
Pulsolith l.
Q-switched Nd:YAG l.
Q-switched ruby l.
Revitalase erbium cosmetic l.
l. scanning cytometry (LSC)
l. sclerosis
Selecta 7000 l.
SilkLaser esthetic carbon dioxide l.
Skinlight erbium:YAG l.
SLS l.
Smoothbeam l.
SoftLight l.
Softscan l.
Spectranetics excimer l.
SPTL 1b vascular lesion l.
Surgilase 150 high-powered CO_2 l.
Surgilase Nd:YAG l.
l. system
TEC-2100 postioning l.
THC:YAG l.
l. thermal ablation (LTA)
l. thermal keratoplasty (LTK)
thulium-holmium-chromium:YAG l.
Topaz CO_2 l.
TruPulse CO_2 l.
UltraPulse CO_2 l.
Urolase fiber l.
Vbeam pulsed-dye l.
VersaLight l.
VersaPulse holmium l.
Versatome l.
Visulas Nd:YAG l.
Visx Star 3 excimer l.
Visx Star S2 excimer l.
Vitesse Cos l.
l. welding
Xanar 20 Ambulase CO_2 l.
xenon-chloride l.
XTRAC l.
YAG l.
yttrium-aluminum-garnet l.
Zeiss Visulas 690s l.

laser-assisted
l.-a. balloon angioplasty (LABA)
l.-a. microvascular anastomosis
l.-a. spinal endoscopy (LASE)
l.-a. uvulopalatoplasty (LAUP)

laser-induced
l.-i. interstitial thermotherapy
l.-i. thermography (LITT)
l.-i. thermotherapy (LITT)
LaserOptic
Indigo L.
laser-polarized
l.-p. helium MRI
l.-p. helium MR imaging
Laserprobe-PLR Plus
Laserscope laser
LaserSonics
L. EndoBlade laser
L. Nd:YAG Laserblade laser
L. Surgiblade laser
Laserthermia laser
LaserTripter MDL 3000 laser
Lasertrolysis laser
LaserTweezers
LASH
left anterosuperior hemiblock
Lasix renography
last
l. image hold (LIH)
l. normal vertebra (LNV)
Lastec System angioplasty laser
lata
fascia l.
snapping fascia l.
latae
tensor fasciae l.
Latarjet
nerve of L.
late
l. central nervous system toxicity
l. effect of normal tissue
(LENT)
l. false aneurysm
l. fetal death
l. film
l. flattening IUGR
l. graft occlusion
l. normal tissue sequela
l. phase
l. systolic bulge
l. systolic retraction
l. venous filling
late-effect
l.-e. analysis
l.-e. toxicity score
latent
l. coccidioidomycosis
l. empyema
l. image
l. membrane protein-1
l. pleurisy
late-onset
l.-o. dwarfism
l.-o. metachromatic leukodystrophy

late-phase
    l.-p. image
    l.-p. termination

lateral
    l. aneurysm
    l. anterior drawer stress view
    l. arcuate ligament
    l. aspect
    l. band
    l. basal segmental bronchus
    l. bending injury
    l. bending view
    l. border
    l. breast-prone image
    l. capsular sign
    l. cephalometric radiograph
    l. cervical spine film
    l. collateral ligament (LCL)
    l. collateral ligament complex
    l. column calcaneal fracture
    l. compartment
    l. compartment impaction
    l. compartment traumatic bony
      injury
    l. conal fascia
    l. condylar humeral fracture
    l. condyle
    l. corticospinal tract
    l. costotransverse ligament
    l. crus
    l. cystourethrogram
    l. decubitus film
    l. decubitus position
    l. decubitus radiograph
    l. decubitus view
    l. disc herniation
    l. divergence angle (LDA)
    l. elbow tendinosis
    l. entrapment
    l. epicondylar bursa
    l. epicondylitis
    exaggerated craniocaudal l. (XCCL)
    l. extension view
    l. facial cleft
    l. femoral notch
    l. femoral sulcus
    l. fissure
    l. flexion-extension radiograph
    l. flexion view
    l. geniculate body
    l. gutter
    l. horn
    l. hypopharyngeal pouch (LHP)
    l. impingement
    l. joint line
    l. joint space
    l. left anterior oblique position
    l. lemniscus tract
    l. lobe of prostate

    l. lumbar meningocele
    l. lumbar support
    l. malleolar fracture
    l. malleolus
    l. margin of esophagogastric
      junction
    l. mass
    l. meniscal uncovering
    l. myocardial infarct
    l. oblique axial projection
    l. oblique fascia
    l. oblique jaw radiograph
    l. oblique view
    l. occipital sulcus
    l. occipitotemporal gyrus
    l. opposed beam
    l. part of occipital bone
    l. patellofemoral angle
    l. placenta previa
    l. plantar metatarsal angle
    l. precordium
    l. process of talus
    l. pterygoid muscle
    l. pterygoid tendinous attachment
    l. pyelography
    l. ramus radiograph
    l. recess
    l. recess stenosis
    l. recess syndrome
    l. rectus muscle
    l. recumbent position
    l. reflection of colon
    l. resolution
    l. reticular formation
    l. root
    l. rotatory ankle instability
    l. sagittal image
    l. semicircular canal
    l. sesamoid bone
    l. shelf
    l. sinus
    l. skull radiograph
    l. spinothalamic tract
    l. spring ligament of foot
    l. subluxation
    l. talar dome
    l. talar dome injury
    l. talar process
    l. talocalcaneal angle
    l. talocalcaneal ligament
    l. talometatarsal angle
    l. tarsometatarsal angle
    l. temporal epileptogenic lesion
    l. thoracic meningocele
    l. tibial plateau fracture
    l. tilt stress ankle view
    l. tomography
    l. transcranial projection
    l. transfacial projection

L

lateral (*continued*)
 l. tug
 l. ulnar collateral ligament (LUCL)
 l. umbilical fold
 l. ventricle
 l. ventricle of cerebrum
 l. ventricle trigone
 l. wall refractive shadowing
 l. web
 l. wedge fracture
lateralis
 ampulla ossea l.
 interdigitation of vastus l.
 meniscus l.
 proboscis l.
 sinus l.
 stria longitudinalis l.
 stria olfactoria l.
 vastus l.
laterality
lateralization deficit
lateralizing
 l. finding
 l. sign
laterally displaced fracture
laterocervical region
lateroconal fascia
lateromedial
 l. oblique projection
 l. oblique view
latex
 Spli-Prest l.
LaTIS endovascular laser system
latissimus dorsi muscle
latitude film
lattice
 l. index
 l. relaxation time
 l. vibration
 l. work
Laubry-Pezzi syndrome
Laue pattern
Lauge-Hansen ankle fracture
 classification
Laugier fracture
LAUP
 laser-assisted uvulopalatoplasty
Laurin
 L. angle
 L. x-ray view
Lauth ligament
lavage
 bronchoalveolar l. (BAL)
 cavity l.
 oral colonic l. (OCL)
law
 Angström l.
 Avogadro l.
 Beer l.

 Bergonie-Tribondeau l.
 Bragg l.
 Coulomb l.
 Courvoisier l.
 Curie l.
 Doerner-Hoskins distribution l.
 Faraday l.
 Fick l.
 Gibbs-Donnan l.
 Good Samaritan l.
 Hilton l.
 Le Borgne l.
 Lenz l.
 Ohm l.
 Poiseuille l.
 L. position
 Rayleigh scattering l.
 transformer l.
 L. view
 Wolff l.
Lawrence
 L. lateral proximal humerus view
 L. method
 L. position
lawrencium (Lr)
laxative
 bulk l.
laxity
 chronic ligament complex l.
 joint l.
 ligamentous l.
 varus stress l.
layer
 basal l.
 Bekhterev l.
 boundary l.
 bright l.
 circumferential echodense l.
 echodense l.
 echo-free l.
 fibrofatty l.
 fluid-blood l.
 half-life l.
 half-value l. (HVL)
 hypoechoic l.
 inner bright l.
 intermediate signal intensity l.
 parietal l.
 seromuscular l.
 sonolucent l.
 subserous l.
 10th-value l.
 visceral l.
layered gallstones
layering
 l. calcification
 calcium l.
 l. debris
 l. effusion

l. of contrast material
l. of gallstones
Lazarus sign
Lazorthes
posterior thalamic artery of L.
L/B
lesion-brain
L/B ratio
LBBB
left bundle-branch block
LBCD
left border of cardiac dullness
LBD
lamellar body density
LBO
large bowel obstruction
L/C
lesion-countersite ratio
LCA
left coronary angiography
left coronary artery
LCB
low-concentration barium
LCCM
low-concentration contrast medium
LCD
liquid crystal display
low-contrast detail
LC-DCP
low-contact dynamic compression plate
LCDD
light-chain deposition disease
LCH
Langerhans cell histiocytosis
LCIS
lobular carcinoma in situ
LCL
lateral collateral ligament
LCNEC
large cell neuroendocrine carcinoma
LCP
Legg-Calvé-Perthes disease
LCP disease
LCR
low-contrast resolution
LCS
laser correlational spectroscopy
LCT
liquid crystal thermography
LCU
laparoscopic contact ultrasonography
LDA
lateral divergence angle
left descending artery
LDD
low-dose dobutamine
LDD-gated SPECT
LDF
laser Doppler flowmetry

LDLT
living-donor liver transplant
Le
L. Borgne law
L. Fort amputation
L. Fort fibular fracture
L. Fort I, II, III fracture
L. Fort mandibular fracture
L. Fort-Wagstaffe fracture
LE
lupus erythematosus
lead
l. apron shield
bipolar l.
chest l.
l. collimation
l. encephalopathy
esophageal l.
l. eye shield
l. gonad shield
intracardiac l.
l. line
pacemaker l.
pacing l.
l. pellet marker
l. pin
l. point
precordial l.
radioactive l.
leading edge
lead-pipe
l.-p. fracture
l.-p. rigidity
lead-rubber apron
lead-time bias
leaf, *pl.* **leaves**
l. of diaphragm
l. of mesentery
leafless tree appearance
leaflet
anterior motion of posterior mitral
valve l.
anterior tricuspid valve l.
apposition of l.'s
arching of mitral valve l.
bowing of mitral valve l.
coapted l.
commissural l.
doming of l.
floating l.
l. function
hammocking of mitral valve l.
heart valve l.
mitral l.
l. motion
myxomatous valve l.
noncalcified mitral l.
posterior mitral valve l. (PMVL)
posterior tricuspid l.

L

leaflet (*continued*)
    pseudomitral l.
    redundant aortic valve l.
    redundant mitral valve l.
    l. retraction
    l. separation
    septal l.
    spoonlike protrusion of l.
    systolic prolapse of mitral valve l.
    valve l.
leaflike villus
leak
    air l.
    aortic paravalvular l.
    ascites due to bile l.
    baffle l.
    biliary l.
    blood l.
    calibrated l.
    capillary l.
    cerebrospinal fluid l.
    chyle l.
    contained l.
    current l.
    distal l. (type I)
    femoral l.
    generalized capillary l.
    interatrial baffle l.
    interstitial pneumonia air l.
    light l.
    Luschka duct l.
    lymphatic l.
    mitral l.
    paraprosthetic l.
    paravalvular l.
    periprosthetic l.
    perivalvular l.
    spontaneous cerebrospinal fluid l.
    transient chyle l.
leakage
    anastomotic l.
    bile l.
    blood-tumor barrier l.
    chylous l.
    contrast medium l.
    injection l.
    paraprosthetic l.
    radiation l.
    silicone implant l.
leaking
    l. abdominal aortic aneurysm
    l. vein
leaky
    l. lung syndrome (LLS)
    l. valve
lean mass
LEAP
    low-energy all-purpose
    LEAP collimator

leather bottle stomach
leave-alone lesion
leaves (*pl. of* leaf)
Leclercq test
LE-CTV
    lower extremity CT venography
ledge
    eccentric l.
left
    l. anterior chest wall
    l. anterior descending (LAD)
    l. anterior descending artery
    l. anterior fascicular block (LAFB)
    l. anterior hemiblock
    l. anterior internal diameter (LAID)
    l. anterior oblique (LAO)
    l. anterior oblique position
    l. anterior oblique projection
    l. anterior oblique projection
      ventriculogram
    l. anterior oblique view
    l. anterosuperior hemiblock (LASH)
    l. apexcardiogram, calibrated
      displacement (LACD)
    l. atrial active emptying fraction
    l. atrial appendage (LAA)
    l. atrial cannulation
    l. atrial chamber
    l. atrial end-diastolic pressure
    l. atrial enlargement (LAE)
    l. atrial function
    l. atrial hypertrophy
    l. atrial maximal volume
    l. atrial myxoma
    l. atrial pressure (LAP)
    l. atrioventricular groove artery
    l. atrium
    l. atrium-aortic root ratio (LA/AR)
    l. auricle
    l. auricular appendage
    l. axillary artery catheterization
    l. axis deviation (LAD)
    l. border of cardiac dullness
      (LBCD)
    l. border of heart
    l. brain
    l. bundle branch
    l. bundle-branch block (LBBB)
    l. bundle-branch hemiblock
    l. circumflex
    l. circumflex coronary artery
    l. colon
    l. colonic flexure
    l. common carotid artery
    l. common femoral artery
    l. coronary angiography (LCA)
    l. coronary artery (LCA)
    l. coronary cusp
    l. coronary plexus

l. coronary sinus
l. crus
l. descending artery (LDA)
l. gastric artery
l. gutter
l. heart catheterization
l. heart syndrome
l. hemisphere
l. hepatic vein (LHV)
l. iliac system
l. intercostal space (LICS)
l. internal carotid artery (LICA)
l. internal mammary artery (LIMA)
l. internal mammary artery
  anastomosis
l. lateral projection
l. lobe of liver
l. lower extremity (LLE)
l. lower lobe (LLL)
l. lower lobe lesion
l. lower quadrant (LLQ)
l. main coronary artery (LMCA)
l. mainstem bronchus
l. mediastinum
l. middle lobe (LML)
l. pleural apical hematoma cap
l. posterior oblique (LPO)
l. posterior oblique position
l. posterior oblique projection
l. primary bronchus
l. pulmonary artery (LPA)
l. pulmonary cusp
l. pulmonary vein (LPV)
l. respiratory nerve
l. retroaortic renal vein
l. sternal border
l. subclavian central venous pressure
  (LSCVP)
l. subphrenic space
l. upper lobe (LUL)
l. upper lobe lesion
l. upper quadrant (LUQ)
l. ventricle
l. ventricular afterload
l. ventricular aneurysm (LVA)
l. ventricular angiography
l. ventricular apex
l. ventricular assist device (LVAD)
l. ventricular asynergy
l. ventricular cardiomyopathy
l. ventricular cavity pressure
l. ventricular chamber
l. ventricular chamber volume
l. ventricular configuration
l. ventricular contraction pattern
l. ventricular diastolic dimension
  (LVdd)
l. ventricular dilation
l. ventricular dysfunction (LVD)

l. ventricular ejection fraction (LVEF)
l. ventricular ejection time (LVET)
l. ventricular end-diastolic dimension
  (LVEDD)
l. ventricular end-diastolic pressure
  (LVEDP)
l. ventricular end-diastolic volume
l. ventricular end-diastolic volume
  index (LVEDI)
l. ventricular end-systolic dimension
  (LVESD)
l. ventricular end-systolic volume
  index (LVESVI)
l. ventricular failure
l. ventricular fast filling time
l. ventricular filling pressure
l. ventricular fractional shortening
  index
l. ventricular free wall (LVFW)
l. ventricular functional shortening
  (LVFS)
l. ventricular function wall motion
l. ventricular gated blood pool scan
l. ventricular hypertrophy (LVH)
l. ventricular hypertrophy with strain
l. ventricular hypoplasia
l. ventricular inflow tract obstruction
l. ventricular inflow volume (LVIV)
l. ventricular internal diameter
  (LVID)
l. ventricular internal diastolic
  dimension (LVIDd)
l. ventricular internal dimension at
  end-systole (LVIDs)
l. ventricular loading
l. ventricular mass (LVM)
l. ventricular mass index (LVMI)
l. ventricular maximal volume
l. ventricular muscle
l. ventricular noncompaction
l. ventricular outflow pressure
  gradient
l. ventricular outflow tract (LVOT)
l. ventricular outflow tract
  obstruction (LVOTO)
l. ventricular outflow volume
  (LVOV)
l. ventricular peak systolic pressure
l. ventricular posterior wall (LVPW)
l. ventricular posterosuperior process
l. ventricular preload
l. ventricular pressure (LVP)
l. ventricular regional wall motion
l. ventricular regional wall motion
  abnormality
l. ventricular slow filling time
l. ventricular strain pattern
l. ventricular stroke volume
l. ventricular stroke work (LVSW)

L

left (*continued*)
    l. ventricular stroke work index (LVSWI)
    l. ventricular support system
    l. ventricular systolic (LVs)
    l. ventricular systolic/diastolic function
    l. ventricular systolic functional reserve
    l. ventricular systolic pump function
    l. ventricular systolic time interval ratio
    l. ventricular wall (LVW)
    l. ventriculogram (LVG)

left-dominant coronary anatomy

left-handedness
    ventricular l.-h.

left-right asymmetry

left-sided
    l.-s. empyema
    l.-s. heart failure
    l.-s. heart pressure
    l.-s. pleural effusion

left-sidedness
    bilateral l.-s.

left-side-down
    l.-s.-d. decubitus position
    l.-s.-d. decubitus scan

left-to-right
    l.-t.-r. flow
    l.-t.-r. shift
    l.-t.-r. shunting of blood

leg
    l. axis
    baker's l.
    bayonet l.
    bowed l.
    champagne-bottle l.'s
    deep vein system of l.
    l. edema
    postphlebitic l.
    scissoring of l.'s
    l. shortening
    tennis l.

Legg-Calvé-Perthes disease (LCP)

Leggiero hydrophilic coated microcatheter

Legionella pneumophilia

Legionnaires disease

leg-length discrepancy (LLD)

LEGP
    low-energy general purpose

LEHR
    low-energy high-resolution

Leichtenstern sign

Leigh
    L. disease
    L. syndrome

leiomyoblastoma

leiomyoma
    benign metastasizing l.
    degenerated uterine l.
    epithelioid l.
    esophageal l.
    fundal l.
    gastric l.
    kidney l.
    multiple vascular l.'s
    pedunculated l.
    renal l.
    small bowel l.
    stomach l.
    urinary bladder l.
    uterine l.
    vascular l.

leiomyomatosis
    diffuse l.
    esophageal l.

leiomyomatous kidney hamartoma

leiomyosarcoma
    duodenal l.
    esophageal l.
    gastric l.
    intramural l.
    intravascular l.
    jejunal l.
    retroperitoneal l.
    right atrial extension of uterine l.
    small bowel l.
    stomach l.
    uterine l.

Leksell
    L. cobalt-60 Gamma knife
    L. D-shaped stereotactic frame
    L. gamma unit
    L. stereotactic system

Leksell-Elekta stereotactic frame

LEL
    low-energy laser

Lemierre syndrome

lemnisci (*pl. of* lemniscus)

lemniscus, *pl.* **lemnisci**
    medial l.

lemon sign

Lenard ray tube

length
    basic cycle l. (BCL)
    basic drive cycle l. (BDCL)
    Beatson combined ankle l.
    cervical l.
    crown-heel l.
    crown-rump l. (CRL)
    CSF systole l.
    echo-train l. (ETL)
    effective path l. (EPL)
    femur l.
    fetal femoral l.

focal l.
humeral l.
jet l.
limb l.
metacarpal l.
metacarpophalangeal l.
path l.
pulse l.
pyloric channel l.
radial l.
sinus cycle l. (SCL)
subcutaneous fat l.
track cone l.
urethral l.

length-biased sampling
length-time bias
Lennox-Gastaut syndrome
Lenoir facet
lens

acoustic l.
catadioptric l.
right-angled telescopic l.
Thorpe plastic l.

lens-sparing external beam radiation
therapy
LENT

late effect of normal tissue
LENT score
LENT scoring system

lenticular

l. area
l. bone
l. carcinoma
l. fasciculus
l. loop
l. nucleus

lenticulostriate

l. artery
l. supply
l. vasculopathy (LSV)
l. vessel

lentiform

l. bone
l. nucleus

lentigines
Lenz law
Leonardo software fusion
workstation
leontiasis ossea
leopard skin demyelination
lepidic growth
leptocyte
leptocytosis
leptofibril
leptomeningeal

l. anastomosis
l. angiomatosis
l. arachnoid cyst
l. artery

l. carcinoma
l. disease
l. fibrosis
l. ivy sign
l. metastasis
l. process

leptomeninges
leptomeningitis
leptomeningoencephalitis
leptomyelolipoma
Lequesne

center-edge angle of L.

Léri

melorheostosis of L.
L. pleonosteosis
L. sign

Leriche syndrome
Léri-Weill syndrome
LES

lower esophageal sphincter

Lesch-Nyhan syndrome
Lesgaft

L. hernia
L. triangle

lesion

ABCS joint and bone l.'s
acute cerebellar hemispheric l.'s
admixture l.
adrenal l.
afferent nerve l.
ALPSA l.
anechoic l.
angiocentric immunoproliferative
l.
angiocentric lymphoproliferative l.
angulated l.
anterior cranial base l.
anterior labroligamentous periosteal
sleeve avulsion l.
anterior parietal l.
anterochiasmatic l.
Antopol-Goldman l.
anular constricting l.
aortic arch l.
aortic valve l.
apical l.
apophysial l.
appendiceal l.
apple-core l.
Armanni-Ebstein l.
atheromatous l.
atherosclerotic l.
atrophic brain l.
Baehr-Lohlein l.
Bankart l.
barrel-shaped l.
benign fibrous bone l.
benign lymphoepithelial l.
benign lymphoproliferative l.

L

lesion (*continued*)
    benign vascular l.
    Bennett l.
    bifurcation l.
    bilateral l.'s
    bilobate polypoid l.
    biparietal l.
    bird's-nest l.
    black star breast l.
    blastic l.
    bleeding l.
    blistering l.
    blowout bone l.
    Blumenthal l.
    bone marrow l.
    Bracht-Wachter l.
    brain l.
    brain-infective l.
    brainstem l.
    breast l.
    Brown-Séquard l.
    bubbling l.
    bubbly bone l.
    bulbourethral gland l.
    bull's-eye l.
    butterfly l.
    calcified l.
    callosal l.
    candidate l.
    capsular drop l.
    cardiac valvular l.
    carinal l.
    carpet l.
    cartilaginous l.
    cavernous sinus l.
    caviar l.
    cavitary lung l.
    cavitary pulmonary l.
    cavitary small bowel l.
    central medullary bone l.
    centrilobular l.
    cerebral l.
    cerebrospinal fluid-containing l.
    cervical cord l.
    chest wall l.
    Chiari I-IV l.
    chiasmal l.
    cholesterol-containing brain l.
    circular l.
    circumscribed l.
    cochlear l.
    coin l.
    cold l.
    collar-button chest l.
    colonic apple-core l.
    colonic carpet l.
    colonic saddle l.
    complete nerve l.
    complex sclerosing l. (CSL)

    concentric l.
    condylomatous atypia l.
    congenital cystic neck l.
    l. conspicuity
    constricting esophageal l.
    conus medullaris l.
    convexity l.
    cookie bite l.
    cookie cutter l.
    coordinates for target l.
    cord epidural extramedullary l.
    cord intramedullary l.
    coronary artery l.
    corpus callosum ring-enhancing l.
    cortical bone l.
    corticospinal pathway l.
    Cowper gland l.
    critical l.
    culprit l.
    cyclops l.
    cystic epididymis l.
    cystic intracranial fetal l.
    cystic liver l.
    cystic splenic l.
    deep-seated l.
    dendritic l.
    de novo l.
    dense enhancing brain l.
    dense lung l.
    desmoid l.
    destructive bone l.
    destructive discovertebral l.
    l. detectability
    diaphysial l.
    Dieulafoy l.
    differential diagnosis bone l.
    difficult-to-treat vascular l.
    diffuse ulcerative l.
    disc l.
    discrete l.
    dominant hemisphere l.
    don't-touch l.
    dorsal root entry zone l.
    doughnut l.
    DREZ l.
    dumbbell l.
    Duret l.
    dysplasia-associated l.
    Ebstein l.
    eccentric medullary bone l.
    eccentric restenosis l.
    echogenic solid l.
    ellipsoid l.
    encapsulated fat-containing l.
    encephaloclastic l.
    endobronchial l.
    enhancing brain l.
    epicortical l.
    epididymis l.

epidural extramedullary l.
epileptogenic l.
esophageal apple-core l.
Essex-Lopresti l.
excitatory l.
expanding cavernous sinus brain l.
expansile lytic l.
expansile multilocular bone l.
expansile rib l.
expansile unilocular well-demarcated
  bone l.
extraaxial CNS l.
extraaxial low-attenuation l.
extracranial mass l.
extrahepatic l.
extramedullary compressive l.
extrapancreatic l.
extrapleural l.
extratemporal structural l.
extratesticular l.
extrathoracic l.
extrinsic l.
falx cerebri l.
fast-flow l.
fat-containing breast l.
fatty metastatic l.
fibrohistiocytic l.
fibromuscular l.
fibroosseous l.
fibrous bone l.
fibrous GI tract polypoid l.
finger lucent l.
fingertip l.
florid duct l.
flow-compromising l.
flow-limiting l.
focal articular cartilage l.
focal cold liver l.
focal hemispheric l.
focal hot liver l.
focal hypoechoic l.
focal ischemic l.
focal parenchymal brain l.
focal splenic l.
frank l.
friable l.
frondy l.
frontal lobe l.
full-thickness chondral l.
gallium-67-avid l.
GARD l.
gastric intramural-extramucosal l.
geographic l.
Ghon primary l.
Gill l.
GLAD l.
glenoid articular rim disruption l.
glenolabral articular disruption l.
GLOM l.

glomerular l.
grapelike multilocular cystic l.
greater sphenoid wing l.
gross l.
ground-glass l.
HAGL l.
hamartomatous l.
hemisphere l.
hemispheric demyelinating l.
hemodynamically significant l.
hemorrhagic l.
herald patch l.
high cervical spinal cord l.
high-density l.
high-grade obstructive l.
high-grade squamous intraepithelial
  l. (HGSIL)
high-intensity l.
high pontile l.
high-probability l.
high-signal l.
Hill-Sachs shoulder l.
hole-within-hole bone l.
holoprosencephaly l.
homogeneous l.
hot l.
hourglass-shaped l.
hyperdense brain l.
hyperintense periventricular brain l.
hypermetabolic l.
hyperplastic l.
hypoattenuating l.
hypodense basal ganglion brain l.
hypodense mesencephalic low-density
  brain l.
hypointense sella l.
l. hypometabolism
hypothalamic l.
iceberg l.
iliac l.
impaction l.
indiscriminate l.
indolent l.
infectious bubbly bone l.
infiltrating l.
inflammatory l.
infranuclear l.
internal auditory canal enhancing l.
intraaxial brain l.
intracerebral l.
intraconal l.
intracortical l.
intracranial mass l.
intracranial vascular l.
intradural extramedullary l.
intramammary l.
intramedullary cord l.
intramedullary space-occupying l.
intramedullary spinal l.

L

lesion (*continued*)

intramural-extramucosal stomach l.
intraocular l.
intraosseous bone l.
intraperitoneal l.
intrascrotal l.
intrasellar l.
intraspinal l.
intrinsic stenotic l.
intrinsic stomach wall l.
invasive l.
irregularly shaped l.
ischemic l.
ischiorectal fossa l.
isointense l.
Janeway l.
jet l.
juxtacortical bone l.
Kidner l.
kissing l.'s
lacrimal gland l.
lateral temporal epileptogenic l.
leave-alone l.
left lower lobe l.
left upper lobe l.
lipomatous l.
liver l.
local glomerular l.
l. localization
localized l.
Löhlein-Baehr l.
low-attenuation l.
low-density mesencephalic l.
lower motor neuron l.
low-grade squamous intraepithelial l.
  (LGSIL, LSIL)
lucent finger l.
lucent lung l.
lumbar spine l.
Lynch and Crues type 2 l.
lytic bone l.
macroorchidism l.
macroscopic placental l.
magnetic resonance-detected white
  matter l.
malacic l.
malignant osseous l.
Mallory-Weiss l.
mammographically suspicious l.
mass l.
masslike l.
medial longitudinal fasciculus l.
median nerve l.
mediastinal l.
melanocytic l.
mesencephalic low-density brain l.
mesencephalodiencephalic l.
mesenteric vascular l.
mesial temporal epileptogenic l.

metabolic l.
metachronous l.
metastatic l.
microcrust formation l.
micropapillary l.
midbrain l.
midline l.
miliary l.
mixed fat-water breast density l.
mixed sclerotic and lytic bone l.
MLF l.
Mongolian spotlike l.
monomelic bone l.
Monteggia l.
mucinous l.
mucosal l.
mulberry eye l.
multicentric lytic l.
multifocal enhancing brain l.
multilocular cystic l.
multiple lucent lung l.'s
multiple lytic bone l.'s
multiple osteosclerotic l.'s
multiple parotid gland l.'s
multiple stenotic l.'s
muscular l.
musculoskeletal l.
nail bed l.
napkin-ring anular l.
necrotic l.
needle localization of breast l.
neoplastic l.
neurogenic l.
neurologic bladder l.
neurovascular l.
nidus of l.
nodular l.
nondominant hemisphere l.
nonenhancing l.
nonexpansile multilocular bone l.
nonexpansile unilocular bone l.
noninvasive l.
nonmeningiomatous malignant l.
nonneoplastic l.
nonpalpable breast l.
nonproliferative l.
nonspecific punctate white
  matter l.
nontumorous l.
nucleus ambiguus l.
nucleus basalis l.
obstructive l.
occipital l.
occlusive l.
occult l.
ocular l.
onionskin l.
optic nerve l.
organic l.

osseous l.
ossified l.
osteoblastic l.
osteocartilaginous l.
osteochondral l.
osteolytic l.
osteosclerotic l.
ostial l.
outcropping of l.
pagetoid l.
papillary l.
papular l.
papulonecrotic l.
paradiscal l.
paralabral l.
paraorbital l.
parasagittal l.
parasellar region l.
parasellar vascular l.
parietal cortex l.
parietal lobe l.
parietooccipital l.
parosteal bone l.
partial l.
patch l.
pathologic l.
pedunculated l.
perforative l.
periapical l.
peripheral nerve l.
periventricular l.
permeative l.
Perthes l.
Perthes-Bankart l.
phlyctenula l.
phosphaturic intraosseous l.
photon-deficient bone l.
photopenic l.
pinguecula l.
plaquelike l.
pleural l.
POLPSA l.
polyostotic bone l.
polypoid l.
pontile l.
popcornlike reticulated l.
portal vein l.
posterior column l.
posterior compartment l.
posterior fossa l.
posterior fossa-foramen magnum l.
posterior language area l.
posterior vertebral element blowout l.
posttraumatic l.
prechiasmal optic nerve l.
presacral cystic l.
pretectal l.
primary l.
proliferative l.

prostate hypoechoic l.
pseudotumoral l.
pulmonary l.
punched-out lytic bone l.
punctate l.
purulent l.
questionable l.
radial sclerosing l.
radiodense l.
radiofrequency l.
radiographic stability of l.
radiolucent l.
radiopaque l.
reactive fibrous l.
reactive lymphoid l.
rectal l.
rectosigmoid polypoid l.
recurrent l.
regurgitant l.
remote lower motor neuron l.
renal mass l.
resectable l.
reticulonodular l.
retrochiasmal l.
retroglandular l.
reverse Hill-Sachs l.
rheumatic l.
rib l.
right lower lobe l.
right upper lobe l.
rim-enhancing l.
ring l.
ring-enhancing brain l.
ringlike l.
ring-wall l.
root entry zone l.
rotator cuff l.
rounded l.
round lucent l.
saddle l.
satellite l.
scar l.
scirrhous l.
sclerosing l.
sclerotic l.
secondary l.
segmental bronchus l.
serial l.'s
sessile l.
shagreen l.
sharply demarcated circumferential
  l.
sinonasal l.
sinusoidal l.
skeletal l.
skip l.
SLAP l.
slow-flow l.
slowly developing l.

L

lesion (*continued*)
  small bowel cavitary l.
  solid splenic l.
  solid thymic l.
  solitary cold l.
  solitary osteosclerotic l.
  solitary rib l.
  solitary sternal l.
  sonolucent cystic l.
  space-occupying intracranial l.
  spheric l.
  spicular scirrhous l.
  spinal cord l.
  spleen l.
  splenic l.
  spontaneous l.
  squamous intraepithelial l. (SIL)
  stacked ovoid l.
  stellate border breast l.
  Stener gamekeeper's thumb l.
  stenoobstructive l.
  stenotic l.
  sternal l.
  Sterner l.
  striatal l.
  structural l.
  subareolar l.
  subchondral l.
  subcortical intracranial l.
  subcortical low-intensity l.
  submucosal l.
  subtentorial l.
  subtotal l.
  superficial l.
  superior labral anteroposterior l.
  supraaortic l.
  supranuclear l.
  suprasellar low-density l.
  supratentorial l.
  suspicious l.
  swan-neck tubular l.
  synchronous l.
  systemic l.
  tandem l.
  target lung l.
  teardrop-shaped l.
  tectal l.
  telangiectatic l.
  temporal lobe l.
  tentorium cerebelli l.
  testicular cystic l.
  thalamic l.
  thoracic inlet l.
  tight l.
  total l.
  trabeculated bone l.
  transfer l.
  transverse cord l.
  trophic l.
  true-negative l.
  tuberculous l.
  tubular l.
  tumorlike l.
  tumor-mimicking breast l.
  ulcerative l.
  ulnar nerve l.
  umbilical cord l.
  uncommitted metaphysial l.
  unilateral l.
  unilocular cystic l.
  unilocular well-demarcated bone
    defect expansile l.
  unresectable l.
  unstable l.
  upper motor neuron l.
  valvular regurgitant l.
  vascular l.
  vasculitic l.
  vegetative l.
  vertebral expansile l.
  visceral l.
  Waldeyer throat ring l.
  wedge-shaped l.
  well-circumscribed l.
  well-defined l.
  white matter l.
  white star breast l.
  wide-field l.
  wire-loop l.
  Wolin meniscoid l.
  X, Y, and Z coordinates for
    target l.
lesion-background ratio
lesion-brain (L/B)
lesion-countersite ratio (L/C)
lesion-muscle ratio
lesion-nonlesion count ratio
lesion-normal tissue ratio
lesion-to-cerebrospinal fluid noise
lesion-to-white-matter contrast
lesion-to-white matter noise
LESP
  lower esophageal sphincter pressure
lesser
  l. arc injury
  l. atrophy
  l. curvature of stomach
  l. curvature ulcer
  l. metatarsophalangeal joint
  l. muscle
  l. omentum
  l. pancreas
  l. pelvis
  l. peritoneal sac
  l. petrosal
  l. sac abscess

l. sac hernia
l. sac of peritoneal cavity
l. saphenous system
l. saphenous vein
l. sciatic foramen
l. sciatic notch
l. trochanter
l. trochanteric fracture
l. trochanter of femur
l. tubercle
l. tuberosity

Lester Jones bypass tube
LET
linear energy transfer
lethal
l. bone dysplasia
l. dose
l. dwarfism
l. midline granuloma
l. musculoskeletal dysplasia
l. myocardial injury
l. neoplasia
lettering artifact
leucine radical
leucocyte (*var. of* leukocyte)
leucocytopenia (*var. of* leukopenia)
leucodystrophy (*var. of* leukodystrophy)
leucoencephalitis (*var. of* leukoencephalitis)
leucoencephalopathy (*var. of* leukoencephalopathy)
leucopenia (*var. of* leukopenia)
leucoplakia (*var. of* leukoplakia)
LEUHR
low-energy ultrahigh resolution
LEUHR fan-beam collimator
LEUHR parallel-hole collimator
leukemia
acute basophilic l.
acute lymphoblastic l.
acute lymphocytic l.
acute monoblastic l.
acute myeloblastic l.
acute myelocytic l.
acute myelogenous l. (AML)
acute myeloid l.
acute promyelocytic l.
chronic lymphocytic l.
chronic myeloid l.
chronic myelomonocytic l. (CMML)
chronic phase chronic myelogenous l.
hemorrhagic l.
Philadelphia chromosome-negative chronic myelogenous l.
Philadelphia chromosome-negative chronic myelomonocytic l.
plasma cell l.

Rieder cell l.
T-cell acute lymphoblastic l.
T-cell-type acute lymphoblastic l.
leukemic bone line
leukemid
leukemogenesis
leukemoid
leukoaraiosis (LA)
leukocoria, leukokoria
leukocyte, leucocyte
agranular l.
autologous labeled l.
basophilic l.
endothelial l.
eosinophilic l.
gallium-67-labeled l.
granular l.
heterophilic l.
indium-111-labeled l.
^{111}In-oxime-labeled l.
mast l.
motile l.
neutrophilic l.
nongranular l.
nonmotile l.
polymorphonuclear l.
polynuclear neutrophilic l.
radiolabeled l.
technetium 99m l.
technetium-99m-labeled l.
l. uptake
leukodystrophy, leucodystrophy
adrenal l.
autosomal dominant l.
congenital l.
global cell l.
infantile-onset l.
late-onset metachromatic l.
metachromatic l.
primary l.
sporadic l.
leukoencephalitis, leucoencephalitis
acute hemorrhagic l.
radiation l.
leukoencephalopathy, leucoencephalopathy
Cree l.
diffuse necrotizing l.
disseminated necrotizing l.
hereditary diffuse l.
heroin vapor l.
multifocal l.
necrotizing l.
periventricular l.
postviral l.
progressive multifocal l. (PML)
radiation-induced l.
spongiform l.
toxic l.

L

leukokoria (*var. of* leukocoria)
leukomalacia
    periventricular l. (PVL)
    radiation-induced l.
leukopenia, leucocytopenia, leucopenia
    radiofrequency radiogenic l.
    radiogenic l.
leukoplakia, leucoplakia
leukoreduction filter
LeukoScan
    L. imaging agent
    technetium 99m HMPAO mixed
       leukocyte L.
leukostasis
    pulmonary l.
Leur-par collimator
LeuTech radiolabeled imaging agent
levator
    l. ani
    l. muscle
    l. palpebrae superioris
    l. scapulae
    l. span
    l. veli palatini
LeVeen
    L. plaque cracker
    L. RF probe
level
    air-fluid l.
    attenuation l.
    contrast window l.
    C-reactive protein l.
    debris-fluid l.
    energy l.
    fat-fluid l.
    fluid l.
    fluid-fluid l.
    gas-fluid l.
    intracapsular fat-fluid l.
    intrasinus air-fluid l.
    l. I obstetric ultrasound
    pontile-medullary l.
    protein-fat fluid l.
    significance l.
    stairstep air-fluid l.
    supraventricular l.
    window l.
    zero reference l.
    Zielke derotation l.
level-dependent
    blood oxygenation l.-d.
    (BOLD)
3-level Haar wavelet decomposition
Levenberg-Marquardt method
Levine tube
levoangiocardiogram
levocardia
levocardiogram
levodopa

levogram
levo phase
levoposition
levorotatory scoliosis
levoscoliosis
levotransposition
levoversion
Levovist
    L. imaging agent
    L. myocardial contrast
       echocardiography
Lewis
    L. angle
    L. antibody
    L. position
Lewy body disease
Leydig
    L. cell adenoma
    L. cell tumor
Leyla arm
LFOV
    large field of view
LFUS
    low-frequency ultrasound
LGL
    Lown-Ganong-Levine
    LGL syndrome
LGSIL
    low-grade squamous intraepithelial
    lesion
LHBT
    long head of biceps tendon
    LHBT tenosynovitis
Lhermitte-Duclos
    L.-D. disease
    L.-D. syndrome
Lhermitte-Duclos-Cowden syndrome
LHP
    lateral hypopharyngeal pouch
LHR
    local host response
LHV
    left hepatic vein
Libman-Sacks endocarditis disease
LICA
    left internal carotid artery
lichenoides
    tuberculosis l.
    tuberculosis cutis l.
Lichtenstein-Jaffe disease
licorice powder
LICS
    left intercostal space
LICU
    laparoscopic intracorporeal ultrasound
LID
    low-iodine diet
lidocaine-adrenaline solution
lidofenin

lie

L. classification
fetal l.
horizontal l.
longitudinal l.
posterior l.
transverse l.
unusual fetal l.

Liebel-Flarsheim CT 9000 contrast delivery system

Lieberkühn crypt

Liebermeister groove

Liebow

usual interstitial pneumonia of L.

lienis

sustentaculum l.

lienography

lienophrenic ligament

lienorenal ligament

Lieutaud trigone

LiF

lithium fluoride
LiF thermoluminescence dosimeter
LiF thermoluminescence dosimetry

LifeJet catheter

Life-Lung fluorescence endoscopy system

Life-Pack 5 cardiac monitor

lifestyle-limiting claudication

life-threatening

l.-t. hemorrhage
l.-t. pneumothorax

lifetime regimen

lift

gallbladder l.
heave and l.
sternal l.

ligament

accessory atlantoaxial l.
acromioclavicular l.
acromiocoracoid l.
adipose l.
alar l.
anococcygeal l.
anterior cruciate l. (ACL)
anterior fibular l.
anterior talofibular l.
anterior tibiofibular l.
anterior tibiotalar l.
anteroinferior tibiofibular l.
anular l.
apical l.
Arantius l.
arcuate l.
arterial l.
ATF l.
atlantal l.
attenuated l.
auricular l.
avulsed l.

axis l.
Bardinet l.
Barkow l.
beak l.
Bellini l.
Berry l.
Bertin l.
Bichat l.
bifurcate l.
Bigelow l.
Botallo l.
Bourgery l.
broad l.
Brodie l.
Burns l.
calcaneoclavicular l.
calcaneocuboid l. (CCL)
calcaneofibular l. (CFL)
calcaneonavicular l.
calcaneotibial l.
Caldani l.
Campbell l.
Camper l.
capsular l.
Carcassonne l.
cardinal l.
caroticoclinoid l.
carpometacarpal l.
Casser l.
casserian l.
caudal l.
ceratocricoid l.
cervical mover l.
checkrein l.
cholecystoduodenal l.
chondroxiphoid l.
ciliary l.
Civinini l.
Clado l.
Cleland l.
clinoid l.
Cloquet l.
coccygeal l.
collateral l.
Colles l.
congenital laxity of l.
conjugate l.
conoid l.
conus l.
Cooper suspensory l.
coracoacromial l.
coracoclavicular l.
coracohumeral l.
corniculopharyngeal l.
coronary l.
costoclavicular l.
costocolic l.
costotransverse l.
costoxiphoid l.

L

ligament (*continued*)

cotyloid l.
Cowper l.
cricopharyngeal l.
cricothyroid l.
cricotracheal l.
cruciate l.
cruciatum cruris l.
cruciform l.
Cruveilhier l.
cuboideonavicular l.
cuneocuboid l.
cuneonavicular l.
cystoduodenal l.
deep collateral l.
deltoid l.
Denonvilliers l.
dentate l.
denticulate l.
diaphragmatic l.
dorsal metacarpal l.
dorsal wrist l.
Douglas l.
duodenal l.
duodenorenal l.
epicondyloolecranon l.
epihyal l.
extracapsular l.
extrinsic l.
fabellofibular l.
falciform l.
fallopian l.
femoral l.
Ferrein l.
fibular collateral l.
fibulotalar l.
fibulotalocalcaneal l.
flaval l.
floating l.
Flood l.
FTC l.
fundiform l.
gastrocolic l.
gastrodiaphragmatic l.
gastrohepatic l.
gastrolienal l.
gastropancreatic l.
gastrophrenic l.
gastrosplenic l.
genital l.
genitoinguinal l.
Gerdy l.
Gillette suspensory l.
Gimbernat l.
gingivodental l.
glenohumeral l.
glenoid l.
glossoepiglottic l.
Grayson l.

Günzberg l.
Haines-McDougall medial sesamoid l.
hammock l.
Helmholtz axis l.
Henle l.
Hensing l.
hepatic l.
hepatocolic l.
hepatocystocolic l.
hepatoduodenal l.
hepatoesophageal l.
hepatogastric l.
hepatogastroduodenal l.
hepatophrenic l.
hepatorenal l.
hepatoumbilical l.
Hesselbach l.
Hey l.
Holl l.
Hueck l.
humeral avulsion of glenohumeral l. (HAGL)
Humphry l.
Hunter l.
Huschke l.
hyalocapsular l.
hyoepiglottic l.
iliofemoral l.
iliolumbar l.
iliopectineal l.
iliopubic l.
iliotibial l.
iliotrochanteric l.
inferior dorsal radioulnar l.
inferior pulmonary l.
infrapatellar l.
infundibuloovarian l.
infundibulopelvic l.
inguinal l.
intercapital l.
intercarpal l.
interclavicular l.
interclinoid l.
intercornual l.
intercuneiform l.
interdigital l.
interfoveolar l.
intermetatarsal l.
internal collateral l.
interosseous sacroiliac l.
interosseous talocalcaneal l.
intersesamoid l.
interspinal l.
intertransverse l.
intervertebral l.
intraarticular l.
intrascapular l.
intrinsic l.

ischiocapsular l.
ischiofemoral l.
Jarjavay l.
jugal l.
Krause l.
laciniate l.
lacunar l.
Landsmeer l.
Lannelongue l.
lateral arcuate l.
lateral collateral l. (LCL)
lateral costotransverse l.
lateral talocalcaneal l.
lateral ulnar collateral l. (LUCL)
Lauth l.
lienophrenic l.
lienorenal l.
limited proteoglycan matrix of l.
Lisfranc l.
Lockwood l.
longitudinal l.
lumbocostal l.
lunotriquetral interosseus l.
Luschka l.
Mackenrodt l.
macroscopic hemorrhage l.
Maissiat l.
Mauchart l.
Meckel l.
medial collateral l. (MCL)
median arcuate l.
median cruciate l.
median umbilical l.
meniscofemoral l.
meniscotibial l.
metacarpoglenoid l.
metacarpophalangeal l.
microscopic hemorrhage of l.
mucosal suspensory l.
natatory l.
naviculocuneiform l.
nuchal l.
occipitoatlantoaxial l.
occipitoaxial l.
odontoid l.
l. of epididymis
l.'s of Henry and Wrisberg
l. of ovary
l. of Scarpa
l. of Treitz
opacification of posterior longitudinal l.
orbicular l.
Osborne l.
ossification of posterior longitudinal l. (OPLL)
ossified posterior longitudinal l.
ovarian suspensory l.
palmar metacarpal l.

palmar radiocarpal l.
pectinate l.
pelvic ring l.
pericardioperitoneal l.
pericardiophrenic l.
periodontal l.
peritoneal part of inguinal l.
Petit l.
Pétrequin l.
petroclinoid l.
phalangeal glenoid l.
phrenicocolic l.
phrenicoesophageal l.
phrenicogastric l.
phrenicolienal l.
phrenicosplenic l.
pisohamate l.
pisometacarpal l.
pisounciform l.
plantar l.
popliteal l.
posterior cruciate l. (PCL)
posterior longitudinal l. (PLL)
posterior talofibular l.
posterior tibiotalar l.
posteroinferior tibiofibular l.
posterooblique l.
Poupart inguinal l.
pterygomandibular l.
pterygospinous l.
PTF l.
pubocapsular l.
pubocervical l.
pubofemoral l.
puboprostatic l.
pubovesical l.
pulmonary l.
quadrate l.
radial collateral l.
radial metacarpal l.
radiate sternocostal l.
radiocarpal l.
radiolunotriquetral l.
radioscaphocapitate l.
radioscaphoid l.
radioscapholunate l.
reflected edge of Poupart l.
reflected inguinal l.
l. reflecting edge
retinacular l.
Retzius l.
rhomboid l.
right triangular l.
ring l.
Robert l.
round l.
Rouvière l.
sacrodural l.
sacrospinous l.

L

ligament (*continued*)

    sacrotuberous l.
    Santorini l.
    Sappey l.
    scapholunate l.
    scaphotriquetral l.
    Schlemm l.
    serous l.
    sesamoid l.
    sesamophalangeal l.
    sheath l.
    l. shelving edge
    shelving edge of Poupart l.
    short radiolunate l.
    Simonart l.
    Soemmerring l.
    sphenomandibular l.
    spinoglenoid l.
    spinous tarsus l.
    spiral l.
    splenocolic l.
    splenorenal l.
    spring l.
    Stanley cervical l.
    stellate l.
    sternoclavicular l.
    sternopericardial l.
    stretched-out l.
    Struthers l.
    stylohyoid l.
    stylomandibular l.
    stylomaxillary l.
    superficial dorsal sacrococcygeal l.
    superficial posterior sacrococcygeal l.
    superficial transverse metacarpal l.
    superficial transverse metatarsal l.
    superior costotransverse l.
    superior pubic l.
    superior transverse scapular l.
    suprascapular l.
    supraspinous l.
    suspensory l.
    sutural l.
    syndesmotic l.
    synovial l.
    talocalcaneal l.
    talofibular l.
    talonavicular l.
    tarsal l.
    tarsometatarsal l.
    l. tear
    tectoral l.
    temporomandibular l.
    Teutleben l.
    Thompson l.
    thyroepiglottic l.
    thyrohyoid l.
    tibial collateral l.

    tibial sesamoid l.
    tibiocalcaneal l.
    tibiofibular l.
    tibionavicular l.
    torn meniscotibial l.
    transverse atlantal l.
    transverse axial l.
    transverse carpal l.
    transverse cervical l.
    transverse crural l.
    transverse genicular l.
    transverse humeral l.
    transverse intertarsal l.
    transverse metacarpal l.
    transverse metatarsal l.
    transverse perineal l.
    transverse tibiofibular l.
    trapezoid l.
    triangular l.
    triquetrohamate l.
    triquetroscaphoid l.
    Tuffier inferior l.
    ulnar collateral l. (UCL)
    ulnocarpal l.
    ulnolunate l.
    ulnotriquetral l.
    umbilical l.
    urachal l.
    uterine l.
    uterosacral l.
    uterovesical l.
    vaginal l.
    venous l.
    ventral sacrococcygeal l.
    ventral sacroiliac l.
    ventricular l.
    vertebropelvic l.
    vesicosacral l.
    vesicoumbilical l.
    vesicouterine l.
    vestibular l.
    vocal l.
    volar carpal l.
    Walther oblique l.
    Weitbrecht l.
    Winslow l.
    Wrisberg l.
    xiphocostal l.
    xiphoid l.
    Y-shaped l.
    Zaglas l.
    Zinn l.

ligamentous

    l. ankylosis
    l. attachment
    l. bouncing
    l. box
    l. calcification
    l. complex

l. disruption
l. impingement
l. insertion
l. instability
l. laxity
l. luxation
l. strain
l. support
l. thickening
l. trauma

ligamentous-muscular hypertrophy
ligamentum

l. arteriosum
l. flavum
l. flavum hypertrophy
l. flavum thickening
l. mucosum
l. nuchae
l. patellae
l. teres
l. venosum fissure

ligand

l. agent
kit l.
^{99m}Tc-labeled l.

ligation

Doppler-guided hemorrhoid artery l.
(DGHAL)
Hunter aneurysm l.
thoracic duct l.

light

l. bulb appearance
hot l.
infrared l.
invisible l.
l. leak
l. microscopy
l. pink lung
l. scanning
l. sedation
stray l.
structured l.
l. therapy
Wood l.

light-chain deposition disease (LCDD)
light-induced

l.-i. autofluorescence spectroscopy
l.-i. fluorescence endoscope

light-reflection rheography
LightSheer SC diode laser
LightSpeed

L. multidetector CT scanner
L. QXi CT scanner
L. Ultra CT system

Lightstic 180, 360 fiberoptic laser
Lightwood syndrome
LIH

last image hold

likelihood ratio

LILI

low-intensity laser irradiation

Lilienfelds position
Liliequist membrane
LILT

low-intensity laser therapy

LIMA

left internal mammary artery
LIMA anastomosis

limb

l. absence
l. bone length ratio
l. bud
chronic lymphedematous l.
l. girdle
l. holder
l. kinking
l. length
l. of anterior capsule
l. of bifurcation graft
l. perfusion
l. reduction
l. reduction abnormality
l. reduction anomaly
Roux-en-Y l.
l. venography
vertebral, anal, cardiac, tracheal,
esophageal, renal, l. (VACTERL)

limb-body wall complex
limb-girdle muscular dystrophy
limbi (*pl. of* limbus)
limbic

l. lobe
l. region
l. system

limb-length

l.-l. asymmetry
l.-l. discrepancy (LLD)
l.-l. inequality

limb-lengthening procedure
limb-threatening ischemia
limbus, *pl.* **limbi**

l. fossae ovalis
l. of Vieussens
l. suture
l. vertebra

limit

eye exposure l.
Nyquist l.
quantum l.
tracking l.

limitation

beam l.
biophysical l.
infarct size l.
l. of joint motion
l. of MR imaging
l. of ultrasound
positive beam l. (PBL)

L

limited
    l. examination
    l. film
    l. imaging
    l. oxidative capacity
    l. proteoglycan matrix of ligament
    Sirtex Medical L.
    l. view
limited-cut plane
limited-slice computed tomography
limited-stage
    l.-s. diffuse large cell lymphoma
    l.-s. DLCL
limiting membrane
limitus
    hallux l.
LINAC
   linear accelerator
   LINAC radiosurgery
   Varian LINAC
   X-band LINAC
Lindegaard ratio
line
    absence of innominate l.
    absorption l.
    acanthomeatal l.
    acetabular l.
    AC-PC l.
    air-fluid l.
    Andren-von Rosen l.
    aneuploid cell l.
    anorectal l.
    anterior axillary l. (AAL)
    anterior humeral l.
    anterior junction l.
    aortic vent suction l.
    Arrow PICC l.
    l. artifact
    auricular l.
    axillary l.
    azygoesophageal l.
    basilar l.
    bimastoid l.
    black pleural l.
    Blumensaat anterior cruciate
      ligament l.
    Bolton nasion l.
    branching l.
    calcification l.
    Camper l.
    canthomeatal l.
    Cantlie l.
    cement l.
    central sacral l. (CSL)
    central venous pressure l.
    Chamberlain l.
    Chaussier l.
    clinoparietal l.
    Conradi l.

Correra l.
costoclavicular l.
costophrenic septal l.
Crampton l.
Cremin M l.
crescent hip l.
curved radiolucent l.
curvilinear subpleural l.
Cyma l.
Daubenton l.
demarcation l.
dentate l.
digastric l.
displaced left paraspinal l.
divisionary l.
Ellis l.
Ellis-Garland l.
epiphysial l.
fat-density l.
Feiss l.
Fischgold bimastoid l.
Fischgold biventer l.
Fleischner l.
l. focus principle
fracture l.
Fränkel white l.
Frankfort l.
F T l.
gallbladder-vena cava l.
gas density l.
gaussian l.
glabelloalveolar l.
glabellomeatal l.
gluteal l.
Granger l.
growth arrest l.
Gubler l.
Hampton l.
Harris l.
Hawkins l.
Hickman l.
Hilgenreiner l.
His l.
humeral l.
ilioischial l.
iliopectineal l.
l. imaging
infraorbital l.
infraorbitomeatal l. (IOML)
innominate absence of l.
l. integral concept
interlobar septal l.
interpupillary l.
intralobular l.
intravenous infusion l.
isodose l.
isoelectric l.
isopotential l.
joint l.

junction l.
Kerley A, B, C l.
Kilian l.
Köhler l.
Langer l.
Lanz l.
lateral joint l.
lead l.
leukemic bone l.
linguine l.
Linton l.
Looser l.
lorentzian l.
lower lung l.
low-intensity l.
lucent l.
Mach l.
McGregor l.
McKee l.
McRae l.
medial joint l.
median l.
Mees l.
Merkel cell carcinoma cell l.
Meyer l.
midaxillary l.
midclavicular l. (MCL)
midhumeral l.
midscapular l.
midspinal l.
midsternal l.
Moyer l.
Nélaton l.
oblique prescription l.
obturator l.
l. of Gennari
l. of response (LOR)
l. of Retzius
Ogston l.
Ohngren l.
omental l.
orbitomeatal l.
orthogonal tag l.
l. pair
parallel M l.'s
parallel pitch l.'s
paramedian l.
paraspinal l.
pectinate l.
peripheral intravenous infusion l.
peripherally inserted central catheter
l.
Perkin l.
Perkins-Ombredanne l.
photon therapy beam l.
PICC l.
l. placement
pleural l.
pleuroesophageal l.

popliteal l.
posterior axillary l.
posterior cervical l.
posterior junction l.
posterior nipple l. (PNL)
pronator quadratus l.
properitoneal fat l.
psoas l.
pubococcygcal l. (PCL)
radiocapitellar l.
radiolucent crescent l.
raster l.
reference l.
Reid l.
resonance l.
Richter-Monroe l.
Rolando l.
sacrococcygeal inferior pubic point
l.
Sappey l.
l. saturation
l. scanning
Schoemaker congenital hip
dislocation l.
sclerotic l.
scorbutic white l.
semilunar l.
septal l.
l. shadow
l. shape
Shenton l.
Simpson white l.
skin l.
Skinner pelvic menstruation l.
soleal l.
spectral l.
spinographic l.
spinolaminar l. (SLL)
l. spread function (LSF)
subchondral fracture l.
subclavian l.
subcutaneous fat l.
subpleural curvilinear l.
suture l.
transcondylar l.
transverse lucent metaphysial l.
trough l.
Trümmerfeld scurvy l.
twining l.
Ullmann l.
ventral venous pressure l.
vertebral body l.
visualization of Z l.
Wagner l.
water density l.
Wegner l.
white l.
l. width
zero l.

L

linea, *pl.* **lineae**
    l. alba
    l. semilunaris
lineae (*pl. of* linea)
lineage
    M4-M5 l.
linear
    l. absorption coefficient
    l. accelerator (LINAC)
    l. accelerator isocenter motion
    l. accelerator unit
    l. actuator
    l. amplifier
    l. artifact
    l. atelectasis
    l. attenuation
    l. attenuation coefficient
    l. band of maximal radiolucency
    l. branching microcalcification
    l. calcification
    l. combination model software
    l. compartmental system
    l. defect
    l. degenerative signal intensity
    l. density
    l. echo
    l. electrode array
    l. emphysema
    l. energy transfer (LET)
    l. erosion
    l. focus
    l. focus within cyst wall
    l. gradient
    l. high signal intensity
    l. infiltrate
    l. interpolation
    l. interpolator
    l. interstitial disease pattern
    l. low signal
    l. lucency
    l. margin
    l. marking
    l. measure
    l. opacity
    l. phased array
    l. phosphate
    l. photon
    l. polarization
    l. prediction
    l. prediction with singular value decomposition
    l. radiopacity
    l. regression analysis
    l. scan imaging
    l. scanning
    l. sebaceous nevus syndrome
    l. shadow
    l. skull fracture
    l. stenosis
    l. structure
    l. tomography
    l. transducer
    l. ulcer
linear-array
    l.-a. CCD scanner
    l.-a. echoendoscope
    l.-a. hydrophone assembly
    l.-a. transducer
    l.-a. transrectal ultrasound probe
linearity
    absolute l.
    gradient l.
    intrinsic spatial l.
    lung l.
    pulmonary l.
    scintillation camera l.
linearization
    perceptual l.
linearly polarized coil
linear-quadratic (LQ)
linebacker's arm
line-pair measurement
line-shape sensitivity
lingual
    l. artery
    l. bone
    l. goiter
    l. gyrus
    l. nerve
    l. root
    l. thyroid
    l. tonsil
linguine
    l. line
    l. sign
lingula, *pl.* **lingulae**
    l. pulmonis
    right middle lobe l.
lingulae (*pl. of* lingula)
lingular
    l. bronchus
    l. collapse
    l. division of left lung
    l. infiltrate
    l. mandibular bony defect (LMBD)
    l. nodule
    l. orifice
    l. pneumonia
lining
    mucosal l.
linitis
    l. plastica
    l. plastica carcinoma
link
    musculotendinous-osseous l.
Linsman water test
Linton line
Lintro-Scan

liothyronine sodium
lip
>cleft l.
>hilar kidney l.
>median cleft l.
>l. of hilum
>l. of lateral sulcus
>osteophytic bone l.
>posterior l.
>rhombic l.
>l. ring artifact

LIP
>lymphocytic interstitial pneumonia
>lymphocytic interstitial pneumonitis
>lymphoid interstitial pneumonia
>lymphoid interstitial pneumonitis

lipid
>l. artifact
>l. cholecystitis
>l. content of storage fat
>l. cyst
>l. embolus
>l. fraction relaxation rate
>l. lake
>necrotic l.
>l. signal
>l. zone

lipid-laden
>l.-l. foamy macrophage
>l.-l. plaque

lipid-lowering therapy
lipidoses (*pl. of* lipidosis)
lipidosis, *pl.* **lipidoses**
>cerebroside l.
>sphingomyelin l.

lipid-polarized helium MR imaging
lipid-rich material
lipid-sensitive
>l.-s. MR
>l.-s. MR imaging

Lipiodol
>L. embolization
>L. myelographic imaging agent
>L. Ultra-Fluid

liplike projection of cartilage
lipoblastic meningioma
lipoblastoma
lipocalcinogranulomatosis
lipodystrophy
>intestinal l.
>mesenteric l.

lipofibroadenoma
>breast l.

lipofuscinosis
>neuronal ceroid l.

lipogenic tumor
lipogranuloma
>sclerosing l.

lipogranulomatosis
>disseminated l.

lipohemarthrosis
lipohyalinosis
lipoid
>l. adrenal hyperplasia
>l. dermatoarthritis
>l. endogenous pneumonia
>l. granulomatosis
>l. pneumonitis

lipoleiomyoma
lipoma, *pl.* **lipomas**
>l. arborescens
>bone l.
>brain l.
>breast l.
>cardiac l.
>corpus callosum l.
>diffuse synovial l.
>epidural l.
>GI tract l.
>hepatic l.
>hilar l.
>infiltrating l.
>intracranial l.
>intradural l.
>intramedullary l.
>intraosseous l.
>intratentorial l.
>intrathecal l.
>liver l.
>mediastinal l.
>pericallosal l.
>soft tissue l.
>spinal l.
>spine l.
>subpial l.
>synovial diffuse l.

lipomas (*pl. of* lipoma)
lipomatosa
>macrodystrophia l.

lipomatosis
>central sinus l.
>epidural l.
>esophageal l.
>mediastinal l.
>l. mediastinum
>multiple symmetric l.
>pancreatic l.
>pelvic l.
>peripelvic l.
>renal sinus l.
>sinus l.
>soft tissue l.

lipomatous
>l. hypertrophy
>l. hypertrophy of interatrial septum
>l. lesion
>l. polyp

L

lipomatous (*continued*)
    l. tissue
    l. tumor
lipomyelomeningocele
lipomyeloschisis
liponecrosis
    l. macrocystica calcificans
    l. microcystica calcificans
lipophilic
    l. cationic diphosphine
    l. compound
    l. dye
    l. imaging agent
    l. indium oxine
    l. sequestration system
lipoplasty
    ultrasound-assisted l. (UAL)
LipoProfile
liposarcoma
    dedifferentiated l.
    metastatic pleomorphic l.
    myxoid l.
    myxomatous l.
    pleomorphic l.
    retroperitoneal l.
    round cell l.
    well-differentiated l.
liposarcomatous differentiation
liposclerotic mesenteritis
liposculpture
    3D superficial l.
liposome
    antibody-conjugated paramagnetic l.
      (ACPL)
    mannan-coated l.
liposome-based contrast agent
Lipowitz metal
Lippes loop
lipping
    osteophytic l.
Lippman-Cobb
    L.-C. angle
    L.-C. method
LIQ
    lower inner quadrant
liquefaction
    l. degeneration
    l. necrosis
liquefactive emphysema
liquid
    l. barium suspension
    l. bolus
    l. calcium
    l. crystal contact thermography
    l. crystal display (LCD)
    l. crystal display projector
    l. crystal thermography (LCT)
    l. embolic agent
    l. food dysphagia

    l. nylon
    l. pleural effusion
    l. scintillation analysis
    l. scintillation spectrometer
    l. scintillation spectrometry
    l. scintillator
Lisch nodule
Lisfranc
    L. amputation
    L. Charcot joint
    L. dislocation
    L. fracture
    L. injury
    L. ligament
Lissauer
    L. column
    L. tract
lissencephalia (*var. of* lissencephaly)
lissencephaly, lissencephalia
    cobblestone l.
list
    l. mode data collection
    l. mode lithium
Listeria
    L. encephalitis
    L. monocytogenesis
listerial
    l. infection
    l. rhombencephalitis
Lister tubercle
lithiasis
    gallbladder l.
    intraglandular calcified l.
    renal l.
lithium
    l. 7
    l. fluoride (LiF)
    list mode l.
lithoclast miniature pneumatic drill
lithogenic
    l. bile
    l. index
lithokelyphopedion, lithokelyphopedium
lithokelyphopedium (*var. of*
  lithokelyphopedion)
litholysis
litholytic agent
lithopedion, lithopedium
lithopedium (*var. of* lithopedion)
Lithostar nonimmersion lithotriptor
lithotomy position
lithotresis
    ultrasonic l.
lithotripsy, lithotrity
    biliary l.
    Candela l.
    electrohydraulic l. (EHL)
    electrohydraulic shock wave l.
      (ESWL)

endoscopic l.
extracorporeal shock wave l. (ESWL)
laser biliary l.
microexplosion l.
pulsed-dye laser l.
rotational contact l.
ultrasonic l.

lithotriptor
DoLi S extracorporeal shock wave l.
Dornier compact l.
Dornier HM3, HM4 l.
Lithostar nonimmersion l.
Modulith SL 20 l.
Pulsolith laser l.
Siemens Lithostar l.
Sonolith Praktis l.
Swiss lithoclast intracorporeal l.
Wolf Piezolith 2200 l.

lithotrite
Kensey-Nash l.

lithotrity (*var. of* lithotripsy)

LithoTron

LITT
laser-induced thermography
laser-induced thermotherapy
LITT applicator

little
l. finger
L. Leaguer's shoulder

littoral cell angioma

Littré
L. gland
L. hernia

Litvack Advanced Interventional Systems (LAIS)

Litzmann obliquity

livedo reticularis

liver
l. abscess
l. agenesis
alcoholic fatty l.
amiodarone l.
l. angiosarcoma
l. bed
biliary cirrhotic l.
brimstone l.
bronze l.
l. calcification
l. capillary hemangioma
l. capsule
cardiac impression on l.
caudate lobe of l.
l. cell adenoma
centrilobular region of l.
Chinese fluke l.
l. cirrhosis
cirrhotic l.
l. coil

l. cyst
degenerative l.
degraded l.
diaphragmatic surface of l.
l. dome
l. echinococcosis
echogenic l.
l. edema
l. edge
enlarged l.
European Association for Study of the L.
extracorporeal l
l. failure
fat-spared area in fatty l.
fatty l.
l. fissure
l. flap
floating l.
l. fluke
focal fatty infiltration of l.
frosted l.
graft-versus-host disease of l.
l. granuloma
l. hemangiosarcoma
hobnail l.
l. hydatid disease
hyperperfusion abnormality of l.
hypoechoic l.
l. impression
infantile hemangioendothelioma of l.
intracorporeal l.
l., kidneys, and spleen (LKS)
l. laceration
large-droplet fatty l.
left lobe of l.
l. lesion
l. lipoma
l. lobe
l. lymphoma
l. mass
l. metastasis
nodular l.
nodule-in-nodule l.
noncirrhotic l.
nutmeg appearance of l.
l. parenchyma
l. phylogeny
polycystic l.
polylobar l.
prominent l.
pyogenic l.
quadrate lobe of l.
right lobe of l.
l. scan
l. scintigraphy
l. scintiphotography
l. segment
shrunken l.

L

liver (*continued*)
    small-droplet fatty l.
    l. span
    l. spoked wheel pattern
    stasis l.
    l. steatosis
    tramline effect in l.
    l. transplant
    l. trauma
    undersurface of l.
    visceral surface of l.
    wandering l.
    waxy l.
liver-aorta (L/A)
liverlike lung
liver-lung scan
Liverpool silicosis
liver-specific
    l.-s. contrast ultrasound imaging
    l.-s. MRI contrast agent
liver-spleen
    l.-s. imaging
    l.-s. overlap
    l.-s. scan
liver-to-aorta peak ratio
liver-to-liver peak (L/LP)
liver-to-muscle contrast ratio
liver-to-spleen attenuation ratio
Livierato sign
living-donor liver transplant (LDLT)
Livingston triangle
LKS
    liver, kidneys, and spleen
LLD
    leg-length discrepancy
    limb-length discrepancy
LLE
    left lower extremity
LLL
    left lower lobe
L-loop
    L-l. heart
    L-l. ventricular situs
L-looping
L/LP
    liver-to-liver peak
    L/LP ratio
LLQ
    left lower quadrant
LLS
    leaky lung syndrome
L-malposition of aorta
LMBD
    lingular mandibular bony defect
LMCA
    left main coronary artery
L-methylmethionine
    [11]C L-m.

LML
    left middle lobe
LMR
    localized magnetic resonance
    Biosense-guided LMR
LMWH
    low molecular weight heparin
LN
    lymph node
    Imagent LN
LNV
    last normal vertebra
load
    combination flow and pressure l.
    exercise l.
    iodine l.
    osmotic l.
    predominant flow l.
    rotatory l.
loading
    axial weight l.
    coil l.
    contrast l.
    fracture callus l.
    left ventricular l.
    longitudinal l.
    peripheral l.
    spike l.
    l. technique
    uniform l.
lobar
    l. breast anatomy
    l. bronchus
    l. cavitation
    l. consolidation
    l. dysmorphism
    l. emphysema
    l. holoprosencephaly
    l. hyperinflation
    l. intracerebral hemorrhage
    l. lung atrophy
    l. nephronia
    l. pneumonia
    l. renal infarct
    l. resorption atelectasis
    l. sclerosis
lobation
    fetal kidney l.
    persistent cortical kidney l.
    persistent renal l.
lobatum
    hepar l.
lobatus
    ren l.
lobe
    accessory l.
    anterior tip of temporal l.
    association cortex of parietal l.
    calciform l.

caudate l.
collapsed l.
cuneiform l.
fetal l.
flocculonodular l.
frontal l.
hepatic l.
hot caudate l.
hyperexpanded l.
inferior l.
insular l.
left lower l. (LLL)
left middle l. (LML)
left upper l. (LUL)
limbic l.
liver l.
lower l.
medial temporal l.
middle l.
occipital l.
l. of azygos vein
l. of kidney
orbital aspect of frontal l.
parietal l.
polyalveolar l.
prominent pyramidal thyroid l.
pulmonary l.
pyramidal l.
ratio of caudate to right
  hepatic l.
Riedel l.
right lower l. (RLL)
right middle l. (RML)
right upper l. (RUL)
Rokitansky l.
sequestered l.
spigelian l.
succenturiate placental l.
superior l.
temporal l.
thyroid l.
uncus of temporal l.
upper l.
wedge-shaped l.

lobectomy
anterior temporal l. (ATL)
sleeve l.

lobster-claw deformity

lobular
l. alveolar pattern
l. architecture
l. atelectasis
l. breast calcification
l. breast microcalcification
l. bronchiole
l. carcinoma
l. carcinoma in situ (LCIS)
l. neoplasia
l. pneumonia

lobulate (*var. of* lobulated)
l. margin

lobulated, lobulate
l. border
l. contour
l. filling defect
l. kidney
l. mass
l. paratracheal mediastinum
l. saccular appearance
l. shape
l. tumor

lobulation
fetal l.

lobule
breast l.
fat l.
inferior parietal l.
inferior temporal l.
lung l.
l. of epididymis
paracentral l.
primary pulmonary l.
pulmonary l.
Reid l.
secondary pulmonary l.
splenic l.

LOCA
low-osmolar contrast agent

local
l. bone blood flow
l. bulge of kidney contour
l. bulge of renal contour
l. cavus
l. compression fracture
l. decompression fracture
l. edema
l. glomerular lesion
l. gradient coil
l. host response (LHR)
l. irradiation
l. metastasis
l. misregistration
l. nodal disease
l. recurrence
l. recurrence-free survival
l. streptokinase infusion

LocaLisa cardiac navigation system

localization
anatomic l.
autologous white cell l.
autoradiographic l.
CT-directed hook-wire l.
fluoroscopic l.
g-probe l.
l. grid
lesion l.
magnetic resonance imaging-guided
  wire l.

L

localization (*continued*)
    MRI-guided wire l.
    needle l.
    needle-hookwire l.
    off-axis point l.
    pelvic film for IUD l.
    placental l.
    point l.
    preoperative l.
    radiopharmaceutical l.
    radiotherapy l.
    sagittal l.
    seizure l.
    stereotactic l.
    surface coil l.
    l. technique
    voxel l.
    l. window
    wire l.

localization-compression grid plate
localized
    l. angiofollicular lymph node
    hyperplasia
    l. caliectasis
    l. coarctation
    l. edema
    l. expansion
    l. fibrous mesothelioma
    l. fibrous tumor of pleura
    l. H-1 spectroscopy
    l. hyperintensity
    l. ileus
    l. intimal flap
    l. lesion
    l. lucent lung
    l. lymphangioma
    l. magnetic resonance (LMR)
    l. mass effect
    l. myeloma
    l. necrosis
    l. obstructive emphysema
    l. osteopenia
    l. osteoporosis
    l. pleural thickening
    l. pleura tumor
    l. proton magnetic resonance
    spectroscopy
    l. pure ground-glass opacity
    l. shimming
    l. single-voxel proton spectrum
    l. uptake
localizer
    axial l.
    breast l.
    Homer needle/wire l.
    picket fence stereotactic l.
    T1-weighted axial l.
localizing
    l. image

    l. imaging
    l. probe
    l. sign
locally
    l. advanced breast cancer
    l. invasive tumor
location
    juxtadiaphragmatic l.
loci (*pl. of* locus)
lock
    air l.
    field l.
    suture l.
locked
    l. facet
    l. knee
    l. nuclear magnetization
locked-in syndrome
locking
    adiabatic off-resonance spin l.
    l. disc
lock-washer configuration
Lockwood ligament
LOCM
    low-osmolar contrast medium
locomotor pattern
locoregional
    l. breast cancer
    l. breast carcinoma
    l. control
    l. disease
    l. field radiotherapy
    l. hyperthermia
    l. lymph node
    l. recurrence
locular
loculated
    l. empyema
    l. hydropneumothorax
    l. pleural effusion
    l. pleural fluid
    l. ventricle
loculation
    dumbbell l.
    intraosseous l.
loculi (*pl. of* loculus)
loculus, *pl.* **loculi**
locus, *pl.* **loci**
    quantitative trait l.
    scanning l.
Löffler
    L. fibroplastic endocarditis
    L. pneumonia
    L. syndrome
Löfgren syndrome
log
    l. amplifier
    l. roll
logetronography

Logic 700 MR transducer
log-rank test
Löhlein-Baehr lesion
Löhlein diameter
loiasis
lollipop tree appearance
long
    l. axial oblique view
    l. axis
    l. axis of bone
    l. axis of kidney
    l. axis of spleen
    l. bone
    l. dural tail
    l. echo-train fast spin-echo sequence
    l. fiber
    l. finger
    l. head
    l. head of biceps
    l. head of biceps tendon (LHBT)
    l. oblique fracture
    l. segmental diaphysial uptake bone
      scintigraphy
    l. smooth esophageal narrowing
    l. smooth narrowing esophagus
    l. TE MR spectroscopy
    l. tract
    l. tract sign
    l. TR/TE
    l. TR/TE sequence
    l. ultrashort T2-suppressed echo
      time
    l. wavelength photo label
long-axis
    l.-a. acquisition
    l.-a. parasternal view
    l.-a. ray
    l.-a. slice
long-bone
    l.-b. fracture
    l.-b. pseudarthrosis
    l.-b. survey
long-bore collimator
long-chain fatty acid
longitudinal
    l. acoustic wave
    l. arch
    l. arteriography
    l. axis
    l. band
    l. blood supply
    l. B-mode
    l. esophageal fold
    l. esophageal stricture
    l. fasciculus
    l. fissure
    l. image
    l. lie
    l. ligament

l. loading
l. magnetization
l. muscle
l. narrowing
l. oval pelvis
l. raphe
l. recovery time
l. relaxation
l. relaxation time
l. relaxivity
l. renal ectopia
l. ridge
l. scan
l. section imaging
l. section tomography
l. split biceps tendon
l. suture
l. tear of brevis tendon
l. tenia musculature
l. tibial fatigue fracture
l. transarticular derangement
l. ultrasonic biometry
l. ultrasound view
longitudinalis medialis fasciculus
long-scale
    l.-s. contrast
    l.-s. imaging agent
long-taper stiff-shaft Glidewire
long-term
    l.-t. nonprogressor
    l.-t. patency
    l.-t. sequela
    l.-t. venous instrumentation
longus
    abductor pollicis l. (APL)
    adductor l.
    l. colli muscle
    extensor carpi radialis l. (ECRL)
    extensor digiti l.
    extensor digitorum l. (EDL)
    extensor hallucis l. (EHL)
    extensor pollicis l. (EPL)
    flexor digitorum l. (FDL)
    flexor hallucis l.
    flexor pollicis l.
    palmaris l.
    peroneus l.
lookup table (LUT)
loop
    access l.
    afferent l.
    air-filled l.
    alpha sigmoid l.
    bowel l.
    C l.
    capillary l.
    cervical l.
    cine l.
    closed conducting l.

L

loop (*continued*)
    colonic l.
    conductive l.
    contiguous l.'s
    Cope l.
    Cordonnier ureteroileal l.
    dextro l.
    diathermic l.
    dilated bowel l.
    l. distribution
    double reverse alpha
      sigmoid l.
    duodenal l.
    duodenal C l.
    efferent l.
    flow-volume l.
    frontal plane l.
    gamma transverse colon l.
    Gerdy interatrial l.
    Gerdy interauricular l.
    l. graft
    herniated bowel l.
    horizontal plane l.
    Hutson l.
    ileal l.
    intestinal l.
    J l.
    jejunal l.
    lenticular l.
    Lippes l.
    malrotation of bowel l.
    matted small bowel l.
    Meyer l.
    Meyer-Archambault l.
    nonrotation of bowel l.
    N-shaped sigmoid l.
    l. of Henle
    l. ostomy bridge
    P l.
    peduncular l.
    pressure-volume l.
    puborectalis l.
    reentrant l.
    Roux l.
    rubber vessel l.
    sagittal plane l.
    sentinel l.
    separation of bowel l.
    sigmoid l.
    small bowel l.
    Stoerck l.
    subclavian l.
    T l.
    thickened bowel l.
    transverse colon l.
    unopacified bowel l.
    vector l.
    ventricular l.
    vessel l.
    Vieussens l.
    Waltman l.

2-loop ileal J pouch
loopless antenna
loopogram imaging
loopography
    ileal l.
loose
    l. fracture
    l. intraarticular body
    l. mesenchymal tissue
    l. osteochondral fragment
    l. shoulder
Looser
    L. line
    L. transformation zone
lopamidol
LOQ
    lower outer quadrant
LOR
    line of response
Lorad
    L. digital breast imager
    L. full-field digital mammography
      system
    L. StereoGuide
Lorain-Lévi dwarfism
lordosis
    cervical l.
    gentle l.
    lumbar l.
    reversal of cervical l.
    spinal l.
    thoracic l.
lordotic
    l. aspect
    l. curve
    l. pelvis
    l. position
    l. view
lorentzian
    l. curve
    l. field mapping
    l. line
    l. line saturation
Lorenz position
lorry driver's fracture
LoSo Prep bowel preparation
loss
    l. coincidence
    dead time l.
    electron equilibrium l.
    global tissue l.
    high-velocity signal l.
    l. of bone mass
    l. of definition
    l. of distinction
    l. of elasticity of cartilage
    l. of parallelism of facet joint

l. of sigmoid curve
l. of thoracic kyphosis
percentage signal intensity l.
segmental bone l.
signal l.
single collision energy l.
time-of-flight signal l.
TOF signal l.
transformer l.
volume l.

lossless image data compression
lossy image data compression
lost intrauterine device
lotus position
Louis

L. angle
sternal angle of L.

Louis-Bar syndrome
lovers' knot
low

l. attenuation
l. back injury
l. back pain
l. back syndrome
l. cardiac output
l. conus medullaris
l. density
l. field MRI
l. field-strength MR imaging
l. flip-angle gradient-echo imaging
l. frame rate
l. frame-rate run
l. interobserver variation
l. lung volume
l. metastatic potential
l. molecular weight heparin
 (LMWH)
l. normal
l. osmolality
l. pitch
l. right atrium (LRA)
l. septal right atrium
l. signal intensity
l. signal-intensity artifact
l. signal intensity fibrous band
l. signal-intensity fibrous septum
l. signal intensity peripheral band
l. signal-intensity replacement
l. signal intensity synchondrosis
l. signal intensity tumor
l. small bowel obstruction
l. urethral pressure (LUP)
l. yield

low-amplitude internal echo
low-angle

l.-a. scattering
l.-a. shot technique

low-attenuation

l.-a. lesion

l.-a. mediastinal mass
l.-a. pulsation artifact

Low-Beers

L.-B. position
L.-B. projection
L.-B. view

low-compliance fixed-diameter balloon
low-concentration

l. c. barium (LCB)
l.-c. contrast medium (LCCM)

low-contact dynamic compression plate
 (LC-DCP)
low-contrast

l.-c. detail (LCD)
l.-c. detectability
l.-c. film
l.-c. resolution (LCR)
l.-c. structure

low-density

l.-d. mesencephalic lesion
l.-d. rim
l.-d. ring
l.-d. structure

low-dose

l.-d. dobutamine (LDD)
l.-d. film
l.-d. film mammographic technique
l.-d. hepatic multidetector computed
 tomography
l.-d. mammography
l.-d. screen-film technique

low-dose/high-dose protocol
Löwenberg canal
low-energy

l.-e. all-purpose (LEAP)
l.-e. collimator
l.-e. fracture
l.-e. general purpose (LEGP)
l.-e. high-resolution (LEHR)
l.-e. laser (LEL)
l.-e. photon attenuation measurement
l.-e. radiofrequency conduction
 hyperthermia treatment
l.-e. ultrahigh resolution (LEUHR)

lower

l. basilar aneurysm
l. esophageal mucosal ring
l. esophageal narrowing
l. esophageal sphincter (LES)
l. esophageal sphincter dysfunction
l. esophageal sphincter pressure
 (LESP)
l. extremity
l. extremity arterial tree
l. extremity CT venography
 (LE-CTV)
l. extremity imaging
l. field-strength MRI scanner
l. field visual sector

L

lower (*continued*)
    l. gastrointestinal hemorrhage
    l. inner quadrant (LIQ)
    l. limb venography
    l. limb venography imaging
    l. lobe
    l. lobe lung mass
    l. lobe of lung
    l. lobe pneumonia
    l. lobe reticulation
    l. lung field
    l. lung line
    l. moiety ureter
    l. motor neuron
    l. motor neuron lesion
    l. outer quadrant (LOQ)
    l. pole
    l. pole collecting system
    l. pole of kidney
    l. pole of patella
    l. pole of ureter
    l. pulmonary lobe atelectasis
    l. right quadrant (LRQ)
    l. station
    l. sternal border
    l. tract
    L. tubercle
lower-energy image
Lowe syndrome
low-field
    l.-f. magnetic resonance
    l.-f. MR angiography
    l.-f. MRI system
    l.-f. MR scanner
    l.-f. open scanner
low-flow syndrome
low-flux polysufone membrane
low-frequency
    l.-f. scatter
    l.-f. ultrasound (LFUS)
low-grade
    l.-g. astrocytoma
    l.-g. central osteosarcoma
    l.-g. glioma
    l.-g. malignancy
    l.-g. neoplasia
    l.-g. squamous intraepithelial lesion
    (LGSIL, LSIL)
low-intensity
    l.-i. laser irradiation (LILI)
    l.-i. laser therapy (LILT)
    l.-i. line
    l.-i. pulsed ultrasound
low-iodine diet (LID)
low-level echo
low-lying placenta
Lown-Ganong-Levine (LGL)
    L.-G.-L. Syndrome
low-osmolality contrast agent

low-osmolar
    l.-o. contrast agent (LOCA)
    l.-o. contrast medium (LOCM)
low-output heart failure
low-pass
    l.-p. 3-dimensional postfiltering
    l.-p. filter
    l.-p. filtering
low-photon energy
low-pressure
    l.-p. cardiac tamponade
    l.-p. hydrocephalus
    l.-p. mercury arc amp
low-profile
    l.-p. IUGR
    l.-p. mitral valve
low-resistance spectral waveform
low-resolution imaging
low-risk single-stone former
low-signal mass
Lowsley lobar anatomy
low-temperature diffraction
low-T humerus fracture
low-velocity flow
LP
    lumbar puncture
    lymphomatous polyposis
LPA
    left pulmonary artery
L-PAM
    l-phenylalanine mustard
l-phenylalanine mustard (L-PAM)
LPI
    laser projection imaging
    LPI laser system
LPO
    left posterior oblique
    LPO position
LPSM
    laparoscopic port-site metastasis
LP^2 stainless steel delivery system
LPV
    left pulmonary vein
LQ
    linear-quadratic
    LQ ratio
Lr
    lawrencium
LRA
    low right atrium
L-radiation
LRQ
    lower right quadrant
LSC
    laser scanning cytometry
LSCVP
    left subclavian central venous pressure
LSF
    line spread function

LSIL
  low-grade squamous intraepithelial
    lesion
LSO
  lutetium oxyorthosilicate
    LSO crystal scintillator material
L5-S1 projection
LSR
  lanthanide shift reagent
LSS
  lumbosacral spine
LSV
  lenticulostriate vasculopathy
LTA
  laser thermal ablation
    MRI-guided LTA
LTK
  laser thermal keratoplasty
L-transposition
LTRC
  Lung Tissue Resource Consortium
**LTX3000 lumbar rehabilitation
  system**
l-tyrosine imaging agent
Lu
  lutetium
lucency
    area of l.
    artifactual l.
    interspersed l.
    linear l.
    pulmonary l.
    sandlike l.
    slitlike residual l.
lucent
    l. band
    l. calculus
    l. center
    l. defect
    l. finger lesion
    l. halo
    l. hilar notch
    l. interval
    l. line
    l. lung lesion
lucent-centered calcification
Lucite
    L. beam
    L. beam spoiler
LUCL
  lateral ulnar collateral ligament
Ludovici angle
Ludwig
    L. angina
    L. angle
    L. plane
luetic
    l. aortic aneurysm
    l. aortitis

    l. arteritis
    l. diaphysitis
luftsichel sign
LUL
  left upper lobe
Luma cervical imaging system
lumazenil
    ^{11}C l.
lumbago
lumbales
    vertebra l.
lumbar
    l. aortography
    l. arteriography
    l. artery
    l. curvature
    l. disc
    l. facet angle
    l. fascia
    l. flexion and extension study
    l. hernia
    l. kidney
    l. kyphosis
    l. lordosis
    l. lordotic curve
    l. lymph node
    l. myelogram
    l. myelography
    l. nerve root
    l. part of diaphragm
    l. plexus
    l. pneumoencephalography
    l. puncture (LP)
    l. rib
    l. root avulsion
    l. scoliosis
    l. spinal canal
    l. spinal stenosis
    l. spine
    l spine dimension
    l. spine fracture
    l. spine lesion
    l. spine view
    l. sympathetic block
    l. synovial cyst
    l. transverse process
    l. vertebra
    l. vertebral body index
lumbarization
lumbarized spine
lumbocostal ligament
lumbocostoabdominal triangle
lumboperitoneal shunting
lumborum
    quadratus l.
lumbosacral
    l. agenesis
    l. canal
    l. dermal sinus

L

lumbosacral (*continued*)
l. disc
l. intervertebral disc herniation
l. joint angle
l. kyphosis
l. lateral recess
l. myelography
l. plexus
l. projection
l. series
l. spine (LSS)
l. spine depth
l. spine strain
l. trunk
lumbrical tendon
lumbricoides
Ascaris l.
lumen, *pl.* **lumina,** *pl.* **lumens**
aortic l.
arterial l.
l. assessment
attenuated l.
bile duct l.
bowel l.
bronchial l.
carotid l.
clot-filled l.
cloverleaf-shaped l.
crescentic l.
cystic duct l.
l. delineation
l. diameter
dilated small bowel l.
double l.
double-barrel l.
D-shaped vessel l.
duct l.
duodenal l.
eccentrically placed l.
elliptic l.
esophageal l.
false l.
gastric l.
gastroduodenal l.
in-stent l.
intestinal l.
midgroove portion of l.
occluded l.
patent l.
scalloped bowel l.
slitlike l.
slit-shaped vessel l.
star-shaped vessel l.
tracheal l.
true l.
vascular l.
lumen-intima interface
8-lumen manometric catheter
lumenogram (*var. of* luminogram)

lumenographic technique
lumens (*pl. of* lumen)
lumina (*pl. of* lumen)
luminal
l. area
l. caliber
l. defect
l. dimension
l. distention
l. encroachment
l. irregularity
l. narrowing
l. plaque
l. plug
l. silhouette
l. stenosis
l. thrombosis
l. wall
luminance
view-box l.
luminescence
pulsed optically stimulated l.
(POSL)
Luminexx
L. biliary stent
L. self-expanding stent
luminiferous
luminogram, lumenogram
air l.
luminous intensity
Lumiscan LS 85 scanner
Lumisys 20 digital x-ray scanner
lumpectomy bed
lump kidney
lumpy appearance of lung
LUNA
laparoscopic uterosacral nerve
ablation
lunar
L. DPX densitometer
L. Expert densitometer
L. scanner
lunate
avascular necrosis of l.
l. bone
l. dislocation
l. facet
l. fracture
l. tilt
lunate-shaped trachea
lunate-triquetral coalition
lunatomalacia
Lunderquist exchange guidewire
Lunderquist-Ring guidewire
lung
l. abscess
acquired unilateral hyperlucent l.
l. adenocarcinoma
l. agenesis

air conditioner l.
air-filled l.
airless l.
l. airspace
amiodarone l.
l. amyloidosis
l. apex
l. aplasia
l. arch
l. architecture
arc welder's l.
artificial l.
atelectatic l.
azygos lobe of l.
l. base
l. base infiltrate
bauxite fibrosis of l.
Bible printer's l.
bilateral hyperlucent l.'s
bird breeder's l.
bird fancier's l.
bird handler's l.
black l.
blunt border of l.
brown induration of l.
bubbly l.
budgerigar fancier's l.
l. calculus
l. capacity
l. carcinoma
l. cavity
cheese handler's l.
cheese washer's l.
chest fluke l.
cluster-of-grapes l.
coal miner's l.
coal worker's l.
l. coccidioidomycosis
coffee worker's l.
coin lesion of l.
collapsed l.
l. compliance
l. connectivity test
consolidated l.
contralateral l.
l. contusion
convexity of l.
corundum smelter's l.
l. count curve
l. cylindroma
l. cyst
cystic l.
dark l.
l. decortication
l. density
dependent l.
drowned l.
dusty l.
dynamic l.

l. echinococcosis
eclipse effect l.
l. edema
l. emphysema
emphysematous l.
empty collapsed l.
endstage l.
expanded l.
l. expansion
farmer's l.
fibroid l.
fibroma of l.
fibrosis of l.
l. field
fishmeal worker's l.
l. fissure
fissure of l.
l. fluke
folded l.
l. fungus ball
furrier's l.
gangrene of l.
grain handler's l.
l. granuloma
graphite fibrosis of l.
gray l.
l. hamartoma
hardened l.
harvester's l.
hazy opaque l.
l. hemangioma
l. hemorrhage
hemorrhagic consolidation of l.
hen worker's l.
l. hepatization
l. hilum
l. histoplasmosis
honeycomb l.
horizontal fissure of l.
horseshoe l.
humidifier l.
hyperlucent l.
hypersensitivity l.
hypogenetic l.
hypoinflation of l.
hypolucency of l.
l. hypoplasia
hypoplastic l.
idiopathic unilateral hyperlucent l.
l. imaging
immature l.
l. infarct
inferior lobe of l.
l. infiltrate distribution
l. inflammation
l. interstitium
l. laceration
light pink l.
l. linearity

L

565

lung (*continued*)
    lingular division of left l.
    liverlike l.
    l. lobule
    localized lucent l.
    lower lobe of l.
    lumpy appearance of l.
    l. lymphangiectasis
    l. lymphangioma
    l. lymphoid hyperplasia
    l. lymphoma
    malignant epithelioid
      leiomyoblastoma of l.
    MALT worker's l.
    maple bark-stripper's l.
    l. marking
    mason's l.
    l. mass
    meat wrapper's l.
    l. metastasis
    middle lobe of l.
    miller's l.
    miner's l.
    mottled gray l.
    mushroom worker's l.
    native l.
    l. necrosis
    neoplasm of l.
    l. nodularity
    l. nodule
    nondependent l.
    oblique fissure of l.
    l. opacity
    l. overexpansion
    l. overinflation
    l. paragonimiasis
    parakeet fancier's l.
    l. parenchyma
    l. parenchyma consolidation
    partial collapse of l.
    l. perfusion
    l. perfusion defect
    l. perfusion radionuclide
    l. periphery
    physiologically immature l.
    pigeon fancier's l.
    polycystic l.
    l. popcorn calcification
    postperfusion l.
    l. pseudocavitation
    l. pseudolymphoma
    pump l.
    l. reexpansion
    reperfusion injury of postischemic l.
    l. resistance-related protein
    right l.
    l. root
    rounded border of l.
    rudimentary l.

    l. sarcoid
    l. scan
    l. scintigraphy
    l. segmentation
    septic l.
    sequestered lobe of l.
    sharp border of l.
    shock l.
    l. shock
    shrunken l.
    silicotic fibrosis of l.
    silo-filler's l.
    silver finisher's l.
    silver polisher's l.
    smoker's l.
    solid edema of l.
    l. starfish scar
    static l.
    l. stiffness
    stiff noncompliant l.
    l. stone
    stretched l.
    structurally immature l.
    subsegment of l.
    superior lobe of l.
    surface tension of l.
    l. talcosis
    L. Tissue Resource Consortium
      (LTRC)
    l. torsion
    l. transplant
    transverse fissure of l.
    true unilateral hyperlucent l.
    l. tuberculoma
    l. tumor
    l. underinflation
    underventilated l.
    unilateral hyperlucent l.
    upper lobe of l.
    uremic l.
    vanishing l.
    l. varix
    l. volume
    l. volume loop flow
    l. washout
    welder's l.
    well-inflated l.
    wet l.
    l. window
    l. zone
lung-heart ratio of thallium-201 activity
lung-mediastinum interface
lunocapitate bone
lunohamate arthritis
lunotriquetral
    l. interosseus ligament
    l. joint
lunula, *pl.* **lunulae**

lunulae (*pl. of* lunula)
LUP
    low urethral pressure
lupus
    l. cerebritis
    drug-induced erythematous l.
    l. erythematosus (LE)
LUQ
    left upper quadrant
Luque rod
LUS
    laparoscopic ultrasound
Luschka
    L. bursa
    L. crypt
    L. duct leak
    foramen of L.
    L. joint
    L. ligament
    L. muscle
    sinuvertebral nerve of L.
lusoria
    arteria l.
    dysphagia l.
LUT
    lookup table
luteal
    l. cyst
    l. phase
    l. phase defect
luteinized
    l. unruptured follicle
    l. unruptured follicle syndrome
Lutembacher
    L. complex
    L. syndrome
luteoma
lutetium (Lu)
    l. oxyorthosilicate (LSO)
    l. oxyorthosilicate-based PET
    scanner
    l. tantalate
lux (LX, lx)
luxated bone
luxation
    ligamentous l.
Luxtec fiberoptic system
luxury
    l. perfusion
    l. perfusion syndrome
Luys body
LVA
    left ventricular aneurysm
LVAD
    left ventricular assist device
LVD
    left ventricular dysfunction
LVdd
    left ventricular diastolic dimension

LVEDD
    left ventricular end-diastolic dimension
LVEDI
    left ventricular end-diastolic volume
    index
LVEDP
    left ventricular end-diastolic pressure
LVEF
    left ventricular ejection fraction
    exercise 1st-pass LVEF
LVESD
    left ventricular end-systolic dimension
LVESVI
    left ventricular end-systolic volume
    index
LVET
    left ventricular ejection time
LVFS
    left ventricular functional shortening
LVFW
    left ventricular free wall
LVG
    left ventriculogram
LVH
    left ventricular hypertrophy
LVID
    left ventricular internal diameter
LVIDd
    left ventricular internal diastolic
    dimension
LVIDs
    left ventricular internal dimension at
    end-systole
LVIV
    left ventricular inflow volume
LVM
    left ventricular mass
LVMI
    left ventricular mass index
LVOT
    left ventricular outflow tract
    LVOT flow rate
LVOTO
    left ventricular outflow tract
    obstruction
LVOV
    left ventricular outflow volume
LVP
    left ventricular pressure
LVPW
    left ventricular posterior wall
LVs
    left ventricular systolic
    LVs system
LVSW
    left ventricular stroke work
LVSWI
    left ventricular stroke work
    index

L

LVW
    left ventricular wall
LX, lx
    lux
    LX EchoSpeed 1.5T CV/i, NVi MR
      system
    LX 20 laser
    LX 8.3 software
lye stricture
Lyme carditis
lymph
    l. capillary
    l. duct
    l. gland
    l. node (LN)
    l. node amyloidosis
    l. node dissection
    l. node eggshell calcification
    l. node enlargement
    l. node imaging
    l. node involvement
    l. node metastasis
    l. node-revealing solution
    l. node sinus
    l. node station
    l. node syndrome
    l. node tissue
    l. plexus
    l. vessel of prostate
lymphadenectomy
lymphadenitis
    cervical tuberculous l.
    cryptococcal l.
    granulomatous l.
    nonspecific granulomatous l.
    regional granulomatous l.
    subacute necrotizing l.
    tuberculous l.
lymphadenography
lymphadenopathy
    amyloid l.
    angioblastic l.
    angioimmunoblastic l.
    axillary l.
    benign l.
    cervical l.
    intraabdominal l.
    mediastinal l.
    mesenteric l.
    peripancreatic l.
    persistent generalized l.
    reactive l.
    retrocrural l.
    retroperitoneal l.
    secondary axillary l.
    superficial l.
    l. syndrome
    tuberculous l.

lymphangeitis (*var. of* lymphangitis)
lymphangiectasia (*var. of* lymphangiectasis)
lymphangiectasis, lymphangiectasia
    acquired intestinal l.
    congenital l.
    generalized l.
    intestinal l.
    lung l.
    primary pulmonary l.
    pulmonary l.
    pulmonary cystic l.
    secondary l.
    submucosal l.
    subserosal l.
lymphangiitis (*var. of* lymphangitis)
lymphangiogram (LAG)
lymphangiographic imaging agent
lymphangiography
    bipedal l.
    contrast l.
    high-resolution magnetic resonance l.
      (HR-MRL)
    l. imaging
    magnetic resonance l. (MRL)
    pedal l.
lymphangiohemangioma
lymphangioleiomyomatosis (LAM)
lymphangioma
    capillary l.
    cardiac l.
    cavernous l.
    diffuse l.
    localized l.
    lung l.
    l. mesentery
    neck l.
    orbital l.
    pancreatic cystic l.
    pericardial l.
    retroperitoneal l.
    simple capillary l.
lymphangiomatosis
    pulmonary l.
lymphangitic
    l. carcinomatosis
    l. metastasis
lymphangitis, lymphangiitis, lymphangeitis
lymphatic
    l. canal
    l. carcinomatosis
    l. channel
    l. collecting vessel
    l. cortex
    l. development
    dilated l.'s
    l. drainage pattern
    l. duct
    l. dysplasia

l. edema
l. hypoplasia
l. imaging
l. leak
l. malformation
l. mapping
l. medulla
l. metastasis
l. needle disruption
l. network
l. obstruction
paracervical l.'s
patulous l.'s
prominent septal l.'s
pulmonary l.'s
l. reflux
l. sac
l. sarcoma
subpleural l.'s
thoracic l.'s
l. tissue
l. trunk
l. tuberculosis
l. tumor spread
l. valve
l. vessel invasion

lymphatica
pseudopolyposis l.

**lymphaticovenous secondary
edema**

lymphaticum
angioma l.

Lymphazurin imaging agent

lymphedema
Meige l.
Nonne-Milroy l.
postmastectomy l.
primary l.
secondary l.

lymphoblastic lymphoma

lymphoblastoma

lymphocapillary vessel

lymphocele
renal transplant l.

lymphocyte-rich tumor

lymphocytic
l. hypophysitis
l. interstitial pneumonia (LIP)
l. interstitial pneumonitis (LIP)
l. plasmacytoid lymphoma
l. poorly differentiated lymphoma
l. well-differentiated lymphoma

lymphoepithelial
l. carcinoma
l. cyst
l. parotid tumor

lymphoepithelioma
salivary gland l.

lymphogenous
l. dissemination
l. embolus
l. metastasis

lymphogranuloma venereum

lymphography
computed tomographic l.
contrast material-enhanced
    intravenous l.
indirect computed tomographic l.
magnetic resonance l.
MR l.
pedal l.
percutaneous transhepatic l. (pTL)
time-lapse quantitative computed
    tomographic l.

lymphohematogenous dissemination

lymphohistiocytosis
familial l.
hemophagocytic l. (HLH)

lymphoid
l. follicle
l. hamartoma
l. hyperplasia
l. hypophysitis
l. interstitial pneumonia (LIP)
l. interstitial pneumonitis (LIP)
l. polyp
l. tumor

lymphoma
abdominal l.
acute lymphoblastic l.
adult T-cell l.
African Burkitt l.
aggressive good prognosis
    non-Hodgkin l.
aggressive histology l.
anaplastic large cell l. (ALCL)
angioimmunoblastic
    lymphadenopathy-like T-cell l.
angioimmunoblastic T-cell l.
    (ATCL)
angiotropic large cell l.
B-cell monocytoid l.
B-cell non-Hodkin l.
bone l.
brain l.
breast l.
Burkitt l.
Burkitt-like l.
butterfly l.
B-zone small lymphocytic l.
Castleman l.
centroblastic l.
centrocytic l.
cerebral l.
cleaved cell l.
CNS l.

L

lymphoma (*continued*)
    cobblestone appearance of l.
    colorectal l.
    convoluted T-cell l.
    cutaneous B-cell l. (CBCL)
    cutaneous T-cell l. (CTCL)
    diffuse aggressive l.
    diffuse intermediate lymphocytic l.
    diffuse large cell l. (DLCL)
    diffuse mixed small and large
      cell l.
    diffuse small cell lymphocytic l.
    dural arachnoid l.
    enteropathy-associated T-cell l.
    epidural l.
    extranodal follicular l.
    extranodal non-Hodgkin l.
    follicular B-cell l.
    follicular center cell l.
    follicular mixed small cleaved l.
    follicular predominantly large
      cell l.
    follicular predominantly small
      cell l.
    fulminant cerebral l.
    gallium scintigraphy of l.
    gastric l.
    gastrointestinal l.
    giant follicle l.
    granulomatous l.
    hepatic non-Hodgkin l.
    histiocytic bone l.
    histiocytic brain l.
    histiocytic chest l.
    Hodgkin l.
    human immunodeficiency
      virus-associated non-Hodgkin l.
    immunoblastic large cell l.
    infiltrative l.
    intracerebral l.
    kidney l.
    large B-cell l.
    large cell thyroid l.
    large cleaved cell l.
    limited-stage diffuse large cell l.
    liver l.
    lung l.
    lymphoblastic l.
    lymphocytic plasmacytoid l.
    lymphocytic poorly differentiated l.
    lymphocytic well-differentiated l.
    lymphoplasmacytoid l.
    macroglobulinemic l.
    malignant l.
    MALT l.
    mantle cell l. (MCL)
    marginal zone l. (MZL)
    marginal zone B-cell l.

    mediastinal l.
    mesencephalic cerebral l.
    mesenterial Castleman l.
    mesenteric l.
    metastatic testicular l.
    mixed lymphocytic-histiocytic l.
    mixed small and large cell l.
    monocytoid B-cell l.
    mucosa-associated lymphoid tissue l.
      (MALToma)
    multifocal l.
    noncleaved cell l.
    non-Hodgkin l. (NHL)
    orbital l.
    osseous l.
    pancreatic l.
    peripheral l.
    perirenal l.
    plasmablastic l.
    pleomorphic T-cell l.
    polypoid l.
    primary adrenal l.
    primary bone l.
    primary brain l.
    primary central nervous system l.
    primary cerebral non-Hodgkin l.
    primary CNS l.
    primary cutaneous large B-cell l.
      (PCLBCL)
    primary extranodal l.
    primary gastric non-Hodgkin l.
    primary refractory Burkitt l.
    primary splenic l. (PSL)
    primary uterine l.
    pulmonary l.
    pyothorax-associated pleural l.
    recurrent l.
    renal l.
    retroperitoneal l.
    Revised European American L.
      (REAL)
    secondary brain l.
    secondary cutaneous large B-cell l.
      (SCLBCL)
    sinonasal l.
    skeletal l.
    small B-cell l.
    small lymphatic l.
    small lymphocytic T-cell l.
    spinal epidural l.
    splenic B-cell l.
    splenic marginal l.
    sporadic Burkitt l.
    l. staging
    subcutaneous panniculitis-like T-cell
      l. (SPTL)
    systemic brain l.
    T-cell lymphoblastic l.

thymic l.
thyroid l.
true histiocytic l.
T-zone l.
ulcerative l.
undefined l.
undifferentiated non-Hodgkin l.
urinary bladder l.
uterine cervical l.
vitreous l.
Waldeyer ring l.

lymphomatoid granulomatosis
lymphomatosis
lymphomatosum
cystadenoma l.
papillary cystadenoma l.

lymphomatous
l. lymph node
l. mass
l. polyposis (LP)

lymphonodular hyperplasia
lymphoplasmacytic infiltrate
lymphoplasmacytoid lymphoma
lymphopneumatosis
peritoneal l.

lymphoproliferative disorder
lymphoreticular tissue
LymphoScan
L. imaging agent
L. nuclear imaging system
L. nuclear imaging system scanner
L. Tc99m-labeled murine antibody
fragment

lymphoscintigraphy
cutaneous l.
internal mammary l.
radiocolloid l.

lymphovascular
lymphovenous grafting
Lynch and Crues type 2 lesion
lyoluminescence
lyophilized
Lyra laser
lysate
Lyser
trapezoid bone of L.

Lysholm
L. grid
L. method

lysis
acute tumor l.
bony l.
clot l.
cystic l.
follicle l.
ultrasonic l.

lysosomal storage disorder
lytic
l. area
l. area bone flap
l. bone lesion
l. change
l. lesion of skull
l. osteolysis
l. osteosarcoma
l. pattern

L

m
    meter
        Artoscan M
        M pattern
        M shell
mA, ma
    milliamperage
    milliampere
M2A
    M2A imaging capsule endoscopy
    M2A swallowable imaging
        capsule
MAA
    macroaggregated albumin
        ^{99m}Tc MAA
        MAA study
MACE
    major adverse cardiac event
maceration
    clot m.
Macewen sign
Mach
    M. band
    M. band effect
    M. line
machine
    Acoma portable x ray m.
    Aestiva/5 MRI anesthesia m.
    cobalt megavoltage m.
    2D B-mode ultrasound m.
    Echospeed 1.5T MR m.
    focused segmented ultrasound m.
    m. injection
    neutron therapy m.
    panoramic rotating m.
    parallel virtual m. (PVM)
Mackenrodt ligament
Mackenzie point
Macklin effect
Macleod syndrome
macrencephalia (var. of macrencephaly)
macrencephaly, macrencephalia
macroadenoma
    pituitary m.
    prolactin-secreting pituitary m.
macroaggregated
    m. albumin (MAA)
    m. albumin imaging agent
macroangiography
macrocalcification
macrocirculation
macrocolon
macrocyst
    adrenocortical m.

macrocystic
    m. adenoma
    m. encephalomalacia
    m. neoplasia
    m. pilocytic cerebellar astrocytoma
    m. serous cystadenoma
macrocytic anemia
macrodacryocystography
macrodystrophia lipomatosa
macrofistulous arteriovenous
    communication
macroglobulinemic lymphoma
macrolobular cirrhosis
macrolobulated
macromolecular
    m. content
    m. contrast-enhanced MR imaging
    m. contrast medium (MMCM)
    m. drug
    m. hydration effect
    m. imaging agent
macronodular pattern
macronodule
    mesenteric m.
macroorchidism lesion
macrophage
    m. inflammatory protein (MIP)
    lipid-laden foamy m.
    m. scavenger receptor
    tumor-associated m.
macroradiography
    Buckland-Wright m.
macroreentrant circuit
macroscopic
    m. hemorrhage ligament
    m. magnetic moment
    m. magnetization vector
    m. placental lesion
Macrotec imaging agent
macrovesicular steatosis
MacSpect real-time NMR workstation
macula, pl. maculae
maculae (pl. of macula)
macule
    coal m.
maculopathy bull's-eye magnet
maculosa
    atrophia m.
Maddahi method of calculating right
    ventricular ejection fraction
Madelung
    M. deformity
    M. neck
Madura foot

M

maduromycosis
Maffucci syndrome
MAG
    mercaptoacetyltriglycine
magenblase
Magendie foramen
magenstrasse
MagForce nanoparticle
Maggi biopsy needle
magic
    m. angle effect
    m. angle effect artifact
    m. angle phenomenon
    m. angle spinning imaging
    m. angle spinning NMR
    M. S/P Wallstent
MagicView workstation
Magilligan technique for measuring
  neutral anteversion
MAG3 Lasix renal scan
Maglinte catheter
magna
    abnormal cisterna m.
    arteria radicularis anterior m.
    chorda m.
    cisterna m.
    coxa m.
    mega cisterna m.
Magnascanner
    Picker M.
Magna-SL scanner
Magnes
    M. biomagnetometer
    M. biomagnetometer system
    M. 2500 whole-blood scanner
    M. 2500 whole-head imaging
magnesium
    m. chloride
    m. contrast medium
magnet
    air-core m.
    beam-bending m.
    m. compression anastomosis
    cryostable m.
    doughnut m.
    Eindhoven m.
    Fe-Ex orogastric tube m.
    GE Signa 1.5T m.
    Gyroscan NT 10 m.
    Gyroscan 1.5T superconducting m.
    high-field m.
    Horizon LX 1.5T superconducting
     m.
    hybrid m.
    large-bore m.
    maculopathy bull's-eye m.
    Magnetom SP4000 m.
    Magnex m.

    m. mode
    nonenclosed m.
    open m.
    Oxford m.
    pancake MRI m.
    passively shimmed superconducting
     m.
    permanent m.
    Philips Gyroscan ACS NT
     superconducting m.
    poor shimming of MRI m.
    m. rate
    resistive m.
    m. response
    shimmed m.
    short-bore m.
    m. stability
    superconducting m.
    superconductive m.
    1.0T, 1.5T superconducting m.
    tubular m.
    Walker m.
magnetic
    m. anisotropy
    m. bolus tracking
    m. chemotherapy
    m. circuit
    m. dipole
    m. dipole-dipole coupling
    m. dipole moment
    m. disc
    m. domain
    m. field gradient (MFG)
    m. field perturbation
    m. field strength
    m. flux
    m. flux density
    m. focal plane
    m. fringe field
    m. induction
    m. induction device
    m. interaction
    m. inversion
    m. iron oxide particle (MIOP)
    m. line of force
    m. material
    m. nucleus
    m. particulate
    m. permeability
    m. pole
    m. radiation exposure
    m. resonance (MR)
    m. resonance angiography (MRA)
    m. resonance angiography-directed
     bypass procedure
    m. resonance arthrography
    m. resonance catheter imaging
    m. resonance cholangiogram (MRC)

m. resonance cholangiography with HASTE

m. resonance cholangiopancreatography (MRCP)

m. resonance-compatible pedal ergometer

m. resonance dacryocystography

m. resonance depiction

m. resonance-detected white matter lesion

m. resonance detection

m. resonance diffusion imaging

m. resonance digital subtraction angiography (MRDSA)

m. resonance discriminator of osseous metastasis

m. resonance elastography (MRE)

m. resonance enhancement pattern

m. resonance epidurography

m. resonance hydrographic technique

m. resonance imaging (MRI)

m. resonance imaging-compatible piezoelectric power drill

m. resonance imaging-guided focused ultrasound sector transducer

m. resonance imaging-guided wire localization

m. resonance lymphangiography (MRL)

m. resonance lymphography

m. resonance mammography (MRM)

m. resonance multispectral color image

m. resonance myelography

m. resonance needle tracking

m. resonance neurography (MRN)

m. resonance pancreatography (MRP)

m. resonance pelvimetry

m. resonance perfusion imaging

m. resonance phase velocity mapping

m. resonance phlebography

m. resonance receptor agent

m. resonance sialography

m. resonance signal

m. resonance simulator

m. resonance spectroscopic imaging (MRSI)

m. resonance spectroscopy (MRS)

m. resonance spin incoherence

m. resonance tomography (MRT)

m. resonance urography (MRU)

m. resonance user interface (MRUI)

m. resonance user interface software

m. resonance venogram (MRV)

m. resonance venography (MRV)

m. resonance volume estimation

m. retentivity

m. servomotor

m. shielding

m. source imaging (MSI)

m. stimulation

m. surgery system

m. susceptibility

m. susceptibility artifact

m. susceptibility-weighted image

m. tape storage

magnetic-assisted intervention (MAI)

magnetism

nuclear m.

magnetite (Fe₃O₄)

m. albumin imaging agent (Fe_3O_4)

magnetization

m. and spin-lock transfer imaging

complementary spatial modulation of m. (CSPAMM)

equilibrium m.

locked nuclear m.

longitudinal m.

net tissue m.

net transverse m.

m. precession angle

rephased transverse m.

residual m.

resting m.

spatial modulation of m. (SPAMM)

SSFP m.

steady-state free precession m.

tissue m.

m. transfer (MT)

m. transfer contrast (MTC)

m. transfer effect

m. transfer gradient-echo image

m. transfer ratio (MTR)

m. transfer technique

m. transfer weighted imaging

transverse m.

magnetization-prepared (MP)

m.-p. contrast-enhanced breath-hold volume-targeted imaging

m.-p. rapid acquisition gradient echo (MP-RAGE)

m.-p. rapid acquisition gradient-echo sequence

m.-p. rapid gradient echo-water excitation (MP-RAGE-WE)

magnetoacoustic

m. imaging

m. MRI

magnetoencephalogram (MEG)

magnetoencephalography (MEG)

M

magnetogyric ratio
magnetohydrodynamic effect
Magnetom
    M. Espree open MRI unit
    M. Open system
    M. Sonata 1.5T MR system
    M. SP4000 magnet
    M. SP MRI imager
    M. SP63 scanner
    M. Symphony MR scanner
    M. Symphony whole-body scanner
    M. Trio 3T unlimited MRI system
    M. 1.5T scanner
    M. Vision MR unit
    M. Vision scanner
    M. Vision 1.5T MR imaging
       system
magnetometer probe
magneton
    Bohr m.
    electron m.
magnetooptical disc (MOD)
magnetopharmaceutical
magnetoresistive sensor circuit
Magnevist
    M. gadopentate dimeglumine
    M. imaging agent
Magnex
    M. Alpha MR system
    M. magnet
    M. MR scanner
magnification
    m. and spot compression
    m. angiography
    electronic m.
    m. error
    m. factor
    film-screen m.
    m. hard copy
    high-resolution m.
    m. mammography
    m. radiography
    signal m.
    spot m.
    ultrahigh m.
    m. view
magnitude
    m. calculation
    m. image
    m. of obliquity
    m. reconstruction
    vector m.
magnum
    M. biopsy instrument
    foramen m.
    vertebra m.
    visibility of foramen m.
magnus
    adductor m.

Mahaim
    M. and James fiber
    M. bundle
MAI
    magnetic-assisted intervention
    Mycobacterium avium-intracellulare
main
    m. bundle
    m. energy substrate
    m. fissure
    m. glow peak
    m. magnetic field inhomogeneity
       artifact
    m. pancreatic duct (MPD)
    m. papillary duct (MPD)
    m. portal vein peak velocity
       (MPPv)
    m. pulmonary artery (MPA)
    m. timing event (MTE)
    m. tumor
mainline granulomatosis
mainstem
    m. bronchus
    m. carina
    m. coronary artery
Mainster retina laser
maintenance
    m. immunosuppressive treatment
       (MIST)
    m. of flow
Mainz pouch
Maisonneuve
    M. fibular fracture
    M. injury
    M. sign
Maissiat
    M. band
    M. ligament
Majestik shielded angiographic
  needle
major
    m. adverse cardiac event
       (MACE)
    m. aortopulmonary collateral
       artery
    m. bronchus
    m. calyx
    m. duodenal papilla
    m. fissure
    m. fracture fragment
    globus m.
    m. muscle
    psoas m.
    rhomboid m.
    teres m.
majus
    omentum m.
malabsorption
Malacarne antrum

malacic lesion
malacoplakia, malakoplakia
    renal parenchymal m.
maladie de Roger
malakoplakia (*var. of* malacoplakia)
malaligned atrioventricular septal defect
malalignment
    patellar m.
    rotational m.
    subtle m.
malangulation
malar
    m. bone
    m. eminence
    m. fracture
    m. lymph node
malarial granuloma
malayi
    Brugia m.
Malcolm-Lynn C-RXF cervical retractor
  frame
maldescended testis
maldevelopment
    pubic bone m.
maldistribution of ventilation and
  perfusion
male
    m. genital tract calcification
    m. pelvis
    m. Turner syndrome
    m. urethra
Malecot nephrostomy catheter
malformation
    adenomatoid m.
    angiographically occult intracranial
      vascular m. (AOIVM)
    angiographically occult vascular m.
      (AOVM)
    angiographically visualized vascular
      m. (AVVM)
    anorectal m.
    aortic arch m.
    Arnold-Chiari m.
    arterial m.
    arteriovenous m. (AVM)
    arteriovenous brain m.
    arteriovenous colon m.
    arteriovenous cord m.
    arteriovenous kidney m.
    bronchopulmonary foregut m.
      (BPFM)
    capillary m.
    capillary-lymphatic m. (CLM)
    cardiovascular m.
    cavernous m.
    cerebral arteriovenous m.
    cerebrovascular m.
    Chiari I-II m.
    cloacal m.

    computer-assisted resection of
      cerebral arteriovenous m.
    congenital cystic adenomatoid m.
      (CCAM)
    congenital heart m.
    congenital vascular m. (CVM)
    coronary artery m.
    cryptic vascular m. (CVM)
    cystic adenomatoid m.
    dancer's foot m.
    Dandy-Walker m.
    DeMyer system of cerebral m.
    Dieulafoy vascular m.
    diffuse m.
    dural arteriovenous m.
    Ebstein m.
    endocardial cushion m.
    extremity m.
    familial cavernous m.
    fast-flow m.
    fetal cystic adenomatoid m.
    fetal hand m.
    focal m.
    frontal arteriovenous m.
    frontoparietal arteriovenous m.
    fusiform m.
    galenic venous m.
    glomus-type arteriovenous m.
    hindbrain m.
    intracerebral arteriovenous m.
    intracerebral vascular m.
    intracranial arteriovenous m.
    intramedullary arteriovenous m.
    intramuscular venous m.
    intraosseous arteriovenous m.
    intraosseous vascular m.
    Joubert m.
    lymphatic m.
    Michel m.
    microarteriovenous m.
    mixed venous-lymphatic m.
    molar tooth midbrain-hindbrain m.
    Mondini m.
    mural-type vein of Galen m.
    neural axis vascular m.
    occult cerebrovascular m. (OCVM)
    occult vascular brain m.
    pseudo-Dandy-Walker m.
    pulmonary arterial m.
    pulmonary arteriovenous m. (PAVM)
    retromedullary arteriovenous m.
    saccular m.
    septal m.
    sink-trap m.
    slow flow vascular m.
    spinal cord m. (SCM)
    spinal vascular m.
    split cord m. (SCM)
    split spinal cord m. (SSCM)

M

malformation (*continued*)
  subpial arteriovenous m.
  telencephalic m.
  valve m.
  vascular m.
  vein of Galen m.
  venous vascular m.
  Wyburn-Mason arteriovenous
    m.
malformed phlebectasia
Malgaigne pelvic fracture
malignancy
  adrenal m.
  aggressive m.
  borderline m.
  epithelial m.
  extrapelvic m.
  extrathymic m.
  gastrointestinal m.
  high-grade m.
  low-grade m.
  metastatic m.
  mimicker of m.
  myeloid m.
  nonepithelial parenchymal m.
  pelvic m.
  periprosthetic m.
  primary pulmonary m.
  secondary m.
  sinonasal m.
  submucosal m.
  synchronous primary m.
  m. threshold
  uroepithelial m.
  urogenital m.
  vulvar m.
malignant
  m. acetabular osteolysis
  m. adrenal mass
  m. airway obstruction
  m. ascites
  m. bone aneurysm
  m. brain edema
  m. breast calcification
  m. chondrosarcoma
  m. degeneration
  m. duodenal tumor
  m. ependymoma
  m. epitheliod mesothelioma
  m. epithelioid leiomyoblastoma of
    lung
  m. external otitis
  m. fibroosseous histiocytoma
  m. fibrous histiocytoma (MFH)
  m. fibrous histiocytoma of bone
    (MFH-B)
  m. fibroxanthoma
  m. gastric ulcer
  m. giant cell tumor

  m. glioma
  m. hemangioendothelioma
  m. hypercalcemia
  m. hyperthermia
  m. lymphoma
  m. mediastinal teratoid tumor
  m. melanoma gallium imaging
  m. melanoma of soft part
  m. melanoma staging
  m. meningioma
  m. mesenchymal tumor
  m. myeloid sarcoma
  m. myoepithelioma
  m. nephrosclerosis
  m. osseous lesion
  m. osteoid
  m. osteopetrosis
  m. ovarian germ cell tumor
  m. ovarian teratoma tumor
  m. peripheral nerve sheath tumor
    (MPNST)
  m. phenylketonuria
  m. pheochromocytoma
  m. pleomorphic adenoma
  m. pleural effusion
  m. pleural implant
  m. pleural mesothelioma
  m. pulmonary mesothelioma
  m. salivary gland tumor
  m. schwannoma
  m. small bowel tumor
  m. teratoma
  m. thymoma
  m. transformation
  m. urethral neoplasia
  m. vertebral compression fracture
malignum
  adenoma m.
Mallampati score
mallearis
  stria m.
mallei (*pl. of* malleus)
malleolar
  m. fossa
  m. fracture
malleoli (*pl. of* malleolus)
malleolus, *pl.* **malleoli**
  m. bone
  lateral m.
  medial m.
mallet
  m. finger
  m. fracture
mallet-finger deformity
malleus, *pl.* **mallei**
Mallinckrodt
  M. Institute of Radiology
    guidelines
  M. scanner

Mallory-Weiss
>M.-W. esophageal tear
>M.-W. lesion
>M.-W. mucosal tear
>M.-W. syndrome

Malmo mammographic screening trial
malocclusion
malomaxillary suture
Maloney endootoprobe laser
malperfused
malperfusion syndrome
malpighian
>m. body
>m. body of spleen
>m. cell tumor
>m. follicle
>m. vesicle

malposition
>cardiac m.
>m. of branch pulmonary artery

malpositioned
>m. fetus
>m. heart
>m. testis

malrotation
>complete small bowel m.
>intestinal tract m.
>kidney m.
>midgut volvulus with m.
>m. of bowel loop
>m. of intestine
>partial small bowel m.
>renal m.
>small bowel m.

MALT
>mucosa-associated lymphoid tissue
>MALT lymphoma
>MALT worker's lung

MALToma
>mucosa-associated lymphoid tissue
>lymphoma

malum perforans pedis
malunion of fracture fragment
malunited fracture
Malvern 2600 Sizer laser diffraction scanner
mamillary
>m. body
>m. suture
>m. system

mamillothalamic fasciculus
Mamm-Aire heart failure
Mammalock needle
mammaplasty, mammoplasty, mastoplasty
>augmentation m.
>postreduction m.

mammary
>m. artery
>m. calculus

>m. cyst
>m. duct
>m. duct ectasia
>m. duct obstruction
>m. ductogram
>m. ductogram imaging
>m. dysplasia
>m. galactogram
>m. galactogram imaging
>m. gland
>m. implant
>m. parenchyma
>m. tissue
>m. tumorigenesis

Mammex TR computer-aided mammography diagnosis system
mammillare (*var. of* mammillary)
mammillary, mammillare
Mammo
>M. Mask dedicated viewer
>M. Mask illuminator
>M. Plus mammography system
>M. QC mammography

mammogram
>CAD-evaluated m.
>digitized contact m.
>false-negative m.
>film-based screening m.
>true-negative m.
>x-ray m.

mammographic
>m. evaluation of breast mass
>m. feature
>m. guidance
>m. measurement
>m. phantom
>m. technique
>m. view box

mammographically
>m. occult carcinoma
>m. suspicious lesion

mammographic-histopathologic correlation
mammography
>baseline m.
>computed tomography laser m. (CTLM)
>contoured tilting compression m.
>contrast-enhanced near-infrared laser m.
>contrast subtraction m.
>diagnostic m.
>digital subtraction m. (DSM)
>dual-energy m.
>dynamic computed tomography m.
>Egan m.
>evaluation of mass m.
>film-screen m.
>full-field digital m.
>high-resolution CT m.

M

mammography (*continued*)
    low-dose m.
    magnetic resonance m. (MRM)
    magnification m.
    Mammomat B m.
    Mammo QC m.
    microfocal spot m.
    near-infrared optical m.
    NIR optical m.
    nonmagnified m.
    orthogonal projection m.
    positron emission m. (PEM)
    M. Quality Control Manual
    M. Quality Standards Act (MQSA)
    radionuclide m.
    screen-film m.
    screening m.
    Senographe Essential mobile m.
    Senographe 500T, 600T, 700T, 800T m.
    single-view oblique m.
    spot compression magnification m.
    stage-matched intervention on repeat m.
    step-oblique m.
    stereotactic m.
    m. technique
    ultrahigh-magnification m. (UHMM)
    ultrasound-augmented m.
    2-view film-screen m.
    x-ray m.
Mammo-Lume
Mammomat B mammography
mammoPET breast apparatus
mammoplasia
mammoplasty (*var. of* mammaplasty)
MammoReader
    M. computer-aided dectection system
    M. mammogram device
    M. mammography system
Mammorex
MammoSite
    M. radiation therapy
    M. radiation therapy system catheter
    M. RTS
Mammospot
Mammotest
    M. breast biopsy system
    M. unit
Mammotome
    Biopsys M.
    M. ultrasound system
Mammotrax
Mammoviewer
management
    real-time position m. (RPM)
managing
    high-resolution storage phosphor m.

Manchester
    M. LDR implant system
    M. ovoid
mandible, mandibula, mandibulum
    alveolar border of m.
    ascending ramus of m.
    coronoid of m.
    genial tubercle of m.
    m. hypoplasia
    m. osteolysis
    symphysis of m.
mandibula, *pl.* **mandibulae** (*var. of* mandible)
mandibulae (*pl. of* mandibula)
mandibular
    m. angle
    m. canal
    m. capitulum
    m. condyle
    m. disc
    m. division
    m. foramen
    m. fossa
    m. fracture
    m. lymph node
    m. nerve
    m. ramus
    m. triangle
mandibularis
    torus m.
mandibulofacial dysostosis
mandibulum (*var. of* mandible)
mandril
maneuver
    Adson m.
    circumduction-adduction shoulder m.
    core-warming m.
    costoclavicular m.
    flexion m.
    Fogarty m.
    Hampton m.
    Heineke-Mikulicz m.
    hyperabduction m.
    jugular compression m.
    Kocher m.
    manual Matas m.
    Müller esophageal varices m.
    Osler m.
    Phalen m.
    pull m.
    push m.
    Rivero-Carvallo m.
    scalene m.
    squatting m.
    temporal artery tap m.
    transabdominal left lateral retroperitoneal m.
    Valsalva m.

mangafodipir
    m. trisodium
    m. trisodium agent
    m. trisodium-enhanced MR
      imaging
mangafodipir-enhanced MRCP
manganese (Mn)
    m. chloride
    m. chloride contrast medium
    m. citrate
    m. dipyridoxyl diphosphate
    m. imaging agent
    m. sulfate
    m. tetrasodium-meso-tetra
manganese-BOPTA
**manganese-containing contrast
agent**
manifestation
    imaging m.
manifold
    3-stopcock m.
manipulation
    deformable m.
    rigid m.
Mankin method
manmade environmental radiation
mannan-coated liposome
Mann-Bollman fistula
**mannitol and saline imaging
agent**
Mannkopf sign
manofluorography (MFG)
manometer
manometric
    m. measurement
    m. pattern
manometry
    anal m.
    aneroid m.
    anorectal m.
    biliary m.
    ERCP m.
    esophageal m.
    rectosigmoid m.
    sphincter of Oddi m.
mansori
    Schistosoma m.
mantle
    anechoic m.
    m. block
    brain m.
    m. cell lymphoma (MCL)
    cement m.
    cerebral m.
    m. complex
    m. field
    m. field irradiation
    hypoechoic m.
    m. radiotherapy

manual
    m. compression
    m. injection
    Mammography Quality Control M.
    m. Matas maneuver
    m. muscle testing
    m. pressure over carotid sinus
    m. subtraction film
manubria (*pl. of* manubrium)
manubriosternalis
    symphysis m.
    synchondrosis m.
manubriosternal joint
manubrium, *pl.* **manubria**
    m. hypersegmentation
map
    acceleration m.
    ADC m.
    anisotropy m.
    blackout m.
    bladder m.
    bull's-eye polar m.
    cerebral blood volume m.
    computed perfusion m.
    cylindrical projection m.
    decimalized variance m.
    end-diastolic polar m.
    end-systolic polar m.
    functional m.
    geometry factor m.
    polar m.
    polar blackout m.
    sestamibi polar m.
    spheric m.
    trace m.
    ventilation m.
MAP
    mean arterial pressure
MAPCA
    multiple aortopulmonary collateral
    arteries
**map-guided partial endocardial
ventriculotomy**
maple
    m. bark disease
    m. bark-stripper's lung
    m. syrup urine disease
maplike skull
mapping
    activation sequence m.
    advanced cardiac m.
    body surface laplacian m. (BSLM)
    body surface potential m.
    BO field m.
    brain electrical activity m.
      (BEAM)
    cardiac m.
    catheter m.
    color-flow m.

M

mapping (*continued*)
    contour m.
    cortical m.
    2D m.
    digital road m.
    direction-encoded color m.
    Doppler color-flow m.
    2D pulsatility index m.
    2D resistance index m.
    eddy current m.
    electrophysiologic m.
    endocardial activation m.
    endocardial catheter m.
    epicardial m.
    functional anatomic m.
    homology m.
    Hough transform m.
    intramural m.
    intraoperative electrocortical
      stimulation m.
    intraoperative lymphatic m.
    k-space velocity m.
    lorentzian field m.
    lymphatic m.
    magnetic resonance phase velocity
      m.
    moving slice velocity m.
    MRI m.
    MR velocity m.
    m. of cerebral sulcus
    m. of defect
    pace m.
    parallel analogue m.
    phase difference m.
    phase-shift velocity m.
    precordial m.
    quantitative multilevel m.
    radiocolloid m.
    retrograde atrial activation m.
    saphenous vein m.
    sentinel lymph node m.
    sinus rhythm m.
    spastic m.
    spatial m.
    susceptibility m.
    texture m.
    thermal m.
    vein m.
    velocity m.
    volumetric magnetic resonance brain
      m.

marantic
    m. clot
    m. endocarditis

marble
    m. bone
    m. bone disease

marbling of pancreatic parenchyma

Marcacci muscle

march
    m. foot
    m. fracture

Marchiafava-Bignami disease

Marchiafava-Micheli syndrome

Marconi/Elscint MxTwin CT

Marcus Gunn syndrome

Marex MRI system

Marfan syndrome

margin
    anterior vertebral body m.
    bandlike m.
    beveled m.
    blurring of disc m.
    cardiac m.
    circumscribed m.
    colon m.
    convex posterior m.
    cortical m.
    costal m.
    costodiaphragmatic m.
    depression of renal m.
    disc m.
    enhancing ventricular m.
    fluffy m.
    ill-defined m.
    indistinct endometrial m.
    infraorbital m. (IOM)
    inking the m.
    ipsilateral m.
    m. irregularity
    linear m.
    lobulate m.
    medial talar m.
    m. necrosis
    m. of apposition
    m. of scapula
    overhanging m.
    periarticular m.
    pleural m.
    posterior disc m.
    psoas m.
    scapular m.
    sclerotic m.
    sharp lateral m.
    spicular m.
    stomach m.
    subcostal m.
    superomedial m.
    supraorbital m. (SOM)
    tumor m.
    vertebral body m.

marginal
    m. branch
    m. branch of left circumflex
      coronary artery
    m. branch of right coronary artery
    m. circumflex artery
    m. erosion

m. exostosis
m. fracture
m. gyrus
m. kidney depression
obtuse m. (OM)
m. osteophyte
m. osteophyte formation
m. placenta
m. placenta previa
m. ridge
m. sclerosis
m. serration
m. sinus
m. spur
m. spurring
m. syndesmophyte
m. ulcer
m. vein
m. zone
m. zone B-cell lymphoma
m. zone lymphoma (MZL)

Marie-Bamberger disease
Marie-Strümpell disease
Marimastat
Marine-Lenhart syndrome
Marinesco-Sjögren syndrome
marked
m. hypoechogenicity shadowing
m. sclerosis
m. shunting of blood
markedly accentuated pulmonic component
marker
anatomic m.
external fiducial m.
fiducial skin m.
implanted imaging opaque m.
isotope-tagged m.
lead pellet m.
metallic m.
MicroMark tissue m.
molecular m.
needle m.
nipple m.
m. of metabolism
Pinnacle R/O II radiopaque m.
radioactive string m.
radiopaque gold m.
round lead m.
Sitzmarks radiopaque m.
spherical fiducial m.
m. transit imaging
m. transit study
tumor m.
marker-channel diagram
marking
absence of haustral m.
absence of vascular m.
accentuation of m.

bronchopulmonary m.
bronchovascular m.
bronchovesicular m.
coarse bronchovascular m.
confluence of vascular m.'s
convolutional m.
crowding of bronchovascular m.'s
digital m.
haustral m.
increased interstitial m.
increased pulmonary vascular m.
interstitial m.
linear m.
lung m.
peribronchial m.
perihilar m.
pullback arterial m.
pulmonary arterial m.
pulmonary vascular m.
sulcal m.
sutural m.
vascular m.

Markov
M. chain
M. chain Monte Carlo technique
M. random field
Mark V Plus automatic injector
Marlex band
Marmor-Lynn fracture
Maroteaux-Lamy syndrome
marrow
aberrant bone m.
m. agent bone scintigraphy
m. blush
bone m.
bright fatty m.
m. canal
cancellous hemopoietic m.
m. cavity
central nidus of high-intensity m.
choked m.
m. dosimetry
m. edema pattern
epiphysial hemopoietic m.
m. fat signal intensity
fatty m.
functional m.
hemopoietically active bone m.
hemopoietic bone m.
high signal intensity yellow m.
hypercellular reconverted bone m.
m. hyperstimulation pattern
hypocellular m.
m. infarct
m. infiltrate
m. infiltration
island of red m.
peripheral hemopoietic intermediate
signal-intensity m.

M

marrow (*continued*)
    red m.
    shunting of tracer to bone m.
    m. signal change
    m. space
    sternal m.
    m. transplant
    uptake in bone m.
    yellow m.
Marshall vein
marshmallow bolus
Martin-Bell syndrome
Martin disease
Martinez universal interstitial template
Martorell
    M. aortic arch syndrome
    M. hypertensive ulcer
    M. sign
mAs
    milliampere seconds
MAS
    midaortic syndrome
    MAS in FAS
masculine pelvis
masculinizing tumor
mask
    convolution m.
    m. data
    ISAH stereotactic immobilizing m.
    Orfit m.
    particle m.
    m. threshold
    m. ventilation
mask-based approach
masking
    unsharp m.
    white m.
Mason radial fracture classification
mason's lung
masquerading effect
mass
    abdominopelvic m.
    m. absorption coefficient
    adrenal m.
    adrenal cystic m.
    air-containing neck m.
    airless m.
    anechoic m.
    anterior mediastinal m.
    aortopulmonary window m.
    appendiceal m.
    apperceptive m.
    m. attenuation coefficient
    avascular brain m.
    avascular kidney m.
    avascular renal m.
    m. balance
    benign adrenal m.
    bilateral fetal chest m.'s

bilateral renal m.'s
bilobate m.
brain m.
calcified brain m.
calcified intracranial m.
calcified kidney m.
calcified renal m.
cardiophrenic right-angle m.
carotid space m.
cavitary m.
cerebellar cystic m.
circumscribed m.
m. collision stopping power
complex solid and cystic m.
congenital nasal m.
conglomerate m.
conical m.
cord intradural extramedullary m.
cordlike m.
critical m.
cystic abdominal m.
cystic breast m.
cystic teratomatous m.
m. defect
dense brain m.
dense cerebral m.
dirty m.
discoid chest m.
discrete m.
doughy m.
dumbbell brain m.
dysplasia with associated lesion or
    m. (DALM)
echogenic m.
m. effect
elongated m.
encapsulated m.
endobronchial m.
m. energy equivalence
enhancing m.
epidermoid m.
epidural m.
exophytic m.
expanding intracranial m.
expansile m.
external ear m.
extracardiac m.
extradural m.
extramedullary m.
extraosseous m.
extraovarian m.
extrapleural m.
extratesticular m.
extrauterine pelvic m.
extravascular m.
fallopian tube m.
fat-containing m.
fat-density m.
fetal abdominal cystic m.

fibrin m.
firm m.
fixed m.
fleecy m.
fluctuant m.
fluid-filled kidney m.
focal m.
freely movable m.
friable m.
fusiform m.
glenoid ovoid m.
glenolabral ovoid m. (GLOM)
groin m.
heterodense soft tissue m.
heterogeneous breast m.
high-signal m.
hilar m.
homogeneous intrasellar m.
hyperattenuated intrasellar m.
hyperdense m.
hyperechoic breast m.
hyperintense m.
hypervascular mediastinal m.
hypoattenuating m.
hypodense m.
ideal body m. (IBM)
ileocecal m.
ill-defined m.
m. imaging
indurated m.
inflammatory polypoid m.
inguinal m.
injection m.
inner ear m.
interbronchial m.
intermediate signal-intensity m.
intraabdominal m.
intracardiac m.
intracaval fat m.
intracavity m.
intracranial m.
intracystic solid m.
intraductal solid m.
intradural extramedullary m.
intraluminal stomach m.
intramedullary m.
intrasellar brain m.
intrathoracic fetal m.
intrathoracic low-attenuation m.
intravascular m.
intraventricular m.
irregular m.
isodense m.
isoechoic breast m.
jugular foraminal m.
kidney sinus m.
kinetic energy released per unit m.
  (Kerma)
lacrimal m.

large solid adrenal m.
lateral m.
lean m.
left ventricular m. (LVM)
m. lesion
liver m.
lobulated m.
loss of bone m.
low attenuation mediastinal m.
lower lobe lung m.
low-signal m.
lung m.
lymphomatous m.
malignant adrenal m.
mammographic evaluation of breast
  m.
masticator space m.
mediastinal high-attenuation m.
mesenteric m.
middle ear m.
middle mediastinal m.
mixed-attenuation m.
mixed-density m.
mixed echogenic solid m.
mixed-signal m.
mixed solid-cystic m.
mobile intraluminal gallbladder m.
molar m.
mulberry-like m.
multilobulated m.
multiloculated m.
mushroom-shaped m.
myocardial m.
nasal vault m.
nasopharyngeal m.
nodular m.
noncalcified nodular m.
nonhemorrhagic m.
nonhomogeneous hyperdense m.
nonopaque intraluminal m.
nonpulsatile abdominal m.
m. number
omental m.
orbital superolateral quadrant m.
oval m.
ovarian m.
pancreatic m.
paraaortic m.
paracardiac m.
paranasal sinus m.
parasagittal intracranial m.
parasellar brain m.
paraspinal soft tissue m.
paravertebrally situated pelvic tumor
  m.
paravertebrally situated thoracic
  tumor m.
paucilocular cystic m.
pedunculated m.

M

mass (*continued*)
    pelvic cystic m.
    periosseous soft tissue m.
    perirenal m.
    peritoneal m.
    perivascular m.
    petrous apex dumbbell m.
    pharyngeal space m.
    phlegmonous m.
    phosphaturic m.
    photopenic m.
    pineal m.
    pleural m.
    polypoid calcified irregular m.
    porta hepatis low-density m.
    posterior mediastinal m.
    prepubertal testicular m.
    presacral m.
    prevertebral space m.
    promontory m.
    pulmonary m.
    pulsating m.
    radiopaque m.
    red cell m. (RCM)
    relativistic m.
    renal sinus m.
    reniform m.
    retrobulbar m.
    retrocardiac m.
    retroperitoneal residual tumor m.
    retropharyngeal space m.
    retrosternal m.
    right cardiophrenic angle m.
    right ventricular m. (RVM)
    ring-enhancing m.
    saccular m.
    scrotal m.
    sellar m.
    soft tissue density m.
    solid m.
    solitary m.
    sonolucent cystic m.
    space-occupying m.
    m. spectrometer
    spheric m.
    spicular m.
    stellate m.
    stony m.
    subareolar m.
    subinsular m.
    suprasellar m.
    suspicious m.
    teratomatous m.
    thalamic-hypothalamic m.
    thymic m.
    m. thymus
    thyroid m.
    tissue m.

    torsed ovarian m.
    tubal m.
    tuboovarian m.
    tubular fluid-density adnexal m.
    tumor m.
    umbilical m.
    uncinate process m.
    unilateral adrenal m.
    unilateral fetal chest m.
    unilateral kidney m.
    urinary bladder extrinsic m.
    urinary bladder wall m.
    uterine m.
    ventricular m.
    water density m.
    wedge-shaped m.
    well-circumscribed breast m.
    well-defined m.
    woody m.

Massachusetts General Hospital utility multiprogramming system

mass-effect hydrocephalus

masseteric enlargement

masseter muscle

massive
    m. aortic regurgitation
    m. ascites
    m. collapse
    m. embolus
    m. exsanguinating hemorrhage
    m. fibrosis
    m. hepatic necrosis
    m. herniated disc
    m. infiltrate
    m. osteolysis
    m. ovarian edema
    m. pleural effusion
    m. pneumonia
    m. pulmonary hemorrhagic edema

massively enlarged heart

masslike
    m. configuration
    m. lesion

Masson body

mast
    m. cell
    m. cell-enhancing activity
    m. cell reticulosis
    m. leukocyte

MAST
    military antishock trousers
    motion artifact suppression technique
    MAST suit

mastectomy
    non-skin-sparing m. (non-SSM)
    simple m.
    skin-sparing m.

master knot of Henry

masticator
>   m. muscle
>   m. space
>   m. space infection
>   m. space mass

mastitis
>   m. fibrosa cystica
>   m. obliterans

mastocytosis
>   bone m.
>   GI tract m.
>   systemic m.

mastoid
>   m. antrum
>   m. bone
>   m. canal
>   m. complex
>   m. fontanelle
>   m. foramen
>   m. lymph node
>   m. polytomography
>   m. process
>   m. sinus
>   m. suture

mastopathy
>   diabetic m.
>   fibrous m.

mastoplasia
>   cystic m.

mastoplasty (*var. of* mammaplasty)
match
>   nontransmural m.
>   transmural m.
>   triple m.

matched peripheral dose (MPD)
matching
>   atlas m.
>   electron-photon field m.
>   general pattern m.
>   impedance m.
>   m. network

matchline wedge
mater
>   dura m.

material
>   anthracotic m.
>   atheromatous m.
>   ballistic m.
>   byproduct m.
>   coffee-grounds m.
>   collection of contrast m.
>   columnization of contrast m.
>   contrast m.
>   dental contrast m.
>   embolic m.
>   extraneous m.
>   fecal m.
>   ferromagnetic m.
>   flow of contrast m.

>   inspissated m.
>   Interpore bone replacement m.
>   intravenous administration of contrast
>   m.
>   iodinated contrast m.
>   layering of contrast m.
>   lipid-rich m.
>   LSO crystal scintillator m.
>   magnetic m.
>   nonferrous m.
>   nonionic contrast m.
>   opaque m.
> ^{103}Pd radioactive m.
>   PET target m.
>   phosphaturic m.
>   radioactive m.
>   m. spin echocardiogram total
>   volume imaging
>   superabsorbent polymer embolic m.
>   tagging m.
>   target m.
>   trophoblastic m.
>   uptake of radioactive m.
>   vessel cutoff of contrast m.

maternal
>   m. lake
>   m. placenta

**Mathews classification of olecranon
   fracture**
matrices (*pl. of* **matrix**)
matrix, *pl.* **matrices**
>   acquisition m.
>   bone tumor m.
>   calcific m.
>   m. calculus
>   cartilage m.
>   chondroid m.
>   data m.
>   decision m.
>   demineralized bone m. (DBM)
>   extracellular m.
>   germinal bleed m.
>   m. image
>   m. injury
>   k-space m.
>   M. LR3300 laser imaging
>   m. metalloprotease-3 (MMP-3)
>   m. mineralization
>   nuclear m.
>   osteoid m.
>   proteoglycan m.
>   quantization m. (QM)
>   reduced-acquisition m. (RAM)
>   m. size
>   solid m.
>   m. stone
>   stromal m.
>   transformation m.
>   tumor m.

M

matted small bowel loop
matter
- cortical gray m.
- cortical white m.
- cytotoxic edema of gray m.
- gray m. (GM)
- heterotopic gray m.
- infratentorial gray m.
- normal-appearing white m. (NAWM)
- particulate m.
- periaqueductal gray m.
- perilesional white m.
- peritrigonal white m.
- periventricular gray m.
- periventricular white m.
- pulverized plaque particulate m.
- PVG m.
- scalloped appearance of white m.
- shearing of white m.
- subcortical gray m.
- supratentorial gray m.
- supratentorial white m.
- vanishing white m.
- white m.

maturation
- bone m.
- disc m.
- m. index
- pulmonary structural m.
- skeletal m.

mature
- m. bone
- m. mediastinal teratoma
- m. ovarian cystic teratoma
- m. pancreatic pseudocyst
- m. pouch
- m. pseudocyst of pancreas
- skeletally m.
- m. vertebra

maturity
- m. of fetus
- skeletal m.

Mauchart ligament
MAVIS
- mobile artery and vein imaging system

Maxicamera
maxilla, *pl.* **maxillae**
- anterior nasal spine of m.

maxillae (*pl. of* maxilla)
maxillary
- m. antrum
- m. artery
- m. bone
- m. canal
- m. division
- m. fracture

- m. nerve anatomy
- m. process
- m. sinus
- m. sinus carcinoma
- m. sinus hypoplasia
- m. sinus opacification
- m. sinus papilloma
- m. sinus puncture
- m. sinus radiograph
- m. spine

maxillectomy
maxillofacial
- m. fracture
- m. imaging

Maxima II TENS unit
maximal (*var. of* maximum)
maximization
maximum, maximal
- m. amplitude constant
- m. anteroposterior diameter
- m. density (D_{max})
- m. depth
- m. diameter to minimum diameter ratio
- m. entropy processing
- m. estimated gradient
- m. inflation pressure
- m. inflation time
- m. intensity
- m. midexpiratory flow (MMEF)
- m. midexpiratory flow rate (MMFR)
- ordered subset expectation m. (OSEM)
- m. permissible body burden
- m. permissible concentration
- m. permissible dose (MPD)
- m. predicted heart rate (MPHR)
- m. radiographic distention
- m. short-axis diameter (MSAD)
- m. slew rate ramp
- m. tolerated dose (MTD)
- m. transaortic jet velocity
- m. venous outflow (MVO)
- m. ventricular elastance
- m. volume of left atrium
- m. voluntary ventilation (MVV)
- m. walking time

maximum-intensity
- m.-i. pixel (MIP)
- m.-i. projection (MIP)
- m.-i. projection and source image
- m.-i. projection imaging
- m.-i. sliding thin-slab projection

maximus
- gluteus m.

Max Plus MR scanner
Maxwell
- M. coil

M. 3D field simulator
M. pair
M. theory of radiation
maxwellian distribution
Mayer
M. position
M. view
Mayer-Rokitansky-Küster-Hauser syndrome
May-Hegglin anomaly
Mayneord F factor
May-Thurner syndrome
Mazabraud syndrome
Mazur ankle evaluation classification
MB
muscle-brain
MB fraction
M-band myeloma
MBF
myocardial blood flow
MBS-MRA
minimum basis set magnetic resonance angiography
MCA
middle cerebral artery
multichannel analyzer
multiple congenital anomalies
MCAT
myocardial contrast appearance time
McBurney point
McCabe-Fletcher classification
McCallum patch
McCune-Albright syndrome
MCD
mean central dose
molecular coincidence detection
multicentric Castleman disease
MCD imaging
MCDK
multicystic dysplastic kidney
MCE
myocardial contrast echocardiography
MCFSR
mean circumferential fiber shortening rate
McGinn-White sign
McGregor line
mCi
millicurie
MCi
megacurie
mCi-hr
millicurie-hour
McIlwain tissue chopper
MCK
multicystic kidney
McKee line
McKusick-Kaufman syndrome

McKusick-type
M.-t. metaphysial chondrodysplasia
M.-t. metaphysial dysplasia
MCL
mantle cell lymphoma
medial collateral ligament
midclavicular line
MCL bursa
McLain-Weinstein spinal tumor classification
MCLC
medial collateral ligament complex
MCLS
mucocutaneous lymph node syndrome
McMurray test
McNamara coaxial catheter infusion set
MCP
metacarpophalangeal
MCP joint
MCPJ
metacarpophalangeal joint
MCPT
Monte Carlo photon transport
MCPT simulation
McRae line
MCS
middle coronary sinus
MCT
mean circulation time
MCTC
metrizamide computed tomography cisternography
MCTD
mixed connective tissue disease
MCU
micturating cystourethrogram
MDAC
multiplying digital-to-analogue converter
MDCT
multidetector CT
MDCTU
multidetector computed tomography urography
MDD
medical device directive
MD-Gastroview imaging agent
MDP
methylene diphosphonate
TechneScan MDP
technetium 99m MDP
MDP-Bracco
MDS
myelodysplastic syndrome
MDS coil
MDS-2000 microwave irradiator
MDT
minimal deformation target

M

MEA
microwave endometrial ablation
Meadows syndrome
meal
barium m.
Boyden test m.
cornflake, milk, and sugar m.
double-contrast barium m.
dual-labeled solid and liquid m.
Ewald test m.
fatty m.
isotope m.
motor test m.
opaque m.
retention m.
small bowel m.
test m.
mean
m. ankle-brachial systolic pressure index
m. aortic flow velocity
m. aortic pressure
m. arterial pressure (MAP)
m. blood pressure
m. body weight
m. brachial artery pressure
m. cardiac vector
m. central dose (MCD)
m. circulation time (MCT)
m. circulatory filling pressure
m. circumferential fiber shortening rate (MCFSR)
m. corpuscular volume
m. deviation
m. diameter overframing
m. diffusivity
m. examination time
m. free path
m. gonad dose
m. left atrial pressure
m. mitral valve gradient
m. optical density
m. perfusate temperature
m. posterior wall velocity
m. pulmonary artery pressure (MPAP)
m. pulmonary artery wedge pressure
m. pulmonary capillary pressure (MPCP)
m. pulmonary flow velocity
m. pulmonary transit time
m. right atrial pressure
m. sac diameter (MSD)
m. systolic gradient
m. transit time (MTT)
m. venous pulsation
m. wall motion score
m. wall motion score index

Meary metatarsotalar angle
measles pneumonia
measurable endpoint
measure
linear m.
measurement
ankle-brachial pressure m.
antegrade perfusion pressure m. (APPM)
appendicular bone mass m.
attenuation m.
automated cardiac flow m. (ACM)
blood flow m.
body composition m.
bolus passage perfusion m.
bone density m.
breath pentane m.
cardiac output m.
cerebrospinal fluid flow m.
Cerenkov m.
Cobb m.
densitometric m.
2-dimensional cine phase-contrast flow m.
diode m.
Dixon fat fraction m.
end-diastolic velocity m.
m. error
excitation function m.
fat-fraction m.
fetal foot length m.
fetal long bone m.
flow cytometric DNA m.
gestational sac m.
Hausdorff m.
high-sensitivity m.
hilum m.
histomorphometric m.
indicator dilution method for cardiac output m.
intercomparison m.
m. in vivo
line-pair m.
low-energy photon attenuation m.
mammographic m.
manometric m.
microbubble concentration m.
morphometric m.
National Council on Radiation Protection and M. (NCRP)
nondynamometric trunk strength m.
nutation angle m.
occlusion m.
orbit m.
phase-contrast flow m.
phase-sensitive flow m.
photon attenuation m.
polarographic needle electrode m.
pQCT m.

pressure m.
pulsatility m.
pulse-echo distance m.
quantitative diffusion m.
quantitative regional myocardial
  flow m.
regional washout m.
renal length m.
rocking curve m.
root-mean-squared gradient m.
segmental correction using x-ray m.
segmental pressure m.
semiquantitative m.
signal intensity m.
TCD m.
temperature distribution m.
thermodilution method of cardiac
  output m.
thyroid uptake m.
time-of-flight flow m.
time-velocity m.
topographic m.
transcutaneous oxygen pressure m.
  ($tcPO_2$)
true conjugate m.
U1-NA cephalometric m.
whole-brain magnetization transfer
  m.
Wits m.
xenon CT m.
Z score in bone mineral density m.

meatal segment
meatus, *pl.* **meatus**
  acoustic m.
  external auditory m.
  internal auditory m.
  nasal m.
meat wrapper's lung
mebrofenin
  technetium 99m m.
mechanical
  m. augmentation
  m. axis
  m. biliary obstruction
  m. compound scan
  m. counterpulsation
  m. duct obstruction
  m. extrahepatic obstruction
  m. genu varus
  m. ileus
  m. insufflation
  m. insult
  m. intestinal obstruction
  m. potential energy
  m. respiratory tract obstruction
  m. sector scanner
  m. small bowel obstruction
  m. thrombectomy
  m. thrombolysis

m. valve
m. ventilation
m. wall shear stress
mechanically
  m. activated implant
  m. detachable platinum coil
  m. sealed
mechanics
  body m.
  intramural m.
mechanism
  blood clotting m.
  central extensor m. (CEM)
  check-valve m.
  compensatory m.
  contrecoup m.
  deglutition m.
  excitotoxic m.
  extensor m.
  flap-valve m.
  Frank-Starling m.
  heart rate reserve m.
  homing m.
  humeral m.
  internal retention m.
  iron-transporting protein m.
  Laplace m.
  m. of injury
  osseous pinch m.
  pinchcock m.
  propulsive m.
  sinus m.
  sodium-potassium ATPase-dependent
    exchange m.
  sphincteric m.
  swallowing m.
  Taylor-Blackwood m.
  ventricular escape m.
  watershed m.
Mecholyl test
Meckel
  M. band
  M. cavity
  M. diverticulitis
  M. diverticulum
  M. ligament
  M. plane
  M. scan
  M. syndrome
Meckel-Gruber syndrome
meclofenamic acid
meconium
  m. aspiration
  m. aspiration syndrome
  m. ileus
  m. ileus equivalent
  m. peristalsis
  m. peritonitis
  m. plug

M

meconium (*continued*)
  m. plug syndrome
  m. pseudocyst
Meddars cardiac catheterization analysis
  system
Medelec DMG 50 Teflon-coated
  monopolar electrode
Medgraphics body plethysmograph
media (*pl. of* medium)
media-adventitia interface
medial
  m. and lateral support structures of
    knee
  m. angle
  m. arch
  m. arteriosclerosis
  m. aspect
  m. basal segmental bronchus
  m. border
  m. calcific sclerosis
  m. carpal capsule
  m. collateral ligament (MCL)
  m. collateral ligament calcification
  m. collateral ligament complex
    (MCLC)
  m. column calcaneal fracture
  m. compartment
  m. condyle
  m. crus
  m. cuneiform bone
  m. cystic necrosis
  m. dissection
  m. eminence
  m. end of clavicle osteolysis
  m. epicondylar bursa
  m. epicondyle
  m. epicondyle fracture
  m. epicondylitis
  m. extension
  m. femoral buttressing
  m. fibroplasia
  m. geniculate body
  m. geniculate fascia
  m. hyperplasia
  m. joint line
  m. joint space
  m. lemniscus
  m. longitudinal fasciculus
    (MLF)
  m. longitudinal fasciculus lesion
  m. malleolar fracture
  m. malleolus
  m. malleolus periostitis
  m. oblique axial projection
  m. oblique view
  m. occipitotemporal gyrus
  m. papillary muscle
  m. physis
  m. plantar artery

  m. plica
  m. plica of knee
  m. posterior choroidal (MPCh)
  m. pterygoid muscle
  m. rectus muscle
  m. rotation
  m. sesamoid bone
  m. shelf
  m. supraclavicular node
  m. talar dome injury
  m. talar margin
  m. talar osteochondral injury
  m. temporal lobe
  m. tibial stress syndrome
  m. traction spur
  m. umbilical fold
  m. wall fracture
mediales (*pl. of* medialis)
medialis, *pl.* **mediales**
  meniscus m.
  stria olfactoria m.
  vastus m.
medially
median
  m. antebrachial vein
  m. arcuate ligament
  m. arcuate ligament of diaphragm
  m. arcuate ligament syndrome
  m. bar
  m. cleft lip
  m. cruciate ligament
  m. facial cleft
  m. lethal dose
  m. level echo
  m. line
  m. lip cleft
  m. lobe of prostate
  multiples of m.
  m. nerve
  m. nerve entrapment
  m. nerve lesion
  m. palatine suture
  m. raphe
  m. raphe plane
  m. sacral artery
  m. sagittal plane
  m. septum
  m. umbilical ligament
mediastinal
  m. abscess
  m. adenopathy
  m. air
  m. angiolipoma
  m. arterial variant
  m. border
  m. bronchogenic cyst
  m. bulk
  m. collagenosis
  m. contour

m. cross-sectional imaging
m. crunch
m. dermoid
m. deviation
m. displacement
m. dorsal enteric cyst
m. duplication cyst
m. dysgerminoma
m. emphysema
m. fat
m. fat edema
m. fibrosis
m. fistula
m. germinoma
m. granuloma
m. hematoma
m. hemorrhage
m. hernia
m. high-attenuation mass
m. invasion
m. lesion
m. lipoma
m. lipomatosis
m. lung surface
m. lymphadenopathy
m. lymph node enlargement
m. lymphoma
m. node
m. panniculitis
m. parathyroid adenoma
m. pleura
m. pleurisy
m. prominence
m. pseudomass
m. retraction
m. seminoma
m. septum
m. seroma
m. shift
m. structure
m. teratocarcinoma
m. teratoid tumor
m. teratoma
m. thickening
m. thyroid tissue
m. tube
m. uptake
m. vein
m. viscus
m. wedge
m. widening
m. window

mediastinitis
acute m.
fibrosing m.
granulomatous m.
idiopathic fibrous m.
sclerosing m.

mediastinogram

mediastinography
gas m.
gaseous m.
opaque m.

mediastinoscopy

mediastinum
anterior m.
deviated m.
epidermoid m.
inferior m.
left m.
lipomatosis m.
lobulated paratracheal m.
middle m.
posterior m.
right m.
seminoma m.
superior m.
teratoid m.
m. testis
widened m.

medical
m. asepsis
BioSphere M.
m. cyclotron
m. device directive (MDD)
m. holography
m. internal radiation dose (MIRD)
m. internal radiation dosimetry
(MIRD)
m. ultrasound 3-dimensional portable
with advanced communication
(MUSTPAC)

medicamentosa
thyrotoxicosis m.

medicine
Brain Imaging Council of the
Society of Nuclear M.
complementary and alternative m.
(CAM)
Digital Imaging and Communications
in M. (DICOM)
Fellow of the American College of
Nuclear M.
nuclear m.
photonic m.

Medigraphics analyzer

Medilase angioscope-laser delivery system

MedImage scanner

Medinvent

**mediobasal hypothalamus luteinizing
hormone-releasing hormone**

mediodens (*var. of* mesiodens)

mediolateral
m. aspect
m. flow direction
m. oblique (MLO)
m. oblique projection
m. oblique view

M

mediolateral (*continued*)
    m. radiocarpal angle
    m. stress
medionecrosis
    cystic m.
medionodular cirrhosis
mediopatellar
MediPort catheter
Medison scanner
Medi-tech
    M.-t. catheter
    M.-t. ureteral stent system
Mediterranean fever
medium, *pl.* **media**
    barium sulfate contrast m.
    benzoic acid contrast m.
    bismuth contrast m.
    brominized oil contrast m.
    bullet kit culture m.
    m. caliber
    cerebral contrast m.
    contrast m. (CM)
    delayed excretion of contrast m.
    m. detachment pressure
    diatrizoic acid contrast m.
    endogenous adenosine contrast m.
    Entero Vu contrast m.
    EntroEase oral radiopaque
      contrast m.
    ethiodized oil contrast m.
    ethyliodophenylundecyl contrast m.
    extraluminal contrast m.
    FDDNP PET scan contrast m.
    galactose contrast m.
    Gd-DOTA contrast m.
    glucaric acid-labeled contrast m.
    hand injection of contrast m.
    high-concentration contrast m.
      (HCCM)
    high-osmolar contrast m.
      (HOCM)
    hyperconcentration of contrast m.
    Imagopaque contrast m.
    intravascular contrast m.
    intravenous contrast m.
    iodide contrast m.
    iodinated intravascular contrast m.
    iodinated radiologic contrast m.
      (IRCM)
    iodine-containing contrast m.
    iodixanol contrast m.
    iodophendylate contrast m.
    ioglunide contrast m.
    ioglycamic acid contrast m.
    Iomeron 150, 250, 300, 350
      contrast m.
    ionic dimer contrast m.
    ionic monomeric contrast m.
    ionic paramagnetic contrast m.
    iopromide contrast m.
    iotroxamide contrast m.
    ioxaglic acid contrast m.
    ioxithalamate contrast m.
    isoefamate contrast m.
    Isopaque contrast m.
    isosmolar contrast m. (IOCM)
    low-concentration contrast m.
      (LCCM)
    low-osmolar contrast m.
      (LOCM)
    macromolecular contrast m.
      (MMCM)
    magnesium contrast m.
    manganese chloride contrast m.
    meglumine salts contrast m.
    methylglucamine contrast m.
    Micropaque contrast m.
    MultiHance contrast m.
    nephrotoxic contrast m.
    Niopam contrast m.
    nonionic dimer contrast m.
    nonionic water-soluble contrast m.
    oil-soluble contrast m. (OSCM)
    opaque m.
    potassium bromide contrast m.
    ProHance contrast m.
    radiochromic dosimetry m.
    radiologic contrast m.
    radiolucent m.
    radiopaque contrast m. (ROCM)
    rectal contrast m.
    Resovist MR contrast m.
    Solutrast 200, 250, 300, 370
      contrast m.
    sonicated saline contrast m.
    tantalum-178 contrast m.
    Telebrix contrast m.
    tetraiodophenolphthalein contrast m.
    thorium dioxide radiopaque m.
    topical water-soluble contrast m.
    triiodobenzoic acid contrast m.
    Triosil contrast m.
    tunica m.
    Uromiro contrast m.
    water-soluble contrast m.
      (WSCM)
    Xenetix 250, 300, 350 contrast m.
medium-energy
    m.-e. collimator
    m.-e. high-resolution (MEHR)
medium-sized bronchus
medius
    digitus m.
    gluteus m.
    scalenus m.
MedNova
    M. Neuroshield
    M. stent

Medos Hakim programmable valve
Medrad
    M. automated power injector
    M. contrast medium injector
    M. MRInnervu endorectal colon
      probe coil
    M. power angiographic injector
medronate scan
Medsonic plethysmography
Medspec
    M. MR imaging system
    M. MR imaging system
      scanner
    M. 30/80 tesla MR scanner
Med-Tec VacLoc immobilization
  system
Medtronic
    M. catheter
    M. Minix
    M. Pulsor Intrasound
    M. radiofrequency receiver
    M. Talent prosthesis
medulla, *pl.* **medullae**
    adrenal m.
    hyperechoic renal m.
    lymphatic m.
    m. oblongata
    ovarian m.
    renal m.
    rostral m.
    spinal m.
medullae (*pl. of* medulla)
medullare
    corpus m.
    osteoma m.
medullaris
    artery of conus m.
    conus arteriosus m.
    m. hypoplasia
    low conus m.
medullary
    m. artery
    m. bone
    m. bone infarct
    m. breast carcinoma
    m. calcification
    m. canal
    m. cavity
    m. compression
    m. cone
    m. cord
    m. cystic disease
    m. lamina
    m. nephrocalcinosis
    m. nephrogram
    m. pyramid
    m. rod
    m. sinus
    m. sponge

    m. sponge kidney
    m. tegmentum
    m. thyroid carcinoma
    m. vein
    m. venous anatomy
medullary-type adenocarcinoma
medulloblastoma
    desmoplastic m.
    m. metastasis
    vermian m.
medusae
    caput m.
Medusa hairlike opacity
Medweb clinical reporting system
MedX
    M. camera
    M. scanner
Mees line
mefenamic acid
MEG
    magnetoencephalogram
    magnetoencephalography
megabulb
    jugular m.
megabulbus
    duodenum m.
megacalyces (*pl. of* megacalyx)
megacalycosis
megacalyx, *pl.* **megacalyces**
    congenital m.
mega cisterna magna
megacolon
    acquired m.
    aganglionic m.
    congenital m.
    m. dilation
    functional m.
    idiopathic m.
    toxic m.
megacurie (MCi)
megacystic microcolon
megacystis, megalocystis
    m.
megacystis-microcolon-intestinal
  hypoperistalsis syndrome
megaduodenum
megaelectron volt (MeV)
megaesophagus of achalasia
megahertz (MHz)
Megalink stent
megalocornea
megalocystis (*var. of* megacystis)
megaloencephaly
    unilateral m.
megalosplenia (*var. of* splenomegaly)
megalothymus
megaloureter (*var. of* megaureter)
megalourethra
megarectum

M

595

megaureter, megaloureter
  congential m.
  primary congenital m.
megavolt (MV)
  m. therapy
megavoltage
  m. grid
  m. grid therapy
  m. radiation
  m. radiation therapy
  m. radiotherapy
  m. treatment beam
  m. x-ray therapy
meglumine
  m. acetrizoate
  Cholografin m.
  m. diatrizoate
  m. diatrizoate imaging agent
  gadoterate m.
  iocarmate m.
  iodipamide m.
  m. iodipamide imaging agent
  iodoxamate m.
  m. iotroxate imaging agent
  ioxaglate m.
  m. salts contrast medium
megophthalmos
MEHR
  medium-energy high-resolution
  MEHR collimator
meibomian
  m. cyst
  m. gland carcinoma
Meiboom-Gill sequence
Meige lymphedema
Meigs
  M. capillary
  M. syndrome
Meigs-Cass syndrome
Meigs-Salmon syndrome
Meissner plexus
melanin-containing tumor
melanocytic lesion
melanocytoma
  meningeal m.
melanotic
  m. carcinoma
  m. neuroectodermal tumor
  m. neuroectodermal tumor of
  infancy (MNTI)
  m. whitlow
MELAS
  mitochondrial encephalomyopathy with
  lactic acidosis and strokelike
  episode
mellitus
  diabetes m. (type 1, 2)
Melnick-Needles syndrome

**Melone distal radius fracture
  classification**
melorheostosis
  m. of Léri
  soft tissue pathoanatomy in m.
Melrose solution
melting
  m. ice cube sign
  m. sign
Meltzer sign
membranacea
  placenta m.
membrane
  amnionic m.
  atlantooccipital m.
  axonal m.
  Bichat m.
  m. closure time
  cricothyroid m.
  glial limiting m.
  glomerular basement m. (GBM)
  hourglass m.
  interosseous m. (IOM)
  intertwin m.
  intraluminal m.
  intrauterine m.
  Liliequist m.
  limiting m.
  low-flux polysufone m.
  microporous m.
  mucous m.
  obturator m.
  m. of bone
  m. oxygenator
  m. permeability
  m. phosphate
  prostate-specific m.
  rolling m.
  serous m.
  Shrapnell m.
  synovial m.
  Transwell m.
  umbo of tympanic m.
  vernix m.
membranous
  m. bronchiole
  m. glomerulonephritis
  m. labyrinth
  m. obstruction of inferior vena
  cava
  m. pregnancy
  m. septum
  m. subaortic stenosis
  m. subvalvular aortic stenosis
  m. tendon
  m. urethra
  m. ventricular septal defect
  m. viscerocranium

Memorial
    M. Symptom Assessment Scale
    M. Symptom Assessment
      Scale-Physical
memory
    Aloka color Doppler real-time 2D
      blood flow imaging with cine m.
    random access m. (RAM)
    thermal shape m.
Memotherm nitinol self-expandable stent
MEMP
    multiecho multiplane
      contiguous slice MEMP
MEN
    multiple endocrine neoplasia
Mendelson syndrome
Ménétrier disease
Mengert index
Menghini Surecut bone biopsy needle
Ménière
    M. disease
    M. syndrome
meningeal
    m. artery
    m. artery groove
    m. cell tumor
    m. diverticulum
    m. enhancement
    m. fibroma
    m. fibrosis
    m. hemangiopericytoma
    m. hemorrhage
    m. infiltrate
    m. inflammation
    m. melanocytoma
    m. sarcoma
    m. tuberculosis
    m. vasculature
    m. vein
meninges (*pl. of* meninx)
meningioangiomatosis
meningioma
    angioplastic m.
    atypical m.
    cavernous sinus m.
    cerebellopontine angle m.
    clival m.
    convexity m.
    cystic intraparenchymal m.
    ectopic m.
    endotheliomatous m.
    m. en plaque
    extracranial m.
    falcine m.
    falcotentorial m.
    fibroblastic m.
    fibrous m.
    globular m.

intraosseous m.
intraparenchymal m.
intraventricular m.
lipoblastic m.
malignant m.
meningothelial m.
meningotheliomatous m.
multicentric m.
m. of cribriform plate
m. of posterior fossa
olfactory groove m.
optic nerve sheath m.
parasagittal m.
perioptic m.
posterior fossa m.
psammoma body m.
psammomatous m.
pulmonary m.
sphenoid ridge m.
sphenoid wing m.
sphenoorbital m.
spinal m.
subfrontal m.
suprasellar m.
temporal m.
tentorial m.
transitional m.
tuberculum sellae m.
meningiomatosis
meningitides (*pl. of* meningitis)
meningitidis
    Neisseria m.
meningitis, *pl.* **meningitides**
    bacterial m.
    carcinomatous m.
    coccidioidomycosis m.
    cryptococcal m.
    fungous m.
    neonatal m.
    tuberculous m.
    viral m.
meningocele
    anterior sacral m.
    anterior thoracic m.
    cervical m.
    cranial m.
    dorsal m.
    lateral lumbar m.
    lateral thoracic m.
    occipital m.
    occult intrasacral m.
    sacral m.
    simple m.
    traumatic m.
meningoencephalitis
meningoencephalocele
    ethmoidal m.
    sphenopharyngeal m.

M

meningofacial angiomatosis
meningohypophysial
    m. artery
    m. trunk
meningomyelocele
meningothelial-like nodule
meningothelial meningioma
meningotheliomatous meningioma
meningovascular syphilis
meninx, *pl.* **meninges**
    m. of brain
    m. of spinal cord
meniscal
    m. cleft
    m. cyst
    m. degeneration
    m. fragmentation
    m. horn
    m. injury
    m. ossicle
menisci (*pl. of* meniscus)
meniscocapsular
    m. attachment
    m. junction
    m. separation
meniscocondylar coordination
meniscofemoral
    m. attachment
    m. ligament
meniscosynovial junction
meniscotibial
    m. attachment
    m. ligament
    m. separation
meniscus, *pl.* **menisci**
    articular m.
    m. articularis
    discoid lateral m.
    diverging m.
    dysplastic m.
    fibrocartilaginous m.
    free-floating m.
    m. lateralis
    m. medialis
    pleural m.
    radiohumeral m.
    m. sign
    m. tear
meniscus-shaped calcification
Menkes
    M. kinky hair disease
    M. syndrome
Mennell sign
mental
    m. canal
    m. foramen
    m. spine
mentoanterior

mentooccipital diameter
mentoparietal diameter
Mentor prostatic biopsy needle
mentum, *gen.* **menti**
Menzel olivopontocerebellar
  degeneration
meralgia paresthetica
mercaptoacetyltriglycine (MAG)
Mercator
    M. atrial high-density array
      catheter
    M. projection
merchant
    M. angle
    M. patella view
Mercuhydrin
mercurihydroxypropane
1-mercuri-2-hydroxypropane (MHP)
mercury
    m. arc lamp
    m. artifact
    m. vapor lamp
Merge Mammo imaging software
Meridian echocardiography
Merkel
    M. cell carcinoma
    M. cell carcinoma cell line
Merland perimedullary arteriovenous
  fistula classification
merlin
mermaid
    m. deformity
    m. syndrome
meroacrania
merosin
merosin-deficient congenital muscular
  dystrophy
MERRF
    myoclonic epilepsy and ragged red
    fibers
mertiatide
    technetium 99m m.
mesalamine enema
mesaraic (*var. of* mesenteric)
mesareic (*var. of* mesenteric)
mesatipellic pelvis
mesencephalic
    m. artery
    m. cerebral lymphoma
    m. cistern
    m. cistern effacement
    m. infarct
    m. low-density brain lesion
    m. reticular formation
    m. tract
    m. vein
mesencephalitis
mesencephalodiencephalic lesion

[handwritten note: mmHg]

mesencephalon aqueduct
mesenchymal
- m. abnormality
- m. chondrosarcoma
- m. liver hamartoma
- m. neoplasia
- m. tissue
- m. tumor

mesenchymoma
- atrial m.
- benign m.
- chest wall m.

mesenterial
- m. Castleman lymphoma
- m. sarcoma

mesenteric, mesaraic, mesareic
- m. adenitis
- m. adenitis-ileitis complex
- m. adenopathy
- m. angiography
- m. apoplexy
- m. arterial thrombosis
- m. arteriography
- m. artery
- m. artery occlusion
- m. attachment
- m. border
- m. calcification
- m. cyst
- m. fat stranding
- m. fibromatosis
- m. fibrosis
- m. fistula
- m. infarct
- m. ischemia
- m. lipodystrophy
- m. lymphadenopathy
- m. lymph node pathology
- m. lymphoma
- m. macronodule
- m. mass
- m. metastasis
- m. node
- m. panniculitis
- m. phlegmon
- m. pregnancy
- m. rupture
- m. sclerosis
- m. tear
- m. thromboembolism (MTE)
- m. tissue
- m. triangle
- m. tuberculosis
- m. vascular insufficiency
- m. vascular lesion
- m. vasculitis
- m. vein
- m. vein occlusion
- m. venous thrombosis
- m. vessel
- m. Weber-Christian disease

mesentericoparietal fossa
mesenteritis
- chronic fibrosing m.
- fibrosing m.
- liposclerotic m.
- retractile m.
- sclerosing m.

mesenterium commune
mesenteroaxial volvulus
mesentery
- fan-shaped m.
- fatty m.
- intestinal m.
- ischemic m.
- leaf of m.
- lymphangioma m.
- root of m.
- small intestine m.
- ventral m.
- Weber-Christian m.

mesh
- stent m.
- tantalum m.
- tubular wire m.

mesial
- m. aspect
- m. frontal cortex
- m. frontal focus
- m. hemisphere
- m. hyperperfusion
- m. temporal epileptogenic lesion
- m. temporal sclerosis

mesiodens, mediodens
mesiodistal plane
mesoappendix
mesoblastic nephroma
mesocardia
mesocaval shunt
mesocephalic head shape
mesocolic
- m. band
- m. shelf
- m. vessel

mesocolon
- m. fat
- sigmoid m.
- transverse m.

mesocuneiform bone
mesoderm
- extraembryonic m.

mesodermal
- m. dysplasia
- m. sarcoma

mesomelia

M

mesomelic
    m. dwarfism
    m. dysplasia
mesometanephric carcinoma
mesonephric kidney
mesonephroi (*pl. of* mesonephros)
mesonephros, *pl.* **mesonephroi**
mesoporphyrine
    Bid-Gd m.
mesorectum
mesosigmoid colon
mesosternum
mesothelial cyst
mesothelioma
    asbestos-related m.
    atrioventricular node m.
    benign m.
    cystic m.
    diffuse malignant peritoneal m.
    epithelioid malignant m.
    fibrosing m.
    localized fibrous m.
    malignant epitheliod m.
    malignant pleural m.
    malignant pulmonary m.
    peritoneal m.
    pleural m.
    well-differentiated papillary m.
mesothorium
mesotympanum
mesoversion of heart
mesylate
    fenoldopam m.
metabolic
    m. alteration
    m. bone disease
    m. bone disorder
    m. bone series
    m. bone survey
    m. calculus
    m. cardiomyopathy
    m. cirrhosis
    m. demyelination
    m. lesion
    m. rate of oxygen
    m. response
    m. stone
    m. tracer uptake
metabolically inert area
metabolism
    calcium m.
    carbon m.
    cerebral m.
    evaluation of glucose m.
    fat m.
    fatty acid m.
    hepatic m.
    marker of m.
    myocardial m.

    oxidative m.
    phosphorus m.
metacarpal
    base of m.
    m. bone
    m. fracture
    m. index
    m. length
    m. sign
metacarpi (*pl. of* metacarpus)
metacarpoglenoid ligament
metacarpophalangeal (MCP)
    m. articulation
    m. bone marrow development
    m. joint (MCPJ)
    m. length
    m. ligament
metacarpus, *pl.* **metacarpi**
metachromatic leukodystrophy
metachronous
    m. lesion
    m. metastasis
    m. transitional cell carcinoma
metadiaphysial
metadiaphysis
metaiodobenzylguanidine (MIBG)
    ^{123}I m.
    iodine-123 m. (I-123 MIBG)
    iodine-131 m.
    radioiodinated m.
metal
    m. chelate complex
    Co-Cr-W-Ni alloy implant m.
    lanthanide m.
    m. line-pair phantom
    Lipowitz m.
    m. oxide semiconductor (MOS)
    m. oxide semiconductor field effect
      transistor (MOSFET)
    paramagnetic transition m.
    radioactive m.
    m. technetium target
    transition m.
metallic
    m. artifact
    m. biliary endoprosthesis
    m. cage
    m. debris
    m. density
    m. distal end of tube
    m. echo
    m. foreign body (MFB)
    m. fragment
    m. hookwire
    m. marker
    m. needle
    m. otologic implant
    m. pointer
    m. rod fixation

m. screw
m. staple
m. stent
m. suture
m. track of bullet
metallic-tip cannula
metalloporphyrin
metalloprotease
metalloprotease-3
matrix m.-3 (MMP-3)
metalloproteinase
tissue inhibitor of m.
metanephric
m. diverticulum
m. vesicle
metanephroi (*pl. of* metanephros)
metanephros, *pl.* **metanephroi**
metaphyseal (*var. of* metaphysial)
metaphyses (*pl. of* metaphysis)
metaphysial, metaphyseal
m. abscess
m. chondrodysplasia
m. dysostosis
m. dysplasia
m. extension
m. fibrous defect
m. flare
m. fracture
m. lucent band
m. metaphysis
metaphysial-diaphysial
m.-d. angle
m.-d. junction
m.-d. low signal intensity red
marrow inhomogeneity
metaphysial-epiphysial angle
metaphysis, *pl.* **metaphyses**
agnogenic myeloid m.
autoparenchymatous m.
celomic m.
columnar m.
frayed m.
fundic m.
humeral m.
intestinal m.
metaphysial m.
myeloid m.
primary myeloid m.
secondary myeloid m.
squamous m.
subphysial m.
metaplasia
agnogenic myeloid m.
apocrine m.
articular m.
cartilaginous m.
gastric m.
intestinal m.
keratinizing squamous m.

monarticular synovium-based
cartilage m.
osseous m.
osteocartilaginous m.
squamous m.
metaplastic
m. carcinoma
m. polyp
metapneumonic
m. empyema
m. pleurisy
metastable
m. radionuclide
m. state
m. trap
metastases (*pl. of* metastasis)
metastasis, *pl.* **metastases**
adnexal m.
adrenal m.
aggressive m.
aortic node m.
atrial m.
axillary node m.
blastic m.
bone marrow m.
brain m.
breast m.
calcareous m.
calcified ovarian m.
calcifying m.
carcinomatous cavitary m.
cardiac m.
cavitary m.
cavitating lung m.
celiac lymph node m.
cerebral m.
choroidal m.
clivus m.
cutaneous m.
cystic nodal m.
diffuse skeletal m.
disseminated m.
distant m.
drop m.
dural m.
echogenic liver m.
endobronchial m.
extracapsular m.
extrahepatic m. (EHM)
extraocular muscle m.
extraskeletal m.
extrathoracic m.
gallbladder m.
gastric m.
gingival m.
hematogenous m.
hemorrhagic m.
hepatic m.
hypervascular liver m.

M

metastasis (*continued*)
inguinal lymph node m.
intracranial m.
intramedullary spinal cord m.
intramuscular m.
in-transit m.
intraparenchymal m.
intrathecal drop m.
kidney m.
laparoscopic port-site m.
  (LPSM)
leptomeningeal m.
liver m.
local m.
lung m.
lymphangitic m.
lymphatic m.
lymph node m.
lymphogenous m.
magnetic resonance discriminator of
  osseous m.
medulloblastoma m.
mesenteric m.
metachronous m.
metatarsal m.
micronodular m.
MR discriminator of osseous m.
muscle m.
necrotic hepatic m.
neuroendocrine hepatic m.
nodal m.
occult bone m.
omental m.
orbital m.
osseous m.
osteoblastic m.
osteogenic m.
osteolytic osseous m.
ovarian m.
overcalling m.
pancreatic m.
paracardiac m.
parasellar m.
parenchymatous brain m.
peritoneal m.
placental m.
pleural m.
port-site m.
pulmonary m.
pulsating m.
renal m.
satellite m.
skeletal muscle m.
skip m.
skull m.
small bowel m.
solitary sternal m.
sphenoid sinus m.
spinal cord m.

splenic m.
subcutaneous m.
testicular m.
thyroid m.
m. to pancreas
tumor, nodal involvement, m.
  (TNM)
uterine sarcoma m.
Virchow m.
visceral m.
white m.
widespread m.

metastasizing fibroleiomyoma

metastatic
m. adenocarcinoma
m. adenocarcinoma in serosal
  surface
m. adenopathy
m. axillary involvement
m. bone survey
m. carcinoid syndrome
m. disease
m. efficiency index
m. focus
m. lesion
m. lymph node
m. malignancy
m. myocardial tumor
m. neuroblastoma
m. osteosarcoma
m. pleomorphic liposarcoma
m. polyp
m. renal neoplasia
m. rhabdomyosarcoma
m. seeding
m. site
m. soft tissue calcification
m. testicular lymphoma
m. urothelial carcinoma

metasynchronous tumor

metatarsal (MT)
m. angle
angle of declination of m.
m. axis
m. bone
m. fracture
m. head
m. head width (MHW)
m. injury
m. joint
m. length ratio
m. metastasis
m. parabola
m. synostosis

metatarsi (*pl. of* metatarsus)
metatarsocalcaneal angle
metatarsocuneiform
m. joint
m. joint fusion

metatarsophalangeal (MTP)
    m. bone marrow development
    m. capsule
    m. joint
    m. joint arthritis
    m. joint fusion
metatarsotalar angle
metatarsus, *pl.* **metatarsi**
    m. adductocavus deformity
    m. adductovarus deformity
    m. adductus
    m. adductus angle
    m. adductus deformity
    m. atavicus deformity
    m. latus deformity
    m. primus varus angle (MPVA)
    m. primus varus deformity
    m. valgus
    m. varus
metatrophic
    m. dwarfism
    m. dysplasia
metencephalon
meter (m)
    analogue rate m.
    attenuation in phantom m.
    counting rate m.
    dose area product m.
    exposure m.
    Gammex RMI DAP m.
    Geiger-Müller survey m.
    kVp m.
    m.'s per second (mps)
    photovolt pH m.
    rate m.
    roentgen m.
    roentgens per hour at 1 m.
meter-candle
methemoglobin effect
methiodal sodium imaging agent
methionine
    ^{11}C m.
method
    acoustic reflection m.
    Agatston calcium scoring m.
    AIPH m.
    Andren m.
    area-length m.
    Arelin m.
    autoattenuation correction m.
    automated airway tree segmentation m.
    Ball m.
    Bauer-Kirby disc diffusion m.
    Bayler-Pinneau m.
    Benassi m.
    Benedict-Talbot body surface area m.
    Bertel m.

Bigliani and Morrison m.
black blood m.
Blackett-Healy m.
blood oxygen level-dependent fMRI m.
border detection m. (BDM)
Borell and Fernström m.
Born m.
Brasdor m.
Bull m.
Caldwell m.
calibration m.
Cameron m.
CHESS m.
chunk acquisition and reconstruction m. (CHARM)
Clauss m.
Cleaves m.
Cobb m.
Colbert m.
column extraction m.
computer m.
deconvolution m.
Demons m.
destroy and replace m.
2DFT m.
double-echo m.
downstream sampling m.
dual-balloon m.
2-dye m.
echo-planar imaging m.
electrocardiographic trigger m.
ellipsoid m.
empirical m.
error diffusion m.
extraction m.
FBP m.
Ferguson m.
FI m.
Fick m.
filtered back-projection m.
fractal-based m.
Friedman m.
full-scan m.
Gaynor-Hart m.
Gerota m.
gradient-echo m.
Graf m.
Grashey m.
Greulich and Pyle m.
Haas m.
Hawkins m.
Hickey m.
inflow/outflow m.
in vivo m.
IPSP neuron evaluation m.
isocenter shift m.
isodose shift m.
Joliot m.

M

method (*continued*)
    Kauppi m.
    Kety-Schmidt m.
    keyhole m.
    Kumar, Welti and Ernst m.
    KWE m.
    Lawrence m.
    Levenberg-Marquardt m.
    Lippman-Cobb m.
    Lysholm m.
    Mankin m.
    Meyerding anterior displacement of vertebral body m.
    Monte Carlo m.
    multiple-line scanning m.
    multiple sensitive-point m.
    multisection m.
    neutron/gamma transmission m.
    m. of Larsen
    m. of perpendiculars
    m. of Scarpa
    paddlewheel m.
    parallax m.
    Pearson m.
    Pelizzari surface matching m.
    Pfeiffer-Comberg intraorbital foreign body localization m.
    phase-inversion m.
    phase-unwrapping m.
    Pirie m.
    pixel count m.
    Porcher m.
    Powell m.
    pulse-echo m.
    radioimmunoassay m.
    radiotracer foil m.
    Ranawat m.
    ray-casting m.
    receiver operating characteristic m.
    ROC m.
    rotational m.
    Sansregret m.
    segmentation m.
    selective excitation m.
    selective saturation m.
    SENSE m.
    sensitivity encoding m.
    Settegast m.
    short-cannula coaxial m.
    simulated annealing m.
    spin-label m.
    spin-warp m.
    spiral imaging m.
    Strickler m.
    sum-peak m.
    surface coil m.
    surface normal overlap m.
    Sweet m.
    Thom m.

    thresholding m.
    time-of-flight m.
    triangulation m.
    TRICKS m.
    ultrashort m.
    under-scan m.
    Valdini m.
    variable projection m.
    vertebral body ratio m.
    volume-ratio m.
    Wolf m.
    Zimmer m.
methodology
    Gehan m.
methoxy-17-alpha-iodvinyl estradiol (Z-MIVE)
methoxyisobutylisonitrile (MIBI)
    m. SPECT
    technetium 99m m. (^{99m}Tc MIBI, Tc-99m MIBI)
methoxystaurosporine
    ^{11}C m.
methyl
    m. methacrylate bead
    m. methacrylate bead implant
    m. methacrylate imaging agent
    m. proton
methyl-ABV
methylcellulose gel
methylene
    m. blue enema
    m. diphosphonate (MDP)
    m. diphosphonate concentration
methylglucamine
    m. contrast medium
    m. diatrizoate
    iodipamide m.
methylsulfate
    neostigmine m.
metopic suture
MET-PET
    ^{11}C-methionine positron emission tomography
    MET-PET scan
metrics
    histogram-derived m.
metrizamide
    m. computed tomography cisternography (MCTC)
    m. CT cisternogram
    m. imaging agent
    m. myelography
    m. myelography computed tomography
    m. ventriculogram
metrizoate imaging agent
metrizoic acid
metrography
metroperitoneal fistula

metroplasty
metrosalpingography
Metz spatially varying filter
MeV
    megaelectron volt
    million electron volts
Mewissen infusion catheter
Meyer
    M. dysplasia
    M. line
    M. loop
    supratubercular ridge of M.
Meyer-Archambault loop
Meyerding anterior displacement of
  vertebral body method
Meyer-McKeever tibial fracture
  classification
Meynet node
mf
    microfarad
MFB
    metallic foreign body
MFG
    magnetic field gradient
    manofluorography
MFH
    malignant fibrous histiocytoma
      giant cell-type MFH
      inflammatory MFH
      myxoid MFH
      postirradiation MFH
      storiform-pleomorphic MFH
MFH-B
    malignant fibrous histiocytoma of bone
MG
    multigeometry
    Millennium MG
mHCC
    moderately differentiated hepatocellular
    carcinoma
MHP
    1-mercuri-2-hydroxypropane
MH-908 slim ultrasonic probe
MHV
    middle hepatic vein
MHW
    metatarsal head width
MHz
    megahertz
MI
    myocardial infarct
      inferior wall MI
MIBG
    metaiodobenzylguanidine
      MIBG scintigraphy
      MIBG SPECT scan
      MIBG washout
MIBI
    methoxyisobutylisonitrile

MIC
    minimal inhibitory concentration
      MIC gastroenteric tube
      MIC transgastric jejunal feeding
      tube
micaceous
mica pneumoconiosis
mice (*pl. of* mouse)
micelle
    fluorescent m.
Michaelis
    M. complex
    rhomboid of M.
Michaelis-Gutmann body
Michel
    M. anomaly
    M. aplasia
    M. deformity
    M. malformation
Michels classification
Mickey
    M. Mouse appearance
    M. Mouse ears pelvis
MIC-Key low-profile transgastric jejunal
  feeding tube
Mick seed applicator
Mi/Cr
    myoinositol-creatine ratio
micrencephalia (*var. of* micrencephaly)
micrencephaly, micrencephalia,
  microencephaly
micro
    m. CT imaging
    m. CT-20 scanner
microabscess
    m. of spleen
    splenic m.
microadenoma
    adrenocorticotropin m.
    ectopic intracavernous pituitary m.
    pituitary m.
microaggregated albumin
microanalyzer
    electronic m. (EMA)
microaneurysm
    Charcot-Bouchard intracerebral m.
    retinal m.
microangioarchitecture
microangiogram
microangiography
microangiopathy
    diabetic m.
    mineralizing m.
    thrombotic m.
microangioscopy
microarchitecture
    bone m.
microarteriography
microarteriovenous malformation

M

microatelectasis
microautoradiography
micro-AVM
    single-shot embolization of m.-AVM
microballoon
    Rand m.
microbubble
    m. concentration measurement
    m. contrast enhancement
    intranasal m.
    sonicated albumin m.
    targeted monolayer coated m.
microbubble-based contrast agent
microbubble-enhanced CDUS
microcalcification
    breast m.
    m. cluster
    coarse m.
    ductal breast m.
    granular m.
    linear branching m.
    lobular breast m.
    pleomorphic m.
    psammomatous m.
    sole cluster of m.
    subtle m.
microcalculi (*pl. of* microcalculus)
microcalculus, *pl.* **microcalculi**
microcardia
Micro-Cast collimator
microcatheter
    AngiOptic m.
    ball-tip m.
    Cardima Pathfinder m.
    Equinox balloon m.
    Excel-14 m.
    Excelsior m.
    F m.
    Flow Rider m.
    Hieshima m.
    Leggiero hydrophilic coated m.
    Microferret m.
    Rapid Transit m.
    Renegade Hi-Flo m.
    Tracer m.
    Tracker 10 m.
microcavitation
microcephalia (*var. of* microcephaly)
microcephaly, microcephalia
microcinematography
microcirculation
    m. abnormality
    pulmonary m.
microcirculatory blood flow
microcluster
    biodegradable magnetic m.
microcoil
    complex platinum m.
    Dacron-coated m.

    Hilal m.
    Intercept esophagus m.
    Intercept prostate m.
    Intercept urethra m.
    platinum m.
microcolon
    megacystic m.
microcomputed tomography
microconidia (*pl. of* microconidium)
microconidium, *pl.* **microconidia**
microcrust formation lesion
microcurie
microcyst
    milk-of-calcium m.
microcystic
    m. adenoma
    m. degeneration
    m. encephalomalacia
    m. formation
    m. lumbar spine
    m. pancreatic tumor
    m. pilocytic cerebellar astrocytoma
microcystica
microcytosis
microdactylia (*var. of* microdactyly)
microdactyly, microdactylia
microdistribution
    heterogeneous m.
microdosimetry
microembolism
    cerebral m.
microembolization
    ferromagnetic m.
microembolus
    tumor m.
microencephaly (*var. of* micrencephaly)
microendoscope
    ophthalmic laser m.
    (OLM)
microenvironment
    bone marrow m.
microerosion
microexplosion lithotripsy
microextension
microfarad (mf)
Microferret microcatheter
microfibrillar collagen
microfilament
microfixation plate
microfluidization
microfocal
    m. direct magnification in vitro
    x-ray tube
    m. spot mammography
microform of holoprosencephaly
microfracture
    subchondral m.
    trabecular m.
microgastria

microglandular adenosis
microglioma
microglobulin labeling
micrognathia
Micro-Guide
microguidewire
    hydromer-coated m.
microhamartoma
    biliary m.
microhemorrhage
microimaging
microinfarct
microkymatotherapy
microlaparoscope
    Imagyn m.
Microlase transpupillary diode laser
microlattice
    cerebral vascular m.
microlesion
Microlight 830 laser
microlith
microlithiasis
    alveolar m.
    pulmonary alveolar m.
    testicular m.
microlobular cirrhosis
microlobulation
micromanometer-tipped catheter
MicroMark tissue marker
micromelia
    bowed m.
    extreme m.
micromelic
    m. dwarfism
    m. dysplasia
micrometallic artifact
micrometastasis
    systemic m.
micrometer
MicroMewi multiple-sidehole infusion catheter
micro-MRI with FIESTA
micron
micronester platinum embolization coil
micronodular
    m. cirrhosis
    m. infiltrate
    m. metastasis
    m. pattern
micronodularity
micronodule
    centrilobular m.
    peribronchial m.
    subpleural m.
micron-resolution retinal image in vivo

micropapillary
    m. carcinoma
    m. DCIS
    m. lesion
    m. tumor
Micropaque contrast medium
microperforation
micropipet (*var. of* micropipette)
micropipette, micropipet
microplate reader
microporous membrane
Microprobe laser
microprolactinoma
micropuncture needle
microradiogram
microradiography
microreceiver
microreentrant circuit
microroentgen
microsatellite instability (MSI)
microscintigraphy
microscope
    multimode imaging confocal optical m. (MIMCOM)
    projection x-ray m.
    scanning acoustic m. (SAM)
    scanning electron m. (SEM)
    video-rate 2-photon laser scanning m.
    x-ray tomographic m. (XTM)
microscopic, microscopical
    m. air bubble
    m. angiogenesis grading system
    m. cortical dysplasia
    m. hemorrhage of ligament
    m. imaging
    m. polyangiitis
microscopical (*var. of* microscopic)
microscopy
    darkfield m.
    differential interference contrast m.
    3D magnetic resonance m.
    electron m.
    fluorescence resonance energy transfer m.
    immune electron m.
    interferometric synthetic aperture m. (ISAM)
    in vivo m.
    light m.
    polarized light m.
    ultrasound backscatter m. (UBM)
microsecond pulsed flashlamp-pumped dye laser
microSelectron-HDR
microSelectron rapid delivery system
microsnare
microsomia
    hemifacial m.

M

microsphere
    acrylic m.
    calibrated tris-acryl gelatin m.
    Contour SE m.
    degradable starch m.
    EmboGold m.
    Embosphere m.
    ferromagnetic m.
    hollow albumin m.
    human albumin m.
    m. perfusion scintigraphy
    silicone m.
    sodium acrylate and vinyl alcohol
      copolymer m.
    stainless steel m.
    superabsorbent polymer m.
      (SAP-MS)
    superparamagnetic m.
    technetium 99m human albumin m.
    tris-acryl gelatin m. (TAGM,
      TGMS)
    ^{90}Y m.
    ytterbium-90 m.
    yttrium-90 m.
microstructural
    m. architecture
    m. change
microstructure
    3-dimensional trabecular bone m.
microtear
Microtek ScanMaker 9600XL scanner
microtomography
    view m.
MicroTrach
    Heimlich M.
Microtrast
microtrauma
    cumulative m.
    repetitive m.
microtron accelerator
microtubule
microvascular
    m. circulation
    m. decompression
    m. disease
    m. retrieval
microvasculature
    pulmonary m.
microvenoarteriolar fistula
microvesicular fat
microvessel
    m. density
    intraparenchymal m.
microvolt
microwave
    m. cardiac ablation system
    m. coagulation therapy
    m. endometrial ablation (MEA)
    m. hyperthermia

    m. hyperthermia treatment
    m. imaging
    m. nonsurgical treatment
    m. tumor coagulation
micturating
    m. cystourethrogram (MCU)
    m. cystourethrography
micturition cystourethrography
mid
    m. left sternal border
    m. marginal branch
midabdominal wall
midaortic
    m. arch
    m. syndrome (MAS)
midarterial phase
midaxillary line
midbody of vertebra
midbrain
    m. aqueduct
    m. function
    m. lesion
    m. reticular formation (MRF)
    m. tegmentum
    m. tremor
midbrain-hindbrain junction
midcarpal
    m. compartment
    m. dislocation
    m. instability
    m. joint
    m. joint cavity
midcircumflex
midclavicular
    m. line (MCL)
    m. plane
midcolon
midcoronal
    m. oblique image
    m. plane
middiastole
middistal
middle
    m. aortic syndrome
    m. cardiac vein
    m. cerebral artery (MCA)
    m. cerebral artery bifurcation
    m. cerebral artery fenestration
    m. cerebral artery infarct
    m. cerebral artery occlusion
    m. coronary sinus (MCS)
    m. cranial fossa
    m. cuneiform bone
    m. ear
    m. ear choristoma
    m. ear mass
    m. ear neoplasia
    m. extrahepatic bile duct
    m. facet of subtalar joint

m. field-strength MR imaging
m. finger
m. fossa syndrome
m. frontal gyrus
m. hepatic vein (MHV)
m. hypoattenuated appearance
m. lobe
m. lobe bronchus
m. lobe of lung
m. lobe syndrome
m. mediastinal mass
m. mediastinum
m. meningeal artery
m. meningeal artery groove
m. muscle
m. palatine suture
m. perforating collagen bundle
m. pole
m. pulmonary lobe atelectasis
m. 3rd of thoracic esophagus
m. 3rd shaft
m. rectal vein
m. temporal gyrus
m. turbinate bone
middle-caliber needle
middorsal
midepigastrium
midesophageal diverticulum
midesophagus
midexpiratory tidal flow
midface
fetal m.
m. fracture
m. retrusion
midfacial fracture
midfemur
midfoot fracture
midfrontal
m. plane
m. plane coronal section
midget MRI scanner
midgraft stenosis
midgroove portion of lumen
midgut
m. volvulus
m. volvulus with malrotation
midhumeral line
midinfrared laser
midinguinal point
midlateral course
midline
m. cerebellum
m. cystic structure
m. echoencephalograph
m. granuloma
m. herniation of disc
m. incense presentation
infracolic m.
m. lesion

m. longitudinal pontile cleft
m. malignant reticulosis
m. mucosa-sparing block
m. of brain cyst
m. parasagittal focus
m. shift
midlung
m. field
m. zone
midpalmar
m. abscess
m. space
midpapillary short axis
midpatellar tendon
midpelvis
midplane
m. depth
m. sagittal image
midpole
midportion
midsagittal
m. diameter (MSD)
m. MR image
m. MR imaging
m. plane
midscapular line
midshaft fracture
midshunt peak velocity (MSPv)
midsigmoid colon
midspinal line
midsternal
m. area
m. line
midsternum
midsystolic
m. buckling of mitral valve
m. notching of velocity spectrum
m. retraction
midtarsal
m. injury
m. joint (MTJ)
midthalamic plane
midthigh amputation
midthoracic spine
midventricular short-axis slice
midwaist scaphoid fracture
midzonal necrosis
midzone
Miescher granulomatosis
Mignon granuloma
migrainous scintillation
migration
m. abnormality
bowel m.
catheter m.
coil m.
m. disorder
embolus m.
gallstone m.

M

mm Hg

migration (*continued*)
    hallux m.
    m. index
    neuronal m.
    m. of acetabular cup
    placenta m.
    sesamoid m.
    stent m.
    tissue m.
migrational
    m. anomaly
    m. pattern
migratory
    m. patchy infiltrate
    m. pneumonia
MII
    multichannel intraluminal impedance
Mikity-Wilson syndrome
Mikulicz
    M. angle
    M. disease
    M. syndrome
Milch
    M. classification of humeral fracture
    M. elbow fracture classification (I, II)
mild
    m. cognitive impairment
    m. edema
    m. head injury
    m. recess
    m. subcostal retraction
    m. traumatic brain injury
mildly enlarged heart
Miles operation
miliary
    m. aneurysm
    m. embolus
    m. granuloma
    m. lesion
    m. lung disease
    m. node
    m. nodule
    m. parenchymal disease
    m. pattern
    m. pulmonary tuberculosis
military antishock trousers (MAST)
milk
    m. leg syndrome
    m. of calcium
    m. tooth
milk-alkali syndrome
milking effect
milkmaid's
    m. elbow
    m. elbow dislocation
milkman
    M. pseudofracture
    M. syndrome

milkman's fracture
milk-of-calcium
    m.-o.-c. calcification
    m.-o.-c. microcyst
    m.-o.-c. urinary tract cyst
milky effusion
Millar catheter-tip transducer
Millennium
    M. MG
    M. VG SPECT system
miller
    M. double mushroom biliary stent
    M. index
    M. position
Miller-Abbott tube
Miller-Dieker syndrome
miller's lung
milliamperage (mA, ma)
milliampere (mA)
    m. seconds (mAs)
milliampere-impulse
millicurie (mCi)
millicurie-hour (mCi-hr)
millimeter
millimole (mmol)
million electron volts (MeV)
millirad (mrad)
millirem (mrem)
milliroentgen
millisecond (msec)
millivolt (mV)
Milroy disease
Milwaukee shoulder syndrome
MIMCOM
    multimode imaging confocal optical microscope
mimic
MIMIC
    multivane intensity modulation compensator
mimicked
mimicker of malignancy
mimicking
mimosa pattern
Minaar classification of coalition
minced rib
mind-body interaction
mineralization
    bone m.
    matrix m.
    stippled m.
mineralizing microangiopathy
mineralocorticoid secretion
mineral oil imaging agent
miner's lung
miniature
    m. imaging
    m. stomach
    m. uterine cavity

miniaturized mitral valve
mini-balloon system
Mini 6000 C-arm
minicholecystostomy
minicoil
minification
minimal
    m. deformation target (MDT)
    m. inhibitory concentration (MIC)
    m. interstitial thickening
    m. luminal diameter (MLD)
    m. peripheral dose
    m. port diameter (MPD)
    m. volume
minimally
    m. attenuating medical-grade
      foam
    m. displaced fracture
    m. invasive access set
    m. invasive endovascular stent
      placement
    m. invasive osteoplasty
    m. invasive saline-enhanced RFA
minimi
    flexor digiti m.
    opponens digiti m.
minimicroaggregated albumin colloid
minimizing bias
minimum
    m. basis set magnetic resonance
      angiography (MBS-MRA)
    m. blood pressure
    m. pixel density
    m. tolerance dose
minimum-intensity
    m.-i. projection image
    m.-i. projection imaging
    m.-i. sliding thin-slab projection
minimus
    digitus pedis m.
    gluteus m.
    scalenus m.
minipuncture sheath
Minix
    Medtronic M.
Mink-Deutsch classification
Minnesota tube
minor
    bursa omentalis m.
    m. calyx
    m. duodenal papilla
    m. fissure
    globus m.
    m. muscle
    rhomboid m.
    M. sign
    teres m.
minora
Minot-von Willebrand syndrome

minus
    omentum m.
minuscule
minus-density artifact
minute
    m. bleeding ulcer
    blood volume per m.
    cycles per m. (cpm)
    rotations per m.
    m. ventilation
    m. vessel
    m. volume
minute-sequence study
MION
    monocrystalline iron oxide nanoparticle
MIOP
    magnetic iron oxide particle
MIP
    macrophage inflammatory protein
    maximum-intensity pixel
    maximum-intensity projection
    MIP image
    MIP image processing
    MIP reconstruction
MIR
    multiple isomorphous replacements
    MIR guidelines
    MIR intrauterine tandem
    MIR system
mirabile
    rete m.
Miraluma
    M. injection
    M. nuclear scan of breast
    M. scan
MIRD
    medical internal radiation dose
    medical internal radiation dosimetry
Mirizzi syndrome
mirror
    beam-splitting m.
    m. image
    m. imaging
    polygon m.
mirrored FISP
mirror-image
    m.-i. aneurysm
    m.-i. artifact
    m.-i. brachiocephalic branching
    m.-i. dextrocardia
    m.-i. interpretation
    m.-i. reversal
mirrorlike echo
MIS
    mitral insufficiency
misalign
misalignment
    cytoskeletal m.
    neurofilamentous m.

M

miscible pool
miscommunication
    neural m.
Miser tube
misery perfusion
misinterpretation
misleading
    m. image
    m. imaging
mismapping
    phase m.
mismatch
    diffusion-perfusion m.
    FDG-blood flow m.
    flow-function m.
    perfusion-metabolism reverse m.
    ventilation-perfusion m.
    V/Q m.
mismatched defect
misplaced thoracentesis
misregistration
    anatomic m.
    m. artifact
    chemical-shift m.
    local m.
    oblique flow m.
    respiratory m.
missed
    m. bronchogenic carcinoma
    m. testicular torsion
missile
    m. effect
    m. wound
missing pulse steady-state free precession
  sequence
MIST
    maintenance immunosuppressive
    treatment
    MIST therapy system
mistiness of pericolonic fat
Mitchell classification
Mitek bone anchor
mitochondrial
    m. ATP production
    m. encephalomyopathy
    m. encephalomyopathy with lactic
    acidosis and strokelike episode
    (MELAS)
    m. function
    m. genome
    m. respiratory chain disorder
    m. uncoupler
mitosis-karyorrhexis index (MKI)
mitral
    m. apparatus
    m. arcade
    m. component
    m. configuration of cardiac
    shadow

    m. deceleration slope
    m. flow velocity index
    m. inflow velocity
    m. insufficiency (MIS)
    m. leaflet
    m. leak
    m. orifice
    m. regurgitant signal area
    m. regurgitation (MR)
    m. regurgitation artifact
    m. ring calcification
    m. stenosis (MS)
    m. valve
    m. valve anulus
    m. valve area (MVA)
    m. valve atresia
    m. valve calcification
    m. valve commissure
    m. valve cusp
    m. valve deformity
    m. valve echocardiography
    m. valve echogram
    m. valve flow
    m. valve gradient
    m. valve incompetence
    m. valve leaflet systolic prolapse
    m. valve leaflet tip
    m. valve myxomatous degeneration
    m. valve opening (MVO)
    m. valve orifice (MVO)
    m. valve prolapse (MVP)
    m. valve regurgitation
    m. valve replacement (MVR)
    m. valve ring
    m. valve septal separation
    m. valve stenosis (MVS)
    m. valve systolic anterior motion
mitralization
Mitsuyasu staging system
mixed
    m. aneurysm
    m. connective tissue disease
    (MCTD)
    m. echogenic solid mass
    m. fat-water breast density lesion
    m. fat-water lesion density
    m. gonadal dysgenesis
    m. hernia
    m. IUGR
    m. lymphocytic-histiocytic
    lymphoma
    m. lytic and sclerotic pattern
    m. müllerian tumor
    m. petal-fugal flow
    m. rheumatoid and degenerative
    arthritis
    m. sclerotic and lytic bone lesion
    m. sclerotic osteolysis
    m. small and large cell lymphoma

m. solid-cystic mass
m. tissue disease
m. venous blood
m. venous-lymphatic malformation
m. venous saturation

mixed-attenuation mass
mixed-cell sarcoma
mixed-density mass
mixed-echo appearance
mixed-signal mass
mixing
intracardiac m.
mixture
barium m.
Ingenor silicone m.
injectable procoagulant m.
MKI
mitosis-karyorrhexis index
MLC
multileaf collimator
MLD
minimal luminal diameter
ML-700 daylight processor
MLF
medial longitudinal fasciculus
MLF lesion
MLO
mediolateral oblique
MLS
multiple-line scan
MLSI
multiple line-scan imaging
ML-Ultra balloon stent
MMCM
macromolecular contrast medium
MMEF
maximum midexpiratory flow
MMFR
maximum midexpiratory flow
rate
M4-M5 lineage
M-mode
motion mode
time-motion mode
M-m. cardiography
M-m. display
M-m. echocardiogram imaging
M-m. echocardiography
M-m. echophonocardiography
M-m. scanning
M-m. sector transducer
M-m. time-motion scan
M-m. ultrasound
mmol
millimole
MMP-3
matrix metalloprotease-3
MMR
mobile mass x-ray

M1-M5 segment of middle cerebral artery
Mn
manganese
MnDPDP-enhanced MRI
MNTI
melanotic neuroectodermal tumor of infancy
^{99}Mo, Mo-99
molybdenum 99
Mo
molybdenum
MoAb
monoclonal antibody
^{131}I-labeled human MoAb
radiolabeled MoAb
Moberg-Gedda fracture
Mobetron
M. electron beam system
M. intraoperative radiation therapy treatment system
mobile
m. artery and vein imaging system (MAVIS)
cecum m.
cor m.
m. duodenum
m. fat ball
m. fluoroscopy
m. gallbladder
m. imaging procedure
m. intraluminal gallbladder mass
m. magnetic resonance
m. mass x-ray (MMR)
m. radiography
m. spiral computed tomography scanner
m. thrombus
m. without recapture
m. with recapture
mobility film
Mobin-Uddin
M.-U. umbrella endoluminal device
M.-U. vena cava filter
MobiTrak
M. automated table
M. moving table
MOD
magnetooptical disc
Multi-Operatory Dentalaser
modality
cross-sectional m.
diagnostic m.
imaging m.
multislice m.
neuroimaging m.
optimal m.
m. performed procedure step (MPPS)

M

modality (*continued*)
  radiation-free imaging m.
  tomographic m.
modal velocity
mode
  AAI rate-responsive m.
  m. abandonment
  active m.
  asynchronous transfer m. (ATM)
  blink m.
  brightness m.
  byte m.
  cine m.
  coincidence detection m.
  continuous m.
  decay m.
  dispersion m.
  dual-demand pacing m.
  electron-capture decay m.
  full 3-dimensional m.
  full-to-empty VAD m.
  fundamental Doppler m.
  high spatial resolution m.
  high temporal resolution m.
  imaginary m.
  inactive m.
  magnet m.
  modified 2-dimensional acquisition
    m.
  multiplanar m.
  multislice m.
  noncommitted m.
  pulsed m.
  roadmapping m.
  semicommitted m.
  sequential m.
  step-and-shoot m.
  stimulated echo acquisition m.
    (STEAM)
  stimulation m.
  motion m. (M-mode)
  time-motion m. (M-mode)
  triggered flow m.
  triggered pacing m.
  underdrive m.
  unipolar pacing m.
  volume m.
  volume-rendered m.
model
  Diomed 630 PDT laser m.
  pharmacokinetic m.
modeling
  compartmental m.
  3D m.
  electromagnetic m.
  Monte Carlo m.
  thermal m.
  tracer kinetic m.

  ultrasonographic m.
  vascular and airway m.
moderately
  m. differentiated adenocarcinoma
  m. differentiated hepatocellular
    carcinoma (mHCC)
  m. dilated ureter
moderate sedation
moderate-sized-volume joint effusion
moderator band
modest caliber
Modic disc abnormality classification
modification
  thiol m.
modified
  m. Bagshawe protocol
  m. barium swallow
  m. Bernoulli equation
  m. bird-cage coil
  m. Blalock-Taussig shunt patency
  m. 2-dimensional acquisition
    mode
  m. electron beam CT scanner
  m. linear accelerator
  m. linear accelerator radiosurgery
  m. look-locker sequence
  m. projection
  m. SENSE (mSENSE)
  m. Simpson rule
  m. stage exercise
  m. vessel image processor
    software
modioli (*pl. of* modiolus)
modiolus, *pl.* **modioli**
modular stent-graft
modulation
  amplitude m.
  brightness m.
  image m.
  object m.
  off-center m.
  print reflectance m.
  specific m.
  m. transfer function (MTF)
module
  detecting m.
  E-TOF detecting m.
  tube geometry m.
Modulith SL 20 lithotriptor
modulus image
mogul
  cardiac m.
  m. of heart
  3rd cardiac m.
Mohn-Wriedt brachydactyly
Mohr syndrome
moiety
  upper pole m.

moiré
> m. fringe
> m. fringe artifact
> m. pattern
> m. photography

molal solution

molar
> m. mass
> m. pregnancy
> m. tooth
> m. tooth appearance
> m. tooth configuration
> m. tooth fracture
> m. tooth midbrain-hindbrain malformation
> m. volume

mold
> filter m.

molded immobilizer

molding
> atheroma m.
> m. of skull

molecular
> m. coincidence detection (MCD)
> m. diffusion
> m. imaging
> m. marker
> m. recognition unit (MRU)
> m. vibration
> m. weight dependence of relaxation

molecularly targeted therapy

molecule
> accessory adhesion m.
> cleaved polyprotein precursor m.
> costimulatory m.
> homing m.
> intracellular adhesion m.
> signaling lymphocytic activation m.

molecule-1
> vascular cell adhesion m.-1 (VCAM-1)

molle
> fibroma m.
> heloma m.
> papilloma m.

molluscum
> fibroma m.
> m. fibrosum

Molnar disc

Molteno
> M. double-plate drainage device
> M. single-plate drainage device

molybdenum (Mo)
> m. 99 (^{99}Mo, Mo-99)
> m. anode
> m. target
> m. target tube

molybdenum-99
> m.-99 breakthrough test
> m.-99 generator

molybdenum-molybdenum target-filter combination

molybdenum-rhodium target-filter combination

molybdenum-technetium generator

moment
> macroscopic magnetic m.
> magnetic dipole m.
> nuclear magnetic m.
> quadrupole m.
> zeroth m.

momentum
> angular m.

monarticular
> m. process
> m. synovium-based cartilage metaplasia

Mönckeberg
> M. arteriosclerosis
> M. calcification
> M. degeneration

Mondini
> M. anomaly
> M. dysplasia
> M. malformation

Mondor disease

Mongolian spotlike lesion

mongoloid feature

moniliasis

moniliform ectasia

monitor
> actocardiotocograph m.
> Acuson V5M m.
> air m.
> Appraise m.
> beam m.
> Biotrack coagulation m.
> blood perfusion m. (BPM)
> Brilliance 109 MP PC m.
> cardiac m.
> CardioBeeper CB-12L cardiac m.
> Doppler blood flow m.
> Doppler ultrasonic fetal heart m.
> FreeDop Doppler m.
> gray-scale m.
> HeartView CT cardiac m.
> Life-Pack 5 cardiac m.
> MyoTrac 2 EMG m.
> N-Cat N-500 tonometric blood pressure m.
> Nicolet Elite Doppler m.
> onLine ABG m.
> OxiFirst fetal oxygen m.
> Polar Vantage XL heart rate m.
> Propaq Encore vital signs m.
> Pulse Pro heart rate m.

M

monitor (*continued*)
    radiation beam m.
    tonometric blood pressure m.
    m. unit
monitoring
    electrode m.
    periprocedural m.
    photoplethysmographic m.
    ultrasound m.
    video electroencephalography m.
    whole-body dose m.
monoamine oxidase
monoarticular
monochorionic
monochorionic-diamniotic twin pregnancy
monochorionic-monoamniotic
    m.-m. twin
    m.-m. twin pregnancy
monochromatic
    m. ray
    m. synchrotron
    m. synchrotron radiation
    m. x-ray
    m. x-ray beam
monochromatization
monoclonal
    m. antibody (MoAb, MoAb)
    m. antibody imaging agent
    m. gammopathy
monocrystalline iron oxide nanoparticle (MION)
monocuspid tilting-disc valve
monocyte colony-stimulating factor
monocytogenesis
    Listeria m.
monocytoid B-cell lymphoma
monodermal dermoid
monodisc
monodisperse iodinated macromolecular blood pool agent
monoenergetic radiation
Monoject hypodermic needle
monomalleolar fracture
monomelic bone lesion
monomer
    ionic m.
    nonionic triiodinated m.
mononuclear
    autologous bone marrow m. (ABMMN)
monophalangic great toe
monophasic
monophosphate
    carbovir m.
    cyclic adenosine m.
    cyclic guanosine m.
monopolar
    m. electrode
    m. radiofrequency electrocautery

Monopty
    M. core biopsy
    M. needle
monoradicular filling defect
Monorail
    Carotid-Wallstent M.
    M. Wallstent self-expanding stent
monorchia (*var. of* monorchism)
monorchism, monorchia
monosegmental image reconstruction
monosomy X
monostotic
    m. fibrous dysplasia
    m. Paget disease
monotherapy
monoventricle
monoxide
    carbon m.
    ^{11}C carbon m.
monozygotic twin
Monro
    M. aqueduct
    M. bursa
    foramen of M.
    M. obstruction
Monroe-Kellie doctrine
mons pubis
Monte
    M. Carlo calculation
    M. Carlo method
    M. Carlo modeling
    M. Carlo photon transport (MCPT)
    M. Carlo photon transport simulation
    M. Carlo technique
Monteggia
    M. dislocation
    M. fracture
    M. fracture-dislocation
    M. lesion
Montercaux fracture
Montgomery gland
Moore fracture
morcellation, morcellement
morcellator
    Diva laparoscopic m.
morcellement (*var. of* morcellation)
morcellized bone
Morgagni
    M. appendix
    column of M.
    M. crypt
    M. foramen
    M. hernia
    M. hydatid
    hyperostosis of M.
    M. lacuna

M. nodule
sinus of M.
M. syndrome
tubercle of M.
M. ventricle
Morgagni-Adams-Stokes syndrome
morgagnian cyst
Morison pouch
morphine-augmented study
morphine sulfate scintigraphy
morphologic, morphological
 m. and physiologic image
  coregistration
 m. correlation
 m. criterion
 m. filtering
 m. growth
 m. imaging
 m. left ventricle
 m. MRI
morphological (*var. of* morphologic)
morphologically normal
morphology
 disc m.
 enhancement m.
 joint m.
 ovarian m.
 residuum m.
 spine m.
morphometric
 m. measurement
 m. x-ray absorptiometry
morphometry
 MRI m.
 pelvic m.
Morquio
 M. sign
 M. syndrome
Morquio-Brailsford syndrome
morrhuate
 sodium m.
Morris point
mortality rate ratio
mortise
 ankle m.
 ball-and-socket ankle m.
 cuneiform m.
 diaphysial cortical m.
 m. joint
 m. of bone
 m. projection
 m. radiograph
 m. view
Morton
 M. neuroma
 M. plane
 M. toe
morula
morula-like epithelial cell

MOS
 metal oxide semiconductor
  MOS capacitor
mosaic
 m. artifact
 m. attenuation pattern
 m. detector configuration
 m. duodenal mucosal pattern
 m. jet signal
 m. oligemia
 m. pattern of lung attenuation
 m. perfusion
Moschcowitz test
MOSFET
 metal oxide semiconductor field effect
 transistor
Mossbauer spectrometer
Mosse syndrome
Moss gastrostomy tube
mossy fiber
Motarjeme catheter
moth-eaten
 m.-e. appearance
 m.-e. bone destruction
 m.-e. pattern
motile leukocyte
motility
 antroduodenal m.
 colonic m.
 m. disorder
 esophageal m.
 ileal m.
 jejunal m.
 m. of Golden
 small bowel m.
 m. study
motion
 akinetic segmental wall m.
 anterior wall m.
 apical wall m.
 m. artifact
 m. artifact suppression technique
  (MAST)
 m. averaging
 m. blur
 bowel m.
 brisk wall m.
 brownian water m.
 cardiac wall m.
 catheter tip m.
 chest wall paradoxic m.
 CSF oscillatory m.
 cusp m.
 m. degradation
 discernible venous m.
 dyskinetic segmental wall m.
 forceful parasternal m.
 m. gating
 heaving precordial m.

M

motion (*continued*)
    hyperkinetic segmental wall m.
    hypokinetic segmental wall m.
    incoherent m.
    inferior wall m.
    intravoxel coherent m.
    intravoxel incoherent m. (IVIM)
    isotropic m.
    leaflet m.
    left ventricular function wall m.
    left ventricular regional wall m.
    limitation of joint m.
    linear accelerator isocenter m.
    mitral valve systolic anterior m.
    m. mode (M-mode)
    nonoscillatory m.
    paradoxic leaflet m.
    paradoxic septal m.
    parasternal m.
    patient m.
    m. pattern
    phantom simulating cardiac m.
    photoreceptor m.
    posterior wall m.
    posterolateral wall m.
    precessional m.
    random m.
    rapid oscillatory m.
    regional hypokinetic wall m.
    respiratory m.
    rocking precordial m.
    rotational m.
    scapulothoracic m.
    segmental wall m.
    septal wall m.
    stationary zero-order m.
    sustained anterior parasternal m.
    swirling m.
    systolic anterior m. (SAM)
    through-slice m.
    time m. (TM)
    translational m.
    trifid precordial m.
    m. unsharpness
    venous m.
    ventricular wall m.
    vibratory m.
    visible anterior m.
    wall m.
    within-view m.
motional narrowing
motion-compensating format converter
motion-compensation gradient pulse
motion-free
    m.-f. imaging
    m.-f. positioning
motion-induced phase shift
motion-insensitive
    fast inversion-recovery m.-i. (FIRM)

motion-nulling gradient
motion-related blurring
motion-sensitive spin-echo sequence
    mechanical wave
motion-triggered cine kinematic MR image
motoneuron, motor neuron
motor
    m. alexia
    m. area
    m. branch
    m. cortex
    m. impairment
    m. neuron
    m. nucleus
    programmable stepper m.
    m. reinnervation
    m. root
    m. test meal
    m. tract
    m. urge incontinence
    m. vehicle injury
    versive m.
motorcyclist's knee
MOTSA
    multiple overlapping thin-slab
    acquisition
Mott body
mottle
    photon m.
    quantum m.
    radiographic m.
mottled
    m. appearance
    m. calcification
    m. density
    m. distribution
    m. echotexture
    m. gas collection
    m. gray lung
    m. hepatic uptake
    m. infiltrate
    m. liver uptake
    m. pattern
    m. radioactivity
    m. thickening
mottling
    diffuse m.
    m. of renal parenchyma
Mouchet fracture
mound
    infraumbilical m.
Mounier-Kuhn syndrome
Mountain View transducer
Mourits criterion
mouse, *pl.* **mice**
    peritoneal m.
mouse-ear
    m.-e. appearance
    m.-e. erosion

mouth
    tapir m.
mouthpiece
    E-Z-Guar m.
movable, moveable
    m. core guidewire
    m. heart
    m. kidney
    m. vertebra
moveable (*var. of* movable)
movement
    arcuate m.
    m. artifact
    bowel m.
    choreiform m.
    fetal m.
    fetal breathing m. (FBM)
    fiducial m.
    m. pattern
    pendulum m.
    propulsive m.
    spontaneous fetal m.
    systolic anterior m.
    table m.
movement-related cortical potential
mover
    smooth m.
moving
    m. bed infusion tracking
        MRA
    m. platform posturography
    m. slice velocity mapping
    m. slot radiography
    m. table technique
    m. tabletop MR imaging
moyamoya
    m. disease
    m. syndrome
    m. vascularity
Moyer line
Moynahan syndrome
MP
    magnetization-prepared
        MP inversion pulse
MPA
    main pulmonary artery
MPAP
    mean pulmonary artery pressure
    multipurpose access port
MPCh
    medial posterior choroidal
MPCP
    mean pulmonary capillary
        pressure
MPD
    main pancreatic duct
    main papillary duct
    matched peripheral dose
    maximum permissible dose

methylene diphosphonate
    minimal port diameter
    multiplanar display
MPGR
    multiplanar gradient recall
        MPGR technique
MPHR
    maximum predicted heart rate
MPI
    myocardial perfusion imaging
MPNST
    malignant peripheral nerve sheath
        tumor
mPower PET scanner
MPPS
    modality performed procedure step
MPPv
    main portal vein peak velocity
MPR
    multiplanar reformatting
        MPR view
MP-RAGE
    magnetization-prepared rapid acquisition
        gradient echo
        MP-RAGE protocol
        MP-RAGE technique
MP-RAGE-WE
    magnetization-prepared rapid gradient
        echo-water excitation
mps
    meters per second
MPS
    mucolipidosis
    mucopolysaccharidosis
    MPS (type I-IV)
MPVA
    metatarsus primus varus angle
MPVR
    multiplanar volume reformation
MQSA
    Mammography Quality Standards Act
MR
    magnetic resonance
    mitral regurgitation
        MR arthrography
        BP MR
        MR catheter imaging and
            spectroscopy system scanner
        chemical-selective fat-saturation
            MR
        MR colonographic technique
        MR colonography
        combined multisection
            diffuse-weighted and
            hemodynamically weighted
            echo-planar MR
        continuous arterial spin-labeling
            perfusion MR
        contrast-enhanced MR

M

MR (*continued*)
  MR coronary ateriography
  MR discriminator of osseous
    metastasis
  echo FLASH MR
  MR echo-planar imaging
  MR enteroclysis imaging
  MR flow quantification study
  MR hydrography
  MR imaging-guided endovascular
    device tracking
  lipid-sensitive MR
  MR lymphography
  oxygenation-sensitive functional MR
  MR proton spectroscopy
  renal artery stenosis screening MR
  MR SmartPrep
  MR spectroscopy data
  1st-pass myocardial perfusion MR
  MR velocity mapping

MRA
  magnetic resonance angiography
    body coil-based contrast-enchanced
      MRA
    bolus-chase stepping-table 3D
      MRA
    contrast-enhanced MRA
    3D MRA
    MRA imaging
    inflow MRA
    moving bed infusion tracking MRA
    multiphase MRA
    phase-contrast MRA (PC-MRA)
    stepping-table MRA
    time-resolved CE MRA
    ultrafast contrast-enhanced MRA
    MRA using 3D k-space reordering
    whole-body MRA

mrad
  millirad

MRC
  magnetic resonance cholangiogram

MR-compatible
  MR-c. incubator
  MR-c. power injector
  MR-c. ventilator

MRCP
  magnetic resonance
    cholangiopancreatography
    breath-hold MRCP
    kinematic MRCP
    mangafodipir-enhanced MRCP
    secretin-enhanced dynamic MRCP
    MRCP using HASTE with
      phased-array coil

MRDSA
  magnetic resonance digital subtraction
    angiography
    2D MRDSA

MRE
  magnetic resonance elastography
mrem
  millirem
MRF
  midbrain reticular formation
MR-guided
  MR-g. focused ultrasound surgery
  MR-g. laser-induced thermotherapy
  MR-g. lumbar sympathicolysis
MRI
  magnetic resonance imaging
    A-FAIR MRI
    black blood coronary arterial wall
      MRI
    body-coil MRI
    BOLD contrast functional MRI
    breath-hold contrast-enhanced
      MRI
    cardiac MRI
    catheter-based interventional MRI
    chondroitin sulfate iron
      colloid-enhanced MRI
    contrast-enhanced MRI
    coregistered MRI
    coronal FLAIR MRI
    MRI CSF flow study
    diffusion MRI
    diffusion-tensor MRI
    digital reformatting knee MRI
    double-dose delayed-contrast MRI
    dual-echo chemical shift
      gradient-echo MRI
    dynamic contrast MRI
    dynamic contrast-enhanced MRI
    electrocardiogram-gated MRI
    endoluminal MRI
    Excelart short-bore MRI
    extremity MRI (E-MRI)
    functional MRI
    Gd-DTPA-enhanced turbo FLASH
      MRI
    gradient subsystem in MRI
    HASTE MRI
    high-resolution magnetic resonance
      imaging (HR-MRI)
    intradiscal administration of
      gadolinium followed by MRI
    intravascular MRI
    intravenously enhanced MRI
    in utero MRI
    iPlan BOLD MRI
    laser-polarized helium MRI
    low field MRI
    magnetoacoustic MRI
    MRI mapping
    MnDPDP-enhanced MRI
    morphologic MRI
    MRI morphometry

multinuclear MRI
multiplanar MRI
nonaccelerated MRI
nonproton MRI
Opart MRI
open MRI
opposed-phase MRI
OrthOne 1-tesla extremity MRI
oxygen-enhanced MRI
parallel MRI
perfusion MRI
perfusion-weighted MRI
phase-contrast cine MRI
phased-array MRI
MRI prescan
MRI probehead
Propeller MRI
proton density-weighted MRI
MRI pulse sequence
MRI segmentation
selective partial inversion-recovery
  MRI
SENSE MRI
MRI severity scale score
subtraction ictal SPECT coregistered
  to MRI (SISCOM)
susceptibility contrast-weighted
  MRI
3T MRI
target-specific MRI
T1, T2 quantitative MRI
MRI thermometry
ultrafast MRI
vagus nerve stimulation-synchronized
  blood oxygen level-dependent
  functional MRI
velocity-encoded cine MRI
MRI-compatible electrode
MRI-guided
  MRI-g. breast biopsy
  MRI-g. focused ultrasound
    transducer
  MRI-g. laser-induced interstitial
    imaging
  MRI-g. laser-induced interstitial
    thermotherapy
  MRI-g. laser thermal ablation
  MRI-g. LTA
  MRI-g. periradicular nerve root
    infiltration therapy
  MRI-g. wire localization
MRL
  magnetic resonance lymphangiography
MRM
  magnetic resonance mammography
MRN
  magnetic resonance neurography
MRP
  magnetic resonance pancreatography

MRS
  magnetic resonance spectroscopy
    proton MRS
    slice-point MRS
MRSI
  magnetic resonance spectroscopic
    imaging
MRT
  magnetic resonance tomography
**MR-trackable intramyocardial injection
catheter**
MRU
  magnetic resonance urography
  molecular recognition unit
    ThromboScan MRU
MRUI
  magnetic resonance user interface
    MRUI software
MRV
  magnetic resonance venogram
  magnetic resonance venography
MS
  mitral stenosis
  multiple sclerosis
MSA
  multiple-system atrophy
    MSA syndrome
MSAD
  maximum short-axis diameter
  multiple-scan average dose
3M scanner
MS-325 contrast agent
MSCT
  multislice spiral CT
    aortic valve calcium quantification
      with MSCT
    MSCT technique
MSCTA
  multislice computed tomographic
    angiography
MSCV
  multislice cardiovolume
MSD
  mean sac diameter
  midsagittal diameter
MSDI
  multigated spectral Doppler imaging
    simultaneous MSDI
msec
  millisecond
M1-segment aneurysm
mSENSE
  modified SENSE
MS-EPI
  multishot echo-planar imaging
M-shaped
  M-s. mitral valve pattern
  M-s. pattern of mitral
    valve

M

MSI
   magnetic source imaging
   microsatellite instability
     3D MSI
MSK
   musculoskeletal
     MSK radiology
MSPv
   midshunt peak velocity
^{87m}Sr
   strontium 87m
MT
   magnetization transfer
   metatarsal
     half-dose enhanced MRI with MT
     MT prepulse
     MT saturation
     triple-dose gadolinium-enhanced MR imaging without MT
^{99m}Tc, Tc-99m
   technetium 99m
     ^{99m}Tc aggregated albumin imaging agent
     ^{99m}Tc albumin colloid imaging agent
     ^{99m}Tc albumin microsphere imaging agent
     ^{99m}Tc biciromab imaging agent
     ^{99m}Tc bicisate imaging agent
     ^{99m}Tc Ceretec
     ^{99m}Tc Ceretec bind
     ^{99m}Tc ciprofloxacin
     ^{99m}Tc depreotide
     ^{99m}Tc depreotide scintigraphy
     ^{99m}Tc dimer captosuccinic acid imaging agent
     ^{99m}Tc disofenin imaging agent
     ^{99m}TcDMSA
     ^{99m}TcECD
     ^{99m}Tc ethyl cysteinate dimer
     ^{99m}Tc exametazime imaging agent
     ^{99m}Tc furifosmin imaging agent
     ^{99m}Tc galactosyl human serum albumin imaging agent
     ^{99m}Tc glucarate imaging agent
     ^{99m}Tc gluceptate imaging agent
     ^{99m}Tc glucoheptanoate
     ^{99m}Tc glucoheptanoate scintimammography
     ^{99m}Tc GSA imaging agent
     ^{99m}Tc HIG scintigraphy
     ^{99m}TcHMPAO
     ^{99m}Tc HMPAO hyperfixation
     ^{99m}Tc HMPAO-labeled leukocyte total-body scan
     ^{99m}Tc HMPAO uptake
     ^{99m}TcHSA

     ^{99m}Tc human polyclonal immunoglobulin G scintigraphy
     ^{99m}Tc human serum albumin imaging agent
     ^{99m}Tc human serum albumin scintigraphy
     ^{99m}Tc L-ethyl cysteinate dimer
     ^{99m}Tc lidofenin imaging agent
     ^{99m}TcMAA
     ^{99m}Tc MAA rhinoscintigraphy
     ^{99m}Tc MDP skeletal scintigram
     ^{99m}Tc MDP uptake
     ^{99m}Tc mebrofenin imaging agent
     ^{99m}Tc medronate imaging agent
     ^{99m}Tc mertiatide imaging agent
     ^{99m}Tc MIBI radiopharmaceutical
     ^{99m}Tc microaggregated albumin imaging agent
     ^{99m}Tc Myoview myocardial perfusion imaging
     ^{99m}Tc oxidronate imaging agent
     ^{99m}Tc pentetate calcium trisodium imaging agent
     ^{99m}Tc pentetate sodium imaging agent
     ^{99m}Tc pertechnetate thyroid
     ^{99m}Tc phosphate
     ^{99m}Tc polyphosphate compound radiopharmaceutical
     ^{99m}Tc polyphosphate imaging agent
     ^{99m}Tc pyrophosphate
     ^{99m}Tc pyrophosphate imaging agent
     ^{99m}Tc red blood cell SPECT
     ^{99m}Tc sestamibi
     ^{99m}Tc sestamibi imaging agent
     ^{99m}Tc sodium pertechnetate imaging agent
     ^{99m}Tc succimer imaging agent
     ^{99m}Tc sulfur colloid (^{99m}Tc SC)
     ^{99m}Tc sulfur colloid imaging agent
     ^{99m}Tc teboroxime imaging agent
     ^{99m}Tc tetrofosmin imaging agent
     ^{99m}Tc WBC scan
MTC
   magnetization transfer contrast
^{99m}Tc-bis-dimethylphosphonoethane
^{99m}Tc-depreotide
^{99m}Tc-DMSA
   technetium 99m dimercaptosuccinic acid
     ^{99m}Tc-DMSA scanning
     ^{99m}Tc-DMSA scintigraphy
MTC-Dox-Spheres
^{99m}Tc-DTPA
   technetium 99m diethylenetriamine pentaacetic acid

^{99m}Tc-ECD
 technetium 99m ethyl cysteinate dimer
  ^{99m}Tc-ECD radiopharmaceutical
^{99m}Tc-glucoheptanate
^{99m}Tc-hexamethylpropyleneamine oxime
^{99m}Tc-HMPAO
 technetium 99m
  hexamethylpropyleneamine oxime
  ^{99m}Tc-HMPAO cerebral perfusion
   SPECT imaging
  ^{99m}Tc-HMPAO radiopharmaceutical
  ^{99m}Tc-HMPAO radiotracer
  ^{99m}Tc-HMPAOSPECT
^{99m}Tc-iminodiacetic acid derivative radiopharmaceutical
^{99m}Tc-labeled
 technetium-99m-labeled
  ^{99m}Tc-labeled anti-E-selectin Fab
   fragment
  ^{99m}Tc-labeled antigranulocyte
   antibody
  ^{99m}Tc-labeled cerebral perfusion
   imaging agent
  ^{99m}Tc-labeled denatured autologous
   RBC imaging
  ^{99m}Tc-labeled iminodiacetic acid
  ^{99m}Tc-labeled ligand
  ^{99m}Tc-labeled macroaggregated
   albumin scan
  ^{99m}Tc-labeled octreotide
  ^{99m}Tc-labeled phosphate analogue
  ^{99m}Tc-labeledRBC
  ^{99m}Tc-labeled somatostatin
  ^{99m}Tc-labeledWBC
  ^{99m}Tc-labeled white blood cell
   scintigraphy
^{99m}Tc-MAG3
 technetium 99m mercapto acetyl
  triglycine
  ^{99m}Tc-MAG3 radiopharmaceutical
^{99m}Tc-methoxyisobutylisonitrile scintigraphy
^{99m}Tc-N-NOEt neutral myocardial perfusion imaging agent
^{99m}Tc-PYP
 technetium 99m pyrophosphate
  ^{99m}Tc-PYP scintigraphy
99mTc-RBC
 technetium 99m red blood cell
  denatured ^{99m}Tc-RBC
  heat-damaged ^{99m}Tc-RBC
^{99m}Tc-tagged RBC
MTD
 maximum tolerated dose
MTE
 main timing event
 mesenteric thromboembolism

MTF
 modulation transfer function
MTJ
 midtarsal joint
MTP
 metatarsophalangeal
  MTP joint
  semiflexed MTP
MTR
 magnetization transfer ratio
MTSA
 multiple thin-slab acquisition
MTT
 mean transit time
m-tyrosine
mu
 m. heavy-chain disease
 m. rhythm
mucicarmine stain
mucin-hypersecreting carcinoma
mucinous
 m. adenocarcinoma
 m. adenoma
 m. breast carcinoma
 m. bronchoalveolar carcinoma
 m. bronchogram
 m. cyst
 m. cyst adenocarcinoma
 m. cystadenoma
 m. degeneration
 m. ductal ectasia of pancreas
 m. ductectatic tumor of pancreas
 m. lesion
 m. ovarian cystadenocarcinoma
 m. ovarian tumor
 m. pancreatic cystic neoplasia
mucin-producing
 m.-p. adenocarcinoma
 m.-p. carcinoma
muckiness of pericolonic fat
mucocele
 appendix m.
 breast m.
 bronchial m.
 erosive m.
 frontal sinus m.
 frontoethmoidal m.
 orbital m.
 paranasal sinus m.
mucociliary transport
mucocutaneous
 m. junction
 m. lymph node syndrome (MCLS)
mucoepidermoid
 m. carcinoma
 m. carcinoma parotitis
mucoid
 m. degeneration of umbilical cord

mucoid (*continued*)
    m. impaction
    m. impaction of bronchus
    m. plugging of airway
    m. umbilical cord degeneration
mucolipidoses (*pl. of* mucolipidosis)
mucolipidosis (MPS), *pl.* **mucolipidoses**
    m. IV
mucopolysaccharidoses (*pl. of*
  mucopolysaccharidosis)
mucopolysaccharidosis (MPS), *pl.*
  mucopolysaccharidoses
mucopyocele
mucosa, *pl.* **mucosae**
    bowel m.
    bronchial m.
    buccal m.
    burned-out m.
    cobblestone m.
    colorectal m.
    ectopic gastric m.
    endocervical m.
    friable m.
    frothy colonic m.
    gastric m.
    isoeffective bronchial m.
    muscularis mucosae
    outpocketing of m.
    polypoid m.
    prolapsed antral m.
    prolapsed gastric m.
    sloughed m.
    unstable m.
mucosa-associated
    m.-a. lymphoid tissue (MALT)
    m.-a. lymphoid tissue lymphoma
    (MALToma)
mucosae (*pl. of* mucosa)
mucosal
    m. abnormality
    m. bridge
    m. crinkling
    m. destruction
    m. esophageal nodule
    m. esophageal tumor
    m. fold
    m. fold pattern
    m. ganglioneurofibromatosis
    m. gland
    m. hyperplasia
    m. inflammation
    m. island
    m. lesion
    m. lining
    m. mass collecting system
    m. necrosis
    m. prolapse syndrome
    m. relief radiography
    m. ring

    m. space
    m. suspensory ligament
    m. thickening
    m. ulcer
mucosa-sparing block
mucosum
    ligamentum m.
mucous
    m. bronchogram
    m. carcinoma
    m. cell hyperplasia
    m. degeneration
    m. fistula
    m. hypersecretion
    m. lake
    m. lake of stomach
    m. membrane
    m. membrane hyperemia
    m. plug
    m. plugging
    m. polyp
    m. pseudomass
    m. retention cyst
mucus-filled small airway
mud
    biliary m.
MUGA
    multigated acquisition
    multiple gated acquisitions
    MUGA cardiac blood pool
     imaging
    MUGA scan
    1st-pass MUGA
Muir-Torre syndrome
mulberry
    m. calculus
    m. eye lesion
    m. gallstone
    m. ovary
mulberry-like mass
mulberry-type
    m.-t. calcification
    m.-t. classification
Mulder sign
Müller
    M. canal
    M. esophageal varices maneuver
    M. fiber
    M. humerus fracture
     classification
    M. muscle
    M. sign
    M. test
    M. tray
müllerian
    m. duct
    m. duct anomaly
    m. duct cyst
    m. mucinous borderline tumor

multangular
    m. bone
    m. ridge fracture
multiaccess catheter
multiarc LINAC radiosurgery
multiaxial classification
multibreath washout study
multicentric
    m. angiofollicular lymph node
    m. basal cell carcinoma
    m. carcinoid tumor
    m. Castleman disease (MCD)
    m. fibromatosis
    m. germinoma
    m. glioblastoma
    m. invasive lobular carcinoma
    m. lytic lesion
    m. malignant glioma
    m. meningioma
    m. osteosarcoma
    m. primary breast cancer
    m. reticulohistiocytosis
multicentricity
multichannel
    m. analyzer (MCA)
    m. intraluminal impedance (MII)
    m. pelvic phased-array coil
    m. RF system
multicoil
    phased-array m.
multicolor flow cytometry
multicompartment clearance
multicoupled loop-gap resonator
multicrystal
    m. BGO ring system
    m. gamma camera
multicystic
    m. acoustic neuroma
    m. dysgenetic kidney
    m. dysplasia
    m. dysplastic kidney (MCDK)
    m. encephalomalacia
    m. kidney (MCK)
multidetector
    m. computed tomography
    m. computed tomography urography
    (MDCTU)
    m. CT (MDCT)
    m. CTA
    m. CT scanner
    m. helical CT
    m. helical scanner
    m. helical scanning
    m. system
multidetector-row
    m.-r. CT
    m.-r. CT scan
    m.-r. helical computed tomography
multidimensional adaptive filtering

MultiDop P, T, X transcranial Doppler device
multidose vial
multidrug-resistant
    m.-r. protein
    m.-r. tuberculosis
multiecho
    m. axial image
    m. coronal image
    m. imaging
    m. multiplane (MEMP)
    preinversion m.
    m. sequence
    standard m.
multielectrode catheter
multielemental neutron activation analysis
multiexponential relaxation
multifactorial etiology
multifield beam
multifocal
    m. aggressive infiltrate
    m. anaplastic astrocytoma
    m. area of hyperintensity
    m. autonomic adenoma
    m. brain tumor
    m. breast carcinoma
    m. enhancing brain lesion
    m. fibrosclerosis
    m. glioblastoma multiforme
    m. hemorrhage
    m. infarct
    m. invasive lobular carcinoma
    m. leukoencephalopathy
    m. lymphoma
    m. nephroblastomatosis
    m. osteosarcoma
    m. papillary thyroid carcinoma
    m. residual focus
    m. short stenosis
    m. subperitoneal sclerosis
    m. systemic tuberculosis
    m. traumatic axonal injury
multifollicular ovary
multiformat camera
multiformatted imaging
multiforme
    glioblastoma m. (GBM)
    multifocal glioblastoma m.
multiform ventricular complex
multigated
    m. acquisition (MUGA)
    m. angiography
    m. Doppler
    m. pulsed Doppler flow system
    m. spectral Doppler analysis
    software
    m. spectral Doppler imaging
    (MSDI)

M

multigeometry (MG)
MultiHance
    M. contrast medium
    M. imaging agent
multihole collimator
multi-illuminant color correction
multiinfarct dementia
multiinterval
multilamellar periosteal reaction
multilaminar body
multileaf
    m. collimating system
    m. collimator (MLC)
multilevel fusion
multiline scanning technique
Multi-Link
    M.-L. Penta stent
    M.-L. Terra stent
multilobular
    m. cirrhosis
    m. configuration
multilobulated mass
multilocular
    m. cystic lesion
    m. cystic nephroma
    m. renal cyst
multiloculated mass
multilog effect
multimodal image fusion technique
multimodality
    m. imaging
    m. therapy
multimode imaging confocal optical
  microscope (MIMCOM)
multinodular, multinodulate
    m. goiter
    m. struma
    m. thyroid
multinodulate (*var. of* multinodular)
multinuclear MRI
Multi-Operatory Dentalaser (MOD)
multiorgan imaging
multiparametric color composite display
multiparticle cyclotron
multipartite
    m. fracture
    m. patella
multipennate muscle
multipharmaceutical chemoembolization
  solution
multiphase MRA
multiphase-multisection T2-weighted MR
  imaging
multiphasic
    m. contrast injection
    m. helical CT
    m. multislice MRI technique
    m. multislice spin-echo imaging
      technique

    m. perfusion computed tomography
    m. renal computerized tomography
multiplanar
    m. compression
    m. display (MPD)
    m. endorectal ultrasound
    m. gradient-echo software
    m. gradient recall (MPGR)
    m. gradient-recalled echo
    m. gradient refocus
    m. gradient refocused sequence
    m. mode
    m. MRI
    m. MR imaging
    phase-offset m. (POMP)
    phase-ordered m. (POMP)
    m. reconstruction
    m. reformatted radiographic and
      digitally reconstructed radiographic
      imaging
    m. reformatting (MPR)
    m. reformatting view
    m. scanning
    m. transducer
    m. transesophageal echocardiography
    m. volume reformation (MPVR)
    m. volume-reformatted image
multiplane
    m. dosage calculation
    multiecho m. (MEMP)
multiple
    m. accessory spleens
    m. aortopulmonary collateral arteries
      (MAPCA)
    m. averaging
    m. bile duct hamartomas
    m. blocks
    m. bull's-eye lesions of bowel
      wall
    m. chords
    m. colon filling defects
    m. concentric GI rings
    m. congenital anomalies (MCA)
    m. congenital fibromatosis
    m. cortical infarcts
    m. ectopic thyroid
    m. emboli
    m. enchondromatosis
    m. endocrine neoplasia (MEN)
    m. endocrine neoplasia syndrome
    m. epiphysial dysplasia
    m. fetuses
    m. fibroxanthomas
    m. focal lesions of spinal cord
    m. foci
    m. fractures
    m. gated acquisitions (MUGA)
    m. gated acquisition scans
    m. gated blood pool imaging

m. gated blood pool scans
m. gestations
m. idiopathic hemorrhagic sarcomas
m. intestinal neoplasia
m. isomorphous replacements (MIR)
m. line-scan imaging (MLSI)
m. loops of small bowel
m. lucent lung lesions
m. lung nodules
m. lytic bone lesions
m. mucosal neuromas syndrome
m. mural dilations
m. myeloma
m.'s of median
m. osteochondromatosis
m. osteolysis
m. osteosclerotic lesions
m. overlapping thin-slab acquisition (MOTSA)
m. parotid gland lesions
m. peripheral papillomas
m. planar gradient-recalled images
m. pleural densities
m. polyposis
m. polyps
m. pregnancies
m. pterygium syndrome
m. pulmonary calcifications
m. pulmonary cysts
m. pulmonary necrobiotic nodules
m. quantum coherence
m. recurrent inversion injuries
m. sclerosis (MS)
m. sclerotic osteosarcomas
m. sclerotic plaques
m. sensitive-point method
m. sensitive points
m. small bowel filling defects
m. small bowel stenoses
m. small bowel ulcers
m. spin echoes
m. stenotic lesions
m. stenotic lesions of small bowel
m. stones
m. symmetric lipomatosis
m. system atrophy syndrome
m. thin-slab acquisition (MTSA)
m. thin-walled lung cavities
m. thyroid cysts
m. traumas
m. vascular leiomyomas
multiple-beam interface spacing
multiple-coil array
multiple-echo
m.-e. imaging
m.-e. single shot
multiple-electrode probe system
multiple-exposure volumetric holography

multiple-gland disease
multiple-headed gamma camera
multiple-injection protocol
multiple-jointed
m.-j. digitizer
m.-j. digitizer scanner
multiple-lesion osteosclerosis
multiple-line
m.-l. scan (MLS)
m.-l. scanning method
multiple-organ failure
multiple-plane imaging
multiple-projection biplane angiography
multiple-sample clearance
multiple-scan average dose (MSAD)
multiple-sidehole
m.-s. infusion catheter
m.-s. infusion system
multiple-slice
m.-s. acquisition
m. s. imaging
multiple-suture synostosis
multiple-system atrophy (MSA)
multiplex
dysostosis m.
dysplasia epiphysialis m.
multiplexing
multiplying digital-to-analogue converter (MDAC)
multiply tuned coil
Multi-Pro biopsy needle
multipurpose
m. access port (MPAP)
m. catheter
multiray fracture
multireader E-MRI assessment
multirod collimator
multiscalar
multiscale image detail contrast amplification (Musica)
multisection
m. diffusion-weighted magnetic resonance imaging
m. gradient-echo echo-planar imaging
m. method
m. multirepetition acquisition
multisectional dose-volume histogram
multisegment
m. disease
m. reconstruction
multisegmental image reconstruction
multisensor
m. structured light-range digitizer
m. structured light-range digitizer scanner
multiseptate appearance
multiseptated gallbladder

M

multishot
>m. echo-planar imaging (MS-EPI)
>m. echo-shifted gradient-echo EPI sequence
>m. spin-echo/echo-planar imaging

multisideport infusion catheter

multislab magnetic resonance angiography

multislice
>m. acquisition
>m. cardiovolume (MSCV)
>m. computed tomographic angiography (MSCTA)
>m. CT
>m. CT scanner
>2D m.
>ECG-gated m.
>m. FLASH 2D
>m. flow-related enhancement
>m. full line scan
>m. modality
>m. mode
>m. modified KWE direct Fourier imaging
>m. spin-echo sequence
>m. spin-echo technique
>m. spiral computed tomography
>m. spiral CT (MSCT)
>m. spiral weighting
>m. 1st-pass myocardial perfusion imaging

multislit catheter

multispectral diffuse transillumination

multispin relaxation

Multistar
>M. angiographic unit
>M. Top Plus DSA system

multisweep
>high-resolution m. (HRMS)

multitargeted antifolate

multitime point imaging

multitracer
>m. imaging
>m. study

multivane intensity modulation compensator (MIMIC)

multivariant regressional analysis

multivoxel imaging

multiwire proportional chamber

multizone transmit-receive focus

mummy restraint

mural
>m. aneurysm
>m. arch
>m. architecture
>m. change
>m. clot
>m. CNS nodule
>m. defect

m. degeneration
m. dilation
m. endomyocardial fibrosis
m. fibrosing alveolitis
m. hematoma
m. infiltrate
m. kidney
m. leaflet of mitral valve
m. nodulation
m. pregnancy
m. stratification
m. thickening
m. thrombus
m. thrombus formation

mural-type vein of Galen malformation

murine Peyer patch

murmur

muscarinic receptor

muscle
>abductor digiti quinti m.
>abductor hallucis m.
>abductor pollicis brevis m.
>accessory m.
>adductor magnus m.
>Aeby m.
>Albinus m.
>anconeus m.
>anomalous m.
>anterior papillary m. (APM)
>antigravity m.
>m. artifact
>auricular m.
>axillary m.
>BBC m.'s
>2-bellied m.
>belly of m.
>biceps, brachialis, coracobrachialis m.'s
>biceps femoris m.
>bipennate m.
>Bochdalek m.
>Bovero m.
>Bowman m.
>brachioradialis m.
>Braune m.
>Brücke m.
>bulbocavernosus m.
>m. bulk
>cardiac m.
>Casser m.
>casserian m.
>cervical m.
>Chassaignac m.
>circular m.
>Coiter m.
>conal papillary m.
>cone of extraocular m.
>m. contracture
>Crampton m.

cricopharyngeus m.
dartos m.
deep m.
detrusor m.
digastric m.
dorsal m.
Dupré m.
Duverney m.
ECRB m.
ECRL m.
ECU m.
EDB m.
EDC m.
EDL m.
EDQ m.
EIP m.
EPB m.
EPL m.
extensor carpi radialis brevis m.
extensor carpi radialis longus m.
extensor carpi ulnaris m.
extensor digiti quinti m.
extensor digitorum brevis m.
extensor digitorum communis m.
extensor digitorum longus m.
extensor hallucis longus m.
extensor indicis m.
extensor pollicis brevis m.
extensor pollicis longus m.
external oblique m.
extraocular m.
extrinsic foot m.
fast-twitch m.
FDI m.
FDL m.
FDQB m.
FDS m.
m. fiber (type I, II)
m. fiber wasting
fibrosed m.
fixator m.
flexor carpi radialis m.
flexor digiti quinti brevis m.
flexor digitorum longus m.
flexor digitorum profundus m.
flexor digitorum superficialis m.
flexor hallucis brevis m.
Folius m.
frontotemporal m.
fused papillary m.
Gantzer m.
gastrocnemius m.
Gavard m.
genioglossus m.
gluteus maximus m.
Guthrie m.
Hilton m.
Horner m.
Houston m.

hyoglossus m.
hyperintense m.
m. hyperintensity
ileococcygeus m.
iliocostal m.
iliopsoas m.
m. infarct
infarcted heart m.
inferior gemellus m.
infraspinatus m.
innermost intercostal m.
intercostal m.
internal intercostal m.
interosseous m.
interspinal m.
intertransverse m.
intraauricular m.
intrinsic foot m.
m. irritability
ischiocavernosus m.
Klein m.
Lancisi m.
lateral pterygoid m.
lateral rectus m.
latissimus dorsi m.
left ventricular m.
lesser m.
levator m.
longitudinal m.
longus colli m.
Luschka m.
major m.
Marcacci m.
masseter m.
masticator m.
medial papillary m.
medial pterygoid m.
medial rectus m.
m. metastasis
middle m.
minor m.
Müller m.
multipennate m.
mylohyoid m.
myocardial m.
nonstriated m.
oblique m.
obturator internus m.
occipitofrontalis m.
Ochsner m.
Oddi m.
ODQ m.
Oehl m.
m. of deglutition
omohyoid m.
opponens digiti quinti m.
opposing m.'s
organic m.
m. ossification

M

muscle (*continued*)
    palatal m.
    papillary m.
    paralaryngeal m.
    paraspinal m.
    Passavant m.
    pectineal m.
    pectoralis major m.
    pectoralis minor m.
    peroneal m.
    peroneus quartus m.
    pharyngeal m.
    Phillips m.
    piriform m.
    piriformis m.
    plantaris m.
    platysma m.
    posterior papillary m. (PPM)
    postural m.
    Pozzi m.
    psoas m.
    pterygoid m.
    pterygomasseteric m.
    pubococcygeus m.
    pupillary constrictor m.
    pyloric m.
    quadrate m.
    quadriceps m.
    reactive disease of
      smooth m.
    m. recruitment pattern
    rectus m.
    Reisseisen m.
    retractor bulbi m.
    retronuchal m.
    rhomboideus major m.
    ribbon m.
    rider's m.
    Riolan m.
    rotator cuff m.
    Rouget m.
    round m.
    Ruysch m.
    sacrospinalis m.
    Santorini m.
    m. sarcoma
    sartorius m.
    scalenus anterior m.
    scalenus minimus m.
    Sebileau m.
    semimembranosus m.
    semispinal m.
    semitendinous m.
    septal papillary m.
    serratus anterior m.
    m. sheath
    short m.
    shoulder m.
    Sibson m.

    skeletal m.
    slow-twitch m.
    smooth m.
    Soemmerring m.
    soleus m.
    somatic m.
    m. spasm
    sphenomandibularis m.
    m. spindle
    spindle-shaped m.
    sternalis m.
    sternohyoid m.
    sternothyroid m.
    m. strain
    strap m.
    striated m.
    styloglossus m.
    stylohyoid m.
    subaortic m.
    subclavius m.
    subscapularis m.
    sucking m.
    superficial m.
    supinator m.
    supraspinatus m.
    synergic m.
    tailor's m.
    temporalis m.
    tendinous part of epicranius m.
    tensor veli palatini m.
    Theile m.
    thenar m.
    thigh m.
    m. tissue
    Tod m.
    Toynbee m.
    transversus abdominis m.
    trapezius m.
    Treitz m.
    triangular m.
    trigonal m.
    true back m.
    unipennate m.
    m. uptake
    Valsalva m.
    vascular smooth m.
    vastus medialis m.
    ventral m.
    vertical m.
    visceral m.
    vocal m.
    vocalis m.
    voluntary m.
    Wilson m.
    wrinkler m.
muscle-brain (MB)
muscle-crushing injury
muscle-eye-brain disease
muscle-fat interface

muscular
> m. atrioventricular septum
> m. branch
> m. bridge
> m. crus
> m. crus of diaphragm
> m. degeneration
> m. dystrophy
> m. hypertrophy
> m. insufficiency
> m. lesion
> m. ring esophagus
> m. slip
> m. subaortic stenosis
> m. tube
> m. twig
> m. ventricular septal defect

muscularis
> m. mucosae
> m. propria

musculature
> axial m.
> cervical m.
> longitudinal tenia m.
> paraspinous m.
> paravertebral m.
> scalene m.

musculi (*pl. of* musculus)
musculoaponeurotic
> m. fibroma
> m. fibromatosis

musculocutaneous sarcoidosis
musculofascial pedicle
musculophrenic
> m. artery
> m. branch
> m. vessel

musculoskeletal (MSK)
> m. imaging
> m. imaging study
> m. lesion
> m. radiography
> m. system
> m. tumor
> M. Tumor Society

musculotendinous
> m. cuff
> m. junction
> m. retraction
> m. unit

musculotendinous-osseous link
musculotubal canal
musculus, *pl.* **musculi**
> m. uvulae

mushroom
> m. appearance
> m. picker's disease
> m. shape
> m. worker's lung

mushroom-shaped mass
Musica
> multiscale image detail contrast amplification

Musset sign
mustard
> l-phenylalanine m. (L-PAM)
> nitrogen m.

MUSTPAC
> medical ultrasound 3-dimensional portable with advanced communication
> MUSTPAC ultrasound imaging

mutagenicity
mutant
mutation
> point m.
> reel-in m.

mutational dysostosis
mutilans
> arthritis m.

muzzle velocity
mV
> millivolt

MV
> megavolt

MVA
> mitral valve area

MVO
> maximum venous outflow
> mitral valve opening
> mitral valve orifice

MVP
> mitral valve prolapse

MVR
> mitral valve replacement

MVS
> mitral valve stenosis

MVV
> maximum voluntary ventilation

myasthenia gravis
mycalamide A
mycetoma
> m. formation
> kidney m.

mycobacteria (*pl. of* Mycobacterium)
Mycobacterium, *pl.* **mycobacteria**
> *M. avium-intracellulare* (MAI)
> nontuberculous *M.*

mycophenolic acid
mycoplasma
> m. pneumonia
> m. pneumonitis

mycosis
mycotic
> m. aortic aneurysm
> m. brain aneurysm
> m. intracranial aneurysm
> m. lung infection

M

mycotic (*continued*)
   m. plaque
   m. pneumonia
   m. sinusitis
   m. thrombus
myelencephalon
myelin
   m. ball
   m. ball formation
   m. base protein
   m. edema
   m. sheath
myelination, myelinization
   delayed m.
   nerve fiber m.
   optic pathway m.
myelinization (*var. of* myelination)
myelinolysis
   central pontile m.
   extrapontine m.
   pontile m.
myelinopathy
   spongiform m.
   vacuolating m.
myelitis
   acute transverse m.
   radiation m.
   subacute necrotizing m.
   transverse m.
myeloblastoma
myelocele
myelocisternoencephalography
myelo-CT
myelocystocele
myelocystography
myelodysplasia
myelodysplastic syndrome (MDS)
myelodyspoiesis
myelofibrosis
   acute m.
   idiopathic m.
   m. osteosclerosis
myelogenesis
myelogram
   cervical m.
   lumbar m.
myelographic imaging agent
myelography
   air m.
   cervical m.
   complete m.
   computed m.
   computed tomographic metrizamide
    m. (CTMM)
   computer-assisted m. (CAM)
   CT m.
   extraarachnoid m.
   Hypaque m.
   m. imaging

   lumbar m.
   lumbosacral m.
   magnetic resonance m.
   metrizamide m.
   oil m.
   opaque m.
   oxygen m.
   Pantopaque m.
   positive contrast m.
   thoracic m.
   water-soluble m.
myeloid
   m. hyperplasia
   m. malignancy
   m. metaphysis
myelolipoma
   adrenal m.
   extraadrenal m.
myeloma
   amyloidosis of multiple m.
   endothelial m.
   indolent m.
   localized m.
   M-band m.
   multiple m.
   nonsecretory multiple m.
   plasmablastic m.
   sclerosing m.
   solitary bone m.
   spinal plasma cell m.
myelomalacia
   cystic m.
myelomatosis
   nonsecretory m.
myelomeningocele
myelopathy
   acute posttraumatic m.
   carcinomatous m.
   cervical spondylotic m. (CSM)
   cystic m.
   delayed posttraumatic m.
   necrotizing m.
   paracarcinomatous m.
   posttraumatic ascending m.
   posttraumatic cystic m.
   progressive posttraumatic m.
   radiation m.
   spondylotic m.
   subacute necrotizing m.
myelophthisic splenomegaly
myeloproliferative disorder
myeloschisis
myelosclerosis
myelosuppression
myelotomography
myelotoxicity
myenteric
   m. plexus
   m. plexus of Auerbach

Myerson sign
mylohyoid
    m. muscle
    m. ridge
myoblastoma
    granular breast cell m.
    granular lung cell m.
    granular sella cell m.
myocardia (*pl. of* myocardium)
myocardial
    m. band
    m. blood flow (MBF)
    m. blush
    m. bridge
    m. calcification
    m. cellular degeneration
    m. cellular hypertrophy
    m. centroid
    m. contractile function
    m. contractility
    m. contracture
    m. contrast appearance time
      (MCAT)
    m. contrast echocardiography
      (MCE)
    m. contusion
    m. depression
    m. dilation
    m. disarray
    m. fiber
    m. fibrous degeneration
    m. function assessment
    m. hibernation
    m. I-123 MIBG imaging
    m. incompetence
    m. infarct (MI)
    m. infarct imaging
    m. infarct recovery index
    m. infiltration
    m. inflammation
    m. insufficiency
    m. insult
    m. irritability
    m. ischemia
    m. jeopardy index
    m. mass
    m. metabolism
    m. muscle
    m. necrosis
    m. O_2 demand index
    m. oxygen consumption
    m. perfusion
    m. perfusion echocardiography
    m. perfusion imaging (MPI)
    m. perfusion imaging Q complex
    m. perfusion reserve
    m. perfusion scan
    m. perfusion scintigraphy
    m. perfusion tomography

    m. preservation
    m. protection
    m. recovery
    m. reperfusion injury
    m. revascularization
    m. rupture
    m. scar
    m. stunning
    m. tagging
    m. texture analysis
    m. thallium imaging
    m. thickening
    m. tissue viability
    m. twist
    m. uptake
    m. wall
    m. work
myocardiopathy
myocarditis
    fibroid m.
    fragmentation m.
myocardium, *pl.* **myocardia**
    asynergic m.
    calcification of m.
    collateral-dependent m.
    dilated m.
    hibernating m.
    hypertrophied m.
    hypokinetic m.
    infarcted m.
    inferoapical aspect of m.
    ischemic reperfused m.
    ischemic viable m.
    jeopardized m.
    necrotic m.
    noninfarcted m.
    nonperfused m.
    perfused m.
    recovery period of m.
    refractory period of m.
    reperfused m.
    rupture of m.
    salvage of m.
    senile m.
    sparkling appearance of m.
    stunned m.
    thinned m.
    ventricular m.
    viable m.
myocardium-to-abdomen count ratio
myoclonic epilepsy and ragged red
  fibers (MERRF)
myocutaneous
    transverse rectus abdominis m.
      (TRAM)
myocyte
    cardiac m.
    m. membrane purinoceptor
myoepithelial sialadenitis

M

myoepithelioma
  malignant m.
myofascial
  m. disruption
  m. pain-dysfunction
  syndrome
myofibrillar disintegration
myofibril volume fraction
myofibroblastoma
  giant m.
  intranodal m.
myofibrohistiocytic proliferation
myofibromatosis
  infantile m.
myogenesis
myoid hamartoma
myoinositol-creatine ratio (Mi/Cr)
myointimal
  m. hyperplasia
  m. proliferation
myoma
  complicated m.
  intramural m.
  pedunculated subserous m.
  serosal m.
  submucous m.
  uncomplicated m.
  uterine m.
myometrial
  m. contraction
  m. septum
myometrium
  uterine m.
myonecrosis
  calcific m.
myoneural junction
myopathy
  alcoholic m.
  carcinomatous m.
  statin-induced m.
  systemic sclerosis-related m.
  uremic m.
myosarcoma
Myoscint
  M. imaging
  M. imaging agent
MyoSight imaging system
myosin
  ^{111}In murine monoclonal antibody
  Fab to m.
myosis
  endolymphatic stromal m.
myositis
  brucellar m.

eye m.
granulomatous m.
m. ossificans circumscripta
m. ossificans progressiva
m. ossificans traumatica
viral m.
myostatic contracture
myotendinous
  m. junction
  m. junction rupture
  m. strain
Myotherm XP cardioplegia delivery system
MyoTrac 2 EMG monitor
myotube
Myoview imaging agent
myxadenoma
myxedema
  m. of heart
  pretibial m.
myxoglobulosis
myxoid
  m. cyst
  m. degenerative change
  m. extraskeletal chondrosarcoma
  m. liposarcoma
  m. malignant fibrous histiocytoma
  m. MFH
myxolipoma
myxoma
  atrial m.
  biatrial m.
  cardiac m.
  complex m.
  familial m.
  heart m.
  intramuscular m.
  left atrial m.
  odontogenic m.
  m. of heart
  pedunculated uterine m.
  vascular m.
  ventricular m.
myxomatodes
  fibroma m.
myxomatous
  m. liposarcoma
  m. proliferation
  m. tumor
  m. valve leaflet
myxomembranous colitis
myxopapillary ependymoma
MZL
  marginal zone lymphoma

N
  nitrogen
^{13}N, N-13
  nitrogen 13
    ^{13}N ammonia radioactive
      tracer
    ^{13}N ammonia uptake
^{14}N, N-14
  nitrogen 14
^{15}N, N-15
  nitrogen 15
^{23}Na, Na-23
  sodium 23
    ^{23}Na magnetic resonance imaging
    ^{23}Na MR imaging with short echo
      time
^{24}Na, Na-24
  sodium 24
NAA
  N-acetyl aspartate
nabothian
  n. cyst
  n. follicle
***N*-acetyl aspartate (NAA)**
Naclerio
  V-sign of N.
nadir
  untransformed n.
naevus (*var. of* nevus)
Naffziger sign
Nägele
  N. obliquity
  N. pelvis
NaI
  sodium iodide
  NaI detector
nail
  n. bed lesion
  body of n.
  Gamma n.
  intramedullary n.
  Jewett n.
  orthopaedic n.
  n. plate
  n. plate avulsion
  n. plate device
  Smith-Petersen n.
  spoon-shaped n.
  triflanged n.
  Zickel supracondylar n.
nailing
  elastic stable intramedullary n.
    (ESIN)
nail-patella syndrome
Nakata index

naked facet sign
naloxone imaging agent
Namaqualand spondyloepiphysial
  dysplasia (NSED)
nanocolloid
  technetium 99m n.
nanocurie (nCi)
nanogram (ng)
nanoparticle
  colloidal gold n.
  gadolinium-rich n.
  iodinated n.
  MagForce n.
  monocrystalline iron oxide n.
    (MION)
nanoparticulate imaging
  agent
naphthalene
  fluorine-18
    2-dialkylamino-6-acylmalononitrile
    substituted n. (FDDNP)
napkin-ring
  n.-r. anular lesion
  n.-r. anular stenosis
  n.-r. anular tumor
  n.-r. trachea
Napoleon hat sign
Narcomatic flowmetry
nares (*pl. of* naris)
naris, *pl.* **nares**
NARP
  neuropathy, ataxia and retinitis
    pigmentosa
narrow
  n. anteroposterior diameter
  n. beam
  n. caliber
  n. chest
  n. collimation
  n. gating tolerance
narrow-band spectral-selective
  radiofrequency pulse
narrow-beam half-thickness
narrowed
  n. orifice
  n. valve
narrowing
  airway n.
  antral stomach n.
  arterial n.
  arteriolar n.
  artificial lumen n.
  n. asymmetry
  atherosclerotic n.
  beaklike n.

narrowing (*continued*)
    bile duct n.
    bird-beak configuration or n.
    bronchiolar n.
    carinal angle n.
    circumferential n.
    colonic n.
    concentric n.
    degenerative n.
    diffuse n.
    discrete n.
    disc space n.
    duodenal n.
    eccentric n.
    esophageal n.
    n. exchange
    focal esophageal n.
    gastric n.
    glottic n.
    high-grade n.
    intervertebral disc n.
    joint space n.
    large airway n.
    longitudinal n.
    long smooth esophageal n.
    lower esophageal n.
    luminal n.
    motional n.
    nasopharyngeal n.
    neural foraminal n.
    n. of artery
    n. of bronchiolar passage
    n. of forefoot
    n. of spinal canal
    n. of thecal sac
    oropharyngeal n.
    pancompartmental joint space n.
    rectal n.
    residual luminal n.
    retropharyngeal n.
    segmental bronchus n.
    smooth esophageal n.
    stomach n.
    subcritical n.
    subglottic n.
    supraglottic n.
    symmetric n.
    tracheal n.
    vallecular n.

nasal
    n. airway resistance
    n. bone
    n. bridge
    n. canal
    n. cavity
    n. cavity wall
    n. concha
    n. fracture
    n. intubation

    n. meatus
    n. mucociliary clearance function
    n. part of pharynx
    n. polyp
    n. septum
    n. septum hematoma
    n. sinus
    n. spine
    n. suture
    n. tip deformity
    n. turbinate
    n. vault mass
    n. vestibule
nasal-to-plasma radioactivity ratio
nascent stage
NASH
    nonalcoholic steatohepatitis
nasi
    agger n.
nasion
    Bolton n.
    n. recession
nasobregmatic arc
nasociliary nerve
nasoenteric tube
nasoethmoid fracture
nasofrontal
    n. duct
    n. suture
nasogastric (NG)
    n. intubation
    n. tube (NGT)
nasojejunal feeding tube
nasolabial
    n. cyst
    n. lymph node
nasolacrimal
    n. canal
    n. drainage system obstruction
      (NDSO)
    n. duct
nasomaxillary
    n. fracture
    n. suture
nasooccipital arc
nasoorbital fracture
nasopalatal fissure
nasopalatine canal
nasopharyngeal
    n. atresia
    n. carcinoma (NPC)
    n. carcinoma in situ
    n. craniopharyngioma
    n. hematoma
    n. mass
    n. mucous retention cyst
    n. narrowing
    n. reflux
    n. squamous cell carcinoma

nasopharyngography
nasopharynx
nasotracheal
    n. intubation
    n. tube
natal cleft
natatory ligament
natiform skull
national
    N. Council on Radiation Protection and Measurement (NCRP)
    N. Heart, Lung, and Blood Institute
    N. Institute of Neurological and Communicative Disorders
    N. Institute of Neurological Disorders and Stroke (NINDS)
    N. Institute of Standards and Technology
    N. Institutes of Health stroke scale (NIHSS)
    N. Polyp Study
    N. Radiological Protection Board (NRPB)
native
    n. aorta
    n. aortic valve
    n. aortic valve closure
    n. atherosclerosis
    n. coronary artery
    n. image
    n. kidney
    n. kidney renal artery stenosis
    n. kidney renal vein thrombosis
    n. lung
    n. tissue harmonic imaging (NTHI)
    n. ventricle
    n. vessel
natural
    n. active acquired immunity
    n. killer (NK)
    n. neon gas
    n. radiation
    n. radioactivity
Naumoff syndrome
Navarre drainage catheter
navel
    n. ring artifact
    n. string
Navi Ball guidance system
navicular
    n. body
    n. body fracture
    n. bone
    carpal n.
    n. hand fracture
    ossific nucleus of n.

    n. projection
    protrusion of n.
    target n.
    tarsal n.
    n. to 1st metatarsal angle
    n. tuberosity
    n. view
naviculare
    os n.
navicularis
    fossa n.
naviculocapitate fracture
naviculocunciform
    n. joint
    n. ligament
navigable echo signal
navigated spin-echo diffusion-weighted MR imaging
navigation
    computer-assisted intracranial n.
    electromagnetic n.
navigator
    N. computer workstation
    n. echo
    n. echo-based real-time respiratory gating and triggering
    n. echo motion correction technique
    n. pulse
    n. shift
navigator-guided motion correction
Navigus cranial electrode system
Navi-Star ablation catheter
Navitrack computer-assisted surgery system
NAWM
    normal-appearing white matter
    NAWM metabolite concentration
NBCA
    N-butyl cyanoacrylate
***N*-butyl cyanoacrylate (NBCA)**
***N*-butyl-2-cyanoacrylate embolization**
NB200 vascular access device
N/C
    nuclear-to-cytoplasmic ratio
N-Cat N-500 tonometric blood pressure monitor
NCCT
    noncontrast head CT
nCi
    nanocurie
NCP
    noncontrast phase
    implanted NCP
NCPF
    noncirrhotic portal fibrosis
NCRP
    National Council on Radiation Protection and Measurement

N

2nd
2nd branchial arch
2nd branchial cleft cyst
2nd cranial nerve
2nd cuneiform bone
2nd diagonal branch
2nd echo image
2nd harmonic imaging
2nd malignant neoplasia (SMN)
2nd portion of duodenum
2nd primary carcinoma
2nd primary tumor
2nd trimester
2nd ventricle of cerebrum
2nd-degree
2nd-d. AV block
2nd-d. heart block
2nd-look arthroscopy
2nd-order
2nd-o. chorda
2nd-o. compensation
2nd-o. correction
2nd-o. reflection
2nd-o. subtraction
NDP-K
nucleoside diphosphate kinase
NDSO
nasolacrimal drainage system
obstruction
2nd-trimester
2nd-t. gestational dating
2nd-t. placenta
Nd:YAG
neodymium:yttrium-aluminum-garnet
Nd:YAG CTLC
Nd:YAG laser catheter
Nd:YLF
neodymium:yttrium-lithium fluoride
Nd:YLF laser
near
n. field
n. infrared (NIR)
near-anatomic
n.-a. position
n.-a. position of joint
near-field effect
near-infrared
n.-i. optical mammography
n.-i. spectroscopy (NIRS)
near-isotropic reformatted image
near-normal radiotracer uptake
near-resonance spin-lock contrast
near-water
n.-w. attenuation
n.-w. density
NEC
noise effective count
necessity
fracture of n.

neck
anatomic n.
aneurysmal n.
aneurysm remnant n.
bone n.
n. coil
dental n.
n. emphysema
femoral n.
n. fracture
n. germ cell tumor
hyperextension of n.
n. lymphangioma
Madelung n.
n. of aneurysm
n. of bladder
n. of femur
n. of gallbladder
n. of pancreas
n. of rib
n. of talus
pancreatic n.
n. phantom
posterior triangle of n.
potato tumor of n.
selective occlusion of ancurysmal n.
surgical n.
n. teratoma
uterine wry n.
vesical n.
webbed n.
neck-shaft angle (NSA)
neck-space anatomy
necrobiotic nodule
necrolytic
necroses (*pl. of* necrosis)
necrosis, *pl.* **necroses**
acute cortical n.
acute laminar n.
acute native kidney tubular n.
acute renal transplant tubular n.
acute sclerosing hyaline n. (ASHN)
acute tubular n. (ATN)
alcoholic avascular n.
alveolar septal n.
aortic idiopathic n.
arteriolar n.
aseptic n.
asphyxia-related renal n.
avascular n. (AVN)
avascular bone n.
avascular cortical infarction n.
avascular femoral head n.
avascular tarsal scaphoid n.
avascular vertebral body n.
bilateral cortical n.
biliary piecemeal n.
bloodless zone of n.
bony n.

bowel n.
breast fat n.
bridging n.
caseous n.
central caseous n.
centrilobular n.
chemotherapy-induced n.
coagulation n.
colliquative n.
colonic n.
comedo n.
contraction band n.
cortical kidney n.
diffuse n.
dirty n.
embolic n.
encapsulated fat n.
epiphysial ischemic n.
Erdheim cystic medial n.
fascial margin n.
fat n.
fatty n.
fibrinoid n.
fibrosing piecemeal n.
Ficat stage of avascular n.
focal fat n.
focal hepatic n.
frank n.
heart muscle n.
hemorrhagic n.
hepatic n.
hyaline n.
idiopathic avascular n.
indurative n.
intestinal n.
intratumoral n.
ischemic n.
laminar brain n.
liquefaction n.
localized n.
lung n.
margin n.
massive hepatic n.
medial cystic n.
midzonal n.
mucosal n.
myocardial n.
nontraumatic avascular n.
Paget quiet n.
pancreatic n.
papillary n.
peripheral n.
piecemeal n.
postbiopsy fat n.
postpartum pituitary n.
postsurgical fat n.
posttraumatic aseptic n.
posttraumatic fat n.
pressure n.

progressive emphysematous n.
punctate n.
radiation n.
radiation-induced n. (RIN)
radiation-induced cerebral n.
radium n.
renal allograft n.
renal cortical n.
renal papillary n.
renal tubular n.
septal n.
septic n.
soft tissue n.
strangulation n.
stromal n.
subacute hepatic n.
subcapsular hepatic n.
subcutaneous fat n.
subendocardial n.
submassive hepatic n.
superficial n.
total n.
tracheobronchial mucosal n.
transmural n.
traumatic fat n.
tubular n.
tumor n.
vascular n.
ventricular muscle n.
Zenker n.

necrotic

n. bone
n. bone pseudocyst
n. debris
n. flap
n. hepatic metastasis
n. inflammation
n. lesion
n. lipid
n. myocardium
n. renal cell carcinoma
n. sequestrum
n. tissue
n. tumor
n. ulcer

necrotizing

n. aspergillosis
n. emphysema
n. enterocolitis
n. external otitis
n. fasciitis
n. gastritis
n. glomerulonephritis
n. granulomatous disease
n. leukoencephalopathy
n. myelopathy
n. pancreatitis
n. pneumonia
n. respiratory granulomatosis

N

necrotizing (*continued*)
    n. thrombosis
    n. ulcerative gingivitis (NUG)
NECT
    nonenhanced computed tomography
NED
    no evidence of disease
needle
    Abrams biopsy n.
    abscission n.
    Accucore II biopsy n.
    Amplatz angiography n.
    Arrow Fischell EVAN N.
    aspiration biopsy n.
    automated biopsy n.
    Bauer-Temno biopsy n.
    B-D bone marrow biopsy n.
    beveled n.
    Bierman n.
    BioPince n.
    biopsy n.
    n. biopsy
    Biopty cut n.
    blood-containment n.
    blunt-end sialogram n.
    Brockenbrough n.
    BV2 n.
    cesium n.
    Chiba n.
    coaxial sheath cut-biopsy n.
    coaxial Temno n.
    Colapinto n.
    Conrad-Crosby bone marrow biopsy n.
    Cope biopsy n.
    core bone biopsy n.
    Cournand arteriography n.
    Cournand-Grino angiography n.
    n. deviation
    Dos Santos aortography n.
    dumbbell n.
    Echo-Coat ultrasound biopsy n.
    Echo Tip trocar n.
    E-Z-EM cut-biopsy n.
    flexible biopsy n.
    Franseen n.
    full-intensity n.
    Greene n.
    half-intensity n.
    Hawkins-Akins n.
    Hawkins breast lesion localization n.
    Hawkins 1-stick n.
    Homerlok n.
    Homer Mammalok n.
    n. hydrophone
    iridium n.
    Kopans n.
    Kormed liver biopsy n.
    larger-caliber cutting n.

    n. localization
    n. localization of breast lesion
    Maggi biopsy n.
    Majestik shielded angiographic n.
    Mammalock n.
    n. marker
    Menghini Surecut bone biopsy n.
    Mentor prostatic biopsy n.
    metallic n.
    micropuncture n.
    middle-caliber n.
    Monoject hypodermic n.
    Monopty n.
    Multi-Pro biopsy n.
    nonferromagnetic n.
    Ostycut bone biopsy n.
    PercuCut cut-biopsy n.
    percutaneous access n.
    pronged Franseen-type-point n.
    n. pyelography
    Quick-Core biopsy n.
    Quincke spinal n.
    ^{226}Ra n.
    Rosch-Uchida n.
    Ross n.
    scalp vein n.
    Seldinger n.
    self-aspirating cut-biopsy n.
    sheath n.
    sialography n.
    single-wall n.
    skinny n.
    small-caliber n.
    Sos Pulse-Vu bloodless entry n.
    spinal n.
    spring-loaded biopsy n.
    Temno II cutting n.
    T-fastener delivery n.
    thin-walled guiding n.
    TLA n.
    translumbar aortography n.
    Tuohy aortography n.
    n. visualization
    Westcott n.
    Whitacre spinal n.
    Yueh centesis n.
2-needle biopsy technique
needle-guided excisional biopsy
needle-hookwire localization
needle-localized breast biopsy (NLBB)
needle-shaped breast calcification
needle-tip bioimpedance
needle-wire system
Neel temperature
Neer
    N. classification of shoulder fracture
    N. impingement sign
    N. lateral shoulder view
    N. transscapular view

Neer-Horowitz
>   N.-H. classification of humeral
>   fracture
>   N.-H. humerus fracture classification

NEFA
>   nonesterified fatty acid
>   NEFA scintigraphy

Neff percutaneous access set

negative
>   breakpoint cluster region n.
>   n. EMA result
>   n. factor
>   n. image
>   n. image pulmonary edema
>   n. Mach band
>   n. mucin result
>   n. predictive value (NPV)
>   pulmonary edema photographic n.
>   n. puncture result
>   replication error n.
>   n. tropism
>   true n.
>   n. ulnar variance

negative-contrast
>   n.-c. effect
>   n.-c. imaging agent
>   n.-c. left atriography

negative-ion cyclotron

negatron emission

negligible pressure gradient

Neisseria meningitidis

Nélaton
>   N. dislocation
>   N. fold
>   N. line

Nelson syndrome

NEMD
>   nonspecific esophageal motility disorder

neoadjuvant
>   n. chemoradiation therapy
>   n. chemotherapy
>   n. hormonal therapy
>   n. radiotherapy

neoangiogenesis

neoaorta

neoaortic valve

neobladder
>   ileal n.

neocerebellum

neocholangiole

neocortex

neodensity

neodymium:YAG laser therapy

neodymium:yttrium-aluminum-garnet
>   **(Nd:YAG)**
>   n:y.-a.-g. laser

neodymium:yttrium-lithium fluoride
>   **(Nd:YLF)**

neofissure

neogalactosyl albumin

neointima formation

neointimal
>   n. hyperplasia
>   n. proliferation

Neo-Iopax

neonatal
>   n. adrenal ultrasound
>   n. ascites
>   n. cardiac failure
>   n. choroid plexus hemorrhage
>   n. cystic pulmonary emphysema
>   n. encephalopathy
>   n. heart failure
>   n. hepatitis
>   n. hepatitis/cholestasis syndrome
>   n. herpes
>   n. hyperthyroidism
>   n. intracerebellar hemorrhage
>   n. intracranial hemorrhage
>   n. intracranial ischemia
>   n. intraventricular hemorrhage
>   n. lupus syndrome
>   n. meningitis
>   n. morphologic imaging
>   n. omphalitis
>   n. osteomyelitis
>   n. pneumonia
>   n. radiography
>   n. subdural hemorrhage
>   n. transfontanellar brain ultrasound
>   n. wet lung disease

neonate
>   n. encephalomalacia
>   n. mediastinal shift

neonatorum
>   edema n.

neon particle protocol

neopallium

neoplasia
>   adrenocortical n.
>   benign n.
>   bone n.
>   breast n.
>   bronchopulmonary n.
>   cavitating n.
>   cervical intraepithelial n.
>   choroid plexus n.
>   colonic n.
>   connective tissue n.
>   cranial nerve n.
>   cystic splenic n.
>   ductectatic mucinous cystic n.
>   encapsulated n.
>   epithelial n.
>   esophageal n.
>   exophytic n.
>   external ear n.
>   extrinsic n.

N

neoplasia (*continued*)
    firm n.
    focally decreased renal n.
    functioning n.
    gestational trophoblastic n.
    gonadal n.
    granulosa-theca n.
    hepatic n.
    interdigital n.
    intracranial n.
    intraductal papillary mucinous n.
      (IPMN)
    intrahepatic biliary n.
    intramedullary compartment n.
    lethal n.
    lobular n.
    low-grade n.
    macrocystic n.
    malignant urethral n.
    mesenchymal n.
    metastatic renal n.
    middle ear n.
    mucinous pancreatic cystic n.
    multiple endocrine n. (MEN)
    multiple intestinal n.
    2nd malignant n. (SMN)
    neuroepithelial n.
    NK cell n.
    osteocartilaginous parasellar n.
    ovarian n.
    pancreatic n.
    papillary epithelial n.
    papillary pancreatic cystic n.
    pearly n.
    pineal gland n.
    primary n.
    skeletal n.
    soft tissue n.
    spheric n.
    supratentorial n.
    T-cell n.
    thoracic spine n.
    thymic n.
    transitional cell n.
    trochlear nerve n.
    vaginal intraepithelial n.
    vulvar intraepithelial n.
    well-circumscribed n.
neoplasm
    bone-forming n.
    fibrotic n.
    germ cell n.
    hemorrhagic n.
    hyperdense n.
    intraventricular n.
    nerve sheath n.
    n. of lung
    periprosthetic n.
    primary malignant n.

    pulmonary n.
    radiation-induced n.
    recurrent n.
    retroperitoneal n.
    sinonasal n.
    splenic n.
    synchronous n.
    thymic epithelial n.
    tracheal n.
    vascular n.
neoplastic
    n. aneurysm
    n. calcification
    n. C-cell hyperplasia
    n. cyst
    n. destruction of spinal
      element
    n. fracture
    n. invasion
    n. lesion
    n. process
    n. stenosis
    n. tissue
Neoprobe
    N. 1000, 1500 portable radioisotope
      detector
    N. radioactivity detector
neopterin
neorectum
Neoscan
NeoSpect diagnostic imaging agent
neosphincter
neostigmine methylsulfate
NeoTect imaging agent
neoterminal ileum
neovagina
neovascularity
    tumor n.
neovascularization
    choroidal n. (CNV)
neovasculature
    tumor n.
nepheline pneumoconiosis
nephritic calculus
nephritis
    acute diffuse bacterial n.
    acute focal bacterial n.
    acute interstitial n. (AIN)
    bacterial n.
    Balkan n.
    chronic hereditary n.
    diffuse bacterial n.
    focal bacterial n.
    glomerular n.
    interstitial n.
    nephrocalcinosis n.
    radiation n.
    salt-losing n.
    tubulointerstitial n.

nephroblastoma
    classic n.
    cystic partially differentiated n.
    polycystic n.
nephroblastomatosis
    multifocal n.
    panlobar n.
    superficial diffuse n.
nephrocalcinosis
    cortical n.
    medullary n.
    n. nephritis
    renal cortical n.
nephrogenetic (*var. of* nephrogenic)
nephrogenic, nephrogenetic
    n. bladder adenoma
    n. diabetes insipidus
    n. phase
    n. systemic fibrosis
nephrogram
    cortical rim n.
    delayed unilateral n.
    increasingly dense n.
    medullary n.
    obstructive n.
    rim n.
    n. rim
    segmental n.
    shell n.
    n. shock
    soap-bubble n.
    spotted n.
    striated angiographic n.
    sunburst n.
    Swiss cheese n.
    tubular n.
nephrographic
    generalized n. (GNG)
    n. phase
nephrography
    isotope n.
nephrolithiasis
nephrolithotomy
    percutaneous n. (PCNL)
nephroma
    congenital mesoblastic n.
    cystic n.
    mesoblastic n.
    multilocular cystic n.
NephroMax balloon catheter
nephronia
    lobar n.
nephron-sparing surgery
nephropathia (*var. of* nephropathy)
nephropathic cystinosis
nephropathy, nephropathia
    allograft n.
    analgesic n.
    Balkan n.

    contrast-induced n. (CIN)
    contrast medium-induced n.
    diabetic n.
    HIV n.
    ischemic n.
    obstructive n.
    radiation n.
    radiocontrast-induced n.
    radiographic contrast medium-induced
      n.
    reflux n.
    urate n.
    uric acid n.
nephrophthisis
    juvenile n.
nephroptosia (*var. of* nephroptosis)
nephroptosis, nephroptosia
nephropyelography
nephropyosis (*var. of* pyonephrosis)
nephrosclerosis
    arterial n.
    benign n.
    malignant n.
    senile n.
nephroscope
    Alken-Marberger n.
    flexible n.
    percutaneous n.
    Wickham-Miller n.
nephroscopic fulguration
nephroscopy
nephrosis
    congenital Finnish n.
nephrosonography
nephrostogram
    n. imaging
    postprocedure n.
nephrostolithotomy
    calyceal n.
    percutaneous n.
nephrostomy
    n. bag
    n. catheter
    circle wire n.
    Cope loop n.
    percutaneous n.
    n. puncture
    single-stick n.
    n. track
nephrotic
    n. edema
    n. syndrome
nephrotomogram
nephrotomography
    n. imaging
    infusion n.
nephrotoxic contrast medium
nephrotoxicity
    contrast medium n.

N

nephrotoxicity (*continued*)
    cyclosporin n.
    drug-induced n.
nephroureteral
    n. stent
    n. stent system
nephroureterectomy
nephroureterostomy stent
nephrourography
nephrouroradiology
Neptune trident appearance
neptunium 59 (^{59}Np, Np-59)
NER
    no evidence of recurrence
NERD
    no evidence of recurrent disease
Nernst equation
nerve
    accessory n.
    acoustic n.
    afferent digital n.
    cluneal n.
    cochlear n.
    VIII n. complex
    cranial n.
    dorsal ramus of spinal n.
    efferent digital n.
    n. entrapment
    excrescentic thickening of optic n.
    facial n.
    femoral n.
    N. Fiber Analyzer GDx
    n. fiber myelination
    frontal n.
    fusiform enlargement of optic n.
    greater superficial petrosal n.
    hypoglossal n.
    inferior alveolar n.
    n. injury
    intercostal n.
    intercostobrachial n.
    interosseous n.
    lacrimal n.
    laryngeal n.
    left respiratory n.
    lingual n.
    mandibular n.
    median n.
    nasociliary n.
    2nd cranial n.
    n. of Latarjet
    ophthalmic n.
    peripheral n.
    periradicular n.
    peroneal n.
    petrosal n.
    pinched n.
    n. plexus
    posterior interosseous n. (PIN)

    recurrent laryngeal n.
    recurrent meningeal n.
    n. root
    n. root avulsion
    n. root axillary pouch
    n. root compression
    n. root edema
    n. root embarrassment
    n. root impingement
    n. root irritability
    n. root of cauda equina
    n. root sheath
    n. root sheath effacement
    n. root sleeve
    n. root tumor
    rostral cervical n.
    sacral n.
    saphenous n.
    n. sheath neoplasm
    n. sheath tumor
    spinal accessory n.
    subcostal n.
    supraspinatus n.
    sural n.
    4th cranial n.
    5th cranial n.
    trigeminal n.
    trochlear n.
    n. trunk
    vestibular division of 8th cranial n.
    vestibulocochlear n.
    vidian n.
nervus intermedius
nesidioblastoma
nesidioblastosis
nest
    junctional n.
nester coil
net
    n. magnetization factor
    n. magnetization vector
    n. shunt
    n. tissue magnetization
    n. transverse magnetization
network
    articular n.
    artificial neural n.
    hypertrophic duct n.
    lymphatic n.
    matching n.
    neural n.
    vascular n.
    venous n.
neural
    n. arch cleft
    n. arch fracture
    n. axis vascular malformation
    n. blockade
    n. canal

n. crest origin
n. crest tissue
n. fibrolipoma
n. foramen
n. foramen remodeling
n. foraminal narrowing
n. foraminal stenosis
n. groove
n. miscommunication
n. network
n. pathway
n. placode
n. sheath
n. tube
n. tube defect (NTD)
n. tuberculosis
n. vertebral arch

neuralgia
postherpetic n.
sphenopalatine n.

neural-origin bone tumor

neuraxis
n. radiation therapy
n. staging

neuraxonal dystrophy

neurenteric
n. canal
n. cyst
n. fistula

neurilemmoma (*var. of* neurilemoma)

neurilemoma, neurilemmoma
abdominal n.
intradermal n.

neurinoma

neuritic
n. plaquing
n. senile plaque

neuritides (*pl. of* neuritis)

neuritis, *pl.* **neuritides**
axial n.
brachial plexus n.
friction n.
optic n.

neuro
N. Lobe software
N. SPGR software

Neuroacryl tissue adhesive
neuroangiography
neuroarthropathy
neuroaugmentation
neuroblastoma
adrenal n.
cerebral n.
cervical n.
chest wall n.
dumbbell-type n.
Hutchinson-type n.
intracranial n.
intraventricular n.

metastatic n.
olfactory n.
stage 4S n.
n. staging
thoracic n.

neuroblockage
neurocentral synchondrosis
neurocutaneous syndrome
neurocysticercosis
neurocytoma
central n.
intraventricular n.

neurodegenerative disease
neurodiagnostic
n. imaging
n. scanner

NeuroEcho software
neuroectodermal
n. dysplasia
n. origin
n. tumor

neuroendocrine
n. hepatic metastasis
n. small cell carcinoma
n. tumor

neuroendoscopy
**neuroendovascular interventional
  procedure**
neuroenteric cyst
neuroepithelial neoplasia
neurofibrillary tangle
neurofibroma
aryepiglottic fold n.
craniofacial plexiform n.
dumbbell n.
extraspinal n.
paraspinal n.
plexiform n.

neurofibromatosis
abortive n.
central n.
incomplete n.
kidney n.
peripheral n.
segmental n.
n. (type 1, 2) (NF1, NF2)
n. with bilateral acoustic neuromas

neurofibrosarcoma
neurofilament
neurofilamentous misalignment
NeuroFOCUS scanner
neurogenetic (*var. of* neurogenic)
neurogenic, neurogenetic, neurogenous
n. bladder
n. deficit
n. disorder
n. fracture
n. intestinal obstruction
n. lesion

N

neurogenic (*continued*)
    n. pulmonary edema
    n. sarcoma
    n. shock
    n. tumor
neurogenous (*var. of* neurogenic)
neuroglial tumor
neurogram
neurography
    magnetic resonance n. (MRN)
neuroimaging
    3D n.
    functional n.
    n. modality
    3-tesla n.
neurointerventional radiology
NeuroLink II data acquisition system
Neurolite imaging agent
neurologic, neurological
    n. bladder lesion
    n. sequela
    n. soft sign
neurological (*var. of* neurologic)
neurology
    American Academy of N. (AAN)
neurolymphomatosis
neuroma, *pl.* **neuromata,**
 pl. **neuromas**
    acoustic n.
    digital n.
    interdigital n.
    Morton n.
    multicystic acoustic n.
    neurofibromatosis with bilateral
      acoustic n.'s
    postamputation n.
    posttraumatic n.
neuromas (*pl. of* neuroma)
neuromata (*pl. of* neuroma)
neuromatosa
    elephantiasis n.
neuromeningeal trunk
neuromorphometric
neuromorphometry
neuromuscular
    n. junction
    n. system electric induction
neuromyelitis optica
neuromyopathy
    carcinomatous n.
neuron, neurone
    lower motor n.
    motor n.
    nigrostriatal dopaminergic n.
    pyramidal n.
    upper motor n.
neuronal
    n. cell-origin tumor
    n. ceroid lipofuscinosis

    n. cytotoxic edema
    n. migration
    n. plasticity
    n. proliferation
neuronavigation
neurone (*var. of* neuron)
neuroorthopaedic syndrome
neurootologist
Neuropack 4, 8 EMG
neuropathic
    n. ankle
    n. arthropathy
    n. Charcot foot
    n. fracture
    n. midfoot deformity
    n. osteoarthropathy
    n. pain
    n. tarsometatarsal joint
neuropathicum
neuropathologic correlation
neuropathy
    n., ataxia and retinitis pigmentosa
     (NARP)
    autonomic n.
    compression n.
    diabetic n.
    entrapment n.
    optic n.
    radiation-related optic n. (RON)
neuropore
neuroradiologic
    n. correlation
    n. examination
    n. imaging
neuroradiology
    American Society of N.
    interventional n.
    pediatric n.
neuroreceptor
neuroroentgenography
neurosarcoidosis
neurosarcoma
NeuroScan 3D imager
neurosecretory granule
Neurosector
    N. ultrasound
    N. ultrasound system
Neuroshield
    N. distal protection device
    MedNova N.
neurosonogram
neurosonography
neurosonology
neurospectroscopy
neurotized melanocytic nevus
neurotomography
neurotoxic effect
neurotransmission
    dopaminergic n.

neurotransmitter
  excitatory n.
  n. imaging
  inhibitory n.
  n. precursor
neurotrophic
  n. fracture
  n. imaging agent
  n. joint
neurovascular
  n. bundle (NVB)
  n. compression
  n. lesion
neurovegetative disturbance
neurulation
neutral
  adduction to n.
  n. amyloid probe
  n. hip position
  n. ulnar variance
neutralization plate
neutrino
  electron n.
neutron
  n. absorption process
  n. activation analysis
  n. beam
  n. bombardment
  epithermal n.
  fast n.
  n. irradiation
  n. number
  n. radiation
  n. radiography
  slow n.
  n. therapy
  n. therapy machine
  thermal n.
neutron-atomic number ratio
neutron-deficient
  n.-d. nucleus
  n.-d. short-lived isotope
neutron/gamma
  n./g. transmission
  n./g. transmission method
  n./g. transmission therapy
neutron-rich biomedical tracer
neutropenia
  chemotherapy-induced n.
neutropenic enterocolitis
neutrophilic leukocyte
nevi (*pl. of* nevus)
Neviaser frozen shoulder classification
nevoid
  n. basal cell carcinoma
  n. basal cell carcinoma syndrome
nevus, *pl.* **nevi**
  neurotized melanocytic n.
  n. verrucosus

new
  n. bone formation
  N. York Heart Association (NYHA)
newborn hernia
Newman
  N. classification of radial neck and
    head fractures
  N. radial fracture classification
new-onset seizure
NewTom
  N. CT scanner
  N. VG cone beam tomography
Newton guidewire
Newvicon camera tube
NEX
  number of excitations
NexStent
NF1
  neurofibromatosis (type 1)
NF2
  neurofibromatosis (type 2)
  Wishart-Lee-Abbott NF2
ng
  nanogram
NG
  nasogastric
NGT
  nasogastric tube
NHL
  non-Hodgkin lymphoma
niche
  Haudek n.
nickel-titanium (NiTi)
  n.-t. naval ordnance laboratory
    (nitinol)
Nicoladoni-Branham sign
Nicolet
  N. Elite Doppler monitor
  N. Elite Doppler ultrasound
  N. NMR spectrometer
Nicoll bone
nicotinamide
  n. imaging agent
  n. radiosensitizer
Nidek
  N. EC-5000 excimer laser
  N. EC-5000 excimer laser system
nidi (*pl. of* nidus)
nidus, *pl.* **nidi**
  n. angle
  arteriovenous malformation n.
  central n.
  n. demarcation
  n. of lesion
  n. patency
  thrombus n.
  tumor n.
Niemann-Pick disease
Niemeier gallbladder perforation

N

Nievergelt
>N. disease
>N. syndrome

Niewenglowski ray
NightHawk Radiology Services
nightstick fracture
nigra
>substantia n.

nigricans
>acanthosis n.

nigrostriatal
>n. dopaminergic neuron
>n. dopaminergic pathway

Nihon Kohden Neurofax electroencephalograph
NIHSS
>National Institutes of Health stroke scale
>NIHSS score

Nijmegen breakage syndrome
nimodipine
>n. imaging agent
>intraarterial superselective n.

NINDS
>National Institute of Neurological Disorders and Stroke

niobium
>zirconium with n. 95

niobium/titanium superconductor
Niopam
>N. contrast medium
>N. imaging agent

NIP
>nonspecific interstitial pneumonia

nipple
>adenoma of n.
>aortic n.
>deep to n.
>n. marker
>out-of-profile n.
>n. retraction
>n. ring artifact
>n. sector
>n. shadow

nipple-areola complex
nipplelike
>n. common bile duct
>n. osteophyte formation

NIPS
>noninvasive programmed electrical stimulation

NIR
>near infrared
>NIR contrast agent
>NIR optical mammography
>NIR stent

NIRS
>near-infrared spectroscopy

Nishimoto Sangyo scanner

Nissen
>N. antireflux operation
>N. fundoplication
>N. fundoplication of stomach procedure

NiTi
>nickel-titanium
>NiTi alloy stent

nitinol
>n. guidewire
>n. inferior vena cava filter
>n. Symphony stent
>n. U-clip
>n. wire core

niton
nitrate
>organic n.

Nitrex
>N. ev3 guidewire
>N. nitinol guidewire

nitric oxide
nitrocellulose film
nitrogen (N)
>n. 13 (^{13}N, N-13)
>n. 14 (^{14}N, N-14)
>n. 15 (^{15}N, N-15)
>n. mustard
>n. washout

nitrogen-13 ammonia imaging agent
nitroxide-stable free radical
NK
>natural killer
>NK cell neoplasia

NLBB
>needle-localized breast biopsy

***N*-methylspiperone**
***N*-methylspiroperidol (NMS)**
>^{11}C *N*-m.

NMR
>nuclear magnetic resonance
>continuous-wave NMR
>2D NMR
>NMR LipoProfile test
>magic angle spinning NMR
>NMR magnetometer probe
>pulse NMR
>pulsed-electron paramagnetic NMR
>NMR quadrature detection array
>NMR scan
>NMR signal
>NMR spectrometer
>surface coil NMR

NMS
>*N*-methylspiroperidol

no
>n. discernible finding
>n. evidence of disease (NED)
>n. evidence of recurrence (NER)

n. evidence of recurrent disease
(NERD)

n. frequency wrap

noble

n. gas

n. gas in magnetic resonance study

N. position

Nocardia **brain abscess**

nocardial osteomyelitis

nocardiosis

no-carrier-added

n.-c.-a. ^{18}F imaging agent

n.-c.-a. radionuclide

nociceptive pain

nociceptor

ectopic firing n.

nocturnal polysomnography

nodal

n. bed

n. conduction

n. disease

n. fibrosis

n. impulse

n. metastasis

n. point

n. premature contraction

n. rhythm

n. rupture

n. staging

n. station

n. tissue

node

abdominal lymph n.

accessory lymph n.

anorectal lymph n.

aortic lymph n.

aortic window n.

apical lymph n.

appendicular lymph n.

Aschoff n.

Aschoff-Tawara n.

atrioventricular n.

auricular lymph n.

AV n.

axillary lymph n. (ALN)

azygos lymph n.

benign n.

bifurcation lymph n.

Bouchard n.

brachial lymph n.

brachiocephalic lymph n.

bronchopulmonary lymph n.

buccinator lymph n.

n. calcification

calcified lymph n.

cardiac n.

cartilaginous n.

caval lymph n.

celiac lymph n.

central lymph n.

cervical paratracheal lymph n.

cervicoabdominal n.

Cloquet inguinal lymph n.

common iliac lymph n.

companion lymph n.

coronary n.

cubital lymph n.

cystic lymph n.

cystic metastatic n.

delphian lymph n.

deltopectoral lymph n.

diaphragmatic lymph n.

Dürck n.

eggshell calcification of lymph n.

epicolic lymph n.

epigastric lymph n.

epitrochlear lymph n.

Ewald n.

external iliac lymph n.

fibular lymph n.

Flack sinuatrial n.

foraminal n.

gastric lymph n.

gastroduodenal lymph n.

gastroepiploic lymph n.

gastrohepatic ligament n.

gastroomental lymph n.

Ghon n.

giant hyperplasia lymph n.

gluteal lymph n.

gouty n.

Haygarth n.

Heberden n.

hemal n.

hemolymph n.

Hensen n.

hepatic lymph n.

hilar lymph n.

ileocolic lymph n.

iliac circumflex lymph n.

ilioinguinal lymph n.

image-intensifier n.

infraclavicular n.

infrahyoid lymph n.

inguinal lymph n.

intercostal lymph n.

interiliac lymph n.

internal mammary n. (IMN)

internal mammary lymph n.

interpectoral lymph n.

intramammary lymph n.

in-transit n.

intraparenchymal lymph n.

intrapulmonary lymph n. (IPLN)

jugular lymph n.

jugulodigastric n.

juguloomohyoid lymph n.

juxtaintestinal n.

node (*continued*)

Keith n.
Keith-Flack sinuatrial n.
Koch sinuatrial n.
lacunar n.
locoregional lymph n.
lumbar lymph n.
lymph n. (LN)
lymphomatous lymph n.
malar lymph n.
mandibular lymph n.
mastoid lymph n.
medial supraclavicular n.
mediastinal n.
mesenteric n.
metastatic lymph n.
Meynet n.
miliary n.
multicentric angiofollicular lymph n.
nasolabial lymph n.
nontumor-involved n.
obturator lymph n.
occipital lymph n.
Osler n.
pancreatic lymph n.
pancreaticoduodenal lymph n.
pancreaticolienal lymph n.
pancreaticosplenic n.
paraaortic lymph n.
paracolic lymph n.
paramammary lymph n.
pararectal lymph n.
parasternal lymph n.
paratracheal lymph n.
parauterine lymph n.
paravaginal lymph n.
paravesicular lymph n.
parietal lymph n.
parotid lymph n.
Parrot n.
pectoral lymph n.
pelvic lymph n.
periaortic lymph n.
peribronchial lymph n.
pericardial lymph n.
pericholedochal n.
perisplenic n.
phrenic lymph n.
popliteal n.
porta hepatis n.
postaortic lymph n.
postcaval lymph n.
posterior mediastinal n.
postvesicular lymph n.
potato n.
preaortic lymph n.
precaval lymph n.
prececal lymph n.
prelaryngeal n.

prepericardial lymph n.
pretracheal lymph n.
prevertebral lymph n.
prevesicular lymph n.
pulmonary juxtaesophageal lymph n.
pyloric lymph n.
Ranvier n.
rectal lymph n.
regional lymph n.
retroaortic lymph n.
retroauricular lymph n.
retrocecal lymph n.
retrocrural n.
retroperitoneal n.
retropharyngeal lymph n.
retropyloric n.
retrorectal lymph n.
right hilar lymph n.
Rosenmüller n.
Rotter n.
Rouvière n.
SA n.
sacral lymph n.
satellite n.
scalene n.
Schmorl n.
sentinel lymph n. (SLN)
sick sinus n.
sigmoid lymph n.
signal n.
singer's n.
sinoauricular n.
sinuatrial n. (SAN)
sinus n.
Sister Mary Joseph n.
solitary lymph n.
spinal accessory lymph n.
splenic lymph n.
subcarinal lymph n.
subcentimeter n.
submandibular lymph n.
submental lymph n.
subpyloric n.
subscapular lymph n.
superficial inguinal lymph n.
supraclavicular lymph n.
suprapyloric n.
supratrochlear n.
syphilitic n.
Tawara atrioventricular n.
thyroid lymph n.
tibial n.
tracheal lymph n.
tracheobronchial lymph n.
Troisier n.
tumor-bearing lymph n.
vesicular lymph n.
vestigial left sinuatrial n.
Virchow sentinel n.

Virchow-Troisier n.
visceral lymph n.
node-negative carcinoma
node-positive carcinoma
nodosa
periarteritis n.
polyarteritis n. (PAN, PN)
salpingitis isthmica n.
nodoventricular
n. bypass fiber
n. pathway
n. tachycardia
nodular
n. adrenal hyperplasia
n. aneurysm
n. appearance
n. density
n. enhancement
n. goiter
n. hyperintense focus
n. induration of temporal artery
n. irregularity
n. lesion
n. liver
n. liver regeneration
n. lung disease
n. lymphoid hyperplasia
n. mass
n. obstruction
n. opacity
n. pattern
n. proliferation
n. pulmonary parenchymatous
opacity
n. regenerative hyperplasia (NRH)
n. sclerosis Hodgkin disease
n. subepidermal fibrosis
n. synovitis
n. thyroid disease
nodularity
calcified n.
coarse n.
lung n.
noncalcified n.
pulmonary n.
surface n.
tendon n.
vein n.
nodulation
mural n.
nodule
acinar n.
adenomatous n.
airspace n.
Albini n.
aortic valve n.
Arantius n.
Aschoff n.
autonomous thyroid n. (ATN)

Bianchi n.
calcified lung n.
Caplan n.
cartilaginous n.
cavitating lung n.
centrilobular n.
cerebral n.
circumscribed n.
cirrhotic n.
coalescent n.
colloid n.
conglomerate pulmonary n.
cortical n.
Cruveilhier n.
cutaneous n.
Dalen-Fuchs n.
discordant thyroid n.
discrete pulmonary n.
dysplastic liver n.
eccentric enhancing n.
echogenic n.
enhancing n.
esophageal mucosal n.
fibrocartilaginous n.
fibrous n.
fluffy pulmonary n.
Fränkel typhus n.
functioning n.
Gamna n.
Gamna-Gandy n.
Gaucher n.
glial n.
ground-glass n.
n. halo
hemorrhagic lung n.
heterotopic n.
hot pulmonary n.
hyperechoic renal n.
hyperfunctioning thyroid n.
hypermetabolic n
hypointense n.
interstitial n.
intrapulmonary n.
intrasplenic n.
kaolin lung n.
Kerckring n.
Koeppe n.
laryngeal n.
lingular n.
Lisch n.
lung n.
meningothelial-like n.
miliary n.
Morgagni n.
mucosal esophageal n.
multiple lung n.'s
multiple pulmonary necrobiotic n.'s
mural CNS n.
necrobiotic n.

N

nodule (*continued*)
    noncavitary n.
    nondelineated n.
    nonenhancing n.
    nonfunctioning thyroid n.
    ossific n.
    peripheral n.
    pleura-based lung n.
    pleural n.
    pneumoconiotic n.
    prostatic hyperplastic n.
    pulmonary n.
    regenerative liver n.
    rheumatoid n.
    Rokitansky n.
    satellite n.
    Scheuermann n.
    Schmorl n.
    semiautonomous n.
    shaggy lung n.
    silicotic n.
    singer's n.
    Sister Mary Joseph n.
    solitary metastatic lung n.
    solitary pulmonary n. (SPN)
    solitary pulmonary necrobiotic n.
    subcutaneous n.
    subpleural n.
    surfer's n.
    tendon n.
    thyroid adenoma n.
    thyroid colloid n.
    tobacco n.
    toxic n.
    toxic autonomous n.
    tuberculous n.
    typhoid n.
    typhus n.
    warm n.
nodule-in-nodule
    n.-i.-n. appearance
    n.-i.-n. liver
noduli (*pl. of* nodulus)
nodulus, *pl.* **noduli**
nodus arcus venae azygos
nofetumomab diagnostic imaging agent
noire
    atrophie n.
noise
    digitalization n.
    echogenic n.
    n. effective count (NEC)
    n. equivalent quantum
    gaussian n.
    gradient switching n.
    image n.
    lesion-to-cerebrospinal fluid n.
    lesion-to-white matter n.
    pixel n.

    quantum n.
    radiographic n.
    Rayleigh n.
    n. reconstruction kernel
    n. spike artifact
    statistical n.
    structured n.
    subtractive n.
    systematic n.
    thermal n.
    total image n.
Nölke position
NOMI
    nonocclusive mesenteric ischemia
nomifensine
nominal
    n. single dose
    n. standard dose
nomogram
nomosSTAT serial tomotherapy
nonablative heating
nonaccelerated MRI
nonaccidental injury
nonalcoholic steatohepatitis (NASH)
nonanaplastic glioma
nonaneurysmal perimesencephalic subarachnoid hemorrhage
nonarrhythmic myocardial infarct
nonarticular radial head fracture
nonatherosclerotic disease
nonattenuation-corrected
    n.-c. image
    n.-c. slice
    n.-c. SPECT imaging
nonavid infarct imaging
nonaxial beam technique
nonbony union
noncalcareous renal calculus
noncalcified
    n. carcinoma
    n. coronary stenosis
    n. fibroadenoma
    n. mitral leaflet
    n. nodularity
    n. nodular mass
    n. ocular process
noncardiac
    n. angiography
    n. pulmonary edema
noncardiogenic pulmonary edema
noncaseating
    n. granuloma
    n. tubercle
noncavitary
    n. nodule
    n. tuberculoma
nonchromaffin paraganglioma
noncircularity degree

noncirrhotic
    n. liver
    n. portal fibrosis (NCPF)
nonclassifiable interstitial pneumonia
noncleaved cell lymphoma
non-CNS PNET
noncoaxial catheter tip position
noncoiled umbilical cord
noncollagenous pneumoconiosis
noncollinear direction
noncolonic structure
noncommitted mode
noncommunicating
    n. cyst
    n. hydrocephalus
noncompaction
    left ventricular n.
noncompliant plaque
noncontact imaging technology
noncontiguous
    n. expiratory HRCT
    n. fracture
noncontractile scar tissue
noncontrast
    n. CT scan
    n. head CT (NCCT)
    n. phase (NCP)
noncontrast-enhanced angiography
noncoplanar
    n. arc technique
    n. beam technique
    n. therapy beam
noncoronary
    n. cusp
    n. sinus
noncritical
    n. soft tissue
    n. stenosis
noncytotoxic drug
nondeciduate placenta
nondecremental
nondelineated nodule
nondependent lung
nondetachable
    n. balloon
    n. balloon catheter
nondilated system
nondisplaced fracture
nondissociative instability
nondominant
    n. hemisphere lesion
    n. putaminal hemorrhage
    n. vessel
nondynamometric trunk strength measurement
non-ECG-assisted multidetector row CT
nonechogenic tumor
nonembolic infarct

nonenclosed magnet
nonenhanced
    n. computed tomography (NECT)
    n. CT
    n. CT scan
nonenhancing
    n. lesion
    n. nodule
nonepithelial parenchymal malignancy
nonesterified
    n. fatty acid (NEFA)
    n. fatty acid scintigraphy
nonexpansile
    n. multilocular bone lesion
    n. osteolysis
    n. unilocular bone lesion
    n. well-demarcated multilocular bone defect
    n. well-demarcated unilocular bone defect
nonfamilial intestinal pseudoobstruction
nonferromagnetic
    n. needle
    n. positioning device
nonferrous material
nonfetal
    n. complication
    n. uterine condition
nonfilarial chylocele
nonfilling venous segment
nonflow-compensated sequence
nonforeshortened angiographic view
nonfunctional extraadrenal paraganglioma
nonfunctioning
    n. gallbladder
    n. heart valve
    n. islet cell tumor
    n. kidney
    n. parathyroid cyst
    n. pituitary adenoma
    n. thyroid nodule
nonfusion of cranial suture
nongangrenous cholecystitis
nongated CT scan
nonglial brain tumor
nongranular leukocyte
nonhemorrhagic
    n. infarct
    n. ischemia
    n. mass
non-Hodgkin lymphoma (NHL)
nonhomogeneous
    n. consolidation
    n. enhancement
    n. hyperdense mass
nonhyperfunctioning adrenal adenoma
nonhypoxic ischemic encephalopathy
nonidiosyncratic anaphylactoid reaction

N

nonimmune
    n. fetal hydrops
    n. hydrops fetalis
noninducible tachycardia
noninfarcted
    n. myocardium
    n. segment
noninfarct zone
noninflammatory joint effusion
noninvasive
    n. angiogram
    n. aspergillosis
    n. imaging
    n. imaging study
    n. lesion
    n. programmed electrical stimulation (NIPS)
    n. technique
    n. thermometry
    n. thymoma
    n. ultrasound
    n. vascular assessment
nonionic
    n. contrast material
    n. dimer contrast medium
    n. iodinated contrast agent
    n. paramagnetic contrast imaging agent
    n. triiodinated monomer
    n. water-soluble contrast medium
nonionizing radiation
nonischemic congestive cardiomyopathy
nonisotropic gradient
nonketotic hyperosmolar coma
nonlethal
    n. dwarfism
    n. dysplasia
    n. myocardial ischemic injury
nonlinear
    n. excitation profile
    n. sampling
nonlinearity
nonlingular
    n. branch
    n. branch of upper lobe bronchus
nonlocalized ischemia
nonmagnetization transfer gradient-refocused echo image
nonmagnified
    n. image
    n. mammography
nonmeningiomatous malignant lesion
nonmetastasizing fibrosarcoma
nonmotile leukocyte
nonmucinous adenocarcinoma
Nonne-Milroy lymphedema
nonneoplastic
    n. cyst

    n. lesion
    n. tumor
nonnephrotoxic contrast agent
nonnipple sector
nonnodular
    n. fibrosis
    n. silicosis
nonnucleoside reverse transcriptase inhibitor
nonobstructive
    n. atelectasis
    n. cardiomyopathy
    n. hydrocephalus
    n. ileus
nonocclusive
    n. mesenteric arterial insufficiency
    n. mesenteric ischemia (NOMI)
nonodontogenic
nonolfactory cortex
nononcogenic
nonopaque
    n. calculus
    n. intraluminal mass
    n. stone
nonorthogonal plane
nonoscillatory motion
nonossifying fibroma
nonosteogenic fibroma
nonpalpable breast lesion
nonperfused myocardium
nonphysial fracture
nonplanar
    n. configuration
    n. slice
nonpolar crevice
nonpregnant horn of bicornuate uterus
nonproductive cough
nonprogessor
    long-term n.
nonproliferative lesion
nonproton MRI
nonpulsatile abdominal mass
nonpyogenic infection
nonradiopaque
    n. foreign body
    n. stone
nonreplantable amputation
nonresonance Raman spectroscopy
nonrheumatic
    n. aortic insufficiency
    n. valvular aortic stenosis
nonrhizomelic chondrodysplasia punctata
non-rib-bearing vertebra
nonrotational burst fracture
nonrotation of bowel loop
nonsecretor
nonsecretory
    n. multiple myeloma
    n. myelomatosis

nonsegmental area of opacification
nonselective
    n. angiography
    n. pulse
nonseminomatous testicular germ cell tumor
nonseptate
nonseptic embolic brain infarct
non-skin-sparing mastectomy (non-SSM)
non-small-cell
    n.-s.-c. carcinoma (NSCC)
    n.-s.-c. lung carcinoma (NSCLC)
nonspecific
    n. accumulation
    n. bowel gas pattern
    n. change
    n. conglomerate
    n. esophageal motility disorder (NEMD)
    n. finding
    n. granulomatous lymphadenitis
    n. interstitial pneumonia (NIP, NSIP)
    n. lymphocytic thyroiditis
    n. punctate white matter lesion
non-SSM
    non-skin-sparing mastectomy
nonstanding lateral oblique view
nonstress
    n. fetal test
    n. test (NST)
nonstriated muscle
nonsubperiosteal cortical defect
nonsubtracted image
nonsubtraction
    n. image
    n. imaging
nonsuppurative
    n. ascending cholangitis
    n. destructive cholangitis
nonsurgical ablative therapy
nonsyndromic
    n. bicoronal synostosis
    n. focal cerebellar dysplasia
    n. unicoronal synostosis
nontarget embolization
nonteratomatous ovarian cyst
nonthromboembolic
    n. condition
    n. pulmonary disease
nonthrombogenic
nonthrombotic pulmonary embolism
nontoxic goiter
nontrabeculated atrium
nontransmural
    n. match
    n. myocardial infarct
nontraumatic
    n. avascular necrosis

    n. DCO
    n. epidural hemorrhage
    n. rhabdomyolysis
nontriggered phase-contrast MR angiography
nontuberculous *Mycobacterium*
nontumoral hemorrhage
nontumor-involved node
nontumorous lesion
nontunneled catheter
nonuniform
    n. attenuation
    n. excitation
    n. rotational defect (NURD)
nonuniformity
nonunion
    atrophic n.
    bony n.
    fibrous n.
    fracture n.
    hypertrophic n.
    n. of fracture fragments
    torsion wedge n.
nonunited fracture
nonvalved conduit
nonvascular intervention
nonviable
    n. fetus
    n. gestation
    n. scar
    n. tissue
nonviral vector
nonvisualization
    n. of fetal stomach
    n. of gallbladder
    n. of spleen
nonweightbearing view
Noonan syndrome
noose keyhole pull-away sign
no-reflow phenomenon
Norland
    N. bone densitometry
    N. pQCT XCT2000 scanner
    N. XR26 bone densitometer
normal
    n. anatomic position
    n. anatomic variation
    n. anteroposterior view
    n. axis
    n. bladder caliber
    borderline n.
    n. calcification
    n. chest film
    n. echogenicity
    n. fold urethrogram
    n. gestation
    n. hemodynamic liver parameter
    high n.
    n. lordotic curve

normal (*continued*)
    low n.
    n. lower esophageal sphincter resting pressure
    n. male sex chromosome (XY)
    morphologically n.
    n. ossification
    n. ovarian surface epithelium (NOSE)
    n. perfusion pressure breakthrough
    n. planar MR anatomy
    n. range
    n. renal parenchyma
    n. sinus rhythm
    n. spleen weight
    upper limits of n.
    n. variant
    n. variant fluorodeoxyglucose uptake distribution
    n. variant of Ga-67 uptake
    n. whole-body fluorodeoxyglucose distribution
normal-appearing
    n.-a. bronchus
    n.-a. white matter (NAWM)
normal-caliber
    n.-c. bowel
    n.-c. duct
normalization
    interictal n.
    spatial n.
normalized
    n. average glandular dose
    n. cross-section
    n. plateau slope
    n. to plasma activity
normal-pressure hydrocephalus
normal-region pixel
normochromia
normoglycemia
normotensive hydrocephalus
normoxia
Norrie disease
North American Symptomatic Carotid Artery Endarterectomy Trial
NOS
    not otherwise specified
nose
    anteater n.
    beak-shaped n.
    external n.
    n. ring artifact
NOSE
    normal ovarian surface epithelium
nose-chin position
nose-forehead position
notable cerebral insult
notch
    anacrotic n.

    angular n.
    antegonial n.
    aortic n.
    apical n.
    auricular n.
    cardiac n.
    cerebellar n.
    clavicular n.
    coracoid n.
    costal n.
    craniofacial n.
    dicrotic n.
    digastric n.
    ethmoidal n.
    fibular n.
    Frankfort mandibular n.
    n. from gastric sling fiber
    frontal n.
    greater sciatic n.
    greater sigmoid n.
    interclavicular n.
    intercondylar n.
    interpeduncular n.
    intervertebral n.
    lateral femoral n.
    lesser sciatic n.
    lucent hilar n.
    n. projection
    radial sigmoid n.
    sacrosciatic n.
    scapular n.
    sciatic n.
    semilunar n.
    septal n.
    sigmoid n.
    spinoglenoid n.
    splenic n.
    sternal n.
    suprasternal n.
    trochlear n.
    ulnar n.
    n. view
notched
    n. aortic knob
    n. vertebra
notching
    cortical n.
    n. of pulmonic valve
    pelvic n.
    rib n.
    n. ureter
    ureteral n.
Nothnagel syndrome
no-threshold
    n.-t. body
    n.-t. concept
notochordal
    n. canal
    n. process

notochord remnant
not otherwise specified (NOS)
Novacor left ventricular assist system
Novadaq SPY intraoperative imaging
  system
NovaLine Litho-S DUV excimer
  laser
Novalis radiosurgery system
NovaPulse CO_2 laser
novel agent
Novopaque
Novus Medical Image Card
nozzle effect
^{59}Np, Np-59
  neptunium 59
NPC
  nasopharyngeal carcinoma
NPV
  negative predictive value
NRH
  nodular regenerative hyperplasia
NRPB
  National Radiological Protection
  Board
NSA
  neck-shaft angle
  number of signals averaged
    NSA of femur
NSCC
  non-small-cell carcinoma
NSCLC
  non-small-cell lung carcinoma
NSED
  Namaqualand spondyloepiphysial
  dysplasia
N-shaped sigmoid loop
NSIP
  nonspecific interstitial pneumonia
NST
  nonstress test
NT
  nuchal translucency
NTD
  neural tube defect
NTHI
  native tissue harmonic imaging
NTP
  nucleoside triphosphate
nuchae
    ligamentum n.
nuchal
    n. cord
    n. cyst
    n. ligament
    n. plane
    n. rigidity
    n. skin thickening
    n. translucency (NT)
nuchofrontal projection

Nuck
    N. canal
    N. diverticulum
nuclear
    n. aggregation
    n. angiography
    n. anular differentiation
    n. atom
    n. bone imaging
    n. cardiovascular imaging
    n. chemistry
    n. decay
    n. disintegration
    n. electric quadripole relaxation
    n. emulsion
    n. enema
    n. energy
    n. fission
    n. force
    n. fusion
    n. gated blood pool imaging
    n. gated blood pool testing
    n. genome
    n. hepatobiliary imaging
    n. herniation
    n. magnetic LipoProfile device
    n. magnetic moment
    n. magnetic resonance (NMR)
    n. magnetic resonance Fourier
    transform
    n. magnetic resonance image
    n. magnetic resonance imaging
    n. magnetic resonance phantom
    n. magnetic resonance relaxation
    rate enhancement
    n. magnetic resonance scan
    n. magnetic resonance scanning
    sequence
    n. magnetic resonance signal
    intensity
    n. magnetic resonance spectography
    n. magnetic resonance spectral
    parameter
    n. magnetic resonance spectrometer
    n. magnetic resonance spectroscopy
    n. magnetic resonance spectrum
    n. magnetic resonance tomography
    n. magnetism
    n. matrix
    n. matrix protein
    n. medicine
    n. medicine camera
    n. medicine imaging
    n. medicine information system
    n medicine technologist
    n. Overhauser effect
    n. particle
    n. perfusion imaging
    n. pleomorphism

N

nuclear (*continued*)
    n. polarization
    n. probe
    n. pulse amplifier
    n. reaction
    n. reactor
    N. Regulatory Commission
    n. renal scintigraphy
    n. scanner
    n. scanning
    n. signal
    n. spin
    n. spin quantum number
    n. structure
nuclear-to-cytoplasmic ratio (N/C)
nuclei (*pl. of* nucleus)
nucleide
nucleiform, nucleoid
nucleography
nucleoid (*var. of* nucleiform)
nucleon number
nucleoside
    n. diphosphate kinase (NDP-K)
    n. phosphonate
    n. triphosphate (NTP)
nucleotide scan
Nucletron
    N. applicator
    N. MicroSelectron/LDR remote afterloader
nucleus, *pl.* **nuclei,** *pl.* **nucleuses**
    n. ambiguus lesion
    arcuate n.
    basal n.
    n. basalis lesion
    caudate n.
    cranial n.
    dentate n.
    dorsomedial n.
    head of caudate n.
    inferior syndrome of red n.
    Köllicker n.
    lenticular n.
    lentiform n.
    magnetic n.
    motor n.
    neutron-deficient n.
    oculomotor-trochlear n.
    n. of Cajal
    n. of Darkschewitsch
    n. of solitary tract
    ossific n.
    parafascicular n.
    pretectal n.
    n. pulposus herniation
    quadripolar n.
    residual n.
    sensory n.
    6th n.
    ventral cochlear n.
nucleuses (*pl. of* nucleus)
nuclide
    n. analysis
    daughter n.
    n. generator
    isobar n.
    isomer n.
    isotone n.
    isotope n.
    parent n.
    radioactive n.
NUG
    necrotizing ulcerative gingivitis
nulled
nulling
    gradient moment n. (GMN)
null point
NuLytely bowel preparation
number
    average gradient n.
    body atomic n.
    clonogen n.
    CT n.
    effective atomic n.
    Euler n.
    Hounsfield n.
    Huckman n.
    imaginary n.
    mass n.
    neutron n.
    nuclear spin quantum n.
    nucleon n.
    n. of excitations (NEX)
    n. of signals averaged (NSA)
    n. profile
    quantum n.
    Reynolds n. (R_e, Re)
    S n.
    spin quantum n.
numerary renal anomaly
nummular pneumonia
NURD
    nonuniform rotational defect
Nurick
    N. classification of spondylosis
    N. spondylosis classification
nursemaid's elbow
nutation
    n. angle
    n. angle measurement
nutcracker
    n. esophagus
    n. fracture
    n. phenomenon
    n. syndrome

nutmeg appearance of liver
nutrient
    n. artery growth
    n. artery of femur
    n. artery of fibula
    n. foramen
Nutriflex tube
nutrition
    total parenteral n. (TPN)
nutritional
    n. anemia
    n. cirrhosis
Nuvolase 660 laser

NVB
    neurovascular bundle
NYHA
    New York Heart Association
        NYHA congestive heart failure
        classification
nylon
    n. catheter
    liquid n.
Nyquist
    N. criterion
    N. frequency
    N. limit
    N. sampling theorem

N

O_2
oxygen
O_2 consumption index
^{15}O, O-15
oxygen 15
^{16}O, O-16
oxygen 16
^{17}O, O-17
oxygen 17
^{18}O, O-18
oxygen 18
OA
osteoarthritis
OAF
off-axis factor
OAR
off-axis ratio
OAR malleolar rule
O-arm multidimensional surgical imager
oasis
O. thrombectomy catheter
O. thrombectomy system
O. triple-lumen catheter
oat cell carcinoma
OAV
oculoauriculovertebral
object
o. coordinate system
high-density o.
o. modulation
side-by-side o.'s
unidentified bright o. (UBO)
object-based
o.-b. interpolation
o.-b. visualization
object-film distance (OFD)
object-plane blur
oblique
o. angle reconstruction
o. annihilation photon pair
o. axial MR imaging
o. coronal plane
o. diameter
o. film
o. fissure
o. fissure of lung
o. flow misregistration
o. lateral jaw radiograph
o. lateral projection
left anterior o. (LAO)
left posterior o. (LPO)
o. magnetic resonance imaging

mediolateral o. (MLO)
o. muscle
o. pericardial sinus
o. position
o. prescription line
o. radiograph
o. ridge
right anterior o. (RAO)
right posterior o. (RPO)
o. sagittal EKG-gated spin-echo magnetic resonance imaging
o. sagittal sequence
o. slice
o. spiral fracture
superior o.
T2-weighted fast spin-echo coronal o.
o. vein
o. vein of left atrium
o. view
obliquely
o. oriented axon
o. oriented fiber
obliquity
degree of neck o.
Litzmann o.
magnitude of o.
Nägele o.
pelvic o.
Roederer o.
varying degrees of o.
obliquus
vastus medialis o. (VMO)
obliterans
arteriosclerosis o. (ASO)
bronchiolitis o. (BO)
bronchiolitis fibrosa o.
endarteritis o.
mastitis o.
postinfectious bronchiolitis o.
thromboangiitis o.
obliterated costophrenic angle
obliterating endarteritis
obliteration
balloon-occluded transvenous o.
subdeltoid fat plane o.
obliterative
o. arteriosclerosis
o. bronchiolitis
o. cardiomyopathy
o. inflammation
oblongata
medulla o.

O

O'Brien
> O. classification of radial fracture
> O. radial fracture classification

OBS
> organic brain syndrome

obscuration arteriosclerosis

observation
> fluoroscopic o.

observed maximal uptake

observer variation

obstetric, obstetrical
> o. hemorrhage
> o. sonography
> o. ultrasound

obstetrical (*var. of* obstetric)

Obstétrique
> Fédération Internationale de Gynécologie O. (International Federation of Gynecology) (FIGO)

obstipation

obstructed shunt tube

obstructing embolus arteriosclerosis

obstruction
> acute abdominal o.
> adynamic intestinal o.
> airway o.
> aortic arch o.
> aortic outflow o.
> aortic valve o.
> aortoiliac o.
> aqueductal o.
> arachnoid villus o.
> arterial o.
> ball-valve o.
> benign biliary o. (BBO)
> bilateral o.
> bile flow o.
> biliary tract o.
> biliary tree o.
> bladder outlet o.
> bowel o.
> bronchial o.
> bronchiolar o.
> cardiac o.
> catheter o.
> central venous o.
> cerebrospinal fluid o.
> chronic airway o. (CAO)
> closed-loop intestinal o.
> colonic o.
> common bile duct o.
> complete bowel o.
> congenital duodenal o.
> congenital left-sided outflow o.
> congenital pelviureteric junction o.
> congenital subpulmonic o.
> congenital ureteric o.

cystic duct o.
distal common bile duct o.
duct o.
duodenal o.
duodenal-gastric outlet o.
efferent loop o.
ejaculatory duct o.
embolic o.
endobronchial o.
esophageal o.
extrahepatic biliary o.
extrathoracic o.
extrinsic malignant o.
false colonic o.
fecal o.
fetal bowel o.
fetal renal o.
fixed airway o.
fixed coronary o.
flow-dependent o.
food bolus o.
foreign body upper airway o.
functional o.
functional ureteral o.
gastric outlet o.
gastrointestinal tract o.
genital tract outflow o.
hepatic venous outflow o.
high-grade o.
high small bowel o.
hilar o.
hydrocephalic o.
idiopathic o.
ileal o.
iliac vein o.
incomplete o.
increased pulmonary o.
inferior vena cava o.
infravesical o.
intermittent o.
interposed colon segment o.
intestinal o.
intrapancreatic o.
intrathoracic upper airway o.
intraventricular o.
intravesical o.
irreversible airway o.
jejunal o.
large bowel o. (LBO)
left ventricular inflow tract o.
left ventricular outflow tract o. (LVOTO)
low small bowel o.
lymphatic o.
malignant airway o.
mammary duct o.
mechanical biliary o.
mechanical duct o.
mechanical extrahepatic o.

mechanical intestinal o.
mechanical respiratory tract o.
mechanical small bowel o.
Monro o.
nasolacrimal drainage system o.
  (NDSO)
neurogenic intestinal o.
nodular o.
otic o.
outflow o.
outlet o.
pancreatic duct o.
paralytic colonic o.
partial small bowel o.
pelvic venous o.
porta hepatis o.
posttransplantation ureteric o.
posttuberculous o.
postural ureteric o.
preocclusive o.
primary acquired nasolacrimal
  duct o. (PANDO)
prostatic o.
pulmonary artery o.
pulmonary outflow o.
pulmonary vascular o.
pulmonary venous o. (PVO)
pyloric outlet o.
pyloroduodenal o.
rectal o.
renal o.
respiratory tract o.
right ventricular outflow o.
Rigler triad of small bowel o.
secondary o.
segmental biliary o.
sequence o.
simple mechanical o.
small bowel o. (SBO)
strangulated o.
strangulating o.
subclavian artery o.
subpulmonic o.
subrectus o.
subvalvular aortic o.
subvalvular diffuse muscular o.
superior vena cava o. (SVCO)
suprapancreatic o.
supravesical o.
thrombotic o.
transient shunt o.
tubal o.
UPJ o.
upper airway o.
ureteral renal transplant o.
ureteropelvic junction o.
ureterovesical junction o.
urethral o.
urinary o.

urinary tract o.
vascular o.
venous outflow o.
ventricular o.
vesical outlet o.

obstructive
  o. abnormality
  o. airway disease
  o. arterial disease
  o. atelectasis
  o. biliary cirrhosis
  o. calculus
  o. component
  o. dysfunctional ileitis
  o. emphysema
  o. hydrocephalus
  o. hypertrophic cardiomyopathy
  o. hypopnea
  o. lesion
  o. lung disease
  o. nephrogram
  o. nephropathy
  o. pancreatitis
  o. plaque
  o. pneumonia
  o. pulmonary arterial hypertension
  o. pulmonary disease (OPD)
  o. pulmonary overinflation
  o. renal dysplasia
  o. shock
  o. thrombus
  o. uropathy
  o. ventilatory defect

obtundation
obturating embolus
obturator
  o. avulsion fracture
  o. externus
  o. foramen
  o. hernia
  o. internus
  o. internus fascia
  o. internus muscle
  o. internus tendon
  o. line
  o. lymph node
  o. membrane
  o. nodal chain
  o. sign

obtuse
  o. marginal (OM)
  o. marginal branch (OMB)
  o. marginal coronary
    artery

occipital
  o. artery
  o. bone
  o. bossing
  o. cephalocele

O

occipital (*continued*)
- o. condyle
- o. condyle fracture
- o. condyle hypoplasia
- o. condyle invasion
- o. eminence
- o. encephalocele
- o. fissure
- o. focus
- o. fontanelle
- o. gyrus
- o. horn
- o. hypometabolism
- o. lesion
- o. lobe
- o. lobe infarct
- o. lymph node
- o. meningocele
- o. plane
- o. pole
- o. protuberance
- o. sinus
- o. suture
- o. tip
- o. vessel
- o. view
- o. view of skull

occipitalization
- atlas o.

occipitoanterior

occipitoatlantoaxial
- o. anomaly
- o. fusion
- o. ligament

occipitoaxial, occipitoaxoid
- o. joint
- o. ligament

occipitoaxoid (*var. of* occipitoaxial)

occipitocervical
- o. angle
- o. articulation
- o. fusion
- o. junction
- o. plate

occipitofrontal
- o. diameter (OFD)
- o. fasciculus

occipitofrontalis muscle

occipitomastoid suture

occipitomental
- o. diameter
- o. projection

occipitoparietal
- o. infarct
- o. suture

occipitopontine tract

occipitoposterior

occipitosphenoid suture

occipitotemporal
- o. convolution
- o. gyrus
- o. sulcus

occiput

occluded
- o. compartment
- o. graft
- o. lumen

occluder
- ameroid o.
- CardioSEAL o.
- clamshell double umbrella o.
- Flo-Rester vessel o.
- radiolucent plastic o.
- Rashkind o.

occluding
- o. agent
- o. spring embolus

occlusal
- o. facet
- o. film
- o. plane
- o. radiograph
- o. segment
- o. surface

occlusion
- angiographic o.
- o. angiography
- aqueductal o.
- arterial o.
- atrial septal defect o.
- balloon o.
- balloon test o.
- basilar o.
- bilateral o.
- carotid artery o. (CAO)
- carotid-cavernous fistula o.
- celiac axis o.
- cerebral sinovenous o.
- complete o.
- coronary o.
- deep venous o.
- diathermic vascular o.
- ductus arteriosus o.
- dural sinus o.
- embolic o.
- fallopian tube o.
- graft o.
- infrapopliteal artery o.
- intermittent o.
- internal carotid artery o.
- intracranial vascular o.
- late graft o.
- o. measurement
- mesenteric artery o.
- mesenteric vein o.
- middle cerebral artery o.

o. of artery
parent artery o.
parent vessel o.
percutaneous thermal o.
pulmonary arterial o.
selective test o.
side-branch o.
snowplow o.
subclavian artery o.
subclavian vein o.
subtotal o.
superficial femoral artery o.
tandem ICA/MCA o.
tapering o.
test balloon o.
thermal o.
thrombotic o.
top of carotid T o.
total o.
transrenal ureteric o.
transvenous o.
traumatogenic o.
tubal o.
unilateral o.
ureteral o.
vascular brain o.
vein graft o.
venous o.
vertebral artery o.
vertebrobasilar o.
vertebrobasilar artery o.
vessel o.

occlusive
o. arterial thrombus
o. carotid disease
o. cerebrovascular disease
o. cerebrovascular insult
o. drain
o. dressing
o. ileus
o. impedance phlebography
o. lesion
o. mesenteric infarct

occult
o. blood
o. bone metastasis
o. bronchial carcinoid
o. cerebrovascular malformation (OCVM)
o. detection
o. hydrocephalus
o. intrasacral meningocele
o. lesion
o. lesion of breast
o. osseous fracture
o. osseous injury
o. papillary carcinoma
o. pericardial constriction

o. phosphaturic mesenchymal tumor
o. primary tumor of testis
radiographically o.
o. residual herniated disc
radiographically o.
o. sacral fracture
o. spinal dysraphism
o. subluxation
o. thyroid carcinoma
o. vascular brain malformation

occulta
spina bifida o. (SBO)

occultum
cranium bifidum o.

occupational
o. lung disease
o. nuclear radiation

OCD
osteochondral defect

OCG
oral cholecystogram
OCG imaging

ochronosis

Ochsner muscle

OCL
oral colonic lavage
OCL bowel preparation

O'Connor finger dexterity test

OCR
off-center ratio

OCT
optic coherence tomography

octagonal configuration

Octane postprocessing workstation

OctreoScan
O. 111 radioactive imaging agent
O. system

octreotide
o. imaging
o. imaging agent
^{111}In o.
^{99m}Tc-labeled o.
o. paraganglioma scintigraphy
o. tumor localization scan

ocular
o. adnexa
o. globe topography
o. implant
o. lesion
o. magnification system
o. pneumoplethysmography (OPG)
o. radiation therapy (ORT)
o. rhabdomyosarcoma
o. sarcoidosis
o. trauma

OcuLight SL diode laser

oculoauriculovertebral (OAV)

O

oculocerebrorenal dystrophy
oculomotor apparatus
oculomotor-trochlear
  nucleus
oculopharyngeal dystrophy
oculoplethysmography
  (OPG)
oculoplethysmography/carotid
  phonoangiography (OPG/CPA)
oculopneumoplethysmography
oculosubcutaneous syndrome of
  Yuge
oculosympathetic paresis
OCVM
  occult cerebrovascular
    malformation
odd-echo dephasing
Oddi
  O. muscle
  sphincter of O.
odds ratio
Odelca camera unit
O'Donoghue unhappy
  triad
odontogenic
  o. cyst
  o. fibromyxoma
  o. keratocyst
  o. myxoma
  o. tumor
odontoid
  o. bone
  o. condyle fracture
  o. dysplasia
  o. erosion
  o. fracture (type I-III)
  o. ligament
  pannus deformity of o.
  o. process
  o. vertebra
  o. view
odontoideum
  os o.
odontoma
odontoradiograph
ODQ
  opponens digiti quinti
    ODQ muscle
ODT
  optic Doppler tomography
odynophagia
OEF
  oxygen extraction fraction
Oehl muscle
O₂ER, OER
  oxygen extraction rate
OFD
  object-film distance
  occipitofrontal diameter

off-axis
  o.-a. dose inhomogeneity
  o.-a. factor (OAF)
  o.-a. point localization
  o.-a. ratio (OAR)
  o.-a. rotational acquisition
off-center
  o.-c. cut
  o.-c. modulation
  o.-c. ratio (OCR)
off-lateral projection
off-resonance
  3D rotating delivery of excitation
    o.-r.
  rotating delivery of excitation o.-r.
    (RODEO)
  o.-r. saturation
  o.-r. saturation pulse imaging
  o.-r. spin-locking
off-resonant spin
offset
  chemical-shift spatial o.
  E-zero o.
  o. fan beam
  focal osseous o.
  o. frequency
  quarter-detector o.
  o. radiofrequency spin echo
  resonance o.
Ogden
  O. classification of epiphysial
    fracture
  O. epiphysial fracture
    classification
Ogilvie syndrome
Ogston line
Ohio
  O. infuser
  O. Nuclear Delta 50 FS, 2000
    scanner
Ohm law
Ohngren line
OHP
  orthogonal-hole test pattern
OI
  osteogenesis imperfecta
OIH
  orthoiodohippurate
    iodine-131 OIH
oil
  brominated o.
  chloriodized o.
  o. cyst
  o. embolus
  o. emulsion imaging
    agent
  ethiodized o.
  iodized poppy seed o.
  iophendylate o.

o. myelography
silicone o.
oil-aspiration pneumonia
oil-retention enema (ORE)
oil-soluble contrast medium
(OSCM)
oil-water phantom
oily contrast agent
okadaic acid
Okuda
O. hepatic compromise (stage
I-III)
O. transhepatic obliteration of
varix
old
o. hemorrhage
o. myocardial infarct
olecranon
o. bursa
o. bursitis
o. fossa
o. process
o. tip fracture
oleoperitoneography
oleothorax
Olerud and Molander fracture
classification
olfactoriae
striae o.
olfactory
o. area
o. bulb
o. canal
o. groove meningioma
o. gyrus
o. neuroblastoma
o. sulcus
o. tract
o. tubercle
oligemia
mosaic o.
oligemia-related cyanotic
CHD
oligoastrocytoma
anaplastic mixed o.
recurrent vermian o.
oligodactylia (*var. of* oligodactyly)
oligodactyly, oligodactylia
oligodendroglia
oligodendroglioma
bifrontal o.'s
subependymal o.
oligohydramnios
oligomeganephronia
oligonucleotide
antisense o.
o. probe
radiolabeled antisense o.
olisthesis

olivary
o. degeneration
o. hypertrophy
olive
amiculum of o.
inferior o.
posterior o.
Oliver-Cardarelli sign
olivopontocerebellar
o. atrophy
o. degeneration (OPCD)
Ollier disease
OLM
ophthalmic laser microendoscope
Olshevsky tube
Olympus
O. CF-1T100L colonoscope
O. CF-200Z colonoscope
O. CHF-BP30 transduodenal
choledochofiberscope
O. endoscopic ultrasound
O. endoscopic ultrasound scanner
O. ENF-P2 laryngoscope
O. EU-M30 system
O. EVIS Q-200V endoscope
O. Gastrocamera GTF-A
O. GF-UM2, GF-UM3
echoendoscope
O. GIF-1T10 echoendoscope
O. JF1T10 fiberoptic duodenoscope
O. JF-UM20 echoendoscope
O. MH-908 slim ultrasonic
probe
O. OSF sigmoidoscope
O. SIF-100 video enteroscope
O. S20-20R transendoscopic
ultrasound probe
O. TJF-100 endoscope
O. VU-M2 echoendoscope
O. XIF-UM3 echoendoscope
O. XQ230 gastroscope
OM
obtuse marginal
orbitomeatal
OM artery
OMB
obtuse marginal branch
Omenn syndrome
omenta (*pl. of* omentum)
omental
o. band
o. bursa
o. cake
o. carcinomatosis
o. cyst
o. infarct
o. line
o. mass
o. metastasis

O

omental (*continued*)
   o. smudging
   o. tuberosity
omentoportography
omentum, *pl.* **omenta**
   colic o.
   gastric o.
   gastrocolic o.
   gastrohepatic o.
   gastrosplenic o.
   greater o.
   incarcerated o.
   lesser o.
   o. majus
   o. minus
   pancreaticosplenic o.
   sigmoid o.
   splenogastric o.
Omni
   O. Flex biliary stent
   O. Flush 3F, 4F, 5F catheter
   O. Selective 0-3 catheter
Omnilink/Megalink balloon-expanded stent
Omnipaque
   O. 140, 180, 240, 300, 350 imaging agent
   O. injection
OmniPulse-MAX holmium laser
Omniscan imaging agent
Omniscience valve
Omnisense
   O. multisite QUS device
   O. 7000S bone sonometer
omohyoid muscle
omovertebral bone
omphalic
omphalitis
   neonatal o.
omphalocele
   infraumbilical o.
omphaloma
omphalomesenteric
   o. artery
   o. duct
   o. duct cyst
   o. remnant
omphalopagus twin
onchocerciasis
oncocalyx
oncocytic
   o. papilloma
   o. thyroid adenoma
oncocytoma
   pituitary o.
oncogenesis
   radiation o.
oncogenic osteomalacia

oncologist
   radiation o.
oncology
   picture archiving and communication systems in radiation o.
   radiation o.
on-column preparation
OncoRad OV103
OncoScint
   O. CR103
   O. CR/OV breast imaging agent
   O. OV103
   O. PR
oncosis
OncoTrac
oncotropic
OneStep paracentesis drainage catheter
onionlike laminar structure
onion peel appearance
onion-shaped dilation of duodenum
onionskin
   o. appearance
   o. configuration of collagenous fiber
   o. lesion
   o. periosteal reaction
onlay graft
online
   o. ABG monitor
   o. portal imaging
Onodi cell
on-off phenomenon
onset
on-the-fly random correction
onychoosteodysplasia
   familial o.
Onyx-015 genetically engineered adenovirus
oocyte retrieval
oophorectomy
oophoroma folliculare
oophorus
   cumulus o.
opacification
   arterial o.
   collecting system o.
   contrast o.
   early segmental o.
   extravesical o.
   ground-glass o. (GGO)
   hemithorax o.
   insufficient venous o.
   maxillary sinus o.
   nonsegmental area of o.
   o. of posterior longitudinal ligament
   pedal artery o.
opacified
opacifying
   o. gallstone
   o. injection

opacity
    abnormal lung o.
    airspace o.
    asymmetric lung o.
    basilar reticular o.
    branching centrilobar o.
    bubbly o.
    centrilobar o.
    chronic diffuse confluent lung o.
    chronic multifocal ill-defined
     lung o.
    coarse linear o.
    coarse reticular o.
    conglomerate o.
    dependent o.
    diffuse airspace o.
    generalized hazy o.
    granular o.
    ground-glass o.
    hazy o.
    homogeneous o.
    interstitial o.
    linear o.
    localized pure ground-glass o.
    lung o.
    Medusa hairlike o.
    nodular o.
    nodular pulmonary parenchymatous
     o.
    parenchymatous o.
    patchy alveolar o.
    pleura-based area of increased o.
    o. profusion
    pulmonary o.
    pure ground-glass o. (pGGO)
    reticular o.
    rounded o.
    tree-in-bud o.
    tubular o.
    uterine o.
    whole-lung o.
opaque
    o. arthrography
    o. branching structure
    o. calculus
    o. enema
    o. foreign body
    o. material
    o. meal
    o. mediastinography
    o. medium
    o. myelography
    o. powder
    o. stone
    o. synovium
    o. wire suture
Opart MRI
OPCD
    olivopontocerebellar degeneration

OPD
    obstructive pulmonary disease
**Opdima digital mammography
system**
**OPD-Scan optical path difference
scanning system**
open
    o. beam
    o. bronchus sign
    o. dislocation
    o. fontanelle
    o. fracture
    o. magnet
    o. magnetic resonance defecography
    o. MRI
    o. MRI system
    o. neural tube defect
    o. pneumothorax
    o. reading frame (ORF)
    o. reduction
    o. reduction and internal fixation
     (ORIF)
    o. ring sign
    o. tuberculosis
open-architecture system
open-book fracture
open-break fracture
**open-configuration magnetic resonance
system**
open-cord tendon implant
open-ended guidewire
opening
    aortic o.
    aortic valve o.
    breast cup o.
    buttonhole o.
    caval o.
    esophageal o.
    mitral valve o. (MVO)
    peripherally inserted central catheter
     occlusion line o. (PICCOLO)
    o. slope
    tubal fimbrial o.
    valvular o.
open-mouth
    o.-m. odontoid view
    o.-m. projection
OpenPACS system
opera-glass hand
operating voltage
operation
    3D connect o.
    Doppler o.
    Fontan o.
    Miles o.
    Nissen antireflux o.
    pulsed-mode o.
    Senning o.
    Whipple o.

O

operative
    o. arteriography
    o. cholangiogram
operator-dependent positioning
operator exposure
operator-related difference
opercula (*pl. of* operculum)
opercular
    o. cortex
    o. segment of middle cerebral
      artery
operculofrontal artery
operculum, *pl.* **opercula**
    cerebral o.
    frontal o.
    parietal o.
    sylvian o.
    temporal o.
OPES
    oropharyngoesophageal scintigraphy
OPG
    ocular pneumoplethysmography
    oculoplethysmography
    ophthalmoplethysmography
OPG/CPA
    oculoplethysmography/carotid
      phonoangiography
ophenoxic acid
ophthalmic
    o. artery
    o. biometry by ultrasound
      echography
    o. laser microendoscope (OLM)
    o. nerve
    o. vein
ophthalmopathy
    euthyroid o.
    Graves o.
    thyroid o.
ophthalmoplegia
ophthalmoplethysmography (OPG)
ophthalmoscope
    Panoramic 200 nonmydriatic o.
ophthalmoscopy
    scanning laser o.
opisthion
opisthotonic position
Opitz thrombophlebitic splenomegaly
OPLL
    ossification of posterior longitudinal
      ligament
      thoracic OPLL
Opmilas
    O. CO_2 multipurpose laser
    O. 144 Plus laser system
Oppenheim sign
opponens
    o. digiti minimi
    o. digiti quinti (ODQ)

    o. digiti quinti muscle
    o. pollicis
opportunistic lung cavity infection
opposed
    o. GRE image
    o. loop-pair quadrature NMR coil
opposed-phase
    o.-p. GRE MR imaging
    o.-p. MRI
    o.-p. sequence
    o.-p. T1-weighted image
opposing
    o. articular surfaces
    o. muscles
    o. pleural surfaces
opsonized
Opta
    O. 5 angioplasty balloon
    O. balloon stent-graft
OptEase permanent vena cava filter
optic, optical
    o. alexia
    o. canal
    o. chiasm
    o. chiasm disease
    o. coherence tomography (OCT)
    o. complex tumor
    o. density
    o. Doppler tomography (ODT)
    o. excrescentic thickening
    o. foramen
    o. glioma pathway
    o. globe
    o. glove
    o. isomer
    o. nerve atrophy
    o. nerve compression
    o. nerve drusen
    o. nerve enlargement
    o. nerve fusiform thickening
    o. nerve glioma
    o. nerve hypoplasia
    o. nerve lesion
    o. nerve sheath meningioma
    o. neuritis
    o. neuropathy
    o. papilla
    o. pathway myelination
    o. radiation
    o. recess
    o. strut
    o. surface imaging (OSI)
optica
    neuromyelitis o.
optical (*var. of* optic)
    O. Biopsy System laser
    O. Path Difference-Scan optical
      device
Opticath catheter

opticochiasmatic cistern
Opti-Flow dialysis catheter
optimal
o. angle imaging
o. dose
o. imaging plane
o. modality
o. visualization
optimally positioned view
OptiMARK contrast agent
optimization
acquisition o.
interactive gradient o.
o. parameter
sequence o.
optimum dose
option
postreconstruction filtering o.
optional target-to-background ratio
Optiplanimat automated unit
Optiplast
O. balloon dilation catheter
O. Centurion balloon
OptiQue catheter
Optiray 10, 240, 300, 320, 350 imaging agent
Optison sterile injectable sonography contrast agent
Optispike dispensing pin
Optistar MR contrast delivery system
Optistat power injector
OptiVision laser
optoacoustic imaging
ora, *pl.* **orae** (also *pl. of* os)
Orabilex
oracle
O. McgaSonics catheter
O. Micro Plus catheter
O. PTCA catheter
orae (*pl. of* ora)
Oragrafin
O. calcium imaging agent
O. sodium imaging agent
oral
o. candidiasis
o. cavity tumor
o. cephalocele
o. cholecystogram (OCG)
o. cholecystogram imaging
o. cholecystography
o. colonic lavage (OCL)
o. contrast imaging agent
o. enhanced CT scan
o. fissure
o. intubation
o. magnetic particle
o. part of pharynx
o. radiology
o. urography

orange
acridine o.
orbicular
o. bone
o. ligament
orbicularis
zona o.
orbit
angular process of o.
o. artifact
body contour o.
bony o.
egg-shaped o.
electron o.
floor of o.
o. measurement
Rhese view of o.
orbitae
aditus o.
orbital
o. abscess
o. amyloidosis
o. aneurysm
o. angiography
o. apex
o. apex syndrome
o. aspect of frontal lobe
o. base
o. blood cyst
o. blowout fracture
o. bone
o. canal
o. capillary hemangioma
o. cavity
o. cellulitis
o. childhood tumor
o. chocolate cyst
o. dermoid cyst
o. edema
o. electron
o. emphysema
o. exenteration
o. fissure
o. floor fracture
o. granulocytic sarcoma
o. gyrus
o. infection
o. juvenile pilocytic astrocytoma
o. lymphangioma
o. lymphoma
o. mass compression
o. metastasis
o. mucocele
o. plane
o. plate
o. pseudotumor
o. rhabdomyosarcoma
o. rim
o. rim stepoff

O

orbital (*continued*)
 o. sarcoidosis
 o. schwannoma
 o. space
 o. superolateral quadrant
 mass
 o. teratoma
 o. trauma
 o. varix
 o. varix of ophthalmic vein
 o. wall
orbitofrontal
 o. cortex
 o. dominance
orbitography
orbitomeatal (OM)
 o. line
 o. plane
orbitopathy
 thyroid o.
 thyroid-associated o.
orbitosphenoid bone
orbitotomy
 Krönlein o.
Orbix x-ray unit
Orca C-arm fluoroscopy
orchiditis (*var. of* orchitis)
orchitis, orchiditis
order
 phase-encoding o.
ordered
 o. phase encoding
 o. subset expectation maximum
 (OSEM)
ORE
 oil-retention enema
OR1 electronic system
ORF
 open reading frame
Orfit mask
organ
 accessory o.
 adjacent o.
 anulospiral o.
 o.'s at risk
 o. capsule
 circumventricular o.
 Corti o.
 critical o.
 extraperitoneal o.
 floating o.
 hollow o.
 o. ischemia
 o. piping
 pole of o.
 retroperitoneal o.
 rudimentary o.
 sanctuary o.
 secondary retroperitoneal o.

 target o.
 o. tolerance dose (OTD)
 o. transplant
 Zuckerkandl o.
organ-confined prostate cancer
organelle
 sphere o.
organic
 o. acid disorder
 o. acidemia
 o. anion transporter polypeptide
 o. brain syndrome (OBS)
 o. free radical
 o. granulomatosis
 o. lesion
 o. muscle
 o. nitrate
organification
 o. defect
 o. status
organified radioiodine
organization
 AIDS service o.
organized
 o. hematoma
 o. thrombus
organizer
 embryonic o.
 isthmic o.
organizing
 o. focal pneumonia
 o. interstitial pneumonia
organoaxial
 o. rotation
 o. volvulus
organogenesis
organoid structure
organomegaly
organ-sparing treatment approach
organ-specific
 o.-s. concentration
 o.-s. scintigraphic imaging
Oriental
 O. cholangiohepatitis
 O. lung fluke
orientation
 angle of o.
 axial o.
 coronal o.
 cruciate o.
 disc to magnetic field o.
 disturbed o.
 sagittal o.
 scan o.
 slice o.
 spatial o.
 temporal o.
 transverse o.
 true short-axis o.

ORIF
> open reduction and internal fixation

orifice
> anal o.
> aortic o.
> atrioventricular nodal o.
> cardiac o.
> coronary o.
> double coronary o.
> esophagogastric o.
> external urethral o.
> gastroduodenal o.
> hypoplastic tricuspid o.
> ileocecal o.
> inferior vena cava o.
> internal urethral o.
> lingular o.
> mitral o.
> mitral valve o. (MVO)
> narrowed o.
> pharyngeal o.
> pulmonary o.
> pyloric o.
> rectal o.
> regurgitant o.
> segmental bronchus o.
> slitlike o.
> tricuspid o.
> ureteral o.
> urethral o.
> vaginal o.
> valvular o.

orifice-anulus ratio

origin
> aberrant o.
> anomalous o.
> brown fat o.
> fever of unknown o. (FUO)
> histiocytic bone tumor o.
> neural crest o.
> neuroectodermal o.
> o. of artery
> o. of vessel
> primary tumor of o.
> spatial o.

Ormond disease
orodigitofacial syndrome
oroendotracheal tube
orofacial fistula
orogastric tube
oropharyngeal
> o. airway
> o. dysfunction
> o. dysphagia
> o. emptying
> o. narrowing

oropharyngoesophageal scintigraphy (OPES)
oropharynx

orotracheal intubation
ORT
> ocular radiation therapy

Orthicon
> O. camera
> O. tube

orthocephalic
orthodeoxia
orthodiagram
orthodiagraph
orthodiagraphy
orthodiascopy
orthogonal
> o. angiographic projection
> o. C-arm fluoroscopy
> o. plane
> o. projection mammography
> o. radiofrequency coil
> o. radiograph
> o. tag line
> o. view
> o. view on angiography

orthogonal-hole test pattern (OHP)
orthogonally
orthoiodohippurate (OIH)
> iodine-123 o.
> iodine-131 o.

OrthOne 1-tesla extremity MRI
OrthOneXT dedicated MRI system
orthonormal diameter
orthopaedic, orthopedic
> o. nail
> o. pin
> o. plate
> o. rod
> o. screw
> o. staple

orthopantogram imaging
orthopantograph
orthopantomograph panoramic digital radiography unit
orthopedic (*var. of* orthopaedic)
orthoroentgenogram
orthoroentgenography
orthoscope
orthostatic
> o. back pain
> o. headache

orthostereoscope
orthotic plate
orthotopic
> o. heart transplant
> o. liver transplant
> o. total heart replacement
> o. ureter
> o. ureterocele

orthovoltage
> o. radiation therapy
> o. radiotherapy

O

Ortner syndrome
Ortolani
    O. sign
    O. test
os, *pl.* **ora,** *pl.* **ossa (bone)**
    o. acetabulum
    o. acromiale
    o. calcis
    o. calcis bone
    coronary sinus o.
    o. coxae
    o. cuboides secondarium
    external o.
    o. fabella
    o. infundibulum
    internal cervical o.
    o. naviculare
    o. odontoideum
    o. peroneum
    o. peroneum syndrome
    o. pubis
    o. styloideum
    o. supranaviculare
    o. supratrochleare dorsale
    o. sustentaculum
    o. terminale
    o. tibiale externum
    o. trigonum
    o. trigonum syndrome
Osborne ligament
Oscar ultrasonic bone cement removal system
oscillating
    o. Bucky
    o. electron
    o. gradient
    o. grid
    o. magnetic field
oscillation
    resonant frequency of o.
oscillatory shear rate
oscillography
oscilloscope
    cathode ray o. (CRO)
    o. tuning station
OSCM
    oil-soluble contrast medium
OSEM
    ordered subset expectation maximum
Osgood-Schlatter disease
O shell
OSI
    optic surface imaging
Osler
    O. disease
    O. maneuver
    O. node
    O. sign
    O. triad

Osler-Libman-Sacks syndrome
Osler-Weber-Rendu
    O.-W.-R. syndrome
    O.-W.-R. telangiectasia
Osm
    osmole
osmium
osmolality
    low o.
osmole (Osm)
osmotic
    o. edema
    o. effect
    o. gradient
    o. load
ossa (*pl. of* os)
ossea
    facies o.
    leontiasis o.
ossei
    globuli o.
    vertex cranii o.
osseocartilaginous
    o. arch
    o. thoracic cage
osseoligamentous arch
osseous, osteal
    o. abnormality
    o. activity
    o. and soft tissue sarcomas (OSTS)
    o. bone contusion
    o. bridge
    o. cervical spine injury
    o. coalition
    o. defect
    o. destructive process
    o. dysplasia
    o. graft
    o. hemangioendothelioma
    o. hemangioma
    o. hydatidosis
    o. instability
    o. labrum
    o. labyrinth
    o. lacuna
    o. lesion
    o. lymphoma
    o. metaplasia
    o. metastasis
    o. metastatic disease
    o. patellar outgrowth
    o. pinch mechanism
    o. polyp
    o. rarefaction
    o. remodeling
    o. spiral lamina
    o. structure
    o. survey

o. trauma
o. tumor of soft tissue
o. union

ossicle
accessory o.
Kerckring o.
meniscal o.
Riolan o.

ossiferous

ossific
o. nodule
o. nucleus
o. nucleus of navicular

ossificans
fasciitis o.
labyrinthitis o.
panniculitis o.
pseudomalignant myositis o.
subacute myositis o.

ossification
abnormal o.
o. center
diaphysial o.
diffuse pulmonary o.
disc o.
dural o.
ectopic o.
enchondral o.
extraarticular posterior o.
flowing anterior vertebra o.
heterotopic scar o.
intracartilaginous o.
intramembranous o.
irregular enchondral o.
joint-restricting o.
muscle o.
normal o.
o. of cartilaginous structure
o. of posterior longitudinal ligament (OPLL)
paravertebral o.
periarticular heterotopic o. (PHO)
peripheral o.
primary center of o.
scar o.
secondary center of o.
soft tissue o.
spine o.
unilateral o.
o. variant
vertebral arch ligament o.

ossified
o. body
o. cartilage
o. lesion
o. posterior longitudinal ligament
o. scar

ossiform

ossifying
o. bone fibroma
o. cochleitis
o. epiphysis
o. ischiopubic synchondrosis
o. skull fibroma

ossium
fibrogenesis imperfecta o.
fragilitas o.

osteal (*var. of* osseous)

osteitis, ostitis
o. condensans ilii
o. deformans
diffuse periapical sclerosing o.
o. fibrosa circumscripta
o. fibrosa cystica
o. fibrosa disseminata
o. pubis
radiation o.
septic cortical o.

ostemia

ostempyesis

OsteoAnalyzer bone densitometry device

osteoarthritic
o. cartilage
o. change
o. spur

osteoarthritis (OA)
degenerative o.
early o.
erosive o.
facet o.
generalized o.
o. grade
o. grading classification
hand o.
inflammatory o.
interphalangeal o.
posttraumatic o.
premature o.
traumatic o.

osteoarthropathy
hypertrophic pulmonary o.
neuropathic o.
primary hypertrophic o.
pulmonary o.
pulmonary hypertrophic o. (PHOA)

osteoarthrosis

osteoarticular

osteoblastic
o. activity
o. bone regeneration
o. lesion
o. metastasis
o. osteosarcoma
o. presentation
o. reaction
o. tumor

O

osteoblastoma
    benign o.
    expansile o.
osteocartilaginous
    o. defect
    o. exostosis
    o. lesion
    o. metaplasia
    o. parasellar neoplasia
    o. spur
    o. tissue
    o. tumor
osteochondral
    o. defect (OCD)
    o. fracture fragment
    o. injury
    o. lesion
    o. lesion of talus
    o. loose body
    o. separation of epiphysis
    o. slice fracture
osteochondritis dissecans
osteochondrodysplasia
osteochondrodystrophia deformans
osteochondrodystrophy
osteochondrofibroma
osteochondrolysis
osteochondroma
    benign o.
    coat hanger o.
    epiphysial o.
    soft tissue o.
    solitary o.
osteochondromatosis
    bursal o.
    multiple o.
    synovial o.
    tenosynovial o.
    tumefactive synovial o.
osteochondromyxoma
osteochondrophyte
osteochondroplastica
    tracheobronchopathia o.
    tracheopathia o.
osteochondrosarcoma
osteochondrosis
    o. deformans juvenilis
    o. dissecans
    intervertebral o.
    spinal o.
    vertebral o.
osteoclasia (*var. of* osteoclasis)
osteoclasis, osteoclasia
osteoclastic
    o. erosion
    o. resorption
osteoclast-mediated bone resorption
osteoclastoma

osteocondensation
osteoconductive polymer
osteocyte
osteocytoma
osteodentin
osteodermia
osteodermopathia hypertrophicans
osteodiastasis
osteodystrophia (*var. of* osteodystrophy)
    o. fibrosa
osteodystrophy, osteodystrophia
    Albright hereditary o.
    azotemic o.
    congenital renal o.
    fibrous o.
    renal o.
osteoenchondroma
osteofibroma
osteofibromatosis
    cystic o.
osteofibrous dysplasia
osteogenesis
    distraction o.
    o. imperfecta (OI)
    o. imperfecta tarda
osteogenetic (*var. of* osteogenic)
osteogenic, osteogenetic
    o. bone fibroma
    o. metastasis
    o. sarcoma
Osteo-Gram bone density test
osteoid
    calcified o.
    o. carcinoma
    o. formation
    malignant o.
    o. matrix
    o. osteoma
    o. seam
    tumor o.
osteoid-origin tumor
osteolipochondroma
osteolipoma
osteolucency
osteolysis
    blade-of-grass o.
    candle-flame o.
    carpotarsal o.
    distal clavicle o. (DCO)
    essential o.
    expansile o.
    idiopathic multicentric o.
    lytic o.
    malignant acetabular o.
    mandible o.
    massive o.
    medial end of clavicle o.
    mixed sclerotic o.

multiple o.
nonexpansile o.
o. on both sides of joint
periprosthetic o.
sacral o.
scalloping o.
skull o.
temporomandibular joint o.
trabeculated o.
o. tuft
unilocular o.

osteolytic

o. lesion
o. osseous metastasis

osteoma

cancellous osteoid o.
choroidal o.
compact o.
cortical osteoid o.
costal o.
o. cutis
o. durum
o. eburncum
fibrous o.
giant osteoid o.
intracapsular osteoid o.
ivory o.
juxtaarticular osteoid o.
o. medullare
osteoid o.
parosteal o.
peripheral o.
soft tissue o.
o. spongiosum
spongy o.
subperiosteal osteoid o.
trabecular o.
tropical ulcer o.
ulcer o.

osteomalacia

axial o.
hematogenous o.
hypophosphatemic o.
oncogenic o.
renal tubular o.
senile o.
tumor-induced o.

osteomalacic pelvis
osteomatoid
osteomatosis
osteomesopyknosis
osteomyelitic sinus
osteomyelitis

Ackerman criteria for o.
active o.
acute hematogenous o. (AHO)
bacterial o.
brucellar o.

caseous granulomatous o.
central vertebral o.
childhood o.
chronic recurrent multifocal o.
 (CRMO)
chronic sclerosing o.
cystic tuberculous o.
discovertebral o.
early o.
Garré sclerosing o.
neonatal o.
nocardial o.
puncture wound o.
pyogenic o.
recurrent multifocal o.
rib o.
sacral o.
Salmonella vertebral o.
o. scintigraphy
sclerosing nonsuppurative o.
sneaker o.
spinal o.
subligamentous vertebral o.
synovitis, acne, pustulosis,
 hyperostosis, o. (SAPHO)
tuberculous o.
vertebral o.

osteomyelofibrosis
osteomyelography
osteonal bone
osteonecrosis

bisphosphonate-related o.
idiopathic o.
radiation o.
spontaneous o.
steroid-induced o.

osteopathia (*var. of* ostcopathy)

o. condensans disseminata
o. striata

osteopathy, osteopathia
osteopenia

localized o.

osteopenic bone
osteopetrosis

autosomal dominant benign form
 of o.
cranial o.
malignant o.

osteophyte

anterior o.
bony o.
bridging o.
cervical o.
discogenic o.
floating o.
o. formation
fringe of o.
horseshoe o.

O

osteophyte (*continued*)
    impinging o.
    jagged o.
    marginal o.
    posterior o.
    spinal o.
osteophytic
    o. bone lip
    o. bridge
    o. defect
    o. lipping
    o. proliferation
    o. spurring
osteophytosis in fluorosis
osteoplastica
    tracheopathia o.
osteoplastic flap
osteoplasty
    anterolateral o.
    minimally invasive o.
    percutaneous o.
osteopoikilosis
osteoporosis
    aggressive o.
    o. circumscripta
    o. circumscripta cranii
    corticosteroid-induced o.
    disuse o.
    ground-glass o.
    juvenile o.
    localized o.
    o. of bone
    partial transient o.
    periarticular o.
    picture-framing o.
    postmenopausal o.
    posttraumatic o.
    regional migratory o.
    regional transient o.
    senile o.
    transient regional o.
osteoporotic
    o. bone
    o. compression fracture
osteoradiologist
osteoradiology
osteoradionecrosis
osteosarcoma
    cardiac o.
    central o.
    chondroblastic o.
    classic o.
    conventional o.
    costal o.
    dedifferentiated parosteal o.
    epithelioid o.
    extraosseous o.
    extraskeletal o.

    extremity o.
    fibroblastic o.
    gnathic o.
    high-grade surface o.
    intracortical o.
    intramedullary o.
    intraosseous low-grade o.
    juxtacortical o.
    low-grade central o.
    lytic o.
    metastatic o.
    multicentric o.
    multifocal o.
    multiple sclerotic o.'s
    o. of jaw
    osteoblastic o.
    parosteal o.
    periosteal o.
    postirradiation o.
    sacral o.
    sclerosing o.
    sclerotic o.
    secondary o.
    small cell o.
    surface o.
    telangiectatic o.
osteosarcomatosis
osteosarcomatous
osteosclerosis
    constitutional o.
    diffuse o.
    multiple-lesion o.
    myelofibrosis o.
    solitary o.
    subchondral o.
    o. tuft
    o. vertebral sarcoidosis
osteosclerotic lesion
osteosis, ostosis
osteospongioma
Osteosynthesefragen
    Arbeitsgemeinschaft für O. (AO)
osteosynthesis
    biologic o.
osteothrombosis
osteotomy
    femoral varus derotational o.
    high tibial o.
    Pemberton o.
    periacetabular o.
    sagittal ramus o. (SRO)
    Steele triple innominate
    o.'s
OsteoView
    O. desktop hand x-ray system
    Digital O. 2000
    O. digital bone densitometer
    O. 2000 digital imaging system

ostia (*pl. of* ostium)
ostial
    o. cannulation
    o. lesion
    o. renal artery stenosis
ostiomeatal
    o. complex
    o. unit
ostitic lesion of sternum
ostitis (*var. of* osteitis)
ostium, *pl.* **ostia**
    o. abdominale tubae uterinae
    aneurysmal o.
    aortic o.
    artery o.
    atrioventricular nodal o.
    conus branch o.
    coronary artery o.
    coronary sinus o.
    fistula o.
    o. primum
    o. primum atrial septal defect
    o. secundum
    o. secundum atrial septal defect
ostosis (*var. of* osteosis)
Ostreg spinal marker system
OSTS
    osseous and soft tissue sarcomas
Ostwald solubility coefficient
Ostycut bone biopsy needle
OTD
    organ tolerance dose
otic
    o. capsule
    o. ganglion
    o. obstruction
otitis
    malignant external o.
    necrotizing external o.
OtoLAM laser
otologic implant
otomastoiditis
otosclerosis
    cochlear o.
    fenestral o.
    retrofenestral o.
    stapedial o.
otospongiosis
Ottawa ankle rule
Otto
    O. disease
    O. pelvis
Otto-Kobak pelvis
OURQ
    outer upper right quadrant
out
    rule o. (R/O)
    silhouetted o.

outcropping of lesion
outer
    o. anular/posterior longitudinal
      ligament complex
    o. border of uterus
    o. canthus
    o. isoattenuated striated mural
      appearance
    o. table of skull
    o. table thickening
    o. upper right quadrant (OURQ)
outer-air
    o.-a. region
    o.-a. segmentation
outflow
    double o.
    o. effect
    hepatic venous o.
    hypoplastic subpulmonic o.
    maximum venous o. (MVO)
    o. obstruction
    o. of ventricle
    subpulmonic o.
    swan-neck shape of ventricular o.
    o. tract
    o. tract gradient
outgrowth
    osseous patellar o.
outlet
    cervical o.
    o. impingement
    o. obstruction
    pelvic o.
    pyloric o.
    thoracic o.
    ventricular o.
    o. view
    o. view radiograph
    widened thoracic o.
outline
    absent kidney o.
    double o.
    gastric o.
    renal o.
    trabeculated o.
out-of-field count
out-of-phase
    o.-o.-p. gradient echo
    o.-o.-p. GRE imaging
out-of-profile nipple
out-of-slice artifact
outpocketing of mucosa
outpouching
    aneurysmal o.
    saccular o.
output
    adequate cardiac o.
    o. amplitude

O

output (*continued*)
 augmented cardiac o.
 cardiac o.
 Dow method for measuring cardiac o.
 Fick method for measuring cardiac o.
 Gorlin method for measuring cardiac o.
 Hamilton-Stewart formula for measuring cardiac o.
 inadequate cardiac o.
 instrument o.
 low cardiac o.
 o. point
 pulmonary o.
 reduced systemic cardiac o.
 stroke o.
 systemic o.
 thermodilution cardiac o.
 ventricular o.
outrigger arm
outside-to-inside segmentation
OV103
 OncoRad OV103
 OncoScint OV103
ova (*pl. of* ovum)
Ovadia-Beals tibial plafond fracture classification
oval
 o. aneurysm
 o. aneurysm with bleb
 o. mass
 o. shape
 o. window
ovalbumin
ovale
 centrum o.
 foramen o.
 patent foramen o. (PFO)
ovalis
 anulus o.
 fossa o.
 limbus fossae o.
ovarian
 o. abscess
 o. anatomy
 o. artery
 o. carcinoma
 o. choriocarcinoma
 o. cortex
 o. cystadenofibroma
 o. cystadenoma
 o. cystic teratoma
 o. dermoid
 o. dermoid cyst
 o. Doppler signal
 o. dysgenesis
 o. dysgerminoma

 o. edema
 o. epithelial tumor
 o. fibroma
 o. fishnet weave pattern
 o. follicular cyst
 o. fossa
 o. germ cell tumor
 o. gland
 o. hemorrhage
 o. hernia
 o. hyperstimulation syndrome
 o. image signature cyst
 o. mass
 o. medulla
 o. mesonephroid tumor
 o. metastasis
 o. morphology
 o. neoplasia
 o. pregnancy
 o. remnant syndrome
 o. retention cyst
 o. serous cystadenocarcinoma
 o. size
 o. suspensory ligament
 o. torsion
 o. vascular pedicle sign
 o. vein
 o. vein embolization
 o. vein syndrome
 o. vein thrombosis
 o. venography
 o. volume
ovarii
 struma o.
 testiculoma o.
ovarioabdominal pregnancy
ovary
 atrophied o.
 clear cell neoplasm of o.
 cystic o.
 embryonic o.
 fibroma-thecoma tumor of o.
 hilar cell tumor of o.
 hyperstimulation of o.
 ligament of o.
 mulberry o.
 multifollicular o.
 palpable postmenopausal o.
 pearly white o.
 polycystic o.
 postmenopausal o.
 sclerocystic o.
 stromal carcinoid tumor of o.
 suspensory ligament of o.
 teratoblastoma of o.
 teratocarcinoma of o.
 thecoma of o.
 transposition of o.'s

overaeration
overall treatment time
overcalling
    o. metastasis
    o. pneumonia
overcirculation
    pulmonary vessel o.
    o. vascularity
overcouch
    o. exposure
    o. tube
    o. view
overcoverage
overdamping
overdevelopment
    bone o.
overdiagnostic bias
overdistension (*var. of* overdistention)
overdistention, overdistension
    alveolar o.
    o. of alveolar population
    pulmonary o.
overdrainage
overdrive suppression
overembolize
overexpansion
    lung o.
    pulmonary o.
overexposure
overframing
    horizontal o.
    mean diameter o.
    subtotal o.
overgrowth
    bony o.
    cuticular o.
    epiphysial o.
    fibrocartilaginous o.
    vertebral body o.
overhanging
    o. border
    o. margin
Overhauser effect
overhead
    o. film
    o. oblique view
overinflation
    lung o.
    obstructive pulmonary o.
    pulmonary o.
    unilateral o.
overlap
    liver-spleen o.
    o. shadow
    o. syndrome
overlapping
    o. finger
    o. fracture
    o. image

    o. rib
    o. suture
overlay
    anatomic o.
    o. plate
    venous o.
overload
    acute hemodynamic o.
    cardiac o.
    chronic hemodynamic o.
    diastolic o.
    fluid o.
    pressure o.
    right ventricular o.
    systolic ventricular o.
    transfusional iron o.
    volume o.
overlying
    o. attenuation artifact
    o. bowel contents
    o. bowel gas
    o. bowel shadow
    o. branching pattern
overpenetrated film
overread
overrelaxation factor
override
    aortic o.
overriding
    o. aorta
    o. great artery
    o. of fracture fragment
    o. suture of fontanelle
    o. toe
oversampled
over-the-wire
    o.-t.-w. coronary stent
    o.-t.-w. design
    o.-t.-w. Greenfield filter
overuse injury
overventilation
    alveolar o.
overview angiogram
overvoltage
oviductal pregnancy
ovoid
    afterloading tandem and o.
    o. heart
    o. high signal intensity
    Manchester o.
    o. ossification center
    o. shape
    tandem and o.
ovulation
    incessant o.
    o. induction
ovulatory
    o. failure
    o. phase

O

ovum, *pl.* **ova**
    aspiration of ova
Owen view
owl's-eye appearance
oxalosis
    bone o.
    kidney o.
    primary o.
Oxford
    O. magnet
    O. 2T large-bore imaging system
      scanner
ox heart
oxidase
    cytochrome o. (COX)
    cytochrome c o.
    monoamine o.
oxidation
    Baeyer-Villiger o.
    o. state
oxidative metabolism
oxide
    deuterium o.
    nitric o.
    superparamagnetic iron o. (SPIO)
    ultrasmall superparamagnetic iron o.
      (USPIO)
oxidized complex
oxidronate
    technetium 99m o.
OxiFirst fetal oxygen monitor
Oxilan imaging agent
oxime
    hexamethylpropyleneamine o.
      (HMPAO)
    ^{99m}Tc-hexamethylpropyleneamine o.
    technetium 99m
      hexamethylpropyleneamine o.
      (^{99m}Tc-HMPAO)
oximetry
    pulse o.
oxine
    ^{111}In o.
    indium o.
    lipophilic indium o.
oxycephalia (*var. of* oxycephaly)
oxycephaly, oxycephalia
oxygen
    o. 15 (^{15}O, O-15)
    o. 16 (^{16}O, O-16)

o. 17 (^{17}O, O-17)
o. 18 (^{18}O, O-18)
activation-induced uncoupling of
  cerebral o.
cerebral metabolic rate of o.
  (CMRO$_2$)
cistern o.
o. cisternography
o. consumption (QO$_2$)
o. effect
o. enhancement ratio
o. extraction fraction (OEF)
o. extraction rate (OER,
  O$_2$ER)
o. imaging agent
metabolic rate of o.
o. myelography
regional cerebral metabolic rate for
  o. (rCMRO$_2$)
o. saturation
oxygenated perfluorocarbon blood
substitute
oxygenation
    extracorporeal membrane o.
    tissue o.
oxygenation-sensitive
    o.-s. functional MR
    o.-s. functional MR imaging
oxygenator
    bubble o.
    disc o.
    extracorporeal membrane o.
    film o.
    membrane o.
    rotating disc o.
    screen o.
oxygen-dependent emphysema
oxygen-enhanced
    o.-e. lung MR imaging
    o.-e. MRI
oxygen-17 NMR spectroscopy
oxygen-supersaturated water
Oxyguard endoscopy biteblock
oxyorthosilicate
    gadolinium o.
    lutetium o. (LSO)
oxyphilic adenoma
oxysulphide
    gadolinium o.
oyster-pearl breast calcification

P
> phosphorus
>> P glocoprotein (P-gp)
>> P loop
>> P pulmonale pattern
>> P wave-QRS wave ratio (P/QRS)

³¹P, P-31
> phosphorus 31
>> ³¹P spectroscopy

³²P, P-32
> phosphorus 32

P/A
> perimeter-area
>> P/A ratio

PA
> posteroanterior
>> PA and lateral films
>> PA position
>> PA projection

Pa
> protactinium

Paas disease

pacchionian
> p. body
> p. depression
> p. granulation

pace
> p. mapping
> P. Plus System scanner
> P. technique

PACE
> prospective acquisition
> correction

pacemaker
> p. artifact
> bipolar p.
> p. effect
> epicardial p.
> implanted p.
> intravascular p.
> p. lead
> p. wire

pachydermoperiostosis
pachyfibril
pachygyria
pachymeningitis
pachymeninx
pachymetry
> ultrasonic p.

pachypleuritis
pacing
> p. artifact
> p. box
> p. lead

Packard Merlin life-monitoring system
packed beads
packing
> edge p.
> endosaccular p.
> p., extraction, and calculation technique
> p. fraction

PACS
> picture archival communication system
> picture archiving and communication system
>> PACS PathSpeed MR imaging
>> PACS workstation

pad
> decubitus p.
> p. effect
> electrical grounding p.
> fibrocartilaginous p.
> fly-swatterlike p.
> Sat P.
> p. sign of aortic insufficiency
> standoff p.
> thickened heel p.
> UltraEase ultrasound p.
> ultrasound p.
> wireless handheld Web p.

padding
> antral p.
> zero p.

paddle
> compression p.
> spot compression p.

paddlewheel
> p. method
> p. reformation

PADP-PAWP
> pulmonary artery diastolic pressure and pulmonary artery wedge pressure

PAEDP
> pulmonary artery end-diastolic pressure

Page kidney
Paget
> P. abscess
> P. carcinoma
> P. disease of bone
> P. jaw disease
> P. osteitis deformans
> P. quiet necrosis

P

pagetic
pagetoid
> p. bone
> p. epidermal involvement
> p. lesion

Paget-von Schroetter syndrome
PAH
> paraaminohippurate
> pulmonary arterial hypertension

pain
> focal back p.
> low back p.
> neuropathic p.
> nociceptive p.
> orthostatic back p.
> periumbilical p.
> phantom limb p.
> p. provocation response

painful
> p. disc derangement
> p. osmotic demyelination syndrome

painless
> p. hematuria
> p. jaundice
> p. thyroiditis
> p. torsion

paint brush striation
pair
> electron-positron p.
> exon-specific primer p.
> line p.
> Maxwell p.
> oblique annihilation photon p.
> p. production
> transaxial annihilation photon p.

paired
> p. inferior vena cava
> p. parietal branches
> p. visceral branches

Pais fracture
palatal muscle
palate
palatina
> uvula p.

palatine
> p. bone
> p. canal
> p. foramen
> p. ridge
> p. root
> p. shelf
> p. suture
> p. tonsil

palatini
> levator veli p.
> tensor veli p.

palatoethmoidal suture
palatoglossus
palatograph

palatography
palatomaxillary
> p. canal
> p. suture

palatomyograph
palatopharyngeal fold
palatopharyngeus
palatovaginal canal
paleopathologic and radiologic studies
palisade formation
palladium (Pd)
> p. 103 (^{103}Pd, Pd-103)
> p. imaging agent
> p. implant

palliative
> p. debulking
> p. esophagostomy
> p. irradiation
> p. radiation therapy

pallidotomy
pallidus
> globus p.

Pallister-Hall syndrome
palmar
> p. angulation
> p. aponeurosis
> p. arterial arch
> p. cutaneous vein
> p. displacement
> p. fascia
> p. fasciitis
> p. fibromatosis
> p. ganglion
> p. interosseus
> p. metacarpal ligament
> p. plate
> p. radiocarpal ligament
> p. slope
> p. surface
> p. tilt
> p. wrist

palmaris
> p. brevis
> p. longus
> p. longus tendon

palmatae
> plicae p.

Palmaz
> P. Genesis balloon-expanded stent
> P. large balloon-expanded stent
> P. medium balloon-expanded stent
> P. P564, PS424 stent
> P. P394 stainless steel
>   balloon-expandable stent
> P. 424, 784 stent

Palmaz-Schatz long medium
  balloon-expanded stent
palmitate
> ^{11}C p.

palmitic acid
palmoplantar pustulosis
Palomar SLP1000 diode
Palomo varicocelectomy procedure
palpable
    p. aortic ejection sound
    p. postmenopausal ovary
    p. presystolic bulge
    p. pulmonic ejection sound
Palpagraph breast mapping device
palpation-guided approach
palpatory T-stage prostate carcinoma
palpebra, *pl.* **palpebrae**
palpebrae (*pl. of* palpebra)
palpebral
    p. fissure
    p. raphe
palsy
    dyskinetic cerebral p.
    Erb p.
    progressive supranuclear p.
    recurrent laryngeal nerve p.
    waiter's tip p.
PAM
    pulmonary artery mean pressure
pamidronate
    p. disodium
    p. therapy
pampiniform plexus
PAN, PN
    polyarteritis nodosa
panacinar emphysema
panaortic
panaortitis
panbronchiolitis
    diffuse p.
pancake
    p. appearance
    p. compression
    p. kidney
    p. MRI magnet
pancarpal destructive arthritis
panchamber
    p. enlargement
    p. hypertrophy
Pancoast
    P. syndrome
    P. tumor
pancolitis
pancompartmental joint space narrowing
pancreas, *pl.* **pancreata**
    aberrant p.
    accessory p.
    anterior surface of p.
    anular p.
    Aselli p.
    body of p.
    calcified p.
    degeneration of p.

    p. divisum
    dorsal p.
    ectopic p.
    fat-spared area in p.
    p. gland
    head of p.
    heterotopic p.
    intraductal papillary mucinous tumor
      of p.
    lesser p.
    mature pseudocyst of p.
    metastasis to p.
    mucinous ductal ectasia of p.
    mucinous ductectatic tumor of p.
    neck of p.
    posterior surface of p.
    tail of p.
    p. transplant
    p. ultrasonography imaging
    uncinate process of p.
    ventral p.
pancreata (*pl. of* pancreas)
pancreatic
    p. abscess
    p. angiography
    p. arteriography
    p. ascites
    p. atrophy
    p. calcification
    p. calculus
    p. carcinoma
    p. cholera syndrome
    p. cutaneous fistula
    p. cyst
    p. cystadenocarcinoma
    p. cystadenoma
    p. cystic fibrosis
    p. cystic lymphangioma
    p. degeneration
    p. disease
    p. dorsal anlage
    p. duct
    p. ductal adenocarcinoma
    p. duct branch
    p. duct dilation
    p. duct obstruction
    p. duct sphincter
    p. duct stent
    p. fluid collection
    p. hamartoma
    p. head
    p. hemorrhage
    p. islet cell tumor
    p. lipomatosis
    p. lymph node
    p. lymphoma
    p. macrocystic adenoma
    p. mass
    p. metastasis

P

pancreatic (*continued*)
    p. microcystic adenoma
    p. neck
    p. necrosis
    p. neoplasia
    p. parenchymatous phase
      (PPP)
    p. phlegmon
    p. pseudocyst
    p. pseudocyst drainage
    p. reflux
    p. scan
    p. trauma
    p. vein
pancreatic-enteric continuity
pancreaticobiliary
    p. common channel
    p. disease
    p. ductal junction
    p. function variant
    p. sphincter
    p. tract
    p. ultrasound
pancreaticoblastoma, pancreatoblastoma
pancreaticoduodenal, pancreatoduodenal
    p. artery
    p. lymph node
pancreaticoduodenectomy,
  pancreatoduodenectomy
pancreaticohepatic, pancreatohepatic
    p. syndrome
pancreaticolienal, pancreatolienal
    p. lymph node
pancreaticopleural, pancreatopleural
    p. fistula
pancreaticosplenic, pancreatosplenic
    p. node
    p. omentum
pancreaticus
    hemosuccus p.
pancreatitis
    acute p.
    autoimmune p. (AIP)
    chronic calcifying p.
    chronic obstructive p.
    diffuse p.
    edematous p.
    focal p.
    necrotizing p.
    obstructive p.
    phlegmonous p.
    p. pseudoaneurysm
    Santiani-Stone classification of p.
    suppurative p.
    tropical p.
pancreatoblastoma (*var. of*
  pancreaticoblastoma)
pancreatocholangiogram
    retrograde p.

pancreatoduodenal (*var. of*
  pancreaticoduodenal)
pancreatoduodenectomy (*var. of*
  pancreaticoduodenectomy)
pancreatogram
pancreatography
    endoscopic retrograde p.
    p. imaging
    intraoperative p.
    magnetic resonance p. (MRP)
    percutaneous p.
    retrograde p.
pancreatohepatic (*var. of*
  pancreaticohepatic)
pancreatolienal (*var. of* pancreaticolienal)
pancreatolithiasis
pancreatopleural (*var. of*
  pancreaticopleural)
pancreatosplenic (*var. of*
  pancreaticosplenic)
pancytopenia-dysmelia syndrome
panda appearance
Pander island
PANDO
    primary acquired nasolacrimal duct
    obstruction
panduriform placenta
panencephalitis
    progressive rubella p.
    sclerosing p.
    subacute sclerosing p. (SSPE)
panfacial fracture
panhypopituitarism
panlobar nephroblastomatosis
panlobular emphysema
panmyelopathy
panmyelosis
Panner disease
panni (*pl. of* pannus)
panniculitis
    mediastinal p.
    mesenteric p.
    p. ossificans
    systemic nodular p.
pannus, *pl.* **panni**
    p. deformity
    p. deformity of odontoid
    p. formation
    p. of synovium
    retrodental p.
    synovial p.
panography
panoral radiography
panoramic
    p. CT scan
    p. image
    p. imaging
    P. 200 nonmydriatic ophthalmoscope
    p. radiograph

p. radiography
p. rotating machine
p. surface projection
p. tomography
p. view
p. x-ray film
Panorex view
pansinusitis
pansystolic mitral regurgitation
pantalar fusion
pantaloon
    p. embolus
    p. hernia
pantomogram
pantomograph
pantomographic view
pantomography
    concentric p.
    eccentric p.
Pantopaque
    P. cisternography
    P. imaging agent
    P. myelography
PAOD
    peripheral arterial occlusive
    disease
PAP
    pulmonary alveolar proteinosis
    pulmonary artery pressure
Papavasiliou classification of olecranon
  fracture
paper-doll fetus
paper strip tracing
Papile classification
papilla, *pl.* **papillae**
    aberrant p.
    acoustic p.
    bile p.
    circumvallate p.
    duodenal p.
    major duodenal p.
    minor duodenal p.
    p. of columnar epithelium
    p. of Vater
    p. of Vater enlargement
    p. of Vater stenosis
    optic p.
    renal p.
    Santorini p.
    sloughed p.
    smudged p.
    urethral p.
papillae (*pl. of* papilla)
papillary, papillate
    p. adenoma of large intestine
    p. apocrine change
    p. bile duct stenosis
    p. breast carcinoma
    p. cystadenoma lymphomatosum

p. cystic adenoma
p. DCIS
p. duct of Bellini
p. epididymal cystadenoma
p. epithelial neoplasia
p. excrescence
p. fibroelastoma
p. lesion
p. microcarcinoma of thyroid
p. muscle
p. muscle infarct
p. muscle rupture
p. muscle uptake
p. necrosis
p. pancreatic cystic
  neoplasia
p. projection
p. proliferation
p. renal cell carcinoma
p. serous adenocarcinoma
p. serous carcinoma
p. thyroid carcinoma
p. tumor
papillate (*var. of* papillary)
papilledema
papillocarcinoma
papillogram
papilloma
    p. acuminatum
    basal cell p.
    benign intraductal p.
    breast p.
    choroid plexus p.
    cockscomb p.
    cylindrical p.
    p. diffusum
    ductal p.
    p. durum
    exophytic p.
    fibroepithelial p.
    fungiform p.
    glandular p.
    hard p.
    Hopmann p.
    p. inguinale
    intraductal p.
    inverted p.
    large duct p.
    laryngeal p.
    maxillary sinus p.
    p. molle
    multiple peripheral p.'s
    p. of bladder
    p. of 4th ventricle
    oncocytic p.
    penile squamous p.
    schneiderian p.
    sinonasal inverted p.
    soft p.

P

papilloma (*continued*)
    solitary pulmonary glandular p.
    squamous cell p.
    tonsillar p.
    transitional urethral cell p.
    villous p.
papillomatosis
    intraductal breast p.
    invasive p.
    juvenile breast p.
    juvenile laryngeal p.
    laryngeal p.
    pulmonary p.
    recurrent respiratory p.
    tracheobronchial p.
papillomatous growth
papillomavirus
    human p. (HPV)
Papillon-Lèfevre syndrome
Papillon technique
papillotomy
    endoscopic p.
papular lesion
papule
    Gottron p.
papulonecrotic lesion
PAPVR
    partial anomalous pulmonary venous return
papyracea
    lamina p.
papyraceus
    fetus p.
PAR
    plain abdominal radiography
paraaminobenzoic acid
paraaminohippurate (PAH)
paraaminohippuric acid
paraaminosalicylic acid (PAS)
paraanastomotic aneurysm repair
paraaortic
    p. lymph node
    p. mass
paraarticular
    p. bone remodeling
    p. calcification
parabola
    digital p.
    metatarsal p.
parabolic velocity profile
paracarcinomatous myelopathy
paracardiac
    p. mass
    p. metastasis
    p. tumor
paracardiac-type total anomalous venous return
paracecal appendix

paracentesis
    abdominal p.
    subxiphoid p.
paracentral
    p. artery
    p. gyrus
    p. lobule
paracervical lymphatics
parachute
    p. deformity of mitral valve
    p. mitral valve deformity
paracicatricial emphysema
paracoccidioidal granuloma
paracolic
    p. abscess
    p. gutter
    p. lymph node
paracorporeal heart
paracortical hyperplasia
paracostal
paracystic pouch
paracytic infection
paradigm
    block p.
    coregistration p.
    event-related p.
paradiscal lesion
paradoxic, paradoxical
    p. bronchospasm
    p. cerebral embolus
    p. colon dilation
    p. embolization
    p. enhancement
    p. headache
    p. leaflet motion
    p. middle turbinate
    p. septal motion
    p. suppression
paradoxical (*var. of* paradoxic)
paradoxus
    pulsus p.
paraduodenal
    p. fold
    p. fossa
    p. hernia
    p. recess
paraesophageal
    p. hiatal hernia
    p. varix
paraesophagogastric devascularization
parafascicular
    p. nucleus
    p. thalamotomy
paraffin-embedded tissue
paraffinoma
paraganglioma
    adrenal p.
    cardiac p.
    cervical p.

chromaffin p.
extraadrenal p.
functional p.
gangliocytic p.
nonchromaffin p.
nonfunctional extraadrenal p.
thoracic p.
paragangliomatosis
paraglenoid cyst
paragonimiasis
brain p.
lung p.
paragranuloma
parahiatal hernia
parahilar
parahippocampal gyrus
paraileostomal hernia
parainfluenza
p. virus
p. virus pneumonia
paraisopropyliminodiacetic
p. acid (PIPIDA)
p. acid technetium-99m hepatobiliary scan
parakeet fancier's lung
paralabral
p. cyst
p. lesion
paralanguage
paralaryngeal
p. muscle
p. space
parallax
p. method
p. view
parallel
p. analogue mapping
p. and spiral flow patterns
p. array
p. cine
p. data acquisition coils
p. imaging
p. line equal spacebar phantom
p. line equal spacing (PLES)
p. mean translation
p. M lines
p. MRI
p. pitch lines
p. rays
p. reception
p. tag planes
p. transmission
p. virtual machine (PVM)
parallel-hole
p.-h. collimated imaging
p.-h. collimation
p.-h. medium-sensitivity collimator
p.-h. scintigram

parallelism
p. of articular surface
p. of facet joint
parallel-opposed
p.-o. beams
p.-o. unmodified ports
parallel-tagged MR image
paralyses (*pl. of* paralysis)
paralysis, *pl.* **paralyses**
diaphragmatic p.
hemidiaphragmatic p.
hernia p.
Klumpke p.
p. of diaphragm
phrenic nerve p.
thyrotoxic periodic p. (TPP)
transient p.
vocal cord p.
paralytic
p. chest
p. colonic obstruction
p. ileus
paralytica
dysphagia p.
paramagnetic
p. artifact
p. cation
p. contrast agent
p. contrast-enhanced MR study
p. contrast enhancement
p. effect
p. enhancement accentuation
p. enhancement accentuation by chemical-shift imaging
p. influence
p. lanthanide
p. shift
p. shift relaxation
p. trace element
p. transition metal
paramagnetism
apparent p.
collective p.
paramalleolar artery
paramammary lymph node
paramedian
p. infarct
p. line
p. pontile reticular formation (PPRF)
p. position
p. sagittal plane
p. section
p. thalamic artery
p. thalamoperduncular artery
p. triangle
paramediastinal gland
parameningeal rhabdomyosarcoma
parameniscal cyst

P

paramesonephric
    p. duct
    p. duct cyst
parameter
    clinical p.
    extrinsic cellular p.
    growth p.
    hematologic p.
    intrinsic cellular p.
    kinetic perfusion p.
    normal hemodynamic liver p.
    nuclear magnetic resonance spectral
      p.
    optimization p.
    physiologic p.
    rendering p.
    scan p.
    sonographic p.
    thermal treatment p.
    timing p.
    ventricular function p.
parametrectomy
    radical p.
parametria (*pl. of* parametrium)
parametrial fat
parametric image
parametrium, *pl.* **parametria**
paranasal
    p. sinus
    p. sinus carcinoma
    p. sinus fracture
    p. sinusitis
    p. sinus mass
    p. sinus mucocele
paraneoplastic
    p. cerebellar degeneration
    p. encephalitis
    p. process
    p. syndrome
    p. thromboembolism
paraorbital lesion
paraosteoarthropathy
paraovarian (*var. of* parovarian)
paraparesis
parapatellar plica
parapelvic
    p. cyst
    p. gutter
parapharyngeal
    p. abscess
    p. space
    p. space cyst
paraphyses (*pl. of* paraphysis)
paraphysis, *pl.* **paraphyses**
parapneumonic effusion
paraprosthetic
    p. leak
    p. leakage
paraprosthetic-enteric fistula

pararectal
    p. abscess
    p. fossa
    p. lymph node
    p. pouch
pararenal
    p. abscess
    p. aortic aneurysm
    p. aortic atherosclerosis
    p. space
parasagittal
    p. depression
    p. image
    p. intracranial mass
    p. lesion
    p. meningioma
    p. plane
parasellar
    p. brain mass
    p. cistern
    p. dermoid tumor
    p. metastasis
    p. region lesion
    p. vascular lesion
paraseptal
    p. emphysema
    p. position
parasinoidal
parasitic
    p. fetus
    p. infiltrate
parasitized collateral
paraspinal
    p. abnormality
    p. abscess
    p. calcification
    p. empyema
    p. interface
    p. line
    p. muscle
    p. neurofibroma
    p. pleural stripe
    p. soft tissue mass
    p. soft tissue shadowing
    p. vein
paraspinous
    p. musculature
    p. tumor
parasternal
    p. bulge
    p. long-axis view
    p. long-axis view echocardiography
    p. lymph node
    p. motion
    p. scanning
    p. short-axis view
    p. short-axis view echocardiography
    p. view of heart
    p. window

parastomal hernia
parastriate cortex
parasympathetic
    p. fiber
    p. ganglion tumor
    p. nervous system
parasymphysial fracture
paraterminal gyrus
paratesticular
    p. rhabdomyosarcoma
    p. tumor
parathyroid
    p. adenoma
    p. carcinoma
    p. cyst
    ectopic p.
    p. gland
    p. hormone (PTH)
    p. hyperplasia
    p. insufficiency
    p. scintigraphy
    technetium 99m sestamibi p.
    p. tumor
    p. ultrasonography imaging
    p. vein
parathyroidectomy
    radioguided p.
paratracheal
    p. adenopathy
    p. convexity
    p. density
    p. lymph node
    p. region
    p. soft tissue
    p. space
    p. tissue stripe
paratrooper's fracture
paratubal serous cyst
paratumoral injection
paraumbilical
    p. anterior abdominal wall
    p. vein
paraureteral diverticulum
paraurethral
    p. canal
    p. cyst
    p. duct
    p. gland
parauterine lymph node
paravaginal
    p. lymph node
    p. soft tissue
paravalvular
    p. leak
    p. regurgitation
paravertebral
    p. ganglion
    p. groove
    p. gutter

    p. musculature
    p. nerve plexus
    p. ossification
    p. scanning
    p. venous plexus
paravertebrally
    p. situated pelvic tumor mass
    p. situated thoracic tumor
    mass
paravesical
    p. fossa
    p. pouch
paravesicular lymph node
parcellation of structure
parchment
    p. heart
    p. right ventricle
parenchyma
    bleeding into brain p.
    brain p.
    breast p.
    cerebral p.
    computerized texture analysis of
      lung nodules and lung p.
    hepatic p.
    liver p.
    lung p.
    mammary p.
    marbling of pancreatic p.
    mottling of renal p.
    normal renal p.
    pulmonary p.
    renal p.
    spinal cord p.
    testicular p.
parenchymal (*var. of* parenchymatous)
parenchymatous, parenchymal,
  parenchymous
    p. atrophy
    p. blastoma
    p. blood
    p. brain metastasis
    p. breast pattern
    p. cerebellar degeneration
    p. change
    p. cone
    p. consolidation
    p. echogenicity
    p. enhancement
    p. extension
    p. fibrous band
    p. goiter
    p. hematoma
    p. hemorrhage
    p. infarct
    p. infection
    p. inflammation
    p. interstitium
    p. laceration

P

parenchymatous (*continued*)
    p. lung band
    p. lung disease
    p. opacity
    p. peliosis hepatis
    p. phase
    p. phase image
    p. pneumonia
    p. renal disease
    p. scarring
    p. tissue
    p. tracer accumulation
    p. transit
parenchymography
    endoscopic retrograde p. (ERP)
parenchymous (*var. of* parenchymatous)
parent
    p. artery occlusion
    p. element
    p. isotope
    p. nuclide
    p. radionuclide
    p. vein
    p. vessel
    p. vessel occlusion
parenterally acquired human immunodeficiency virus
parentheses-like calcification
Parenti-Fraccaro disease
paresis
    oculosympathetic p.
    vocal cord p.
paresthetica
    meralgia p.
Parham-Martin band
parietal
    p. association area
    p. band
    p. bone
    p. bone thinning
    p. boss
    p. cephalohematoma
    p. convexity
    p. cortex
    p. cortex lesion
    p. diameter
    p. eminence
    p. encephalocele
    p. extension
    p. extension of infundibular septum
    p. eye field (PEF)
    p. fistula
    p. foramen
    p. gyrus
    p. layer
    p. lobe
    p. lobe gray matter cytosolic choline pathogenetic mechanism of myocardial fibrosis

    p. lobe lesion
    p. lymph node
    p. middle cerebral artery
    p. operculum
    p. pelvic fascia
    p. pericardial calcification
    p. pericardium
    p. peritoneum
    p. pleura
    p. pleural scarring
    p. pregnancy
    p. presentation
    p. suture
parietography
    gastric p.
parietomastoid suture
parietooccipital
    p. area
    p. branch of posterior cerebellar artery
    p. lesion
    p. region
    p. sulcus
    p. suture
parietoorbital projection
parietotemporal
    p. area
    p. suture
Parinaud syndrome
Paris ultrasound system
park
    p. bench position
    P. Medical Systems scanner
Parkes-Weber syndrome (PWS)
Parkinson disease
parkinsonian syndrome
parkinsonism
    vascular p.
Parks
    P. bidirectional Doppler flowmeter
    P. 800 bidirectional Doppler flowmetry
parosteal
    p. bone lesion
    p. chondrosarcoma
    p. osteoma
    p. osteosarcoma
    p. soft tissue angiosarcoma
parotid
    p. abscess
    p. cyst
    p. duct
    p. gland
    p. gland sialography
    p. lymph node
    p. pleomorphic adenoma
    p. pneumatocele
    p. space
    p. tumor

parotidectomy
    superficial p.
parotiditis (*var. of* parotitis)
parotitis, parotiditis
    adenoid cystic carcinoma p.
    benign mixed tumor p.
    cylindroma p.
    mucoepidermoid carcinoma p.
    pleomorphic adenoma p.
parovarian, paraovarian
    p. cyst
    p. varicosity
paroxysmal
    p. auricular tachycardia
    p. AV block
    p. change
    p. pulmonary edema
parrot
    frontal bossing of P.
    P. node
parrot-beak
    p.-b. labral tear
    p.-b. meniscus tear
    p.-b. pattern
parry fracture
Parry-Romberg syndrome
pars, *pl.* **partes**
    p. flaccida cholesteatoma
    p. infravaginalis gubernaculi
    p. interarticularis
    p. interarticularis defect
    p. interarticularis fracture
    pedicle and p.
    p. tensa cholesteatoma
Parsons
    3rd intercondylar tubercle of P.
    P. tubercle
part
    fetal small p.
    malignant melanoma of soft p.
    presenting p.
partes (*pl. of* pars)
1-, 2-, 3-, 4-part fracture
partial
    p. anomalous pulmonary venous
      connection
    p. anomalous pulmonary venous
      return (PAPVR)
    p. atrioventricular canal defect
    p. brain irradiation
    p. brain radiation therapy
    p. bursal surface tear
    p. collapse of lung
    p. complex seizure
    p. corpus callosum agenesis
    p. dislocation
    p. dislodgement
    p. external biliary diversion
    p. flip-angle fast-scan technique

    p. Fourier imaging
    p. Fourier technique
    p. heart block
    p. k-space sampling
    p. lesion
    p. liquid ventilation
    p. liquid ventilation with perflubron
    p. obliteration of lateral ventricle
    p. pericardial abscess
    p. pericardial absence
    p. placenta previa
    p. saturation
    p. saturation pulse sequence
    p. saturation spin echo
    p. saturation technique
    p. small bowel malrotation
    p. small bowel obstruction
    p. thickening
    p. transient osteoporosis
    p. transposition of great artery
    p. tubular appearance
    p. ureter duplication
    p. volume averaging
    p. volume effect artifact
partialis
    situs inversus p.
partially
    p. polycystic kidney
    p. relaxed Fourier transform (PRFT)
partial-ring bismuth germanate-crystal
  scanner
partial-thickness split tear
particle
    accelerated p.
    p. accelerator
    alpha p.
    p. approach
    p. beam radiation therapy
    beta p.
    bone p.
    calcium/oxyanion-containing p.
    charged p.
    dextran-coated p.
    Embosphere p.
    gelatin sponge p.
    gold p.
    heavy charged p.
    p. identification
    p. image velocimetry (PIV)
    Ivalon p.
    large colloidal p.
    magnetic iron oxide p. (MIOP)
    p. mask
    nuclear p.
    oral magnetic p.
    polyvinyl alcohol p.
    PVA p.
    p. size determination
    Spongel gelatin sponge p.

P

particle (*continued*)
    submicron magnetic p.
    superparamagnetic iron oxide p.
    viral p.
    Zimmermann elementary p.
particulate
    p. arterial embolization
    p. debris
    p. echo
    p. embolic agent
    magnetic p.
    p. matter
partition
    atrial p.
    p. coefficient
    gastric p.
partitioning
    recursive p.
parturient canal
parturition
parvus
    p. et tardus waveform
    pulsus tardus et p.
PAS
    paraaminosalicylic acid
    pulmonary artery systolic
    PAS pressure
pascal of force
PASH
    pseudoangiomatous stromal hyperplasia
Pasonage-Turner syndrome
PASP/SASP
    pulmonary artery systolic
    pressure/systemic artery systolic
    pressure
    PASP/SASP ratio
pass
    p. coaxially
    interleaved imaging p.
passage
    adiabatic fast p.
    adiabatic rapid p. (ARP)
    biliary p.
    free air p.
    narrowing of bronchiolar p.
    p. pressure
Passager nitinol self-expandable stent
Passavant
    P. bar
    P. muscle
    P. ridge
passive
    p. acquired immunity
    p. atelectasis
    p. chest expansion
    p. clot
    p. edema
    p. epicardial restraint
    p. filling

    p. hepatic congestion
    p. hyperemia
    p. loss of correlation effect
    p. pneumonia
    p. shielding
    p. shimming
    p. track detector
    p. vascular congestion
    p. venous distention
passively
    p. congested lung tissue
    p. shimmed superconducting magnet
PASTA
    partial articular supraspinatus tendon
    avulsion
    PASTA imaging
paste
    ferric ammonium citrate-cellulose p.
pastil, pastille
    p. radiometer
    Sabouraud p.
pastille (*var. of* pastil)
PASV
    pressure-activated safety valve
    PASV catheter
    PASV technology
Patau syndrome
patch
    ash leaf p.
    blood p.
    p. crinkling
    p. electrode
    epidural blood p.
    p. kinking
    p. lesion
    McCallum p.
    murine Peyer p.
    Peyer p.
    pigskin p.
    sclerotic calvarial p.
    subcutaneous p.
patch-graft
    p.-g. aortoplasty
    p.-g. reconstruction
patchy
    p. alveolar opacity
    p. area of consolidation
    p. area of density
    p. area of pneumonia
    p. atelectasis
    p. atrophy of renal cortex
    p. colonic ulcer
    p. distribution of tracer
    p. edema
    p. migratory infiltrate
    p. zone
patella, *pl.* **patellae**
    p. alta
    apex of head of p.

p. baja
bipartite p.
dislocation of p.
floating p.
half-moon p.
high-lying p.
high-riding p.
ligamentum patellae
lower pole of p.
multipartite p.
pebble-shaped p.
skyline view of p.
squared p.
subluxation of p. (SLP)
subluxing p.
undersurface of p.

patellae (*pl. of* patella)
patéllae
chondromalacia p.
patellar
p. bursa
p. bursitis
p. button
p. cartilage thickness
p. chondromalacia
p. contour
p. dislocation
p. edge
p. entrapment
p. fat-pad
p. fossa
p. fracture
p. groove
p. ligament-to-patella ratio
p. malalignment
p. plica
p. pole
p. retinaculum
p. shaving
p. shelf
p. skyline view
p. sleeve fracture
p. subluxation
p. tendinopathy
p. tendinosis
p. tendon
p. tilt
patellectomy
patelliform
patellofemoral
p. angle
p. articular cartilage
p. articulation
p. compartment
p. congruence
p. disorder
p. incongruity
p. index
p. joint

p. joint space
p. realignment
patelloquadriceps tendon
patency
p. and valvular reflux of deep vein
arterial p.
coronary artery bypass graft p.
ductus arteriosus p.
ductus venosus p.
graft p.
long-term p.
modified Blalock-Taussig shunt p.
nidus p.
p. of artery
p. of vein graft
p. of vessel
p. rate
short-term p.
shunt p.
p. trifurcation
vascular p.
vein p.
patent
p. bifurcation
p. ductus arteriosus (PDA)
p. foramen ovale (PFO)
p. lumen
p. stent
p. urachus
p. vessel
widely p.
Paterson-Parker system
path
p. length
mean free p.
puncture p.
water p.
pathogenic factor
pathognomonic
p. finding
p. imaging characteristic
p. sign
pathologic, pathological
p. correlation
p. dislocation
p. fracture
p. intracranial calcification
p. lesion
p. marrow infiltration
pathological (*var. of* pathologic)
pathology
acute aortic p.
coronary p.
mesenteric lymph node p.
radiographic p.
pathophysiologic change
pathway
amygdalofugal p.
anomalous p.

P

pathway (*continued*)
    antegrade fast p.
    anterior internodal p.
    atrio-His p.
    cerebellar p.
    cerebropontocerebellar p.
    cerebrospinal fluid p.
    corticobulbar p.
    corticopontocerebellar p.
    corticospinal motor p.
    dentatoolivary p.
    dual atrioventricular node p.'s
    Embden-Meyerhof glycolytic p.
    hepatobiliary p.
    interhemispheric p.
    neural p.
    nigrostriatal dopaminergic p.
    nodoventricular p.
    optic glioma p.
    reticulocortical p.
    retrovestibular neural p.
    septal accessory p.
    striatal output p.
    synaptic p.
    Thorel p.

patient
    p. motion
    p. motion artifact
    p. volume

Patlak plot

pattern
    abnormal lung p.
    acinar p.
    activation p.
    airspace filling p.
    airway p.
    alveolar p.
    anhaustral colonic gas p.
    anular tear p.
    arborization p.
    architectural p.
    arterial deficiency p.
    attenuation p.
    atypical vessel colposcopic p.
    balance p.
    ballerina-foot p.
    basket-weave p.
    bat's-wing p.
    beam p.
    benign-appearing p.
    bigeminal p.
    blood flow p.
    bony trabecular p.
    bowel gas p.
    branching p.
    broken bough p.
    bronchiectatic p.
    bronchopneumonia p.
    bronchovascular p.

    bubbly p.
    butterfly p.
    cavitating p.
    centrum semiovale p.
    cerebral cortical gyral p.
    circadian p.
    coarse p.
    cobblestone p.
    cobweb p.
    coiled spring p.
    collimator plugging p.
    colonic urticaria p.
    combined lineonodular radigraphic
      lung p.
    comedo p.
    concertina p.
    contractile p.
    contrast enhancement p.
    convolutional p.
    corduroy cloth p.
    corkscrew p.
    corkscrew-type flow p.
    crazy paving p.
    cribriform p.
    cross-sectional p.
    cystic p.
    degenerative nuclear p.
    diffraction p.
    diffuse contrast agent distribution p.
    dissemination p.
    divergent spiculated p.
    dot-and-dash p.
    3D physiologic flow p.
    ductal p.
    early repolarization p.
    echo p.
    echodense p.
    echolucent p.
    edema p.
    enhancement p. (type I-IV)
    esophageal achalasia p.
    even distribution p.
    extended p.
    feathery p.
    fernlike p.
    fibrotic cavitating p.
    fibrous nodular p.
    filigree p.
    fine peripheral reticular p.
    finger-in-glove p.
    fingerprint p.
    fleur-de-lis p.
    flip-flop p.
    focal p.
    fold p.
    folial p.
    follicular p.
    fragmented p.
    gas p.

gastric mucosal p.
geographic p.
ground-glass p.
gyriform p.
hairbrush p.
hanging-fruit p.
haustral p.
helical p.
hemodynamic p.
hepatic echo p.
herringbone p.
heterogeneous internal echo p.
heterogeneous perfusion p.
hierarchical scanning p.
hole p.
homogeneous echo p.
homogeneous MR p.
honeycomb p.
hourglass p.
infiltration p.
inhomogeneous echo p.
interstitial lung p.
interstitial tear p.
intestinal gas p.
intraaneurysmal inflow p.
intraaneurysmal outflow p.
inverse follicle p.
juvenile T-wave p.
kidney mass growth p.
lacelike trabecular p.
ladderlike p.
Laue p.
left ventricular contraction p.
left ventricular strain p.
linear interstitial disease p.
liver spoked wheel p.
lobular alveolar p.
locomotor p.
lymphatic drainage p.
lytic p.
M p.
macronodular p.
magnetic resonance enhancement p.
manometric p.
marrow edema p.
marrow hyperstimulation p.
micronodular p.
migrational p.
miliary p.
mimosa p.
mixed lytic and sclerotic p.
moiré p.
mosaic attenuation p.
mosaic duodenal mucosal p.
moth-eaten p.
motion p.
mottled p.
movement p.
M-shaped mitral valve p.

mucosal fold p.
muscle recruitment p.
nodular p.
nonspecific bowel gas p.
p. of destruction
p. of spread
orthogonal-hole test p. (OHP)
ovarian fishnet weave p.
overlying branching p.
parallel and spiral flow p.'s
parenchymatous breast p.
parrot-beak p.
peribronchial p.
permeative p.
phlebographic p.
pin p.
PLES bar p.
pneumoencephalographic p.
postembolization angiographic p.
P pulmonale p.
primary inflammatory complex
  radiographic p.
proliferative p.
prominent ductal p.
pseudohomogeneous edema p.
pseudoinfarct p.
pseudomantle zone p.
pulmonary flow p.
pulmonary vascular p.
pulsatile flow p.
pulsation p.
QR p.
4-quadrant bar p.
quantum mottling p.
railroad track p.
ray p.
recurrence p.
relief p.
restrictive p.
reticular interstitial disease p.
reticular lung p.
reticulogranular p.
reticulonodular p.
reverberating flow p.
reverse crescent p.
rheologic p.
right ventricular strain p.
ringlike p.
rosary bead p.
rugal p.
salt-and-pepper chromatin p.
sawtooth excretory p.
sclerotic p.
segmental alveolar p.
seizure p.
sheetlike growth p.
shish kabob p.
sigmoid hair p.
signet ring p.

P

697

pattern (*continued*)
  sinus p.
  slice-of-sausage breast p.
  small bowel mucosal p.
  snowflake p.
  snowstorm breast p.
  solid p.
  speckled p.
  SPECT perfusion p.
  spectral p.
  spike-and-dome p.
  spiral flow p.
  spoiler gradient p.
  spoked wheel p.
  star test p.
  stellate p.
  storiform p.
  storiform-pleomorphic p.
  strain p.
  sulcal p.
  sunburst gyral p.
  surface convexity p.
  Tabar p.
  tagging p.
  task-rest p.
  temporal sawtooth p.
  thermal convection p.
  tigroid p.
  trabecular p.
  tram-track p.
  transducer beam p.
  tree-in-bud p.
  trigeminal p.
  triple signal p.
  tubular gas p.
  typical cobblestone p.
  V p.
  variegated p.
  ventricular contraction p.
  vesicular p.
  whirllike p.
  white branching linear p.
  Wolfe DY, NI, P1, P2 p.
  Wolfe mammographic
    parenchymatous p.
  zebra stripe p.
patulous
  p. cardia
  p. esophagogastric region
  p. hiatus
  p. lymphatics
PAU
  penetrating atherosclerotic
  ulcer
pauciarticular
paucilocular
  p. cystic mass
  p. tumor
pauciostotic

paucity
  alveolar p.
  p. of bowel gas
Pauli exclusion principle
Pauly point
pause
  asystolic p.
  compensatory p.
  postextrasystolic p.
  sinus p.
Pauwel
  P. angle
  P. femoral neck fracture
    classification
paving
  crazy p.
paving-stone degeneration
PAVM
  pulmonary arteriovenous malformation
Pawlik
  P. triangle
  P. trigone
Pawlow
  P. position
  P. projection
PAWP
  pulmonary artery wedge pressure
Payr sign
PBD
  percutaneous biliary drainage
PBF
  pulmonary blood flow
PBI
  protein-bound iodine
PBL
  positive beam limitation
PBPI
  penile-brachial pressure index
PBT
  pulmonary barotrauma
PBV
  pulmonary blood volume
PBVI
  pulmonary blood volume index
PC
  posterior commissure
    PC MR angiography
PCA
  posterior cerebral artery
  posterior communicating artery
PCC
  peripheral cholangiocarcinoma
PCCT
  phase-contrast x-ray computed
    tomography
PCD
  percutaneous catheter drainage
pCi
  picocurie

PCIS
  postcardiac injury syndrome
PCL
  posterior cruciate ligament
  pubococcygeal line
PCLBCL
  primary cutaneous large B-cell
  lymphoma
PC-MRA
  phase-contrast MRA
PCNL
  percutaneous nephrolithotomy
PCOD
  polycystic ovarian disease
PCOS
  polycystic ovary syndrome
PCP
  Pneumocystis carinii pneumonia
  pulmonary capillary pressure
PCPA
  postcatheterization pseudoaneurysm
PCRA
  percutaneous coronary rotational
  atherectomy
PCS
  proximal coronary sinus
PCWP
  pulmonary capillary wedge pressure
Pd
  palladium
^{103}**Pd, Pd-103**
  palladium 103
    ^{103}Pd isotope
    ^{103}Pd prostatic implant
    ^{103}Pd radioactive material
PDA
  patent ductus arteriosus
  poorly differentiated adenocarcinoma
  posterior descending artery
PDD
  percentage depth dose
  progressive diaphysial dysplasia
pDEXA
  peripheral dual-energy x-ray
  absorptiometry
    pDEXA peripheral bone
    densitometer
PDI
  power Doppler imaging
PDR
  pulsed dose rate
PDS
  power Doppler sonography
PDT
  photodynamic therapy
PE
  pericardial effusion
  polyethylene
  pulmonary edema

pulmonary embolus
  PE catheter
Peacock system
peak
  p. airway pressure
  p. amplitude
  p. aortic flow velocity
  p. area
  p. arterial frame
  backscatter p.
  Bragg ionization p.
  carotid pulse p.
  p. count density
  p. diastolic gradient
  diffraction p.
  p. dP/dt
  p. early diastolic filling velocity
  early systolic p. (ESP)
  p. ejection rate (PER)
  p. expiratory flow (PEF)
  p. filling
  p. filling rate (PFR)
  p. fitting
  p. flow variability
  p. flush flow
  frequency-related p.
  full energy p.
  p. identification
  p. inflation pressure
  p. instantaneous gradient
  juxtaphrenic p.
  kilovolt p. (kVp)
  p. late diastolic filling velocity
  liver-to-liver p. (L/LP)
  main glow p.
  p. of maximum enhancement (PME)
  p. parenchymatous activity
  photon p.
  pressure p.
  p. pressure gradient
  p. profile
  p. pulmonary flow velocity
  recirculation p.
  p. regurgitant flow velocity
  p. regurgitant wave pressure
  p. repetition frequency
  p. right ventricular-right atrial
  systolic gradient
  p. scatter factor
  p. shape
  single p.
  p. skin radiation dose
  spread Bragg p.
  p. systolic and diastolic ratio
  p. systolic aortic pressure
  p. systolic gradient
  p. systolic velocity (PSV)
  temporal p.
  time to p. (TTP)

P

peak (*continued*)
  p. transmitted velocity
  p. velocity of blood flow
peak-to-peak pressure gradient
pearl
  keratin p.
  p. necklace gallbladder
  scrotal p.
pearlescent solid tumor
pearl-like breast calcification
pearly
  p. body
  p. CNS tumor
  p. neoplasia
  p. white ovary
pear-shaped
  p.-s. defect
  p.-s. heart
  p.-s. urinary bladder
  p.-s. uterus
Pearson
  P. attachment
  P. correlation coefficient
  P. method
  P. position
  P. syndrome
pea-size
pebble-shaped patella
PEC
  perivascular epithelioid cell
Pecquet
  cistern of P.
pecten pubis
pectinate
  p. ligament
  p. line
pectineal, pectineus
  p. muscle
pectineus (*var. of* pectineal)
pectora (*pl. of* pectus)
pectoral
  p. girdle
  p. heart
  p. lymph node
  p. ridge
pectoralis
  p. major muscle
  p. major syndrome
  p. minor muscle
pectoris (*gen. of* pectus)
pectus, *pl.* **pectora,** *gen.* **pectoris**
  angina pectoris
  p. carinatum deformity
  p. excavatum
  p. excavatum deformity
  p. recurvatum
pedal
  p. artery opacification
  p. bone

  p. lymphangiography
  p. lymphography
pedes (*pl. of* pes)
pedestal sign
pediatric
  p. biplane TEE probe
  p. bronchiolitis
  p. fibroxanthoma
  p. hemangioma
  P. Ingesta Scan metal detector
  p. neuroradiology
  p. nuclear medicine imaging
  p. primary brain tumor
  p. radiology
  p. scintigraphy
  p. solid tumor
pedicle
  p. and pars
  p. bone graft
  p. erosion
  p. finger
  p. flap
  p. fracture
  internal mammary artery p.
  musculofascial p.
  p. of vertebra
  phrenic p.
  p. plate
  pulmonary p.
  p. sclerosis
  p. signal intensity
  spinal p.
  splaying of p.
  p. targeting
  vascular p.
pedicolaminar fracture-dislocation
pedicular renal artery stenosis
pedis (*gen. of* pes)
pedobarography
  dynamic p.
PEDRI
  proton-electron double-resonance
  imaging
peduncle
  cerebellar p.
  cerebral p.
  inferior cerebellar p.
peduncular
  p. loop
  p. segment of superior cerebellar
  artery
pedunculated
  p. leiomyoma
  p. lesion
  p. mass
  p. polyp
  p. subserous myoma
  p. thrombus
  p. uterine fibroid

p. uterine myxoma
p. vesical tumor
pedunculation
peel
pleural p.
peel-away sheath
PEF
parietal eye field
peak expiratory flow
peg
cerebellar p.
rete p.
PEG
percutaneous endoscopic gastrostomy
pneumoencephalogram
pneumoencephalography
polyethylene glycol
Pegasus PIV laser
Pegasys workstation
PEHO
progressive encephalopathy with edema,
hypsarrhythmia, and optic atrophy
PEHO syndrome
PEI
percutaneous ethanol injection
PEI 1-shot technique
PEI 2-shot technique
PELA
peripheral excimer laser angioplasty
peliosis
spleen p.
Pelizaeus-Merzbacher disease
Pelizzari surface matching method
Pellegrini-Stieda
P.-S. calcification
P.-S. disease
pellet
alanine-silicone p.
p. artifact
radiopaque p.
pellucidum
cavum septum p.
septum p.
pelvem
aditus ad p.
pelves (*pl. of* pelvis)
pelvic
p. abscess
p. aneurysm
p. arteriography
p. artery
p. bone
p. brim
p. canal
p. chocolate cyst
p. collateral vessel
p. colon
p. congestion syndrome
p. cystic mass

p. diameter
p. diaphragm
p. exenteration
p. exostosis
p. fascia
p. femoral angle
p. fibrolipomatosis
p. film for IUD localization
p. floor
p. fluid
p. fracture frame
p. girdle
p. infection
p. inflammatory disease
p. inlet
p. insufficiency fracture
p. kidney
p. lipomatosis
p. lymph node
p. malignancy
p. mass complex
p. mass frequency
p. morphometry
p. notching
p. obliquity
p. organ prolapse (POP)
p. outlet
p. peritoneal surface
p. peritoneum
p. phased-array coil
p. plane
p. plexus
p. rim fracture
p. ring
p. ring fracture
p. ring ligament
p. sidewall
p. sonography
p. space
p. spot
p. spur syndrome
p. steal
p. steal test
p. straddle fracture
p. teardrop
p. ultrasound
p. ultrasound CT scan
p. unleveling
p. vascular trauma
p. vein thrombosis
p. venous obstruction
p. venous stenosis
p. view
p. viscus
p. wall
pelvicaliceal (*var. of* pelvicalyceal)
pelvicaliectasis
pelvicalyceal, pelvicaliceal
p. change

P

pelvicalyceal (*continued*)
    p. dilation
    p. distention
    p. effacement
    p. system
pelvicephalography (*var. of* cephalopelvimetry)
pelviectasis
pelvimetry
    magnetic resonance p.
    planographic p.
    radiographic p.
    stereoscopic p.
pelviography
pelvioplasty (*var. of* pyeloplasty)
pelvioradiography, pelviradiography
pelvioscopy, pelvoscopy
pelviradiography
pelviroentgenography
pelvis, *pl.* **pelves**
    aditus p.
    android p.
    anthropoid p.
    assimilation p.
    beaked p.
    bifid p.
    bifid renal p.
    bony p.
    brachypellic p.
    brim of p.
    champagne glass p.
    contracted p.
    cordiform p.
    Deventer p.
    diameter obliqua p.
    diameter transversa p.
    dolichopellic p.
    dwarf p.
    elephant ears p.
    extrarenal renal p.
    false p.
    female p.
    flat p.
    frozen p.
    funnel-shaped p.
    goblet-shaped p.
    greater p.
    gynecoid p.
    hardened p.
    heart-shaped p.
    intrarenal p.
    inverted p.
    juvenile p.
    Kilian p.
    kyphoscoliotic p.
    kyphotic p.
    lesser p.
    longitudinal oval p.
    lordotic p.

    male p.
    masculine p.
    mesatipellic p.
    Mickey Mouse ears p.
    Nägele p.
    p. of kidney
    osteomalacic p.
    Otto p.
    Otto-Kobak p.
    platypellic p.
    postmenarchal female p.
    pseudoosteomalacic p.
    rachitic p.
    renal p.
    reniform p.
    Rokitansky p.
    scoliotic p.
    small p.
    spider p.
    spondylolisthetic p.
    tombstone p.
    transverse oval p.
    trident p.
    true p.
    windswept p.
    wine glass p.
pelviureteric junction (PUJ)
pelviureterography (*var. of* pyelography)
pelviureteroradiography (*var. of* pyelography)
pelvocaliectasis
pelvocephalography (*var. of* cephalopelvimetry)
pelvoscopy (*var. of* pelvioscopy)
PEM
    positron emission mammography
Pemberton osteotomy
Pena-Shokeir syndrome
pencil
    p. dosimeter
    p. electron beam
pencil-beam
    p.-b. approach
    p.-b. navigator echo
pencil-in-cup
    p.-i.-c. appearance
    p.-i.-c. deformity
penciling
    p. deformity
    p. of distal clavicle
    p. of rib
    p. of terminal tuft
pencil-like deformity
pencil-point metatarsal deformity
pendent positioning
pendetide
    indium-111 capromab p.
    ^{111}In satumomab p.
    satumomab p.
Pendred syndrome

PenduLaser
    Kaplan P. 115
pendulous
    p. heart
    p. pouch
    p. reference axis (PRA)
    p. urethra
pendulum
    cor p.
    p. movement
penes (*pl. of* penis)
penetrability
penetrating
    p. aortic ulcer
    p. atherosclerotic ulcer (PAU)
    p. fracture
    p. head injury
    p. lung injury
    p. trauma
    p. TRD
    p. wound
penetration
    acoustic p.
    bowel wall p.
    p. fraction
    insufficient acoustic p.
    lack of acoustic p.
    radiographic p.
    rectal p.
penetrometer
    Benoist p.
penial (*var. of* penile)
penile, penial
    p. artery
    p. bulb
    p. fibromatosis
    p. implant
    p. plaque
    p. raphe
    p. sonography
    p. squamous papilloma
    p. urethra
    p. vein
    p. vessel
penile-brachial pressure index (PBPI)
penis, *pl.* **penises,** *pl.* **penes**
    bulb of p.
    bulbospongiosus muscle of p.
    clubbed p.
    concealed p.
    corpus cavernosum p.
    corpus spongiosum p.
    crus of p.
    deep fascia of p.
    dorsal artery of p.
    dorsal nerve of p.
    dorsum of p.
    double p.
    glans p.

    hypoplastic p.
    ischiospongiosus muscle of p.
    root of p.
    suspensory ligament of p.
    webbed p.
peniscopy
penises (*pl. of* penis)
penoscrotal
PenRad mammography clinical reporting system
Penta balloon
pentacene
pentagastrin imaging agent
pentalogy
    Cantrell p.
    p. of Fallot
pentavalent DMSA imaging agent
Pentax ELLB 6000, 6500 ultrasound gastroscope
Pentax-Hitachi FG32UA endosonographic system
pentetate
    [111]In imciromab p.
pentetic acid imaging agent
pentetreotide
    p. imaging agent
    [111]In p.
    indium-111 p.
    p. tumor localization scan
pentose cycle
penultimate section
penumbra
    dosimetric p.
    hemodynamic p.
    ischemic p.
    p. zone
PEP
    preejection period
pepper
    P. syndrome
    P. tumor
peppermint oil imaging agent
pepper-pot pitting
pepsic (*var. of* peptic)
peptic, pepsic
    p. esophagitis
    p. stricture
    p. ulcer
    p. ulcer disease (PUD)
peptide
    anionic neutrophil-activating p. (ANAP)
    p. imaging agent
    p. receptor scintigraphy
PER
    peak ejection rate
percentage
    p. classification
    p. depth dose (PDD)
    p. signal intensity loss

P

Perception scanner
perceptual linearization
perched facet joint
Percheron
    artery of P.
perchlorate
    potassium p.
    sodium p.
    p. washout test
Perclose
    P. arterial closure device
    P. closer
    P. diagnostic device
    P. PVS suture system
    P. therapeutic device
percreta
    placenta p.
PercuCut cut-biopsy needle
Percuflex stent
percussion sensitivity
Percusurg distal protection device
percutaneous
    p. abscess drainage
    p. access needle
    p. antegrade biliary drainage
    p. antegrade pyelography
    p. antegrade urography
    p. arterial closure device
    p. automated discectomy
    p. biliary drainage (PBD)
    p. bone biopsy
    p. catheter drainage (PCD)
    p. cavity drainage catheter
    p. cecostomy
    p. cementoplasty
    p. cervical cordotomy
    p. chemical ablation
    p. cholecystocholedochostomy
    p. cholecystotomy catheter
    p. choledochoscopy
    p. coronary revascularization
    p. coronary rotational atherectomy (PCRA)
    p. dilation of biliary duct
    p. dissolution of thrombus
    p. electrical nerve stimulation
    p. embolectomy
    p. embolotherapy
    p. endofluoroscopy
    p. endoluminal placement
    p. endometrial drug delivery
    p. endopyelotomy
    p. endoscopic gastrostomy (PEG)
    p. endoscopy
    p. ethanol injection (PEI)
    p. ethanol injection therapy
    p. ethanol instillation
    p. ethanol sclerotherapy
    p. excimer laser coronary angioplasty

p. femoral arteriography
p. gastroenterostomy
p. hepaticojejunostomy
p. hepatobiliary cholangiography
p. interventional radiology
p. intraaortic balloon
p. intraaortic balloon counterpulsation
p. intracoronary angioscopy imaging
p. mechanical thrombectomy (PMT)
p. microwave coagulation therapy
p. nephrolithotomy (PCNL)
p. nephroscope
p. nephrostolithotomy
p. nephrostomy
p. nonvascular abdominal intervention
p. osteoplasty
p. pancreatography
p. pericardioscopy
p. peritoneovenous shunt creation
p. pin insertion
p. radiofrequency catheter ablation
p. retrograde transfemoral technique
p. splenoportography
p. stent
p. suture-mediated arteriotomy closure device
p. thermal occlusion
p. transcatheter therapy
p. transhepatic biliary drainage (PTBD)
p. transhepatic cholangial drainage (PTCD)
p. transhepatic cholangiogram (PTC, PTCA, PTHC)
p. transhepatic cholangiography (PTC, PTCA)
p. transhepatic cholecystostomy
p. transhepatic decompression
p. transhepatic endoluminal biliary biopsy
p. transhepatic liver biopsy
p. transhepatic lymphography (pTL)
p. transhepatic portography
p. transluminal angioplasty (PTA)
p. transluminal angioplasty balloon
p. transluminal balloon dilation
p. transluminal coronary angioplasty (PTCA)
p. transluminal coronary recanalization technique
p. transluminal renal angioplasty (PTRA)
p. transluminal septal myocardial ablation (PTSMA)
p. transluminal therapeutic intervention
p. transperineal seed implantation
p. transthoracic needle biopsy (PTNB)
p. transtracheal bronchography

p. tube insertion
p. tumor treatment
p. ultrasound-guided thrombin injection
p. umbilical blood sampling
p. vascular surgical device
p. vertebroplasty
percutaneously cannulated
Perez sign
Perflex stainless steel balloon-expandable stent
perflubron
    p. imaging agent
    partial liquid ventilation with p.
perfluorocarbon-exposed sonicated dextrose albumin (PESDA)
perfluorocarbon imaging agent
perfluorochemical
perfluorooctyl bromide (PFOB)
perflutren lipid microsphere injectable suspension
perforans
perforated
    p. aortic cusp
    p. appendicitis
    p. cholecystitis
    p. diverticulum
    p. gangrenous appendix
    p. hollow viscus
    p. ulcer
perforating
    p. aneurysm
    p. artery
    p. branch
    p. colorectal carcinoma
    p. fracture
    p. vein
    p. wound
perforation
    bladder p.
    bowel p.
    cardiac p.
    colonic p.
    common bile duct spontaneous p.
    cystic duct p.
    duodenal ulcer p.
    esophageal p.
    gallbladder p.
    iatrogenic esophageal p.
    idiopathic gastric p.
    intestinal p.
    Niemeier gallbladder p.
    renal transplant GI tract p.
    septal p.
    spontaneous p.
    transseptal p.
    ulcer p.
    ureteral p.

vascular p.
ventricular p.
perforative lesion
perforator
    incompetent p.
    septal p.
    p. vessel
Performa mammography system
perfusate vessel
perfused
    p. myocardium
    p. needle applicator
    p. twin
perfusion
    p. abnormality
    adequate coronary p.
    p. agent
    p. and ventilation lung imaging
    antegrade p.
    blood p.
    brain p.
    capillary p.
    continuous hyperthermic peritoneal p.
    p. CT
    decreased distal p.
    diminished airway p.
    diminished systemic p.
    gated stress myocardial p.
    p. gradient
    hepatic arterial p.
    homogeneous p.
    hypothermic p.
    impaired renal p.
    increment of p.
    p. index
    inhomogeneous p.
    intraperitoneal hyperthermic p. (IPHP)
    isolated hepatic p.
    isolated hepatic portal and arterial p.
    isolation p.
    limb p.
    lung p.
    p. lung scan
    luxury p.
    maldistribution of ventilation and p.
    p. measurement technique
    misery p.
    mosaic p.
    p. MRI
    p. MR imaging
    myocardial p.
    peripheral p.
    poor p.
    p. pressure
    pulsatile p.
    quantitative cardiac p.
    regional cerebral p.
    regional pulmonary p.
    regional vascular p.

P

perfusion (*continued*)
   renal p.
   resting p.
   retrograde cardiac p.
   p. scintigraphy
   1st-pass cardiac p.
   p. study
   p. time
   tissue p.
   total liver p.
   unilateral lung p.
perfusion-metabolism reverse mismatch
perfusion-weighted
   p.-w. imaging (PWI)
   p.-w. MRI
periacetabular osteotomy
periadventitial fibrosis
perialveolar fibrosis
periampullary
   p. carcinoma
   p. diverticulum
   p. duodenal tumor
perianal
   p. abscess
   p. hematoma
periaortic
   p. area
   p. fibrosis
   p. lymph node
   p. mediastinal hematoma
periaortitis
   chronic p.
periapical
   p. cemental dysplasia
   p. film
   p. granuloma
   p. lesion
   p. radiograph
periappendiceal
   p. abscess
   p. structure
periaqueductal
   p. gray matter
   p. hemorrhage
periareolar fistula
periarteriolar lymphoid sheath
periarteritis nodosa
periarthritis
   adhesive p.
periarticular
   p. calcification
   p. fluid collection
   p. fracture
   p. heterotopic ossification (PHO)
   p. margin
   p. osteoporosis
   p. tissue
periauricular region
peribiliary cyst

peribronchial
   p. alveolar space
   p. connective tissue
   p. cuffing
   p. distribution
   p. fibrosis
   p. hemorrhage
   p. infiltrate
   p. lymph node
   p. marking
   p. micronodule
   p. pattern
   p. thickening
peribronchovascular interstitial compartment
peribursal fat
pericalyceal cyst
pericallosal
   p. artery
   p. lipoma
   p. vein
   p. vessel
pericapsular fat infiltrate
pericardia (*pl. of* pericardium)
pericardiac
   p. fat
   p. pleura
pericardiacophrenic vein
pericardial
   p. aorta
   p. calcareous deposit
   p. calcification
   p. cavity
   p. chyle with tamponade
   p. cyst
   p. cystic echinococcosis
   p. defect
   p. diaphragmatic adhesion
   p. disease
   p. duplication cyst
   p. effusion (PE)
   p. empyema
   p. fat-pad
   p. flap
   p. fluid
   p. fold
   p. friction rub
   p. halo
   p. hematoma
   p. infusion
   p. knock sound
   p. lymphangioma
   p. lymph node
   p. reserve volume
   p. sac
   p. silhouette
   p. sinus
   p. sleeve recess
   p. space

p. tamponade
p. vein
p. window
pericardicentesis (*var. of*
pericardiocentesis)
pericardiectomy
pericardiocentesis, pericardicentesis
hand-carried ultrasound-guided p.
pericardioperitoneal
p. canal
p. ligament
pericardiophrenic ligament
pericardioscopy
percutaneous p.
pericarditis
bread-and-butter p.
constrictive p.
diffuse p.
hemorrhagic p.
postmeningococcal p.
radiation-induced p.
pericardium, *pl.* **pericardia**
adherent p.
autologous p.
calcified p.
congenitally absent p.
crus p.
diaphragmatic p.
p. fibrosum
fibrous p.
inelastic p.
parietal p.
rheumatic adherent p.
roughened state of p.
serous p.
shaggy p.
soldier's patch of p.
visceral p.
pericarinal injury
pericatheter
p. thrombosis
p. thrombus
pericaval
pericavernous
pericecal abscess
pericentral fibrosis
pericerebral fluid
pericholecystic
p. abscess
p. edema
p. fluid
p. fluid collection
pericholedochal
p. node
p. varix
perichondral, perichondrial
p. bone
p. cell seeding
p. ring

perichondrial (*var. of* perichondral)
perichondrium
pericicatricial emphysema
pericolic
p. abscess
p. haziness
pericolonic
p. abscess
p. fat
p. fluid
pericranii
sinus p.
pericyst
pericystic edema
pericytoma
peridental space
peridiaphragmatic hematoma
peridiploid
peridiverticulitis
periductal
p. calcification
p. fibrosis
peridural fibrosis
periesophageal fluid
perifascial fluidlike collection
perifocal
p. edema
p. emphysema
perigastric
p. deformity
p. fat
perigestational hemorrhage
perigraft
p. fluid
p. hematoma
p. seroma
perihepatic
p. abscess
p. space
perihepatitis
focal p.
perihilar
p. area
p. batwing infiltrate
p. density
p. fat
p. fibrosis
p. lung disease
p. marking
p. pulmonary edema
p. region
periileal
periinfarcted zone
periinfarction
p. block
p. conduction defect
p. ischemia
p. zone
perilabral sulcus

P

perilesional
p. edema
p. white matter
perilobular
p. connective tissue
p. duct
perilunate fracture-dislocation
perimedial
p. dysplasia
p. renal artery fibroplasia
perimedullary
perimembranous ventricular septal defect
perimeniscal capsular plexus
perimesencephalic
p. cistern
p. nonaneurysmal subarachnoid hemorrhage
perimeter-area (P/A)
perimetry testing
perimuscular
p. fibrosis
p. plexus
perinatal
p. anoxia
p. asphyxia
p. injury
perinea (*pl. of* perineum)
perineal
p. descent
p. fascia
p. sinus
p. space
perineogram imaging
perineoplastic edema
perineovaginal fistula
perinephric
p. air injection
p. fat
p. fluid collection
p. hematoma
p. space
p. space hemorrhage
p. urinoma
perinephritic abscess
perineum, *pl.* **perinea**
perineural
p. arachnoid cyst
p. disease
p. extension
p. fat
p. fibroblastoma
p. fibroblastoma tumor
p. fibrosis
p. glial proliferation
p. invasion
p. sacral cyst
p. tumor spread
perinuclear halo

period
antegrade refractory p.
diastasis heart p.
diastolic filling p.
effective refractory p. (ERP)
embryonic p.
fetal p.
functional refractory p. (FRP)
immediate postictal p.
isoelectric p.
isovolumic p.
phase-encoding p.
postbiopsy p.
preejection p. (PEP)
radiofrequency p.
rapid filling p.
raster p.
reduced ventricular filling p.
relative refractory p. (RRP)
retrograde refractory p.
roentgen-equivalent-man p. (REMP)
systolic ejection p. (SEP)
total atrial refractory p. (TARP)
ventricular effective refractory p. (VERP)
window p.
periodic
p. acid-Schiff
p. sharp wave (PSW)
p. synchronous discharge (PSD)
periodically rotated overlapping parallel lines with enhanced reconstruction
periodicity
circadian p.
periodontal
p. disease
p. ligament
periodontitis
perioptic meningioma
periorbital
p. bidirectional Doppler
p. directional Doppler ultrasonography
p. edema
periosseous soft tissue mass
periostea (*pl. of* periosteum)
periosteal
p. artery
p. bone
p. bone collar
p. cloaking
p. creep
p. desmoid
p. dysplasia
p. elevation
p. fibroma
p. fibrosarcoma
p. ganglion

p. new bone formation
p. osteosarcoma
p. reaction
p. resorption
p. sarcoma
periosteitis (*var. of* periostitis)
periosteum, *pl.* **periostea**
p. of rib
periostitis, periosteitis
exuberant p.
florid reactive p.
medial malleolus p.
periotic bone
peripancreatic
p. artery
p. fluid collection
p. lymphadenopathy
peripartum dilated cardiomyopathy
peripelvic
p. collateral vessel
p. cyst
p. fat proliferation
p. lipomatosis
peripheral
p. airspace disease
p. arterial occlusive disease
(PAOD)
p. arteriography
p. arteriosclerosis
p. artery
p. artery aneurysm
p. blood
p. blood flow
p. bolus chase
p. border
p. bronchogenic carcinoma
p. cholangiocarcinoma (PCC)
p. chondrosarcoma
p. circulation
p. circulatory vasoconstriction
p. consolidation
p. cutaneous vasoconstriction
p. directional atherectomy
p. dual-energy x-ray absorptiometry
(pDEXA)
p. embolus
p. excimer laser angioplasty (PELA)
p. expansion
p. fracture
p. hemopoietic intermediate
signal-intensity marrow
p. hypoperfusion
p. infiltrate
p. interstitium
p. intravenous infusion line
p. laser angioplasty
p. lesion enhancement
p. loading
p. lung disease

p. lymphoma
p. meniscocapsular tear
p. MR angiography
p. necrosis
p. nerve
p. nerve decompression
p. nerve injury
p. nerve lesion
p. nervous system
p. neuroectodermal tumor
p. neurofibromatosis
p. nodule
p. ossification
p. ossifying fibroma
p. osteoma
p. parenchymatous atelectasis
p. perfusion
p. perimeniscal capillary ingrowth
p. pneumonia
p. pseudoaneurysm
p. puddling
p. pulmonary artery stenosis
(PPAS)
p. pulse gating
p. quantitative computed tomography
(pQCT)
p. runoff
p. skeleton
p. small airway study
p. synovitis
p. texture
p. vascular disease (PVD)
p. vascular imaging
p. vascular occlusive disease
(PVOD)
p. vascular resistance (PVR)
p. vasculature
p. vasogenic edema
p. venography
p. vessel
p. zone (PZ)
peripherally
p. inserted central catheter
(PICC)
p. inserted central catheter line
p. inserted central catheter occlusion
line opening (PICCOLO)
periphery
echogenic p.
lung p.
p. of anulus
periportal
p. area
p. cirrhosis
p. collar
p. fibrosis
p. sinusoidal dilation
p. tracking
p. tracking of blood

P

periprocedural monitoring
periprosthetic
    p. abscess
    p. bone resorption
    p. fracture
    p. infection
    p. leak
    p. malignancy
    p. neoplasm
    p. osteolysis
    p. uptake
periradicular
    p. nerve
    p. sheath
perirectal
    p. abscess
    p. fat
perirenal
    p. abscess
    p. air study
    p. bleeding
    p. compartment
    p. fat
    p. hematoma
    p. hemorrhage
    p. insufflation
    p. lymphoma
    p. mass
    p. septum
    p. space (PRS)
perirolandic parietal cortex
perisigmoid colon
perisinusoidal space
perisplenic node
peristalsis
    abnormal esophageal p.
    absence of primary p.
    absent p.
    accelerated p.
    antegrade p.
    bowel p.
    decreased p.
    esophageal p.
    hyperactive p.
    increased p.
    meconium p.
    primary esophageal p.
    retrograde p.
    reversed p.
    secondary p.
    small bowel p.
    ureteral seesaw p.
    uterine p.
    visible p.
    yo-yo esophageal p.
    yo-yo ureteral p.
peristaltic
    p. activity
    p. contraction

    p. rush
    p. sequence
    p. wave
peristriate cortex
perisylvian cortex
peritendinitis, peritenonitis, peritenontitis
peritendinous
    p. adhesion
    p. calcification
peritenonitis
peritenontitis (*var. of* peritendinitis)
perithyroid vein
peritonea (*pl. of* peritoneum)
peritoneal
    p. abscess
    p. attachment
    p. band
    p. carcinomatosis
    p. cavity
    p. cavity fluid
    p. desmoid tumor
    p. dialysis catheter
    p. effusion
    p. enhancement
    p. fold
    p. gutter
    p. hernia
    p. inclusion cyst
    p. lymphopneumatosis
    p. mass
    p. mesothelioma
    p. metastasis
    p. metastatic implant
    p. mouse
    p. part of inguinal ligament
    p. recess
    p. sac
    p. scintigraphy
    p. seeding
    p. shunting
    p. sign
    p. soiling
    p. space
    p. thickening
    p. tuberculosis
peritoneal-venous shunt patency test
peritonei
    carcinomatosis p.
    gliomatosis p.
    pseudomyxoma p.
peritoneocele
peritoneogram imaging
peritoneography
    CT/MR p.
peritoneopericardial diaphragmatic
  hernia
peritoneopleural communication
peritoneoscintigraphy
peritoneovenous shunt (PVS)

peritoneum, *pl.* **peritonea**
   parietal p.
   pelvic p.
   visceral p.
peritonitis
   bacterial p.
   bile p.
   p. carcinomatosa
   chemical p.
   meconium p.
   sclerosing encapsulating p.
   tuberculous p.
peritrigonal white matter
peritrochanteric fracture
peritubular vascular bed
peritumoral
   p. cyst
   p. edema
   p. enhancement
   p. injection
   p. tissue
periumbilical
   p. pain
   p. swelling
periungual fibroma
periureteral fibrosis
periurethral gland
perivalvular
   p. leak
   p. pseudoaneurysm
perivascular
   p. cloaking
   p. cuffing
   p. distribution
   p. edema
   p. epithelioid cell
    (PEC)
   p. fibrosis
   p. infiltrate
   p. mass
   p. pseudorosette
   p. space
periventricular
   p. blush
   p. bright signal
   p. calcification
   p. echogenicity (PVE)
   p. gray (PVG)
   p. gray matter
   p. halo
   p. hemorrhagic infarct
   p. hypodensity
   p. lesion
   p. leukoencephalopathy
   p. leukomalacia (PVL)
   p. plaque
   p. white matter
perivenular fibrosis
perivesical

Perkin line
Perkins-Ombredanne line
permanent
   p. brachytherapy
   p. callus
   p. interstitial implant
   p. magnet
   p. stoma
PermCath
   Quinton P.
permeability
   capillary p.
   p. constant
   constant p.
   Crone-Renkin index of p.
   magnetic p.
   membrane p.
   pulmonary capillary p.
   p. surface
   tumor capillary p.
permeation
permeative
   p. bone destruction
   p. lesion
   p. pattern
permutation
peroneal
   p. artery
   p. bone
   p. muscle
   p. nerve
   p. retinaculum
   p. sign
   p. tendon injury
   p. tendon subluxation
   p. tenosynovitis
   p. thrombus
   p. trochlea
   p. tubercle
   p. vein
   p. vessel
peroneal-to-anterior compartment
  ratio
peroneum
   os p.
peroneus
   p. brevis tendon
   p. longus
   p. longus muscle avulsion
   p. longus tendon
   p. quartus muscle
   p. tertius
   p. tertius tendon
peroral
   p. cone radiation therapy
   p. cyanosis
   p. implantation
   p. retrograde pancreaticobiliary
    ductography

P

peroxidase
    tracer horseradish p.
peroxyl
perpendicular
    p. mean translation
    method of p.'s
Persantine
    P. imaging agent
    P. thallium imaging
persistent
    p. bronchopleural fistula
    p. common atrioventricular canal
    p. cortical kidney lobation
    p. ductus arteriosus
    p. fetal circulation
    p. generalized lymphadenopathy
    p. hyperparathyroidism
    p. left inferior vena cava
    p. left superior vena cava
    p. loop sign
    p. metopic suture
    p. ossiculum terminale
    p. ostium atrioventriculare commune
    p. primitive trigeminal artery
    p. pulmonary hypertension
    p. pylorospasm
    p. renal lobation
    p. sciatic artery
    p. splenomegaly
    p. truncus arteriosus (PTA)
personal ionization chamber
perspective volume rendering (PVR)
Pertechnegas
pertechnetate (TcO₄)
    free p.
    p. scintigraphy
    sodium p.
    technetium 99m p.
Perthes
    P. disease
    P. epiphysis
    P. lesion
Perthes-Bankart lesion
perturbation
    cytoskeletal p.
    magnetic field p.
    radiation dose p.
perturbing magnetic field
pertussoid eosinophilic pneumonia
perversus
    situs p.
pervious duct of Botallo
pes, *pl.* **pedes,** *gen.* **pedis**
    p. abductus
    p. adductus
    p. anserine bursa
    p. anserinus
    p. anserinus bursitis
    p. arcuatus

    p. arcuatus clawfoot deformity
    p. calcaneocavus
    p. calcaneovalgus
    p. calcaneus
    calcar pedis
    p. calvaneovalgus
    p. cavovalgus
    p. cavovarus
    p. cavus
    p. cavus clawfoot deformity
    p. contortus
    digitus pedis
    dorsalis pedis
    dorsum pedis
    p. equinovalgus
    p. equinovarus
    p. equinus
    p. malleus valgus
    malum perforans pedis
    p. planovalgus
    p. planovalgus deformity
    p. plantigrade planus
    p. planus deformity
    pollex pedis
    p. pronation
    p. pronatus
    p. varus
PESDA
    perfluorocarbon-exposed sonicated
    dextrose albumin
pestis
    Yersinia p.
PET
    positron emission tomography
    PET balloon
    cardiac PET
    PET compound
    PET full-ring scanner
    PET lung imaging
    PET measurement of dopamine
      receptor availability
    PET metabolic imaging
    PET myocardial fatty acid imaging
    PET perfusion metabolism imaging
    PET radioligand
    PET radiopharmaceutical
    PET scan
    PET target material
    tyrphostin radiotracer for PET
petal-fugal flow
PET/CT scanner
petiole
petit
    P. ligament
    p. mal seizure
    P. sinus
PET/MRI fusion
Pétrequin ligament
petrobasilar suture

petroclinoid ligament
petromastoid
petrosal
  p. bone
  p. cerebellum
  p. foramen
  p. ganglion
  greater p.
  lesser p.
  p. nerve
  p. sinus
  p. vein
petrositis
  apical p.
petrosphenobasilar suture
petrosphenoid
petrosphenooccipital
  p. suture
  p. suture of Gruber
petrosquamosal
petrous
  p. apex
  p. apex dumbbell mass
  p. carotid canal
  p. carotid canal stenosis
  p. ICA
  p. pyramid
  p. pyramid scalloping
  p. ridge
  p. segment of internal carotid
    artery
  p. temporal bone
  p. tip
PETT
  positron emission transaxial
    tomography
  positron emission transverse
    tomography
  PETT imaging
  PETT VI PET scanner
Peutz-Jeghers
  P.-J. gastrointestinal
    polyposis
  P.-J. polyp
  P.-J. syndrome
Peyer patch
Peyronie disease
PF3, PF4
  platelet factor 3, 4
PFA
  platelet function analyzer
PFA-100 system
Pfaundler-Hurler
  P.-H. disease
  P.-H. syndrome
Pfeiffer
  P. acrocephalosyndactyly
  P. disease
  P. syndrome

**Pfeiffer-Comberg intraorbital foreign
  body localization method**
PFFD
  proximal focal femoral
    deficiency
PFIC
  progressive familial intrahepatic
    cholestasis
Pfizer 200 FS, 400 scanner
PFO
  patent foramen ovale
PFOB
  perfluorooctyl bromide
PFR
  peak filling rate
pGGO
  pure ground-glass opacity
P-gp
  P glocoprotein
PGSE
  pulsed-gradient spin echo
PHA
  proper hepatic artery
  pulse-height analyzer
PHACES
  posterior fossa malformations, facial
    hemangiomas, arterial anomalies,
    cardiac anomalies and aortic
    coarctation, eye anomalies, and
    sternal clefting and/or supraumbilical
    raphe
  PHACES syndrome
phacomatosis, phakomatosis
phagedenic ulcer
phagocyte
phakomatoses
phakomatosis (*var. of* phacomatosis)
phalangeal
  p. bone
  p. branch
  p. diaphysial fracture
  p. glenoid ligament
  p. herniation
  p. preponderance
  p. shortening
phalanges (*pl. of* phalanx)
phalanx, *pl.* **phalanges**
  base of p.
  drumstick p.
  hourglass p.
  ivory p.
  p. of foot
  p. of hand
  rectangular p.
Phalen
  P. maneuver
  P. position
phantogeusia
  global p.

P

phantom
    Alderson anthropomorphic p.
    anthropomorphic p.
    attenuation in p. (AIPH)
    p. bone
    p. breast tumor
    cat p.
    chest p.
    computer-simulated p.
    Derenzo p.
    p. dosimetry
    flood p.
    gelatin p.
    Hine-Duley p.
    Hoffman brain p.
    p. image
    Jaszczak p.
    p. limb pain
    p. limb syndrome
    p. lung tumor
    mammographic p.
    metal line-pair p.
    neck p.
    nuclear magnetic resonance p.
    oil-water p.
    parallel line equal
      spacebar p.
    p. pregnancy
    p. radiograph
    reference p.
    Rollo p.
    p. simulating cardiac motion
    p. study
    velocity evaluation p.
    wax p.
phantosmia
    birhinal p.
    unirhinal p.
pharmacoangiography
pharmacodynamics
pharmacokinetic model
pharmacologic, pharmacological
    p. dilation
    p. stress
    p. stress dual-isotope myocardial
      perfusion SPECT
    p. stress echocardiography
pharmacological (*var. of*
  pharmacologic)
pharmacomechanical thrombolysis
pharmacoradiologic disimpaction of
  esophageal foreign body
pharmacoradiology
pharmacovigilance
PharmaSeed palladium-103
  seed
pharyngeal
    p. abscess
    p. area

    p. artery
    p. canal
    p. muscle
    p. orifice
    p. plexus
    p. pouch
    p. recess
    p. space mass
    p. tonsil
    p. wall carcinoma
pharynges (*pl. of* pharynx)
pharyngobasilar fascia
pharyngoesophageal
    p. diverticulum
    p. function
    p. pouch
    p. sphincter
pharyngoesophagogram
pharyngoesophagography
pharyngography
pharyngotonsillitis
pharyngotympanic tube
pharynx, *pl.* **pharynges**
    p. cross-section
    laryngeal part of p.
    nasal part of p.
    oral part of p.
    postcricoid p.
phase
    accelerated p.
    accumulation p.
    p. analysis
    p. angle
    arterial p.
    blastic p.
    blood pool p.
    p. cancellation
    cardiac p.
    chronic p.
    p. coherence
    p. contrast
    p. correction
    corticomedullary p.
    p. cycling
    p. delay
    delayed p.
    diastolic depolarization p.
    p. difference mapping
    p. discontinuity artifact
    p. effect
    p. encoding
    equilibrium p.
    excretory p.
    expiratory p.
    fat-water out of p.
    p. filtering
    follicular p.
    Fournier p.
    p. gain

hepatic arterial p.
p. identification
p. image
inspiratory p.
p. instability
interictal p.
late p.
levo p.
luteal p.
midarterial p.
p. mismapping
nephrogenic p.
nephrographic p.
noncontrast p. (NCP)
ovulatory p.
pancreatic parenchymatous p. (PPP)
parenchymatous p.
plateau p.
portal venous p. (PVP)
portal venous dominant p.
prolonged expiratory p.
prolonged inspiratory p.
pyelogram p.
rapid early repolarization p.
rapid ventricular filling p.
p. relation
p. sampling ratio (PSR)
p. shift
spent p.
static bone p.
thallium redistribution p.
vascular p.
venous p.
ventilation scintigraphy equilibrium p.
wash-in p.
washout p.
zero p.

2-phase
2-p. computed tomographic imaging
2-p. CT imaging
2-p. helical computed tomography
2-p. helical CT

3-phase
3-p. bone scan
3-p. bone scintigraphy (TPBS)
3-p. current
3-p. generator
3-p. imaging
3-p. system
3-p. technetium study
3-p. voltage supply
3-p. whole-body bone imaging
phase-angle display redundancy
4-phase bone scintigraphy
phase-contrast
p.-c. angiography
p.-c. cine MRI
p.-c. flow measurement
p.-c. MRA (PC-MRA)

p.-c. sequence
p.-c. venography
p.-c. x-ray computed tomography (PCCT)
phase-corrected GRE image
phased-array
p.-a. body coil MR imaging
p.-a. MRI
p.-a. multicoil
p.-a. multicoil imaging
p.-a. probe
p.-a. scanner
p.-a. surface coil
p.-a. surface coil MR imaging
p.-a. torso coil
p.-a. transducer
phase-dependent spectroscopic imaging
phase-encoded
p.-e. pulse
p.-e. time-reduced acquisition sequence
p.-e. time-reduced acquisition sequence imaging
phase-encoding
p.-e. direction
p.-e. gradient
p.-e. motion artifact
p.-e. order
p.-e. period
p.-e. step
phase-inversion
p.-i. harmonic imaging
p.-i. method
phase-offset multiplanar (POMP)
phase-ordered multiplanar (POMP)
phase-preserving reconstruction
phase-sensitive
p.-s. detector
p.-s. flow measurement
p.-s. gradient echo MR imaging
phase-shift
p.-s. artifact
p.-s. effect
p.-s. velocity mapping
phase-shifting interferometry
phase-specific action
phase-unwrapping method
phase-velocity
p.-v. image
p.-v. imaging
phasic
p. contraction
p. pressure
phasicity
phasing-in time
pHCC
poorly differentiated hepatocellular carcinoma
Phemister triad

P

phenazopyridine
phenobarbital
    p. biliary atresia
    p. imaging agent
phenoltetrachlorophthalein
phenomena (*pl. of* phenomenon)
**phenomenologic effective surface
  potential**
phenomenon, *pl.* **phenomena**
    Ashman p.
    Austin Flint p.
    autoimmune p.
    Bancaud p.
    Bell p.
    common cavity p.
    crankshaft p.
    Cushing p.
    dip p.
    embolic p.
    extinction p.
    flare p.
    flip-flop p.
    flow p.
    fogging p.
    Friedreich p.
    Gärtner p.
    glove p.
    ground-glass p.
    Hurst p.
    interference p.
    irradiation p.
    jet p.
    Jod-Basedow p.
    Katz-Wachtel p.
    kindling p.
    magic angle p.
    no-reflow p.
    nutcracker p.
    on-off p.
    pivot-shift p.
    Raynaud p.
    resonance p.
    R-on-T p.
    Schiff-Sherrington p.
    seizure p.
    shine-through p.
    signal flare p.
    spin-phase p.
    staircase p.
    steal p.
    step-down, step-up p.
    stunning p.
    treppe p.
    truncation p.
    unilateral Raynaud p.
    vacuum disc p.
    vascular p.
    vertebral steal p.
    Wenckebach p.

phenotype
phenoxyacetic acid
phentetiothalein
phenylketonuria (PKU)
    malignant p.
phenyloxazolyl
pheochromocytoma
    adrenal p.
    bladder p.
    cardiac p.
    extraadrenal p.
    malignant p.
    p. rule of 10
Philadelphia
    P. chromosome
    P. chromosome-negative chronic
      myelogenous leukemia
    P. chromosome-negative chronic
      myelomonocytic leukemia
Philips
    P. DVI 1 system
    P. Gyroscan ACS-NT, NT5, NT15,
      S5, T5 scanner
    P. Gyroscan ACS-NT
      superconducting magnet
    P. Integris 5000 digital subtraction
      angiography system
    P. linear accelerator
    P. 1.5 NT-Intera scanner
    P. 1.5T NT MR scanner
    P. Tomoscan 350, SR 6000 CT
      scanner
    P. 4.7T small-bore system scanner
Philips/ADAC cardiac imaging program
Phillips muscle
phlebectasia
    malformed p.
phlebectatic peliosis hepatis
phlebitis
    postvenography p.
phlebogram
    ascending contrast MR p.
    direct puncture MR p.
    impedance MR p.
phlebograph
phlebographic pattern
phlebography
    ascending contrast p.
    cervical magnetic resonance p.
    (CMRP)
    direct puncture p.
    impedance p.
    magnetic resonance p.
    occlusive impedance p.
phlebolith
phlebolith-like calcification
phleborheography (PRG)
phlebosclerosis
phlebostasis

phlebostenosis
phlebothrombosis
phlegmasia cerulea dolens
phlegmon
> Holz p.
> mesenteric p.
> pancreatic p.

phlegmonous
> p. absccss
> p. gastritis
> p. mass
> p. pancreatitis

phlyctenula, *pl.* **phlyctenulae**
> p. lesion

phlyctenulae (*pl. of* phlyctenula)
PHO
> periarticular heterotopic ossification

PHOA
> pulmonary hypertrophic osteoarthropathy

phocomelia, phocomely
phocomely (*var. of* phocomelia)
phonation study
phonoangiography
> carotid p.
> oculoplethysmography/carotid p.
> (OPG/CPA)

phonocardiography
phonophotography
**PhorMax CR desktop workstation
system**
phosphatase
> tartrate-resistant acid p.

phosphatase-1
> fas-associated p.-1

phosphate
> chromium p.
> p. enema
> linear p.
> membrane p.
> ^{99m}Tc p.
> phosphorus-32 sodium p.
> potassium titanyl p. (KTP)
> sodium p.
> technetium 99m p.

phosphate-inducing tumor
phosphate-wasting tumor
phosphaturic
> p. intraosseous lesion
> p. mass
> p. material
> p. mesenchymal tumor

phosphomonoester (PME)
> p. signal

phosphonate
> ethylenediamine tetramethylene p.
> nucleoside p.
> samarium-153 ethylenediamine
> tetramethylene p. (Sm-153
> EDTMP)

phosphor
> cesium iodide input p.
> fluorescent p.
> photostimulable p. (PSP)
> p. plate

phosphorated
phosphorescence
phosphorescent
**phosphoric acid imaging
agent**
phosphorus (P)
> p. 31 (^{31}P, P-31)
> p. 32 (^{32}P)
> colloidal chromic p.
> p. imaging agent
> inorganic p.
> p. isotope
> labeled p.
> p. magnetic resonance spectroscopy
> (P-MRS)
> p. metabolism
> radioactive p.

phosphorus-31 (^{31}P, P-31)
> p. 31 magnetic resonance
> spectroscopy

phosphorus-32 (^{32}P, P-32)
> p.-32 intracavitary irradiation
> p.-32 sodium phosphate

phosphorylase
> purine nucleoside p.
> thymidine p. (TP)

Phospho-Soda enema
Phosphotec
Phosphotope oral solution
photechic effect
photic
photo
> analogue p.
> p. cell
> p. plotter film
> p. transformation

photoacoustic ultrasound
photoactinic
photoaffinity
photoaging
photoangioplasty
photocathode
photocell plethysmography
photochemotherapy
> extracorporeal p.

photochromogen
photocoagulation
> interstitial laser p.
> intraoperative laser p.
> krypton laser p.

photocoagulator
> xenon arc p.

photodeficient region
photodensitometry

P

photodetector
    CCD p.
photodiode
photodisintegration
photodisplay unit
photodisruption
photodynamic therapy (PDT)
photoechoic effect
photoelasticity
photoelectric
    p. absorption
    p. effect
    p. emission
    p. interaction
    p. system
photoelectron
photoexcitation
photoflow
photofluorogram
photofluorographic
photofluorography
photofluoroscope
photogastroscope
PhotoGenica V-Star laser
photographic
    p. effect
    p. radiometer
photography
    CT bone window p.
    moiré p.
    raster stereo p.
photolysis
    FLASH p.
photometer
    HemoCue p.
photomicrograph
    cystic hyperplasia p.
photomultiplier (PM)
    p. gain adjustment
    p. tube (PMT)
photon
    annihilation p.
    p. attenuation
    p. attenuation measurement
    p. cataract removal system
    Compton scattering p.
    p. correlation spectroscopy
    p. deficiency
    degraded p.
    p. densitometry
    p. density
    dual p.
    p. energy
    p. fluence
    p. flux
    gamma p.
    p. interaction depth
    linear p.
    p. mottle

    p. peak
    p. radiosurgery system (PRS)
    p. radiosurgical therapy
    soft p.
    p. starvation
    p. theory of radiation
    p. therapy beam line
photon-deficient
    p.-d. area
    p.-d. bone lesion
    p.-d. bone lesion scintigraphy
photoneutron
photonic medicine
photon-neutron mixed-beam radiation therapy
photonuclear
    p. effect
    p. reaction
photooptical detection
photopeak
    p. breadth
    p. fraction
photopenia
    postexternal radiotherapy p.
    radiotherapy p.
photopenic
    p. area
    p. defect
    p. lesion
    p. mass
    p. region
Photopic Imaging ultrasound system
photoplethysmographic
    p. digit
    p. monitoring
photoplethysmography
PhotoPoint
    P. laser
    P. photodynamic therapy
photoprotein
photoradiation therapy (PRT)
photoradiometer
photoreceptor
    p. fractional velocity error
    p. motion
photorecording
photoroentgenography
photoscan
photoscanner
photospectrum
    technetium 99m p.
photostimulable
    p. luminescence intensity
    p. phosphor (PSP)
    p. phosphor computed radiography
    p. phosphor dental radiography
    p. phosphor digital imaging
    p. phosphor plate
phototherapeutic keratectomy (PTK)

photothermal sclerosis
phototimer
phototoxic
phototoxicity
phototube output circuit
photovolt pH meter
PHP
    pseudohypoparathyroidism
phrenic
    p. ampulla
    p. artery
    p. lymph node
    p. nerve injury
    p. nerve paralysis
    p. pedicle
phrenicocolic, phrenocolic
    p. ligament
phrenicoesophageal, phrenoesophageal
    p. ligament
phrenicogastric (*var. of* phrenogastric)
    p. ligament
phrenicolienal ligament
phrenicosplenic (*var. of*
  phrenosplenic)
    p. ligament
phrenocolic (*var. of* phrenicocolic)
phrenoesophageal (*var. of*
  phrenicoesophageal)
phrenogastric, phrenicogastric
phrenopericardial angle
phrenosplenic, phrenicosplenic
phrenovertebral junction
phrygian
    p. cap
    p. cap deformity
phrynoderma
phthalocyanine
phthinoid chest
phthisis bulbi
phyllode
phyllodes
    cystosarcoma p.
    p. tumor
phylogeny
    liver p.
physial
    p. bar
    p. bony bridging
    p. cartilage
    p. closure
    p. damage
    p. distraction
    p. injury
    p. plate fracture
physical half-life
physician
    Fellow of the American College of
      Nuclear P.'s
physicochemical characterization

physics
    radiation p.
physiologic, physiological
    p. atrophy
    p. herniation
    p. high activity
    p. hyperplasia
    p. hypertrophy
    p. imaging
    p. ovarian cyst
    p. parameter
    p. regurgitation
    p. shunt flow
    p. sphincter
    p. uptake
    p. uterine blush
physiological (*var. of* physiologic)
physiologically immature lung
physis
    distal tibial p.
    fibular p.
    fused p.
    medial p.
    unfused p.
phytobezoar
pia arachnoid
pial
    p. AVM
    p. vessel
piano key sign
PIB
    Pittsburgh Compound B
    PIB imaging agent
PICA
    posteroinferior cerebellar artery
pica artifact
PICC
    peripherally inserted central catheter
    Groshong NXT PICC
    PICC line
    Vaxcel PICC
PICCOLO
    peripherally inserted central catheter
    occlusion line opening
    PICCOLO study
PICHI
    pulse-inversion contrast harmonic
    imaging
pick
    P. body
    P. bundle
    P. disease
    P. tubular adenoma
picker
    P. Eclipse MR unit
    P. Magnascanner
    P. MR scanner
    P. PQ 5000 helical CT scanner
    P. PQ 2000 spiral CT scanner

P

picker (*continued*)
    P. Prism 3000 PET scanner
    P. Prism 3000XP gamma camera
    P. SPECT attenuation correction
    P. Synerview 600 scanner
    P. system
picket
    p. fence appearance
    p. fence stereotactic localizer
pick-off artifact
pickup tube
picocurie (pCi)
picometer
picomole (pmol)
picosecond (psec)
    p. pulse
picture
    p. archival communication system
      (PACS)
    p. archiving and communication
      system (PACS)
    p. archiving and communication
      systems in radiation oncology
    p. element (pixel)
picture-frame
    p.-f. appearance
    p.-f. pattern of vertebral body
    p.-f. vertebra
picture-frame-like
picture-framing osteoporosis
PIE
    postinfectious encephalomyelitis
    pulmonary interstitial emphysema
piece
    chin-occiput p.
    pole p.
piecemeal necrosis
Piedmont fracture
Pierre-Marie-Bamberger syndrome
Pierre Robin syndrome
piezoelectric
    p. effect
    p. generator
    p. transducer
PiGalileo computer-assisted orthopaedic surgery system
pigeon
    p. chest
    p. fancier's lung
pigeon-breast deformity
Pigg-O-Stat
    P.-O-S. mechanical immobilizer
    P.-O-S. pediatric positioning device
pigmented
    p. basal cell carcinoma
    p. iris hamartoma
    p. villonodular bundle
    p. villonodular synovitis (PVNS)

pigmentosa
    neuropathy, ataxia and retinitis p.
      (NARP)
pigment stone
pigskin patch
pigtail
    p. catheter
    p. stent
PIHI
    pulse-inversion harmonic imaging
pilar, pilary
    p. sheath
    p. tumor
pilaris
    keratosis p.
pilary (*var. of* pilar)
pile
    sentinel p.
pile-up
    pulse p.-u.
pill
    barium p.
    p. esophagitis
    video p.
pillar
    faucial p.
    p. fracture
    p. projection
    tonsillar p.
    p. view
PillCam ESO video camera
pill-induced inflammation
pillion fracture
pillow
    cervical skull p.
    foam vacuum p.
    p. fracture
pilocytic, piloid
    p. astrocytoma
    p. tumor
piloid (*var. of* pilocytic)
pilomatrixoma
pilon ankle fracture
pilonidal
    p. cyst
    p. fistula
    p. sinus
    p. tract
pilorum
    vortices p.
pilosebaceous unit
pilosity
pin
    Hagie p.
    lead p.
    Optispike dispensing p.
    orthopaedic p.
    p. pattern

resorbable p.
revolving Ge-68 p.
track of p.

PIN
positive-intrinsic-negative
posterior interosseous nerve
PIN diode
pincer impingement
pincer-type impingement
pinchcock
p. effect
p. mechanism
pinched nerve
pinch-off syndrome
pincushion distortion
Pindborg tumor
pineal
p. apoplexy
p. body
p. cyst
p. dysgerminoma
p. germ cell tumor
p. germinoma
p. gland
p. gland calcification
p. gland neoplasia
p. gland shift
p. gland teratocarcinoma
p. gland tumor
p. gland tumor classification
p. mass
p. parenchymatous tumor
p. region
p. region tumor
p. teratoma
p. ventricle
pinealoma
ectopic p.
pineoblastoma
pineocytoma
ping-pong
p.-p. ball deformity
p.-p. fracture
p.-p. heart volume
pinguecula lesion
pinhole
bone p.
p. camera
p. collimated imaging
p. collimator
p. image
p. scintigram
p. technique
p. view
pink tetralogy
pinnacle
P. Destination renal guiding sheath
P. R/O II radiopaque marker

Pinnacle₃ radiotherapy planning system
pinning
hip p.
in situ p.
PinPoint stereotactic arm
Pins sign
pion
p. beam
p. dosimetry
PIOPED
prospective investigation of pulmonary embolus diagnosis
PIOPED criterion
Piotrowski sign
PIP
proximal interphalangeal
PIP joint
pipe
endoscopic washing p.
pipestem
p. artery
p. cirrhosis
p. fibrosis
p. ureter
pipestemming of ankle-brachial index
PIPIDA
paraisopropyliminodiacetic acid
PIPIDA hepatobiliary imaging
PIPIDA scan
technetium 99m PIPIDA
piping
organ p.
PIPJ
proximal interphalangeal joint
Pipkin femoral fracture classification
pirate sign
Pirie
P. bone
P. method
P. transoral projection
piriform, pyriform
p. cortex
p. muscle
p. recess
p. sinus
p. sinus carcinoma
piriformis
apertura p.
p. muscle
Pirogoff
P. amputation
P. angle
PISA
proximal isovelocity surface area
pisiform
p. bone
p. fracture

P

pisohamate ligament
pisometacarpal ligament
pisoscaphoid distance
pisotriquetral
    p. articulation
    p. joint
pisounciform, pisouncinate
    p. ligament
pisouncinate (*var. of* pisounciform)
pistol-grip
    p.-g. appearance
    p.-g. femur deformity
pistoning
pistonlike reflux
pit
    anal p.
    articular p.
    auditory p.
    central p.
    colonic p.
    costal p.
    cutaneous p.
    gastric p.
    herniation p.
    p. of stomach
    pitch ratio p.
    postanal p.
    primitive p.
    scan pitch p.
    spiral CT pitch p.
    synovial herniation p.
pitch
    beam p.
    calcaneal p.
    data p.
    high p.
    high-quality p.
    high speech p.
    low p.
    p. ratio
    p. ratio pit
    recon p.
    scan p.
    spiral CT p.
pitchblende
pitfall
    breast prosthesis attenuation p.
Pitressin
pitted cartilage
pitting
    pepper-pot p.
Pittsburgh
    P. Compound B (PIB)
    P. Compound B imaging agent
    P. pneumonia
pituicytoma
pituilith
pituitary
    p. adenoma

    p. adenoma chromophobe
    p. apoplexy
    p. bright spot
    p. cyst
    p. dwarfism
    p. failure
    p. fossa
    p. gland
    p. gland anatomy
    p. gland enlargement
    p. hemosiderosis
    p. hyperplasia
    p. infarct
    p. infundibulum
    p. macroadenoma
    p. microadenoma
    p. oncocytoma
    p. stalk
    p. stalk distortion
    p. stone
    p. tumor
PIV
    particle image velocimetry
pivot
    p. joint
    p. of calcar
pivoting table
pivot-shift
    p.-s. phenomenon
    p.-s. sign
    p.-s. test
pixel
    aliased p.
    p. block
    p. count method
    edge-region p.
    maximum-intensity p. (MIP)
    p. noise
    normal-region p.
    p. shift program
    p. size calibration
    p. value
pixel-specific contrast agent
pixel-wise
Pixsys FlashPoint camera
PKU
    phenylketonuria
placement
    anular p.
    catheter p.
    double-J stent p.
    extragastric p.
    iliac artery stent p.
    intracoronary stent p.
    intragastric p.
    intrapericardial patch lead p.
    line p.
    minimally invasive endovascular
      stent p.

percutaneous endoluminal p.
radiotherapy field p.
shim p.
shunt p.
subanular p.
subject p.
superselective microcatheter p.
transcatheter filter p.
transjugular portosystemic stent-shunt p.
transluminal endovascular stent-graft p.
transpapillary p.

placenta
abnormal adherence of p.
accessory p.
p. accreta
adherent p.
anterofundal p.
anular p.
battledore p.
bilobate p.
p. biopsy
chorioallantoic p.
circummarginate p.
cirsoid p.
deciduate p.
Duncan p.
p. enlargement
extrachorial p.
fetal p.
fundal p.
horseshoe p.
incarcerated p.
p. increta
kidney-shaped p.
low-lying p.
marginal p.
maternal p.
p. membranacea
p. migration
2nd-trimester p.
nondeciduate p.
panduriform p.
p. percreta
premature senescence of p.
p. previa
3rd-trimester p.
retained p.
p. rotation
Schultze p.
1st-trimester p.
p. tumor
vascular space of p.
velamentous p.
villous p.

placentae
abruptio p.

placental
p. abruption
p. circulation

p. disc
p. edema
p. grade
p. hemorrhage
p. infarct
p. localization
p. metastasis
p. polyp
p. septal cyst
p. septum
p. souffle
p. villus

placentation abnormality

placentogram
displacement p. (DPG)

placentography
indirect p.

placode
neural p.
unneurulated neural p.

plafond
p. fracture
tibial p.

plagiocephaly
deformation posterior p.
posterior p.
synostotic posterior p.

plain
p. abdominal radiography
(PAR)
p. film
p. film imaging
p. radiograph
p. tomogram
p. view

plain-paper image

plan
isodose p.
posterior transaxial scan p.

plana
coxa p.
vertebra p.

planar
p. brain scan
p. circular coil
p. configuration
p. detector
p. diagnostic I-231 scintigraphy
p. exercise thallium-201 scintigraphy
p. gated radionuclide
ventriculography
p. left anterior oblique image
p. plate
p. radionuclide imaging
p. spin imaging
p. thallium imaging
p. thallium scan
p. thallium with quantitative analysis
p. view

P

Planck
- P. constant
- P. quantum theory

plane
- AC-PC p.
- Aeby p.
- anatomic p.
- areolar p.
- axial p.
- axiolabiolingual p.
- axiomesiodistal p.
- Baer p.
- biparietal p.
- bite p.
- Blumenbach p.
- Bolton nasion p.
- Broadbent-Bolton p.
- buccolingual p.
- Calvé vertebral p.
- canthomeatal p.
- capsular p.
- 4-chamber p.
- circular p.
- clip-editing p.
- coronal p.
- counts per p.
- cross-sectional p.
- Daubenton p.
- E p.
- eye-ear p.
- facial p.
- fascial p.
- fat p.
- flexion-extension p.
- Frankfort p.
- Frankfort horizontal p.
- frontal biauricular p.
- frontoparallel p.
- German horizontal p.
- gonion-gnathion p.
- Hensen p.
- Hodge p.
- horizontal p.
- imaging p.
- interiliac p.
- internervous p.
- intersphincteric p.
- interspinal p.
- intertubercular p.
- ischiorectal fossa p.
- kx-ky p.
- limited-cut p.
- Ludwig p.
- magnetic focal p.
- Meckel p.
- median raphe p.
- median sagittal p.
- mesiodistal p.
- midclavicular p.
- midcoronal p.
- midfrontal p.
- midsagittal p.
- midthalamic p.
- Morton p.
- nonorthogonal p.
- nuchal p.
- oblique coronal p.
- occipital p.
- occlusal p.
- p. of cleavage
- p. of reference
- optimal imaging p.
- orbital p.
- orbitomeatal p.
- orthogonal p.
- parallel tag p.'s
- paramedian sagittal p.
- parasagittal p.
- pelvic p.
- Poschl p.
- principal p.
- radial p.
- reverse Waters p.
- sagittal p.
- scan p.
- sella-nasion p.
- semicoronal p.
- sensitive p.
- p. sensitivity
- short-axis p.
- slicing p.
- spinous p.
- sternoxiphoid p.
- 1st parallel pelvic p.
- subadventitial p.
- subcostal p.
- subintimal cleavage p.
- supracristal p. (SCP)
- supraorbitomeatal p.
- suprasternal notch p.
- p. suture
- tag p.
- temporal p.
- thalamic p.
- thoracic p.
- 4th parallel pelvic p.
- transaxial scan p.
- transmedial p.
- transpyloric p.
- transtrabecular p.
- transtubercular p. (TTP)
- transumbilical p. (TUP)
- transverse p.
- tumor cleavage p.
- umbilical p.
- valve p.
- varus-valgus p.
- vertical p.

Virchow p.
XY p.
ZY p.
2-plane
2-p. fluorometry
2-p. view
planigram (*var. of* tomogram)
planigraphic principle
planigraphy (*var. of* tomography)
planimeter
planimetry
planing
planithorax
planning
3D radiation treatment p.
radiation therapy p. (RTP)
radiation treatment p. (RTP)
p. target volume (PTV)
planogram (*var. of* tomogram)
planographic pelvimetry
planography (*var. of* tomography)
planovalgus
p. foot
p. foot deformity
pes p.
plantae
quadratus p.
plantar
p. aponeurosis
p. arterial arch
p. aspect
p. axial view
p. bursa
p. calcaneal enthesophyte
p. calcaneal spur
p. capsule
p. compartment
p. compartmental anatomy
p. fasciitis
p. fibromatosis
p. flexion-inversion deformity
p. flexion stress view
p. hyperplasia
p. interossei
p. ligament
p. metatarsal angle
p. metatarsal artery
p. plate
p. shift
p. surface
p. vault
plantaris
p. muscle
p. rupture
p. tendon
tylosis palmaris et p.
plantarward
plantodorsal projection
plant thorn tenosynovitis

planum sphenoidale
planus
pes plantigrade p.
plaque
arterial p.
arteriosclerotic p.
asbestos pleural p.
atheromatous p.
beta amyloid senile p.
p. burden
calcified p.
carotid artery p.
p. cleaving
p. compression
concentric atherosclerotic p.
p. constituent
p. cracker
discrete p.
disrupted p.
eccentric atherosclerotic p.
echogenic p.
echolucent p.
endocardial p.
p. erosion
esophageal p.
p. evaluation
fatty p.
fibrofatty p.
fibrotic p.
fibrous intima p.
fissured atheromatous p.
florid p.
focal pleural p.
p. fracture
fungous p.
gastrointestinal p.
p. hemorrhage
heterogeneous carotid p.
p. histomorphometry
homogeneous carotid p.
Hutchinson p.
hypoechoic p.
iliac p.
infiltrating p.
intraluminal p.
lipid-laden p.
luminal p.
meningioma en p.
multiple sclerotic p.'s
mycotic p.
neuritic senile p.
noncompliant p.
obstructive p.
penile p.
periventricular p.
pleural p.
pleuroparenchymal p.
pulverized p.
Randall p.

P

plaque (*continued*)
p. regression
p. remodeling
residual p.
p. rupture
ruptured p.
sclerotic p.
senile p.
sequential paired opposed p.
  (SPOP)
sessile p.
p. splitting
stenotic p.
talc p.
p. tearing
ulcerated atheromatous p.
ulcerated carotid artery p.
uncalcified pleural p.
unstable p.
p. vaporization
vulnerable coronary p.
plaque-containing artery
plaquelike
p. lesion
p. linear defect
plaquing
p. calcification
neuritic p.
plasm (*var. of* plasma)
plasma, plasm
p. cell granuloma
p. cell leukemia
p. cell pneumonia
p. emission spectroscopy
P. 1000 ICP-AES unit
p. iron turnover
p. radioiron disappearance rate
p. radioiron turnover rate
p. volume
plasmablast
plasmablastic
p. lymphoma
p. myeloma
plasmacytoma
anaplastic p.
endobronchial anaplastic p.
extramedullary p. (EMP)
primary cutaneous p.
primary pulmonary p.
primary solitary endobronchial p.
  (PSEP)
secondary cutaneous p.
solitary bone p. (SBP)
solitary osseous p.
thyroid p.
plasmodium embolus
plaster
x-ray in p. (XIP)
x-ray out of p. (XOP)

plastic
p. bowing fracture
carbon fiber-reinforced p.
p. clot
p. pleurisy
p. Vortex Port system
plastica
linitis p.
plasticity
brain p.
neuronal p.
plate
acetabular reconstruction p.
alar p.
amorphous selenium p.
anal p.
anchor p.
auditory p.
axial p.
basal p.
blade p.
bone fixation p.
bony p.
buttress p.
cap p.
cardiogenic p.
cartilaginous growth p.
cloacal p.
cloverleaf p.
compression p.
condylar p.
connecting p.
cortical p.
cranial fixation p.
cribriform p.
3D p.
dorsal p.
dual p.
epiphysial cartilage p.
epiphysial growth p.
ethmovomerine p.
femoral p.
fenestrated compression p.
fibrocartilaginous volar p.
flat p.
flexor p.
foot p.
Fresnel zone p.
frontal p.
fusion p.
ground p.
growth p.
hilar p.
hyaline cartilage p.
interfragmentary p.
intertrochanteric p.
localization-compression grid p.
low-contact dynamic compression p.
  (LC-DCP)

meningioma of cribriform p.
microfixation p.
nail p.
neutralization p.
occipitocervical p.
orbital p.
orthopaedic p.
orthotic p.
overlay p.
palmar p.
pedicle p.
phosphor p.
photostimulable phosphor p.
planar p.
plantar p.
Plexiglas p.
prechordal p.
PSP imaging p.
pterygoid p.
quadrigeminal p.
quadrilateral p.
p. reader
resorbable p.
selenium p.
septal cartilage p.
sinodural p.
skeletal growth p.
skull p.
Spli-Prest p.
stabilization p.
stainless steel p.
stem base p.
subchondral bone p.
supracondylar p.
tarsal p.
tectal p.
tendon p.
tissue p.
titanium p.
vertebral body p.
volar p.
xeroradiographic selenium p.
Y bone p.
plate-and-screw fixation
plateau
p. phase
tibial p.
p. tibial fracture
platelet
adhesive p.
p. factor 3, 4 (PF3, PF4)
p. fibrin embolus
p. function analyzer (PFA)
radiolabeled p.
platelet-derived endothelial cell growth factor
platelet-rich thrombus
platelike atelectasis

platform
Antares ultrasound p.
positioning p.
spinal imaging p. (SIP)
transcatheter intravascular ring p. (TIRP)
platinocyanoide
barium p.
platinum (Pt)
p. coil
p. coil embolization
p. microcoil
P. Plus guidewire
p. wire
platinum-marked stent
platinum-resistant ovarian carcinoma
platinum-tip guidewire
platybasia
platycephaly
platypellic, platypelloid
p. pelvis
platypelloid (*var. of* platypellic)
platypodia
platysma muscle
platyspondylia, platyspondylisis
platyspondylisis (*var. of* platyspondylia)
play
joint p.
PLC
pulmonary lymphangitic carcinomatosis
pleat
accordion-shaped p.
pleating
p. of ligamentum flavum
p. of small bowel
pledget
gelatin sponge p.
pleomorphic
p. adenoma parotitis
p. calcification
p. liposarcoma
p. lung adenoma
p. microcalcification
p. rhabdomyosarcoma
p. sarcoma
p. T-cell lymphoma
p. type
p. xanthoastrocytoma (PXA)
pleomorphism
nuclear p.
pleonosteosis
Léri p.
PLES
parallel line equal spacing
PLES bar
PLES bar pattern
plesiocurie therapy
plesiography
plesiosectional tomography

P

plesiotherapy
Pletal
plethora-related cyanotic CHD
plethysmograph
    Medgraphics body p.
plethysmography
    air p.
    body box p.
    computer strain-gauge p. (CSGP)
    digital p.
    Doppler ultrasonic velocity detector
      segmental p.
    exercise strain-gauge venous p.
    impedance p. (IPG)
    Medsonic p.
    photocell p.
    segmental bronchus p.
    strain-gauge p.
    thermistor p.
    venous p.
pleura, *pl.* **pleurae**
    cervical p.
    congested p.
    costal p.
    costodiaphragmatic recess of p.
    crus p.
    diaphragmatic p.
    edematous p.
    fibrous tumor p.
    hyaloserositis p.
    inflamed p.
    localized fibrous tumor of p.
    mediastinal p.
    parietal p.
    pericardiac p.
    pulmonary p.
    scarification of p.
    silicotic visceral p.
    solitary fibrous tumor of p. (SFTP)
    visceral p.
    wrinkled p.
pleura-based
    p.-b. area of increased opacity
    p.-b. lung nodule
pleurae (*pl. of* pleura)
pleural
    p. apical hematoma cap
    p. calcification
    p. canal
    p. cavity
    p. change
    p. cupula
    p. cyst
    p. density
    p. disease
    p. effusion
    p. empyema
    p. fibromyxoma

p. fistula
p. flap
p. fluid
p. fluid aspiration
p. fluid collection
p. lesion
p. line
p. margin
p. mass
p. meniscus
p. mesothelioma
p. metastasis
p. nodule
p. peel
p. plaque
p. pseudotumor
p. reaction
p. recess
p. rind
p. sac
p. scarring
p. shunting
p. space
p. stripe
p. thickening
p. tube
pleurisy
    acute p.
    Bends asbestos p.
    blocked p.
    chronic p.
    circumscribed p.
    costal p.
    diaphragmatic p.
    diffuse p.
    double p.
    dry p.
    encysted p.
    exudative p.
    fibrinopurulent p.
    fibrinous p.
    hemorrhagic p.
    ichorous p.
    indurative p.
    interlobar p.
    latent p.
    mediastinal p.
    metapneumonic p.
    plastic p.
    primary p.
    proliferation p.
    pulmonary p.
    pulsating p.
    purulent p.
    sacculated p.
    secondary p.
    septic p.
    serofibrous p.

serous p.
single p.
suppurative p.
typhoid p.
visceral p.
wet p.
pleuritic pneumonia
pleuritis
viral p.
pleurocutaneous fistula
pleurodesis
chemical p.
pleuroesophageal
p. line
p. stripe
pleurography
pleuroparenchymal
p. plaque
p. reflection
pleuropericardial
p. adhesion
p. canal
p. cyst
p. effusion
pleuroperitoneal
p. canal
p. communication
p. fold
pleuropulmonary
p. adhesion
p. blastoma
pleuroscopy
plexiform neurofibroma
Plexiglas plate
plexogenic pulmonary arteriopathy
plexopathy
brachial p.
plexus, *pl.* **plexus, plexuses**
abdominal aortic p.
anterior coronary p.
anterior pulmonary p.
aortic p.
autonomic p.
axillary p.
basilar p.
Batson p.
biliary p.
brachial p.
cardiac p.
carotid p.
cavernous p.
celiac p.
cervical p.
choroid p.
ciliary ganglionic p
coccygeal p.
colic p.
colonic myenteric p.

common carotid p.
coronary p.
cystic p.
dangling choroid p.
deep cardiac p.
deferential p.
enteric p.
epidural venous p.
esophageal p.
Exner p.
extradural vertebral p.
facial p.
femoral p.
gastric p.
gastroesophageal variceal p.
glomus of choroid p.
great cardiac p.
hemorrhoidal p.
hepatic nerve p.
hypogastric p.
ileocolic p.
inferior mesenteric p.
p. injury
intermesenteric p.
left coronary p.
lumbar p.
lumbosacral p.
lymph p.
Meissner p.
myenteric p.
nerve p.
pampiniform p.
paravertebral nerve p.
paravertebral venous p.
pelvic p.
perimeniscal capsular p.
perimuscular p.
pharyngeal p.
posterior coronary p.
posterior pulmonary p.
presacral p.
prostatic venous p.
pterygoid p.
pulmonary p.
rectal p.
retrovertebral p.
right coronary p.
sacral p.
sciatic p.
solar p.
spinal nerve p.
subareolar lymphatic p.
submucosal venous p.
superficial p.
superior hypogastric p.
superior mesenteric p.
tympanic p.
uterovaginal p.

P

plexus (*continued*)
    vaginal p.
    vascular p.
    venous p.
    vertebral venous p.
    vesical venous p.
plexuses (*pl. of* plexus)
plica, *pl.* **plicae**
    plicae circulares
    infrapatellar p.
    medial p.
    plicae palmatae
    parapatellar p.
    patellar p.
    p. resection
    suprapatellar p.
    symptomatic lateral synovial p.
    p. syndrome
    synovial p.
plicae (*pl. of* plica)
plicated dural sheath
plication
    p. defect
    disc p.
    transmesenteric p.
PLIF
    posterior lumbar interbody fusion
P-Link software
PLL
    posterior longitudinal ligament
plot
    box-and-whisker p.
    Patlak p.
    polar p.
plug
    bile p.
    biodegradable collagen p.
    bone p.
    collagen p.
    dermoid p.
    echogenic p.
    fingerlike mucous p.
    p. flow
    gamma-irradiated p.
    hydrogel p.
    interbody bone p.
    Ivalon p.
    keratin p.
    luminal p.
    meconium p.
    mucous p.
    Porstmann Ivalon p.
plugging
    mucous p.
pluglike appearance
Plug-n-View 3D medical imaging software
Plumbicon
plumbline view

Plummer
    P. disease
    P. sign
Plummer-Vinson syndrome
plump vessel
plurality of slices
plural pregnancy
pluridirectional tomography
pluripotential bronchial epithelial stem cell
plus
    GuardWire P.
    Laserprobe-PLR P.
    4096 P. PET scanner
plus-density artifact
plutonism
plutonium
    environmental p.
PM
    photomultiplier
Pm
    promethium
PMC
    primary motor cortex
    PMC activation
PME
    peak of maximum enhancement
    phosphomonoester
    time to PME
PMF
    progressive massive fibrosis
PML
    progressive multifocal leukoencephalopathy
PMMA
    polymethylmethacrylate
pmol
    picomole
PMRA
    pulmonary magnetic resonance angiography
P-MRS
    phosphorus magnetic resonance spectroscopy
PMT
    percutaneous mechanical thrombectomy
    photomultiplier tube
    PMT imaging agent
    PMT robotic fulcrumless tomographic system
PMV
    prolapsed mitral valve
PMVL
    posterior mitral valve leaflet
PN
    polyarteritis nodosa
PNC
    premature nodal contraction

PNET
    primitive neuroectodermal tumor
      non-CNS PNET
pneumatic
    p. bone
    p. reduction of intussusception
pneumatization
pneumatocele
    p. cranii
    extracranial p.
    intracranial p.
    parotid p.
    postinfectious p.
    traumatic p.
pneumatocyst
pneumatoenteric, pneumoenteric
    p. canal
    p. defect
pneumatosis
    p. coli
    cystic p.
    p. cystoides intestinalis
    epidural p.
    gastric p.
    p. sphenoidale
    stomach p.
pneumoalveolography
pneumoangiogram
pneumoangiography
pneumoarthrogram sign
pneumoarthrography
pneumobilia
pneumocardiograph
pneumocardiography
pneumocephalus
    intracranial p.
pneumococcal pneumonia
pneumocolon
pneumoconioses (*pl. of* pneumoconiosis)
pneumoconiosis, pneumonoconiosis, pneumokoniosis, *pl.* **pneumoconioses**
    aluminum p.
    barium p.
    bauxite p.
    p. classification
    coal worker's p. (CWP)
    complicated p.
    fiberglass p.
    fibrogenic p.
    Fuller earth p.
    hard metal p.
    inert dust p.
    kaolin p.
    mica p.
    nepheline p.
    noncollagenous p.
    rheumatoid p.
    sericite p.
    silicate p.

    sillimanite p.
    talc p.
    tungsten carbide p.
    zeolite p.
pneumoconiotic nodule
pneumoconstriction
pneumocystic infection
Pneumocystis
    P. carinii
    P. carinii pneumonia (PCP)
    P. jiroveci pneumonia
pneumocystography
    breast p.
pneumocystosis
    cutaneous p.
pneumocystotomography
pneumoencephalogram (PEG)
pneumoencephalographic pattern
pneumoencephalography (PEG)
    cerebral p.
    fractional p.
    lumbar p.
pneumoencephalomyelogram
pneumoencephalomyelography
pneumoenteric (*var. of* pneumatoenteric)
pneumofasciogram
pneumogastrography
pneumogram
pneumography
    cerebral p.
    retroperitoneal p.
pneumogynogram
pneumohemothorax
pneumohydrothorax (*var. of* hydropneumothorax)
pneumointestinalis
pneumokoniosis (*var. of* pneumoconiosis)
pneumolith
pneumomediastinogram
pneumomediastinography
pneumomediastinum
    postoperative p.
    radiolucent p.
    spontaneous p.
    traumatic p.
pneumomyelography
pneumonectomy chest
pneumonia
    acute eosinophilic p.
    acute interstitial p. (AIP)
    adenovirus p.
    alcoholic p.
    allergic p.
    alveolar p.
    anthrax p.
    aspiration p.
    asthmatic p.
    atypical bronchial p.
    atypical interstitial p.

P

pneumonia (*continued*)
   atypical measles p.
   atypical primary p.
   bacterial p.
   bilateral lower lobe p.
   bilious bronchial p.
   bronchiolitis obliterans with
     organizing p. (BOOP)
   Buhl desquamative p.
   capillary p.
   caseous p.
   catarrhal p.
   cavitating p.
   central p.
   cerebral p.
   cheesy p.
   chelonian p.
   chemical p.
   chemotherapy-induced p.
   chronic interstitial p.
   community-acquired p.
   concomitant p.
   consolidative p.
   contusion p.
   cryptococcal p.
   cryptogenic organizing p.
   deglutition p.
   delayed resolution of p.
   desquamative interstitial p. (DIP)
   diffuse p.
   double p.
   Eaton agent p.
   embolic p.
   endogenous lipid p.
   eosinophilic p.
   ephemeral p.
   exogenous lipoid p.
   extensive bilateral p.
   fibrinous p.
   fibrous p.
   focal organizing p.
   Friedländer p.
   fungous p.
   gangrenous p.
   giant cell interstitial p. (GIP)
   granulomatous p.
   Hecht p.
   hemorrhagic p.
   herpesvirus p.
   HIV p.
   hypersensitivity p.
   hypostatic p.
   idiopathic interstitial p. (IIP)
   incomplete resolution of p.
   indurative p.
   infantile p.
   inhalation p.
   interstitial organizing p.
   interstitial plasma cell p.

   irradiation p.
   lingular p.
   lipoid endogenous p.
   lobar p.
   lobular p.
   Löffler p.
   lower lobe p.
   lymphocytic interstitial p. (LIP)
   lymphoid interstitial p. (LIP)
   massive p.
   measles p.
   migratory p.
   mycoplasma p.
   mycotic p.
   necrotizing p.
   neonatal p.
   nonclassifiable interstitial p.
   nonspecific interstitial p. (NIP,
     NSIP)
   nummular p.
   obstructive p.
   oil-aspiration p.
   organizing focal p.
   organizing interstitial p.
   overcalling p.
   parainfluenza virus p.
   parenchymatous p.
   passive p.
   patchy area of p.
   peripheral p.
   pertussoid eosinophilic p.
   Pittsburgh p.
   plasma cell p.
   pleuritic p.
   pneumococcal p.
   Pneumocystis carinii p. (PCP)
   Pneumocystis jiroveci p.
   postobstructive p.
   posttraumatic p.
   Pseudomonas aeruginosa p.
   purulent p.
   pyogenic p.
   radiation p.
   recurrent p.
   resolving p.
   right-sided p.
   round p.
   SARS-associated coronavirus p.
   secondary p.
   segmental p.
   septic p.
   Staphylococcus aureus p.
   superficial p.
   suppurative p.
   terminal p.
   toxic p.
   traumatic p.
   tuberculous p.
   tularemic p.

unresolved p.
usual interstitial p. (UIP)
varicella p.
viral p.
walking p.
white p.

pneumonic infiltrate

pneumonitis
acute interstitial p.
acute radiation p.
aspiration p.
bacterial p.
basilar p.
chemical p.
Chlamydia p.
chronic p.
diffuse p.
drug-induced p.
early p.
giant cell p.
granulomatous p.
hypersensitivity p.
idiopathic interstitial p.
interstitial p.
lipoid p.
lymphocytic interstitial p. (LIP)
lymphoid interstitial p. (LIP)
mycoplasma p.
radiation p.
subacute p.
unusual interstitial p.
usual interstitial p.
ventilation p.

pneumonocele
pneumonocirrhosis
pneumonoconiosis, pneumonokoniosis
pneumonograph
pneumonography
pneumonokoniosis (*var. of* pneumonoconiosis)
pneumoorbitography
pneumopathy
cobalt p.

pneumopericardium
pneumoperitoneal
pneumoperitoneography
pneumoperitoneum
balanced p.
diagnostic p.
drop test for p.
transabdominal p.

pneumophilia
Legionella p.

pneumoplethysmography
ocular p. (OPG)

pneumopreperitoneum
pneumopyelogram
pneumopyelography
pneumorachicentesis

pneumorachis
pneumoradiography
retroperitoneal p.

pneumoretroperitoneum
pneumoroentgenogram
pneumoroentgenography
pneumoscrotum
pneumotachograph
pneumothorax (PT)
artificial p.
basilar p.
bilateral p.
blowing p.
catamenial p.
closed p.
congenital p.
diagnostic p.
extrapleural p.
induced p.
life-threatening p.
open p.
positive-pressure p.
pressure p.
recurrent p.
simultaneous bilateral spontaneous p. (SBSP)
spontaneous tension p.
subpulmonic p.
sucking p.
tension p.
therapeutic p.
traumatic p.
tuberculous p.
uncomplicated p.
valvular p.

pneumotomography
pneumoventriculogram
pneumoventriculography
PNL
posterior nipple line

Po
polonium

pocket
air p.
p. chamber
p. Doppler
p. dosimeter
infraclavicular p.
p. of Zahn
rectus sheath p.
regurgitant p.
p. shot
subcutaneous p.
subpectoral p.
valve p.

pocketed calculus
pocketing of barium
POD
polycystic ovarian disease

P

POEMS
polyneuropathy, organomegaly,
endocrinopathy, monoclonal
gammopathy, skin changes
POEMS syndrome
POI
postoperative ileus
point
A p.
Addison p.
alveolar p.
apophysial p.
auricular p.
p. Ba
bleeding p.
Bolton craniometric p.
(Bo)
branch p.
breast trigger p.
Cannon p.
Cannon-Boehm p.
cardinal p.
Chauffard p.
choroid p.
Clado p.
coaptation p.
commissural p.
congruent p.
Cope p.
coplanar contour p.
craniometric p.
Crowe pilot p.
D p.
dorsal p.
entry p.
equilibrium p.
Erb p.
frontopolar p.
glenoid p.
Griffith p.
Hartmann p.
ICRU reference p.
p. imaging
interventional reference p.
(IRP)
J p.
Kienböck-Adamson p.
Lanz p.
lead p.
p. localization
Mackenzie p.
McBurney p.
midinguinal p.
Morris p.
multiple sensitive p.'s
p. mutation
p. mutation detection using
exonuclease amplification couple
capture technique

nodal p.
null p.
output p.
Pauly p.
preauricular p.
pressure p.
random p.
reentry p.
Rolando p.
sacrococcygeal inferior pubic p.
(SCIPP)
saddle p.
scanned focal p. (SFP)
p. scanning
seed p.
sensitive p.
p. sensitivity
Sudeck p.
sylvian p.
target p.
time p.
white p.
3-point
3-p. Dixon technique
3-p. Dixon water-fat separation
sequence
pointer
hip p.
metallic p.
shoulder p.
point-in-space stereotactic biopsy
point-resolved
p.-r. spectroscopy (PRESS)
p.-r. spectroscopy localization
technique
4-point restraint
point-spread function (PSF)
point-to-point protocol (PPP)
Poiseuille
P. flow
P. law
poisoning
radiation p.
Poisson
P. distributed activity concentration
P. distribution
P. noise fluctuation
P. ratio
Poisson-Pearson formula
poker spine
Poland
P. epiphysial fracture classification
P. syndrome
polar
p. blackout map
p. coordinate system
p. map
p. plot
P. Vantage XL heart rate monitor

polar-bound water
polarimetry
    scanning laser p.
Polaris
    P. Dx steerable diagnostic catheter
    P. Nd:YAG laser
    P. X steerable diagnostic catheter
polarity-altered
    p.-a. spectral-selective acquisition
    p.-a. spectral-selective acquisition
      imaging
polarization
    cell p.
    chemically induced dynamic nuclear
      p.
    dynamic nuclear p. (DNP)
    linear p.
    nuclear p.
polarized light microscopy
polarographic
    p. needle electrode
    p. needle electrode measurement
Polaroid film
pole
    abapical p.
    cephalic p.
    fetal p.
    p. figure texture analysis
    frontal p.
    germinal p.
    inferior p.
    kidney p.
    lower p.
    magnetic p.
    middle p.
    occipital p.
    p. of organ
    p. of scaphoid bone
    p. of vessel
    patellar p.
    p. piece
    scaphoid p.
    superior p.
    temporal p.
    p. tip
    upper p.
10-pole Butterworth filter
pole-to-pole length of kidney
Polhemus 3D digitizer
polidocanol sclerosing agent
poliosis
polka-dot appearance
pollex pedis
pollicis
    adductor p.
    p. longus tendon
    opponens p.
pollicization
    Riordan finger p.

pollicized ray
polonium (Po)
POLPSA
    posterior labroscapular periosteal
      avulsion
    POLPSA lesion
polyadenopathy
    angiofollicular and plasmacytic p.
Pólya gastrectomy procedure
polyalveolar lobe
polyangiitis
    microscopic p.
polyarcuate diaphragm
polyarteritis nodosa (PAN, PN)
polyarthritis
    juvenile chronic p.
polyarthropathy
polyarticular symmetric tophaceous joint
  inflammation
polychondritis
    relapsing p.
polychromatic
    p. radiation
    p. x-ray
polyclonal antibody
polycycloidal tomography
polycystic
    p. kidney
    p. kidney disease
    p. liver
    p. liver disease
    p. lung
    p. nephroblastoma
    p. ovarian disease (PCOD, POD)
    p. ovary
    p. ovary syndrome (PCOS, POS)
polydactyly
    Wassel classification of thumb p.
      (I-VI)
polydirectional tomography
polyethylene (PE)
    p. catheter
    p. glycol (PEG)
    p. stent
    p. tube
Polyflex stent
polyglycolide
    self-reinforced p.
polygonal elongate cell
polygon mirror
polygyria
polyhydramnios
polylactic acid
polylobar liver
polymastia
polymer
    p. dosimetry
    osteoconductive p.
    sulfonated p.

P

polymer-coated
    hydrophilic p.-c.
polymerization
    fibrin p.
polymerizing agent
polymethylmethacrylate (PMMA)
    p. implant
polymicrogyria
polymorphism
    single-strand conformational p. (SSCP)
polymorphonuclear
    p. cell
    p. leukocyte
polymyalgia rheumatica
polymyositis
Polynesian bronchiectasis
polyneuropathy, organomegaly, endocrinopathy, monoclonal gammopathy, skin changes (POEMS)
polynomial stepwise multilinear regression
polynuclear neutrophilic leukocyte
— **polyostotic** — *metastatic neoplasia*
    p. bone lesion
    p. fibrous dysplasia
polyp
    adenomatous p.
    angiomatous nasal p.
    antral p.
    antrochoanal p.
    bleeding p.
    broad-based p.
    bronchial p.
    cardiac p.
    carpet p.
    cervical p.
    choanal p.
    cholesterol gallbladder p.
    colonic adenomatous p.
    colonic hamartomatous p.
    colorectal p.
    cystic p.
    cyst or p.
    dental p.
    duodenal p.
    endometrial p.
    epithelial colonic p.
    fibrinous p.
    fibroepithelial urethral p.
    fibroid p.
    fibrous urinary tract p.
    fibrovascular p.
    filiform p.
    gallbladder p.
    gastric p.
    hamartomatous gastric p.

Hopmann p.
hydatid p.
hyperplastic adenomatous p.
hyperplastic colon p.
hyperplastic gastric p.
hyperplastic stomach p.
inflammatory colonic p.
inflammatory esophagogastric p.
inflammatory fibroid p.
inflammatory stomach p.
intraluminal p.
juvenile p.
laryngeal p.
lipomatous p.
lymphoid p.
metaplastic p.
metastatic p.
mucous p.
multiple p.'s
nasal p.
osseous p.
pedunculated p.
Peutz-Jeghers p.
placental p.
postinflammatory p.
rectal p.
regenerative gastric p.
retention colon p.
retention stomach p.
sessile p.
sigmoid p.
single p.
p. stalk
tubular p.
tubulovillous p.
uterine fibroid p.
vascular fibrous p.
villoglandular p.
villous stomach p.
polypeptide
    organic anion transporter p.
polypharmacy
polyphase generator
polyphosphate
polyphosphonate
    technetium p.
polypiform (*var. of* polypoid)
polypoid, polypiform
    p. adenoma
    p. calcified irregular mass
    p. carcinoma
    colitis p.
    p. dysplasia
    p. fibroma
    p. fibroma collecting system
    p. filling defect
    p. lesion
    p. lesion of lower esophagus
    p. lymphoid hyperplasia

p. lymphoma
p. mucosa
polyposa
colitis p.
polyposis
attenuated adenomatous p.
diffuse mucosal p.
familial adenomatous p. (FAP)
familial colorectal p.
familial gastrointestinal p.
familial intestinal p.
familial juvenile p.
familial multiple p.
filiform p.
gastric hamartomatous p.
intestinal p.
juvenile p.
lymphomatous p. (LP)
multiple p.
Peutz-Jeghers gastrointestinal p.
postinflammatory p.
sinonasal p.
polypropylene catheter
polyradiculomyelitis
polyradiculoneuropathy
polyradiculopathy
acute inflammatory demyelinating p.
polysomnogram
polysomnography
nocturnal p.
polysplenia syndrome
polytetrafluoroethylene (PTFE)
p. graft
polythelia
polytomogram
polytomographic radiology
polytomography
mastoid p.
polytrauma
Polytron DSA equipment
polyurethane
p. foam embolus
p. stent
polyvinyl
p. alcohol (PVA)
p. alcohol particle
p. alcohol particle embolization
p. butyral (PVB)
p. chloride (PVC)
polyvinylpyrrolidone (PVP)
POMP
phase-offset multiplanar
phase-ordered multiplanar
POMP imaging
Pompe disease
ponderal index
pond fracture
pons, *pl.* **pontes**
bifid p.

caudal p.
infarct of p.
rostral p.
tegmentum of p.
pontes (*pl. of* pons)
ponticulus posticus
pontile, pontine
p. angle
p. angle tumor
p. artery
central p.
p. cistern
p. contusion
p. glioma
p. hemorrhage
p. hydatid cyst
p. infarct
p. isthmus
p. lesion
p. myelinolysis
p. parareticular formation
p. reticular formation
p. tegmentum
pontile-medullary level
pontine (*var. of* pontile)
pontis
basis p.
brachium p.
pontocerebellar
p. fiber
p. glioma
p. hypoplasia
pontomedullary
p. junction
p. separation
p. sulcus
pontomesencephalic
p. junction
p. vein
pool
blood p.
focal p.
gastric p.
miscible p.
vascular blood p.
pooling
genital blood p.
venous p.
poor
p. perfusion
p. sensitivity
p. shimming of MRI magnet
p. vascular reserve
p. visualization
poorly
p. circumscribed tumor
p. concentrated isotope
p. differentiated adenocarcinoma
(PDA)

P

poorly (*continued*)
p. differentiated carcinoma
p. differentiated embryonal cell tumor
p. differentiated hepatocellular carcinoma (pHCC)
POP
pelvic organ prolapse
popcorn calcification
popcornlike
p. appearance
p. calcification
p. reticulated lesion
popliteal
p. artery
p. artery aneurysm
p. artery entrapment syndrome
p. artery occlusive disease
p. artery pulsation artifact
p. artery trifurcation
p. cavity
p. cyst
p. entrapment
p. fossa
p. hiatus
p. ligament
p. line
p. node
p. pulse
p. recess
p. space
p. tendinitis
p. tendon
p. vein
popliteus
p. bursa
p. fossa muscle tendon
poppet
barium-impregnated p.
disc p.
poppyseed-like calcification
population
overdistention of alveolar p.
uneven recruitment of alveolar p.
porcelain
p. aorta
p. gallbladder
Porcher method
porcine
p. gallbladder
p. heart xenograft
porencephalia (*var. of* porencephaly)
porencephalic cyst
porencephaly, porencephalia
acquired p.
agenetic p.
encephaloclastic p.
true p.
pore of Kore

porokeratosis plantaris discreta
poroses (*pl. of* porosis)
porosis, *pl.* **poroses**
cerebral p.
porous
p. bone
p. ingrowth
p. kidney
p. metallic stent
Porstmann Ivalon plug
port
BardPort low-profile p.
BardPort MRI full-size p.
Cordis multipurpose access p.
p. film
implantable infusion p.
implanted p.
injection p.
multipurpose access p. (MPAP)
parallel-opposed unmodified p.'s
radiation p.
radiotherapy p.
simulation of converging p.'s
single p.
subcutaneous implanted injection p.
tangential p.
treatment p.
PORT
postoperative radiotherapy
PORT radiofrequency electrode design
porta, *pl.* **portae**
p. cirrhosis
p. hepatis
p. hepatis defect
p. hepatis low-density mass
p. hepatis node
p. hepatis obstruction
portable
p. C-arm image intensifier fluoroscopy
p. C-arm intensifier
p. chest film
p. imaging procedure
p. radiography
p. view
p. x-ray
portacamera
Port-A-Cath
portacaval, portocaval
p. shunt
p. space
portae (*pl. of* porta)
portal
p. canal
p. decompression
p. fibrosis
p. fissure
p. flow

p. hypertension
p. phased spiral CT scan
p. portography
radiation p.
radiocarpal p.
radiotherapy p.
simulation of tangential p.
p. space
superomedial p.
p. triad
p. vascular bed
p. vein
p. vein aneurysm
p. vein anomaly (type I-V)
p. vein cavernoma
p. vein congestion index
p. vein enhancement
p. vein lesion
p. vein system
p. vein thrombosis (PVT)
p. vein velocity
p. venography
p. venous anastomosis
p. venous dominant phase
p. venous gas
p. venous phase (PVP)
p. venous phase imaging
p. venous pressure (PVP)
p. venous sampling
portal-enhanced computed tomography
portal-systemic (*var. of* portosystemic)
portal-to-portal
p.-t.-p. bridge
p.-t.-p. fibrosis
PortalVision radiation oncology system
port-catheter system
portion
cavernous p.
intrapericardial p.
supraclinoid p.
portio vaginalis
portocaval (*var. of* portacaval)
portogram
portography
arterial p.
computed tomography arterial p.
computed tomography during arterial p.
double-spiral CT arterial p.
percutaneous transhepatic p.
portal p.
splenic p.
transhepatic p.
transjugular p.
umbilical p.
portohepatic
portomesenteric venous thrombosis
portophlebography

portopulmonary shunt
portosplenic thrombosis
portosplenography
portosystemic, portal-systemic
p. anastomosis
p. collateral
p. collateral circulation
p. collateral vessel
p. gradient
p. shunt
portovenography
portovenous
port-site
p.-s. metastasis
p.-s. tumor seeding
POS
polycystic ovary syndrome
Posada fracture
Posadas-Wernicke coccidioidomycosis
Poschl plane
Posicam HZ PET scanner
position
abduction p.
abduction-external rotation p.
ABER p.
adduction p.
Albers-Schönberg p.
Albert p.
anatomic p.
anterior oblique p.
anteroposterior p.
barber-chair p.
bayonet fracture p.
beach-chair p.
Beclere p.
Benassi p.
Bertel p.
bladder neck p.
Broden p.
brow-down p.
brow-up p.
Caldwell p.
cardiac p.
catheter tip p.
central venous line p.
Chassard-Lapiné p.
Cleaves p.
Clements-Nakayama p.
cock-robin p.
conus medullaris p.
cross-table lateral p.
decubitus p.
dorsal decubitus p.
dorsal recumbent p
dorsosacral p.
dwell p.
p. encoding
erect p.
eversion p.

P

position (*continued*)
 extension p.
 Feist-Mankin p.
 fetal p.
 Fick p.
 figure-4 p.
 Fleischner p.
 flexion p.
 Fowler p.
 Friedman p.
 frogleg p.
 Fuchs p.
 full lateral p.
 Grashey p.
 Haas p.
 heart p.
 Hickey p.
 high Fowler p.
 horizontal p.
 infragenicular p.
 infrapulmonary p.
 inlet p.
 inversion p.
 jackknife p.
 Johnson p.
 LAO p.
 Larkin p.
 lateral decubitus p.
 lateral left anterior oblique
  p.
 lateral recumbent p.
 Law p.
 Lawrence p.
 left anterior oblique p.
 left posterior oblique p.
 left-side-down decubitus p.
 Lewis p.
 Lilienfelds p.
 lithotomy p.
 lordotic p.
 Lorenz p.
 lotus p.
 Low-Beers p.
 LPO p.
 Mayer p.
 Miller p.
 near-anatomic p.
 neutral hip p.
 Noble p.
 Nölke p.
 noncoaxial catheter tip p.
 normal anatomic p.
 nose-chin p.
 nose-forehead p.
 oblique p.
 opisthotonic p.
 PA p.
 paramedian p.
 paraseptal p.

 park bench p.
 Pawlow p.
 Pearson p.
 Phalen p.
 prone p.
 pulmonary capillary wedge p.
 3-quarter prone p.
 reclining p.
 rectus p.
 recumbent p.
 reverse Trendelenburg p.
 reverse Waters p.
 right anterior oblique p.
 right posterior oblique p.
 right-side-down decubitus p.
 Schüller p.
 semiaxial p.
 semierect p.
 semi-Fowler p.
 semilateral p.
 semirecumbent p.
 semisupine p.
 semiupright p.
 Settegast p.
 side-lying p.
 Sims p.
 spatial p.
 squatting p.
 Staunig p.
 Stecher p.
 steep Trendelenburg p.
 Stenver p.
 stepping-source p.
 submentovertex p.
 supine head-first p.
 swimmer's p.
 Tarrant p.
 Taylor p.
 tibial sesamoid p.
 Titterington p.
 Towne p.
 Trendelenburg p.
 tripod p.
 Twining p.
 upright p.
 ventral decubitus p.
 verticosubmental p.
 Walcher p.
 Waters p.
 Wigby-Taylor p.
 Zanelli p.
positional
 p. dysfunction
 p. variation
positioner
 basilar block skull p.
 dual lateral hand p.
 dual oblique hand p.
 Waters p.

positioning
- arms-up p.
- automatic endoscopic system for optimal p. (AESOP)
- p. error
- flap p.
- motion-free p.
- operator-dependent p.
- pendent p.
- p. platform

position-related rhabdomyolysis

positive
- p. beam limitation (PBL)
- breakpoint cluster region p.
- p. cephalopelvic disproportion index
- p. contrast encephalography
- p. contrast myelography
- p. electron
- p. end-expiratory pressure
- ER p.
- estrogen-receptor p.
- p. node basin
- p. predictive value (PPV)
- premenopausal hormone receptor p.
- p. ray
- replication error p.
- p. tropism
- true p.
- p. ulnar variance (PUV)
- p. washout test

positive-contrast agent

positive-intrinsic-negative (PIN)
- p.-i.-n. diode

positive-ion cyclotron

positive-pressure pneumothorax

positrocephalogram

positron
- p. coincidence
- p. decay
- p. emission mammography (PEM)
- p. emission tomography (PET)
- p. emission tomography with fluorodeoxyglucose (FDG-PET)
- p. emission transaxial tomography (PETT)
- p. emission transverse tomography (PETT)
- energetic p.
- labeled p.
- p. matter-antimatter annihilation reaction
- p. range
- p. scanning
- p. scintillation camera

positron-emitting radionucleotide

positronium half-life

POSL
- pulsed optically stimulated luminescence
- POSL dosimeter

Possis AngioJet Xpeedior catheter

post
- p. Diamox state
- p. ECT sequela
- p. fatty meal cholecystography
- p. PTCA residual stenosis

postablation

postamputation neuroma

postanal pit

postangioplasty
- p. angiography
- p. aortography
- p. intimal flap
- p. mural thrombosis
- p. restenosis
- p. stenosis

postaortic lymph node

postaugmentation

postaxial

postbeat filtration

postbiopsy
- p. change
- p. eggshell calcification
- p. fat necrosis
- p. period
- p. renal AV fistula
- p. scarring

postbulbar
- p. duodenum
- p. ulcer

postbypass spasm

postcapillary venule

postcaptopril radioisotope study

postcardiac injury syndrome (PCIS)

postcardiotomy lymphocytic splenomegaly

postcatheterization pseudoaneurysm (PCPA)

postcaval
- p. lymph node
- p. ureter

postcentral
- p. gyrus
- p. sulcus

postcerebral infarction epilepsy

postchemoembolization liver abscess

postchemotherapy image

postcontrast
- p. echocardiography
- p. MR imaging

postcricoid
- p. area
- p. carcinoma
- p. defect
- p. pharynx
- p. soft tissue
- p. web

P

postcubital
postdilation arteriography
postdrainage
    p. cystogram
    p. imaging
    p. projection
postductal
    p. aortic coarctation
    p. coarctation of aorta
Postel destructive coxarthrosis
postembolization
    p. angiographic pattern
    p. angiography
    p. syndrome
postenhancement sequence
posterior
    p. abdominal wall
    p. acoustic enhancement
    p. acoustic shadowing
    ampulla ossea p.
    p. anulus
    p. aorta transposition of great
      arteries
    p. arch fracture
    p. aspect
    p. auricular vein
    p. axillary line
    p. border
    p. border of heart
    p. calcaneal bursitis
    p. capsular distance
    p. cardinal vein
    p. central gyrus
    p. central indentation
    p. cerebral artery (PCA)
    p. cerebral territory infarct
    p. cervical line
    p. cervical space
    p. cervical triangle
    p. choroidal artery
    p. cingulate functional impairment
    p. cingulate gyrus
    p. circulation territory
    p. circumflex humeral artery
    p. cistern
    p. colliculus
    p. column deficit
    p. column demyelination
    p. column lesion
    p. column of spine
    p. column syndrome
    p. commissure (PC)
    p. communicating artery (PCA)
    p. communicating artery aneurysm
    p. compartment
    p. compartment lesion
    p. concavity
    p. coronary groove
    p. coronary plexus

    p. cranial fossa
    p. cruciate ligament (PCL)
    p. cruciate ligament injury
    p. cusp
    p. descending artery (PDA)
    p. descending branch
    p. disc margin
    p. element fracture
    p. embryotoxon
    p. epidural fat
    p. fascicular block
    p. fontanelle
    p. fossa circulation
    p. fossa cyst
    p. fossa-foramen magnum lesion
    p. fossa hematoma
    p. fossa lesion
    p. fossa malformations, facial
      hemangiomas, arterial anomalies,
      cardiac anomalies and aortic
      coarctation, eye anomalies, and
      sternal clefting and/or
      supraumbilical raphe (PHACES)
    p. fossa meningioma
    p. fossa tumor
    p. fracture-dislocation
    p. free wall
    p. ghosting artifact
    p. gray column of cord
    p. gray horn
    p. iliac crest
    p. impingement
    p. impingement syndrome
    p. intercostal artery
    p. intercostal branch
    p. interosseous nerve (PIN)
    p. interosseous nerve entrapment
    p. interventricular groove
    p. interventricular sulcus
    p. interventricular vein
    p. intraoccipital synchondrosis
    p. joint syndrome
    p. junction line
    p. labroscapular periosteal avulsion
      (POLPSA)
    p. language area lesion
    p. leaflet prolapse
    p. lie
    p. lip
    p. longitudinal ligament (PLL)
    p. longitudinal ligament tear
    p. lumbar interbody fusion (PLIF)
    p. lumbar vessel
    p. mediastinal mass
    p. mediastinal node
    p. mediastinum
    p. membrane articulation
    p. metatarsal arch
    p. midbody of corpus callosum

p. mitral valve leaflet (PMVL)
p. neck surface coil
p. neural arch
p. nipple line (PNL)
p. olive
p. osteophyte
p. palatine suture
p. papillary muscle (PPM)
p. patch aortoplasty
p. pharyngeal wall carcinoma
p. pituitary fossa
p. pituitary gland ectopia
p. plagiocephaly
p. pleural recess
p. predominance
p. probability
p. projection
p. pulmonary plexus
p. rectus sheath
p. retrocrural approach
p. reversible encephalopathy
  syndrome (PRES)
p. ring fracture
p. root entry zone
p. root ganglion
p. scalloping of vertebra
p. semicircular canal
p. septal space
p. skull view
p. spinal artery
p. spinal cord horn
p. spine fusion (PSF)
p. spinocerebellar tract
p. spur
p. subluxation
superior labral anterior to p.
  (SLAP)
p. surface
p. surface of pancreas
p. surface of prostate
p. talofibular (PTF)
p. talofibular ligament
p. temporal artery
p. terminal vein
p. thalamic artery of Lazorthes
p. tibial artery
tibialis p.
p. tibial pulse
p. tibial tendon (PTT)
p. tibial vein (PTV)
p. tibiotalar ligament
p. tracheal band
p. transaxial scan plan
p. transcaval approach
p. triangle of neck
p. tricuspid leaflet
p. turn of aortic arch
p. urethra
p. urethral injury

p. urethral valve (type I-IV)
  (PUV)
p. urethrovesical angle (PUVA)
p. vagal trunk
p. ventricular branch
p. vertebral element blowout lesion
p. vertebral scalloping
p. wall
p. wall fracture
p. wall motion
p. wall myocardial infarct
p. wall thickness (PWT)
posteroanterior (PA)
p. chest film
p. lordotic projection
p. view
posteroapical
p. defect
p. segment
posterobasal
p. segment
p. segmental bronchus
p. wall myocardial infarct
posteroexternal
posteroinferior
p. cerebellar artery (PICA)
p. iliac spine
p. myocardial infarct
p. tibiofibular ligament
posterointernal
posterolateral
p. aspect
p. capsule
p. compartment
p. corner injury
p. disc herniation
p. fontanelle
p. rotatory instability
p. rotatory subluxation
p. sclerosis
p. segment
p. spinal artery
p. talar process
p. wall
p. wall motion
p. wall myocardial infarct
posteromedial
p. compartment
p. tibia
posteromedian septum
posterooblique
p. ligament
p. view
posteroparietal artery
posterosuperior glenoid impingement
posterotransverse diameter
postevacuation
p. film
p. view

P

743

postexercise
    p. echocardiography
    p. film
    p. image
    p. imaging
    p. index
    p. stunning
postexternal radiotherapy photopenia
postextrasystolic
    p. pause
    p. potentiation
postfiltering
    3D p.
    low-pass 3-dimensional p.
postfire image
postfrontal cortex
postgadolinium scan
postganglionic
    p. gray fiber
    p. sympathetic fiber
postglomerular arteriolar constriction
postglucose loading examination
posthemorrhagic hydrocephalus
posthepatitic cirrhosis
postherpetic neuralgia
postictal cerebral blood flow scan
posticus
    ponticulus p.
postimplant radiation survey
postinfarction
    p. ventricular aneurysm
    p. ventricular septal defect
postinfectious
    p. bronchiectasis
    p. bronchiolitis obliterans
    p. demyelination
    p. encephalitis
    p. encephalomyelitis (PIE)
    p. hydrocephalus
    p. pneumatocele
postinflammatory
    p. adenopathy
    p. polyp
    p. polyposis
    p. pulmonary fibrosis
    p. renal atrophy
    p. scarring
postinjection
    p. attenuation scan
    p. echocardiography
    p. imaging
    p. scan delay
postintraarticular paramagnetic contrast injection T1-weighted image
postirradiation
    p. fibrosis
    p. fracture
    p. MFH
    p. osteosarcoma

    p. vascular insufficiency
postischemic
    p. atrophy
    p. recovery
postlaminectomy
    p. instability
    p. kyphosis
postlumpectomy skin thickening
postlymphangiography
postmastectomy lymphedema
postmaturity syndrome
postmediastinal
postmediastinum
postmenarchal female pelvis
postmeningococcal pericarditis
postmenopausal
    p. adnexal cyst
    p. endometrial thickness
    p. endometrium
    p. estrogen therapy
    p. osteoporosis
    p. ovary
    p. uterine atrophy
postmetrizamide
    p. CT imaging
    p. CT scan
postmyelography CT
postmyocardial
    p. infarct
    p. infarction echocardiography
    p. infarction syndrome
postmyocardiotomy infarct
postmyocarditis dilated cardiomyopathy
postnatal
    p. injury
    p. ultrasound
postnecrotic
    p. cirrhosis
    p. scarring
postobstructive
    p. atelectasis
    p. pneumonia
    p. renal atrophy
postoperative
    p. angiography
    p. breast hematoma
    p. cholangiography
    p. cholangiography imaging
    p. chylothorax
    p. emphysema
    p. ileus (POI)
    p. infection
    p. mediastinal hemorrhage
    p. pneumomediastinum
    p. radiation therapy
    p. radiotherapy (PORT)
    p. resorption atelectasis
    p. scar tissue
    p. seroma

p. skull defect
p. stenosis
p. thoracic deformity
p. view
postorchiectomy paraaortic radiation therapy
postpartum
p. cardiomyopathy
p. pituitary apoplexy
p. pituitary necrosis
p. uterus
postperfusion lung
postpericardiotomy syndrome
postpharyngeal soft tissue
postphlebitic
p. leg
p. valvular incompetence
postpneumonectomy space
postpolio syndrome
postprandial image
postprimary pulmonary tuberculosis
postprocedure nephrostogram
postprocessing
image p.
p. procedure
p. workstation
postprocessor
postpyelonephritis cortical scarring
postradiation
p. calcification
p. fibrosis
postradiotherapy implant survey reading
postreconstruction filtering option
postreduction
p. film
p. mammaplasty
p. view
p. x-ray
postrelease radiography
postrheumatic cusp retraction
postrolandic parietal cortex
postsphenoid bone
poststenotic dilation
poststress
p. ankle-arm Doppler index
p. image
p. stunning
postsurgical
p. change
p. emphysema
p. fat necrosis
p. pseudoaneurysm
p. recurrent ulcer
posttemporal middle cerebral artery
postterm
p. fetus
p. pregnancy

posttherapy change
postthoracotomy change
postthrombolytic coronary reocclusion
posttourniquet occlusion angiography
posttransplant
p. acute renal failure
p. coronary artery disease
p. lymphoproliferative disorder
posttransplantation ureteric obstruction
posttraumatic
p. angulation
p. arthritis
p. ascending myelopathy
p. aseptic necrosis
p. atrophy of bone
p. cavus
p. central spinal cord syrinx
p. chondrolysis
p. cystic myelopathy
p. fat necrosis
p. fibrosis
p. hemorrhage
p. hydrocephalus
p. intradiploic pseudomeningocele
p. lesion
p. neuroma
p. oil cyst
p. osteoarthritis
p. osteoporosis
p. pneumonia
p. pulmonary insufficiency
p. spinal cord cyst
p. subcapsular hepatic fluid collection
p. syringomyelia
posttuberculous obstruction
postulate
Avogadro p.
postulnar bone
postural
p. headache
p. muscle
p. reduction
p. ureteric obstruction
posture
benediction p.
posturography
moving platform p.
postvagotomy
p. dysphagia
p. effect
p. small bowel distention
postvasectomy change in epididymis
postvenography phlebitis
postvesicular lymph node
postviral leukoencephalopathy
postvoid
p. radiography
p. residual (PVR)

P

745

postvoid (*continued*)
    p. residual urine
    p. residual urine volume
    p. view
postvoiding film
postwash imaging
Potain sign
potassium (K)
    p. 38 (^{38}K, K-38)
    p. 39 (^{39}K, K-39)
    p. 40 (^{40}K, K-40)
    p. 42 (^{42}K, K-42)
    p. 43 (^{43}K, K-43)
    p. bromide contrast medium
    p. imaging agent
    p. iodide
    ionic p.
    p. perchlorate
    p. titanyl phosphate (KTP)
    total exchangeable p. (TEK)
potato
    p. node
    p. tumor of neck
potency
    uterine stimulating p. (USP)
potential
    p. difference
    electrostatic p.
    p. energy
    p. gradient
    ionization p.
    low metastatic p.
    movement-related cortical p.
    phenomenologic effective surface p.
    recruitment p.
    resting phase of cardiac action p.
    sorption p.
    upstroke phase of cardiac action p.
    variable tube p.
potentiation
    postextrasystolic p.
potentiator
potentiometer
Pott
    P. abscess
    P. aneurysm
    P. ankle fracture
    P. disease
    P. puffy tumor
potter
    P. dysplasia
    P. facies
    P. polycystic kidney classification
    P. sequence
    P. syndrome
    P. type IV kidney
Potter-Bucky
    P.-B. diaphragm
    P.-B. grid

Potts shunt
pouce flottant
pouch
    antral p.
    apophysial p.
    arachnoid retrocerebellar p.
    axillary p.
    Blake p.
    blind upper esophageal p.
    branchial p.
    Broca pudendal p.
    celomic p.
    collecting venous p.
    deep perineal p.
    diversion p.
    Douglas rectouterine p.
    dural root p.
    endodermal p.
    endorectal ileal p.
    gastric p.
    Hartmann p.
    haustral p.
    Heidenhain p.
    hepatorenal p.
    hernia p.
    hypophysial p.
    ileal S p.
    ileoanal p.
    ileocecal p.
    Indiana p.
    jejunal p.
    Kock p.
    lateral hypopharyngeal p.
     (LHP)
    2-loop ileal J p.
    Mainz p.
    mature p.
    Morison p.
    nerve root axillary p.
    paracystic p.
    pararectal p.
    paravesical p.
    pendulous p.
    pharyngeal p.
    pharyngoesophageal p.
    Prussak p.
    Rathke p.
    rectal p.
    rectouterine p.
    rectovaginal p.
    rectovaginouterine p.
    rectovesical p.
    renal p.
    Seessel p.
    S-shaped p.
    Studer p.
    superficial inguinal p.
    superficial perineal p.
    suprapatellar p.

4th branchial cleft p.
UCLA p.
ultimobranchial p.
uterovesical p.
venous p.
vesicouterine p.
Willis p.
W-shaped ileal p.
Zenker p.
pouchogram
pouchography
evacuation p.
poudrage
thoracoscopic p.
Poupart inguinal ligament
Pourcelot index
powder
barium p.
bone p.
E-Z-EM barium p.
gelatin sponge p.
licorice p.
opaque p.
p. pseudocalcification
tantalum p.
tungsten p.
Powell method
power
backscattered p.
p. Doppler
p. Doppler imaging (PDI)
p. Doppler signal
p. Doppler sonography
(PDS)
p. Doppler ultrasound
p. gain
p. injection
p. injector
mass collision stopping p
p. ratio
resolving p.
scanning p.
p. spectral analysis (PSA)
stopping p.
stroke p.
P. Trak 6000 gradient
POWERstation LNX workstation
PowerVision ultrasound
Pozzi muscle
PPAS
peripheral pulmonary artery
stenosis
PPH
primary pulmonary hypertension
PPM
posterior papillary muscle
PPP
pancreatic parenchymatous phase
point-to-point protocol

PPRF
paramedian pontile reticular formation
PPS
pulses per second
P1-P4 segment of posterior cerebral
artery
PPV
positive predictive value
pQCT
peripheral quantitative computed
tomography
pQCT measurement
pQCT scanner
PQ 5000 CT scanner
P/QRS
P wave-QRS wave ratio
PR
pulmonary regurgitation
OncoScint PR
Pr
praseodymium
PRA
pendulous reference axis
practicable
as low as readily p. (ALARP)
Prader-Willi syndrome
praseodymium (Pr)
PRE
proton relaxation enhancement
preablation
pre-Achilles fat-pad
preacinar arterial wall thickness
preamplifier
preampullary portion of bile
duct
preangioplasty stenosis
preaortic lymph node
preauricular point
preaxial
precancer
precancerous change
precapillary
p. bed
p. lung hypertension
precaptopril radioisotope study
precarcinomatous
precatheterization
precaution
airborne p.
contact p.
standard p.
transmission-based p.
precaval lymph node
prececal lymph node
precentral
p. artery
p. cerebellar vein
p. gyrus
p. sulcus

P

precentroblast
precessing proton
precession
>p. angle
>fast imaging with steady-state p. (FISP)
>fast imaging with steady-state free p.
>free p.
>Larmor p.
>reverse fast imaging with steady-state free p. (PSIF)
>steady-state free p. (SSFP)
>true fast imaging with steady-state p. (trueFISP)

precessional
>p. frequency
>p. motion

precharred fiber
prechemotherapy image
prechiasmal optic nerve lesion
prechordal, prochordal
>p. plate

precipitate evacuation
precipitating event
precipitation
>contrast p.

Precise self-expanding stent
precision
>test-retest p.

precocity
>isosexual p.

precommunicating
>p. segment of anterior cerebral artery
>p. segment of posterior cerebral artery

precontrast
>p. echocardiography
>p. imaging
>p. scan

precordia
precordial
>p. bulge
>p. lead
>p. mapping

precordium
>active p.
>anterior p.
>bulging p.
>lateral p.

precoronal sagittal sinus
precuneus
precursor
>BH4 p.
>bone marrow myeloid p.
>neurotransmitter p.
>p. sign to rupture of aneurysm

predental space

predetector
predicted
>p. cardiac index
>p. maximal uptake
>p. target heart rate

prediction
>linear p.

predictor
predisposition
>hereditary p.

prediverticular
>p. change
>p. disease

prednisone
predominance
>anterior p.
>basilar p.
>posterior p.
>temporal p.

predominant flow load
preductal aortic coarctation
preejection
>p. interval
>p. period (PEP)

preembolization aortography
preemphasis
preenhancement sequence
preepiglottic
>p. soft tissue
>p. space

preesophageal dysphagia
preexcitation
>ventricular p.

preexposure prophylaxis
preferential
>p. diffusivity
>p. flow

prefilled syringe
prefiltering
>3D p.

prefire image
preformed clot
prefragmentation
prefrontal
>p. artery
>p. bone of von Bardeleben
>p. cortex

pregnancy
>abdominal ectopic p.
>ampullar p.
>anembryonic p.
>bigeminal p.
>broad ligament p.
>cervical p.
>combined p.
>compound p.
>compromised p.
>cornual ectopic p.
>diamniotic p.

dichorionic-diamniotic twin p.
ectopic p.
extrauterine p. (EUP)
failed p.
fallopian p.
false p.
gemellary p.
heterotopic p.
hydatid p.
hypervolemia of p.
implantation bleeding in p.
interstitial ectopic p.
intraligamentary p.
intraperitoneal p.
intrauterine p. (IUP)
membranous p.
mesenteric p.
molar p.
monochorionic-diamniotic
  twin p.
monochorionic-monoamniotic
  twin p.
multiple p.'s
mural p.
ovarian p.
ovarioabdominal p.
oviductal p.
parietal p.
phantom p.
plural p.
postterm p.
prevalence of ectopic p.
prolonged p.
pseudointraligamentary p.
ruptured ectopic p.
sarcofetal p.
sarcohysteric p.
selective reduction of p.
sextuplet p.
spurious p
stump p.
tubal p.
tuboabdominal p.
tuboligamentary p.
tuboovarian p.
tubouterine p.
p. tumor
twin ectopic p.
uteroabdominal p.
uterotubal p.
p. wastage
pregnancy-induced uterine blush
pregnant
p. uterus
p. uterus rupture
preinjection echocardiography
preinsular gyrus
preintegration complex
preinterparietal bone

preinvasive
p. carcinoma
p. disease of cervix, vagina, and
  vulva
preinversion multiecho
Preiser disease
prelaryngeal node
preliminary
p. film
p. view
preload
left ventricular p.
p. reserve
preloading radiation survey
premalleolar bursa
premammillary
p. artery
p. branch
premasseteric
p. space
p. space abscess
premature
p. atherosclerosis
p. calcification
p. closure of ductus arteriosus
p. middiastolic closure of mitral
  valve
p. nodal contraction (PNC)
p. osteoarthritis
p. placental senescence
p. senescence of placenta
p. suture synostosis
p. uterine membrane rupture
p. valve closure
p. ventricular contraction
  (PVC)
prematurely closed suture
premaxillary
p. bone
p. suture
premedication
premedullary arteriovenous fistula
**premenopausal hormone receptor
  positive**
premolar tooth
premonitory sign
premotor
p. area
p. coret activation
p. cortex
**premyocardial infarction
  echocardiography**
prenatal
p. diagnosis
p. hypoxic ischemic encephalopathy
p. injury
p. radiation
prenicogastric
preocclusive obstruction

P

preoperative
- p. angiography
- p. imaging
- p. localization
- p. radiotherapy
- p. resting MUGA scan
- p. view

preosteonecrosis marrow edema
prepapillary bile duct
preparation
- bowel p.
- Colyte bowel p.
- crush p.
- dry bowel p.
- Dulcolax bowel p.
- Emulsoil bowel p.
- p. error
- Evac-Q-Kwik bowel p.
- Fleet Phospho-Soda bowel p.
- flow cytometry sample p.
- GoLYTELY bowel p.
- inadequate bowel p.
- international reference p.
- kit p.
- LoSo Prep bowel p.
- NuLytely bowel p.
- OCL bowel p.
- on-column p.
- Tagitol V p.
- touch p.
- Tridrate bowel p.
- wet bowel p.
- X-Prep bowel p.

prepared
prepatellar
- p. bursa
- p. bursitis

prepectoral fascia
prepectorally
prepericardial lymph node
preperitoneal fat
prepiriform cortex
preplacental hemorrhage
preponderance
- phalangeal p.

prepontine
- p. cistern
- p. white epidermoidoma

prepubertal
- p. female breast
- p. testicular mass

prepulse
- MT p.
- shared p.
- spin-lock p.

prepyloric
- p. antrum
- p. atresia

- p. fold
- p. sphincter
- p. ulcer
- p. vein

prereduction
- p. view
- p. x-ray

prerenal
- p. aortic aneurysm
- p. failure
- p. fat

prerupture of aneurysm
PRES
- posterior reversible encephalopathy syndrome

presacral
- p. anomaly
- p. cystic lesion
- p. mass
- p. plexus
- p. space

presaturation
- p. bolus tracking
- fat-selective p.
- p. projection
- p. pulse
- spatial p.
- p. technique

presbyesophagus
presbyophrenia
prescan
- MRI p.

prescapula
presence
- inferred p.

presenile arteriosclerosis
presentation
- breech p.
- brow p.
- cephalic p.
- compound p.
- cord p.
- face p.
- footling p.
- frank breech p.
- midline incense p.
- osteoblastic p.
- parietal p.
- shoulder p.
- transverse p.
- vertex p.

presenting part
preservation
- myocardial p.
- p. of native aortic valve
- sphincter p.
- zone of partial p. (ZPP)

presinusoidal

preslip
    p. change
    p. staging
presphenoid bone
PRESS
    point-resolved spectroscopy
    PRESS sequence
pressor unit
pressure
    acoustic p.
    airway p.
    alveolar p.
    p. amplitude
    ankle-arm p.
    ankle systolic p.
    aortic root p.
    arterial peak systolic p.
    atmospheric p.
    atrial p.
    A-wave p.
    axial p.
    bile duct p.
    blood p.
    bone marrow p. (BMP)
    brachial artery cuff p.
    brachial artery end-diastolic p.
    brachial artery peak systolic p.
    brachial artery pulse p.
    bursting p.
    capillary hydrostatic p.
    capillary wedge p.
    cardiac filling p.
    cardiovascular p.
    catheter bursting p.
    central aortic p.
    central venous p. (CVP)
    cerebral perfusion p. (CPP)
    cerebrospinal fluid p.
    p. collapse
    colloid oncotic p. (COP)
    coronary perfusion p.
    coronary wedge p.
    CT-estimated superimposed
      hydrostatic p.
    p. cuff
    C-wave p.
    damping of catheter tip p.
    diastolic filling p. (DFP)
    diastolic perfusion p.
    distal coronary perfusion p.
    Doppler ankle systolic p.
    Doppler blood p.
    draining with venous p.
    drifting wedge p.
    elevated lower esophageal sphincter
      resting p.
    endocardial p.
    end-systolic p. (ESP)
    p. epiphysis
    p. equalization
    equalized diastolic p.
    p. erosion
    esophageal peristaltic p.
    extravascular p.
    feeding mean arterial p. (FMAP)
    filling p.
    p. fracture
    p. half-time
    p. half-time technique
    hepatic wedge p. (HWP)
    high filling p.
    high interstitial p.
    high wedge p.
    increased central venous p.
    increased intracranial p.
    increased intrapericardial p.
    increased pulmonary arterial p.
    p. injector
    inspiratory increase in venous p.
    interstitial fluid hydrostatic p.
    intracardiac p.
    intracranial p. (ICP)
    intracranial epidural p.
    intracranial pulse p.
    intraductal p.
    intraluminal esophageal p.
    intramuscular fluid p.
    intraocular p.
    intrapericardial p.
    intrapleural p.
    intrapulmonary p.
    intrathoracic p.
    in vivo balloon p.
    jugular venous p.
    labile blood p.
    left atrial p. (LAP)
    left atrial end-diastolic p.
    left-sided heart p.
    left subclavian central venous p.
      (LSCVP)
    left ventricular p. (LVP)
    left ventricular cavity p.
    left ventricular end-diastolic p.
      (LVEDP)
    left ventricular filling p.
    left ventricular peak systolic p.
    lower esophageal sphincter p.
      (LESP)
    low urethral p. (LUP)
    maximum inflation p.
    mean aortic p.
    mean arterial p. (MAP)
    mean blood p.
    mean brachial artery p.
    mean circulatory filling p.
    mean left atrial p.

P

pressure (*continued*)
- mean pulmonary artery p. (MPAP)
- mean pulmonary artery wedge p.
- mean pulmonary capillary p. (MPCP)
- mean right atrial p.
- p. measurement
- medium detachment p.
- minimum blood p.
- p. necrosis
- normal lower esophageal sphincter resting p.
- p. overload
- PAS p.
- passage p.
- p. peak
- peak airway p.
- peak inflation p.
- peak regurgitant wave p.
- peak systolic aortic p.
- perfusion p.
- p. perfusion imaging
- p. perfusion study
- phasic p.
- p. pneumothorax
- p. point
- portal venous p. (PVP)
- positive end-expiratory p.
- pulmonary arterial systolic pressure to systemic arterial systolic p.
- pulmonary arterial wedge p.
- pulmonary artery p. (PAP)
- pulmonary artery diastolic p.
- pulmonary artery diastolic and wedge p.
- pulmonary artery diastolic pressure and pulmonary artery wedge p. (PADP-PAWP)
- pulmonary artery end-diastolic p. (PAEDP)
- pulmonary artery mean p. (PAM)
- pulmonary artery peak systolic p.
- pulmonary artery systolic pressure/ systemic artery systolic p. (PASP/SASP)
- pulmonary artery wedge p. (PAWP)
- pulmonary capillary p. (PCP)
- pulmonary capillary wedge p. (PCWP)
- pulmonary venous wedge p.
- pulmonary wedge p. (PWP)
- pulse p.
- p. reading
- recoil p.
- regional cerebral perfusion p. (rCPP)
- right atrial p. (RAP)
- right-sided heart p.
- right ventricular p. (RVP)
- right ventricular diastolic p.
- right ventricular end-diastolic p.
- right ventricular peak systolic p.
- right ventricular volume p.
- segmental bronchus-lower extremity Doppler p.
- shockwave p.
- stump p.
- subatmospheric p.
- superior vena cava p.
- supersystemic pulmonary artery p.
- systemic diastolic blood p.
- systemic mean arterial p. (SMAP)
- systolic-diastolic blood p.
- torr p.
- transmyocardial perfusion p.
- transpulmonary p. (Ptp)
- venous p.
- ventricular p.
- ventricularization of p.
- V-wave p.
- p. wave
- p. waveform
- wedge hepatic venous p. (WHVP)
- withdrawal p.
- X-wave p.
- Y-wave p.
- Z-point p.

pressure-activated safety valve (PASV)
pressure-controlled intermittent coronary occlusion technique
pressure-detachable silicone balloon
pressure-flow gradient
pressure-gradient wire system
pressure-volume loop
PressureWire sensor
pressurized fluid jet
prestenotic dilation
prestomal ileitis
prestyloid recess
presymptomatic
presynaptic dopaminergic deficit
pretectal
- p. lesion
- p. nucleus

pretendinous
- p. band
- p. cord

pretherapy imaging
pretibial
- p. dimple
- p. myxedema

pre-TIPS gradient
pretracheal
- p. lymph node
- p. space

prevalence of ectopic pregnancy

prevascular space
prevertebral
p. abscess
p. fascia
p. ganglion
p. lymph node
p. soft tissue (PVST)
p. soft tissue swelling
p. space
p. space mass
p. width
prevesicular lymph node
previa
central placenta p.
complete placenta p.
incomplete placenta p.
lateral placenta p.
marginal placenta p.
partial placenta p.
placenta p.
total placenta p.
previable fetus
PRFT
partially relaxed Fourier transform
PRG
phleborheography
prickle cell carcinoma
primae
synchondrosis costae p.
Prima laser
primary
p. achalasia
p. acquired cholesteatoma
p. acquired nasolacrimal duct
obstruction (PANDO)
p. adrenal insufficiency
p. adrenal lymphoma
p. amyloidosis
p. aspergillosis
p. atelectasis
p. auditory cortex
p. beam
p. benign liver tumor
p. biliary cirrhosis
p. bone lymphoma
p. brain lymphoma
cancer of unknown p. (CUP)
carcinoma of unknown p. (CUP)
p. cartilage joint
p. center of ossification
p. central nervous system lymphoma
p. cerebral non-Hodgkin lymphoma
p. chemotherapy
p. CNS cholesteatoma
p. CNS lymphoma
p. CNS tumor classification
p. coccidioidomycosis
p. complex
p. congenital megaureter

p. cutaneous large B-cell lymphoma
(PCLBCL)
p. cutaneous plasmacytoma
p. cyst of spleen
p. demyelination
p. digital acquisition
p. esophageal peristalsis
p. extranodal lymphoma
p. familial xanthomatosis
p. gastric non-Hodgkin lymphoma
p. hepatocellular carcinoma
p. HIV encephalitis
p. hydrocele
p. hydrocephalus
p. hyperparathyroidism
p. hypertrophic osteoarthropathy
p. hypothyroidism
p. implanted tumor
p. inflammatory complex
radiographic pattern
p. intracerebral hematoma
p. intracranial germ cell tumor
p. intraosseous carcinoma
p. irritant
p. left bronchus
p. lesion
p. leukodystrophy
p. lymphedema
p. malignant liver tumor
p. malignant neoplasm
p. motor cortex (PMC)
p. motor strip
p. myeloid metaphysis
p. neoplasia
p. neuroendocrine small cell
carcinoma
p. non-Hodgkin lymphoma of bone
p. optic atrophy
p. ovarian choriocarcinoma
p. oxalosis
p. peristaltic wave
p. pigmented nodular adrenocortical
disease
p. pleurisy
p. progressive cerebellar degeneration
p. pulmonary hemangiopericytoma
p. pulmonary hypertension (PPH)
p. pulmonary lobule
p. pulmonary lymphangiectasis
p. pulmonary malignancy
p. pulmonary malignant fibrous
histiocytoma
p. pulmonary plasmacytoma
p. pulmonary tuberculosis
p. radiation
p. ray
p. refractory Burkitt lymphoma
p. renal tumor
p. retroperitoneal fibrosis

P

primary (*continued*)
p. rhabdomyosarcoma
p. right bronchus
p. sarcoma
p. sclerosing cholangitis
p. sequestrum
p. solitary endobronchial plasmacytoma (PSEP)
p. somesthetic area
p. splenic lymphoma (PSL)
p. subclavian-axillary vein thrombosis
p. temporal bone cholesteatoma
p. thrombus
p. tooth
p. tumor bed
p. tumor of origin
unknown p.
p. uterine lymphoma
p. vasospasm
p. vesical calculus
p. viremia
p. visual cortex
p. vitreous
p. yolk sac
priming effect
primitive
p. acoustic artery
p. bone
p. dislocation
p. gut
p. hindgut
p. hypoglossal artery
p. neuroectodermal tumor (PNET)
p. neuroepithelial tumor
p. pit
p. streak
p. trigeminal artery (PTA)
p. ventricle
p. vertebra
p. yolk sac
primordial
p. follicle
p. tooth cyst
primordium
thyroid p.
Primovist
primum
ostium p.
septum p.
primus
digitus p.
PrinceStar electrophysiologic imaging study system
principal
p. artery of pterygoid canal
p. bronchus
p. eigenvector
p. plane

principle
Dodge p.
Doppler shift p.
Fick p.
Fuchs p.
Grossman p.
Huygens p.
indicator fractionation p.
line focus p.
Pauli exclusion p.
planigraphic p.
tracer p.
uncertainty p.
print reflectance modulation
prion
p. protein (PrP)
p. virus
prior probability
prism
P. 3-head system
p. interpolation
p. method for ventricular volume
PROACT
Prolyse in acute cerebral thromboembolism
PROACT I, II trial
proactinium
probability
absolute emission p.
emission p.
posterior p.
prior p.
probe
Aloka SSD ultrasound system and p.
AngeLase combined mapping-laser p.
P. balloon dilation system
biplane sector p.
bipolar circumactive p. (BICAP)
Bowman p.
Bruel-Kjaer transvaginal ultrasound p.
Cardiac View p.
p. dilation
Doppler flow echocardiographic p.
electrohydraulic p.
electromagnetic flow p.
fiberoptic p.
freehand p.
gamma p.
gamma-detection p.
GE proton head coil p.
handheld Doppler p.
handheld exploring electrode p.
handheld mapping p.
high-frequency miniature p.
hot-tipped laser p.
hybrid p.

hybridization p.
hyperthermia p.
interstitial p.
intraoperative gamma p.
laparoscopic ultrasound p.
laser Doppler flowmetry p.
LeVeen RF p.
linear-array transrectal ultrasound p.
localizing p.
magnetometer p.
MH-908 slim ultrasonic p.
neutral amyloid p.
NMR magnetometer p.
nuclear p.
oligonucleotide p.
Olympus MH-908 slim
 ultrasonic p.
Olympus S20-20R transendoscopic
 ultrasound p.
pediatric biplane TEE p.
phased-array p.
relaxation p.
scintillation p.
shift p.
side-firing p.
sidehole cannulated p.
Teflon p.
transesophageal echocardiography p.
Transonics flow p.
truncated NMR p.
ultrasonic p.
ultrasound p.
USCI p.
Versadopp ultrasonic Doppler p.

PROBE
 proton brain examination
probehead
 MRI p.
probe-surface distance
PROBE-SV
 proton brain exam-single voxel
 PROBE-SV spectrometry
problematic abdominal activity
problem-focused history
proboscis lateralis
Probst
 P. bundle
 P. callosal bundle
probucol
 halofuginone p.
procedure
 artificial pleural effusion p.
 button p.
 Cabrol composite graft p.
 Carson p.
 catheter-directed interventional p.
 Chamberlain p.
 Denker p.
 diagnostic p.

DKS pulmonary artery to ascending
 aorta anastomosis p.
edge-detection p.
Eloesser p.
endoscopic p.
gastric pullthrough p.
Glenn superior vena cava to right
 pulmonary artery anastomosis p.
Guidant Ancure endograft p.
Hofmeister gastrectomy p.
interventional p.
intestinal bypass p.
invasive radiologic vascular p.
Kasai portoenterostomy p.
laryngeal drop p.
limb-lengthening p.
magnetic resonance
 angiography-directed bypass p.
mobile imaging p.
neuroendovascular interventional p.
Nissen fundoplication of stomach p.
Palomo varicocelectomy p.
Pólya gastrectomy p.
portable imaging p.
postprocessing p.
provocative p.
psoas hitch p.
rapid-heating ablation p.
revascularization p.
Roux-en-Y gastrointestinal system p.
segmentation p.
Senning p.
spatial localization p.
2-step p.
stereotactic p.
STING p.
Swenson colonic pullthrough p.
uroradiologic p.
Whipple radical
 pancreatoduodenectomy p.
Proceed vascular interventional CT
process
 accessory p.
 acromion p.
 alar p.
 alveolar consolidative p.
 apical p.
 articular p.
 ascending p.
 auditory p.
 basilar p.
 bony p.
 bremsstrahlung p.
 calcaneal p.
 capitular p.
 carrier-free separation p.
 caudate p.
 clinoid p.
 cochleariform p.

P

process (*continued*)
    condyloid p.
    conoid p.
    consolidative p.
    coracoacromial p.
    coracoid p.
    coronoid p.
    costal p.
    cribriform p.
    cystic p.
    destructive p.
    2D filtering p.
    energy transfer p.
    ensiform p.
    ethmoidal p.
    falciform p.
    fanning of spinous p.
    fibroplastic p.
    frontal p.
    frontonasal p.
    frontosphenoidal p.
    glenoid p.
    inflammatory synovial p.
    intercondylar p.
    interspinal p.
    intravascular clotting p.
    jugular p.
    knobby p.
    lateral talar p.
    left ventricular posterosuperior p.
    leptomeningeal p.
    lumbar transverse p.
    mastoid p.
    maxillary p.
    monarticular p.
    neoplastic p.
    neutron absorption p.
    noncalcified ocular p.
    notochordal p.
    odontoid p.
    olecranon p.
    osseous destructive p.
    paraneoplastic p.
    posterolateral talar p.
    prominent xiphoid p.
    pseudopermeative p.
    pterygoid p.
    radial styloid p.
    sacral p.
    sacralized transverse p.
    Sand p.
    shimming p.
    space-occupying p.
    spinous p.
    SSFP p.
    Stieda p.
    styloid p.
    superior articulating p.
    supracondylar p.

    temporal p.
    p. tomography
    transverse p.
    trigonal p.
    trochlear p.
    ulnar styloid p.
    uncinate p.
    vermiform p.
    vertebral p.
    vertebrospinous p.
    within-slice filtering p.
    xiphoid p.
    zygomatic p.

processing
    digital imaging p. (DIP)
    enterocytic p.
    intrapixel sequential p. (IPSP)
    maximum entropy p.
    MIP image p.
    signal p.

processor
    array p.
    conventional p.
    daylight p.
    fast array p.
    Kodak RP X-OMAT p.
    ML-700 daylight p.
    p. sensitometry
    sequence p.

processor-related artifact
processus vaginalis
prochordal (*var. of* prechordal)
procoagulant
ProCol vascular bioprosthesis
proctogram
    balloon p.
    defecating p.
    video p.
proctographic feature
proctography
    evacuation p.
proctopathy
    radiation p.
proctostat
procurvature deformity
Prodigy bone densitometer
product
    brightness area p. (BAP)
    cleaved polyprotein precursor
      molecule p.
    decay p.
    dose area p. (DAP)
    dose-length p.
    fibrin-split p.
    fission p.
    iodine-labeled p.
    real-time dose area p.
    respiratory burst p.
    spallation p.

production
　　Cerenkov radiation p.
　　fast routine p.
　　lactoferrin p.
　　mitochondrial ATP p.
　　pair p.
　　radionuclide p.
　　radiopharmaceutical p.
　　remote-controlled p.
　　secondary electron p.
　　1-step p.
proencephalon (*var. of* prosencephalon)
Profasi HP
profile
　　autocalibration k-space p.
　　CH20 Kernal and slim 2 p.
　　3D dose p.
　　excitation p.
　　flat time-intensity p.
　　flow velocity p.
　　fluence p.
　　P. mammography system
　　nonlinear excitation p.
　　number p.
　　parabolic velocity p.
　　peak p.
　　projection p.
　　p. ray view
　　rectangular section p.
　　section-sensitivity p.
　　slice sensitivity p. (SSP)
　　ultralow p. (ULP)
　　velocity p.
profilogram
profluens
　　hydrops tubae p.
Proforma catheter
profound hypothermic circulatory arrest
profunda
　　colitis cystica p.
　　p. femoris artery
profundal popliteal collateral index
profundus
　　flexor digitorum p.
　　p. tendon
profusion
　　opacity p.
progeny
　　radon p.
progeria
　　adult p.
progestin receptor
prognathia (*var. of* prognathism)
prognathic dilation
prognathism, prognathia
prognostic score
program
　　Philips/ADAC cardiac imaging p.
　　pixel shift p.

　　Spofford-Christopher oxygen
　　　optimizing p. (SCOOP)
programmable
　　p. stepper motor
　　p. ventricular shunt valve
programmer
　　pulse p.
　　p. wand
progression
　　freedom from p.
　　inexorable p.
　　inflow disease p.
　　interval p.
　　steady-state free p.
　　true fast imaging and steady p.
progressiva
　　encephalopathia subcorticalis p.
　　fibrodysplasia ossificans p.
　　myositis ossificans p.
　　rhinitis gangrenosa p.
progressive
　　p. coccidioidomycosis
　　p. degeneration
　　p. diaphysial dysplasia (PDD)
　　p. dysphagia
　　p. emphysematous necrosis
　　p. encephalopathy with edema,
　　　hypsarrhythmia, and optic atrophy
　　　(PEHO)
　　p. familial cirrhosis
　　p. familial intrahepatic cholestasis
　　　(PFIC)
　　p. hydrocephalus
　　p. interstitial pulmonary fibrosis
　　p. massive fibrosis (PMF)
　　p. multifocal leukoencephalopathy
　　　(PML)
　　p. nodular pulmonary fibrosis
　　p. postpolio muscle atrophy
　　p. posttraumatic myelopathy
　　p. primary tuberculosis
　　p. rubella panencephalitis
　　p. spin saturation
　　p. stroke
　　p. subcortical encephalopathy
　　p. subcortical gliosis
　　p. suppurative cholangitis
　　p. supranuclear palsy
　　p. systemic sclerosis
　　p. uptake
ProHance
　　P. contrast medium
　　P. imaging agent
projectile horn
projection
　　p. angiogram
　　anterior p.
　　anteroposterior lordotic p.
　　AP p.

P

projection (*continued*)
apical lordotic p.
average pixel p. (APP)
axial p.
axillary p.
back p.
ball-catcher p.
base p.
basilar p.
basovertical p.
p. binning
biplane p.
blowout view p.
bony vertebra p.
brow-down p.
brow-up p.
Caldwell p.
carpal tunnel p.
cartographic p.
caudad p.
caudocranial p.
centroid-based maximum-intensity p.
Chassard-Lapiné p.
Chausse III p.
Chaussier p.
coronal maximum-intensity p.
craniocaudal p.
cross-sectional transverse p.
cross-table lateral p.
cylindrical map p.
decubitus p.
3-dimensional stereotactic surface p.
  (3D SSP)
divergent ray p.
dorsoplantar p.
3D stereotactic surface p.
erect fluoro spot p.
fan-beam p.
fast Fourier p. (FFP)
FI p.
p. fiber damage
filtered back p. (FBP)
fingerlike p.
Fletcher p.
flexion-extension p.
p. formula
frogleg lateral p.
frontal p.
FS p.
full-scan p.
full scan with interpolation p.
Granger p.
half-axial anteroposterior p.
half scan with extrapolation p.
Hermodsson tangential p.
intraoral p.
Lambert p.
LAO p.
lateral oblique axial p.

lateral transcranial p.
lateral transfacial p.
lateromedial oblique p.
left anterior oblique p.
left lateral p.
left posterior oblique p.
Low-Beers p.
L5-S1 p.
lumbosacral p.
maximum-intensity p. (MIP)
maximum-intensity sliding thin-slab
  p.
medial oblique axial p.
mediolateral oblique p.
Mercator p.
minimum-intensity sliding thin-slab p.
modified p.
mortise p.
navicular p.
notch p.
nuchofrontal p.
oblique lateral p.
occipitomental p.
off-lateral p.
open-mouth p.
orthogonal angiographic p.
PA p.
panoramic surface p.
papillary p.
parietoorbital p.
Pawlow p.
pillar p.
Pirie transoral p.
plantodorsal p.
postdrainage p.
posterior p.
posteroanterior lordotic p.
presaturation p.
p. profile
radiographic p.
ramp-filtered back p.
ray-sum p.
recumbent lateral p.
reversed Stenvers p.
Rhese p.
right anterior oblique p.
right posterior oblique p.
rotating tomographic p.
Runström p.
saturation inversion p. (SIP)
scaphoid p.
Schüller p.
semiaxial anteroposterior p.
semiaxial transcranial p.
Settegast p.
simulated annealing method p.
skyline p.
sliding thin-slab maximum-intensity
  p. (STS-MIP)

steep left anterior oblique p.
steep Towne p.
Stenvers p.
stereographic p.
stereo right lateral p.
stereotactic surface p. (SSP)
straight lateral p.
stress p.
Stryker notch p.
submentovertex p.
sunrise p.
superoinferior p.
surface p.
swimmer's p.
tangential p.
thin-slab minimum-intensity p.
p. tract imaging
transaxial maximum-intensity p.
transthoracic p.
tunnel p.
underfilled submentovertical p.
under-scan method p.
variable p. (VARPRO)
verticosubmental p.
Vogt bone-free p.
Waters p.
p. x-ray microscope
projectional image
projection-reconstruction
p.-r. imaging
p.-r. technique
projector
cine p.
liquid crystal display 'p.
white light pattern p.
**prolactin-secreting pituitary
  macroadenoma**
prolapse
anterior leaflet p.
billowing mitral valve p.
cord p.
gastroduodenal mucosal p.
gastrojejunal mucosal p.
holosystolic mitral valve p.
intestinal p.
intracranial fat p.
mitral valve p. (MVP)
mitral valve leaflet systolic
  p.
p. of aortic valve
p. of right aortic valve cusp
p. of spleen
p. of umbilical cord
pelvic organ p. (POP)
posterior leaflet p.
rectal p.
systolic p.
tricuspid valve p.
valve p.

prolapsed
p. antral mucosa
p. gastric mucosa
p. mitral valve (PMV)
p. stoma
p. tumor
proliferans
cholecystitis glandularis p.
proliferation
angiofibroblastic p.
p. area
astrocytic p.
benign sclerosing ductal p.
bile duct p.
bizarre parosteal osteochondromatous
  p.
bizarre subparosteal
  osteochondromatous p.
bony p.
collagen tissue p.
connective tissue p.
extranodal p.
fibroplastic p.
glandular p.
intimal p.
myofibrohistiocytic p.
myointimal p.
myxomatous p.
neointimal p.
neuronal p.
nodular p.
p. of bone
p. of fibrous tissue
osteophytic p.
papillary p.
perineural glial p.
peripelvic fat p.
p. pleurisy
p. rate
reactive fibrovascular arachnoid p.
synovial p.
villous p.
proliferative, proliferous
p. bronchiolitis
p. change
p. glomerulonephritis
p. index
p. inflammation
p. lesion
p. pattern
proliferative-phase endometrium
proliferous (*var. of* proliferative)
prolonged
p. ejection time
p. expiratory phase
p. inspiratory phase
p. interval
p. left ventricular impulse
p. pregnancy

P

Prolyse in acute cerebral thromboembolism (PROACT)
promethium (Pm)
prominence
    aortic p.
    bony p.
    hilar p.
    interstitial p.
    mediastinal p.
    p. of bone
    styloid p.
    tibial tubercle p.
    upper lobe vein p.
prominent
    p. ductal pattern
    p. ductal vascular structure
    p. liver
    p. perivascular space
    p. pyramidal thyroid lobe
    p. rim of radiolucency
    p. septal lymphatics
    p. spur
    p. tubercle
    p. uptake
    p. vertebra
    p. xiphoid process
promontoria (*pl. of* promontorium)
promontorium (*var. of* promontory), *pl.* **promontoria**
promontory, promontorium
    p. mass
    sacral p.
pronate
pronation
    hallucal p.
    pes p.
pronation-abduction
    p.-a. fracture
    p.-a. injury
pronation-eversion fracture
pronation-external
    p.-e. rotation
    p.-e. rotation injury
pronator
    p. quadratus
    p. quadratus line
    round p.
    p. sign
    p. teres
    p. teres tendon
pronatus
    pes p.
prone
    p. angled view
    p. film
    p. lateral view
    p. PET breast acquisition
    p. position

pronephros
    rudimentary p.
pronged Franseen-type-point needle
pronunciation
    artifact p.
propagation
    p. speed artifact
    thrombus p.
Propaq Encore vital signs monitor
propeller
    P. FSE technique
    P. MRI
proper
    p. digital nerve branch
    p. hepatic artery (PHA)
properitoneal
    p. fat
    p. fat line
    p. flank stripe
    p. hernia
prophylactic IVC filter
prophylaxes (*pl. of* prophylaxis)
prophylaxis, *pl.* **prophylaxes**
    preexposure p.
propidium iodide
proportion
    aneurysmal p.
proportional
    p. counter
    p. ratio
proportionality
    cephalofacial p.
propria
    lamina p.
    muscularis p.
    substantia p.
    tunica p.
proprius
    extensor indicis p. (EIP)
    extensor quinti p. (EQP)
    p. tendon
proptosis
propulsive
    p. mechanism
    p. movement
propyliodone imaging agent
prosencephalon, proencephalon
ProSound SSD-5500 ultrasound
prospective
    p. acquisition correction (PACE)
    p. analysis
    p. investigation of pulmonary embolus diagnosis (PIOPED)
    p. synchronization
ProSpeed CT scanner
prostaglandin
    p. E_1
    p. E_1 injection
    p. infusion

Prostalase laser system
Prostar-Techstar suture-mediated closure
  device
Prostar XL 8, 10 suture-mediated
  closure device
ProstaScint
    P. monoclonal antibody imaging
      agent
    P. scan
prostate
    p. abscess
    p. anatomy
    p. apex
    apex of p.
    p. calcification
    p. capsule
    p. carcinoma
    floating p.
    p. gland
    p. hypoechoic lesion
    p. implant
    inferolateral surface of p.
    lateral lobe of p.
    lymph vessel of p.
    median lobe of p.
    posterior surface of p.
    p. seeding
    transrectal ultrasound-guided biopsy
      of p.
    transurethral incision of p.
    transurethral resection of p. (TURP)
    visual laser ablation of p. (VLAP)
prostatectomy
    radical perineal p.
    transurethral ultrasound-guided
      laser-induced p. (TULIP)
prostate-specific
    p.-s. antigen (PSA)
    p.-s. antigen density
    p.-s. antigen velocity (PSAV)
    p.-s. membrane
    p.-s. membrane antigen (PSMA)
prostatic
    p. adenoma
    p. bed
    p. calcification
    p. calculus
    p. carcinoma
    p. cyst
    p. duct
    p. fluid
    p. hyperplasia
    p. hyperplastic nodule
    p. hypertrophy
    p. obstruction
    p. sinus
    p. stent
    p. transition zone
    p. urethra (PU)

    p. urethroplasty
    p. utricle
    p. venous plexus
prostaticovesical junction
prostaticus
    utriculus p.
prostatitis
    cavitary p.
    diverticular p.
prostatography
prostheses (*pl. of* prosthesis)
prosthesis, *pl.* **prostheses**
    Angelchik reflux p.
    inguinal mesh p.
    Medtronic Talent p.
    St. Jude Medical aortic valve graft
      p.
    Teflon p.
prosthetic
    p. cup
    p. femoral distal graft
    p. heart valve
    p. implant
    p. joint replacement
    p. mitral valve
    p. valve embolus
prostrema
    area p.
protactinium (Pa)
protect
    Cardiac P.
protection
    p. factor
    International Commission on
      Radiological P. (ICRP)
    myocardial p.
    radiation p.
    region of p.
protective
    p. cold saline infusion
    p. isolation
Protégé
    P. GPS self-expanding nitinol
      stent-biliary system
    P. GPS stent
    P. self-expanding stent
protein
    antibody to Epstein-Barr virus
      transactivator p.
    carrier p.
    chemically modified p.
    CSF 14-3-3 p.
    HIV nucleocapsid p.
    lung resistance-related p.
    macrophage inflammatory p. (MIP)
    multidrug-resistant p.
    myelin base p.
    nuclear matrix p.
    prion p. (PrP)

P

protein (*continued*)
    retinoblastoma p.
    skeletal muscle p.
    whole-body p.
protein-1
    latent membrane p.-1
proteinaceous fluid
proteinase
protein-bound iodine (PBI)
protein-fat fluid level
protein-interacting contrast agent
protein-losing enteropathy
protein-nucleic acid synthesis in tumor cell
proteinosis
    alveolar p.
    pulmonary alveolar p. (PAP)
proteoglycan
    chondroitin sulfate p. 3
    p. matrix
Proteus syndrome
Protg GPS self-expanding nitinol stent
protium
protocol
    autopsy p.
    axial BMD center with agreed joint p.
    axial T1-SE p.
    biphasic injection p.
    Bruce treadmill p.
    Cornell p.
    CT scan with renal stone p.
    default display p.
    2D GRE dynamic p.
    Ellestad p.
    experimental p.
    Heidelberg p.
    helical CT scanning p.
    low-dose/high-dose p.
    modified Bagshawe p.
    MP-RAGE p.
    multiple-injection p.
    neon particle p.
    point-to-point p. (PPP)
    proton relaxometric p.
    single-injection p.
    telomere repeat amplification p. (TRAP)
    telomeric repeat amplification p. (TRAP)
    triple rule-out p.
    UCLA imaging p.
    weight-adjusted dosing p.
ProtoCO$_2$l automated CO$_2$ insufflator
protodensity MR imaging
protodiastolic reversal of blood flow
proton
    p. beam
    p. brain examination (PROBE)

    p. brain exam-single voxel (PROBE-SV)
    p. chemical-shift imaging
    p. density-weighted fast spin-echo image
    p. density-weighted imaging
    p. density-weighted MRI
    p. dipole-dipole interaction
    p. electron dipole-dipole
    excited p.
    high-energy p.
    interstitial water p.
    p. irradiation
    lactate p.
    p. magnetic resonance
    methyl p.
    p. MRS
    p. MR spectroscopic imaging
    p. MR spectroscopy
    p. nuclear magnetic resonance spectroscopy
    p. nuclear magnetic resonance spectrum
    precessing p.
    p. relaxation
    p. relaxation enhancement (PRE)
    p. relaxometric protocol
    p. spin-lattice relaxation time
    p. therapy
proton-density
    p.-d. axial image
    p.-d. axial MR scan
proton-electron double-resonance imaging (PEDRI)
proton-proton magnetization exchange
protoplasmic astrocytoma
protopulmonary bilharziasis
protracted
    p. exposure sensitization
    p. radiation
    p. venous infusion (PVI)
protruded disc
protruding
    p. atheroma
    p. fat
protrusio acetabuli
protrusion
    acetabular p.
    anal p.
    broad-based disc p.
    coil p.
    disc p.
    hip p.
    p. of cystocele
    p. of navicular
    spicular p.
    spoonlike p.
    vascular p.

protuberance
    bony p.
    occipital p.
protuberans
    dermatofibrosarcoma p.
provisional callus
provocable ischemia
provocative procedure
proximal
    p. acinar emphysema
    p. and distal portions of vessel
    p. anterior tibial artery
    p. aorta
    p. articular set angle
    p. aspect
    p. brain shift
    p. carpal row
    p. circumflex artery
    p. coil
    p. colon
    p. convoluted tubule
    p. coronary sinus (PCS)
    p. digital artery
    p. dilation
    p. esophagitis dilation
    p. femoral fracture
    p. femur
    p. fibula
    p. focal femoral deficiency (PFFD)
    p. humeral fracture
    p. interphalangeal (PIP)
    p. interphalangeal articulation
    p. interphalangeal joint (PIPJ)
    p. interphalangeal joint articulation
    p. isovelocity surface area (PISA)
    p. jejunum
    p. left anterior descending artery
    p. loop syndrome
    p. part of dorsal duct
    p. popliteal artery
    p. radioulnar joint
    p. 3rd shaft
    p. reference axis
    p. segment
    p. small bowel
    p. tibia
    p. tibial metaphysial fracture
    p. trochlear groove
    p. tubular adenoma
proximally
proximity
    p. arteriography
    p. injury
    stent p.
PrP
    prion protein
PRS
    perirenal space
    photon radiosurgery system

PRT
    photoradiation therapy
prune belly syndrome
pruned
    p. appearance of pulmonary
      vasculature
    p. hilum
pruned-tree
    p.-t. appearance
    p.-t. appearance of bile duct
pruning
    p. of pancreatic duct branch
    pulmonary artery p.
pruritus
Prussak
    P. pouch
    P. space
PSA
    power spectral analysis
    prostate-specific antigen
    PSA density
psammoma
    p. body
    p. body meningioma
    Virchow p.
psammomatoid ossifying fibroma
psammomatous
    p. calcification
    p. meningioma
    p. microcalcification
psathyrosis
PSAV
    prostate-specific antigen velocity
PSD
    periodic synchronous discharge
psec
    picosecond
P2-segment aneurysm
PSEP
    primary solitary endobronchial
      plasmacytoma
pseudarthrosis, pseudoarthrosis
    long-bone p.
    tibial p.
pseudoacardia
pseudoachondroplasia
pseudoaneurysm
    anastomotic p.
    aortic p.
    arterial p.
    chronic posttraumatic aortic p.
    extrahepatic p.
    femoral artery p.
    p. formation
    heart p.
    hepatic artery p.
    iatrogenic p.
    inguinal p.
    p. of mitral-aortic fibrosa

P

763

pseudoaneurysm (*continued*)
    pancreatitis p.
    peripheral p.
    perivalvular p.
    postcatheterization p. (PCPA)
    postsurgical p.
    renal transplant p.
    saccular p.
    splenic artery p.
    traumatic aortic p.
    uterine artery p.
pseudoangiomatous stromal hyperplasia (PASH)
pseudoangiosarcoma
pseudoarthritis
pseudoarthrosis (*var. of* pseudarthrosis)
pseudoarticulation
pseudoascites
pseudo-AV block
pseudo-Bennett fracture
pseudobulbar affect
pseudocalcification
    powder p.
pseudocalculus bile duct
pseudocapsule
    fibrous p.
    radiopaque p.
pseudocarcinoma
pseudocarcinomatous
pseudocavitation
    lung p.
pseudo-Charcot joint
pseudochylous effusion
pseudocirrhosis
    cholangiodysplastic p.
pseudocoarctation of aorta
pseudocolor B-mode
pseudocryptorchidism
pseudocyst
    adrenal p.
    gelatinous brain p.
    mature pancreatic p.
    meconium p.
    necrotic bone p.
    p. of humerus
    pancreatic p.
    pulmonary p.
    splenic p.
    subarticular p.
    umbilical cord p.
pseudocystic hygroma
pseudo-Dandy-Walker malformation
pseudodefect
pseudodextrocardia
pseudodiaphragm
pseudodiffusion
pseudodisease

pseudodislocation of humerus
pseudodissection
pseudodiverticulosis
    intramural esophageal p.
pseudodiverticulum
    retrograde ureteral p.
    small bowel p.
pseudodynamic MR imaging
pseudoepiphysis
pseudoexstrophy
pseudofollicle
pseudofollicular salpingitis
pseudofracture
    p. artifact
    Milkman p.
pseudogating
    diastolic p.
pseudogestational sac
pseudogland formation
pseudoglioma
pseudogout
pseudogynecomastia
pseudohaustration
pseudohermaphroditism
    female p.
pseudohomogeneous edema pattern
pseudo-Hurler deformity
pseudohypertrophy
pseudohypoparathyroidism (PHP)
pseudoinfarct pattern
pseudointimal
    p. formation
    p. hyperplasia
pseudointraligamentary pregnancy
pseudointussusception
pseudo-Jefferson fracture
pseudojoint
pseudokidney
    p. appearance
    p. sign
pseudolesion
pseudoluxation
pseudolymphoma
    breast p.
    gastric p.
    lung p.
pseudomalignant
    p. myositis ossificans
    p. tumor
pseudomantle zone pattern
pseudomass
    mediastinal p.
    mucous p.
    thymic p.
    transient p.
pseudo-Meigs syndrome
pseudomembrane
    fetal neck p.

pseudomembranous
   p. colitis
   p. inflammation
   p. radiation gastritis
pseudomeningocele
   posttraumatic intradiploic p.
pseudomitral leaflet
Pseudomonas aeruginosa **pneumonia**
pseudomucinous cystadenocarcinoma
pseudomyxoma peritonei
pseudoneoplasm
pseudonephritis
   athlete's p.
pseudoneuroma
pseudoneuropathic joint
pseudoobstruction
   bowel p.
   chronic idiopathic intestinal p.
    (CIIP)
   colonic p.
   familial intestinal p.
   idiopathic intestinal p.
   nonfamilial intestinal p.
pseudoomphalocele
pseudoorbital tumor
pseudoosteomalacic pelvis
pseudopancreatitis
pseudoperiostitis
pseudopermeative process
pseudoplaque
pseudopneumoperitoneum
pseudopod formation
pseudopodia (*pl. of* pseudopodium)
pseudopodium, *pl.* **pseudopodia**
pseudopolyp
pseudopolyposis lymphatica
pseudoporencephaly
pseudo-post Billroth I appearance
pseudopregnancy
pseudopseudohypoparathyroidism
pseudopyogenic granuloma
pseudorosette
   perivascular p.
pseudosac
pseudosacculation
pseudosarcoma
   esophageal p.
pseudosarcomatous
   p. fasciitis
   p. fibromyxoid tumor
pseudosclerosis
   spastic p.
pseudoseizure
pseudosheath
pseudospondylolisthesis
   Junghans p.
pseudostenosis
   sigmoid p.

pseudostone
pseudostricture
   colon p.
pseudosubluxation
   C-spine p.
pseudotear
pseudothickening
pseudothrombophlebitis syndrome
pseudothrombosis
pseudotrabecula
pseudotrochanteric bursitis
pseudotruncus arteriosus
pseudotumor
   abdominal p.
   p. appearance
   atelectatic asbestos p.
   p. cerebri
   fibrosing inflammatory p.
   flexural p.
   hemophilic p.
   inflammatory carotid p.
   inflammatory idiopathic orbital p.
   inflammatory intestinal p.
   intraosseous hemophilic p.
   kidney p.
   orbital p.
   pleural p.
   renal p.
   small bowel p.
   vermian p.
   xanthomatous p.
pseudotumoral lesion
pseudo-Turner syndrome
pseudoulceration
pseudoureterocele
pseudovagina
pseudo-Whipple disease
pseudowidening
   joint space p.
pseudoxanthoma elasticum
pseudo-Zollinger-Ellison syndrome
  (ps-ZES)
PSF
   point-spread function
   posterior spine fusion
PSH-25GT transcranial imaging
  transducer
PSIF
   reverse fast imaging with steady-state
   free precession
PSL
   primary splenic lymphoma
PSMA
   prostate-specific membrane
   antigen
psoas
   p. abscess
   p. fascia

P

psoas (*continued*)
    p. hitch procedure
    p. line
    p. major
    p. margin
    p. muscle
    p. shadow
    p. shadow angle
    p. sign
    p. stripe
psoralen and ultraviolet A (PUVA)
psoriatic arthritis
PSP
    photostimulable phosphor
        PSP imaging plate
PSR
    phase sampling ratio
PSV
    peak systolic velocity
PSW
    periodic sharp wave
psychotherapeutic drug
ps-ZES
    pseudo-Zollinger-Ellison syndrome
PT
    pneumothorax
Pt
    platinum
PTA
    percutaneous transluminal angioplasty
    persistent truncus arteriosus
    primitive trigeminal artery
        suprainguinal PTA
PTBD
    percutaneous transhepatic biliary
        drainage
PTC
    percutaneous transhepatic cholangiogram
    percutaneous transhepatic
        cholangiography
PTCA
    percutaneous transhepatic cholangiogram
    percutaneous transhepatic
        cholangiography
    percutaneous transluminal coronary
        angioplasty
        PTCA Registry
PTCD
    percutaneous transhepatic cholangial
        drainage
pterion
pterional transsylvian approach
p-terphenyl
pterygium colli
pterygoid
    p. artery
    p. bone
    p. canal
    p. chest

    p. fossa
    p. muscle
    p. plate
    p. plexus
    p. process
pterygoideus hamulus
pterygomandibular
    p. ligament
    p. raphe
pterygomasseteric muscle
pterygopalatine
    p. canal
    p. fossa
    p. ganglion
pterygospinous ligament
PTF
    posterior talofibular
        PTF ligament
PTFE
    polytetrafluoroethylene
        PTFE stent
PTH
    parathyroid hormone
PTHC
    percutaneous transhepatic
        cholangiogram
PTK
    phototherapeutic keratectomy
pTL
    percutaneous transhepatic lymphography
PTNB
    percutaneous transthoracic needle
        biopsy
ptoses (*pl. of* ptosis)
ptosis, *pl.* **ptoses**
ptotic kidney
Ptp
    transpulmonary pressure
PTRA
    percutaneous transluminal renal
        angioplasty
PTSMA
    percutaneous transluminal septal
        myocardial ablation
PTT
    posterior tibial tendon
    pulse transit time
PTV
    planning target volume
    posterior tibial vein
ptyalography
PU
    prostatic urethra
        PU catheter
pubescent uterus
pubic
    p. arch
    p. bone
    p. bone maldevelopment

p. crest
p. ramus
p. symphysis
p. tubercle

pubis
mons p.
os p.
osteitis p.
pecten p.
symphysis p.
widened symphysis p.
pubocapsular ligament
pubocervical ligament
pubococcygeal line (PCL)
pubococcygeus muscle
pubofemoral ligament
puboischial area
puboprostatic ligament
puborectalis loop
pubovesical ligament
Puck film changer
PUD
peptic ulcer disease
puddle sign
puddling
p. of contrast
peripheral p.
pudenda
ulcerating granuloma of p.
pudendal
p. blood supply
p. branch
p. canal
p. cleft
p. vein
p. vein reflux
PUJ
pelviureteric junction
pullback
p. across aortic valve
aortic p.
p. arterial marking
p. esophagram
p. imaging
p. pressure gradient
p. pressure recording
p. study
pulley
bone p.
p. of finger
pull maneuver
pull-type gastrostomy tube
pull-up, pullup
gastric p.-u.
pullup (*var. of* pull-up)
pulmoaortic canal
Pulmo CT software
pulmogram
pulmolith

pulmolithiasis
pulmonale
atrium p.
cor p.
pulmonalis
bifurcatio trunci p.
pulmonary, pulmonic
p. abscess
p. acinus
p. adenopathy
p. alveolar microlithiasis
p. alveolar proteinosis (PAP)
p. alveolar space
p. alveolus
p. amyloidoma
p. amyloidosis
p. and cardiac sclerosis
p. angioma
p. aplasia
p. arborization
p. arc
p. area
p. arterial circulation
p. arterial flow insufficiency
p. arterial hypertension (PAH)
p. arterial input impedance
p. arterial malformation
p. arterial marking
p. arterial occlusion
p. arterial resistance index
p. arterial systolic pressure to
systemic arterial systolic pressure
p. arterial vent
p. arterial wedge pressure
p. arteriography
p. arteriolar resistance
p. arteriolar vasoconstriction
p. arteriosclerosis
p. arteriovenous aneurysm
p. arteriovenous fistula
p. arteriovenous malformation (PAVM)
p. arteriovenous shunt
p. artery
p. artery agenesis
p. artery aneurysm
p. artery apoplexy
p. artery atresia
p. artery balloon pump
p. artery bifurcation
p. artery blockage
p. artery-bronchus ratio
p. artery compression ascending
aortic aneurysm
p. artery diastolic and wedge
pressure
p. artery diastolic pressure
p. artery diastolic pressure and
pulmonary artery wedge pressure
(PADP-PAWP)

P

pulmonary (*continued*)
p. artery dilation
p. artery embolization
p. artery end-diastolic pressure (PAEDP)
p. artery hemorrhage
p. artery interruption
p. artery intima
p. artery mean pressure (PAM)
p. artery obstruction
p. artery peak systolic pressure
p. artery pressure (PAP)
p. artery pruning
p. artery sarcoma
p. artery stenosis
p. artery stenting
p. artery systolic (PAS)
p. artery systolic pressure/systemic artery systolic pressure (PASP/SASP)
p. artery to right ventricle diastolic gradient
p. artery wedge angiography
p. artery wedge pressure (PAWP)
p. asbestosis
p. aspergillosis
p. aspiration
p. atelectasis
p. atresia
p. atrium
p. barotrauma (PBT)
p. blastoma
p. bleb
p. blood flow (PBF)
p. blood flow redistribution
p. blood flow study
p. blood volume (PBV)
p. blood volume index (PBVI)
p. bulla
p. calcification
p. candidiasis
p. capillary endothelium
p. capillary hemangiomatosis
p. capillary permeability
p. capillary pressure (PCP)
p. capillary wedge position
p. capillary wedge pressure (PCWP)
p. capillary wedge tracing
p. carcinoid tumor
p. cartilage
p. cavitation
p. cavity
p. cement embolism
p. cirrhosis
p. collagen vascular disease
p. collapse
p. confluence
p. consolidation
p. contusion

p. *Cryptococcus*
p. cyst
p. cystic lymphangiectasis
p. densitometry
p. density
p. dysmaturity
p. edema (PE)
p. edema photographic negative
p. embolic septic disease
p. embolus (PE)
p. failure
p. fibrosis
p. flow pattern
p. function test
p. gas
p. gas exchange
p. hamartoma
p. heart
p. hemorrhage
p. hemosiderosis
p. hilum
p. histoplasmosis
p. hyalinizing granuloma
p. hyperinflation
p. hypertension
p. hypertrophic osteoarthropathy (PHOA)
p. hypoperfusion
p. hypoplasia
p. incompetence
p. infarct
p. infection
p. infiltrate
p. insufficiency
p. interstitial abnormality
p. interstitial disease
p. interstitial emphysema (PIE)
p. interstitial idiopathic fibrosis
p. interstitial thinning
p. interstitium
p. juxtaesophageal lymph node
p. Kaposi sarcoma
p. lesion
p. leukostasis
p. ligament
p. linearity
p. lobe
p. lobule
p. lucency
p. lymphangiectasis
p. lymphangiomatosis
p. lymphangitic carcinomatosis (PLC)
p. lymphatics
p. lymphoid disorder
p. lymphoma
p. magnetic resonance angiography (PMRA)
p. mainline granulomatosis

p. mass
p. meningioma
p. metastasis
p. microcirculation
p. microvasculature
p. neoplasm
p. neuroendocrine cell hyperplasia
p. nodularity
p. nodule
p. nodule enhancement
p. opacity
p. orifice
p. osteoarthropathy
p. outflow gradient
p. outflow obstruction
p. output
p. output flow
p. output index
p. overdistention
p. overexpansion
p. overinflation
p. papillomatosis
p. parenchyma
p. parenchymatous change
p. parenchymatous infection
p. parenchymatous infiltrate
p. parenchymatous injury
p. parenchymatous window
p. pedicle
p. perfusion and ventilation
p. perfusion imaging
p. perfusion MRI contrast agent
p. pleura
p. pleurisy
p. plexus
p. precapillary arteriole
p. pseudocyst
p. quantitative differential function
  study
p. regurgitation (PR)
p. resection
p. sarcoidosis
p. scar
p. scintigraphy
p. sclerosing hemangioma
p. segment
p. sequestration
p. sequestration spectrum
p. shunt
p. sinus
p. sling
p. sling complex
p. squamous cell carcinoma
p. stable echo enhancer
p. stenosis
p. structural maturation
p. subcutaneous encephalitis
  emphysema
p. sulcus

p. talcosis
p. telangiectasia
p. thromboembolic disease
p. thromboembolism
p. thromboembolization
p. thrombosis
p. time-activity curve
p. toxicity
p. trunk
p. trunk bifurcation
p. trunk idiopathic dilation
p. tuberculoma
p. tuberculosis
p. tumor
p. tumor embolus
p. valve (PV)
p. valve anulus
p. valve area
p. valve atresia
p. valve cusp
p. valve deformity
p. valve dysplasia
p. valve gradient
p. valve insufficiency
p. valve regurgitation
p. valve stenosis
p. valve stenosis dilation
p. valvular stenosis
p. varix
p. vascular bed
p. vascular bed impedance
p. vascular congestion
p. vascular disease
p. vascularity
p. vascular marking
p. vascular obstruction
p. vascular pattern
p. vascular redistribution
p. vascular reserve
p. vascular resistance (PVR)
p. vascular resistance index
  (PVRI)
p. vasculature
p. vasoreactivity
p. vein
p. vein apoplexy
p. vein atresia
p. vein fibrosis
p. vein stenosis
p. vein wedge angiography
p. venolobar syndrome
p. venooclusive disease (PVOD)
p. venous congestion (PVC)
p. venous drainage
p. venous hypertension (PVH)
p. venous obstruction (PVO)
p. venous recess
p. venous return
p. venous system

P

pulmonary (*continued*)
    p. venous-systemic air embolus
    p. venous wedge pressure
    p. ventilation imaging
    p. versus systemic flow
    p. vesicle
    p. vessel
    p. vessel overcirculation
    p. wedge pressure (PWP)
pulmonic (*var. of* pulmonary)
pulmonic-systemic flow ratio
pulmonis
    crista p.
    lingula p.
pulp, pulpa
    p. abscess
    p. canal
    p. of finger
    p. space
    splenic p.
    p. stone
pulpa (*var. of* pulp)
pulpal
pulposus
    herniated nucleus p.
     (HNP)
pulsatile
    p. flow pattern
    p. perfusion
pulsatility
    arterial p.
    p. index
    p. measurement
pulsating
    p. current
    p. empyema
    p. mass
    p. metastasis
    p. pleurisy
    p. vein
pulsation
    p. artifact
    capillary p.
    mean venous p.
    p. pattern
pulse
    adiabatic inversion p.
    adiabatic slice-selective
     radiofrequency p.
    p. amplifier
    apical p.
    balanced fast field-echo p.
    brachial p.
    carotid p.
    compensated composite
     spin-lock p.
    composite p.
    dampened obstructive p.
    DANTE-selective p.

depth p.
p. design
diastolic depolarization p.
Doppler p.
p. Doppler interrogation
dorsalis pedis p.
2D spatially selective radiofrequency
  p.
E point of cardiac apex p.
fat-suppression p.
femoral p.
p. flip angle
flow respiratory artifact obliteration
  with directed orthogonal p.'s
  (FRODO)
frequency-selective p.
globally optimized alternating-phase
  rectangular p. (GARP)
gradient p.
p. Holter system
inversion p.
p. labeling
p. length
motion-compensation gradient p.
MP inversion p.
narrow-band spectral-selective
  radiofrequency p.
navigator p.
p. NMR
nonselective p.
p. oximetry
p.'s per second (PPS)
phase-encoded p.
picosecond p.
p. pile-up
popliteal p.
posterior tibial p.
presaturation p.
p. pressure
p. programmer
P. Pro heart rate monitor
radial p.
radiofrequency p.
radiofrequency excitation p.
p. reappearance time
p. repetition frequency
p. repetition time
resting p.
RF p.
saturation p.
section-select p.
selective p.
p. sequence
p. sequence echo-planar imaging
p. shape
small water-hammer p.
spatially selective inversion p.
synchronous carotid arterial p.
tailored p.

tidal wave of carotid arterial p.
time following inversion p.
p. transit time (PTT)
trough of venous p.
twin-peaked p.
velocity-compensating gradient p.
vertical synchronization p.
p. voltage
p. volume recording (PVR)
p. volume waveform
V peak of jugular venous p.
p. width (PW)
p. width variation

PULSEcdc compact gamma camera

pulsed

p. arterial spin labeling
p. arterial spin-labeling sequence
p. Doppler flowmeter
p. Doppler transesophageal
echocardiography
p. Doppler ultrasound
p. Doppler waveform
p. dose rate (PDR)
p. infrared laser
p. L-band ESR spectrometry
p. magnetization transfer MR
imaging
p. metal vapor laser
p. mode
p. nuclear magnetic resonance
p. optically stimulated luminescence
(POSL)
p. pump
p. therapeutic low-intensity
ultrasound
p. wave

pulsed-dye

p.-d. laser
p.-d. laser lithotripsy
p.-d. laser therapy

pulsed-electron

p.-e. paramagnetic imaging
p.-e. paramagnetic NMR

pulsed-gradient

p.-g. spin echo (PGSE)
p.-g. spin-echo echo-planar pulse
sequence
p.-g. spin-echo technique

pulsed-mode operation

pulsed-wave

p.-w. Doppler
p.-w. Doppler echocardiography
p.-w. Doppler recording
p.-w. Doppler ultrasonography
p.-w. spectral color Doppler
signal

pulse-echo

p.-e. distance measurement
p.-e. image

p.-e. imaging
p.-e. method
p.-e. technique

pulse-height

p.-h. analyzer (PHA)
p.-h. spectral analysis

pulse-inversion

p.-i. contrast harmonic imaging
(PICHI)
p.-i. harmonic imaging (PIHI)
p.-i. harmonic ultrasound

PulseMaster laser

6-pulse 3-phase generator

12-pulse 3-phase generator

pulse-spray

P.-S. infusion
P.-S. injector
P.-S. pulsed infusion system
p.-s. technique

Pulse-Spray/PRO infusion catheter

pulsing current

pulsion

p. diverticulum
P. FS laser

Pulsolith

P. laser
P. laser lithotriptor

pulsus

p. alternans
p. paradoxus
p. tardus et parvus

pulverized

p. plaque
p. plaque particulate matter

pulvinar

p. hip joint
p. hyperintensity
p. of thalamus
p. sign
p. sign of vCJD

pump

AutoCAT intraaortic balloon p.
balloon p.
efflux p.
gradient p.
implantable infusion p.
intraaortic balloon p. (IABP)
intraarterial chemotherapy p.
ion p.
p. lung
pulmonary artery balloon p.
pulsed p.

punch

p. biopsy
Sweet sternal p.

punched-out

p.-o. appearance
p.-o. area
p.-o. bony defect

P

punched-out (*continued*)
    p.-o. lytic bone lesion
    p.-o. ulcer
punch-through
puncta (*pl. of* punctum)
punctata
    chondrodysplasia p.
    dysplasia epiphysialis p.
    nonrhizomelic chondrodysplasia
      p.
    rhizomelic chondrodysplasia p.
punctate
    p. calcification
    p. enhancement
    p. hyperintense focus
    p. infiltrate
    p. lesion
    p. necrosis
    p. ulcer
    p. white matter hyperintensity
punctation
PunctSURE vascular access imaging
punctum, *pl.* **puncta**
puncture
    antegrade p.
    cisternal p.
    CT-directed p.
    diagnostic p.
    direct needle p.
    dural p.
    fine-needle p.
    p. fracture
    p. guidance
    lumbar p. (LP)
    maxillary sinus p.
    nephrostomy p.
    p. path
    retrograde nephrostomy p.
    Rickham reservoir p.
    stereotactic p.
    p. transducer
    p. ulcer
    ultrasound-guided nephrostomy
      p.
    p. wound osteomyelitis
pupil
    blown p.
pupillary
    p. constrictor muscle
    p. sign
pupillometer
    Pupilscan II p.
Pupilscan II pupillometer
pure
    p. ground-glass opacity (pGGO)
    p. word alexia
purging
    bone marrow p.
    immunomagnetic p.

purine nucleoside phosphorylase
purinoceptor
    myocyte membrane p.
purity
    radiochemical p.
    radioisotopic p.
    radionuclide p.
    radiopharmaceutical p.
Purkinje fiber
purpose
    low-energy general p. (LEGP)
purpura
    idiopathic thrombocytopenic p.
     (ITP)
pursestringing effect
purulent
    p. lesion
    p. pleurisy
    p. pneumonia
    p. salpingitis
    p. synovitis
pushability
    stent p.
pushable coil
push maneuver
push-pull
    p.-p. ankle stress view
    p.-p. hip view
pustulosis
    palmoplantar p.
pustulotic arthroosteitis
putamen
putaminal hemorrhage
putty kidney
PUV
    positive ulnar variance
    posterior urethral valve (type
     I-IV)
PUVA
    posterior urethrovesical angle
    psoralen and ultraviolet A
      PUVA radiation
      PUVA therapy
PV
    pulmonary valve
PVA
    polyvinyl alcohol
      PVA particle
PVB
    polyvinyl butyral
PVC
    polyvinyl chloride
    premature ventricular contraction
    pulmonary venous congestion
      PVC catheter
PVD
    peripheral vascular disease
PVE
    periventricular echogenicity

PVG
    periventricular gray
        PVG matter
PVH
    pulmonary venous hypertension
PVI
    protracted venous infusion
PVL
    periventricular leukomalacia
PVM
    parallel virtual machine
PVNS
    pigmented villonodular synovitis
PVO
    pulmonary venous obstruction
PVOD
    peripheral vascular occlusive disease
    pulmonary venooclusive disease
PVP
    polyvinylpyrrolidone
    portal venous phase
    portal venous pressure
        PVP image
PVR
    peripheral vascular resistance
    perspective volume rendering
    postvoid residual
    pulmonary vascular resistance
    pulse volume recording
        PVR fly-through viewing
PVRI
    pulmonary vascular resistance index
PVS
    peritoneovenous shunt
PVST
    prevertebral soft tissue
        PVST shadow
PVT
    portal vein thrombosis
PW
    pulse width
PWI
    perfusion-weighted imaging
PWP
    pulmonary wedge pressure
PWS
    Parkes-Weber syndrome
PWT
    posterior wall thickness
PXA
    pleomorphic xanthoastrocytoma
pyarthrosis
pycnodysostosis, pyknodysostosis
pyelectasia (*var. of* pyelectasis)
pyelectasis, pyelectasia
        fetal p.
pyelitis
        p. cystica
        emphysematous p.

pyelocaliceal (*var. of* pyelocalyceal)
pyelocaliectasis (*var. of* caliectasis)
pyelocalyceal, pyelocaliceal
        p. diverticulum
        p. system
pyelofluoroscopy
pyelogenic cyst
pyelogram, pyelouretergram
        dragon p.
        hydrated p.
        infusion p.
        intravenous p. (IVP)
        p. phase
pyelographic appearance time
**pyelography, pelviureteroradiography,
    pyeloureterography, pelviureterography**
        air p.
        antegrade p.
        ascending p.
        p. by elimination
        drip infusion p.
        excretion p.
        excretory intravenous p.
        p. imaging
        infusion p.
        intravenous p. (IVP)
        lateral p.
        needle p.
        percutaneous antegrade p.
        rapid-sequence intravenous
            p.
        respiration p.
        retrograde p.
        washout p.
pyelolymphatic backflow
pyelolysis
pyelonephritis
        acute focal bacterial p.
        acute suppurative p.
        atrophic p.
        chronic atrophic p.
        emphysematous p. (EPN)
        suppurative p.
        xanthogranulomatous p.
pyeloplasty, pelvioplasty
pyelorenal backflow
pyeloscopy
pyelostogram
pyelotomy
        Davis intubated p.
pyelotubular backflow
pyeloureteritis cystica
pyeloureterogram (*var. of* pyelogram)
pyeloureterography (*var. of*
    pyelography)
pyeloureterostomy
pyelovenous backflow
pyemic embolus
pygopagus twin

P

pyknodysostosis (*var. of* pycnodysostosis)
Pyle
    P. disease
    P. dysplasia
pylori (*pl. of* pylorus)
pyloric
    p. antrum
    p. canal
    p. cap
    p. channel
    p. channel length
    p. channel ulcer
    p. diameter
    p. hypertrophy
    p. index
    p. insufficiency
    p. lymph node
    p. muscle
    p. orifice
    p. outlet
    p. outlet obstruction
    p. ring
    p. sphincter
    p. stenosis
    p. stricture
    p. teat
    p. valve
    p. volume
pyloroduodenal
    p. junction
    p. obstruction
pyloroplasty
pylorospasm
    infantile p.
    persistent p.
pylorus, *pl.* **pylori**
    hypertrophic p.
    torus p.
pyocele
pyocephalus
pyoderma granulosa
pyogenetic (*var. of* pyogenic)
pyogenic, pyogenetic, pyogenous
    p. brain abscess
    p. cholangitis
    p. infection
    p. liver
    p. liver abscess
    p. osteomyelitis
    p. pneumonia
    p. spondylodiscitis
pyogenous (*var. of* pyogenic)
pyometra

pyomyositis
pyonephrosis, nephropyosis
pyopneumothorax
pyosalpinx
pyothorax
pyothorax-associated pleural
  lymphoma
pyoureter ectopic ureterocele
PYP
    pyrophosphate
      PYP imaging
      PYP technetium myocardial
        scan
pyramid
    echogenic renal p.
    medullary p.
    p. method for ventricular volume
    petrous p.
    renal medullary p.
pyramidal
    p. bone
    p. eminence
    p. fracture
    p. hemorrhagic zone
    p. layer of cerebral cortex
    p. lobe
    p. neuron
    p. sign
    p. system
    p. tract
pyridine
    ACS-grade p.
pyridone derivative
pyriform (*var. of* piriform)
pyrimidine
    p. analogue
    halogenated p.
pyrogen testing
Pyrolite kit
pyrophosphate (PYP)
    p. arthropathy
    p. crystal
    p. imaging
    ^{99m}Tc p.
    p. scintigraphy
    stannous p.
    technetium 99m p. (^{99m}Tc-PYP,
      Tc99m PYP)
    p. technetium myocardial scan
    technetium stannous p.
    tetrasodium p. (TSPP)
PZ
    peripheral zone

Q
Q angle
Q complex
Q space
QCA
quantitative coronary angiography
quantitative coronary arteriography
Q-catheter catheterization recording system
QCSI
quantitative chemical-shift imaging
QCT
quantitative computed tomography
QCT bone densitometry system
QCT imaging
QCT 3000 system for bone densitometry
QDA
quadratic discriminant analysis
QDE
quantum detection efficiency
QDR-1500, -2000 bone densitometer
QECT
quantitative contrast-enhanced computed tomography
QEEG
quantitative electroencephalography
QGS
quantitative gated SPECT
QHS
quantitative hepatobiliary scintigraphy
QM
quantization matrix
qMRI, QMRI
quantitative magnetic resonance imaging
QO$_2$
oxygen consumption
QPD
quadrature phase detector
QR
quadriradial
QR pattern
QRS
electrocardiographic wave
QRS interval
QRS score
QRS synchronized shock
QRS vector
QRS-T
electrocardiographic angle between QRS and T vectors
QRS-T angle

Q-switched
Q-s. Nd:YAG laser
Q s. ruby laser
Q-switching
QuaDDS-QP2 stent
QuaDDS stent
Quad 7000, 12000 high-field open MRI scanner
quadrangle cartilage
quadrangulation of Frouin
quadrant
q. energy
left lower q. (LLQ)
left upper q. (LUQ)
lower inner q. (LIQ)
lower outer q. (LOQ)
lower right q. (LRQ)
q. of death
outer upper right q. (OURQ)
right lower q. (RLQ)
right upper q. (RUQ)
upper inner q. (UIQ)
upper left q. (ULQ)
upper outer q. (UOQ)
upper right q. (URQ)
quadrantal
4-quadrant bar pattern
quadrate
q. gyrus
q. ligament
q. lobe of liver
q. muscle
quadratic
q. dependence
q. discriminant analysis (QDA)
q. phase gain
quadrature
q. adult head coil
q. body coil
q. cervical spine coil
q. detection
q. excitation
q. phase detector (QPD)
q. phase detector artifact
q. radiofrequency receiver coil
q. setting
q. surface coil MRI system
q. terminal latency surface coil
q. transmit-receive head coil
quadratus
q. femoris
q. femoris fascia
q. lumborum
q. plantae
pronator q.

quad-resonance NMR probe circuit
quadriceps, *pl.* **quadriceps, quadricepses**
    q. apron
    q. femoris
    q. femoris tendon reflex test
    q. muscle
    q. tendon
    q. tendon tear
quadricepses (*pl. of* quadriceps)
quadricuspid
    q. aortic valve
    q. pulmonary valve
quadrigeminal
    q. plate
    q. plate cistern
    q. segment of posterior cerebral
     artery
    q. vein
quadrigeminy
quadrilateral
    q. bone
    q. brim
    q. plate
    q. retinoblastoma
    q. space syndrome
quadrilocular
quadripartite
quadriplegia
quadriplegic
quadripolar
    q. nucleus
    q. signal broadening
quadripole
quadriradial (QR)
quadrisect
quadrisection
quadritubercular
quadruped fracture
quadruple-phase helical computed
  tomography
quadrupole moment
QuaDS drug-eluting stent
quadsegmental image reconstruction
Quain fatty degeneration of heart
qualitative
    q. analysis
    q. assessment
    q. index
    q. study
quality
    q. factor
    image q.
quanta (*pl. of* quantum)
quantification
    acoustic q.
    automated q.
    flow q.
    rapid fluid q.
    shunt q.

quantimeter
quantitation
    absolute function q.
quantitative
    q. amnionic fluid volume
    q. analysis
    q. brain imaging
    q. cardiac perfusion
    q. chemical-shift imaging (QCSI)
    q. computed tomography (QCT)
    q. contrast-enhanced computed
     tomography (QECT)
    q. coronary angiography (QCA)
    q. coronary arteriography (QCA)
    q. CT densitometry
    q. CT during expiration
    q. diffusion measurement
    q. digital radiography
    q. Doppler assessment
    q. electroencephalography
     (QEEG)
    q. exercise thallium-201 variable
    q. fluorescence imaging
    q. gated SPECT (QGS)
    q. hepatobiliary scintigraphy
     (QHS)
    q. image processing system
     (QUIPS)
    q. imaging of perfusion using
     single subtraction
    q. imaging technique
    q. index
    q. Levovist myocardial contrast
     echocardiography
    q. lung perfusion imaging
    q. magnetic resonance imaging
     (qMRI, QMRI)
    q. magnetization transfer
    q. multilevel mapping
    q. proton MR of neonatal brain
    q. regional lung function study
    q. regional myocardial flow
     measurement
    q. scan
    q. spirometrically controlled CT
    q. spirometrically controlled CT
     imaging
    q. track etch autoradiography
    q. trait locus
    q. ultrasound (QUS)
quantity
    spectrophotometric q.
quantization
    q. error
    q. matrix (QM)
    q. matrix scaling
    sequential scalar q. (SSQ)
    vector q.
    wavelet scalar q. (WSQ)

quantum, *pl.* **quanta**
    q. detection efficiency (QDE)
    q. dot
    q. energy
    q. limit
    q. Monorail balloon catheter
    q. mottle
    q. mottle index
    q. mottling pattern
    q. noise
    noise equivalent q.
    q. number
    q. sink
    q. theory
    q. unit
Quant-X color quantification imaging tool
quarter-detector offset
3-quarter prone position
quarti
    apertura lateralis ventriculi q.
    apertura mediana ventriculi q.
    striae medullares ventriculi q.
quartisect
quartz
    q. glass
    q. lamp
quasiaccelerated fractionation
quasielastic laser light-scattering spectroscope
quasiradiographic image
Queckenstedt sign
quellung reaction
Quénu-Muret sign
questionable lesion
QueST stent

quick
    Q. CT9800 scanner
    Q. Spin Sephadex G-50 column
Quick-Core
    Q.-C. biopsy needle
    Q.-C. biopsy system
QuickSeal femoral arterial closure system
quiescence
Quik-Prep
    Quinton Q.-P.
Quimby implant system
Quimby classification of pelvic fracture
Quincke
    Q. sign
    Q. spinal needle
Quintero umbilical artery blood flow (stage 1-4)
quinti
    abductor digiti q. (ADQ)
    extensor digiti q. (EDQ)
    opponens digiti q. (ODQ)
Quinton
    Q. PermCath
    Q. Quik-Prep
QUIPS
    quantitative image processing system
Quotane
quotient
    amnionic head q. (AHQ)
    Rayleigh q.
QUS
    quantitative ultrasound
QUS-2 calcaneal ultrasonometer
Q-wave myocardial infarct
QX/I CT scanner

Q

R
>asplenia syndrome R

RA
>rotational angiography
>Integris 3D RA

Ra
>radium

^{226}Ra, Ra-226
>radium 226
>^{226}Ra needle

RAA
>right atrial appendage

RAB
>remote afterloading brachytherapy

rabbit ear strand

racemose
>r. aneurysm
>r. cyst
>r. cysticercosis

racemosum
>angioma venosum r.

racetrack microtron accelerator

rachioscoliosis

rachischisis of atlas

rachitic
>r. pelvis
>r. rosary

rad
>radiation absorbed dose

RAD
>reactive airway disease
>right axis deviation

radarkymography

radiability

radiable

radiad

radial
>r. anular tear
>r. aplasia
>r. artery to cephalic vein
>fistula
>r. blurring
>r. bone
>r. breast scar
>r. bursa
>r. collateral ligament
>r. deviation
>r. digital artery
>r. drift
>r. epiphysial displacement
>r. facing of metacarpal head
>r. fossa
>r. glial fiber
>r. head
>r. head fracture

>r. head subluxation
>r. height
>r. inclination
>r. length
>r. metacarpal ligament
>r. neck fracture
>r. neck groove
>r. plane
>r. pulse
>r. ray anomaly
>r. ray defect
>r. resistive force
>r. ridge
>r. scar
>r. scarlike mammographic
>appearance
>r. sclerosing lesion
>r. shift
>r. sigmoid notch
>r. split tear
>r. styloid fracture
>r. styloid process
>r. technique
>r. tuberosity
>r. vascular thermal injury
>r. width

radialis
>flexor carpi r. (FCR)
>r. sign

radialized

radian

radiant
>r. energy
>r. intensity

radiata
>corona r.

radiate sternocostal ligament

radiation
>r. absorbed dose (rad)
>adjuvant r.
>afterloading r.
>alpha r.
>r. anemia
>annihilation r.
>r. arteritis
>background r.
>backscattered r.
>r. barrier
>r. beam
>r. beam monitor
>beta r.
>r. biology
>bone injury r.
>braking r.
>bremsstrahlung r.

radiation (*continued*)
 r. burden
 r. burn
 r. carcinogenesis
 r. caries
 r. cataract
 Cerenkov r.
 characteristic r.
 r. chemistry
 r. chimera
 r. colitis
 corpuscular r.
 cosmic r.
 r. counter
 cyclotron r.
 r. cystitis
 r. delivery technology (RDX)
 r. dermatosis
 r. detector
 diagnostic r.
 direct r.
 dose equivalent r.
 R. Dose in Interventional Radiology (RAD-IR)
 r. dose perturbation
 r. dosimetry
 r. dosimetry calculation
 r. dosimetry of ^{18}F-fluorocholine
 r. effect
 r. effect unit
 electromagnetic r.
 r. energy
 r. enhancement
 r. enteritis
 r. enteropathy
 r. erythema
 r. esophagitis
 r. exposure
 external beam r.
 fatal dose of r.
 r. fistula
 fractionated r.
 gamma r.
 r. gastritis
 r. hepatitis
 heterogeneous r.
 high linear energy transfer r.
 homogeneous r.
 r. hormesis
 Huldshinsky r.
 hyperfractionated r.
 hypofractionated r.
 hysterectomy and r. (H&R)
 infrared r.
 r. injury
 r. intensity
 r. interrogation
 interstitial r.
 intracoronary artery r.

ionization r.
ionizing r.
K r.
r. leakage
r. leukoencephalitis
manmade environmental r.
Maxwell theory of r.
megavoltage r.
monochromatic synchrotron r.
monoenergetic r.
r. myelitis
r. myelopathy
natural r.
r. necrosis
r. nephritis
r. nephropathy
neutron r.
nonionizing r.
occupational nuclear r.
r. of Gratiolet
r. oncogenesis
r. oncologist
r. oncology
optic r.
r. osteitis
r. osteonecrosis
photon theory of r.
r. physics
r. pneumonia
r. pneumonitis
r. poisoning
polychromatic r.
r. port
r. portal
prenatal r.
primary r.
r. proctopathy
r. protection
protracted r.
PUVA r.
radiofrequency r.
recoil r.
rectum r.
remnant r.
r. response (RR)
r. risk
Rollier r.
scatter r.
scattered r.
secondary r.
r. seed
r. sensitivity testing
r. sensitizer
r. sickness
solar r.
specific r.
spontaneous r.
r. stenosis
stray r.

superficial r.
supervoltage r.
synchrotron r.
r. syndrome
r. synovectomy
terrestrial r.
therapeutic external r.
r. therapy (RT)
r. therapy planning (RTP)
r. therapy planning system
r. therapy sequela
r. therapy system (RTS)
thermal r.
thorny bone r.
tissue tolerance to r.
r. tolerance dose
total lymphoid r.
r. treatment planning (RTP)
ultraviolet r.
useful beam r.
r. vasculopathy
r. warning symbol
r. weighting factor
white r.
whole-body r. (WBR)
r. window
radiation-associated papillary tumor
radiation-attenuating surgical glove
radiation-equivalent-man (REM)
radiation-free imaging modality
radiation-induced
r.-i. cancer
r.-i. carcinoma
r.-i. cerebral atrophy
r.-i. cerebral necrosis
r.-i. change
r.-i. colitis
r.-i. fibrosis (RIF)
r.-i. infarct
r.-i. ischemia
r.-i. leukoencephalopathy
r.-i. leukomalacia
r.-i. liver disease (RILD)
r.-i. necrosis (RIN)
r.-i. neoplasm
r.-i. pericarditis
r.-i. peripheral nerve tumor
r.-i. pulmonary toxicity
r.-i. sarcoma
r.-i. sclerosing adenosis
r.-i. skin injury
r.-i. ulcer
r.-i. upregulation
r.-i. vasculopathy
radiation-related
r.-r. ischemia
r.-r. ischemic change
r.-r. optic neuropathy (RON)
radiation-treated astrocytoma

radical
biliary r.
free r.
heterocyclic free r.
r. irradiation
leucine r.
nitroxide-stable free r.
organic free r.
r. parametrectomy
r. perineal prostatectomy
stable free r.
r. vulvectomy
radices (*pl. of* radix)
radiciform
radicular
r. artery
r. compression
r. cyst
r. vessel
radiculomedullary artery
radiculomeningeal fistula
radiculomyelitis
radiculopathy
cervical spondylotic r.
radiculospinal artery
radiferous
Radifocus
R. Glidecath
R. Glidewire
R. hydrophilic coated guidewire
radii (*pl. of* radius)
Radinyl
radioactive
r. accumulation
r. aerosol
r. atom
r. bolus
r. brain scan
r. cancer-specific targeting agent
r. cobalt
r. colloid
r. constant
^{11}C palmitic acid r.
r. cyanocobalamin
r. decay
r. disintegration
r. effluent
r. element
r. emission
r. equilibrium
r. fallout
r. fibrinogen imaging
r. fibrinogen scan
r. gallium
r. gas
r. half-life
r. iodide conversion ratio
r. iodinated serum albumin (RISA)
r. iodinated serum albumin scan

radioactive (*continued*)
  r. iodine
  r. iodine ablation
  r. iodine scan
  r. iodine uptake (RAIU)
  r. iron
  r. isotope
  r. isotope imaging agent
  r. label
  r. labeling
  r. lead
  r. material
  r. metal
  r. nuclide
  r. phosphorus
  r. radon
  r. renogram test
  r. seeding
  r. series
  r. sodium
  r. source
  r. stent
  r. string marker
  r. strontium
  r. sulfur
  r. tag
  r. thorium
  r. thyroxine
  r. tracer
  r. water
  r. xenon clearance
  r. xenon gas inhalation
radioactively tagged
radioactivity
  artificial r.
  r. detection
  r. distribution
  induced r.
  mottled r.
  natural r.
  r. per volume
  unit of r.
radioactor
radioaerosol
  r. clearance
  r. imaging study
radioanaphylaxis
radioassay
radioautogram
radioautograph
radioautography
radiobioassay
radiobiologic, radiobiological
radiobiological (*var. of* radiobiologic)
radiobiologist
radiobiology
radiocalcium
radiocapitellar
  r. articulation

  r. joint
  r. joint ganglion
  r. line
radiocarbon
radiocarcinogenesis
radiocardiogram
radiocardiography
radiocarpal
  r. angle
  r. articulation
  r. compartment
  r. dislocation
  r. joint
  r. ligament
  r. portal
radioccipital
radiocephalic
radiocephalpelvimetry
radiocesium
radiochemical
  r. purity
  r. study
radiochemistry
radiochemotherapy
radiochlorine
radiocholangiography
radiocholecystography
radiocholesterol scanning
radiochromatography
radiochromic
  r. dosimetry medium
  r. film
radiocineangiocardiography
radiocineangiography
radiocinematograph
radiocinematography
radiocobalt
radiocolloid
  r. lymphoscintigraphy
  r. mapping
radiocontaminant
radiocontrast
radiocontrast-associated
radiocontrast-induced
  r.-i. injury
  r.-i. nephropathy
radiocurability
radiocurable
radiodense lesion
radiodensity area
radiodermatitis
radiodermatography
radiodiagnosis
radiodiagnostics
radiodiaphane
radiodigital
radioelectrocardiogram
radioelectrocardiograph
radioelectrocardiography

radioelement
    r. solution
    surface application of
        r.
radioencephalogram
radioencephalography
radioenzyme
radioepidermitis
radioepithelitis
radiofibrinogen uptake scan
radiofluorinated
radiofluorine
radiofrequency (RF)
    r. ablation (RFA)
    r. ablation therapy
    r. absorption
    r. balloon
    r. catheter ablation (RFCA)
    r. electromagnetic field
    r. energy
    r. excitation pulse
    r. gangliolysis
    gaussian r.
    r. generator
    r. hyperthermia
    r. lesion
    r. magnetic shield
    r. modification transcatheter
    r. overflow artifact
    r. percutaneous myocardial
      revascularization (RF-PMR)
    r. period
    r. pulse
    r. radiation
    r. radiogenic leukopenia
    r. radiogold
    r. radiographic control
    r. radiographic hallmark
    r. saturation band
    r. screen
    sinc-Hanning r.
    r. spatial distribution problem
      reconstruction artifact
    r. spin echo
    r. spoiling
    r. subsystem
    r. thermal ablation
    r. tongue base reduction
    r. transmitter-receiver
      coil
    r. wave
radiofrequency-spoiled
    r.-s. 3D GRE sequence
    r.-s. Fourier-acquired steady-state
      technique (RF-FAST)
radiogallium
radiogenesis
radiogenic leukopenia
radiogenics

radiogold
    r. colloid
    radiofrequency r.
radiogram
radiogrammetry
radiograph, skiagraph, skiagram,
  roentgenogram, roentgenograph
    axial r.
    biplane r.
    bitewing r.
    cephalometric r.
    Code and Carlson r.
    coned-down r.
    contact r.
    control r.
    conventional r.
    decubitus r.
    digital abdominal r.
    digital chest r.
    digitally reconstructed r. (DRR)
    double-contrast r.
    dual-energy r. (DER)
    erect lateral flexion-extension
      r.
    extraoral r.
    frontal cephalometric r.
    internal oblique r.
    intraoperative r.
    intraoral r.
    lateral cephalometric r.
    lateral decubitus r.
    lateral flexion-extension r.
    lateral oblique jaw r.
    lateral ramus r.
    lateral skull r.
    maxillary sinus r.
    mortise r.
    oblique r.
    oblique lateral jaw r.
    occlusal r.
    orthogonal r.
    outlet view r.
    panoramic r.
    periapical r.
    phantom r.
    plain r.
    scout digital r.
    soft tissue r.
    spot r.
    stress r.
    submental vertex r.
    supine r.
    survey r.
    tangent r.
    Towne projection r.
    transcranial r.
    Trendelenburg r.
    tunnel r.
    Waters view r.

radiographer
radiographic, roentgenographic
    r. and fluoroscopic
    r. baseline
    r. blurring
    r. cephalometry
    r. change
    r. contrast
    r. contrast medium-induced
      nephropathy
    r. control
    r. criterion
    r. density
    r. diagnosis
    r. distention
    r. effect
    r. finding
    r. image
    r. interpretation
    r. mottle
    r. noise
    r. parallel line shadow
    r. pathology
    r. pelvimetry
    r. penetration
    r. pincushion distortion
    r. projection
    r. silhouette
    r. spiculation
    r. stability of lesion
radiographically, roentgenographically
    r. firm synostosis
    r. normal imaging
    r. occult
    r. occult fracture
radiographic-dense breast
radiography, skiagraphy, roentgenography
    abdominal r.
    advanced multiple-beam equalization
      r. (AMBER)
    air-gap r.
    anatomic programmed r. (APR)
    r. and fluoroscopy (R&F)
    barium r.
    bedside r.
    biomedical r.
    body section r.
    cardiac r.
    cassette-based screen-film r.
    computed r.
    computed dental r. (CDR)
    computerized r.
    contrast r.
    dental r.
    diagrammatic r.
    digital video gastrointestinal r.
    direct digital r. (DDR)
    double-contrast r.
    electron r.

    filmless r.
    film-screen r.
    flexion-extension r.
    fluoroscopic programmed r. (FPR)
    gamma r.
    high-resolution low-speed r.
    horizontal beam r.
    interventional r.
    intraoperative r.
    intraoral periapical r.
    magnification r.
    mobile r.
    moving slot r.
    mucosal relief r.
    musculoskeletal r.
    neonatal r.
    neutron r.
    panoral r.
    panoramic r.
    photostimulable phosphor computed r.
    photostimulable phosphor dental r.
    plain abdominal r. (PAR)
    portable r.
    postrelease r.
    postvoid r.
    quantitative digital r.
    rapid serial r.
    scanned projection r. (SPR)
    scanning equalization r.
    sectional r.
    selective r.
    selenium r.
    serial r.
    slit r.
    soft-copy computed r.
    specimen r.
    spot film r.
    stereoscopic r.
    storage phosphor r.
    stress r.
    traction r.
    video digital gastrointestinal r.
radioguided
    r. laparotomy
    r. parathyroidectomy
    r. surgery
radiohepatographic
radiohumeral
    r. articulation
    r. bursitis
    r. meniscus
radioimmunity
radioimmunoassay (RIA)
    r. method
    scintillation proximity r.
radioimmunoconjugate
radioimmunodetection (RAID)
radioimmunodiffusion
radioimmunoguided surgery (RIGS)

radioimmunoimaging
radioimmunolocalization
radioimmunoluminography
radioimmunoprecipitation test
radioimmunoscintigraphy
radioimmunosorbent
radioimmunotherapy
radioinduced sarcoma
radioinduction
radioiodide
radioiodinated
    r. metaiodobenzylguanidine
    r. serum albumin (RISA)
radioiodination
    direct r.
    electrophilic r.
radioiodine
    r. ablation therapy
    organified r.
    r. test
    r. therapy
    r. uptake
radioiron
    r. oral absorption
    r. red cell utilization
radioisotope
    r. calibrator
    r. camera
    carrier-free r.
    cistern r.
    r. cisternography
    r. cisternography imaging
    r. delivery system (RDS)
    r. gallium imaging
    Gd-DTPA r.
    r. indium-labeled white blood cell
      imaging
    r. labeling
    r. lung scan
    r. renogram test
    r. scanner
    r. scintigraphy
    r. stent
    r. synovectomy
    r. technetium imaging
    r. thyroid scanning
    transplutonium r.
    trapping of r.
    r. uptake
    r. voiding cystogram
radioisotope-labeled tracer
radioisotopic purity
radioisotrope ventriculography study
radiolabel
radiolabeled
    r. antibody
    r. antibody imaging
    r. anti-CEA
    r. antisense oligonucleotide

    r. compound
    r. estrogen analogue
    r. fibrinogen
    r. leukocyte
    r. marker substrate
    r. MoAb
    r. MoAb imaging agent
    r. peptide alpha-M2
    r. platelet
    r. thyroxine
    r. tracer
    r. water study
    r. WBC
radiolabeling
    area of increased r.
radiolead
radiolesion
radioligand
    PET r.
radiologic, radiological, roentgenological
    r. anatomy
    r. contrast medium
    r. diagnosis
    r. distortion
    r. guidance
    r. percutaneous gastrostomy (RPG)
    r. sphincter
    r. stigma
    r. technologist
    r. technology
    r. unit
radiological (*var. of* radiologic)
    R. Society of North America
      (RSNA)
radiologic-anatomic correlation
radiologic-histopathologic study
radiologic-pathologic
    r.-p. concordance
    r.-p. correlation
    r.-p. discordance
radiologist, roentgenologist
radiology, roentgenology
    American Board of R.
    American College of R. (ACR)
    British Institute of R. (BIR)
    cardiovascular r.
    chest r.
    computed r.
    dental r.
    diagnostic r.
    r. information system (RIS)
    interventional r.
    intraoral r.
    MSK r.
    neurointerventional r.
    oral r.
    r. outcomes data
    pediatric r.
    percutaneous interventional r.

radiology (*continued*)
    polytomographic r.
    Radiation Dose in Interventional R.
      (RAD-IR)
    radionuclide r.
    skeletal r.
    Society for Computer Applications
      in R. (SCAR)
    Society of Interventional R.
    storage phosphor r.
    r. telephone access system
    therapeutic r.
radiolucency
    linear band of maximal r.
    prominent rim of r.
    relative r.
    soap-bubble r.
radiolucent
    r. area
    r. cleft
    r. crescent line
    r. density
    r. fat
    r. fat halo
    r. focus
    r. gallstone
    r. joint space
    r. lesion
    r. linear filling defect
    r. medium
    r. operating room table extension
    r. plastic occluder
    r. pneumomediastinum
    r. roll
    r. spine frame
    r. stone
radiolunate articulation
radiolunotriquetral ligament
radiolymphoscintigraphy
    intraoperative r.
radiolysis
radiomedullary artery
radiometallography
radiometer, roentgenometer
    pastil r.
    photographic r.
radiometric
    r. analysis
    r. assay
radiometry, roentgenometry
radiomicrometer
radiomimetic
radiomuscular
radiomutation
radion
radionecrosis
    cerebral r.
radioneuritis
Radionics CRW stereotactic head frame

radionitrogen
radionuclear venography
radionucleotide
    positron-emitting r.
radionuclide
    absorption of r.
    r. angiocardiography
    r. angiogram (RNA)
    r. angiography
    r. blood flow study
    r. bone scan
    r. bone scintigraphy
    r. camera
    r. cardiac perfusion study
    r. cardiography
    r. carrier
    carrier-added r.
    carrier-free r.
    r. carrier system
    r. cerebral angiogram
    r. cerebrospinal fluid study
    r. cholescintigraphy
    r. cineangiography
    r. cisternography
    concentration of r.
    r. contamination
    r. cystogram
    r. cystography
    r. ejection fraction
    r. emission tomography
    r. esophageal dead time
    r. esophagram
    r. flow scan
    r. gastrointestinal bleeding study
    r. gated blood pool imaging
    r. gated blood pool scan
    r. generator
    gold-195m r.
    r. inflammation
    inhaled r.
    r. injection
    r. label
    r. liver scan
    lung perfusion r.
    r. mammography
    metastable r.
    r. milk imaging
    r. milk scan
    no-carrier-added r.
    parent r.
    r. production
    r. purity
    r. radiology
    renal r.
    r. renal imaging
    r. renography imaging
    r. scanning
    r. shuntogram
    r. signal

r. stenosis
r. stroke volume
r. synovectomy
r. table
r. tagged red blood cell bleeding scan
r. testicular scintigraphy
r. therapy
r. thyroid imaging
r. thyroid scan
uptake of r.
r. venography
ventilation r.
r. ventriculogram (RNV, RNVG, RVG)
r. ventriculography (RNV, RNVG, RVG)
r. voiding cystourethrography
r. voiding study
radiopacity
linear r.
radiopaque
r. bone cement
r. contrast medium (ROCM)
r. density
r. distal tip
r. drain
r. fluid extravasation
r. foreign body
r. gold marker
r. imaging agent
r. lesion
r. mass
r. pellet
r. pseudocapsule
r. urine
r. vesical calculus
r. wire of counteroccluder buttonhole
r. xenon gas
radioparency
radioparent
radiopathology
radiopelvimetry
radiopharmaceutical
r. ablation
r. agent
brain imaging r.
r. chemistry
r. dacryocystography
diagnostic r.
r. dose
r. dosimetry
r. localization
^{99m}Tc-ECD r.
^{99m}Tc-HMPAO r.
^{99m}Tc-iminodiacetic acid derivative r.
^{99m}Tc-MAG3 r.
99mTc MIBI r.

^{99m}Tc polyphosphate compound r.
PET r.
r. production
r. purity
r. quality control
r. synovectomy
technetium 99m isonitrile r.
r. therapy
trace amount of r.
r. tracer
r. uptake
r. voiding cystogram
r. volume-dilution technique
radiopharmacy
radiophobia
radiophosphate
radiophosphorus
radiophotography
radiophylaxis
radiopotassium
radiopotentiation
radioprotectant
radioprotective agent
radioprotector
radiopulmonography
radioreaction
radioreceptor
radioresistance
radioresistant
radioresponsiveness
radioscaphocapitate ligament
radioscaphoid
r. articulation
r. joint
r. ligament
radioscapholunate ligament
radioscintigraphy
radioscopy
radiosensibility
radiosensitive tumor
radiosensitivity
fibroblast r.
radiosensitization
radiosensitizer
carbogen r.
halogenated thymidine analogue r.
nicotinamide r.
radiosodium
radiospirometry
radiostereoscopy
radiostrontium
radiosulfur
radiosurgery
Bragg peak r.
charged-particle r.
dynamic stereotactic r.
Gamma Knife-stereotactic r. (GK-SRS)
heavy charged-particle Bragg peak r.

radiosurgery (*continued*)
    image-guided r.
    interstitial r.
    LINAC r.
    modified linear accelerator r.
    multiarc LINAC r.
    stereotactic r. (SRS)
    Winston-Lutz for LINAC-based r.
radiotellurium
radiotherapeutic agent
radiotherapeutics
radiotherapist
radiotherapy (RT), roentgenotherapy
    arc r.
    AVM r.
    computer-controlled r.
    computerized r.
    contact r.
    continuous hyperfractionated
      accelerated r.
    3-dimensional conformal r.
    3-dimensional conformation r.
    dynamic r.
    electron beam intraoperative r.
      (EBIORT)
    extended-field r.
    external beam r.
    fast neutron r.
    r. field placement
    fractionated stereotactic r. (FSR)
    fused imaging-guided r. (FIGURA)
    hemibody r.
    high-dose r.
    high-voltage r.
    hyperfractionated r.
    iceberg r.
    intensity-modulated r.
    interstitial r.
    intracavitary r.
    intraoperative r.
    intraoral r.
    intravaginal r.
    inverted-Y field r.
    large-field r.
    r. localization
    locoregional field r.
    mantle r.
    megavoltage r.
    neoadjuvant r.
    orthovoltage r.
    r. photopenia
    r. port
    r. portal
    postoperative r. (PORT)
    preoperative r.
    rotational r.
    salvage r.
    short-distance r.
    skeletal targeted r. (STR)

    split-course accelerated r.
    stereotactic r.
    supervoltage r.
    teletherapy r.
    whole-body r.
    whole-brain r. (WBRT)
    r. with hyperthermia
    r. without hyperthermia
radiothermy
radiothorium
radiothyroidectomy
radiothyroxin
radiotomy
radiotoxemia
radiotoxicity
radiotracer
    r. accumulation
    r. activity
    decreased uptake of r.
    r. deposition
    r. foil method
    increased uptake of r.
    ^{99m}Tc-HMPAO r.
    r. technique
    r. uptake
radiotransparency
radiotransparent
radiotropic
radioulnar
    r. articulation
    r. joint
    r. proximodistal translation
    r. subluxation
    r. surface
radioulnaris
    syndesmosis r.
RAD-IR
    Radiation Dose in Interventional
    Radiology
    RAD-IR study
radium (Ra)
    r. 226 (^{226}Ra, Ra-226)
    r. beam therapy
    r. emanation
    intracavitary r.
    r. necrosis
    r. radioactive source
radius, *pl.* **radii,** *gen.* **radii**
    Bohr r.
    capitulum radii
    r. hypoplasia
    r. of curvature
    sigmoid cavity of r.
    thrombocytopenia-absent r. (TAR)
radix, *pl.* **radices**
RadNet radiology information system
radon (Rn)
    r. 222 (^{222}Rn, Rn-222)
    r. progeny

radioactive r.
   r. seed implantation
RadPICC catheter
RadStat hemostasis device
RADstation radiology workstation
radwaste radioactivity detection
RAE
   right atrial enlargement
Raeder paratrigeminal syndrome
Rael cell
RAGE
   rapid gradient echo
ragged urethra
ragpicker's disease
RAID
   radioimmunodetection
Raider triangle
railroad
   r. track appearance
   r. track calcification
   r. track ductus arteriosus
   r. track pattern
   r. track sign
railway spine
raiser
   stress r.
RAIU
   radioactive iodine uptake
rake ulcer
RAM
   random access memory
   reduced-acquisition matrix
Raman spectroscopy
rami (*pl. of* ramus)
ramification
ramify
ramp
   r. down
   r. filter
   folded step r.
   maximum slew rate r.
   r. reconstruction
   r. time
   r. up
ramp-filtered back projection
ramping
Ramsay
   R. Hunt cerebellar myoclonic
     dyssynergia
   R. Hunt syndrome
ramus, *pl.* **rami**
   dorsal primary r.
   inferior pubic r.
   r. intermedius artery
   r. intermedius artery branch
   ischiopubic r.
   mandibular r.
   r. medialis artery
   r. medialis artery branch

   r. of ischium
   r. of lateral sulcus
   pubic r.
   superior pubic r.
   ventral primary r.
Ranawat method
Randall plaque
Rand microballoon
random
   r. access memory (RAM)
   r. coincidence event
   r. count
   r. error
   r. motion
   r. point
randomized clinical trial (RCT)
Ranfac cholangiographic catheter
range
   absorbed dose r.
   r. ambiguity artifact
   dynamic r.
   emission r.
   frequency r.
   gray-scale r.
   normal r.
   positron r.
   reference r.
   r. resolution
   slew r.
   therapeutic r.
   water r.
range-gated
   r.-g. Doppler spectral flow analysis
   r.-g. pulsed Doppler
ranging
   echo r.
ranine vein
rank
   Spearman r.
Ranke
   R. angle
   R. complex
ranula
Ranvier
   R. groove
   R. node
RAO
   right anterior oblique
RAP
   right atrial pressure
Rapamune
rapamycin
raphe, rhaphe
   abdominal r.
   amnionic r.
   anococcygeal r.
   anogenital r.
   longitudinal r.
   median r.

raphe (*continued*)
palpebral r.
penile r.
posterior fossa malformations, facial hemangiomas, arterial anomalies, cardiac anomalies and aortic coarctation, eye anomalies, and sternal clefting and/or supraumbilical r. (PHACES)
pterygomandibular r.
scrotal r.
tendinous r.
unicuspid with central r.
RAPI
resting ankle pressure index
rapid
r. acquisition with relaxation enhancement (RARE)
r. axial MR imaging
r. biplane angiocardiography
r. deceleration injury
r. dephasing
r. dissolution formula
r. distribution
r. early repolarization phase
r. exchange (RX)
r. filling
r. filling period
r. filling wave (RFW)
r. film changer
r. fluid expansion
r. fluid quantification
r. gantry rotation
r. gastric emptying
r. gradient echo (RAGE)
r. gradient reversal
r. half-Fourier T2-weighted image
r. image transfer
r. inspiratory flow rate
r. oscillatory motion
r. pull-through technique (RPT)
r. scan technique
r. screen
r. sequential CT scan
r. serial radiography
r. telephone access system (RTAS)
r. thoracic compression technique
r. tracer washout
R. Transit catheter
R. Transit microcatheter
r. ventricular filling phase
r. ventricular rate
r. ventricular response
rapid-acquisition
r.-a. computed tomography
r.-a. spin echo (RASE)
r.-a. with gradient echo
rapid-excitation MR imaging
rapid-heating ablation procedure

Rapid-Scan spectrometer
RapidScreen
R. RS-2000 CAD
R. RS-2000 x-ray equipment
rapid-sequence
r.-s. imaging
r.-s. intravenous pyelography
r.-s. IVP
Rappaport classification
RAR
renal-aortic ratio
retinoic acid receptor
RARE
rapid acquisition with relaxation enhancement
RARE sequence
single-shot thick-slab RARE
RARE technique
RARE-derived pulse sequence
rare-earth
r.-e. scintillator
r.-e. screen
rarefaction
bony r.
fluffy r.
r. of cortex
osseous r.
rarefied area
RAS
renal artery stenosis
RASE
rapid-acquisition spin echo
rash
heliotropic periorbital r.
Rashkind
R. double umbrella device
R. occluder
Rasmussen
R. encephalitis
R. mycotic aneurysm
raster
r. frequency
r. line
r. period
r. spacing error
r. stereo photography
rat-bite erosion
ratchet
rate
ACR r.
r. analysis
atrial r.
count r.
digital sampling r.
dipole-dipole relaxation r.
disintegration r.
dose r.
exogenous glucose r.
flow r.

gastric emptying r.
glomerular filtration r. (GFR)
gradient slew r.
high dose r. (HDR)
high frame r.
inspiratory flow r.
instantaneous enhancement r.
intraoperative high dose r. (IOHDR)
lipid fraction relaxation r.
low frame r.
LVOT flow r.
magnet r.
maximum midexpiratory flow r. (MMFR)
maximum predicted heart r. (MPHR)
mean circumferential fiber shortening
  r. (MCFSR)
r. meter
oscillatory shear r.
oxygen extraction r. (OER, O$_2$ER)
patency r.
peak ejection r. (PER)
peak filling r. (PFR)
plasma radioiron disappearance r.
plasma radioiron turnover r.
predicted target heart r.
proliferation r.
pulsed dose r. (PDR)
rapid inspiratory flow r.
rapid ventricular r.
relaxation r.
shear-strain r.
Solomon-Bloembergen theory of
  dipole-dipole relaxation r.
specific absorption r. (SAR)
spirometer flow r.
standby r.
stone-free r.
stroke ejection r.
ST-segment/heart r.
time to peak filling r. (TPFR)
transverse relaxation r.
ultralow-dose r. (ULDR)
valley-to-peak dose r.
variable response r.
ventricular r.

Rathke
R. cleft cyst
R. duct
R. pouch
R. pouch tumor

rating
clinical dementia r.

ratio
adenoidal-nasopharyngeal r.
adrenal-spleen r. (ASR)
ankle-brachial pressure r.
aortic root r.
aortic valve opening to aortic valve
  closing r. (AO/AC)

apnea-bradycardia r.
artery-aortic velocity r.
artery-bronchus r. (ABR)
bicaudate r.
blank-to-trues r.
blood-to-fat contrast r.
blood-to-myocardium contrast r.
bone age r.
bone and limb growth velocity r.
brain Glx-Cr r.
brain-to-background r.
branching r.
bronchus-to-pulmonary artery r.
cardiothoracic r. (CTR)
carpal content r.
carpal height r.
cerebral blood volume to cerebral
  blood flow r. (CBV/CBF)
chemical-shift r.
compression r.
conduction r.
contrast-to-noise r. (C/N, CNR)
conversion r.
cord-subarachnoid space r.
CT r.
diaphysial bone length r.
diastolic velocity r.
differential uptake r.
distention r.
distribution volume r. (DVR)
dome-to-neck r.
dose nonuniformity r. (DNR)
E-A wave r.
end-systolic wall index to
  end-systolic volume r.
escape-peak r.
ESP-ESV r.
Evans r.
false-negative r.
false-positive r.
flattening r.
Grace method of metatarsal length
  r.
gray-to-white matter activity r.
gray-to-white matter contrast r.
gray-to-white matter utilization r.
grid r.
gyromagnetic r.
HC/AC r.
heart count-mediastinum count r.
  (H/M)
heart-lung r. (HLR)
heart-to-background r.
heart-to-lung r. (HLR)
hilar height r.
Holdaway r.
inferoanterior count r.
infundibular systolic-diastolic r.
infundibulum-bulb r.

ratio (*continued*)
Insall r.
Insall-Salvati r.
inspiratory-to-expiratory r. (I/E)
inverse inspiratory-expiratory time r.
iodine-particle r.
isotopic r.
kidney length to body height r. (KBR)
kidney-to-background r.
L/A peak r.
L/B r.
left atrium-aortic root r. (LA/AR)
left ventricular systolic time interval r.
lesion-background r.
lesion-countersite r. (L/C)
lesion-muscle r.
lesion-nonlesion count r.
lesion-normal tissue r.
likelihood r.
limb bone length r.
Lindegaard r.
liver-to-aorta peak r.
liver-to-muscle contrast r.
liver-to-spleen attenuation r.
L/LP r.
LQ r.
magnetization transfer r. (MTR)
magnetogyric r.
maximum diameter to minimum diameter r.
metatarsal length r.
mortality rate r.
myocardium-to-abdomen count r.
myoinositol-creatine r. (Mi/Cr)
nasal-to-plasma radioactivity r.
neutron-atomic number r.
nuclear-to-cytoplasmic r. (N/C)
odds r.
r. of caudate to right hepatic lobe
off-axis r. (OAR)
off-center r. (OCR)
r. of photoelectric to Compton absorption
optional target-to-background r.
orifice-anulus r.
oxygen enhancement r.
P/A r.
PASP/SASP r.
patellar ligament-to-patella r.
peak systolic and diastolic r.
peroneal-to-anterior compartment r.
phase sampling r. (PSR)
pitch r.
Poisson r.
power r.
proportional r.
pulmonary artery-bronchus r.
pulmonic-systemic flow r.
P wave-QRS wave r. (P/QRS)
radioactive iodide conversion r.
renal-aortic r. (RAR)
repetition time to echo time r. (TR/TE)
right ventricular to left ventricular systolic pressure r.
scatter-air r. (SAR)
scatter-maximum r. (SMR)
scatter-primary r.
sensitizer enhancement r.
septum-to-free wall r.
signal intensity r.
signal-to-clutter r.
signal-to-noise r. (S/N, SNR)
SI joint-sacrum r.
spleen-to-liver r.
standardized uptake r. (SUR)
stroke count r.
stroke volume r.
ST-segment/heart r.
systolic-diastolic r. (S/D)
systolic velocity r.
target-to-background r.
target-to-nontarget r.
thallium-to-scalp r.
thermal enhancement r. (TER)
thickness-diameter of ventricle r.
tissue-air r. (TAR)
tissue-maximum r. (TMR)
tissue-phantom r. (TPR)
TME r.
r. transformer
trapezium-metacarpal eburnation r.
tumor-to-background r.
tumor-to-gray matter r.
tumor-to-normal brain r.
tumor-to-normal tissue r. (TNR)
tumor-to-white matter r.
unfavorable neutron-to-proton r.
uptake r.
V/C r.
ventilation-perfusion r.
ventricle-brain r. (VBR)
vessel density r. (VDR)
V/S r.

RatioVision digital fluorescent imaging system
Ratliff avascular necrosis classification
rat-tail
r.-t. common bile duct
r.-t. esophagus
Rau
apophysis of R.
Rauchfuss triangle
rave
fracture en r.

^R**AW, RAW**
    airway resistance
ray
    actinic r.
    alpha r.
    r. amputation
    anode r.
    Becquerel r.
    beta r.
    Bucky r.
    cathode r.
    central r.
    chemical r.
    corresponding r.
    delta r.
    digital r.
    direct r.
    fluorescent r.
    gamma r.
    glass r.
    grenz r.
    H r.
    hard r.
    hypermobile 1st r.
    incident r.
    indirect r.
    infrared r.
    infraroentgen r.
    intermediate r.
    keV gamma r.
    long-axis r.
    monochromatic r.
    Niewenglowski r.
    parallel r.'s
    r. pattern
    pollicized r.
    positive r.
    primary r.
    reflected r.
    roentgen r.
    secondary r.
    scattered r.'s
    soft r.
    r. sum
    terahertz r.
    r. tracing
    ultraviolet r.
    vertical r.
    W r.
ray-casting
    r.-c. method
    r.-c. technique
Rayleigh
    R. noise
    R. quotient
    R. scattering
    R. scattering law
Rayleigh-Tyndall scattering
Raymond-Cestan syndrome

Raynaud
    R. phenomenon
    R. syndrome
ray-sum
    r.-s. projection
    r.-s. view
Ray-Tec x-ray-detectable surgical
    sponge
Rb
    rubidium
⁸²**Rb, Rb-82**
    rubidium 82
⁸²**Rb-based cardiac imaging**
RBBB
    right bundle-branch block
RBC
    red blood cell
        labeled RBC
        ^{99m}Tc-labeled RBC
        ^{99m}Tc-tagged RBC
        UltraTag RBC
RBE
    relative biologic effectiveness
RB-ILD
    respiratory bronchiolitis-associated
        interstitial lung disease
RCA
    retained cortical activity
    right coronary angiography
    right coronary artery
    rotational coronary
        atherectomy
Rcadia COR analyzer (I, II)
rCBF
    regional cerebral blood flow
        rCBF PET scan
rCBV
    regional cerebral blood
        volume
    relative cerebral blood volume
RCC
    renal cell carcinoma (stage I, II, IIIA,
        IIIB, IIIC, IVA, IVB)
RCM
    red cell mass
rCMRO$_2$
    regional cerebral metabolic rate for
        oxygen
rCPP
    regional cerebral perfusion
        pressure
RCT
    randomized clinical trial
3rd
    3rd branchial arch
    3rd cardiac mogul
    3rd inflow
    3rd intercondylar tubercle of
        Parsons

3rd (*continued*)
    3rd portion of duodenum
    3rd projection of Chausse
    3rd trimester
    3rd ventricle
    3rd ventricle of cerebrum
    3rd ventricle tumor
    3rd ventricular hemangioblastoma
3rd-degree
    3rd-d. AV block
    3rd-d. heart block
RDF
    rotary door flap
3rd-order chorda
RDPA
    right descending pulmonary artery
RDS
    radioisotope delivery system
    respiratory distress syndrome
RDS-like deficiency
3rd-space sequestration
3rd-trimester
    3rd-t. gestational dating
    3rd-t. placenta
RDX
    radiation delivery technology
    RDX coronary radiation catheter
      delivery system
^{186}Re
    rhenium 186
    ^{186}Re etidronate
^{188}Re
    rhenium 188
    generator-produced ^{188}Re
RE
    reflux esophagitis
    Biafine RE
Re
    Reynolds number
    rhenium
Re-186
    rhenium 186
Re-188
    rhenium 188
reabsorption
    r. atelectasis
    sodium r.
reaccumulation
reactance
    capacitive r.
    inductive r.
reaction
    allergic r.
    anaphylactic r.
    anaphylactoid r.
    annihilation r.
    arrest r.
    aseptic granulomatous foreign body
      r.

    biomolecular r.
    chemotoxic r.
    choriodecidual r.
    complex periosteal r.
    Crohn-like lymphoid r.
    dependency r.
    desmoid r.
    desmoplastic r.
    dystonic r.
    Eisenmenger r.
    endoergic r.
    exoergic r.
    extrapyramidal r.
    flare r.
    fluffy periosteal r.
    hair-on-end periosteal r.
    hexokinase r.
    hilar r.
    hypersensitivity r.
    idiosyncratic anaphylactoid r.
    inflammatory r.
    interrupted periosteal r.
    Jones-Mote r.
    lamellar periosteal r.
    multilamellar periosteal r.
    nonidiosyncratic anaphylactoid r.
    nuclear r.
    onionskin periosteal r.
    osteoblastic r.
    periosteal r.
    photonuclear r.
    pleural r.
    positron matter-antimatter annihilation
      r.
    quellung r.
    r. recovery time
    sarcoidlike r.
    scar tissue r.
    Schultz r.
    shell-type periosteal r.
    soft tissue r.
    solid periosteal r.
    1st-order r.
    sunburst periosteal r.
    symmetric periosteal r.
    Teflon granulomatous r.
    thermonuclear r.
    vasomotor r.
    vasovagal r.
    r. vial
reactivation tuberculosis
reactive
    r. airway disease (RAD)
    r. airway dysfunction syndrome
    r. arteriole
    r. arthritis
    r. bone sclerosis
    r. cyst cord
    r. disease of smooth muscle

R

r. fibrosis
r. fibrous lesion
r. fibrovascular arachnoid proliferation
r. follicular hyperplasia
r. gliosis
r. hyperemia
r. interface
r. lymphadenopathy
r. lymphoid hyperplasia
r. lymphoid lesion
r. marrow edema
r. remodeling
r. spinal cyst

reactivity
bronchial r.

reactor
breeder r.
fast breeder r.
nuclear r.

reader
AC 3 plate r.
Immuno-mini NJ-2300 microplate r.
microplate r.
R. paratrigeminal syndrome
plate r.

Readi-Cat oral contrast

reading
postradiotherapy implant survey r.
pressure r.
wet r.

readout
r. delay
echo-planar r.
r. gradient
steady-state projection imaging with dynamic echo-train r. (SPIDER)
r. wavelength

ReadyPET support service

reagent
lanthanide shift r. (LSR)
shift r.
splenic r.

REAL
Revised European American Lymphoma
REAL classification

RealHand instrumentation

realignment
intrarun r.
patellofemoral r.

Reality Engine graphics

real signal

real-time
r.-t. assessment
r.-t. biplanar needle tracking
r.-t. chirp Z transformer
r.-t. color Doppler imaging
r.-t. compression
r.-t. CT fluoroscopy
r.-t. 2D blood flow imaging
r.-t. 2-dimensional Doppler flow imaging system
r.-t. display
r.-t. Doppler
r.-t. dose area product
r.-t. 4D ultrasound imaging system
r.-t. echocardiography
r.-t. echo-planar image
r.-t. enhancement
r.-t. format converter
r.-t. magnetic resonance imaging tracking
r.-t. phase-contrast flow
r.-t. position management (RPM)
r.-t. quantitative flow
r. t. respiratory feedback
r.-t. scan
r.-t. scan ultrasound
r.-t. sector scanning
r.-t. sonogram
r.-t. sonography
r.-t. ultrasonography
r.-t. volume rendering

rear endoluminal view

rearfoot varus

rear-projection screen

rebleeding of aneurysm

rebound
r. excitation
r. sign
thymic r.

rebreathing ventilation scan

recalcitrant

recall
multiplanar gradient r. (MPGR)
spoiled gradient r. (SPGR)

recanalization
endovascular photoacoustic r. (EPAR)
fallopian tube r.
r. technique
transcervical fallopian tube r.

recanalized
r. artery
r. duct

recapture
mobile with r.
mobile without r.
stuck with r.
stuck without r.

receive bandwidth

receive-only circular surface coil

receiver
r. coil
r. dead time
Medtronic radiofrequency r.
r. operating characteristic (ROC)

receiver (*continued*)
  r. operating characteristic curve
  r. operating characteristic
    method
recent dislocation
reception
  parallel r.
receptor
  r. binding
  chemokine r. (2, 3, 5)
  chemokine-related r.
  r. expression
  r. imaging
  macrophage scavenger r.
  muscarinic r.
  progestin r.
  retinoic acid r. (RAR)
  T-cell antigen r.
recess
  attic r.
  azygoesophageal r.
  Baumgarten r.
  cecal r.
  cerebellopontine r.
  cochlear r.
  costodiaphragmatic r.
  costomediastinal r.
  costophrenic r.
  duodenojejunal r.
  epitympanic r.
  hepatorenal r.
  ileocecal r.
  inferior duodenal r.
  infraglenoid r.
  intersigmoid r.
  lacrimal r.
  lateral r.
  lumbosacral lateral r.
  mild r.
  optic r.
  paraduodenal r.
  pericardial sleeve r.
  peritoneal r.
  pharyngeal r.
  piriform r.
  pleural r.
  popliteal r.
  posterior pleural r.
  prestyloid r.
  pulmonary venous r.
  rectouterine r.
  rectovesical r.
  retrocecal r.
  retroduodenal r.
  sacciform r.
  sphenoethmoidal r.
  splenorenal r.
  steplike r.
  sublabral r.

  subphrenic r.
  subscapularis r.
  superior azygoesophageal r.
  superior duodenal r.
  twining r.
recession
  nasion r.
  rib r.
reciprocal
  r. agonist-antagonist relaxation
  r. change
  r. depression
  r. rhythm
reciprocating conduction
reciprocity theorem dose
recirculation peak
RECIST
  Response Evaluation Criteria in Solid
    Tumors
Recklinghausen
  R. disease of bone
  R. tumor
reclining position
recoarctation of aorta
recognizer
  exposure data r. (EDR)
recoil
  r. atom
  r. electron
  r. energy
  r. pressure
  r. radiation
recombinant
  r. anti-p185HER2 monoclonal
    antibody
  G/A r.
  H/G r.
  r. human thyroid-stimulating
    hormone
  r. thyrotropin contrast agent
  r. tissue plasminogen activator
recon pitch
reconstitution
  artery r.
  r. of blood flow in artery
  r. via profunda artery
reconstructed
  3D acquired/2D r.
  r. image
  r. radiographic imaging
reconstruction
  ACV r.
  adaptive cardiac volume r.
  analytic r.
  aortic r.
  aortobifemoral r.
  r. artifact
  coronal r.
  coronal tomographic r.

curved r.
curvilinear r.
3D r.
diagnostic r.
3D image r.
Dor r.
dual-segment r.
extended cardiac r.
external gamma dose r.
fan-beam r.
r. field of view (RFOV)
Fourier 2-dimensional projection r.
Fourier transform r.
r. from projection imaging
gated 3D r.
half-scan r.
image r.
image data r.
r. interval
iterative r.
magnitude r.
MIP r.
monosegmental image r.
multiplanar r.
multisegment r.
multisegmental image r.
oblique angle r.
r. of aorta
patch-graft r.
periodically rotated overlapping
  parallel lines with enhanced r.
phase-preserving r.
quadsegmental image r.
ramp r.
renovascular r.
respiratory gated 3D r.
sagittal tomographic r.
segmental correction using spine r.
1-sided image r.
single-pixel r.
spatial r.
r. study
systolic r.
time-reversal method of focal r.
transanular patch r.
trisegmental image r.
r. view
zygomaticomalar r.
reconstructive imaging
reconstructor
dynamic planar r. (DPR)
dynamic spatial r. (DSR)
reconversion
bone marrow r.
recorded detail
recording
color Doppler r.
continuous-wave Doppler r.
pullback pressure r.

pulsed-wave Doppler r.
pulse volume r. (PVR)
segmental limb pressure r.
simultaneous r.
split-screen r.
recovery
arrhythmia-insensitive flow-sensitive
  alternating inversion r. (A-FAIR)
cardiac r.
3D turbo fluid-attenuated inversion r.
fast short tau inversion r.
R. filter
flow-sensitive alternating inversion r.
  (FAIR)
fluid-attenuated inversion r. (FLAIR)
inversion r. (IR)
myocardial r.
R. nitinol filter
r. period of myocardium
postischemic r.
saturation r.
selective partial inversion r. (SPIR)
selective partial inversion
  recovery-fluid attenuated inversion
  r. (SPIR-FLAIR)
selective saturation r.
shape r.
short inversion r.
short tau inversion r. (STIR)
short TI inversion r. (STIR)
silver r.
spectral presaturation with inversion
  r. (SPIR)
r. time
r. time image
total saturation r. (TSR)
turbo short tau inversion r.
turbo short tau/T1 inversion r.
recrudescence
recrudescent tuberculosis
recruitment potential
recta (*pl. of* rectum)
rectal
r. ampulla
r. balloon
r. carcinoma
r. contrast medium
r. dilation
r. distention
r. duplication cyst
r. endoscopic ultrasonography
r. endosonography
r. fascia
r. fisting
r. fistula
r. fold
r. intussusception
r. lesion
r. lymph node

R

rectal (*continued*)
r. multiplane transducer
r. muscle cuff
r. narrowing
r. obstruction
r. orifice
r. penetration
r. plexus
r. polyp
r. pouch
r. prolapse
r. radiation injury
r. sheath hematoma
r. shelf
r. sidewall
r. stenosis
r. stump
r. tear
r. tip
r. valve
r. vault

rectangular
r. disc
r. field of view
r. phalanx
r. section profile

recti
ampulla r.

rectification
full-wave r.
4-valve tube r.

rectifier
full-wave r.
silicon-controlled r. (SCR)
r. subblock
r. tube

rectilinear
r. biphasic waveform for external
defibrillation
r. bone scan
r. bone scan imaging
r. scanner
r. thyroid scan
r. tomography

rectocele
rectogenital septum
rectorectal intussusception
rectosigmoid
r. carcinoma
r. function
r. index
r. junction
r. manometry
r. polypoid lesion

rectouterine
r. fold
r. fossa
r. pouch
r. recess

rectovaginal
r. fistula
r. pouch
r. septum

rectovaginouterine pouch
rectovesical
r. fistula
r. pouch
r. recess
r. septum

rectum, *pl.* **rectums,** *pl.* **recta**
benign lymphoma of r.
Hartmann closure of r.
r. radiation

rectums (*pl. of* rectum)
rectus
r. femoris
r. femoris tendon
gyrus r.
r. muscle
r. muscle hematoma
r. position
r. sheath
r. sheath pocket

recumbent
r. lateral projection
r. position
r. view

recurrence
ipsilateral breast tumor r. (IBTR)
local r.
locoregional r.
no evidence of r. (NER)
r. pattern
tumor r.

recurrent
r. artery of Heubner
r. bronchiectasis
r. canal
r. digital fibroma
r. dislocation
r. embolus
r. fleeting infiltrate
r. high-grade malignant glioma
r. hyperparathyroidism
r. laryngeal nerve
r. laryngeal nerve palsy
r. lateral patellar subluxation
r. lesion
r. lymphoma
r. meningeal nerve
r. multifocal osteomyelitis
r. neoplasm
r. pneumonia
r. pneumothorax
r. pyogenic cholangitis
r. pyogenic hepatitis
r. respiratory papillomatosis
r. sialadenitis

R

r. stricture
r. ulcer
r. vermian oligoastrocytoma
recursive
r. partitioning
r. partitioning analysis
recurvatum
r. deformity
genu r.
pectus r.
red
r. blood cell (RBC)
r. blood cell iron turnover
r. cell aplasia
r. cell ghost
r. cell mass (RCM)
r. infarct
r. marrow
Reddick cystic duct cholangiogram catheter
redirection of inferior vena cava
redistributed thallium scan
redistribution
blood flow r.
flow r.
pulmonary blood flow r.
pulmonary vascular r.
r. study
r. thallium-201 imaging
vascular r.
Redi-Vu teleradiology system
red-out
REDS
remote endoscopic digital spectroscopy
reduced
r. acquisition
r. alveolar ventilation
r. circulation
r. compliance of chamber
r. filling
r. lung volume
r. plasma volume
r. prominence of pulmonary vessel
r. pulmonary compliance
r. signal intensity
r. stroke volume
r. subluxation
r. systemic cardiac output
r. ventricular filling period
reduced-acquisition
r.-a. matrix (RAM)
r.-a. matrix FAST
reducing stent
reduction
anatomic r.
blood viscosity r.
closed r.

concentric r.
congruent r.
r. deformity
3D field echo acquisition with short repetition time and echo r.
electrolytic r.
field echo acquisition with short repetition time and echo r. (FASTER)
fracture r.
gradient moment r. (GMR)
limb r.
open r.
postural r.
radiofrequency tongue base r.
stable r.
redundancy
r. of interposed colon segment
phase-angle display r.
redundant
r. aortic valve leaflet
r. capsule
r. carotid artery
r. mitral valve leaflet
r. scallop of posterior anulus
r. ureter
reefing
capsular r.
r. of medial retinaculum of knee
reel-in mutation
reentrant
r. loop
r. well chamber
reentry
bundle-branch r. (BBR)
r. circuit
functional r.
intraatrial r.
r. point
sinus node r.
reexpansion
lung r.
r. pulmonary edema
reexploration
reference
chemical-shift r.
r. compound
r. coordinate system
distal line of r. (DLR)
r. dose
r. image
r. line
r. phantom
plane of r.
r. range
rotating frame of r.
r. site
r. standard

reference (*continued*)
    sternospinal r.
    r. wave
referral teleradiology
refill
    capillary r.
Refinity Coblation system
reflectance-guided laser selection
reflected
    r. edge of Poupart ligament
    r. inguinal ligament
    r. ray
reflection
    r. coefficient
    2nd-order r.
    pleuroparenchymal r.
    vascular r.
reflectivity
    echo r.
    high r.
reflectometer tuning unit
reflector
    diffuse r.
    specular r.
reflex
    r. arc
    cat's-eye r.
    conditioned r.
    genitourinary r.
    r. ileus
    stapedius r.
    r. sympathetic dystrophy
    r. sympathetic dystrophy syndrome
    white pupil r.
refluoromyelography
reflux
    acid r.
    r. activity
    alkali r.
    r. atrophy
    bile r.
    chylous r.
    congenital vesicoureteral r.
    cortical venous r.
    duodenobiliary r.
    duodenogastric r. (DGR)
    duodenogastroesophageal r.
    duodenopancreatic r.
    enteroesophageal r.
    esophageal r.
    r. esophagitis (RE)
    free r.
    r. gastritis
    gonadal vein r.
    r. (grade I-V)
    hepatojugular r.
    r. ileitis
    intrarenal r.
    lymphatic r.

    nasopharyngeal r.
    r. nephropathy
    r. of barium
    pancreatic r.
    pistonlike r.
    pudendal vein r.
    r. regurgitation
    ventricular r.
    vesicoureteral r. (VUR)
refluxing spastic neurogenic bladder
refocus
    multiplanar gradient r.
refocusing
reformat
reformation
    coronal r.
    curved multiplanar r.
    curved planar r.
    DentaScan multiplanar r.
    image r.
    multiplanar volume r. (MPVR)
    paddlewheel r.
    thin-section secondary r.
reformatted
    r. computed tomography
    r. T1 magnetic resonance image
reformatting
    cardiac oblique r.
    3D r.
    multiplanar r. (MPR)
refraction
refractive shadowing
refractory
    r. congestive heart failure
    r. hepatic hydrothorax
    r. hypertension
    r. period of myocardium
    r. TLE
    r. to treatment
    r. tumor
refractured bone
regeneration
    imperfect r.
    nodular liver r.
    r. of tissue
    osteoblastic bone r.
regenerative
    r. chondrocyte
    r. gastric polyp
    r. liver nodule
regimen
    lifetime r.
region
    Broca r.
    dark r.
    distention of esophagogastric r.
    esophagogastric r.
    hyperechoic r.
    hypermetabolic r.

hypervariable r.
insular r.
isthmic r.
laterocervical r.
limbic r.
r. of activation
r. of interest (ROI)
r. of protection
outer-air r.
paratracheal r.
parietooccipital r.
patulous esophagogastric r.
periauricular r.
perihilar r.
photodeficient r.
photopenic r.
pineal r.
subpial r.

regional

r. asynergy
r. cerebral blood flow (rCBF)
r. cerebral blood flow response
r. cerebral blood volume (rCBV)
r. cerebral metabolic rate for
    oxygen (rCMRO$_2$)
r. cerebral oxygen saturation
r. cerebral perfusion
r. cerebral perfusion pressure (rCPP)
r. colitis
r. contractile reserve
r. difference in aeration
r. dyskinesia
r. dyssynergia
r. ejection fraction
r. ejection fraction imaging
r. enteritis
r. granulomatous lymphadenitis
r. hypokinesis
r. hypokinetic wall motion
r. intraarterial infusion
r. left ventricular function
r. lymphangitic carcinomatosis
r. lymph node
r. mean transit time (rMTT)
r. migratory osteoporosis
r. myocardial blood flow
r. myocardial dysfunction
r. myocardial function
r. myocardial ischemia
r. myocardial mass distribution
r. oxygen extraction fraction (rOEF)
r. perfusion abnormality
r. pulmonary perfusion
r. spread
r. tracer uptake
r. transient osteoporosis
r. transmural ischemia
r. tumor confinement
r. vascular perfusion

r. ventilation
r. wall motion assessment
r. washout measurement

region-of-interest

r.-o.-i. fluoroscopy
r.-o.-i. imaging technique

registered technologist (RT)

registration

r. and alignment of 3D image
automatic image r. (AIR)
combined anatomic r.
2D portal image r.
feasibility of image r.
image r.
intermodality image r.
landmark r.
robust r.
spastic r.
spatial r.
surface r.

registry

PTCA R.

Regnauld

R. degeneration of MTP joint
R. great toe degeneration

regressed

r. adenoidal tissue
r. cyst

regression

r. analysis
caudal r.
plaque r.
polynomial stepwise multilinear r.
spontaneous r.
stepwise r.

regressive remodeling

regrowth delay

regular

r. connective tissue
r. wedge delay

regularization

Tikhonov r.

regulation

volume r.

regurgitant

r. flow delay
r. fraction
r. jet
r. lesion
r. lesion delay
r. orifice
r. orifice area (ROA)
r. pandiastolic flow
r. pocket
r. stream
r. stroke volume (RSV)
r. systolic flow
r. valve
r. velocity

R

regurgitation
    aortic r.
    congenital aortic r.
    congenital mitral r. (CMR)
    Dexter-Grossman classification of
      mitral r.
    Doppler tricuspid r.
    factitious r.
    Grossman scale for r.
    ischemically mediated mitral r.
    massive aortic r.
    mitral r. (MR)
    mitral valve r.
    pansystolic mitral r.
    paravalvular r.
    physiologic r.
    pulmonary r. (PR)
    pulmonary valve r.
    reflux r.
    semilunar aortic valve r.
    semilunar pulmonic valve r.
    silent r.
    syphilitic aortic r.
    transient tricuspid r.
    tricuspid orifice r.
    tricuspid valve r.
    valvular r. (VR)

Reichert
    R. canal
    R. flexible sigmoidoscope

Reichert-Mundinger-Fischer stereotactic frame

Reid
    R. baseline
    R. line
    R. lobule

Reil
    R. band
    R. island

reimplantation
    r. lung response
    r. technique

reinfarction

reinjection thallium stress examination

Reinke space

reinnervation
    motor r.
    sympathetic r.

reintimalization

reirradiation

Reisseisen muscle

Reiter
    R. syndrome
    R. syndrome arthritis

[188]**Re-labeled self-expanding nitinol stent**

relapse
    bone marrow r.
    solitary r.
    testicular r.

relapsing
    r. course
    r. polychondritis

relation
    end-diastolic pressure-volume r.
    end-systolic pressure-volume r.
    force-frequency r.
    force-length r.
    force-velocity r.
    Frank-Starling r.
    phase r.

relationship
    atlantoaxial r.
    complex anatomic r.
    dentoskeletal r.
    dose-time r.
    dose-volume r.
    globe-orbit r.
    Karplus r.
    Reynolds r.
    tumor cell-host bone r.

relative
    r. biologic effectiveness (RBE)
    r. cerebral blood flow
    r. cerebral blood volume (rCBV)
    r. conversion factor
    r. dose intensity
    r. error
    r. hypoxia
    r. mitral stenosis
    r. peak height
    r. radiolucency
    r. refractory period (RRP)
    r. regional blood flow (rrBF)
    r. shunt flow
    r. value scale

relativistic mass

relaxation
    absent lower esophageal
      sphincter r.
    r. atelectasis
    r. enhancement technique
    esophageal sphincter r.
    ferromagnetic r.
    incomplete lower esophageal
      sphincter r.
    isovolumic r.
    longitudinal r.
    molecular weight dependence of r.
    multiexponential r.
    multispin r.
    nuclear electric quadripole r.
    paramagnetic shift r.
    r. probe
    proton r.
    r. rate
    r. rate frequency dependence
    reciprocal agonist-antagonist r.
    sinusoidal r.

spin-lattice r.
spin-spin r.
r. time
tissue-based T2 r.
transverse r.
T1, T2 star r.
relaxed lower esophageal sphincter
relaxlvity
r. data
longitudinal r.
transverse r.
relaxometer
Bruker PC-10 r.
Bruker TC-10 r.
IBM field-cycling research r.
relaxometry
time-efficient T2 r.
tissue r.
relaxor
ferroelectric r.
releasing factor
relief pattern
rcloading
anode tube r.
REM
radiation-equivalent-man
roentgen-equivalent-man
remasking
remineralization
remitting course
remnant
r. ablation
cystic duct r.
ductal r.
gastric r.
heart r.
notochord r.
omphalomesenteric r.
r radiation
r. stomach
thyroglossal duct r.
thyroid r.
remodeling
balloon r.
bone r.
bony r.
cord r.
coronary r.
craniofacial r.
intimal r.
neural foramen r.
osseous r.
paraarticular bone r.
plaque r.
reactive r.
regressive r.
stress-induced r.
r. technique
thrombus r.

remote
r. afterloading brachytherapy (RAB)
r. afterloading system
r. endoscopic digital spectroscopy (REDS)
r. ischemia
r lower motor neuron lesion
remote-controlled
r.-c. implantation of radioactive source
r.-c. production
removal
brachytherapy implant r.
REMP
roentgen-equivalent-man period
remyclinization
Renaissance 3D workstation
renal
r. abscess
r. adenocarcinoma
r. agenesis
r. allograft
r. allograft necrosis
r. amyloidosis
r. angiography
r. angiography imaging
r. angiomyolipoma
r. anomaly
r. anticoagulant-related bleeding
r. aortography
r. arteriography
r. arteriosclerosis
r. artery
r. artery aneurysm
r. artery dissection
r. artcry fibromuscular dysplasia
r. artery hypertension
r. artery revascularization
r. artery stenosis (RAS)
r. artery stenosis screening MR
r. artery transplant thrombosis
r. axis
r. calcification
r. calculus
r. calyx
r. capsule
r. carbuncle
r. carcinosarcoma
r. cell carcinoma (stage I, II, IIIA, IIIB, IIIC, IVA, IVB) (RCC)
r. cholesterol embolus
r. choristoma
r. clearance
r. cocktail
r. colic
r. collecting structure
r. collecting system

R

renal (*continued*)
   r. collecting system atony
   r. column
   r. cortex
   r. cortical adenoma
   r. cortical isotope scanning agent
   r. cortical necrosis
   r. cortical nephrocalcinosis
   r. cortical scintigraphy
   r. CT imaging
   r. cystic disease
   r. cyst imaging
   r. cyst study
   r. diverticulum
   r. Doppler
   r. duplex imaging
   r. duplex scan
   r. duplication
   r. dwarfism
   r. dysfunction
   r. ectopia
   r. edema
   r. failure
   r. fascia
   r. flow curve
   r. function differential
   r. function impairment
   r. function study
   r. fungal infection
   r. fungus ball
   r. gallium scintigraphy
   r. glomerulus
   r. graft infarct
   r. hamartoma
   r. helical CT
   r. hemangiopericytoma
   r. hilar vessel
   r. hilum
   r. image
   r. impression
   r. infarct
   r. inflammation
   r. injury
   r. insufficiency
   r. interstitium
   r. isthmus
   r. labyrinth
   r. leiomyoma
   r. length measurement
   r. lithiasis
   r. lymphoma
   r. malrotation
   r. mass lesion
   r. medulla
   r. medullary pyramid
   r. metastasis
   r. obstruction
   r. osteodystrophy
   r. outline

   r. papilla
   r. papillary necrosis
   r. parenchyma
   r. parenchymal blush
   r. parenchymal malacoplakia
   r. pelvic fibrolipomatosis
   r. pelvis
   r. pelvis tumor
   r. perfusion
   r. perfusion imaging
   r. pouch
   r. proximal tubular dysfunction
   r. pseudotumor
   r. radionuclide
   r. reflux atrophy
   r. resistive index
   r. scarring
   r. sclerosis
   r. shadow
   r. shutdown
   r. sinus
   r. sinus complex
   r. sinus cyst
   r. sinus echo
   r. sinus fat
   r. sinus lipomatosis
   r. sinus mass
   r. size
   r. stone
   r. stone mineral composition
   r. surface
   r. transplant
   r. transplant GI tract perforation
   r. transplant hypertension
   r. transplant lymphocele
   r. transplant pseudoaneurysm
   r. transplant urine extravasation
   r. trauma
   r. tuberculosis
   r. tubular degeneration
   r. tubular dysgenesis
   r. tubular ectasia
   r. tubular necrosis
   r. tubular osteomalacia
   r. tubule
   r. tumor
   r. ultrasonography imaging
   r. ultrasound
   r. vascular
   r. vascular anatomy
   r. vascular damage
   r. vein
   r. vein renin assay
   r. vein thrombosis (RVT)
   r. vein transplant thrombosis
   r. venogram
   r. venography
   vertebral, anal, tracheal, esophageal,
     r. (VATER)

renal-aortic ratio (RAR)
rendered
>   volume r.

rendering
>   3D surface r.
>   r. parameter
>   perspective volume r. (PVR)
>   real-time volume r.
>   shaded surface r.
>   transparent r.
>   volume r.

Renegade Hi-Flo microcatheter
reniform
>   r. contour
>   r. mass
>   r. pelvis

renin-angiotensin-dependent outer cortex
reninculus
reninoma
renin-secreting tumor
ren lobatus
RenoCal-76
renocystogram
Renografin-60, -76 imaging agent
renogram
>   captopril r.
>   r. curve
>   diuresis r.
>   F-15 r.
>   r. imaging
>   isotope r.

renography
>   ACE inhibition r.
>   acetazolamide r.
>   diuretic r.
>   DTPA r.
>   emission r.
>   enalaprilat-enhanced r.
>   exercise r.
>   furosemide r.
>   Lasix r.
>   technetium 99m MAG3 r.

Reno-M-30, -60
renovascular, renal vascular
>   r. anatomy
>   r. damage
>   r. disease
>   r. hypertension (RVH)
>   r. reconstruction
>   r. stent

Renovist
>   R. II imaging agent
>   R. II injector

Renovue-Dip imaging agent
Renovue-65 imaging agent
rent
>   fascial r.

reocclusion
>   postthrombolytic coronary r.

reordering
>   MRA using 3D k-space r.
>   r. of phase encoding

REP
>   roentgen-equivalent-physical

repair
>   endovascular aneurysm r. (EVAR)
>   paraanastomotic aneurysm r.

reparative giant cell granuloma
repeat
>   variable number tandem r.

repeated free induction decay
reperfused
>   r. artery
>   r. myocardium

reperfusion
>   r. hyperemia
>   r. injury of postischemic lung
>   r. lung edema
>   r. therapy

repetition
>   r. time (RT)
>   r. time to echo time ratio
>   (TR/TE)

repetitive
>   r. anterior subluxation of tibia
>   r. microtrauma
>   r. osseous impingement
>   r. pulse sequence
>   r. seizures
>   r. strain injury (RSI)
>   r. stress injury (RSI)

rephased transverse magnetization
rephasing
>   echo r.
>   even-echo r.
>   field-echo sequence with even-echo
>   r. (FEER)
>   field even-echo r. (FEER)
>   r. gradient
>   gradient moment r. (GMR)
>   gradient motion r. (GMR)

replacement
>   aortic root r.
>   aortic valve r. (AVR)
>   bipolar hip r.
>   r. bone
>   r. fibrosis
>   hip r.
>   low signal-intensity r.
>   mitral valve r. (MVR)
>   multiple isomorphous r.'s (MIR)
>   orthotopic total heart r.
>   prosthetic joint r.
>   valve r.

replacing oblique view
replantable amputation
replantation of finger
replanted digit

replication
    r. error negative
    r. error positive
repolarization
    cardiac r.
    ventricular r. (T wave)
report
    unusual occurrence r. (UOR)
reporting
    structured platform-independent data
      entry and r. (SPIDER)
reproducibility index
reproducible baseline
reproduction
    colorimetric color r.
reproductive tract embryology
reprogramming therapy
requirement
    increased myocardial oxygen r.
rerotation
    varus r.
reroute
resampling
    volumetric r.
rescue
    autologous bone marrow r.
    bone marrow r.
research
    Academy of Radiology R. (ARR)
    Advanced Diagnostic R. (ADR)
resectability
resectable
    r. colorectal carcinoma
    r. lesion
resecting fracture
resection
    abdominoperineal r. (APR)
    absolute curative r.
    absolute noncurative r.
    atrial septal r.
    r. cavity
    colosigmoid r.
    computer-assisted stereotactic r.
    en bloc r.
    extraarticular r.
    gross total r.
    Hartmann perforated sigmoid
      diverticulitis r.
    r. of mobile aortic arch atheroma
    plica r.
    pulmonary r.
    rim r.
    subtotal gastric r.
    transurethral r. (TUR)
    wedge r.
resectoscope
    Iglesias fiberoptic r.
reserve
    blood flow r.

    brain perfusion r.
    cardiac r.
    r. cardiac function
    contractile r.
    coronary flow r. (CFR)
    diastolic r.
    r. force
    fractional flow r. (FFR)
    left ventricular systolic functional
      r.
    myocardial perfusion r.
    poor vascular r.
    preload r.
    pulmonary vascular r.
    regional contractile r.
    stenotic flow r. (SFR)
    systolic r.
    vascular r.
    ventricular r.
reservoir
    r. effect
    ICV r.
    shunt r.
residua (*pl. of* residuum)
residual
    r. aneurysmal sac
    r. barium
    r. calcification
    r. cement
    r. ductal tissue
    fibrocalcific r.
    fibrocystic r.
    fibrotic r.
    r. focus
    gastric r.
    r. gradient
    r. imaging agent
    r. interstitial change
    r. limb-shaped change
    r. luminal narrowing
    r. magnetization
    r. metal fragment shaving
    r. nucleus
    r. plaque
    postvoid r. (PVR)
    r. stone
    r. stress analysis
    r. urine
    r. urine accumulation
    r. volume (RV)
    r. volume/total lung capacity
residue
    fecal r.
residuum, *pl.* **residua**
    r. morphology
resilient artery
resin
    IRA-400 r.
    r. sphere

resistance
acquired radiation r.
airway r. (RAW, ^{R}AW)
arteriolar r.
r. blood flow
calculated r.
coronary vascular r.
decreased peripheral vascular r.
decreased systemic r.
drug-induced drug r.
efferent arteriolar r.
end-organ r.
expiratory r.
fixed pulmonary valvular r.
increased cerebrovascular r.
increased outflow r.
increased peripheral r.
increased pulmonary vascular r.
index of runoff r.
nasal airway r.
peripheral vascular r. (PVR)
pulmonary arteriolar r.
pulmonary vascular r. (PVR)
systemic vascular r. (SVR)
total peripheral r. (TPR)
total pulmonary r. (TPR)
vascular systemic r.
r. wire heater
Wood unit index of r.

resistive
r. exercise table
r. index
r. index angiography
r. magnet

resistivity
conductor r.

resistor

resolution
anatomic r.
angle variation r.
anisotropic r.
axial r.
contrast r.
depth r.
r. element
energy r.
fibrotic r.
high temporal r.
image spatial r.
in-plane spatial r.
interval r.
intrinsic energy r.
isotropic r.
lateral r.
low-contrast r. (LCR)
low-energy ultrahigh r. (LEUHR)
range r.
spatial r.
r. stage

submillimeter r.
temporal r.
ultrahigh r. (UHR)
R. ultrasonic catheter
wide-aperture kinematic table with
  isotropic r. (WakiTrak)

Resolve nonlocking draining catheter

resolving
r. ischemic neurologic defect
r. pneumonia
r. power
r. time

resonance
advanced nuclear medical r.
  (ANMR)
bandbox r.
biphasic magnetic r.
r. capture
computerized tomography/magnetic r.
  (CT/MR)
cough r.
cracked-pot r.
dielectric r.
electron paramagnetic r. (EPR)
electron spin r. (ESR)
fast-scan magnetic r.
field-focusing nuclear magnetic r.
  (FONAR)
focused nuclear magnetic r.
r. frequency
functional magnetic r. (fMR)
gated inflow magnetic r.
r. generator
high-resolution magnetic r. (HR-MR)
lactate r.
r. line
localized magnetic r. (LMR)
low-field magnetic r.
magnetic r. (MR)
mobile magnetic r.
nuclear magnetic r. (NMR)
r. offset
r. phenomenon
proton magnetic r.
pulsed nuclear magnetic r.
skodaic r.
split water r.
tagging cine-magnetic r.
topical magnetic r. (TMR)
T1-weighted magnetic r.
ultrahigh-field magnetic r.
velocity-encoded cine-magnetic r.
  (VEC-MR)

resonant frequency of oscillation

resonator
birdcage r.
bridged loop-gap r.
crossed-loop r.
detunable elliptic transmission line r.

R

resonator (*continued*)
    Faraday shielded r.
    flexible surface coil-type r. (FSCR)
    multicoupled loop-gap r.
resorbable
    r. pin
    r. plate
    r. rod
    r. screw
resorcinol spray
resorption
    r. atelectasis
    bone r.
    bony r.
    cortical bone r.
    dependent edema fluid r.
    fluid r.
    r. lacuna
    osteoclastic r.
    osteoclast-mediated bone r.
    periosteal r.
    periprosthetic bone r.
    r. phase of healing
    subarticular bone r.
    subchondral bone r.
    subperiosteal bone r.
    terminal tuft r.
    total r.
    trabecular bone r.
resorptive atelectasis
Resovist MR contrast medium
respiration
    cardiac gated r.
    r. pyelography
    shallow r.
respiratory
    r. atrium
    r. bronchiolar dilation
    r. bronchiole
    r. bronchiolitis
    r. bronchiolitis-associated interstitial lung disease (RB-ILD)
    r. burst
    r. burst product
    r. capacity
    r. chain complex (I-VI)
    r. compensation
    r. compromise
    r. decompensation
    r. diaphragm
    r. distress syndrome (RDS)
    r. disturbance of acid base
    r. effort
    r. embarrassment
    r. failure
    r. frequency
    r. gated 3D reconstruction
    r. gated imaging
    r. gating

    r. insufficiency
    r. misregistration
    r. modulation of vascular impedance
    r. motion
    r. motion artifact
    r. muscle weakness
    r. ordered phase encoding (ROPE)
    r. sorted phase encoding
    r. spasm
    r. system
    r. tract
    r. tract infection
    r. tract obstruction
    r. trigger
    r. triggered fast SE technique
    r. triggered fat-saturated axial image
    r. triggering
    r. volume
    r. zoonosis
respiratory-esophageal fistula
response
    abnormal ejection fraction r.
    autoimmune r.
    blood flow r.
    blood oxygenation level-dependent r.
    blood pressure r.
    BOLD r.
    cardioinhibitory r.
    cell-mediated immune r.
    clinical complete r.
    clinical partial r.
    controlled ventricular r.
    r. criterion
    deconditioned exercise r.
    desmoplastic r.
    end-organ r.
    R. Evaluation Criteria in Solid Tumors (RECIST)
    graft-versus-tumor r.
    healing flare r.
    hemodynamic r.
    high-rate ventricular r.
    immune r.
    line of r. (LOR)
    local host r. (LHR)
    magnet r.
    metabolic r.
    pain provocation r.
    radiation r. (RR)
    rapid ventricular r.
    regional cerebral blood flow r.
    reimplantation lung r.
    slow ventricular r.
    synovial inflammatory r.
    therapeutic r.
    vasoactive r.
    vasoconstrictor r.
    vasodepressor r.
    vasodilatory r.

ventricular r.
whole-body inflammatory r.
responsiveness
airway r.
rest
r. and exercise gated nuclear
  angiography
cervical r.
glial r.
r. image acquisition
knee r.
restenosis
in-stent r.
postangioplasty r.
restiform body
restiforme
corpus r.
resting
r. ankle-arm pressure index
r. ankle pressure index (RAPI)
r. electrocardiogram
r. end-systolic wall stress
r. energy expenditure
r. forefoot supination angle
r. heart
r. injection
r. left ventricular ejection fraction
r. left ventricular function
r. lower esophageal sphincter
r. magnetization
r. MUGA imaging
r. myocardial echocardiography
r. myocardial perfusion imaging
r. perfusion
r. phase of cardiac action potential
r. pulse
r. redistribution examination
r. redistribution imaging
r. redistribution thallium-201
  scintigraphy
r. regional myocardial blood flow
r. regional myocardial hypoperfusion
r. right ventricular function
r. thallium-201 myocardial imaging
restoration of flow
restraint
r. calipers
foam-padded Velcro r.
mummy r.
passive epicardial r.
4-point r.
restricted water diffusion
restriction
cortical diffusion r.
intrauterine growth r.
unilateral flow r.
restrictive
r. abnormality
r. bulboventricular foramen

r. cardiomyopathy
r. hemodynamic syndrome
r. lung disease
r. myocardial disease
r. pattern
r. pulmonary emphysema
r. ventilatory defect
restrictor
beam r.
restructuring
result
concordant r.
false-negative r.
false-positive r.
negative EMA r.
negative mucin r.
negative puncture r.
suboptimal r.
true-positive r.
retained
r. barium
r. common bile duct stone
r. cortical activity (RCA)
r. dead fetus
r. fetal lung fluid
r. foreign body
r. gallstone
r. gastric antrum
r. placenta
r. products of conception (RPOC)
r. root
r. secretion
r. surgical sponge
r. urine
retardation
asymmetric intrauterine growth r.
fetal growth r.
growth r.
intrauterine growth r. (IUGR)
rete
r. mirabile
r. peg
r. ridge
r. testis
retention
CO_2 r.
r. colon polyp
r. cyst
r. enema
fluid r.
r. index
r. meal
r. of barium
r. of food
r. of secretion
r. of stool
r. stomach polyp
uptake and r.
water r.

retentivity
    magnetic r.
Reteplase
rethrombosis
reticula (*pl. of* reticulum)
reticular, reticulated
    r. abnormality
    r. activating formation
    r. activating substance
    r. connective tissue
    r. formation of brainstem
    gray r.
    r. infiltrate
    r. interstitial disease pattern
    r. lung pattern
    r. opacity
    r. type
    r. varicosity
reticularis
    livedo r.
    zona r.
reticulated (*var. of* reticular)
    r. bone
reticulation
    r. artifact
    chronic diffuse r.
    coarse lung r.
    diffuse fine lung r.
    lower lobe r.
    r. with hilar adenopathy
reticulocortical pathway
reticuloendothelial
    r. imaging
    r. imaging agent
    r. system
    r. tumor
reticuloendotheliosis
reticulogranular
    r. appearance
    r. pattern
    r. pulmonary density
reticulohistiocytic granuloma
reticulohistiocytosis
    multicentric r.
reticuloid
    actinic r.
reticulonodular
    r. infiltrate
    r. lesion
    r. lung disease
    r. pattern
reticulosis
    mast cell r.
    midline malignant r.
reticulospinal tract
reticulum, *pl.* **reticula**
    r. bone cell sarcoma
    r. brain cell sarcoma
    hemopoietic r.

retina
    angiomatosis of r.
retinacula (*pl. of* retinaculum)
retinacular
    r. disruption
    r. ligament
retinaculum, *pl.* **retinacula**
    avulsed r.
    cubital tunnel r.
    r. cutis
    extensor r.
    flexor r.
    free-floating r.
    inferior extensor r.
    inferior peroneal r.
    inferior quadriceps r.
    patellar r.
    peroneal r.
    superior extensor r.
    superior peroneal r.
retinal
    r. angiomatosis
    r. anlage tumor
    r. artery
    r. astrocytoma
    r. degeneration
    r. dysplasia
    r. embolus
    r. hemangioblastoma
    r. microaneurysm
retinoblastoma
    familial r.
    r. gene
    r. hereditary human carcinoma
    r. protein
    quadrilateral r.
    trilateral r.
retinocerebellar angiomatosis
retinochoroiditis
retinocortical time
retinocytoma
retinoic acid receptor (RAR)
retinoma
retinopathy
retracted
    r. rib
    r. stoma
retractile
    r. mesenteritis
    r. testis
retraction
    chest wall r.
    clot r.
    costa r.
    fiber r.
    inspiratory r.
    intercostal r. (ICR)
    late systolic r.
    leaflet r.

mediastinal r.
midsystolic r.
mild subcostal r.
musculotendinous r.
nipple r.
postrheumatic cusp r.
sternocleidomastoid r.
sternum r.
substernal r.
superior r.
suprasternal r.
systolic r.
upward r.

retractor
r. bulbi muscle
external r.

retrievable IVC filter
retrieval
r. catheter
microvascular r.
oocyte r.
transvaginal oocyte r.
transvesical oocyte r.

retroaortic
r. lymph node
r. renal vein

retroappendiceal fossa
retroareolar
r. density
r. dysplasia

retroauricular lymph node
retrobulbar
r. fat
r. hemorrhage
r. mass

retrocalcaneal
r. bursa
r. bursitis
r. exostosis
r. spur

retrocardiac
r. area
r. density
r. infiltrate
r. mass
r. space

retrocaval ureter
retrocecal
r. appendix
r. lymph node
r. recess

retrocerebellar
r. arachnoid cyst
r. CSF collection

retrochiasmal lesion
retroclavicular
retrococcygeal air study
retrocrural
r. adenopathy

r. air
r. lymphadenopathy
r. node
r. space

retrodental pannus
retrodiscal, retrodiskal
r. temporomandibular joint pad
inflammation
r. tissue

retrodiskal (*var. of* retrodiscal)
retrodisplaced fracture
retroduodenal recess
retroesophageal
r. aorta
r. arch
r. right subclavian artery
r. vessel

retrofenestral otosclerosis
retroflected (*var. of* retroflexed)
retroflection (*var. of* retroflexion)
retroflexed, retroflected
r. uterus
r. view

retroflexion, retroflection
uterine r.

retrogasserian target
retrogastric space
retroglandular lesion
retrograde
r. angiocardiography
r. arteriography
r. atherectomy
r. atrial activation mapping
r. block
r. blood flow across valve
r. blood velocity
r. cannulation
r. cardiac perfusion
r. cardioangiography
r. cholangiogram
r. coronary sinus infusion
r. cystogram
r. cystography
r. cystourethrography
r. degeneration
r. embolus
r. femoral aortography
r. femoral artery approach
r. femoral artery catheterization
r. filling
r. flow of gastric contents
r. injection
r. jejunoduodenogastric
intussusception
r. left ventriculogram
r. nephrostomy puncture
r. pancreatocholangiogram
r. pancreatography
r. peristalsis

retrograde (*continued*)
  r. pyelography
  r. refractory period
  r. systolic flow
  r. transaxillary aortography
  r. transfemoral aortography
  r. translumbar aortography
  r. transurethral prostatic urethroplasty
  r. ureteral pseudodiverticulum
  r. ureterogram
  r. ureterography
  r. ureteropyelogram
  r. urethrocystography
  r. urethrogram (RUG)
  r. urogram (RU)
  r. urography
  r. venous route
  r. ventriculoatrial conduction
retrohepatic vena cava
retroileal appendix
retroiliac ureter
retrolental fibroplasia
retrolisthesis
  vertebral body r.
retromalleolar
  r. groove
  r. sulcus
retromammary
  r. fascia
  r. fat
  r. fluid collection
  r. space
  r. space view
retromandibular
retromedullary arteriovenous malformation
retromembranous hematoma
retromolar
  r. trigone carcinoma
  r. trigone tumor
retronasal canal
retronuchal muscle
retroorbital space
retropancreatic tunnel
retroparotid space
retropectoral mammary implant
retroperfusion
  coronary sinus r.
  synchronized r.
retroperitoneal
  r. actinomycosis
  r. adenopathy
  r. air
  r. air study
  r. area
  r. calcification
  r. cavity
  r. cyst
  r. drain

  r. fat stripe displacement
  r. fibrosis (RPF)
  r. fistula
  r. gas insufflation
  r. hematoma
  r. hemorrhage
  r. infection
  r. leiomyosarcoma
  r. liposarcoma
  r. lymphadenopathy
  r. lymphangioma
  r. lymphatic vessel
  r. lymphoma
  r. neoplasm
  r. node
  r. organ
  r. pneumography
  r. pneumoradiography
  r. residual tumor mass
  r. space
  r. tumor
  r. tunnel
  r. viscus
retroperitoneum
retropharyngeal
  r. abscess
  r. hematoma
  r. hemorrhage
  r. lymph node
  r. narrowing
  r. soft tissue
  r. space
  r. space mass
retroplacental
  r. hematoma
  r. hemorrhage
retropneumoperitoneum
retropulsed fracture fragment
retropulsion
  vertebral body r.
retropyloric node
retrorectal
  r. cystic hamartoma
  r. lymph node
retrosomatic cleft
retrospective
  r. respiratory gating
  r. review
  r. synchronization
retrosphenoidal space
retrosternal
  r. airspace
  r. area
  r. mass
  r. soft tissue
  r. space
  r. thyroid
retrotorsion
  femoral r.

retrotracheal
r. adenoma
r. goiter
r. soft tissue
r. vessel
retrovascular goiter
retroversion
femoral r.
r. of acetabular cup
retrovertebral plexus
retroverted uterus
retrovesical
r. septum
r. space
retrovestibular neural pathway
retrusion
midface r.
Rett syndrome
return
anomalous pulmonary venous r.
arterial r.
impaired venous r.
infracardiac-type total anomalous
venous r.
interatrial transposition of venous
r.
paracardiac-type total anomalous
venous r.
partial anomalous pulmonary venous
r. (PAPVR)
pulmonary venous r.
supracardiac total anomalous venous
r.
systemic venous r.
r. to baseline
total anomalous pulmonary venous
r. (TAPVR)
venous r.
Retzius
R. foramen
R. ligament
line of R.
space of R.
R. system
R. vein
REV
room's-eye view
revalidation
revascularization
cerebral r.
coronary ostial r.
endosteal r.
foot r.
graft r.
infragenicular r.
infrainguinal r.
myocardial r.
percutaneous coronary r.
r. procedure

radiofrequency percutaneous
myocardial r. (RF-PMR)
renal artery r.
robotic coronary r.
transmyocardial r. (TMR)
revascularized tissue
**Reveal XVI PET/CT imaging
system**
reverberating flow pattern
reverberation
r. artifact
r. echo
reversal
end-systolic r.
gradient r.
mirror-image r.
r. of cervical lordosis
rapid gradient r.
shunt r.
r. sign
reverse
r. Barton fracture
r. Colles fracture
r. crescent pattern
r. distribution
r. fast imaging with steady-state
free precession (PSIF)
r. Hill-Sachs lesion
r. Monteggia fracture
r. pattern of signal intensity
r. peripheral batwing infiltrate
r. pivot shift (RPS)
r. Segond fracture
r. tennis elbow
r. transcriptase inhibitor
r. transport
r. Trendelenburg position
r. Waters plane
r. Waters position
reversed
r. coarctation
r. coarctation of aorta
r. ductus arteriosus
r. greater saphenous vein
r. peristalsis
r. shunt
r. Stenvers projection
r. vein graft
r. vertebral blood flow
reversed-3
r.-3 configuration
r.-3 sign
reversed-S sign
reversible
r. airway disease
r. bronchiectasis
r. ischemic defect
r. ischemic neurologic deficit
r. myocardial ischemia

R

reversible (*continued*)
    r. posterior leukoencephalopathy syndrome (RPLS)
    r. temporary myocardial dysfunction
    r. vasogenic edema
review
    retrospective r.
Revised European American Lymphoma (REAL)
Revitalase erbium cosmetic laser
revolving Ge-68 pin
Reynolds
    R. number (R_e, Re)
    R. relationship
REZ
    root exit zone
R&F
    radiography and fluoroscopy
    R&F camera
RF
    radiofrequency
        RF coil
        RF coil system
        RF pulse
        RF shielding
        RF spin echo
        RF spoiling
RFA
    radiofrequency ablation
        minimally invasive saline-enhanced RFA
        RFA with perfused needle applicator
RFCA
    radiofrequency catheter ablation
RF-FAST
    radiofrequency-spoiled Fourier-acquired steady-state technique
RFOV
    reconstruction field of view
RF-PMR
    radiofrequency percutaneous myocardial revascularization
RF-shielded cupboard
RF-spoiled FAST
RFW
    rapid filling wave
r-glutamyl transpeptidase (r-GT)
r-GT
    r-glutamyl transpeptidase
Rh
    rhodium
rhabdoid
    r. suture
    r. tumor
rhabdomyoblast
rhabdomyolysis
    exertional r.
    nontraumatic r.

    position-related r.
    traumatic r.
rhabdomyoma
    cardiac r.
    r. of heart
rhabdomyosarcoma (RMS), rhabdosarcoma
    abdominal r.
    alveolar r.
    bladder-prostate r.
    botryoid r.
    cardiac r.
    chest wall r.
    childhood r.
    embryonal r.
    extremity r.
    female genital tract r.
    genitourinary r.
    metastatic r.
    ocular r.
    orbital r.
    parameningeal r.
    paratesticular r.
    pleomorphic r.
    primary r.
    truncal r.
rhabdosarcoma (*var. of* rhabdomyosarcoma)
rhaphe (*var. of* raphe)
rhebosis
rhenium (Re)
    r. 186 ([186]Re, Re-186)
    r. 188 ([188]Re, Re-188)
    r. imaging agent
    r. isotope
rhenium-186 etidronate
rheography
    light-reflection r.
rheologic pattern
rheolytic mechanical thrombectomy device
Rhese
    R. projection
    R. view
    R. view of orbit
rheumatic
    r. adherent pericardium
    r. aortic insufficiency
    r. aortic valvular stenosis
    r. granuloma
    r. heart disease
    r. heart valve
    r. lesion
    r. mitral stenosis
    r. tricuspid stenosis
    r. valvular disease
rheumatica
    polymyalgia r.
    synovitis in active polymyalgia r.

rheumatism
    articular r.
    desert r.
    hydroxyapatite r.
rheumatoid
    r. arthritis
    r. factor
    r. lung disease
    r. nodule
    r. pneumoconiosis
    r. spondylitis
rheumatologist
rhinencephalic mamillary body
rhinitis gangrenosa progressiva
rhinoplasty
rhinoscintigraphy
    ^{99m}Tc MAA r.
rhinoscleroma
rhinosinusitis
rhizolysis
rhizomelia
rhizomelic
    r. chondrodysplasia punctata
    r. dysplasia
rhizotomy
    trigeminal r.
rhodium (Rh)
    r. anode
    r. filter
    r. isoimmunization
rhodium-rhodium target-filter
  combination
rhombencephalitis
    listerial r.
rhombencephalon
rhombencephalosynapsis
rhombic lip
rhomboid, rhomboidal
    r. fossa
    r. ligament
    r. major
    r. minor
    r. of Michaelis
rhomboidal (*var. of* rhomboid)
rhomboideus major muscle
rho transformation
RHV
    right hepatic vein
rhythm
    atrial bigeminal r.
    atrioventricular nodal r.
    A-V nodal r.
    bisferious pulse r.
    escape-capture r.
    idioventricular r. (IVR)
    mu r.
    nodal r.
    normal sinus r.
    reciprocal r.

    sinus r.
    transitional r.
    ventricular r.
rhythmic, rhythmical
    r. paradoxic eruption
    r. segmentation
rhythmical (*var. of* rhythmic)
RIA
    radioimmunoassay
    CA15-3 RIA
rib
    angle of r.
    beaded r.
    bed of r.
    bicipital r.
    bifid r.
    bone lesion of r.
    cervical r.
    r. contusion
    cough fracture of r.
    dense r.
    r. detail
    double-exposed r.
    r. dysplasia
    false r.
    floating r.
    r. fracture
    fused r.
    guillotine r.
    gumma of r.
    head of r.
    hyperlucent r.
    hypoplastic horizontal r.
    inferior margin of superior r.
    jail-bar r.
    r. lesion
    lumbar r.
    minced r.
    neck of r.
    r notching
    r. osteomyelitis
    overlapping r.
    penciling of r.
    periosteum of r.
    r. recession
    retracted r.
    r. ribbon
    rudimentary r.
    r. shadowing
    shaft of r.
    short r.
    slipping r.
    1st r.
    sternal r.
    Stiller r.
    superior border of r.
    superior margin of inferior r.
    5th r.
    true r.

R

rib (*continued*)
    r. tubercle
    twisted ribbonlike r.
    vertebral r.
    vertebrocostal r.   *vestigial*
    vertebrosternal r.
    r. view
    wide r.
rib-bearing vertebra
Ribbing disease
ribbon
    r. application
    r. bowel
    hollow r.
    ^{192}Ir r.
    r. muscle
    rib r.
    seed r.
    r. uterus
ribonucleic acid (RNA)
ribosyl
ribothymidine
ribulose
rib-vertebral angle difference
rice joint body
ricelike muscle calcification
Richter
    R. hernia
    R. syndrome
Richter-Monroe line
rickets classification
rickettsial lung infection
Rickham reservoir puncture
rider's
    r. bone
    r. muscle
    r. tendon
ridge
    alveodental r.
    alveolar r.
    apical ectodermal r. (AER)
    basal r.
    bisagittal r.
    bony r.
    broad maxillary r.
    buccogingival r.
    bulbar r.
    cerebral r.
    cranial r.
    cutaneous r.
    dental r.
    dorsal r.
    epicondylar r.
    epidermal r.
    epipericardial r.
    fibrocartilaginous r.
    fibromuscular r.
    ganglion r.
    gastrocnemial r.

    genital r.
    gluteal r.
    humeral r.
    interarticular r.
    interosseous r.
    intertrochanteric r.
    interureteric r.
    longitudinal r.
    marginal r.
    mylohyoid r.
    oblique r.
    palatine r.
    Passavant r.
    pectoral r.
    petrous r.
    radial r.
    rete r.
    sagittal r.
    semicircular r.
    septal r.
    sphenoid r.
    supraaortic r.
    supracondylar r.
    supracoronary r.
    supraorbital r.
    tentorial r.
    transverse r.
    triangular r.
    ulnar r.
    urethral r.
ridged convoluted villus
riding
    r. embolus
    r. stomach
Ridley sinus
Riedel
    R. lobe
    R. struma
    R. thyroiditis
Rieder
    R. cell
    R. cell leukemia
Riemann classification
Rieux hernia
RIF
    radiation-induced fibrosis
right
    r. and left ankle indices
    r. and left atrial phasic volumetric
      function
    r. anterior oblique (RAO)
    r. anterior oblique position
    r. anterior oblique position
      ventriculogram
    r. anterior oblique projection
    r. anterior oblique view
    r. aortic arch
    r. aortic arch with mirror-image
      branching

r. atrial appendage (RAA)
r. atrial chamber
r. atrial cuff
r. atrial enlargement (RAE)
r. atrial extension of uterine leiomyosarcoma
r. atrial hypertrophy
r. atrial pressure (RAP)
r. atrial sarcoma
r. atrium
r. atrium oxygen saturation
r. auricle
r. axis deviation (RAD)
r. border of heart
r. brain
r. bundle branch
r. bundle-branch block (RBBB)
r. cardiophrenic angle mass
r. colon
r. colonic flexure
r. coronary angiography (RCA)
r. coronary artery (RCA)
r. coronary cusp
r. coronary plexus
r. crus
r. descending pulmonary artery (RDPA)
r. femoral artery
r. gutter
r. heart catheterization
r. hemisphere
r. hepatic duct
r. hepatic vein (RHV)
r. hilar lymph node
r. ileocolic artery
r. inferior epigastric artery
r. internal iliac artery
r. internal jugular artery
r. lateral decubitus view
r. lobe bronchus
r. lobe of liver
r. lower lobe (RLL)
r. lower lobe atelectasis
r. lower lobe lesion
r. lower quadrant (RLQ)
r. lung
r. mainstem bronchus
r. mediastinum
r. middle lobe (RML)
r. middle lobe lingula
r. middle lobe syndrome
r. or left lateral decubitus film
r. ovarian artery
r. paratracheal stripe
r. posterior oblique (RPO)
r. posterior oblique position
r. posterior oblique projection
r. primary bronchus
r. pulmonary artery (RPA)

r. pulmonary vein (RPV)
r. subphrenic space
r. triangular ligament
r. upper lobe (RUL)
r. upper lobe lesion
r. upper quadrant (RUQ)
r. ventricle
r. ventricle of heart
r. ventricle-pulmonary artery conduit
r. ventricle-to-ear time
r. ventricle to main pulmonary artery pressure gradient
r. ventricular apex (RVA)
r. ventricular apical electrogram
r. ventricular assist device (RVAD)
r. ventricular branch of right coronary artery
r. ventricular cardiomyopathy
r. ventricular chamber
r. ventricular coil
r. ventricular conduction defect
r. ventricular diastolic pressure
r. ventricular dilation
r. ventricular dimension (RVD)
r. ventricular dysfunction (RVD)
r. ventricular dysplasia
r. ventricular ejection fraction (RVEF)
r. ventricular end-diastolic pressure
r. ventricular end-diastolic volume (RVEDV)
r. ventricular end-systolic volume (RVESV)
r. ventricular enlargement (RVE)
r. ventricular failure
r. ventricular hypertrophy (type A-C)
r. ventricular infarct
r. ventricular inflow view
r. ventricular infundibulum
r. ventricular internal diameter (RVID)
r. ventricular mass (RVM)
r. ventricular outflow obstruction
r. ventricular outflow tract (RVOT)
r. ventricular overload
r. ventricular peak systolic pressure
r. ventricular pressure (RVP)
r. ventricular strain
r. ventricular strain pattern
r. ventricular stroke volume
r. ventricular stroke work (RVSW)
r. ventricular stroke work index (RVSWI)
r. ventricular systolic/diastolic function

right (*continued*)
    r. ventricular to left ventricular
      systolic pressure ratio
    r. ventricular volume pressure
right-angled
    r.-a. chest tube
    r.-a. isosceles triangle board
    r.-a. telescopic lens
right-dominant coronary anatomy
right-handedness
    ventricular r.-h.
right-sided
    r.-s. angiocardiography
    r.-s. aortic arch
    r.-s. cardiomyopathy
    r.-s. empyema
    r.-s. heart failure
    r.-s. heart pressure
    r.-s. pneumonia
right-sidedness
    bilateral r.-s.
right-side-down decubitus position
right-to-left
    r.-t.-l. cardiac shunt
    r.-t.-l. shift
    r.-t.-l. shunting of blood
rightward
rigid
    r. endofluoroscopy
    r. manipulation
    r. ureter
rigidity
    lead-pipe r.
    nuchal r.
rigidus
    hallux r.
RigiScan Plus rigidity assessment
  system
Rigler
    R. sign
    R. triad
    R. triad of small bowel obstruction
RIGS
    radioimmunoguided surgery
    RIGS system
RIGScan CR49 imaging agent
RILD
    radiation-induced liver disease
Riley-Day syndrome
rim
    r. apophysis
    bony glenoid r.
    dark signal-intensity r.
    r. degeneration
    dorsal r.
    r. enhancement
    glenoid r.
    high-density r.
    hypoechoic r.

    intercartilaginous r.
    low-density r.
    r. nephrogram
    nephrogram r.
    r. of capsule
    r. of cartilage
    r. of fascia
    orbital r.
    r. resection
    sclerotic r.
    r. sign
    signal intensity r.
    volar r.
rim-enhancing lesion
rimlike calcium distribution
rim-rent tear
RIN
    radiation-induced necrosis
rind
    pleural r.
rindlike thickening
ring
    abdominal r.
    amnion r.
    anorectal r.
    r. apophysis
    r. apophysis calcification
    arc r.
    r. badge
    R. biliary drainage catheter
    r. blush on cerebral arteriography
    Carpentier r.
    Carpentier-Edwards r.
    cartilaginous r.
    ciliary r.
    common tendinous r.
    concatenation of shadows
    congenital r.
    constriction r.
    cortical r.
    r. detector
    distal esophageal r.
    double-populated detector r.
    drop-lock r.
    Duran r.
    echogenic r.
    r. enhancement
    r. epiphysis
    esophageal mucosal r.
    esophageal muscular r.
    external inguinal r.
    femoral r.
    fibrous r.
    r. finger
    r. fracture
    gestational r.
    R. guidewire
    halo r.
    Ilizarov r.

inguinal r.
internal abdominal r.
internal inguinal r.
Kayser-Fleischer r.
r. lesion
r. ligament
low-density r.
lower esophageal mucosal r.
mitral valve r.
mucosal r.
multiple concentric GI r.'s
r. of bone
r. of Vieussens
pelvic r.
perichondral r.
pyloric r.
r. scanner
Schatzki r.
r. shadow
r. sign
silastic r.
silicone elastomer r.
sodium iodide r.
stereotactic r.
sugar r.
summation of shadows
superficial inguinal r.
supravalvular r.
symptomatic vascular r.
tracheal r.
R. transjugular intrahepatic access
    set
trophoblastic r.
tubal r.
umbilical r.
valve r.
vascular r.
Waldeyer r.
Wimberger r.
ring-and-arc calcification
ring-around-the-artery sign
ring-disrupting fracture
ring-down
    r.-d. artifact
    r.-d. echo
ring-enhancing
    r.-e. brain lesion
    r.-e. mass
ringing
    edge r.
    Gibbs r.
ringlike
    r. appearance
    r. configuration
    r. contraction
    r. lesion
    r. pattern
    r. structure
ringman's shoulder

R

Ring-McLean sump drainage
  set
ring-of-bone concept
ring-shaped form
ring-type
    r.-t. imaging
    r.-t. imaging system
ring-wall lesion
Riolan
    R. arch
    R. artery
    R. muscle
    R. ossicle
Riordan
    R. clubhand classification
    R. finger pollicization
ripple voltage
RIS
    radiology information system
RISA
    radioactive iodinated serum
      albumin
    radioiodinated serum albumin
Riseborough-Radin intercondylar fracture
  classification
rise time
risk
    organs at r.
    radiation r.
risk-adapted CSI
Risser
    R. sign
    R. stage
Ritchie index
Rivero-Carvallo maneuver
Rivinus
    R. canal
    R. duct
RLL
    right lower lobe
RLQ
    right lower quadrant
RML
    right middle lobe
RMS
    rhabdomyosarcoma
rMTT
    regional mean transit time
Rn
    radon
^{222}Rn, Rn-222
    radon 222
RNA
    radionuclide angiogram
    ribonucleic acid
      gated RNA
RNV
    radionuclide ventriculogram
    radionuclide ventriculography

RNVG
    radionuclide ventriculogram
    radionuclide ventriculography
R/O
    rule out
ROA
    regurgitant orifice area
roadmap
roadmapping
    r. mode
    r. technique
Roadrunner NaviGuide
 guidewire
Robert ligament
robertsonian translocation
Roberts syndrome
Robin
    R. anomalad
    R. sequence
Robinow syndrome
robotic
    r. coronary revascularization
    r. mitral valve surgery
robotics-controlled stereotactic
 frame
Robson
    R. modification of Flocks-Kadesky
      system
    R. staging classification
robust
    r. registration
    r. registration technique
ROC
    receiver operating characteristic
    ROC curve
    ROC method
rockerbottom
    r. foot
    r. foot deformity
rocker deformity
rocking
    r. curve measurement
    r. precordial motion
Rockwood acromioclavicular injury
 classification
ROCM
    radiopaque contrast medium
rod
    Alta reconstruction r.
    Alta tibial/humeral r.
    r. eyelet
    Harrington r.
    Hopkins r.
    IM r.
    Isolar r.
    Luque r.
    medullary r.
    orthopaedic r.
    resorbable r.

    r. source
    thermoluminescent dosimeter r.
    TLD r.
rodding
    IM r.
    intramedullary r.
rodent ulcer
RODEO
    rotating delivery of excitation
      off-resonance
    3D RODEO
    RODEO imaging technique
rod-shaped calcification
Roederer obliquity
rOEF
    regional oxygen extraction fraction
roentgen
    r. knife
    r. kymography
    r. meter
    r.'s per hour at 1 meter
    r.'s per second (R/s)
    r. ray
    r. stereophotogrammetric
    r. stereophotogrammetric analysis
     (RSA)
    r. tube
    r. unit (RU)
roentgen-equivalent-man (REM)
    r.-e.-m. period (REMP)
roentgen-equivalent-physical (REP)
roentgenkymogram
roentgenkymograph
roentgenkymography
roentgenogram (*var. of* radiograph)
roentgenograph (*var. of* radiograph)
roentgenographic (*var. of* radiographic)
roentgenographically (*var. of*
 radiographically)
roentgenography (*var. of* radiography)
roentgenological (*var. of* radiologic)
roentgenologist (*var. of* radiologist)
roentgenology (*var. of* radiology)
roentgenometer (*var. of* radiometer)
roentgenometry (*var. of* radiometry)
roentgenoscope
roentgenoscopy
roentgenotherapy (*var. of* radiotherapy)
Rogan teleradiology system
Roger
    R. disease
    maladie de R.
    R. system
    R. ventricular septal defect
ROI
    region of interest
Rokitansky
    R. diverticulum
    R. lobe

R. nodule
R. pelvis
Rokitansky-Aschoff sinus
Rokitansky-Cushing ulcer
Rokitansky-Mayer-Küster-Hauser
 syndrome
Rokus view
rolandic
r. artery
r. cortex
r. fissure
r. sulcus
Rolando
R. angle
R. area
fissure of R.
R. fracture
R. line
R. point
R. tubercle
R. zone
rolandoparietal glioma
roll
log r.
radiolucent r.
rolled-edge deformity
rolled view
roller mark artifact
Rollet stroma
Rollier radiation
rolling
r. hiatal hernia
r. membrane
r. membrane Wallstent cobalt-based
 alloy balloon-expandable stent
roll-off
Rollo phantom
Rolloscope (II)
Romano-Ward syndrome
Romberg sign
Romberg-Wood syndrome
Romhilt-Estes score for left ventricular
 hypertrophy
ROMI
rule out myocardial infarct
RON
radiation-related optic neuropathy
R-on-T phenomenon
roof
acetabular r.
intercondylar r.
r. of 4th ventricle
roofless 4th ventricle diverticulum
room's-eye view (REV)
room shielding
root
anatomic r.
aortic r.
cervical nerve r.

cochlear r.
r. compression
coronary sinus r.
cranial r.
dental r.
dilacerated tooth r.
dilated aortic r.
r. end granuloma
r. entry zone
r. entry zone lesion
r. exit zone (REZ)
extrathecal nerve r.
facial r.
intradural nerve r.
intrathecal r.
lateral r.
lingual r.
lumbar nerve r.
lung r.
motor r.
nerve r.
r. of mesentery
r. of penis
palatine r.
retained r.
sensory r.
r. sleeve
spinal r.
ventral r.
ventricle r.
rootlet
intradural r.
root-mean-squared gradient measurement
ROPE
respiratory ordered phase
 encoding
ropelike cord
ropy
Rosai-Dorfman disease
rosary
r. bead configuration
r. beading
r. beading bone scintigraphy
r. beading esophagus
r. bead pattern
rachitic r.
Rosch hepatic catheter
Rosch-Uchida
R.-U. liver access set
R.-U. needle
R.-U. porta access set (RUPS)
rose
r. bengal dye
r. bengal ^{131}I radioactive
 agent
r. bengal sodium I-131 biliary
 imaging
R. criterion
r. thorn sign

Rose-Bradford kidney
Rosen
    R. curved guidewire
    R. wire
Rosenbach sign
Rosenmüller
    R. fossa
    R. node
    R. valve
Rosenthal
    basal vein of R. (BVR)
    R. canal
    R. fiber
rosette shape
Ross needle
rostra (*pl. of* rostrum)
rostral
    r. body of corpus callosum
    r. brainstem ischemia
    r. cervical nerve
    r. connection
    r. hypothalamus
    r. medulla
    r. pons
    r. spinal cord
    r. terminus
rostrocaudal extent signal abnormality
rostrum, *pl.* **rostra,** *pl.* **rostrums**
    r. of corpus callosum
    r. sphenoidale
rostrums (*pl. of* rostrum)
Rotablator thrombectomy system
rotary
    r. ankle instability
    r. deviation
    r. door flap (RDF)
    r. subluxation of scaphoid
    r. thoracolumbar scoliosis
rotatable pigtail catheter
rotated
    abducted and externally r.
    (ABER)
    r. craniocaudal view
rotate-rotate scan
rotate-stationary scan
rotating
    r. anode
    r. anode tube
    r. delivery of excitation
    off-resonance (RODEO)
    r. delivery of excitation
    off-resonance MR imaging
    r. disc oxygenator
    r. endoprobe
    r. frame
    r. frame of reference
    r. gamma camera
    r. Ge-68 rod source
    r. hemostatic valve

    r. raw cine data
    r. tomographic projection
    r. ultrafast imaging sequence
    (RUFIS)
rotating-frame
    r.-f. imaging
    r.-f. zeugmatography
rotation
    r. angle
    anisotropic r.
    r. anomaly
    axial r.
    center of r. (COR)
    360-degree r.
    degree of head r.
    gantry r.
    instantaneous axis of r. (IAR)
    internal femoral r.
    medial r.
    organoaxial r.
    r.'s per minute
    placenta r.
    pronation-external r.
    rapid gantry r.
    SPECT center of r.
    supination-external r. (SER)
    r. therapy
    tibiotalar r.
    tube position r.
rotational
    r. alignment
    r. angiography (RA)
    r. atherectomy system
    r. burst fracture
    r. contact lithotripsy
    r. coronary atherectomy (RCA)
    r. correlation time
    r. deformity
    r. dislocation
    r. displacement
    r. field
    r. force
    r. frequency
    r. instability
    r. malalignment
    r. method
    r. motion
    r. radiotherapy
    r. scanography
    r. therapy technique
    r. tomography
rotationally invariant imaging
rotation-shearing injury
rotator
    r. cuff
    r. cuff arthropathy
    r. cuff impingement
    r. cuff lesion
    r. cuff muscle

r. cuff tear
r. interval
rotatory
r. instability
r. load
r. load on spine
Rotch sign
Roth spot
Rotograph Plus panoramic dental tomography imaging system
rotography
Rotor syndrome
rotoscoliosis
rotoscoliotic deformity
Rotter node
rotundum
foramen r.
Rouget muscle
rough
r. calcific deposit
r. zone
roughened
r. articular surface
r. cartilage
r. state of pericardium
roughening
cortical r.
round
r. atelectasis
r. bone cell tumor
r. cancer of breast
r. cell liposarcoma
r. cell sarcoma
r. heart
r. lead marker
r. ligament
r. ligament artery
r. ligament of uterus
r. lucent lesion
r. muscle
r. pneumonia
r. pronator
r. shift
r. shoulder deformity
r. ulcer
roundback deformity
rounded
r. appearance
r. atelectasis
r. border of lung
r. convex border
r. lesion
r. opacity
Rous
R. sarcoma
R. tumor
route
hematogenous r.
retrograde venous r.

thoracic duct r.
translumbar aortic r.
urinary excretory r.
routine magnification view
Rouvière
R. ligament
R. node
Roux-en-Y
R.-e.-Y cystojejunostomy
R.-e.-Y gastrointestinal system procedure
R.-e.-Y hepaticojejunostomy
R.-e.-Y limb
R.-e.-Y takedown
Roux loop
Rovighi sign
Rovsing sign
row
carpal r.
distal carpal r.
proximal carpal r.
1st carpal r.
Rowasa enema
Rowe calcaneal fracture classification (type 1a, 1b, 1c, 2a, 2b, 3-5)
Rowe-Lowell fracture-dislocation classification
row-mode sinogram imaging
Royal Flush pigtail catheter
RPA
right pulmonary artery
RPF
retroperitoneal fibrosis
RPG
radiologic percutaneous gastrostomy
RPLS
reversible posterior leukoencephalopathy syndrome
RPM
real-time position management
RPM tracking system
RPO
right posterior oblique
RPOC
retained products of conception
RPS
reverse pivot shift
RPT
rapid pull-through technique
RPV
right pulmonary vein
RR
radiation response
rrBF
relative regional blood flow
RRP
relative refractory period
R/s
roentgens per second

823

RSA
    roentgen stereophotogrammetric
      analysis
RSI
    repetitive strain injury
    repetitive stress injury
RSNA
    Radiological Society of North America
RSV
    regurgitant stroke volume
RT
    radiation therapy
    radiotherapy
    registered technologist
    repetition time
      RT 3200 Advantage ultrasound
      RT 3200 Advantage ultrasound
        scanner
      RT 6800 ultrasound
      RT 6800 ultrasound scanner
RTAS
    rapid telephone access system
R-to-R imaging
RTP
    radiation therapy planning
    radiation treatment planning
      3D RTP
      RTP system
RTS
    radiation therapy system
      MammoSite RTS
RU
    retrograde urogram
    roentgen unit
Ru
    ruthenium
rub
    pericardial friction r.
rubber
    r. drain
    r. vessel loop
rubella
rubidium (Rb)
    r. 82 (^{82}Rb, Rb-82)
    r. chloride imaging agent
rubral tremor
Rubratope
Rubratope-57 imaging agent
Rudick red flag
rudimentary
    r. bone
    r. lung
    r. organ
    r. outlet chamber
    r. pronephros
    r. rib
    r. sinus
    r. ventricle
    r. ventricular chamber

Ruedi-Allgower
    R.-A. tibial plafond fracture
    R.-A. tibial plafond fracture
      classification
ruffled border formation
RUFIS
    rotating ultrafast imaging sequence
RUG
    retrograde urethrogram
ruga, *pl.* **rugae**
    gastric rugae
rugae (*pl. of* ruga)
rugal
    r. fold
    r. pattern
rugger
    r. jersey appearance
    r. jersey sign
    r. jersey spine
    r. jersey vertebra
rugose, rugous
rugous (*var. of* rugose)
RUL
    right upper lobe
rule
    Buffalo malleolar r.
    modified Simpson r.
    OAR malleolar r.
    r. of threes
    r. of twos
    Ottawa ankle r.
    r. out (R/O)
    r. out myocardial infarct (ROMI)
    pheochromocytoma r. of 10
rule-based scheme
ruler
    endocatheter r.
Rumstrom view
run
    high frame-rate r.
    low frame-rate r.
Rundles-Falls syndrome
runner's
    r. bump
    r. knee
runoff
    absent r.
    aortic r.
    aortofemoral r.
    arterial r.
    r. arteriography
    digital r.
    distal r.
    r. film
    inadequate r.
    peripheral r.
    r. resistance index
    single-vessel r.
    suboptimal r.

vessel r.
2-vessel r.
3-vessel r.
Runström projection
Runyon classification
RUPS
    Rosch-Uchida porta access set
RUPS-100 liver access set
rupture
    Achilles tendon r.
    amnion r.
    aneurysmal r.
    aortic r.
    appendix r.
    arch r.
    arterial dilation and r.
    Berry aneurysm r.
    bladder r.
    breast prosthesis r.
    bronchial r.
    bulbomembranous urethral r.
    buttonhole r.
    cardiac r.
    chordae tendineae r.
    chordal r.
    complex extraperitoneal r.
    contained aneurysmal r.
    contained aortic r.
    delayed splenic r.
    diaphragmatic r.
    esophageal r.
    extraperitoneal bladder r.
    forniceal r.
    frank r.
    hemidiaphragm r.
    hepatic capsular r.
    hernia r.
    interventricular septal r.
    intramural esophageal r.
    intraperitoneal bladder r.
    intratendinous r.
    mesenteric r.
    myocardial r.
    myotendinous junction r.
    nodal r.
    r. of myocardium
    papillary muscle r.
    plantaris r.
    plaque r.
    pregnant uterus r.
    premature uterine membrane r.
    silicone implant r.
    simple extraperitoneal r.
    splenic r.
    spontaneous r.
    subbursal r.
    tendon r.
    testicular r.
    tracheobronchial r.

traumatic aortic r.
urinary bladder r.
ventricular free wall r.
ventricular septal r.
vessel r.
ruptured
    r. aneurysm
    r. aortic cusp
    r. capillary
    r. chordae tendineae
    r. disc
    r. ectopic pregnancy
    r. emphysematous bleb
    r. follicle
    r. hollow viscus
    r. pelvic varix
    r. plaque
    r. spleen
    r. thoracic duct
    r. ulcer
RUQ
    right upper quadrant
Rusch catheter
rush
    peristaltic r.
Russell
    R. body
    R. effect
Russell-Rubinstein cerebrovascular
  malformation classification
Russell-Silver
    R.-S. dwarfism
    R.-S. syndrome
Russian spring-summer encephalitis
ruthenium (Ru)
rutherford
    R. clinical stage of peripheral
      vascular disease
    r. unit
Rutherford-Becker claudication category
  (1-5)
Rutner balloon-dilation helical stone
  extractor set
Ruvalcaba-Myhre-Smith syndrome
Ruysch
    R. disease
    R. muscle
RV
    residual volume
RVA
    right ventricular apex
    RVA electrogram
RVAD
    right ventricular assist device
RVD
    right ventricular dimension
    right ventricular dysfunction
RVE
    right ventricular enlargement

R

RVEDV
  right ventricular end-diastolic volume
RVEF
  right ventricular ejection fraction
RVESV
  right ventricular end-systolic volume
RVG
  radionuclide ventriculogram
  radionuclide ventriculography
RVH
  renovascular hypertension
  right ventricular hypertrophy
   (type A-C)
RVID
  right ventricular internal diameter

RVM
  right ventricular mass
RVOT
  right ventricular outflow tract
RVP
  right ventricular pressure
RVSW
  right ventricular stroke work
RVSWI
  right ventricular stroke work index
RVT
  renal vein thrombosis
RX
  rapid exchange
   RX stent delivery system

S
   sulfur
      S contour
      S distortion
      S number
      S shape
      S sign of Golden
      S value
³⁵S
   sulfur 35
S-35
   sulfur 35
S-A
   sinuatrial
      S-A block
SA
   sinuatrial
      SA node
SAAV
   simultaneous acquisition of artery and
   vein
SAB
   sinuatrial block
saber-sheath trachea
saber-shin
      s.-s. appearance
      s.-s. deformity
sabot
      coeur en s.
      s. heart
Sabourand-Noiré instrument
Sabouraud pastil
sac
      abdominal s.
      air s.
      alveolar s.
      amnionic s.
      aneurysmal s.
      aortic s.
      blind s.
      bursal s.
      chorionic s.
      common dural s.
      cystic s.
      decidual s.
      dental s.
      double decidual s.
      dural s.
      embryonic s.
      empty gestational s.
      endolymphatic s.
      enterocele s.
      false s.
      fluid-filled s.

      gestational s. (GS)
      greater peritoneal s.
      heart s.
      hernia s.
      hydronephrotic s.
      indirect hernia s.
      intrauterine s.
      lacrimal s.
      lesser peritoneal s.
      lymphatic s.
      narrowing of thecal s.
      s. of aneurysm
      pericardial s.
      peritoneal s.
      pleural s.
      primary yolk s.
      primitive yolk s.
      pseudogestational s.
      residual aneurysmal s.
      sacral s.
      secondary yolk s.
      spinal s.
      terminal air s.
      thecal s.
      tight dural s.
      wide-mouth s.
      wrapped aneurysmal s.
      yolk s.
sacciform
      s. aneurysm
      s. kidney
      s. recess
saccular
      s. blood vessel
      s. bronchiectasis
      s. cerebral aneurysm
      s. collection
      s. dilation
      s. ectasia
      s. formation
      s. malformation
      s. mass
      s. outpouching
      s. pseudoaneurysm
sacculated pleurisy
sacculation
saccule
sacculocochlear canal
sacculoutricular canal
sacculus ventricularis
Sack-Barabas syndrome
saclike
      s. cavity
      s. space
sacra (*pl. of* sacrum)

sacral
- s. agenesis
- s. ala
- s. aneurysm
- s. bone
- s. bone tumor
- s. canal
- s. chordoma
- s. crest
- s. cyst
- s. dysgenesis
- s. foramen
- s. gutter
- s. hyperintensity
- s. insufficiency fracture (SIF)
- s. lymph node
- s. meningocele
- s. nerve
- s. osteolysis
- s. osteomyelitis
- s. osteosarcoma
- s. plexus
- s. process
- s. promontory
- s. sac
- s. spine
- s. vertebra

sacralization
sacralized transverse process
sacrococcygeal
- s. chordoma
- s. inferior pubic point (SCIPP)
- s. inferior pubic point line
- s. joint
- s. remnant tumor
- s. teratoma

sacrodural ligament
sacrogenital fold
sacrohorizontal angle
sacroiliac (SI)
- s. articulation
- s. disease
- s. fracture
- s. infection
- s. joint
- s. joint fusion
- s. joint widening
- s. sprain
- s. subluxation

sacrolumbar dysgenesis
sacropubic diameter
sacrosciatic
- s. foramen
- s. notch

sacrospinalis muscle
sacrospinous ligament
sacrotuberous ligament
sacrouterine

sacrovertebral angle
sacrum, *pl.* **sacra**
- cornu of s.
- tilted s.

SACT
- sinuatrial conduction time

saddle
- s. clot
- s. coil
- s. embolus
- s. joint
- s. lesion
- s. peristalsis of ureter
- s. point

saddle-shaped
- s.-s. uterine fundus
- s.-s. uterus

Sadowsky breast marking system
SAE
- stimulated acoustic emission

SAECG, SaECG
- signal-averaged electrocardiogram

Saemisch ulcer
Saethre-Chotzen acrocephalosyndactyly
SafeFlo IVC filter
SAFHS
- sonic-accelerated fracture-healing system
- SAFHS 2000
- Exogen 2000 SAFHS

Saf-T-Intima integrated IV catheter
Sage-Salvatore classification I-III of acromioclavicular joint injury
sagging
- s. brain
- s. gallbladder

sagittal
- s. and coronal reconstruction views
- s. canal diameter (SCD)
- s. celloidin section
- s. cranial suture
- s. fast spin-echo T2-weighted MR imaging
- s. fat-suppressed T1-weighted 3D spoiled gradient-echo image
- s. fontanelle
- s. gradient-echo imaging
- s. groove
- s. HR-MR
- s. localization
- s. magnetization transfer view
- s. oblique imaging
- s. orientation
- s. paraffin section
- s. plane
- s. plane fault
- s. plane loop
- s. plane vectorcardiography

s. porta hepatis
s. ramus osteotomy (SRO)
s. ridge
s. roll spondylolisthesis
s. scan
s. scout image
s. sinus
s. slice
s. synostosis
s. thrombosis
s. tomogram
s. tomographic reconstruction
s. transabdominal imaging
s. T1-weighted MR image
s. ultrasound

SAH
subarachnoid hemorrhage

Sahara
S. clinical bone sonometer
S. portable bone densitometer

sail-like tricuspid valve
sail sign
Saint (St.)
S. triad

Sakellarides classification of calcaneal fracture
Saldino-Noonan syndrome
Salem sump tube
salient
saline
s. chaser
s. chaser bolus
s. enema
s. implant
s. infusion sonohysterography (SIS)
s. solution
s. solution flush
s. torch

saline-enhanced
s.-e. MR arthrography
s.-e. MR imaging
s.-e. radiofrequency tissue ablation

salivagram
salivary
s. calculus
s. duct carcinoma
s. gland
s. gland carcinoma
s. gland dysfunction
s. gland function study
s. gland infection
s. gland lymphoepithelioma
s. gland scan
s. gland scintigraphy
s. stone

Salla disease
Salmonella **vertebral osteomyelitis**
salmon-patch hemorrhage
salpinges (*pl. of* salpinx)

salpingitis
chronic interstitial s.
follicular s.
hemorrhagic s.
interstitial s.
s. isthmica nodosa
pseudofollicular s.
purulent s.
tuberculous s.

salpingogram
salpingography
selective osteal s.

salpingopharyngeus
salpingoscopy
salpinx, *pl.* **salpinges**
salt-and-pepper
s.-a.-p. chromatin pattern
s.-a.-p. duodenal erosion

saltans
coxa s.
hallux s.

Salter-Harris
S.-H. classification of epiphysial fracture (group 1-5)
S.-H. growth plate injury classification

Salter-Harris-Rang epiphysial fracture classification (1a, b, c, 2a, b, c, 3a, b, 4a, b, 5-9)
salt-losing nephritis
Saltzman anatomy
salvage
s. of myocardium
s. radiotherapy
s. therapy

salvo of echoes
SAM
scanning acoustic microscope
systolic anterior motion

samarium (Sm)
s. 153 (^{153}Sm, Sm-153)
s. imaging agent
s. scintigraphy

samarium-153
s.-153 ethylenediamine tetramethylene phosphonate (Sm-153 EDTMP)
s.-153 ethylenediamine tetramethylene phosphonic acid therapy

SAMBA
simultaneous areolar mastopexy and breast augmentation
SAMBA imaging system

same-day
s.-d. exercise-rest Tc-99m tetrofosmin myocardial perfusion scintigraphy
s.-d. microsurgical arthroscopic lateral-approach laser-assisted fluoroscopic discectomy

sampling
>angular s.
>asymmetric data s.
>s. error
>Gibbs s.
>length-biased s.
>nonlinear s.
>partial k-space s.
>percutaneous umbilical blood s.
>portal venous s.
>s. window
>zonal s.

SAN
>sinuatrial node

Sanchez-Perez cassette changer

sanctuary
>s. organ
>s. site

sand
>S. process
>s. tumor

sandal-gap deformity
sandbagging fracture
sandbag hazard
Sanders sign
sandlike lucency
sandwich
>s. appearance
>s. configuration
>s. configuration adenopathy
>s. patch closure
>s. sign
>s. technique
>s. vertebra

sandwiched gadolinium
Sanfilippo syndrome
sanguifacient
sanguiferous
sanguification
sanguineous
Sansom sign
Sansregret method
Santavuori-Haltia disease
Santiani-Stone classification of pancreatitis
Santorini
>S. canal
>S. duct
>S. ligament
>S. muscle
>S. papilla

SAPA
>spatial average-pulse average

saphenofemoral junction
saphenous
>s. nerve
>s. system
>s. varix
>s. vein

>s. vein bypass graft
>s. vein incompetence
>s. vein mapping
>s. vein stenosis

SAPHO
>synovitis, acne, pustulosis, hyperostosis, osteomyelitis
>SAPHO syndrome

SAP-MS
>superabsorbent polymer microsphere
>SAP-MS transarterial embolization

saponated cresol solution
Sappey
>S. inferior vein
>S. ligament
>S. line

saprophytic
>s. aspergillosis
>s. colonization

SAR
>scatter-air ratio
>specific absorption rate

sarcocarcinoma
sarcofetal pregnancy
sarcohysteric pregnancy
sarcoid
>s. granuloma
>lung s.
>s. uveitis

sarcoidlike reaction
sarcoidosis
>acinar s.
>alveolar s.
>bone s.
>breast s.
>cardiac s.
>endobronchial s.
>hepatic s.
>musculocutaneous s.
>ocular s.
>orbital s.
>osteosclerosis vertebral s.
>pulmonary s.
>skeletal s.
>spinal cord s.
>spleen s.
>systemic s.
>thoracic s.

sarcoma
>African Kaposi s.
>alveolar soft part s. (ASPS)
>ameloblastic s.
>angiolithic s.
>bone-forming s.
>botryoid s.
>breast s.
>cardiac s.
>cerebellar s.
>cervical s.

clear cell s.
diaphragmatic s.
embryonal liver s.
endobronchial Kaposi s.
endometrial stromal s.
epithelioid s.
Ewing s.
extraosseous Ewing s.
fascicular s.
fibromyxoid s.
giant cell s.
granulocytic s.
hemangioendothelial bone s.
hemangioendothelial liver s.
hepatic anaplastic s.
intrathoracic Kaposi s.
Kaposi s. (KS)
Kupffer cell s.
lymphatic s.
malignant myeloid s.
meningeal s.
mesenterial s.
mesodermal s.
mixed-cell s.
multiple idiopathic hemorrhagic s.'s
muscle s.
neurogenic s.
orbital granulocytic s.
osseous and soft tissue s.'s (OSTS)
osteogenic s.
periosteal s.
pleomorphic s.
primary s.
pulmonary artery s.
pulmonary Kaposi s.
radiation-induced s.
radioinduced s.
reticulum bone cell s.
reticulum brain cell s.
right atrial s.
round cell s.
Rous s.
soft tissue s.
synovial s.
tenosynovial s.
undifferentiated liver s.
vascular s.
vasoablative endothelial s. (VABES)
sarcomatoid
sarcomatosis
diffuse s.
sclerosing osteogenic s.
sarcomatous
sarcomere
SARS
severe acute respiratory syndrome
SARS-associated coronavirus pneumonia
sartorius
s. insertion

s. muscle
s. tendon
SAS
supravalvular aortic stenosis
SA-SD
subacromial-subdeltoid
SA-SD bursitis
Sassouni analysis
satellite
s. cartilaginous focus
s. lesion
s. metastasis
s. node
s. nodule
s. structure
satellite-borne phased array (SBPA)
satellitosis
satiety
early s.
Sat Pad
satumomab
s. pendetide
s. pendetide imaging agent
saturated potassium iodide solution (SSKI)
saturation
s. analysis
aortic oxygen s.
arterial oxygen s.
s. band
s. current
fat s.
frequency-selective fat s.
gaussian line s.
s. index
s. inversion projection (SIP)
jugular venous oxygen s.
line s.
lorentzian line s.
mixed venous s.
MT s.
off-resonance s.
oxygen s.
partial s.
progressive spin s.
s. pulse
s. recovery
s. recovery image
s. recovery sequence
s. recovery technique
regional cerebral oxygen s.
right atrium oxygen s.
selective s.
spatial-spectral prepulses for fat s.
spectral s.
s. stripe
systemic oxygen s.
s. transfer
T1-weighted axial image with fat s.

S

saucerization of vertebra
saucer-shaped excavation
sausage
    s. digit
    s. digit sign
    s. finger
    s. segment effect
sausage-shaped appearance
sausaging of vein
Sauvage filamentous velour graft
SAVANT
    surgical anatomy visualization and
      navigation tool
    SAVANT imaging system
S7 AVE stent
sawtooth
    s. appearance
    s. configuration
    s. edge
    s. excretory pattern
    s. irregularity of bowel contour
    s. sign
    s. ureter
sawtoothlike thickening
SBDX
    scanning-beam digital
      x-ray
SBE
    single-balloon enteroscope
    small bowel enteroscopy
SBF
    systemic blood flow
SBFT
    small bowel followthrough
SBO
    small bowel obstruction
    spina bifida occulta
SBP
    solitary bone plasmacytoma
SBPA
    satellite-borne phased array
SBS
    shaken baby syndrome
SBSP
    simultaneous bilateral spontaneous
      pneumothorax
Sc
    scandium
^{47}Sc, Sc-47
    scandium 47
SCA
    Simpson Coronary AtheroCath
    single-channel analyzer
    superior cerebellar artery
      SCA system
scabbard trachea
SCAD
    spontaneous coronary artery
      dissection

scalar
    s. coupling
    s. effect
scalariform
scale
    abbreviated injury s. (AIS)
    Bloch s.
    color-flame s.
    digital gray s.
    ECOG s.
    Edmonton Symptom Assessment S.
    expanded disability status s.
    extended computed tomography s.
     (ECTS)
    false color s.
    Fletcher dyspnea s.
    Flint colon injury s.
    Glasgow coma s. (GCS)
    Glasgow outcome s. (GOS)
    gray s.
    Hunt and Hess subarachnoid
     hemorrhage s.
    injury severity s. (ISS)
    Memorial Symptom Assessment S.
    National Institutes of Health stroke
     s. (NIHSS)
    relative value s.
    Scandinavian stroke s.
    unified Parkinson disease rating s.
scalene
    s. fat-pad
    s. maneuver
    s. musculature
    s. node
    s. triangle
    s. tubercle
scalenus
    s. anterior
    s. anterior muscle
    s. anticus muscle hypertrophy
    s. anticus syndrome
    s. medius
    s. minimus
    s. minimus muscle
scale-physical
    Memorial Symptom Assessment S.-P.
scaler
    s. counter
    decade s.
scaling
    s. device
    quantization matrix s.
scalloped
    s. appearance
    s. appearance of white matter
    s. border
    s. bowel lumen
    s. commissure
    s. luminal configuration

scalloping
> bone tumor s.
> s. contour
> cortical s.
> endosteal s.
> s. of margin of vertebral body
> s. osteolysis
> petrous pyramid s.
> posterior vertebral s.
> vertebral s.

scalp
> s. branch of external carotid artery
> s. hematoma
> s. hypothermia
> s. injury
> s. vein needle

scalpel
> s. cut
> interactive electronic s.
> ultrasonically activated s.

scan (*see also* **scintiscan**)
> A s.
> abdominal CT s.
> adrenal s.
> aerosol ventilation s.
> A-mode amplitude modulation s.
> attenuation s.
> axial s.
> axial unenhanced CT s.
> B s.
> Becton-Dickinson FAC s.
> bile duct s.
> biphasic helical CT s.
> blank s.
> blood pool radionuclide s.
> B-mode brightness modulation s.
> bone s.
> bone marrow s.
> brain s.
> bremsstrahlung s.
> brightness modulation s.
> C s.
> capillary blockade perfusion
> C-mode s.
> carcinoembryonic antigen s.
> cardiac s.
> CardioTec s.
> CE-FAST s.
> cerebral perfusion SPECT s.
> cine-CT s.
> cine view in MUGA s.
> clearance phase ventilation s.
> ^{11}C-methionine PET s.
> coincidence detection s.
> colloid shift on s.
> color-flow duplex s.
> computed tomography s.
> contiguous s.'s
> s. converter

coregistered s.
coronal s.
coronary artery s. (CAS)
crazy paving pattern on chest
  CT s.
CT s.
s. decrement
s. defect
delayed-phase s.
dental s.
depreotide s.
DEXA s.
diffusion s.
diuretic renal s.
dot s.
double helical CT s.
2D sector s.
dual-B206 isotope myocardial s.
dual-isotope osteomyelitis s.
dual-phase s.
duplex Doppler s.
dynamic CT s.
dynamic emission s.
elbow coronal s.
electromagnetic interference s.
EMI s.
enhanced CT s.
equilibrium MUGA s.
^{18}FDG-PET s.
FDG-PET s.
s. field of view (SFOV)
F-labeled levodopa PET s.
flow portion of bone s.
fluorescent s.
18-fluoro-deoxyglucose PET s.
full-body CT s.
^{67}Ga bone s.
gadolinium s.
gallium s.
gamma s.
gastric emptying s.
gated blood pool s.
3-head s.
Heart CT s.
helical thin-section CT s.
hepatobiliary s.
hepatoiminodiacetic acid s.
HIDA s.
ictal PET s.
ictal SPECT s.
^{125}I fibrinogen s.
indium-111-labeled white blood
  cell s.
indium-111 leukocyte s.
indium-111 zevalin antibody s.
infarct s.
^{111}In pentetreotide s.
Insight Millennium s.
interictal SPECT s.

S

scan (*continued*)
    intravenously enhanced CT s.
    iodine-131 whole-body s.
    isotope bone s.
    isotope lung s.
    kidney s.
    krypton s.
    labeled leukocyte s.
    lacrimal s.
    left-side-down decubitus s.
    left ventricular gated blood pool s.
    liver s.
    liver-lung s.
    liver-spleen s.
    longitudinal s.
    lung s.
    MAG3 Lasix renal s.
    mechanical compound s.
    Meckel s.
    medronate s.
    MET-PET s.
    MIBG SPECT s.
    Miraluma s.
    M-mode time-motion s.
    ^{99m}Tc HMPAO-labeled leukocyte
     total-body s.
    ^{99m}Tc-labeled macroaggregated
     albumin s.
    ^{99m}Tc WBC s.
    MUGA s.
    multidetector-row CT s.
    multiple gated acquisition s.'s
    multiple gated blood pool s.'s
    multiple-line s. (MLS)
    multislice full line s.
    myocardial perfusion s.
    NMR s.
    noncontrast CT s.
    nonenhanced CT s.
    nongated CT s.
    nuclear magnetic resonance s.
    nucleotide s.
    octreotide tumor localization s.
    oral enhanced CT s.
    s. orientation
    pancreatic s.
    panoramic CT s.
    paraisopropyliminodiacetic acid
     technetium-99m hepatobiliary s.
    s. parameter
    pelvic ultrasound CT s.
    pentetreotide tumor localization s.
    perfusion lung s.
    PET s.
    3-phase bone s.
    PIPIDA s.
    s. pitch
    s. pitch pit
    planar brain s.

    planar thallium s.
    s. plane
    portal phased spiral CT s.
    postgadolinium s.
    postictal cerebral blood flow s.
    postinjection attenuation s.
    postmetrizamide CT s.
    precontrast s.
    preoperative resting MUGA s.
    ProstaScint s.
    proton-density axial MR s.
    PYP technetium myocardial s.
    pyrophosphate technetium myocardial
     s.
    quantitative s.
    radioactive brain s.
    radioactive fibrinogen s.
    radioactive iodinated serum albumin s.
    radioactive iodine s.
    radiofibrinogen uptake s.
    radioisotope lung s.
    radionuclide bone s.
    radionuclide flow s.
    radionuclide gated blood pool s.
    radionuclide liver s.
    radionuclide milk s.
    radionuclide tagged red blood cell
     bleeding s.
    radionuclide thyroid s.
    rapid sequential CT s.
    rCBF PET s.
    real-time s.
    rebreathing ventilation s.
    rectilinear bone s.
    rectilinear thyroid s.
    redistributed thallium s.
    renal duplex s.
    rotate-rotate s.
    rotate-stationary s.
    sagittal s.
    salivary gland s.
    scintillation s.
    sector s.
    segmental lung defect s.
    segmenting dual-echo MR
     head s.
    selective excitation line s.
    s. sequence
    Seratec s.
    serial duplex s.'s
    single-pass s.
    single-photon emission computed
     tomography technetium sestamibi s.
    single-sweep s.
    spatially normalized PET and
     SPECT s.'s
    spin-echo s.
    spiral CT s.
    spleen s.

splenic perfusion measurement by dynamic CT s.
s. spot
stacked s.
static emission s.
stereotactic CT s.
stimulation s.
stress thallium s.
strip s.
sulfur colloid s.
suppression s.
survey s.
TcO₄ thyroid s.
teboroxime cardiac s.
TechneLite s.
technetium 99m hepatoiminodiacetic acid s.
technetium 99m methylene diphosphonate s.
technetium 99m phytate s.
technetium 99m tagged red blood cell s.
thallium-201 s.
thallium myocardial s.
thallium single-photon emission computed tomography s.
thorium-201 SPECT s.
thyroid stimulation s.
thyroid suppression s.
thyroid whole-body s.
s. time
tomographic brain s.
transabdominal ultrasound s.
transaxial CT s.
transaxial joint s.
transaxial PET s.
transmission s.
transverse s.
triple-phase bone s.
T2-weighted s.
ultrafast CT s.
unenhanced magnetic resonance imaging s.
uniform phantom s.
venous s.
ventilation lung s.
ventilation-perfusion lung s.
s. volume
volumetric s.
V/Q lung segment s.
washout-phase ventilation s.
water path s.
water signal on magnetic resonance imaging s.
whole-body bone s.
whole-body PET s.
whole-body transmission s.
s. with contrast enhancement
ZeroRad MRI s.

Scandinavian stroke scale
Scanditronix
    S. 1024-7B camera
    S. MLC system
    S. PET scanner
scandium (Sc)
    s. 47 (^{47}Sc, Sc-47)
Scanmaster DX x-ray film digitizer scanner
scannable tumor
scanned
    s. focal point (SFP)
    s. projection radiography (SPR)
scanner (*see also* **scintiscanner**)
    Acuson 128EP s.
    Acuson Sequoia 512 s.
    Acuson XP 10 s.
    Advanced NMR Systems s.
    Agfa Medical s.
    All-Tronics s.
    Aloka ultrasound linear s.
    Aloka ultrasound sector s.
    American Shared-CuraCare s.
    ANMR Insta-scan MR s.
    Aquilion combined CT-fluoroscopy s.
    Aquilion Plus V-detector CT s.
    Artoscan MRI s.
    ATL Mark 600 real-time sector s.
    ATL Neurosector real-time s.
    Aura Laser helical s.
    Aurora MR breast imaging system s.
    Biograph Duo LSO PET/CT s.
    BioSpec MR imaging system s.
    biplane sector s.
    Brilliance 40 s.
    Bruel-Kjaer ultrasound s.
    Bruker s.
    C300 s.
    Canon s.
    Cardio Data MK3 Holter s.
    cardiovascular computed tomographic s.
    Cencit surface s.
    CereTom portable CT s.
    charge-coupled device s.
    cine-CT s.
    C-150 LXP EBT s.
    coincidence imaging s.
    combined CT-fluoroscopy s.
    CPET s.
    CT9000, 9800 s.
    CT body s.
    CTI 933/04 ECAT s.
    CTI 931 PET s.
    CT Max 640 s.
    C-150 XP s.
    dedicated head s.
    dedicated PET s.

S

scanner (*continued*)
Delarnette s.
Diasonics ultrasound s.
Discovery LS, ST⁴ PET/CT s.
Dornier s.
DSR s.
3D surface digitizer s.
dual-probe rectilinear s.
duplex s.
DuPont s.
Eastman Kodak s.
EBT s.
Echospeed Signa LX 1.5T s.
electron beam CT s.
Elscint Excel 905 s.
Elscint MR s.
Elscint Twin CT s.
eMed s.
EMI 7070 s.
EMI brain s.
EMI CT 500 s.
Esaote extremity s.
e-speed EBT s.
Evolution CT s.
Evolution XP s.
Flexart MRI s.
FONAR-360 MRI s.
full-ring s.
Galen Scan s.
gamma ray s.
Gammex RMI s.
gated CT s.
GE Advance PET s.
GE CT Advantage s.
GE CTI 9800 s.
GE CTI single-detector s.
GE CT Max s.
GE CT Pace s.
GE CT/T7 s.
GE CT/T 8800 s.
GE Discovery LS CT/PET s.
GE Genesis CT s.
GE GN s.
GE 9800 high-resolution CT s.
GE HiSpeed Advantage helical
 CT s.
GE HiSpeed single-detector s.
GE Lightspeed CT s.
GE MR Max s.
GE MR Signa s.
GE MR Vectra s.
GE Omega s.
GE Pace CT s.
GE QE s.
GE Signa 4.7 MRI s.
GE Signa 1.5T s.
GE Signa 5.2 with SR-230 3-axis
 EPI gradient upgrade s.
GE Spiral CT s.

GE Vectra MR s.
Gyroscan ACS-NT MRI s.
Gyroscan ACS-NT 1.5T MR s.
Gyroscan Interna s.
Gyroscan S15 s.
Harvard multidetector s.
helical CT s.
Hewlett-Packard s.
high-field open MRI s.
high field-strength s.
HighSpeed CT s.
HiLight Advantage System CT s.
HiSpeed Advantage helical s.
HiSpeed Advantage System CT s.
Hitachi CT s.
Hitachi MR s.
Hitachi Open MRI system s.
Hitachi 0.3T unit s.
Hologic 2000 s.
Hologic QDR 1000W dual-energy
 x-ray absorptiometry s.
Horizon LX s.
Howtek Scanmaster DX s.
IDSI s.
Imatron C-100 EBT s.
Imatron C-150L EBCT s.
Imatron C-1000 UFCT s.
Imatron C-100 Ultrafast CT s.
Imatron C-150XL CT s.
Imatron C-100XP CT s.
Imatron Fastrac C-100 cine x-ray
 CT s.
Imatron Ultrafast CT s.
Indomitable s.
Innervision MR s.
InstaScan s.
integrated CT s.
Integris 3000 s.
Irex Exemplar ultrasound s.
IRIS s.
Konica s.
large-bore 0.6T, 1.5T imaging
 system s.
LightSpeed multidetector CT s.
LightSpeed QXi CT s.
linear-array CCD s.
lower field-strength MRI s.
low-field MR s.
low-field open s.
Lumiscan LS 85 s.
Lumisys 20 digital x-ray s.
Lunar s.
lutetium oxyorthosilicate-based
 PET s.
LymphoScan nuclear imaging
 system s.
3M s.
Magna-SL s.
Magnes 2500 whole-blood s.

Magnetom SP63 s.
Magnetom Symphony MR s.
Magnetom Symphony whole-body s.
Magnetom 1.5T s.
Magnetom Vision s.
Magnex MR s.
Mallinckrodt s.
Malvern 2600 Sizer laser
  diffraction s.
Max Plus MR s.
mechanical sector s.
MedImage s.
Medison s.
Medspec MR imaging system s.
Medspec 30/80 tesla MR s.
MedX s.
micro CT-20 s.
Microtek ScanMaker 9600XL s.
midget MRI s.
mobile spiral computed
  tomography s.
modified electron beam CT s.
mPower PET s.
MR catheter imaging and
  spectroscopy system s.
multidetector CT s.
multidetector helical s.
multiple-jointed digitizer s.
multisensor structured light-range
  digitizer s.
multislice CT s.
neurodiagnostic s.
NeuroFOCUS s.
NewTom CT s.
Nishimoto Sangyo s.
Norland pQCT XCT2000 s.
nuclear s.
Ohio Nuclear Delta 50 FS, 2000 s.
Olympus endoscopic ultrasound s.
Oxford 2T large-bore imaging
  system s.
Pace Plus System s.
Park Medical Systems s.
partial-ring bismuth germanate-crystal
  s.
Perception s.
PET/CT s.
PET full-ring s.
PETT VI PET s.
Pfizer 200 FS, 400 s.
phased-array s.
Philips Gyroscan ACS, NT, NT5,
  NT15, S5, T5 s.
Philips 1.5 NT-Intera s.
Philips 1.5T NT MR s.
Philips Tomoscan 350, SR 6000
  CT s.
Philips 4.7T small-bore system s.
Picker MR s.

Picker PQ 5000 helical CT s.
Picker PQ 2000 spiral CT s.
Picker Prism 3000 PET s.
Picker Synerview 600 s.
4096 Plus PET s.
Posicam HZ PET s.
PQ 5000 CT s.
pQCT s.
ProSpeed CT s.
Quad 7000, 12000 high-field open
  MRI s.
Quick CT9800 s.
QX/I CT s.
radioisotope s.
rectilinear s.
ring s.
RT 3200 Advantage ultrasound s.
RT 6800 ultrasound s.
Scanditronix PET s.
Scanmaster DX x-ray film
  digitizer s.
scintillation s.
SCU-1200, -2200 digital color
  ultrasound s.
SDCT s.
sector s.
SFP s.
Shimadzu CT s.
Shimadzu MR s.
Siemens Biograph s.
Siemens DRH CT s.
Siemens Ecat Exact HR+ CTI
  PET s.
Siemens Magnetom GBS II s.
Siemens Magnetom SP 4000 s.
Siemens Magnetom 1.5T s.
Siemens Magnetom Vision s.
Siemens One Tesla s.
Siemens Plus 4 Volume Zoom
  multidetector s.
Siemens Somaform 512 CT s.
Siemens Somatom DR2, DR3
  whole-body s.
Siemens Somatom Plus CT s.
Siemens Sonoline Elegra
  ultrasound s.
Signa Horizon LX SR 77 gradient
  1.5T MR s.
Signa MRI s.
Signa 1.5T s.
Signa VH/i3.0T MR s.
single-detector helical s.
single-detector row s.
40-slice s.
16-slice CT s.
small-bore s.
SmartPrep s.
Somatom DR CT s.
Somatom Plus-S CT s.

scanner (*continued*)
    spiral CT, XCT s.
    supercam scintillation s.
    Swissray s.
    TCT900S helical CT s.
    Technicare Delta 2020 s.
    Tecmag Libra-S16 system s.
    3T Medspec 30/80 MR s.
    tomographic multiplane s.
    Tomoscan AVEU spiral CT s.
    Tomoscan SR 7000 s.
    Toshiba MR s.
    Toshiba 900S helical CT s.
    Toshiba 900S/XII s.
    Toshiba TCT-80 CT s.
    Toshiba Xpress SX helical CT s.
    Toshiba X-Vigor s.
    Toshiba Xvision s.
    Trionix s.
    ultrafast computed tomography s.
    ultrahigh field-strength whole-body
      MR s.
    Ultramark 9 s.
    ultrasound bone imaging s. (UBIS)
    UM4 real-time sector s.
    Varian CT s.
    Vidar s.
    Vision Ten V-scan s.
    Vision 1.5T Siemens MRI s.
    whole-body GI Signa MRI s.
    whole-body 1.5-Tesla s.
    whole-body 3T MRI system s.
    whole-body 1.5T Siemens Vision s.
    Xpress/SW helical CT s.
    Xpress/SX helical CT s.
    X-Vigor CT s.
scanning
    s. acoustic microscope (SAM)
    s. arm
    body s.
    breath-hold s.
    close-space thin-section s.
    collimation s.
    combined ^{99m}Tc-DMSA and
      ^{99m}Tc-DTPA s.
    continuous s.
    contrast material-enhanced s.
    delayed-phase s.
    diagnostic radioiodine s.
    diffusion-weighted s.
    discontinuous s.
    dual-isotope s.
    electrical impedance s. (EIS)
    s. electron microscope (SEM)
    s. equalization radiography
    external s.
    full-line s.
    gamma s.
    gated equilibrium blood pool s.

high-resolution ultrasound s.
    IDA s.
    interleaved BOLD-fMRI s.
    intraoperative MIBG s.
    laser diffraction s.
    s. laser ophthalmoscopy
    s. laser polarimetry
    light s.
    line s.
    linear s.
    s. locus
    M-mode s.
    ^{99m}Tc-DMSA s.
    multidetector helical s.
    multiplanar s.
    nuclear s.
    parasternal s.
    paravertebral s.
    point s.
    positron s.
    s. power
    radiocholesterol s.
    radioisotope thyroid s.
    radionuclide s.
    real-time sector s.
    sector s.
    sensitive point s.
    spiral CT s.
    spot s.
    subsecond s.
    suprasternal s.
    s. technique
    total body s.
    transabdominal s.
    triplex s.
    whole-body ^{29}FDG s.
    wide-beam s.
    xenon CT s.
scanning-beam
    s.-b. digital system
    s.-b. digital x-ray (SBDX)
scanogram imaging
scanography
    rotational s.
    slit s.
    spot s.
3-Scape real-time 3D imaging
scaphocapitate
    s. joint
    s. syndrome
scaphocephalic head shape
scaphocephaly
scaphoid
    s. bone
    congenital bipartite s.
    s. facet
    s. fat stripe
    s. hand fracture
    s. pole

s. projection
rotary subluxation of s.
s. shape
s. stomach
scaphoid-lunate (*var. of* scapholunate)
scapholunate (SL), scaphoid-lunate
s. advanced collapse (SLAC)
s. arthritic collapse
s. dislocation
s. dissociation
s. joint
s. ligament
s. space
s. widening
scaphotrapeziotrapezoid (STT)
s. joint
scaphotriquetral ligament
scapula, *pl.* **scapulae**
body of s.
high-riding s.
incisura scapulae
inferior tip of s.
levator scapulae
margin of s.
swallowtail malformation of s.
winged s.
scapulae (*pl. of* scapula)
scapular
s. angle
s. body
s. bone
s. flap
s. margin
s. notch
s. snapping
s. winging
scapuloclavicular articulation
scapulocostal syndrome
scapulothoracic
s. joint
s. motion
scapulovertebral border
scar
s. band
s. carcinoma
central pancreatic lesion s.
s. contracture
dense s.
s. emphysema
femoral physial s.
fibrocartilaginous s.
s. formation
infarcted s.
s. lesion
lung starfish s.
myocardial s.
nonviable s.
s. ossification
ossified s.

pulmonary s.
radial s.
radial breast s.
s. tissue
s. tissue entrapment
s. tissue reaction
tumor of liver s.
well-demarcated s.
SCAR
Society for Computer Applications in
Radiology
scarification of pleura
scarified duodenum
Scarpa
canal of S.
S. fascia
S. ganglion
ligament of S.
method of S.
S. triangle
scarred
s. duodenum
s. kidney
scarring
s. adenocarcinoma
apical s.
basilar pleural s.
fibrotic s.
glial s.
interstitial s.
parenchymatous s.
parietal pleural s.
pleural s.
postbiopsy s.
postinflammatory s.
postnecrotic s.
postpyelonephritis
cortical s.
renal s.
selective s.
valvular s.
scatter
s. activity
s. and veiling glare (SVG)
s. compensation
Compton s.
s. correction
s. degradation factor
s. dose
s. fraction
s. graph
s. grid
low-frequency s.
s. radiation
scatter-air ratio (SAR)
scattered
s. air bronchogram
s. coincidence event
s. count

S

scattered (*continued*)
  s. radiation
  s. rays
scatterer
  s. depth
  echogenicity s.
scattergram
scattering
  broad-beam s.
  classic s.
  coherent s.
  collimator s.
  Compton s.
  s. foil
  s. foil compensator
  forward-angle light s.
  image-degrading s.
  low-angle s.
  Rayleigh s.
  Rayleigh-Tyndall s.
  side s.
  small-angle multiple s.
  s. system
  Thomson s.
scatter-maximum ratio (SMR)
scatterplot
scatter-primary ratio
scavenging system
SCD
  sagittal canal diameter
scene
  s. coordinate system
  s. domain
  s. intensity
scene-based
  s.-b. interpolation
  s.-b. visualization
Sceratti goniometer
SCFE
  slipped capital femoral epiphysis
Scharff-Bloom-Richardson
  S.-B.-R. grade
  S.-B.-R. histologic grade
    system
Schatzker fracture classification
Schatzki
  S. ring
  S. view
Schaumann body
Scheibe dysplasia
Scheie syndrome
scheme
  computer-aided diagnosis s.
  cylindrical ablation s.
  decay s.
  gradient s.
  rule-based s.
  single-ablation s.
  zero-filling interpolation s.

Schepelmann sign
Scheuermann
  S. disease
  S. juvenile kyphosis
  S. nodule
Schick sign of tuberculosis
Schiff-Sherrington phenomenon
Schilder disease
Schiller-Duval body
Schistosoma
  S. haematobium
  S. japonicum
  S. mansori
schistosomal bladder carcinoma
schistosomiasis
schizencephaly
Schlemm
  S. canal
  S. ligament
Schlesinger
  S. sign
  S. vein
Schmid disease
Schmid-like metaphysial chondrodysplasia
Schmidt optics system
Schmid-type metaphysial dysplasia
Schmincke tumor
Schmorl
  S. node
  S. nodule
  S. nucleus pulposus disease
Schneider
  S. enteral stent
  S. Guider catheter
schneiderian
  s. carcinoma
  s. papilloma
Schnitzler syndrome
Schoemaker congenital hip dislocation line
Schonander film changer
Schönlein-Henoch syndrome
Schroedinger equation
Schüller
  S. position
  S. projection
  S. view
Schultze
  S. bundle
  S. placenta
Schultz reaction
Schumacher criterion
Schwann
  S. cell
  S. cell of myelin sheath
  S. tumor
schwannoma
  acoustic s.
  benign s.

dumbbell s.
facial s.
geniculate ganglion s.
jugular foramen s.
malignant s.
orbital s.
trigeminal s.
vestibular s.

Schwartz
S. criterion
S. test for patency of deep
saphenous vein

Schwartze sign
Schwartz-Jampel syndrome (SJS)
SCI
spinal cord injury

sciatic
s. endometriosis
s. notch
s. plexus

scimitar
s. deformity
shadow s.
s. sign
s. syndrome
s. vein

scimitar-shaped
s.-s. flap
s.-s. shadow

scintiangiography
scinticisternography
**Scinticore multicrystal scintillation
camera**
scintigram
^{99m}Tc MDP skeletal s.
parallel-hole s.
pinhole s.
spatial resolution s.

scintigraphic
s. angiography
s. balloon
s. balloon topography
s. evidence
s. perfusion defect
s. scan imaging
s. study

scintigraphy
ACE inhibition s.
adrenal s.
antifibrin s.
s. artifact
bleeding s.
blood pool s.
bone marrow s.
brain perfusion s.
captopril-enhanced renal s.
captopril renal s.
cardiac s.
cardiovascular system s.

cerebral s.
cholesterol-based s.
cold defect renal s.
combined ventilation-perfusion s.
cortical s.
dipyridamole thallium-201 s.
dual intracoronary s.
dynamic antral s.
dynamic radionuclide renal s.
early bone s.
endocrine gland s.
exercise myocardial perfusion s.
exercise stress redistribution s.
exercise thallium s.
functional radioiodine s.
^{67}Ga citrate s.
gallium bone s.
gallium lung s.
gallium tumor s.
gastrointestinal s.
gated blood pool s.
genitourinary system s.
GI tract s.
heart s.
hepatic artery perfusion s. (HAPS)
hepatobiliary s.
^{123}I metaiodobenzylguanidine s.
^{111}In antimyosin s.
Infecton s.
In-pentetreotide s.
iodine s.
iodine-131 whole-body s.
iodomethyl-norcholesterol-59 s.
isotope s.
labeled free fatty acid s.
lacrimal s.
liver s.
long segmental diaphysial uptake
bone s.
lung s.
marrow agent bone s.
MIBG s.
microsphere perfusion s.
morphine sulfate s.
^{99m}Tc depreotide s.
^{99m}Tc-DMSA s.
^{99m}Tc HIG s.
^{99m}Tc human polyclonal
immunoglobulin G s.
^{99m}Tc human serum albumin s.
^{99m}Tc-labeled white blood cell s.
^{99m}Tc-methoxyisobutylisonitrile s.
^{99m}Tc-PYP s.
myocardial perfusion s.
NEFA s.
nonesterified fatty acid s.
nuclear renal s.
octreotide paraganglioma s.
oropharyngoesophageal s. (OPES)

S

scintigraphy (*continued*)
    osteomyelitis s.
    parathyroid s.
    pediatric s.
    peptide receptor s.
    perfusion s.
    peritoneal s.
    pertechnetate s.
    3-phase bone s. (TPBS)
    4-phase bone s.
    photon-deficient bone lesion s.
    planar diagnostic I-231 s.
    planar exercise thallium-201 s.
    pulmonary s.
    pyrophosphate s.
    s. quality control
    quantitative hepatobiliary s.
      (QHS)
    radioisotope s.
    radionuclide bone s.
    radionuclide testicular s.
    renal cortical s.
    renal gallium s.
    resting redistribution thallium-201 s.
    rosary beading bone s.
    salivary gland s.
    samarium s.
    same-day exercise-rest Tc-99m
      tetrofosmin myocardial perfusion s.
    selective spleen s.
    sestamibi parathyroid s. (SPS)
    single-photon planar s. (SPPS)
    soft tissue uptake bone s.
    somatostatin receptor s. (SRS)
    source of artifact s.
    SPECT brain perfusion s.
    SPECT thallium s.
    spleen s.
    splenic s.
    split-function s.
    stress perfusion s.
    sulfur colloid s.
    Tc-labeled red blood cell s.
    TcO$_4$ MIBI subtraction s.
    technetium 99m DMSA s.
    technetium 99m heat-denatured RBC
      splenic s.
    thallium-201 myocardial s.
    thallium perfusion s.
    thyroid s.
    thyroid lymph node s.
    time-course fracture s.
    transit s.
    ventilation s.
    ventilation-perfusion pulmonary s.
    vesicoureteral s.
    white blood cell with indium-
      111 s.
scintillascope

scintillation
    s. camera
    s. camera field uniformity
    s. camera geometry
    s. camera linearity
    s. camera linearity differential
    s. camera uniformity differential
    s. counter
    s. counting technique
    s. crystal
    s. detector
    s. imaging
    migrainous s.
    s. probe
    s. proximity radioimmunoassay
    s. scan
    s. scanner
    s. spectrometer
    s. spectrometry
scintillator
    cesium iodide s.
    liquid s.
    rare-earth s.
scintillometer
scintimammography (SMM)
    ^{99m}Tc glucoheptanoate s.
    technetium 99m
      methoxyisobutylisonitrile s.
scintiphoto (*var. of* scintiphotograph)
scintiphotograph, scintiphoto
    combined transmission-emission s.
scintiphotography, scintography
    liver s.
scintirenography
scintiscan (*see also* **scan**)
scintiscanner (*see also* **scanner**)
Scintiview nuclear computer system
scintography (*var. of* scintiphotography)
**Scintron IV nuclear computer
  system**
SCIPP
    sacrococcygeal inferior pubic point
scirrhous
    s. breast carcinoma
    s. infiltrating adenocarcinoma
    s. lesion
    s. tumor
scission
    double-strand s.
    single-strand s.
scissoring of legs
SCIWORA
    spinal cord injury without radiographic
      abnormality
SCL
    sinus cycle length
SCLBCL
    secondary cutaneous large B-cell
    lymphoma

SCLC
small cell lung carcinoma
scleral canal
sclerocystic ovary
scleroderma
complicated s.
diffuse s.
s. of esophagus
ScleroLaser laser system
scleroma
ScleroPLUS
S. HP
S. HP laser system
sclerosant
sclerosed temporal bone
scleroses (*pl. of* sclerosis)
sclerosing
s. adenitis
s. adenosis
s. agent
s. basal cell carcinoma
s. cholangitis
s. duct hyperplasia
s. encapsulating peritonitis
s. hemangioma
s. hepatic carcinoma (SHC)
s. inflammation
s. injection
s. lesion
s. lipogranuloma
s. mediastinitis
s. mesenteritis
s. myeloma
s. nonsuppurative osteomyelitis
s. osteogenic sarcomatosis
s. osteosarcoma
s. panencephalitis
s. stromal tumor
sclerosis, *pl.* **scleroses**
amyotrophic lateral s. (ALS)
aortic s.
arterial s.
arteriocapillary s.
arteriolar s.
Baló concentric s.
bony s.
brainstem multiple s.
calcified s.
chronic subperitoneal s.
congenital hippocampal s.
coronary s.
cyst s.
diaphysial s.
diffuse CNS s.
diffuse myelinoclastic s.
discogenic vertebral s.
disseminated s.
endocardial s.
endoscopic variceal s. (EVS)

endplate s.
esophageal variceal s.
focal bone s.
gastric s.
hepatic s.
hepatoportal s.
hippocampal s.
idiopathic hypertrophic subaortic s.
(IHSS)
incisural s.
Krabbe diffuse s.
laser s.
lobar s.
marginal s.
marked s.
medial calcific s.
mesenteric s.
mesial temporal s.
multifocal subcritoncal s.
multiple s. (MS)
pedicle s.
photothermal s.
posterolateral s.
progressive systemic s.
pulmonary and cardiac s.
reactive bone s.
renal s.
segmental vein s.
subchondral low signal-intensity s.
subendocardial s.
systemic s. (SSc)
temporal bone s.
thick rind s.
tuberous s.
tumefactive multiple s.
unilateral mesial temporal s.
valvular s.
variceal s.
vascular s.
venous s.
sclerostenosis
sclerotherapy
percutaneous ethanol s.
talc s.
sclerotic
s.
s. area
s. band
s. border
s. calvarial bone island
s. calvarial patch
s. coronary artery
s. degeneration
s. kidney
s. lesion
s. line
s. margin
s. osteosarcoma
s. pattern

S

sclerotic (*continued*)
  s. plaque
  s. rim
  s. stomach
sclerotomy
  ab externo laser s.
  ab interno laser s.
SCM
  spinal cord malformation
  split cord malformation
SCNB
  stereotactic core needle biopsy
scoliosis
  adolescent idiopathic s. (AIS)
  Aussies-Isseis unstable s.
  Cobb measurement of s.
  congenital s.
  Dwyer anterior endoscopic correction
    of s.
  Ferguson method for measuring s.
  fixation of s.
  functional s.
  idiopathic s.
  s. index
  juvenile idiopathic s.
  King classification of thoracic s.
  King-Moe classification of s.
  levorotatory s.
  lumbar s.
  S. Research Society
  rotary thoracolumbar s.
  S-shaped s.
  thoracic s.
  thoracolumbar s.
  uncompensated rotary s.
  Winter-King-Moe s.
scoliotic
  s. pelvis
  s. spine
SCOOP
  Spofford-Christopher oxygen optimizing
    program
  SCOOP model polyurethane
    intratracheal catheter
ScopeGuide
  S. magnetic resonance imaging
    device
  S. MRI device
Scopix Laser film
scorbutic white line
score
  Agatston s.
  aortic valve calcium s.
  biophysical profile s. (BPS)
  calcium s.
  coronary artery calcium s.
    (CACS)
  densitometry z s.
  electron beam CT-derived CAC s.

fetal biophysical profile s.
Gleason s.
injury severity s. (ISS)
late-effect toxicity s.
LENT s.
Mallampati s.
mean wall motion s.
MRI severity scale s.
NIHSS s.
prognostic s.
QRS s.
stroke scale s.
summed difference s. (SDS)
summed rest s.
summed stress s.
thallium SPECT s.
total calcium s. (TCS)
volume s.
wall motion s.
scored cartilage
scoring
  calcium s.
  hand and forearm artery s. (level
    I–V)
scotty
  s. dog
  s. dog appearance
  s. dog fracture
  s. dog sign
  s. dog view
scout
  s. digital radiograph
  s. film
  s. image
  s. imaging
  s. sequence
  s. view
SCP
  supracristal plane
SCR
  silicon-controlled rectifier
scrambled image
screen
  s. craze artifact
  fluorescent s.
  guilt s.
  intensifying s.
  Kodak Min-R s.
  Lanex medium s.
  s. oxygenator
  radiofrequency s.
  rapid s.
  rare-earth s.
  rear-projection s.
  Ultra Vision Rapid s.
screener
screen-film
  s.-f. contact
  s.-f. mammography

screening
  biplane s.
  breast cancer s.
  s. mammography
  s. technique
screening-detected abnormality
screen-intensifying factor
screenless mammography film
screen-type film
screw
  bicortical s.
  bone s.
  cancellous s.
  compression plate
   and s.
  dynamic hip s. (DHS)
  s. fixation
  interference s.
  lag s.
  metallic s.
  orthopaedic s.
  resorbable s.
  transfixing s.
  unicortical s.
scriptorius
  calamus s.
scrofula
scroll bone
scrota (*pl. of* scrotum)
scrotal
  s. abscess
  s. anatomy
  s. area
  s. calcification
  s. fasciitis
  s. fibroma
  s. gas
  s. hematocele
  s. hernia
  s. histiocytoma
  s. mass
  s. pearl
  s. raphe
  s. vein
  s. wall thickening
scrotum, *pl.* **scrota,** *pl.*
 scrotums
  acutely symptomatic s.
scrotums (*pl. of* scrotum)
SCT
  Sertoli cell tumor
  spiral computed tomography
  star-cancellation test
SCTA
  spiral computed tomography
  arteriography
**SCU-1200, -2200 digital color
 ultrasound scanner**
Scully tumor

SCV
  subclavian vein
scyphoid
S/D
  systolic-diastolic ratio
SDCT
  single-detector computed tomography
   SDCT scanner
SDD
  surfactant deficiency disorder
SDH
  subdural hemorrhage
  succinate dehydrogenase
SDRI
  small, deep, recent infarct
SDS
  summed difference score
SE
  spin-echo
   SE proton density-weighted
   image
Se
  selenium
75Se, Se-75
  selenium 75
   75Se selenomethionine radioactive
   agent
SEA
  spinal epidural abscess
seagull
  s. joint
  s. sign
seal
  water s.
sealed
  mechanically s.
seal-fin deformity
seam
  osteoid s.
seatbelt
  s. fracture
  s. injury
sea urchin granuloma
sebaceous
  s. adenoma
  s. carcinoma
  s. cyst
  s. gland calcification
sebaceum
  adenoma s.
SEBI
  stereotactic external beam
  irradiation
Sebileau muscle
second
  cycles per s. (cps)
  S. Look breast imaging device
  S. Look CAD system
  meters per s. (mps)

S

second (*continued*)
    milliampere s.'s (mAs)
    frames per second (FPS)
    pulses per s. (PPS)
    roentgens per s. (R/s)
secondarium
    os cuboides s.
secondary
    s. achalasia
    s. acquired cholesteatoma
    s. amenorrhea
    s. amyloidosis
    s. archnoid cyst
    s. atelectasis
    s. axillary adenopathy
    s. axillary lymphadenopathy
    s. biliary cirrhosis
    s. brain lymphoma
    s. bronchus
    s. calcification
    s. cartilaginous joint
    s. center of ossification
    s. central venous thrombosis
    s. chondromatosis
    s. coccidioidomycosis
    s. collimation
    s. contracture
    s. cutaneous large B-cell lymphoma (SCLBCL)
    s. cutaneous plasmacytoma
    s. degeneration
    s. electron
    s. electron production
    s. extravasation
    s. fracture
    s. gliosis
    s. hydrocele
    s. hydrocephalus
    s. hyperparathyroidism
    s. hypoparathyroidism
    s. hypothyroidism
    s. intracranial hypertension (SIH)
    s. lesion
    s. lymphangiectasis
    s. lymphedema
    s. malignancy
    s. myeloid metaphysis
    s. obstruction
    s. osteosarcoma
    s. ovarian tumor
    s. peristalsis
    s. pleurisy
    s. pneumonia
    s. pulmonary lobule
    s. radiation
    s. ray
    s. retroperitoneal fibrosis
    s. retroperitoneal organ
    s. sclerosing cholangitis
    s. sequestrum
    s. sonographic finding
    s. tooth
    s. ulcer
    s. union
    s. venous insufficiency
    s. viremia
    s. wave
    s. yolk sac
secretin
    intraarterial s.
secretin-enhanced dynamic MRCP
secretion
    adrenocortical s.
    bowel s.
    gastric s.
    hyperdense sinus s.
    inspissated s.
    mineralocorticoid s.
    retained s.
    retention of s.
    sinonasal s.
    tubular kidney s.
secretion-filled bronchus
secretory
    s. adenocarcinoma
    s. calcification
    s. capacity
    s. carcinoma
    s. component
secretory-phase endometrium
section
    axial celloidin s.
    celloidin s.
    contiguous interleaved axial s.'s
    coronal s.
    flood s.
    frontal s.
    midfrontal plane coronal s.
    paramedian s.
    penultimate s.
    sagittal celloidin s.
    sagittal paraffin s.
    serial s.'s
    serpiginous s.
    step s.
    thin s.
    s. timing correction
    tomographic s.
    transverse s.
sectional
    s. radiography
    s. segmental anatomy
section-select
    s.-s. flow compensation
    s.-s. pulse
section-sensitivity profile

sector
    s. echocardiography
    lower field visual s.
    nipple s.
    nonnipple s.
    s. scan
    s. scanner
    s. scanning
    Sommer s.
    s. transducer
    s. unit
sector-scan echocardiography imaging
secular equilibrium
secundum
    s. atrial septal defect
    ostium s.
    septum s.
secundus
    digitus s.
sedation
    conscious s.
    deep s.
    light s.
    moderate s.
sedimented calcium
seed
    encapsulated radioactive s.
    gold s.
    I-Plant brachytherapy s.
    PharmaSeed palladium-103 s.
    s. point
    radiation s.
    s. ribbon
    Symmetra I-125 brachytherapy s.
    s. voxel
seeding
    intracranial s.
    metastatic s.
    perichondral cell s.
    peritoneal s.
    port-site tumor s.
    prostate s.
    radioactive s.
    subarachnoid s.
    subependymal s.
    TheraSeed s.
    tumor s.
seeker
    bone s.
seen on end
seesaw peristalsis of ureter
Seessel pouch
see-through image
segment
    aganglionic s.
    akinetic s.
    angulated s.
    anterobasal s.
    anterolateral s.

    aortic s.
    aperistaltic distal ureteral s.
    apical s.
    apicoposterior s.
    arterial s.
    atretic aortic s.
    blind s.
    bronchopulmonary s.
    cardiac s.
    coarcted s.
    contiguous s.'s
    Couinaud liver s. (1-8)
    diaphragmatic s.
    distal s.
    s. distraction
    diversity s.
    duodenal s.
    expansile aortic s.
    hypokinetic s.
    infarcted lung s.
    inferoapical s.
    inferobasal s.
    inferoposterior s.
    intercalated s.
    interleaved inversion readout s.
    interposed colon s.
    intradiaphragmatic aortic s.
    intramuscular aortic s.
    ischemic s.
    Jackson and Huber classification of
      bronchial s.'s
    joint s.
    liver s.
    meatal s.
    nonfilling venous s.
    noninfarcted s.
    occlusal s.
    posteroapical s.
    posterobasal s.
    posterolateral s.
    proximal s.
    pulmonary s.
    redundancy of interposed colon s.
    septal wall s.
    superior s.
    tail-like s.
    variable s.
    vaterian s.
    venous s.
    views per s. (VPS)
segmental
    s. alveolar pattern
    s. asynergy
    s. biliary obstruction
    s. bone defect
    s. bone loss
    s. bowel infarct
    s. branch of artery
    s. bronchiole

S

segmental (*continued*)
 s. bronchus
 s. bronchus consolidation
 s. bronchus defect
 s. bronchus fracture
 s. bronchus ischemia
 s. bronchus lesion
 s. bronchus-lower extremity Doppler
  pressure
 s. bronchus narrowing
 s. bronchus orifice
 s. bronchus perfusion abnormality
 s. bronchus plethysmography
 s. bronchus-renal artery waveform
 s. bronchus symptom
 s. correction using spine
  reconstruction
 s. correction using x-ray
  measurement
 s. demyelination
 s. dyssynergia
 s. hepatectomy
 s. k-space turbo gradient-echo
  breath-hold sequence imaging
 s. limb pressure recording
 s. liver anatomy
 s. lung defect scan
 s. lung density
 s. necrotizing glomerulonephritis
 s. nephrogram
 s. neurofibromatosis
 s. omental infarct
 s. pneumonia
 s. portal hypertension
 s. pressure measurement
 s. renal artery branch
 s. resorption atelectasis
 s. spinal dysgenesis (SSD)
 s. stenosis
 s. transcatheter arterial
  chemoembolization
 s. vein
 s. vein sclerosis
 s. wall motion

segmentation
 anatomy-oriented colon s.
  (AOCS)
 s. anomaly
 automatic lumen edge s.
 automatic lung nodule s.
 barium s.
 GM s.
 inside-to-outside s.
 lung s.
 s. method
 s. method for real-time
  display
 MRI s.
 outer-air s.

 outside-to-inside s.
 s. procedure
 rhythmic s.
 semiautomated cerebrospinal fluid s.
 time-resolved imaging by automatic
  data s. (TRIADS)
 vascular s.

segmented
 s. cine
 s. echo-planar imaging (SEPI)
 s. k-space cardiac tagging
 s. k-space data acquisition
 s. k-space time-of-flight MR
  angiography

segmenting
 s. dual-echo MR head scan
 s. dual-echo MR imaging

Segond fracture

Segre chart

SEH
 spinal epidural hemorrhage

SEI
 subendocardial infarct

Seidelin body

Seidlitz powder test

**Seinsheimer classification of femoral
 fracture**

seizure
 absence s.
 generalized s.
 grand mal s.
 s. localization
 new-onset s.
 partial complex s.
 s. pattern
 petit mal s.
 s. phenomenon
 repetitive s.'s
 s. threshold
 tonic-clonic s.

SELCA
 smooth excimer laser coronary
  angioplasty

Seldinger
 S. angiography
 S. catheterization
 S. needle
 S. percutaneous technique

select
 BimOdal Slice S. (BOSS)

Selecta 7000 laser

selection
 s. bias
 coil s.
 delay time s.
 gradient s.
 guidance system s.
 reflectance-guided laser s.
 slice s.

selective
- s. angiocardiography
- s. arterial injection
- s. arterial magnetic resonance angiography
- s. cannulation
- s. cerebral arteriography
- s. complete lymph node dissection
- s. coronary arteriography
- s. coronary arteriography view
- s. coronary cineangiography
- s. excitation
- s. excitation line scan
- s. excitation method
- s. excitation projection reconstruction imaging
- s. hole burning
- s. internal radiation therapy (SIRT)
- s. irradiation
- s. laser sintering (SLS)
- s. occlusion of aneurysmal neck
- s. osteal salpingography
- s. partial inversion recovery (SPIR)
- s. partial inversion recovery-fluid attenuated inversion recovery (SPIR-FLAIR)
- s. partial inversion-recovery MRI
- s. population inversion (SPI)
- s. population transfer (SPT)
- s. presaturation MR angiography
- s. pulse
- s. radiography
- s. reduction of pregnancy
- s. saturation
- s. saturation method
- s. saturation recovery
- s. scarring
- s. separation
- s. spleen scintigraphy
- s. test occlusion
- s. tubal assessment to refine reproductive therapy (STARRT)
- s. venography
- s. venous magnetic resonance angiography
- s. visceral aortography
- s. visceral arteriography
- s. visualization
- s. vulnerability

selectivity
- spatial s.

Selectron system
Selenia imaging system
selenium (Se)
- s. 75 (^{75}Se, Se-75)
- amorphous s.
- s. drum detector system
- s. imaging agent
- s. plate
- s. radiography

selenium-based digital chest system
selenium-labeled bile acid imaging
selenomethylcholesterol
self-administered cleansing enema
self-aspirating cut-biopsy needle
self-expandable metal stent
self-expanding
- s.-e. covered stent
- s.-e. Easy Wallstent
- s.-e. metallic endoprosthesis
- s.-e. open mesh stent
- s.-e. stent-graft
- s.-e. tulip sheath

self-injury
self-quenched counter tube
self-reinforced polyglycolide
self-retaining Cope loop pigtail catheter
self-reversed parallel-wire balloon technique
self-scattering
self-sealing latex balloon
self-selection bias
self-shielding
sella
- ballooned s.
- empty s.
- s. enlargement
- J-shaped s.
- s. turcica
- s. turcica calcification
- s. turcica diaphragm

sellae
- decalcified dorsum s.
- diaphragma s.
- dorsum s.
- tuberculum s.

sella-nasion plane
sellar
- s. destruction
- s. floor
- s. mass
- s. tomography

Selvester QRS scoring system
SEM
- scanning electron microscope

semialdehyde
- succinic s.

semiautomated
- s. cerebrospinal fluid segmentation
- s. computed tomography angiography

semiautonomous nodule
semiaxial
- s. anteroposterior projection
- s. position
- s. transcranial projection

S

semicircular
s. canal
s. canal hydrops
s. ridge
semicommitted mode
semiconductor
complementary metal oxide s. (CMOS)
s. detector
metal oxide s. (MOS)
semicoronal plane
semidynamic splint
semierect
s. film
s. position
semiflexed MTP
semi-Fowler position
semihorizontal heart
semiinvasive aspergillosis
semilateral position
semiliquid feces
semilobar holoprosencephaly
semilunar
s. aortic valve regurgitation
s. bone
s. bone formation
s. calcification
s. cartilage
s. fold
s. indentation
s. line
s. notch
s. pulmonic valve regurgitation
s. valve
s. valve cusp
semilunaris
hiatus s.
linea s.
semimembranosus
s. bursa
s. muscle
s. tendon
semimembranosus-tibial collateral ligament bursa
seminal
s. colliculus
s. tract
s. vesicle
s. vesicle atrophy
s. vesicle cyst
s. vesicle hypoplasia
s. vesicle invasion (SVI)
s. vesiculography
seminiferous
s. tubule
s. tubule damage
s. tubule ectasia
seminoma
extragonadal s.

mediastinal s.
s. mediastinum
testicular s.
seminomatous tumor
semiopaque
semiovale
centrum s.
semiquantitative
s. measurement
s. technique
semirecumbent position
semispinal muscle
semisupine position
semitendinosus tendon
semitendinous muscle
semiupright
s. position
s. view
semivertical heart
^{77}Se MRI spectroscopy
send-receive phased-array extremity coil
senescence
premature placental s.
senescent
s. aortic stenosis
s. change
s. periventricular hyperintensity
Sengstaken-Blakemore tube
senile
s. amyloidosis
s. ankylosing hyperostosis
s. arteriosclerosis
s. change
s. degeneration
s. emphysema
s. fibroma
s. myocardium
s. nephrosclerosis
s. osteomalacia
s. osteoporosis
s. plaque
s. subcapital fracture
senilis
atrophia cutis s.
coxa s.
Senning
S. operation
S. procedure
senograph
Senographe
S. 2000D digital mammography imaging
S. 2000D digital mammography system
S. DMRt mammography system
S. Essential mobile mammography
S. 500T, 600T, 700T, 800T mammography

senography
SenoScan
>S. full-field digital imaging system
>S. full-field digital mammography
>system
Sens-A-Ray 2000 dental imaging system
sensation
>foreign body s.
>globus s.
>Siemens Somatom S. 64
>Somatom S. 64
SENSE
>sensitivity encoded
>sensitivity encoding
>generalized SENSE
>SENSE method
>modified SENSE (mSENSE)
>SENSE MRI
>time-adaptive SENSE (TSENSE)
>SENSE with half-Fourier single-shot
>turbo spin echo (SShTSE)
sensing
>s. coil
>s. error
sensitive
>s. plane
>s. plane projection reconstruction
>imaging
>s. point
>s. point scanning
>s. volume
sensitivity
>s. analysis
>contrast s.
>C-sign s.
>s. encoded (SENSE)
>s. encoding (SENSE)
>s. encoding method
>index of s.
>line-shape s.
>percussion s.
>plane s.
>point s.
>poor s.
>spectral s.
>uniform s.
sensitization
>protracted exposure s.
sensitizer
>s. enhancement ratio
>radiation s.
sensitizing gradient
sensitometer
>electroluminescent s.
sensitometric
>s. curve
>s. strip
sensitometry
>processor s.

sensomotor (*var. of* sensorimotor)
sensor
>bispectral index s. (BIS)
>electromagnetic position s.
>PressureWire s.
>temperature s.
sensorimotor, sensomotor
>s. cortex
>s. gyrus
sensory
>s. alexia
>s. ganglion
>s. impairment
>s. nucleus
>s. paralytic bladder
>s. root
>s. strip
>s. tract
sentinel
>s. clot sign
>s. fold
>s. fracture
>s. headache
>s. loop
>s. loop sign
>s. lymph node (SLN)
>s. lymph node biopsy (SLNB)
>s. lymph node mapping
>s. node dissection
>s. node localization and biopsy
>s. pile
>s. transoral hemorrhage
SEP
>systolic ejection period
separation
>acromioclavicular joint s.
>aortic cusp s.
>atlantoaxial s.
>atlantooccipital s.
>carrier free s.
>chorioamnionic s.
>chromatographic s.
>collagen fiber s.
>costochondral junction s.
>E point to septal s. (EPSS)
>fat-water signal s.
>fracture fragment s.
>frequency s.
>leaflet s.
>meniscocapsular s.
>meniscotibial s.
>mitral valve septal s.
>s. of bowel loop
>s. of ghosts
>pontomedullary s.
>selective s.
>septal s.
>shoulder s.
>small bowel s.

S

separator tube
Sephadex bead
SEPI
    segmented echo-planar
      imaging
septa (*pl. of* septum)
septal
    s. accessory pathway
    s. amplitude
    s. arcade
    s. area
    s. asymmetry
    s. band
    s. bone
    s. cartilage plate
    s. cirrhosis
    s. cusp
    s. cusp of Calvé
    s. defect
    s. deviation
    s. dip
    s. hyperperfusion
    s. hypertrophy
    s. hypokinesis
    s. hypoperfusion
    s. leaflet
    s. line
    s. malformation
    s. myocardial infarct
    s. necrosis
    s. notch
    s. papillary muscle
    s. perforating branch
    s. perforation
    s. perforator
    s. perforator artery
    s. placenta cyst
    s. ridge
    s. separation
    s. thickening
    s. tricuspid anulus
    s. vein
    s. wall
    s. wall motion
    s. wall segment
    s. wall thickness
septate
    s. appearance
    s. hypertrophy
    s. uterus
septated gallbladder
septation
    gallbladder s.
    s. septal defect
septic
    s. arthritis
    s. bursitis
    s. cholangitis
    s. cortical osteitis

    s. discitis
    s. embolus
    s. lung
    s. necrosis
    s. pleurisy
    s. pneumonia
    s. pulmonary embolus
    s. pulmonary infarct
    s. shock
    s. thrombophlebitis
    s. thrombosis
septomarginal
    s. band
    s. trabecula
septooptic dysplasia
septostomy
    atrial s.
    balloon atrial s.
septum, *pl.* **septa**
    alveolar s.
    anal intermuscular s.
    anteroapical trabecular s.
    aortic s.
    aortopulmonary s.
    atrial s.
    atrioventricular nodal s.
    bronchial s.
    bulbar s.
    canal s.
    cartilaginous s.
    s. cavum vergae
    conal s.
    connective tissue s.
    conus s.
    crural s.
    distal bulbar s.
    dyskinetic s.
    enhancing s.
    epirenal s.
    femoral s.
    fibrous s.
    gingival s.
    infundibular s.
    intact ventricular s.
    interatrial s. (IAS)
    interhaustral s.
    interlobar s.
    interlobular lung s.
    intermuscular s.
    internal intermuscular s.
    interventricular s.
    Kürner s.
    lipomatous hypertrophy of
      interatrial s.
    low signal-intensity fibrous s.
    median s.
    mediastinal s.
    membranous s.
    muscular atrioventricular s.

myometrial s.
nasal s.
s. of Bertin
parietal extension of
  infundibular s.
s. pellucidum
s. pellucidum cavity
perirenal s.
placental s.
posteromedian s.
s. primum
rectogenital s.
rectovaginal s.
rectovesical s.
retrovesical s.
s. secundum
sinus s.
subarachnoid s.
sublobar s.
thickened s.
transverse vaginal s.
s. transversum
s. transversum defect
ventricular s.
septum-to-free wall ratio
sequela, *pl.* **sequelae**
late normal tissue s.
long-term s.
neurologic s.
post ECT s.
radiation therapy s.
significant s.
tissue s.
sequelae (*pl. of* sequela)
sequence
amnion rupture s.
black blood s.
breath-hold fast-recovery fast-SE
  pulse s.
breath-hold fat saturation s.
breath-hold gradient-recalled echo s.
s. bypass graft
cardiac gated PGSE s.
Carr-Purcell s.
Carr-Purcell-Meiboom-Gill s.
cine-FFE breath-hold s.
cine gradient-echo s.
conventional pulse s.
CP s.
CPMG s.
DANTE s.
3DFT-CISS s.
3D gadolinium s.
diffusion pulse s.
diffusion-sensitive s.
diffusion-weighted pulse s.
3-dimensional driven equilibrium s.
3-dimensional gradient-echo
  volumetric s.

3-dimensional multiple gradient-
  recalled echo s.
double inversion recovery s.
3D-spoiled gradient-recalled echo s.
3D time-of-flight magnetic resonance
  angiographic s.
3D transesophageal echocardiographic
  s.
dual-echo s.
dual gradient-recalled echo pulse s.
dysplasia-carcinoma s.
ECG-triggered phase contrast cine
  gradient-echo s.
echo-planar pulse s.
fast FLAIR s.
fast gradient-echo s.
fast multislice phase-sensitive
  inversion recovery s.
FAST pulse s.
fat-suppressed T2-weighted fast
  spin-echo s.
fat-suppression pulse s.
field-echo pulse s.
FIRM s.
FISP pulse s.
flow-compensated gradient-echo s.
fluid-sensitive s.
gradient-echo imaging s.
gradient-echo pulse s.
GRASS pulse s.
Hahn spin-echo s.
HASTE s.
high-resolution volumetric s.
hypervariable s.
in-phase s.
interleaved GRE s.
inversion recovery spin-echo s.
IRSE s.
Klippel-Feil s.
long echo-train fast spin echo s.
long TR/TE s.
magnetization-prepared rapid
  acquisition gradient-echo s.
Meiboom-Gill s.
missing pulse steady-state free
  precession s.
modified look-locker s.
s. monophasic shock
MRI pulse s.
multiecho s.
multiplanar gradient refocused s.
multishot echo-shifted gradient-echo
  EPI s.
multislice spin-echo s.
nonflow-compensated s.
nuclear magnetic resonance scanning
  s.
oblique sagittal s.
s. obstruction

S

853

sequence (*continued*)
    opposed-phase s.
    s. optimization
    partial saturation pulse s.
    peristaltic s.
    phase-contrast s.
    phase-encoded time-reduced
      acquisition s.
    3-point Dixon water-fat
      separation s.
    postenhancement s.
    Potter s.
    preenhancement s.
    PRESS s.
    s. processor
    pulse s.
    pulsed arterial spin-labeling s.
    pulsed-gradient spin-echo echo-planar
      pulse s.
    radiofrequency-spoiled 3D GRE s.
    RARE s.
    RARE-derived pulse s.
    repetitive pulse s.
    Robin s.
    rotating ultrafast imaging s. (RUFIS)
    saturation recovery s.
    scan s.
    scout s.
    Shine-Dalgamo s.
    short repetition time s.
    short T1 inversion recovery pulse s.
    single breath-hold s.
    single-echo versus multiple-echo s.
    single-shot gradient-echo EPI s.
    single-shot PSIR s.
    single-shot spin-echo echo-planar
      pulse s.
    SL-GRE s.
    spin-echo imaging s.
    spin-echo pulse s.
    spin-warp pulse s.
    spiral pulse s.
    SPIR-FLAIR s.
    spoiled gradient-echo pulse s.
    spoiled gradient-recalled echo s.
    steady-state free precession s.
    STEAM s.
    STIR s.
    susceptibility-sensitive s.
    susceptibility-weighted s.
    s. time
    TOF s.
    TONE s.
    turboFLASH s.
    turbo inversion recovery s.
    turbo-IR s.
    turbo-pulse s.
    turbo-SE s.
    turbo-spin echo T2-weighted s.

    T2-weighted combination s.
    T1-weighted coronal fat-suppressed
      fast spin-echo s.
    T2-weighted fat-saturated s.
    T2-weighted pulse s.
    T2-weighted spin-echo s.
    twin reversed arterial perfusion s.
    ultrafast FLASH 2D s.
    velocity-encoded s.
    VIBE s.
    voiding s.
    water-suppression pulse s.
sequencing
    2D TOF pulse s.
sequential
    s. balloon inflation
    s. circulator
    s. determinant
    s. echo-planar imaging
    s. extraction-radiotracer technique
    s. films
    s. image acquisition
    s. line imaging
    s. mode
    s. paired opposed plaque (SPOP)
    s. plane imaging
    s. point imaging
    s. postcontrast MR image
    s. quantitative MR imaging
    s. scalar quantization (SSQ)
    s. 1st-pass imaging
sequestered
    s. disc
    s. lobe
    s. lobe of lung
sequestra (*pl. of* sequestrum)
sequestral
sequestration
    bronchopulmonary s.
    disc s.
    extralobar s.
    extrapulmonary s.
    fluid s.
    intralobar s.
    labeled red blood cell s.
    pulmonary s.
    3rd-space s.
    s. system
sequestrectomy
sequestrum, *pl.* **sequestra**
    associated s.
    bony s.
    kissing sequestra
    necrotic s.
    primary s.
    secondary s.
    tertiary s.
Sequoia ultrasound system
sequoiosis

SER
 supination-external rotation
  SER type I-IV fracture
Seratec scan
serendipity view
serial
 s. change
 s. cholangiograms
 s. contrast MR imaging
 s. CT slices
 s. cut-film technique
 s. diffusion-weighted MR imaging
  and proton MR spectroscopy
 s. duplex imaging
 s. duplex scans
 s. dynamic imaging
 s. film changer
 s. injections
 s. lesions
 s. radiographic surveys
 s. radiography
 s. sections
 s. splinting
 s. subtraction films
serialoangiocardiography
serialograph (*var. of* seriograph)
serialography (*var. of* seriography)
sericite pneumoconiosis
series, *pl.* **series**
 abdominal s.
 acute abdominal s. (AAS)
 barium GI s.
 basophilic s.
 cardiac s.
 decay s.
 diagnostic skull s.
 dynamic s.
 factor analysis of dynamic s.
  (FADS)
 FCS s.
 full cervical spine s.
 gallbladder s. (GBS)
 gallbladder-gastrointestinal s.
 gastrointestinal s.
 GB-GI s.
 intubated small bowel s.
 Kempe s.
 lumbosacral s.
 metabolic bone s.
 radioactive s.
 sinus s.
 small bowel s.
 upper gastrointestinal s.
seriograph, serialograph
seriography, serialography
 s. imaging
serioscopy
SER-IV
 supination-external rotation IV

serofibrinous pericardial
 effusion
serofibrous pleurisy
serohemorrhagic fluid
seroma
 mediastinal s.
 perigraft s.
 postoperative s.
seromuscular layer
seronegative rheumatoid
 arthritis
serosa
 cecal s.
serosal
 s. endometrial implant
 s. myoma
 s. surface
 s. tear
serosanguineous fluid
serous
 s. adenocarcinoma
 s. carcinoma
 s. cystadenocarcinoma
 s. cystadenoma
 s. effusion
 s. intraparenchymatous cyst
 s. ligament
 s. membrane
 s. ovarian tumor
 s. pericardium
 s. pleurisy
serpentine
 s. aneurysm
 s. appearance
 s. asbestos
 s. enhancement
 s. signal void
 s. structure
serpiginosum
 angioma s.
serpiginous
 s. band
 s. low signal-intensity border
 s. luminal filling defect
 s. section
 s. ulcer
serrated
 s. appearance
 s. suture
serration
 esophageal margin s.
 marginal s.
serratus
 s. anterior
 s. anterior muscle
Sertoli cell tumor (SCT)
Sertoli-Leydig cell tumor
serum sickness
Servelle vein

S

server
> AquariusNET 2D/3D medical
> imaging s.

service
> s. class user
> NightHawk Radiology S.'s
> ReadyPET support s.

servomotor
> magnetic s.

servo power amplifier

Servox amplifier

sesamoid
> s. bone
> s. complex
> fibular hallux s.
> s. injury
> s. ligament
> s. migration
> tibial hallux s.

sesamoidometatarsal joint

sesamophalangeal ligament

sessile
> s. adenoma
> s. filling defect
> s. hydatid
> s. lesion
> s. nodular carcinoma
> s. plaque
> s. polyp
> s. tumor

sestamibi
> s. imaging agent
> ^{99m}Tc s.
> s. ^{99m}Tc with dipyridamole stress
> test
> s. parathyroid scintigraphy
> (SPS)
> s. polar map
> s. stress scan imaging
> s. technetium 99m

set
> access s.
> Ackerman bone biopsy s.
> Amplatz dilator s.
> s. angle
> coaxial micropuncture needle s.
> Codman cranioplastic type 1
> slow s.
> Curry intravascular retriever s.
> 3D MRI data s.
> Greene biopsy s.
> Hawkins accordion catheter
> drainage s.
> Hawkins inside-out nephrostomy s.
> Huisman percutaneous drainage s.
> image s.
> McNamara coaxial catheter
> infusion s.
> minimally invasive access s.

> Neff percutaneous access s.
> Ring-McLean sump drainage s.
> Ring transjugular intrahepatic
> access s.
> Rosch-Uchida liver access s.
> Rosch-Uchida porta access s.
> (RUPS)
> RUPS-100 liver access s.
> Rutner balloon-dilation helical stone
> extractor s.
> telescopic bougie s.
> Van Sonnenberg chest drain s.

Sethotope radioactive imaging agent

seton

Settegast
> S. method
> S. position
> S. projection

setting
> discriminator s.
> quadrature s.
> simulation-aided field s.
> soft tissue window s.
> wide window s.
> window-level s.

setting-sun sign

Sever disease

severe acute respiratory syndrome
(SARS)

Severin
> S. grade
> S. radiographic residual hip
> dysplasia classification

SEW
> slice excitation wave

sextuplet pregnancy

Seze
> angles of Lequesne and de S.

SFA
> superficial femoral artery

SFD
> source-film distance

SFOV
> scan field of view

SFP
> scanned focal point
> SFP scanner

S-F Precise stent

SFR
> stenotic flow reserve

SFTP
> solitary fibrous tumor of pleura

shaded
> s. surface display (SSD)
> s. surface display imaging
> s. surface rendering

shading
> s. appearance
> image s.

shadow
- acoustic s.
- bandlike s.
- batwing s.
- bony s.
- s. box
- breast s.
- butterfly breast s.
- calcific s.
- cardiac s.
- cardiomediastinal s.
- cardiothymic s.
- cardiovascular s.
- centrilobular s.
- clean s.
- companion s.
- concatenation of s.'s
- cortical signet ring s.
- discoid s.
- double-arc gallbladder s.
- double-bubble s.
- dumbbell-shaped s.
- edge s.
- effusion s.
- fusiform s.
- gloved-finger s.
- heart s.
- hilar s.
- iliopsoas muscle s.
- kidney s.
- large thymus s.
- line s.
- linear s.
- mitral configuration of cardiac s.
- nipple s.
- overlap s.
- overlying bowel s.
- psoas s.
- PVST s.
- radiographic parallel line s.
- renal s.
- ring s.
- s. scimitar
- scimitar-shaped s.
- s. shield
- snowstorm s.
- soft tissue s.
- sound s.
- spindle-shaped s.
- summation of s.'s
- superimposition of bowel s.
- thymic s.
- toothpaste s.
- tramline s.
- tubular s.
- tumorlike s.
- vascular s.
- wall-echo s. (WES)
- widened heart s.

shadowgram
shadowgraph
shadowgraphy
shadowing
- dirty acoustic s.
- hyperechoic structure with s.
- hypointense signal s.
- interstitial s.
- lateral wall refractive s.
- marked hypoechogenicity s.
- paraspinal soft tissue s.
- posterior acoustic s.
- refractive s.
- rib s.
- s. stone

shaft
- bone s.
- femoral s.
- s. flange
- s. fracture
- hair s.
- middle 3rd s.
- s. of rib
- proximal 3rd s.

shag
- aortic s.

shagging of cardiac border
shaggy
- s. contour to bowel
- s. esophagus
- s. heart border
- s. lung nodule
- s. pericardium

shagreen lesion
shaken
- s. baby syndrome (SBS)
- s. impact injury

shallow
- s. inspiration
- s. inspiratory effort
- s. respiration

shank bone
shape
- aneurysm with simple s.
- baseball bat s.
- brachycephalic head s.
- cardiac s.
- cricket bat s.
- dumbbell s.
- exponential s.
- gaussian line s.
- gooseneck s.
- half-moon s.
- head s.
- heat s.
- horseshoe s.
- hourglass s.
- ice cream cone s.
- irregular s.

S

shape (*continued*)
  line s.
  lobulated s.
  S. Maker system
  mesocephalic head s.
  mushroom s.
  oval s.
  ovoid s.
  peak s.
  pulse s.
  s. recovery
  rosette s.
  S s.
  scaphocephalic head s.
  scaphoid s.
  sickle s.
  spheric s.
  spheroid s.
  vertebral body s.
  wine glass s.
shaper
  beam s.
shaping
  heat s.
shared
  s. coronary artery
  s. prepulse
sharp
  S. angle
  s. border of lung
  s. carina
  s. dissection
  S. fat saturation technique
  s. lateral margin
Sharpey fiber
sharply demarcated circumferential lesion
sharpness
  image s.
Sharp-Purser test
shattered
  s. kidney
  s. spleen
Shaver disease
shaving
  femoral condylar s.
  patellar s.
  residual metal fragment s.
SHC
  sclerosing hepatic carcinoma
shear
  s. fracture
  s. injury
  s. interface
  s. stiffness
  s. strain
  s. stress
shearing
  axonal s.
  s. force

  s. of white matter
  s. white matter injury
shear-strain
  s.-s. deformation
  s.-s. rate
shear-type brain injury
sheath
  Amplatz Teflon s.
  s. and side-arm
  angioplasty s.
  anterior rectus s.
  ArrowFlex s.
  arterial s.
  axillary s.
  bicipital synovial s.
  bicipital tendon s.
  carotid s.
  catheter s.
  caudal s.
  Check-Flo s.
  check-valve s.
  Colapinto s.
  common synovial flexor s.
  Cordis s.
  crural s.
  dentinal s.
  dural s.
  extensor carpi ulnaris s.
  fascial s.
  femoral s.
  fenestrated s.
  fibrous s.
  flexor tendon s.
  giant cell tumor of tendon s.
  guiding s.
  Henle s.
  hockey-stick guiding s.
  intratendon s.
  s. ligament
  minipuncture s.
  muscle s.
  myelin s.
  s. needle
  nerve root s.
  neural s.
  peel-away s.
  periarteriolar lymphoid s.
  periradicular s.
  pilar s.
  Pinnacle Destination renal guiding s.
  plicated dural s.
  posterior rectus s.
  rectus s.
  Schwann cell of myelin s.
  self-expanding tulip s.
  Spectranetics laser s. (SLS)
  straight guiding s.
  synovial s.
  tendon s.

Terumo Pinnacle R/OII radiopaque
    marker introducer s.
transseptal s.
tulip s.
unplicated s.
vascular s.
venous s.
working s.
sheathing canal
Shebele physician reporting
  workstation
Sheehan syndrome
sheet
    amnionic s.
    s. immobilizer
    s. tracking
sheetlike
    s. dysplasia
    s. growth pattern
Sheffield gamma unit
shelf
    Blumer rectal s.
    buccal s.
    dental s.
    lateral s.
    medial s.
    mesocolic s.
    palatine s.
    patellar s.
    rectal s.
    synovial s.
shell
    acetabular s.
    K s.
    L s.
    M s.
    s. nephrogram
    O s.
shelling off of cartilage
shell-like demarcation
shell-of-bone appearance
shell-type periosteal reaction
Shelton femur fracture classification
shelving edge of Poupart ligament
Shenton line
Shepherd fracture
shepherd's
    s. crook configuration
    s. crook deformity
Shepp-Logan filter function
SHG
    sonohysterography
Shibley sign
shibuol
shield
    acrylic syringe s.
    AME PinSite s.
    apron s.
    bismuth breast s.

Faraday s.
lead apron s.
lead eye s.
lead gonad s.
radiofrequency magnetic s.
shadow s.
tungsten eye s.
tungsten syringe s.
shielded gradient coil
shielded/unshielded breast dose
shielding
    active s.
    faulty radiofrequency s.
    gonadal s.
    magnetic s.
    passive s.
    RF s.
    room s.
shift
    anterior capsular s.
    aromatic solvent-induced s. (ASIS)
    chemical s.
    colloid s.
    diamagnetic s.
    distal s.
    Doppler frequency s.
    flow-related phase s.
    intracranial s.
    lanthanide-induced s.
    left-to-right s.
    mediastinal s.
    midline s.
    motion-induced phase s.
    navigator s.
    neonate mediastinal s.
    s. of heart
    s. of ventricle
    paramagnetic s.
    phase s.
    pineal gland s.
    plantar s.
    s. probe
    proximal brain s.
    radial s.
    s. reagent
    reverse pivot s. (RPS)
    right-to-left s.
    round s.
    simple s.
    square brain s.
    ST-segment s.
    superior frontal axis s.
    tracheal s.
    velocity-induced phase s.
    ventricular s.
shim
    s. coil
    s. inhomogeneity
    s. placement

S

Shimadzu
    S. CT scanner
    S. HeadTome Set-031 camera
    S. HeadTome system
    S. MR scanner
shimmed magnet
shimmering
    visual s.
shimming
    active s.
    localized s.
    passive s.
    s. process
shin
    s. bone
    s. splint
Shine-Dalgamo sequence
Shiner radiopaque tube
shine-through
    s.-t. effect
    s.-t. phenomenon
Shirmer test
shish
    s. kabob esophagus
    s. kabob pattern
shiver
    esophageal s.
shock
    anaphylactic s.
    bowel s.
    cardiac s.
    cardiogenic s.
    circulation s.
    distributive s.
    hypovolemic s.
    Joule s.
    s. lung
    lung s.
    nephrogram s.
    neurogenic s.
    obstructive s.
    QRS synchronized s.
    septic s.
    sequence monophasic s.
    vasogenic s.
shockwave pressure
shoemaker's breast
shone
    S. anomaly
    S. syndrome
shoot-through lateral x-ray film
Shope fibroma
short
    s. acquisition window
    s. bone
    s. echo point-resolved spectroscopic
      sequence spectrum
    s. echo time
    s. echo-time chemical-shift imaging

    s. echo-time proton spectroscopy
    s. esophagus-type hiatal hernia
    s. gut syndrome
    s. half-life
    s. head
    s. head of biceps
    s. insular gyrus
    s. inversion recovery
    s. inversion recovery imaging
    s. limb dysplasia
    s. muscle
    s. oblique fracture
    s. radiolunate ligament
    s. repetition time sequence
    s. rib
    s. rib-polydactyly syndrome
    s. tau inversion recovery (STIR)
    s. tau inversion recovery image
    s. TE proton MR spectroscopy
    s. TI inversion recovery (STIR)
    s. T1 inversion recovery imaging
    s. T1 inversion recovery pulse
      sequence
    s. T1 relaxation time
    s. TR-TE
short-axis
    s.-a. acquisition
    s.-a. image
    s.-a. parasternal view
    s.-a. plane
    s.-a. slice
    s.-a. view echocardiography
short-bore magnet
short-cannula coaxial method
short-distance
    s.-d. radiation therapy
    s.-d. radiotherapy
shortened
    fat-suppressed acquisition with TE
      and TR times s.
shortening
    Achilles tendon s.
    circumferential s.
    s. fraction
    fractional myocardial s.
    left ventricular functional s. (LVFS)
    leg s.
    phalangeal s.
    skeleton s.
    suboccipital s.
    systolic fractional s.
    tendon s.
    truncal s.
    T1, T2 s.
    T2-weighted s.
short-increment sensitivity index
short-range isotope
short-scale contrast
short-segment Barrett esophagus (SSBE)

short-term patency
shot
  cusp s.
  fast low-angle s. (FLASH)
  fluid-attenuated inversion
    recovery-fast low-angle s.
    (FLAIR-FLASH)
  guiding s.
  multiple-echo single s.
  pocket s.
  turbo fast low-angle s.
    (turboFLASH)
1-shot echo-planar imaging
shoulder
  s. ankylosis
  s. arthroplasty
  arthrotomography of s.
  baseball s.
  curvilinear threshold of s.
  s. dislocation
  s. dome
  double-contrast arthrotomography
    of s.
  drooping s.
  drop s.
  dynamic ultrasound of s. (DUS)
  s. dystocia
  flail s.
  football player's s.
  frozen s.
  s. girdle
  s. immobilizer
  s. impingement
  s. impingement syndrome
  intrathoracic dislocation of s.
  s. isocenter
  s. joint
  s. joint instability
  knocked-down s.
  s. labral capsular complex
  Little Leaguer's s.
  loose s.
  s. muscle
  s. of heart
  s. pointer
  s. presentation
  ringman's s.
  s. separation
  subcoracoid dislocation of s.
  subglenoid dislocation of s.
  s. surface coil
  swimmer's s.
  tennis s.
shoulder-hand syndrome
shower
  embolic s.
  s. of echoes
Shprintzen velocardiofacial syndrome
shrapnel

Shrapnell membrane
shrinkage
  aneurysm sac s.
  brain s.
  graft s.
  tumor s.
shriveled kidney
shrunken
  s. bladder
  s. folium
  s. gallbladder
  s. liver
  s. lung
SH U 508A contrast agent
shudder
  carotid s.
shunt
  barium sulfate-impregnated s.
  bidirectional s.
  biliopancreatic s.
  Blalock s.
  Blalock-Taussig s.
  cardiac atrial s.
  cardiovascular s.
  cerebral s.
  Cimino AV s.
  Cimino dialysis s.
  cystoatrial s.
  Davidson s.
  Denver s.
  dialysis s.
  direct intrahepatic portacaval s.
    (DIPS)
  distal splenorenal s.
  esophageal s.
  s. evaluation
  s. fraction
  gastrorenal s.
  Glenn s.
  hepatopulmonary s.
  indwelling nonvascular s.
  intracardiac s.
  intrapulmonary s.
  IVC-to-portal vein s.
  jejunoileal s.
  JI s.
  mesocaval s.
  net s.
  s. patency
  peritoneovenous s. (PVS)
  s. placement
  portacaval s.
  portopulmonary s.
  portosystemic s.
  Potts s.
  pulmonary s.
  pulmonary arteriovenous s.
  s. quantification
  s. reservoir

S

shunt (*continued*)
    s. reversal
    reversed s.
    right-to-left cardiac s.
    small bowel s.
    splenorenal s.
    systemic s.
    systemic portal s.
    s. thrombosis
    transjugular intrahepatic
      portosystemic s. (TIPS)
    s. tube
    VA s.
    s. valve
    ventriculoatrial s.
    ventriculoperitoneal s.
    VP s.
    Waterston s.
    Waterston-Cooley s.
    s. with normal left atrium
shunted
    s. blood
    s. hydrocephalus
    s. tracer
shunting
    s. circuit
    hepatic arterioportal s.
    lumboperitoneal s.
    s. of tracer to bone marrow
    peritoneal s.
    pleural s.
    syringosubarachnoid s.
shuntogram
    s. imaging
    radionuclide s.
shuntography
shutdown
    renal s.
shuttering
    white s.
Shwachman syndrome
SI
    sacroiliac
    SI joint
    SI joint-sacrum ratio
Si
    silicon
SIADH
    syndrome of inappropriate antidiuretic
    hormone
sialadenitis, sialoadenitis
    acute suppurative s.
    autoimmune s.
    chronic recurrent s.
    myoepithelial s.
    recurrent s.
sialadenography
sialangiography
sialectasis

sialoadenitis (*var. of* sialadenitis)
sialogram
sialography
    CT s.
    s. imaging
    magnetic resonance s.
    s. needle
    parotid gland s.
    submaxillary s.
sialolithiasis
sialometaplasia
sialometry
sialosis
siboroxime
    technetium 99m s.
Sibson
    S. fascia
    S. groove
    S. muscle
sick
    s. sinus node
    s. sinus syndrome
sickle
    s. cell anemia
    s. cell disease
    s. hemoglobin
    s. shape
sickle-shaped fold
sickling
    intravascular s.
sickness
    decompression s.
    radiation s.
    serum s.
SID
    source-to-image receptor distance
side
    s. branch
    s. effect
    s. fire
    s. lobe artifact
    s. scattering
side-arm
    sheath and s.-a.
sideband
    total suppression of s.
side-branch occlusion
side-by-side
    s.-b.-s. correlation
    s.-b.-s. objects
    s.-b.-s. transposition of great arteries
1-sided image reconstruction
side-exiting
    s.-e. coaxial needle system
    s.-e. guide
side-firing probe
sidehole cannulated probe
side-lying position
sideplate

Sideris buttoned double-disc device
sideropenic dysphagia
siderophore
siderotic
    s. nodule in spleen
    s. splenomegaly
sideswipe fracture
sidewall
    s. impingement
    pelvic s.
    rectal s.
Sidewinder diagnostic catheter
SIE
    stroke in evolution
Siemens
    S. AG system
    S. Biograph scanner
    S. DRH CT scanner
    S. Ecat Exact HR+ CTI PET
    scanner
    S. e.soft workstation
    S. gamma camera
    S. HICOR/BICOR x-ray system
    S. Icon
    S. Lithostar lithotriptor
    S. Magnetom GBS II scanner
    S. Magnetom SP 4000 scanner
    S. Magnetom 1.5T scanner
    S. Magnetom Vision scanner
    S. Magnetom Vision whole-body
    MR device
    S. Mammomat Novation DM
    full-field digital mammography
    system
    S. Mevatron 74 linear accelerator
    S. One Tesla scanner
    S. Orbiter large field-of-view camera
    S. Plus 4 Volume Zoom
    multidetector scanner
    S. Satellite CT evaluation console
    S. Somaform 512 CT scanner
    S. Somatom DR2, DR3 whole-body
    scanner
    S. Somatom nonhelical unit
    S. Somatom Plus CT scanner
    S. Somatom Plus-4 CT system
    S. Somatom Sensation 64
    S. Sonoline Elegra ultrasound
    scanner
    S. Syngo software
    S. 1.5T system
SieScape
    S. imaging technology
    S. ultrasound
sieve bone
sievert (Sv)
SIF
    sacral insufficiency fracture
sigma filter

sigmoid
    s. carcinoma
    s. cavity
    s. cavity of radius
    s. cavity of ulna
    s. colon
    s. colon volvulus
    s. density curve
    s. diverticulitis
    s. diverticulum
    s. flexure
    s. fold
    s. hair pattern
    s. kidney
    s. loop
    s. lymph node
    s. mesocolon
    s. notch
    s. omentum
    s. polyp
    s. pseudostenosis
    s. sinus
    s. sulcus
    s. valve
    s. volvulus (SV)
sigmoidoscope, sigmoscope
    Olympus OSF s.
    Reichert flexible s.
sigmoidoscopy
sigmoid-shaped configuration
sigmoscope (*var. of* sigmoidoscope)
sign
    Aaron s.
    Abrahams s.
    absent bow-tie s.
    absent diaphragm s.
    accordion s.
    air bronchogram s.
    air-crescent s.
    air-meniscus s.
    Allis s.
    Amoss s.
    angel-wing s.
    anteater nose s.
    antecedent s.
    anterior drawer s.
    aortic nipple s.
    apical cap s.
    arrowhead s.
    Aunt Minnie s.
    bamboo spine s.
    banana s.
    Battle s.
    B6 bronchus s.
    beaded septum s.
    beak s.
    Beevor s.
    Bergman s.
    big rib s.

S

sign (*continued*)

bird-of-prey s.
bite s.
blade-of-grass s.
blister of bone s.
Blumberg s.
blush s.
bone bruise s.
bone-in-bone s.
boutonnière deformity s.
bowler hat s.
bowstring s.
bow-tie s.
Bozzolo s.
Bragard s.
Braunwald s.
brim s.
bronchial cuff s.
bronchus s.
Brudzinski s.
Bryant s.
bubble s.
bulging fissure s.
C s.
calcium s.
Cantelli s.
cardinal s.
cardiorespiratory s.
Carman s.
Carnett s.
carotid string s.
Carvallo s.
catheter coiling s.
cervicothoracic s.
Chaddock s.
Chilaiditi s.
Claybrook s.
clockwise whirlpool s.
cobblestone s.
cobra-eye s.
cockade image s.
Codman s.
Cogan lid twitch s.
cogwheel s.
coiled spring s.
collapsing cord s.
collar s.
Collier s.
colon cutoff s.
comb s.
comet s.
comet-tail s.
commemorative s.
Comolli s.
continuous diaphragm s.
contralateral s.
Coopernail s.
cord s.
Corrigan s.

cortical rim s.
cortical ring s.
cortical vein s.
cotton-wool s.
Courvoisier s.
cranial nerve s.
crescent s.
crescent-in-doughnut s.
crowded carpal s.
Cullen s.
Cupid's bow s.
cupula s.
cutoff s.
cystic duct s.
dagger s.
Dance s.
David Letterman s.
Dawbarn s.
deep lateral femoral notch s.
deep sulcus s.
Dejerine s.
Delbet s.
delta s.
Demianoff s.
de Musset s.
dense MCA s.
d'Espine s.
Dorendorf s.
double bleb s.
double bubble s.
double-condom s.
double decidual sac s. (DDSS)
double-density s.
double diaphragm s.
double duct s.
double halo s.
double lesion s.
double line s.
double PCL s.
double ring esophageal s.
double-track s.
double-wall s.
doughnut s.
drooping lily s.
drooping shoulder s.
Drummond s.
Duchenne s.
duct-penetrating s.
Dupuytren s.
Duroziez s.
Ebstein s.
echogenic starburst s.
elbow fat-pad s.
empty delta s.
Erichsen s.
Ewart s.
extrapleural s.
facet osteoarthritis s. (FOS)
falciform ligament s.

fallen fragment s.
fallen lung s.
false localizing s.
fan s.
fat-blood interface s.
fat-pad s.
FBI s.
feeding vessel s.
figure-3 s.
finger-in-glove s.
Finkelstein s.
Fischer s.
fish vertebra s.
fissure s.
flat waist s.
fleck s.
Fleischner s.
flipped meniscus s.
floating viscera s.
floppy thumb s.
fluid-fluid level s.
flush-tank s.
focal neurologic s.
football s.
fragment-in-notch s.
Friedreich s.
Froment s.
frontal lobe s.
Frostberg s.
Gaenslen s.
Galeazzi s.
garland s.
Gerhardt s.
geyser s.
Glasgow s.
gliding s.
gloved-finger s.
Golden S s.
Goldthwait s.
Gordon s.
Gottron s.
Gowers s.
Grey Turner s.
Griesinger s.
Grocco s.
Gunn crossing s.
hair-on-end s.
half-moon s.
halo s.
Hamman s.
Hampton hump s.
harlequin s.
hatchet s.
Hawkins s.
hay-fork s.
heel pad s.
Heim-Kreysig s.
hilar s.
Hildreth s.

Hill s.
Hill-Sachs s.
Hirschberg s.
Hoffmann s.
Hoover s.
Horner s.
hot nose s.
hot spur s.
Howship-Romberg s.
H vertebra s.
hyperdense middle cerebral artery s.
hyperintense ring s.
iliopsoas s.
incomplete ring s.
inferior triangle s.
insular ribbon s.
interface s.
interrupted duct s.
intradecidual s.
intravertebral vacuum cleft s.
inverted Napoleon hat s.
inverted teardrop s.
inverted-V s.
ivory phalanx s.
Jaccoud s.
Jackson s.
juxtaphrenic peak s.
Kanavel s.
Kantor string s.
Karplus s.
Kehr s.
Kellock s.
Kernig s.
Klemm s.
knuckle s.
Kussmaul s.
Lachman s.
Lancisi s.
Landolfi s.
Lasègue s.
lateral capsular s.
lateralizing s.
Lazarus s.
Leichtenstern s.
lemon s.
leptomeningeal ivy s.
Léri s.
linguine s.
Livierato s.
localizing s.
long tract s.
luftsichel s.
Macewen s.
Maisonneuve s.
Mannkopf s.
Martorell s.
McGinn-White s.
melting s.
melting ice cube s.

S

sign (*continued*)

    Meltzer s.
    meniscus s.
    Mennell s.
    metacarpal s.
    Minor s.
    Morquio s.
    Mulder s.
    Müller s.
    Musset s.
    Myerson s.
    Naffziger s.
    naked facet s.
    Napoleon hat s.
    Neer impingement s.
    neurologic soft s.
    Nicoladoni-Branham s.
    noose keyhole pull-away s.
    obturator s.
    Oliver-Cardarelli s.
    open bronchus s.
    open ring s.
    Oppenheim s.
    Ortolani s.
    Osler s.
    ovarian vascular pedicle s.
    pathognomonic s.
    Payr s.
    pedestal s.
    Perez s.
    peritoneal s.
    peroneal s.
    persistent loop s.
    piano key s.
    Pins s.
    Piotrowski s.
    pirate s.
    pivot-shift s.
    Plummer s.
    pneumoarthrogram s.
    Potain s.
    premonitory s.
    pronator s.
    pseudokidney s.
    psoas s.
    puddle s.
    pulvinar s.
    pupillary s.
    pyramidal s.
    Queckenstedt s.
    Quénu-Muret s.
    Quincke s.
    radialis s.
    railroad track s.
    rebound s.
    reversal s.
    reversed-3 s.
    reversed-S s.
    Rigler s.

    rim s.
    ring s.
    ring-around-the-artery s.
    Risser s.
    Romberg s.
    Rosenbach s.
    rose thorn s.
    Rotch s.
    Rovighi s.
    Rovsing s.
    rugger jersey s.
    sail s.
    Sanders s.
    sandwich s.
    Sansom s.
    sausage digit s.
    sawtooth s.
    Schepelmann s.
    Schlesinger s.
    Schwartze s.
    scimitar s.
    scotty dog s.
    seagull s.
    sentinel clot s.
    sentinel loop s.
    setting-sun s.
    Shibley s.
    signet ring s.
    silhouette s.
    Sister Mary Joseph s.
    Skoda s.
    slim carotid artery s.
    sonographic Murphy s.
    Spalding s.
    spinal s.
    spine s.
    split pleura s.
    Spurling s.
    squeeze s.
    steeple s.
    Steinberg s.
    stepladder s.
    stepoff vertebral body s.
    Sternberg s.
    Stewart-Holmes s.
    Stierlin s.
    string s.
    string-of-beads s.
    string-of-pearls s.
    stripe s.
    Strümpell s.
    Strunsky anterior arch of foot s.
    Sumner s.
    superior triangle s.
    swan neck deformity s.
    tail s.
    target s.
    teardrop s.
    Terry Thomas s.

testicular vascular pedicle s.
threads-and-streaks s.
Thurston Holland s.
thymic sail s.
tibialis s.
Tinel s.
toggle s.
tooth s.
Traube s.
tree-in-bud s.
triple bubble s.
triple track s.
Troisier s.
trolley track s.
trough line s.
Trousseau s.
tumbling bullet s.
Turyn back pain s.
twin peak s.
twisted pedicle s.
Uhthoff s.
vacuum phenomenon s.
Vanzetti sciatica s.
Waddell nonorganic back
  pain s.
Wartenberg s.
Wegner s.
Weill s.
Weiss s.
Westermark s.
whirl s.
whirlpool s.
white cerebellum s.
Wimberger bilateral metaphysial s.
windsock s.
yin-yang s.

Signa

S. Advantage system
S. Excite MRI system
S. Horizon LX MRI system
S. Horizon LX SR 77 gradient
  1.5T MR scanner
S. Horizon X-Echo-Speed
S. MR imaging system
S. MRI scanner
S. 1.5T scanner
S. VH/i3.0T MR scanner

signal

abnormal bright s.
s. acquisition
s. attenuation
s. average
s. blooming
BOLD s.
bright s.
s. change
s. characteristic
color Doppler s.
composite s.

D s.
s. dephasing
s. depth
differential s.
Doppler blood flow velocity s.
Doppler ovary s.
s. dropout artifact
s. enhancement
s. fallout
s. flare phenomenon
flow velocity s.
fluid s.
free induction decay s.
gamma s.
gate s.
GE-Amersham merger s.
s. halo
high-intensity transient s. (HITS)
high-pitched s.
hyperintense s.
hypointense marrow s.
imaginary s.
increased echo s.
s. intensity (grade 1-3)
s. intensity inhomogeneity
s. intensity measurement
s. intensity ratio
s. intensity rim
s. intensity-time curve
isointense s.
s. joint
linear low s.
lipid s.
s. loss
magnetic resonance s.
s. magnification
mosaic jet s.
navigable echo s.
NMR s.
s. node
nuclear s.
ovarian Doppler s.
periventricular bright s.
phosphomonoester s.
power Doppler s.
s. processing
pulsed-wave spectral color Doppler
  s.
radionuclide s.
real s.
s. sonographic feature analysis
s. source
SSFP s.
stimulus-correlated water s.
superimposition of s.
s. suppression
symmetric abnormal increased s.
s. time course
s. transducer

S

signal (*continued*)
    s. transduction
    turbulent s.
    T2-weighted s.
    unsuppressed water s.
    velocity-encoded color Doppler s.
    s. void
    weak s.
signal-averaged electrocardiogram (SAECG, SaECG)
signaling lymphocytic activation molecule
signal-to-clutter ratio
signal-to-noise
    s.-t.-n. calculation
    s.-t.-n. ratio (S/N, SNR)
    s.-t.-n. threshold
signature
    echo s.
    gut s.
    tissue s.
    tumor s.
signet
    s. ring cell carcinoma
    s. ring pattern
    s. ring sign
significance level
significant
    s. axis deviation
    s. residual deficit
    s. sequela
SIH
    secondary intracranial hypertension
    spontaneous intracranial hypotension
SIL
    squamous intraepithelial lesion
silastic
    s. collar-reinforced stoma
    s. finger joint
    s. ring
silence
    electrocerebral s. (ECS)
silent
    s. area of brain
    s. cerebral embolus
    s. cerebral infarct
    s. gallstone
    s. ischemic episode
    s. mitral stenosis
    s. myocardial infarct (SMI)
    s. myocardial ischemia
    s. parathyroid adenoma
    s. patent ductus arteriosus
    s. regurgitation
    s. sinus syndrome
silhouette
    cardiac s.
    cardiothymic s.
    cardiovascular s.
    enlarged cardiac s.

    heart s.
    s. imaging
    S. laser system
    luminal s.
    pericardial s.
    radiographic s.
    s. sign
    s. sign of Felson
    s. technique
    widened cardiac s.
silhouetted out
silhouetting
silicate
    gadolinium s.
    s. pneumoconiosis
silicon (Si)
    amorphous s. (a-Si)
    s. diode array
    s. diode dosimeter
    S. Graphics Reality Engine system
silicon-controlled rectifier (SCR)
silicone
    s. caoutchouc
    s. diode
    s. elastomer band
    s. elastomer ring
    s. elastomer rubber ball implant
    s. fluid
    s. granuloma
    s. implant leakage
    s. implant rupture
    s. injection
    s. microsphere
    s. oil
    s. stent
    s. wrist implant
silicoproteinosis
    acute s.
silicosis
    accelerated s.
    chronic simple s.
    complicated s.
    Liverpool s.
    nonnodular s.
    simple s.
silicotic
    s. fibrosis of lung
    s. nodule
    s. visceral pleura
silicotuberculosis
Si(Li) detector
silk
    s. suture
    s. tuft
SilkLaser
    erbium S.
    S. esthetic carbon dioxide laser
Sillence classification of osteogenesis imperfecta

sillimanite pneumoconiosis
silo-filler's
    s.-f. disease
    s.-f. lung
silver (Ag)
    s. finisher's lung
    s. fork fracture
    Grocott methenamine s.
    s. halide film
    hammered s.
    s. iodide
    s. polisher's lung
    s. recovery
    S. Speed guidewire
    s. wire effect
Silverhawk catheter
simian griffe
Simmond disease
Simmons catheter
Simon
    S. focus
    S. nitinol IVC filter
    S. nitinol vena cava filter
Simonart
    S. band
    S. ligament
Sim Plant
simple
    s. block
    s. bolus
    s. bone cyst
    s. breast cyst
    s. capillary lymphangioma
    s. cortical renal cyst
    s. dislocation
    s. extraperitoneal rupture
    s. goiter
    s. mastectomy
    s. mechanical obstruction
    s. meningocele
    s. pulmonary eosinophilia
    s. shift
    s. silicosis
    s. skull fracture
    s. ureterocele
simplex
    carcinoma s.
    xanthoma tuberosum s.
SimpliCT interventional guidance
  system
Simpson
    S. atherectomy
    S. Coronary AtheroCath (SCA)
    S. Coronary AtheroCath system
    S. directional atherectomy catheter
    S. rule method for ventricular
      volume
    S. white line
Sims position

simulated
    s. annealing
    s. annealing method
    s. annealing method projection
    s. echo
    s. equilibrium factor study
simulation
    s. film
    MCPT s.
    Monte Carlo photon transport s.
    s. of converging ports
    s. of tangential portal
simulation-aided field setting
simulator
    AcQsim CT s.
    magnetic resonance s.
    Maxwell 3D field s.
    virtual reality s.
    Ximatron s.
simultaneous
    s. acquisition of artery and vein
      (SAAV)
    s. acquisition of spatial harmonics
      (SMASH)
    s. areolar mastopexy and breast
      augmentation (SAMBA)
    s. balloon inflation
    s. bilateral spontaneous
      pneumothorax (SBSP)
    s. fluoroscopy
    s. MSDI
    s. multifilm tomography
    s. multiple-angle reconstruction
      technique (SMART)
    s. multislice acquisition
    s. recording
    s. slice
    s. thermoradiotherapy
    s. volume imaging
sincalide
    s. cholescintigraphy
    s. imaging agent
sinc-Hanning radiofrequency
sinc interpolation
sincipital cephalocele
Sinding-Larsen-Johansson patellar
  tendinitis disease
sine wave
singer's
    s. node
    s. nodule
Singh osteoporosis index
single
    s. atrium
    s. axis
    s. breath-hold
    s. breath-hold dynamic subtraction
      CT with multidetector row helical
      technology

S

single (*continued*)
    s. breath-hold sequence
    s. collision energy loss
    s. colonic filling defect
    s. fill/void technique
    s. functioning kidney
    s. isocenter
    s. label
    s. peak
    s. pleurisy
    s. polyp
    s. popliteal vein
    s. port
    s. umbilical artery
    s. umbilical artery spectrum
    s. ventricle
    s. x-ray dosimetry
single-ablation scheme
single-balloon enteroscope (SBE)
single-bevel stylet
single-breath view
single-cannula atrial cannulation
single-cavity cochlea
single-channel analyzer (SCA)
single-contrast
    s.-c. arthrography
    s.-c. barium enema
    s.-c. GI examination
    s.-c. study
single-crystal endoprobe
single-curved Cobra catheter
single-detector
    s.-d. computed tomography (SDCT)
    s.-d. CTA
    s.-d. helical CT
    s.-d. helical scanner
    s.-d. row scanner
single-dose gadolinium imaging
single-echo
    s.-e. diffusion imaging
    s.-e. versus multiple-echo sequence
single-energy x-ray absorptiometer (SXA)
single-field hyperthermia technique
single-headed instrument
single-head rotating gamma camera
single-hole collimator
single-injection protocol
single-lumen silicone breast implant
single-lung transplant
single-needle biopsy technique
single-outlet heart
single-pass scan
single-phase current
single-photon
    s.-p. absorptiometry (SPA)
    s.-p. bone densitometry
    s.-p. counting (SPC)
    s.-p. counting system

    s.-p. densitometer
    s.-p. emission computed tomography (SPECT)
    s.-p. emission computed tomography technetium sestamibi scan
    s.-p. emission CT
    s.-p. emission tomography (SPET)
    s.-p. maximum intensity
    s.-p. planar scintigraphy (SPPS)
single-pixel reconstruction
single-plane angiography
single-pole double-throw (SPDT)
single-power injector
single-sample
    s.-s. clearance
    s.-s. technique
single-section 2D image
single-shot
    s.-s. embolization of micro-AVM
    s.-s. fast spin echo (SSFSE)
    s.-s. gradient-echo EPI sequence
    s.-s. gradient echo-planar imaging
    s.-s. imaging technique
    s.-s. MR cholangiogram
    s.-s. PSIR sequence
    s.-s. spin-echo echo-planar pulse sequence
    s.-s. thick-slab RARE
    s.-s. TSE (SShTSE)
single-slice
    s.-s. CTA
    s.-s. 8-echo technique
    s.-s. gradient-echo image
    s.-s. helical CT
    s.-s. long-axis tomogram
    s.-s. spiral CT
single-stick
    s.-s. catheter introduction
    s.-s. nephrostomy
    s.-s. system
single-strand
    s.-s. conformational polymorphism (SSCP)
    s.-s. scission
single-stripe colitis (SSC)
single-suture synostosis
single-sweep scan
single-vessel
    s.-v. disease
    s.-v. runoff
single-view oblique mammography
single-voxel
    s.-v. in vivo proton spectrum
    s.-v. proton brain examination
    s.-v. proton brain spectroscopy imaging
    s.-v. proton MR spectroscopy
    s.-v. stimulated echo acquisition-mode MR spectroscopy

single-wall needle
singular valve decomposition
(SVD)
sinistral portal hypertension
sinistrum
    atrium s.
sink
    s. effect
    quantum s.
sink-trap malformation
sinoatrial (*var. of* sinuatrial)
sinoauricular node
sinodural plate
Sinografin imaging agent
sinogram
sinography
sinonasal
    s. adenocarcinoma
    s. carcinoma
    s. cavity
    s. inverted papilloma
    s. lesion
    s. lymphoma
    s. malignancy
    s. neoplasm
    s. polyposis
    s. psammomatoid ossifying fibroma
    s. secretion
    s. tumor
sinotubular junction
sinovaginal bulb
sintering
    selective laser s. (SLS)
sinuatrial (SA, S-A), sinoatrial
    s. block (SAB)
    s. branch
    s. bundle
    s. conduction time (SACT)
    s. exit block
    s. nodal reentry tachycardia
    s. node (SAN)
    s. node artery
    s. node dysfunction
    s. node infarct
sinus, *pl.* **sinus, sinuses**
    accessory s.
    alternating s.
    aortic valve s.
    s. arrest
    artery of inferior cavernous s.
    (AICS)
    basilar s.
    branchial s.
    bronchial s.
    carotid s.
    cavernous s.
    s. cavity
    cerebral venous s.
    cervical s.

circular s.
cloudy s.
coccygeal s.
coronary s.
costomediastinal s.
costophrenic s.
cranial s.
s. cycle length (SCL)
dilated intercavernous s.
distal coronary s. (DCS)
dorsal dermal s.
dorsal enteric s.
draining s.
dural venous s.
dura mater venous s.
endodermal s.
ethmoid s.
s. fracture
frontal s.
granulomatous lesion of s.
Guérin s.
hair-containing s.
s. histiocytosis
s. hyperplasia
hypoechoic renal s.
s. hypoplasia
s. infection
inferior sagittal s. (ISS)
inflammatory polyp in s.
intercavernous s.
s. irregularity
lactiferous s.
lateral s.
s. lateralis
left coronary s.
s. lipomatosis
lumbosacral dermal s.
lymph node s.
manual pressure over carotid s.
marginal s.
mastoid s.
maxillary s.
s. mechanism
medullary s.
middle coronary s. (MCS)
nasal s.
s. node
s. node artery
s. node automaticity
s. node depression
s. node dysfunction
s. node electrogram
s. node exit block
s. node recovery time (SNRT)
s. node reentry
noncoronary s.
oblique pericardial s.
occipital s.
s. of epididymis

S

sinus (*continued*)
    s. of Morgagni
    s. of pulmonary trunk
    s. of Valsalva
    s. of Valsalva aneurysm
    s. of vena cava
    osteomyelitic s.
    paranasal s.
    s. pattern
    s. pause
    pericardial s.
    s. pericranii
    perineal s.
    Petit s.
    petrosal s.
    pilonidal s.
    piriform s.
    precoronal sagittal s.
    prostatic s.
    proximal coronary s. (PCS)
    pulmonary s.
    renal s.
    s. rhythm
    s. rhythm mapping
    Ridley s.
    Rokitansky-Aschoff s.
    rudimentary s.
    sagittal s.
    s. septum
    s. series
    sigmoid s.
    s. slowing
    sphenoid s.
    sphenoparietal s.
    straight s.
    subeustachian s.
    superior petrous s. (SPS)
    superior sagittal s. (SSS)
    tarsal s.
    s. tarsi syndrome
    thickened s.
    s. thrombosis
    s. tract
    s. tract imaging
    s. tract study
    transverse pericardial s.
    tubercular s.
    umbilical-urachal s.
    urachal s.
    urogenital s.
    s. venosus
    s. venosus atrial septal defect
    venous s.
    vertebral articular s.
sinuses (*pl. of* sinus)
sinusitis
    acute s.
    allergic s.
    bacterial s.

    bronchiectasis-ethmoid s.
    s. cerebritis
    chronic s.
    mycotic s.
    paranasal s.
    sphenoid s.
sinusography
    cerebral s.
sinusoid
    hepatic s.
    s. reference function
sinusoidal
    s. capillary
    s. histiocyte
    s. lesion
    s. relaxation
    s. vascular space
    s. waveform
sinusoidalization
sinuum
    confluens s.
sinuvertebral nerve of Luschka
SIP
    saturation inversion projection
    spinal imaging platform
siphon
    carotid s.
Sipple syndrome
Siremobile Iso-C3d isocentric C-arm
sirenomelia, symmelia
sirolimus
sirolimus-eluting SMART nitinol stent
SIR-Spheres radioactive sphere
SIRT
    selective internal radiation therapy
Sirtex Medical Limited
SIS
    saline infusion sonohysterography
SISCOM
    subtraction ictal SPECT coregistered to MRI
Sisco spectrometer
Sister
    S. Mary Joseph node
    S. Mary Joseph nodule
    S. Mary Joseph sign
site, situs
    anastomotic s.
    binding s.
    bleeding s.
    cancer of unknown primary s.
    catheter exit s.
    cellular binding s.
    donor s.
    extraadrenal s.
    extranodal s.
    fracture s.
    implantation s.
    ipsilateral antegrade s.

metastatic s.
s. of maximum intensity
reference s.
sanctuary s.
spot s.
termination s.
unknown primary s.
Site-Rite II ultrasound system
site-specific labeling
sitting-up
s.-u. view
s.-u. view angiography
situ
adenocarcinoma in s. (ACIS)
carcinoma in s.
ductal carcinoma in s. (DCIS)
in s.
intracystic breast papillary carcinoma in s.
lobular carcinoma in s.
(LCIS)
nasopharyngeal carcinoma in s.
transitional carcinoma in s.
situs, *pl.* **situs** (*var. of* site)
atrial s.
s. atrialis solitus
s. concordance
D-loop ventricular s.
s. inversus
s. inversus partialis
s. inversus totalis
s. inversus viscerum
L-loop ventricular s.
s. perversus
s. transversus
Sitzmarks
S. capsule
S. radiopaque marker
size
abnormal placenta s.
borderline heart s.
decreased placenta s.
effective focal spot s.
embryo s.
s. estimation error
field s.
focal spot s.
gallbladder s.
kernel s.
kidney s.
matrix s.
s. of spinal cord
ovarian s.
renal s.
top normal limits of s.
uterine s.
ventricular s.
vertebral body s.
voxel s.
x-ray beam s.

Sjögren-Larsson syndrome
Sjögren syndrome
S-JRA
systemic juvenile rheumatoid arthritis
SJS
Schwartz-Jampel syndrome
skeletal
s. amyloidosis
s. bed
s. biopsy
s. disruption
s. dysplasia
s. emphysema
s. growth plate
s. hyperostosis
s. hypoplasia
s. infection
s. lesion
s. lymphoma
s. maturation
s. maturity
s. muscle
s. muscle fiber
s. muscle metastasis
s. muscle protein
s. myxoid chondrosarcoma
s. neoplasia
s. radiology
s. sarcoidosis
s. survey
s. system
s. targeted radiotherapy (STR)
s. tuberculosis
skeletally
s. immature
s. mature
skeletography
skeletology
skeleton
appendicular s.
s. appendiculare
articulated s.
axial s.
s. axiale
bony s.
cardiac s.
central s.
fibrous s.
gill arch s.
laryngeal s.
peripheral s.
s. shortening
spidering s.
spiky s
sulcal s.
s. thoracis
visceral s.
skeletonizing
skewness

S

skiagram (*var. of* radiograph)
skiagraph (*var. of* radiograph)
skiagraphy (*var. of* radiography)
skier's
    s. fracture
    s. injury
    s. thumb
ski jump view
Skillern fracture
skimming of magnetic field
skin
    s. bridge
    s. calcification
    s. carcinoma
    s. crease artifact
    s. depth
    s. dose
    s. effect
    s. fold
    s. lesion artifact
    s. line
    s. staple
    s. thickening
skinfold artifact
Skinlight erbium:YAG laser
Skinner pelvic menstruation line
skinny needle
skin-rolling scapular tenderness
skin-sparing
    s.-s. effect
    s.-s. mastectomy
skip
    s. aganglionosis
    s. area
    s. lesion
    s. metastasis
    s. tomography
skodaic resonance
Skoda sign
skull
    abnormally thin s.
    anterior cerebral artery crawling
      under s.
    s. asymmetry
    s. base
    s. base approach
    s. base foramen
    base of s. (BOS)
    s. base tumor
    beaten brass s.
    beaten silver appearance of s.
    button sequestrum of s.
    cloverleaf s.
    dentate suture of s.
    s. film
    s. fracture
    geographic s.
    hair-on-end of s.
    hammered silver s.

    hammer-marked s.
    hot-cross bun s.
    s. hyperostosis
    indented fracture of s.
    inner table of s.
    lacunar s.
    lytic lesion of s.
    maplike s.
    s. metastasis
    molding of s.
    natiform s.
    occipital view of s.
    s. osteolysis
    outer table of s.
    s. plate
    sonolucent s.
    suture of s.
    synchondrosis of s.
    thin s.
    s. volume
    West-Engstler s.
    West lacuna s.
skullcap (*var. of* calvaria)
**SKYLight gantry-free nuclear medicine
  gamma camera**
skyline
    s. projection
    s. view
    s. view of patella
SL
  scapholunate
  spin-lock
    SL joint
    SL technique
slab
    coronal s.
    3D MRA s.
    interleaved axial s.
    s. thickness
slab-MIP
SLAC
  scapholunate advanced collapse
    SLAC wrist
slant-hole collimator
SLAP
  superior labral anterior to posterior
    SLAP lesion
    SLAP tear
slat collimator
SLE
  systemic lupus erythematosus
sleeve
    conjoined root s.'s
    s. fracture
    s. lobectomy
    nerve root s.
    root s.
    Smitt s.
    thoracic root s.

SLE2000 ventilator
slew range
SL-GRE
    spin-lock gradient-echo
        SL-GRE sequence
slice
    angled s.
    apical short-axis s.
    axial s.
    basal short-axis s.
    contiguous s.'s
    coronal s.
    digitized CT s.
    direct s.
    2D sequential s.
    s. efficiency
    s. excitation wave (SEW)
    s. format
    s. fracture
    gated stress myocardial perfusion s.
    s. geometry
    horizontal long-axis s.
    s. interference
    intermediate CT s.
    long-axis s.
    midventricular short-axis s.
    nonattenuation-corrected s.
    nonplanar s.
    oblique s.
    s. orientation
    s. overlap artifact
    plurality of s.'s
    s. profile artifact
    sagittal s.
    s. select gradient
    s. selection
    s. sensitivity profile (SSP)
    serial CT s.'s
    short-axis s.
    simultaneous s.
    STIR s.
    texture s.
    s. thickness
    tissue s.
    tomographic s.
    transaxial s.
    transverse s.
    vertical long-axis s.
    s. volume
4-slice acquisition
16-slice CT scanner
slice-of-sausage breast pattern
slice-point MRS
40-slice scanner
slice-selective excitation
slicing plane
slider crank theory
sliding
    s. board transfer
    s. hiatal hernia
    s. interleaved kY (SLINKY)
    s. thin-slab approach
    s. thin-slab maximum-intensity
        projection (STS-MIP)
    s. thin-slab maximum-intensity
        projection image
    s. thin-slab minimum-intensity
        projection technique
sliding-slab average-intensity projection
  technique
slim carotid artery sign
sling
    cardiac s.
    s. muscle fiber
    pulmonary s.
    s. ring complex
    tendon s.
    vascular s.
SLINKY
    sliding interleaved kY
slip
    s. angle
    diaphragmatic s.
    muscular s.
    s. of tendon
slip-angle spondylolisthesis
slip-in connection
slippage
    epiphysial s.
    film s.
slipped
    s. capital femoral epiphysis (SCFE)
    s. tendon
    s. upper femoral epiphysis (SUFE)
slipping
    s. rib
    s. rib syndrome
slip-ring
    s.-r. camera
    s.-r. CT
    s.-r. gantry system
    s.-r. imaging
    s.-r. technology
slit
    s. collimator
    s. hemorrhage
    s. radiography
    s. scanography
    s. ventricle
    s. ventricle syndrome
slit-lamp biomicroscopy
slitlike
    s. lumen
    s. orifice
    s. residual lucency
slit-shaped vessel lumen
sliver
    bone s.

S

SLL
    spinolaminar line
SLN
    sentinel lymph node
SLNB
    sentinel lymph node biopsy
slope
    acromial s.
    s. blot analysis
    closing s.
    decreased E-to-F s.
    disappearance s.
    downward s.
    D-to-E s.
    E-to-F s.
    flat diastolic s.
    flattened E-to-F s.
    mitral deceleration s.
    normalized plateau s.
    opening s.
    palmar s.
    ST-segment/heart rate s.
    triquetrohamate helicoid s.
    valve opening s.
slot-scan detection system
slot-scanning detector
slotted tube stent
sloughed
    s. mucosa
    s. papilla
    s. urethra syndrome
sloughing ulcer
slow
    s. channel-blocking drug
    s. filling wave
    s. neutron
    s. stroke
    s. ventricular response
slow-exchange soft tissue
slow-flow
    s.-f. giant saccular aneurysm
    s.-f. lesion
    s.-f. vascular anomaly
    s.-f. vascular malformation
slowing
    background s.
    sinus s.
slowly
    s. developing atelectasis
    s. developing lesion
slow-twitch muscle
slow-wave activity
SLP
    subluxation of patella
SLS
    selective laser sintering
    Spectranetics laser sheath
    SLS laser

sludge
    aggregated s.
    s. ball
    biliary s.
    blood s.
    gallbladder s.
    tumefactive biliary s.
sludgelike intraluminal echo
sludging of retinal vein
sluggish flow
slurry
Sm
    samarium
^{153}**Sm, Sm-153**
    samarium 153
SMA
    spinal muscular atrophy
    superior mesenteric artery
        Doppler sonography of SMA
SMAI
    superomedial acetabular
    index
small
    s. adrenal tumor
    s. airway
    s. airway dysfunction
    s. aorta syndrome
    s. B-cell lymphoma
    s. bowel
    s. bowel
    s. bowel adenocarcinoma
    s. bowel adenoma
    s. bowel atresia
    s. bowel benign tumor
    s. bowel carcinoma
    s. bowel cavitary lesion
    s. bowel contents
    s. bowel delayed transit
    s. bowel disease
    s. bowel diverticulum
    s. bowel duplication cyst
    s. bowel enema
    s. bowel enteroscopy (SBE)
    s. bowel filling defect
    s. bowel fold anatomy
    s. bowel fold atrophy
    s. bowel followthrough
    (SBFT)
    s. bowel gas
    s. bowel hemangioma
    s. bowel hematoma
    s. bowel hemorrhage
    s. bowel infarct
    s. bowel leiomyoma
    s. bowel leiomyosarcoma
    s. bowel loop
    s. bowel malignant tumor
    s. bowel malrotation

s. bowel meal
s. bowel metastasis
s. bowel motility
s. bowel mucosal pattern
s. bowel obstruction (SBO)
s. bowel peristalsis
s. bowel pseudodiverticulum
s. bowel pseudotumor
s. bowel separation
s. bowel series
s. bowel shunt
s. bowel transit time
s. bowel volvulus
s. bowel wall thickening
s. cardiac vein
s. cell
s. cell cribriform carcinoma
s. cell lung carcinoma (SCLC)
s. cell osteosarcoma
s. cell undifferentiated carcinoma
s. colonic J-pouch
s., deep, recent infarct (SDRI)
s. feminine aorta
s. field-of-view MR imaging
s. for gestational age fetus
s. gallbladder
s. gut
s. internal auditory canal
s. intestine
s. intestine carcinoma
s. intestine mesentery
s. left colon syndrome
s. LITT applicator
s. lymphatic lymphoma
s. lymphocytic T-cell lymphoma
s. part of fetus
s. pelvis
s. round cell carcinoma
s. saphenous vein
s. spleen
s vertebral body
s. water-hammer pulse
small-angle
s.-a. double-incidence angiogram
s.-a. multiple scattering
small-bore scanner
small-caliber needle
small-droplet fatty liver
small-lunged emphysema
small-particle iron oxide contrast
small-step distraction
small-vessel
s.-v. stroke
s.-v. vasculitis
small-volume tissue ablation
small-voxel acquisition
SMAP
systemic mean arterial pressure

SMART
simultaneous multiple-angle reconstruction technique
SMART Control self-expanding stent
SMART nitinol self-expandable stent
SmartBeam IMRT
SmartNeedle
SmartPrep
S. imaging agent
MR S.
S. scanner
SmartScore CT imaging
SmartSPOT high-resolution digital imaging system
Smartstent
SMAS
superior mesenteric artery syndrome
SMASH
simultaneous acquisition of spatial harmonics
variable-density SMASH
smear fragment
Smelloff-Cutter valve
SMI
silent myocardial infarct
Smith
S. dislocation
S. fracture
S. orthogonal hole test
S. sesamoid position classification
Smith-Lemli-Opitz syndrome
Smith-Petersen nail
Smith-Robinson bone graft
Smitt sleeve
SMM
scintimammography
SMN
2nd malignant neoplasia
smoked glass image
smokelike echo
smoker's
s. bronchiolitis
s. lung
smooth
s. border
s. brain
s. calcific deposit
s. contour
s. esophageal narrowing
s. excimer laser coronary angioplasty (SELCA)
s. hyperplasia
s. mover
s. muscle
s. muscle hypertrophy
s. tapered appearance
s. thickened mucosal fold
Smoothbeam laser

smooth-bordered
smoothed curve fit
smoothing
> gaussian s.
> spatial s.
> temporal s.

smooth-muscle tumor
smooth-walled bladder
SMR
> scatter-maximum ratio

smudged papilla
smudging
> omental s.

SMV
> superior mesenteric vein

Sn
> stannum
> tin

^{113}**Sn, Sn-113**
> tin 113

S/N, SNR
> signal-to-noise ratio

snake graft
snake's head appearance
snapping
> s. fascia lata
> s. hip
> s. hip syndrome
> scapular s.
> s. triceps syndrome

snapshot
> contrast-enhanced dynamic s.
> dynamic s.
> s. fashion

snare
> Amplatz gooseneck s.

sneaker osteomyelitis
Sneddon syndrome
Sneppen fracture of talus
sniff test
Sniper Elite hydrophilic Ni-Ti alloy guidewire
snowboarder's fracture
snowflake-like calcification
snowflake pattern
snowman
> s. abnormality
> s. appearance of heart
> s. configuration
> s. deformity

snowplow
> s. effect
> s. occlusion

snowstorm
> s. appearance
> s. breast pattern
> s. shadow

SNR, S/N
> signal-to-noise ratio

SNRT
> sinus node recovery time

snuffbox
> anatomic s.

Snyder SLAP lesion classification
soap
> calcium bile s.

soap-bubble
> s.-b. appearance
> s.-b. nephrogram
> s.-b. radiolucency

soapsuds enema
society
> American Cancer S. (ACS)
> American Roentgen Ray S. (ARRS)
> American Thoracic S.
> S. for Computer Applications in Radiology (SCAR)
> Musculoskeletal Tumor S.
> S. of Interventional Radiology
> Scoliosis Research S.

socket-stump interface
Socrates telementoring system
sodium
> s. 23 (^{23}Na, Na-23)
> s. 24 (^{24}Na, Na-24)
> acetrizoate s.
> s. acrylate and vinyl alcohol copolymer microsphere
> s. and/or methylglucamine diatrizoate contrast agent
> s. bicarbonate imaging agent
> s. chloride imaging agent
> Chromitope s.
> s. diatrizoate imaging agent
> fluorescein s.
> s. imaging
> s. iodide (NaI)
> s. iodide detector
> s. iodide iodine-131
> s. iodide ring
> s. iodide ring imaging agent
> iodohippurate s.
> s. iodohippurate imaging agent
> iothalamate s.
> s. iothalamate imaging agent
> ioxaglate s.
> ipodate s.
> s. ipodate imaging agent
> liothyronine s.
> s. meglumine ioxaglate contrast agent
> s. metrizoate acid contrast agent
> s. morrhuate
> s. perchlorate
> s. pertechnetate
> s. pertechnetate imaging agent
> s. phosphate
> radioactive s.

s. reabsorption
technetium 99m pertechnetate s.
tetrabromophenolphthalein s.
s. tetradecyl sulfate
tetraiodophenolphthalein s.
total exchangeable s. (TENa)
tyropanoate s.
s. tyropanoate imaging agent
warfarin s.
ytterbium pentetate s.

sodium-2-mercaptoethane sulfonate
sodium-potassium ATPase-dependent
 exchange mechanism
Soemmerring
    S. ligament
    S. muscle
soft
    s. disc herniation
    s. food dysphagia
    s. infiltrate
    s. palate carcinoma
    s. papilloma
    s. photon
    s. pigment stone
    s. ray
    s. tissue
    s. tissue ablation
    s. tissue abnormality
    s. tissue abscess
    s. tissue attenuation value
    s. tissue calcification
    s. tissue canal encroachment
    s. tissue chondroma
    s. tissue contracture
    s. tissue contrast
    s. tissue contusion
    s. tissue convexity
    s. tissue defect
    s. tissue density
    s. tissue density mass
    s. tissue density structure
    s. tissue derangement
    s. tissue distraction
    s. tissue entrapment
    s. tissue envelope
    s. tissue fibroma
    s. tissue ganglion
    s. tissue gas
    s. tissue hemangioma
    s. tissue injury
    s. tissue interposition
    s. tissue kernel
    s. tissue lesion classification
    s. tissue lipoma
    s. tissue lipomatosis
    s. tissue necrosis
    s. tissue neoplasia
    s. tissue ossification
    s. tissue osteochondroma

s. tissue osteoma
s. tissue pathoanatomy in
  melorheostosis
s. tissue radiograph
s. tissue reaction
s. tissue sarcoma
s. tissue shadow
s. tissue stranding
s. tissue stroma
s. tissue swelling
s. tissue tuberculosis
s. tissue tumor
s. tissue uptake bone scintigraphy
s. tissue window
s. tissue window setting
S. Torque uterine catheter

softball sliding injury
soft-copy computed radiography
softening
    s. of brain
    s. of cartilage
SoftLight laser
Softouch catheter
Softscan
    S. laser
    S. laser mammography system
Soft-Tip catheter
Soft-Vu angiographic catheter
software
    autotriggering s.
    BrainVoyager interactive s.
    calcium scoring s.
    CareGraph skin dose-mapping s.
    CT Perfusion 2 s.
    DecThreads s.
    3-dimensional perfusion/motion map
    s.
    FuncTool s.
    GammaPlan s.
    GE Viewer s.
    HeartView cardiac reconstruction s.
    image-processing s.
    IP Plus image-processing s.
    Kodak s.
    linear combination model s.
    LX 8.3 s.
    magnetic resonance user interface s.
    Merge Mammo imaging s.
    modified vessel image processor s.
    MRUI s.
    multigated spectral Doppler
     analysis s.
    multiplanar gradient-echo s.
    NeuroEcho s.
    Neuro Lobe s.
    Neuro SPGR s.
    P-Link s.
    Plug-n-View 3D medical imaging s.
    Pulmo CT s.

S

software (*continued*)
Siemens Syngo s.
Sparc s.
SPOT mobile 3D ultrasound system
and s.
Starlink s.
StereoPlan stereotactic planning s.
TeraRecon s.
VERT s.
ViewMax s.
Vitrea 2 3D CT angiographic s.
Voxel-Man s.
VoxelView s.
software-controlled internal hardware filter
SOG
supraorbital groove
soiling
peritoneal s.
sojourn time
solar
s. plexus
s. radiation
solarization
soldier's
s. heart
s. patch of pericardium
s. spot
soleal
s. line
s. vein
sole cluster of microcalcification
solenoid surface coil
soleus
s. muscle
s. syndrome
solid
s. and cystic pancreatic tumors
s. and papillary pancreatic
carcinoma
s. and pseudopapillary carcinoma
s. bolus challenge
s. bone
s. bony union
s. circumscribed breast carcinoma
s. component
s. consolidation
s. DCIS
s. echo
s. edema
s. edema of lung
s. food dysphagia
s. lesion spleen
s. lesion thymus
s. mass
s. matrix
s. organ transplant
s. ovarian teratoma
s. ovarian tumor

s. pattern
s. periosteal reaction
s. pilocytic astrocytoma
s. primary tumor
s. pseudopapillary tumor
s. splenic lesion
s. thymic lesion
s. viscus
s. viscus injury
solidifying agent
solid-phase extraction tube
solid-rod ureteroscope
solid-state
s.-s. manometry catheter
s.-s. nuclear track detector
solitary
s. adenoma
s. bone cyst
s. bone myeloma
s. bone plasmacytoma (SBP)
s. cold lesion
s. collapsed vertebra
s. dilated duct
s. fibrous tumor of pleura (SFTP)
s. gallstone
s. left IVC
s. lymph node
s. mass
s. metastatic lung nodule
s. osseous plasmacytoma
s. osteochondroma
s. osteosclerosis
s. osteosclerotic lesion
s. pleura tumor
s. pulmonary glandular papilloma
s. pulmonary necrobiotic nodule
s. pulmonary nodule (SPN)
s. rectal ulcer
s. rectal ulcer syndrome
s. relapse
s. rib hot spot
s. rib lesion
s. small bowel filling defect
s. sternal lesion
s. sternal metastasis
solitus
abdominal situs s.
atrial situs s.
cardiac situs s.
situs atrialis s.
visceral situs s.
solium
Taenia s.
Solomon-Bloembergen
S.-B. equation
S.-B. theory of dipole-dipole
relaxation rate
Solomon syndrome
solubilize

solution
> additive s.
> aqueous s.
> Blankophor FFG, SV s.
> Bracco A-C-D s.
> Carnoy s.
> chemoembolization s.
> Hartmann s.
> hyperosmotic s.
> hypertonic s.
> isosmotic water s.
> lidocaine-adrenaline s.
> lymph node-revealing s.
> Melrose s.
> molal s.
> multipharmaceutical
>   chemoembolization s.
> Phosphotope oral s.
> radioelement s.
> saline s.
> saponated cresol s.
> saturated potassium iodide s. (SSKI)
> 100th-normal s.

Solutrast 200, 250, 300, 370 contrast medium
solvent
> s. suppression
> s. water TI frequency dependence

SOM
> supraorbital margin

somatic muscle
Somatom
> S. DR CT scanner
> S. Plus 4 CT
> S. Plus-S CT scanner
> S. Sensation 64
> S. Volume Zoom CT system

somatosensory cortex
somatostatin
> s. imaging agent
> ^{99m}Tc-labeled s.
> s. receptor scintigraphy (SRS)

somatostatinoma
Sommer sector
Sonablate 200 ultrasound system
sonar
sonarography
Sonata imager
Sonazoid contrast agent
Sones
> S. cineangiography technique
> S. selective coronary arteriography

Song covered duodenal stent
SONIA
> Stroke Outcome and Neuroimaging of
>   Intracranial Atherosclerosis
>   SONIA trial

sonic-accelerated fracture-healing system (SAFHS)

sonicated
> s. albumin microbubble
> s. dextrose albumin imaging agent
> s. saline contrast medium

Sonicath Ultra imaging catheter
sonicating transducer
sonication
Sonicator portable ultrasound
sonic effect
SonicWAVE phacoemulsification system
Sonifer sonicating system
SONK
> spontaneous osteonecrosis of knee

Sonnenberg classification of erosive esophagitis
Sonoace 6000 II ultrasound system
sonoangiogram
SonoCT real-time compound imaging
Sonocut ultrasonic aspirator
sonodynamic therapy
sonofluoroscopy
sonogram
> dual transverse linear-array s.
> fatty meal s. (FMS)
> real-time s.
> transabdominal s.

sonograph
sonographer
> American Registry of Diagnostic
>   Medical S.'s

sonographic
> s. assessment
> s. detection
> s. diagnosis
> s. echo
> s. feature analysis
> s. guidance
> s. hip type
> s. measurement of subtalar joint
>   instability
> s. Murphy sign
> s. parameter
> s. planning of oncology treatment
>   (SPOT)

sonography
> abdominal s.
> Acuson computed s.
> Acuson transvaginal s.
> breast s.
> carotid s.
> color-coded duplex s. (CCDS)
> color-coded real-time s.
> color Doppler s. (CDS)
> color-flow Doppler s.
> color power transcranial Doppler s.
> compression s.
> contrast-enhanced transrectal s.
> Doppler s. (DS)
> duplex s.

S

sonography (*continued*)
 duplex pulsed Doppler s.
 dynamic s.
 endoanal s.
 endoluminal s.
 endoscopic s.
 endovaginal s.
 fatty meal s.
 fetal s.
 followup duplex Doppler s.
 freehand interventional s.
 graded compression s.
 gray-scale s.
 hysterosalpingo-contrast s.
 intraaortic endovascular s.
 intraoperative s. (IOS)
 obstetric s.
 pelvic s.
 penile s.
 power Doppler s. (PDS)
 real-time s.
 TCD s.
 thoracic s.
 tissue harmonic s.
 transabdominal color Doppler s.
 transcranial color-coded Doppler s.
 transcranial color-coded duplex s.
  (TCCS)
 transcranial real-time color-flow
  Doppler s.
 transrectal s.
 transvaginal s. (TVS)
 triplex-mode Doppler s.
 s. unit
 velocity-encoded color Doppler s.
 whole-breast s.
**SonoHeart Elite personal hand-carried
 ultrasound system**
sonohysterography (SHG)
 saline infusion s. (SIS)
Sonolayer ultrasound
Sonoline
 S. Antares 4D ultrasound imaging
 S. Elegra ultrasound system
 S. Sierra ultrasound imaging device
Sonolith Praktis lithotriptor
sonolucent
 s. area
 s. cystic lesion
 s. cystic mass
 s. doughnut
 s. halo
 s. layer
 s. skull
 s. zone
sonometer
 Omnisense 7000S bone s.
 Sahara clinical bone s.
 SoundScan 2000 bone s.

 SoundScan Compact bone s.
 UBIS 5000 ultrasound bone s.
sonoporation
SonoRx oral ultrasound contrast agent
SonoSite
 S. digital ultrasound
 S. hand-carried ultrasound
 S. 180 hand-carried ultrasound
  device
 S. iLook 24 ultrasound
 S. MicroMaxx laptop ultrasound
 S. 180Plus ultrasound
 S. pulsed-wave Doppler
 S. Titan ultrasound
 S. 180 ultrasound system
Sonos 2000 ultrasound unit
Sonotron electronic therapeutic device
SonoVue
Sopha DSX1 camera
Sophy
 S. camera
 S. programmable valve
Sorbie calcaneal fracture classification
sorbitol 70% imaging agent
Sorbol heel
sorption
 s. kinetics
 s. potential
sorter
 FACSVantage cell s.
 fluorescence-activated cell s.
  (FACScan)
sorting
 fluorescence-activated cell s.
Sos Pulse-Vu bloodless entry needle
Sotos syndrome
souffle
 funic s.
 placental s.
 systolic mammary s.
sound
 s. beam
 bowel s.'s
 heart s.'s
 palpable aortic ejection s.
 palpable pulmonic ejection s.
 pericardial knock s.
 s. shadow
 speed of s.
 s. transmission
 s. wave
SoundScan
 S. 2000 bone sonometer
 S. Compact bone sonometer
source
 americium radioactive s.
 cobalt radioactive s.
 Cornell high-energy synchrotron s.
  (CHESS)

¹³⁷Cs point s.
diagnostic x-ray camera and
  imaging s.
discrete bleeding s.
dummy s.
external heat-generating s.
fiberoptic light s.
flood s.
gold radioactive s.
heat-generating s.
s. imaging
interstitial heat-generating s.
interstitial radiation s.
intracavitary radiation s.
iodine radioactive s.
s. of artifact scintigraphy
s. of emission
radioactive s.
radium radioactive s.
remote-controlled implantation of
  radioactive s.
rod s.
rotating Ge-68 rod s.
signal s.
yttrium radioactive s.
source-film distance (SFD)
source-skin distance (SSD)
source-surface distance (SSD)
source-to-image receptor distance (SID)
source-to-skin distance (SSD)
source-tray distance (STD)
SPA
  single-photon absorptiometry
  superior parathyroid adenoma
space
  abdominal s.
  acromioclavicular s.
  action s.
  alveolar dead s.
  anatomic dead s.
  antecubital s.
  anterior clear s.
  anterior pararenal s. (APS)
  arachnoid s.
  axillary s.
  Bogros s.
  Bowman s.
  buccal s.
  capsular s.
  carotid s.
  cartilage joint s.
  cavitary s.
  cisternal s.
  coracoclavicular s.
  cortical liquor s.
  Crookes s.
  CY color s.
  dead s.
  s. deficit

dependent s.
disc s.
Disse s.
dorsal subaponeurotic s.
dorsal subcutaneous s.
echo s.
echo-free s.
enlarged presacral s.
enlargement of subarachnoid s.
epicardial s.
epidural s.
episcleral s.
epitympanic s.
extraarachnoid s.
extraaxial s.
extracellular s.
extradural s.
extrapleural s.
fluid s.
foraminal s.
free pericardial s.
gingival s.
hip joint s.
Holzknecht s.
hyperintense marrow s.
increased lateral joint s.
infraglottic s.
inframesocolic s.
intercellular s.
intercondylar joint s.
intercostal s.
interlobar s.
intermetatarsal s.
interosseous s.
interpeduncular s.
interpleural s.
interstitial fluid s.
intervertebral disc s.
intrasynaptic s.
intrathecal s.
intravascular s.
joint s.
lateral joint s.
left intercostal s. (LICS)
left subphrenic s.
marrow s.
masticator s.
medial joint s.
midpalmar s.
mucosal s.
s. of Retzius
s. of Retzius abscess
orbital s.
paralaryngeal s.
parapharyngeal s.
pararenal s.
paratracheal s.
parotid s.
patellofemoral joint s.

space (*continued*)
    pelvic s.
    peribronchial alveolar s.
    pericardial s.
    peridental s.
    perihepatic s.
    perineal s.
    perinephric s.
    perirenal s. (PRS)
    perisinusoidal s.
    peritoneal s.
    perivascular s.
    pleural s.
    popliteal s.
    portacaval s.
    portal s.
    posterior cervical s.
    posterior septal s.
    postpneumonectomy s.
    predental s.
    preepiglottic s.
    premasseteric s.
    presacral s.
    pretracheal s.
    prevascular s.
    prevertebral s.
    prominent perivascular s.
    Prussak s.
    pulmonary alveolar s.
    pulp s.
    Q s.
    radiolucent joint s.
    Reinke s.
    retrocardiac s.
    retrocrural s.
    retrogastric s.
    retromammary s.
    retroorbital s.
    retroparotid s.
    retroperitoneal s.
    retropharyngeal s.
    retrosphenoidal s.
    retrosternal s.
    retrovesical s.
    right subphrenic s.
    saclike s.
    scapholunate s.
    sinusoidal vascular s.
    spatial frequency s.
    subacromial s.
    subarachnoid s.
    subdural s.
    subendothelial s.
    subhepatic s.
    subperitoneal s.
    subphrenic s.
    subpulmonic pleural s.
    subtrapezial s.
    subumbilical s.

    superficial mucosal s.
    supralevator s.
    supratentorial s.
    Talairach stereotactic s.
    thenar s.
    4th intercostal s.
    5th intercostal s.
    tissue s.
    ventricular s.
    Virchow-Robin perivascular s.
    visceral s.
    widened joint s.

SPACE
    spatial and chemical-shift encoded
    excitation

space-occupying
    s.-o. intracranial lesion
    s.-o. mass
    s.-o. process

spacing
    gray-level s.
    interecho s.
    multiple-beam interface s.
    parallel line equal s. (PLES)

spade
    s. field
    s. finger

spadelike
    s. appearance
    s. hand

spade-shaped valvotome
Spalding sign
spall
spallation product
SPAMM
    spatial modulation of magnetization
    SPAMM technique

span
    levator s.
    liver s.
    ventricular s.

Sparc software
sparganosis
    cerebral s.

sparing
    arytenoid s.
    fatty s.
    focal s.

spark
    s. chamber
    s. gap generator

sparkling appearance of myocardium
SPARS
    spatially resolved spectroscopy
sparsity of bone formation
spasm
    arterial s.
    bowel s.
    bronchial smooth muscle s.

catheter-induced coronary artery s.
colonic s.
coronary artery s. (CAS)
cricopharyngeal s.
diffuse arteriolar s.
diffuse esophageal s. (DES)
esophageal s.
hemifacial s.
inspiratory s.
intermittent diffuse esophageal s.
muscle s.
postbypass s.
respiratory s.
vascular s.
venous s.

spasmodic stricture
spastic
s. bowel syndrome
s. colon
s. electron paramagnetic resonance
  imaging
s. equinovarus deformity
s. esophagus
s. heart
s. hindfoot valgus deformity
s. ileus
s. mapping
s. pseudosclerosis
s. registration

spastica
dysphagia s.

spatial
s. and chemical-shift encoded
  excitation (SPACE)
s. average-pulse average (SAPA)
s. average-pulse average intensity
s. average-temporal average
s. average-temporal average intensity
s. dose distribution
s. encoding
s. filter
s. frequency
s. frequency domain
s. frequency error
s. frequency space
s. harmonics
s. localization procedure
s. mapping
s. misregistration artifact
s. modulation of magnetization
  (SPAMM)
s. modulation of magnetization
  image
s. normalization
s. offset image artifact
s. orientation
s. origin
s. peak-temporal average (SPTA)
s. peak-temporal average intensity

s. position
s. presaturation
s. presaturation band
s. reconstruction
s. registration
s. resolution
s. resolution scintigram
s. selectivity
s. smoothing
s. vectorcardiography

spatially
s. normalized PET and SPECT
  scans
s. resolved spectroscopy (SPARS)
s. selective inversion pulse

spatial-spectral prepulses for fat
  saturation
SPBD
spontaneous perforation of biliary
  duct
SPC
single-photon counting
  SPC system
SP6 camera
SPDT
single-pole double-throw
Spearman
S. correlation coefficient
S. rank
S. rank test
spear tackler's spine
special bolus
specific
s. absorption rate (SAR)
s. activity
s. modulation
s. radiation
specificity
specified
not otherwise s. (NOS)
specimen radiography
specious finding
speck finger
speckled pattern
speckling
heterogeneous color s.
SPECT
single-photon emission computed
  tomography
  acetazolamide-enhanced SPECT
  brain perfusion SPECT
  SPECT brain perfusion scintigraphy
  SPECT center of rotation
  cerebral SPECT
  dual-head SPECT
  dual-isotope SPECT
  dynamic volumetric SPECT
  electrocardiogram-gated SPECT
  FDG SPECT

S

SPECT (*continued*)
    GE SPECT
    ictal ^{99m}Tc HMPAO brain
      SPECT
    SPECT imaging
    interictal brain SPECT
    LDD-gated SPECT
    methoxyisobutylisonitrile SPECT
    ^{99m}Tc-HMPAO SPECT
    ^{99m}Tc red blood cell SPECT
    SPECT myocardial perfusion
      imaging
    SPECT perfusion pattern
    pharmacologic stress dual-isotope
      myocardial perfusion SPECT
    SPECT quality control
    quantitative gated SPECT (QGS)
    stress-rest SPECT
    Symbia TruePoint SPECT
    technetium 99m somatostatin
      analogue SPECT
    SPECT thallium scintigraphy
    Trionix SPECT
    SPECT uniformity
spectamine
    s. brain imaging
    ^{123}I brain imaging s.
spectography
    nuclear magnetic resonance s.
spectra (*pl. of* spectrum)
spectral
    s. analysis
    s. broadening
    s. diffusion
    s. Doppler
    s. Doppler imaging
    s. editing
    s. emission
    s. line
    s. noise distribution
    s. pattern
    s. presaturation with inversion
      recovery (SPIR)
    s. saturation
    s. sensitivity
    s. ultrasound
    s. waveform
    s. width
    s. window
spectral-spatial
    s.-s. fat suppression
    s.-s. image
Spectranetics
    S. excimer laser
    S. laser sheath (SLS)
spectrin
Spectris
    S. MR-compatible injector
    S. power injector

spectrofluorometry
spectrometer
    beta ray s.
    Bragg s.
    Bruker AMX 300 NMR s.
    Compton suppression s.
    EDXRF s.
    gamma ray s.
    GE GN300 multinuclear s.
    GE NMR s.
    IBM NMR s.
    liquid scintillation s.
    mass s.
    Mossbauer s.
    Nicolet NMR s.
    NMR s.
    nuclear magnetic resonance s.
    Rapid-Scan s.
    scintillation s.
    Sisco s.
    Varian Associates s.
    Varian NMR s.
    VT multinuclear s.
    x-ray s.
spectrometry
    accelerator mass s. (AMS)
    Fourier transform NMR s.
    inductively coupled plasma atomic
      emission s. (ICP-AES)
    liquid scintillation s.
    PROBE-SV s.
    pulsed L-band ESR s.
    scintillation s.
spectrophotofluorometer
spectrophotometer
    absorption s.
    F-1200,-2000,-4500 fluorescence s.
    U-1100 UV-Vis s.
spectrophotometric
    s. calculation
    s. quantity
spectrophotometry
    atomic absorption s.
    ultraviolet s.
spectroscope
    direct-vision s.
    quasielastic laser light-scattering s.
spectroscopic voxel
spectroscopy
    atomic absorption s.
    brain proton magnetic resonance s.
    carbon-13 s.
    circular dichroism s.
    correlated s. (COSY)
    COSY H-1 MR s.
    CSI s.
    depth-resolved surface s. (DRESS)
    diffusion s.
    2D J-resolved 1H MR s.

double spin-echo proton s.
3D proton MR s.
elastic scattering s.
electrospray ionization mass s.
flame emission s. (FES)
fluorescence s.
fluorine-19 s.
Fourier transform infrared s.
Fourier transform Raman s.
glutamate s.
H-1 MR s.
hydrogen-1, -2, -3 MR s.
image selected in vivo s. (ISIS)
in vivo optical s. (INVOS)
in vivo 31P MR s.
in vivo proton MR s.
INVOS 2100 optical s.
laser correlational s. (LCS)
light-induced autofluorescence s.
localized H-1 s.
localized proton magnetic resonance
   s.
long TE MR s.
magnetic resonance s (MRS)
MR proton s.
near-infrared s. (NIRS)
nonresonance Raman s.
nuclear magnetic resonance s.
oxygen-17 NMR s.
^{31}P s.
phosphorus magnetic resonance s.
   (P-MRS)
phosphorus-31 magnetic resonance s.
photon correlation s.
plasma emission s.
point-resolved s. (PRESS)
proton MR s.
proton nuclear magnetic resonance
   s.
Raman s.
remote endoscopic digital s. (REDS)
^{77}Se MRI s.
serial diffusion-weighted MR
   imaging and proton MR s.
short echo-time proton s.
short TE proton MR s.
single-voxel proton MR s.
single-voxel stimulated echo
   acquisition-mode MR s.
spatially resolved s. (SPARS)
surface coil rotating-frame s.

spectrum, *pl.* **spectrums,** *pl.* **spectra**
absorption x-ray s.
artery s.
chromatic s.
color s.
continuous x-ray s.
Dandy-Walker s.
Dandy-Walker-Blake s.

S. DG-P pediatric cradle
Doppler frequency s.
energy s.
excitation s.
frequency s.
gamma ray s.
gray matter s.
infinitesimal Z s.
infrared s.
invisible s.
localized single-voxel proton s.
midsystolic notching of velocity s.
nuclear magnetic resonance s.
proton nuclear magnetic resonance
   s.
pulmonary sequestration s.
short echo point-resolved
   spectroscopic sequence s.
single umbilical artery s.
single-voxel in vivo proton s.
thermal s.
ultraviolet s.
VACTERL s.
velocity s.
water-suppressed proton s.
Wiener s.
x-ray s.

spectrums (*pl. of* spectrum)
specular
s. echo
s. reflector
speech area
speed
film s.
s. of sound
Spence
axillary tail of S.
tail of S.
Spengler fragment
Spens syndrome
spent phase
spermatic
s. artery
s. calculus
s. cord
s. cord torsion
s. vein
s. venography
spermatoblast (*var. of* spermatogonium)
spermatocele, spermatocyst
spermatocyst (*var. of* spermatocele)
spermatogone (*var. of* spermatogonium)
spermatogonium, spermatogone,
   spermatoblast
sperm granuloma
SPET
single-photon emission tomography
SPGR
spoiled gradient recall

S

S-phase
    S-p. analysis
    S-p. fraction
    S-p. fractionation
sphenocephaly
sphenoethmoidal
    s. encephalocele
    s. recess
    s. suture
sphenoethmoidalis
    synchondrosis s.
sphenofrontal suture
sphenoid, sphenoidal
    s. angle
    s. bone
    s. bone fracture
    s. dysplasia
    s. encephalocele
    s. fontanelle
    s. fossa
    s. ridge
    s. ridge meningioma
    s. ridge tumor
    s. sinus
    s. sinusitis
    s. sinus metastasis
    s. turbinate bone
    s. wing
    s. wing meningioma
sphenoidal (*var. of* sphenoid)
sphenoidale
    planum s.
    pneumatosis s.
    rostrum s.
sphenoidalis
    apertura sinus s.
sphenomalar suture
sphenomandibularis muscle
sphenomandibular ligament
sphenomaxillary
    s. encephalocele
    s. suture
sphenooccipital
    s. chordoma
    s. suture
    s. synchondrosis
sphenoorbital
    s. encephalocele
    s. meningioma
    s. suture
sphenopalatine
    s. canal
    s. foramen
    s. ganglion
    s. neuralgia
sphenoparietal
    s. sinus
    s. sulcus
    s. suture

sphenopetrosa
    synchondrosis s.
sphenopetrosal suture
sphenopharyngeal
    s. canal
    s. encephalocele
    s. meningoencephalocele
sphenosquamous suture
sphenotemporal suture
sphenovomerine suture
sphenozygomatic suture
sphere
    s. organelle
    resin s.
    SIR-Spheres radioactive s.
spheric
    s. disc
    s. kernel
    s. lesion
    s. map
    s. mass
    s. neoplasia
    s. shape
    s. structure
spherical fiducial marker
spheroid, spheroidal
    s. shape
    tumor s.
spheroidal (*var. of* spheroid)
spherule
sphincter
    antral s.
    s. atony
    basal s.
    bicanalicular s.
    Boyden s.
    canalicular s.
    cardiac s.
    cecal s.
    choledochal s.
    colic s.
    cricopharyngeal s.
    duodenal s.
    duodenojejunal s.
    s. dysfunction
    external anal s.
    external urethral s.
    extrinsic s.
    functional s.
    hypertensive lower esophageal s.
    s. incompetence
    inferior esophageal s. (IES)
    lower esophageal s. (LES)
    s. of bile duct
    s. of Oddi
    s. of Oddi manometry
    pancreatic duct s.
    pancreaticobiliary s.
    pharyngoesophageal s.

physiologic s.
prepyloric s.
s. preservation
pyloric s.
radiologic s.
relaxed lower esophageal s.
resting lower esophageal s.
1st duodenal s.
tonically contracted s.
upper esophageal s. (UES)

sphincteric mechanism
sphingomyelinase deficiency
sphingomyelin lipidosis
sphygmography
sphygmomanometer, sphygmometer
sphygmometer (*var. of*
  sphygmomanometer)
SPI
selective population inversion
spicular, spiculated
s. border
s. carcinoma
s. density
s. distortion
s. margin
s. mass
s. protrusion
s. scirrhous lesion

spiculated (*var. of* spicular)
spiculation
radiographic s.
spicule
bony s.
spider
s. angioma
s. finger
s. pelvis
stainless steel s.
s. x-ray view
SPIDER
steady-state projection imaging with
  dynamic echo-train readout
structured platform-independent data
  entry and reporting
spidering skeleton
spiderlike
s. calyx
s. pelvocaliceal system
spiderweb
s. appearance
s. circulation
Spielmeyer-Vogt disease
spigelian
s. fascia
s. hernia
s. lobe
spike
s. averaging
s. loading

s. staple
sterile vent s.
spike-and-dome pattern
spike-related functional MR imaging
spiking
interictal s.
spiky skeleton
spill
ferromagnetic particle s.
ileal s.
spin
s. coupling
s. density
s. dephasing
s. diffusion
s. echo
s. echo using repeated gradient
  echoes
electron s.
s. exchange
s. flip
flowing s.
high s.
incoherent s.
nuclear s.
off-resonant s.
s. quantum number
stationary s.
s. tagging
transverse relaxation of proton s.
uncoupled s.
unsaturated s.
s. vector
spina, *pl.* **spinae**
s. bifida
s. bifida aperta
s. bifida occulta (SBO)
erector spinae
s. ventosa
spinae (*pl. of* spina)
spinal
s. accessory lymph node
s. accessory nerve
s. angiogram
s. angulation
s. anomaly
s. arteriography
s. artery
s. axis
s. axis tumor
s. capillary hemangioblastoma
s. chordoma
s. column stabilization
s. concussion
s. contusion
s. cord
s. cord angiography
s. cord atrophy
s. cord caliber

S

spinal (*continued*)
s. cord canal
s. cord cleft
s. cord compression
s. cord decompression
s. cord depression
s. cord diameter
s. cord ependymoma
s. cord glioma
s. cord hemisection
s. cord infarct
s. cord injury (SCI)
s. cord injury without radiographic abnormality (SCIWORA)
s. cord laceration
s. cord lesion
s. cord malformation (SCM)
s. cord metastasis
s. cord parenchyma
s. cord sarcoidosis
s. cord stroke
s. cord syrinx
s. cord tethering
s. cord transection
s. cord tumor
s. degeneration
s. dermoid
s. diastematomyelia
s. dorsal horn
s. dural arteriovenous fistula
s. dural AVF
s. dysraphism
s. empyema
s. endplate change
s. epidural abscess (SEA)
s. epidural hemorrhage (SEH)
s. epidural lymphoma
s. extension test
s. fixation
s. fixation device
s. fluid
s. fluoroscopy
s. fracture
s. fusion
s. ganglion
s. growth
s. hemiplegia
s. hydatid cyst
s. imaging platform (SIP)
s. infection
s. inflammation
s. instability
s. integrity
s. lipoma
s. lordosis
s. medulla
s. meningioma
s. muscular atrophy (SMA)
s. needle

s. nerve plexus
s. nerve root avulsion
s. nerve root injury
s. osteochondrosis
s. osteomyelitis
s. osteophyte
s. pedicle
s. plasma cell myeloma
s. root
s. sac
s. sign
s. stenosis
s. subarachnoid hemorrhage
s. subdural hemorrhage (SSH)
s. syndesmophyte
s. tap
s. teratoma
s. tophaceous gout
s. tuberculosis
s. vascular malformation
ventral derotating s. (VDS)
s. videofluoroscopy

spinalis
funiculus medullae s.

spindle
aortic s.
s. colonic groove
His s.
muscle s.
ureteral s.

spindle-shaped
s.-s. aneurysm
s.-s. muscle
s.-s. shadow

spindling

spine
alar s.
s. angioreticuloma
angulation of s.
anterior column of s.
anterior maxillary s.
anteroinferior iliac s.
anteroposterior iliac s.
anterosuperior iliac s. (ASIS)
arachnoid loculation of s.
bamboo s.
basilar s.
biomechanically normal s.
caroticojugular s.
cervical s.
cervical fusion of s.
Charcot s.
cleft s.
coccygeal s.
dendritic s.
dens view of cervical s.
dorsal s.
dysraphic s.
epidermoid s.

extension injury of s.
fetal s.
full cervical s. (FCS)
functional unit of s.
s. hyperflexion
iliac s.
intermaxillary s.
ischial s.
kinetic cervical s.
kissing s.'s
s. lipoma
lumbar s.
lumbarized s.
lumbosacral s. (LSS)
maxillary s.
mental s.
microcystic lumbar s.
midthoracic s.
s. morphology
nasal s.
s. ossification
poker s.
posterior column of s.
posteroinferior iliac s.
railway s.
rotatory load on s.
rugger jersey s.
sacral s.
scoliotic s.
s. sign
spear tackler's s.
static cervical s.
thin-plate s.
thoracic s.
thoracolumbar s.
tibial s.
trochanteric s.
vertebral s.
wedge fracture of s.

spin-echo (SE)
    axial single-shot fast s.-e.
    s.-e. cardiac imaging
    dual-echo turbo s.-e.
    ECG-gated s.-e.
    half-Fourier acquisition single-shot
      turbo s.-e. (HASTE)
    s.-e. imaging sequence
    s.-e. magnetic resonance imaging
    s.-e. pilot image
    s.-e. pulse sequence
    s.-e. scan
    s.-e. technique
    time of formation of RF spin-echo
      when adjusted to be different
      from gradient s.-e.
    s.-e. train
    s.-e. T1-weighted image
    s.-e. T1-weighted transaxial MR
      imaging

spinescope
    Clarus s.
spin-label
    s.-l. method
    s.-l. technique
spin-labeling
    arterial s.-l. (ASL)
spin-lattice
    s.-l. relaxation
    s.-l. relaxation time
    s.-l. T1 image
spin-lock (SL)
    s.-l. and magnetization transfer
      imaging
    s.-l. gradient-echo (SL-GRE)
    s.-l. imaging technique
    s.-l. prepulse
spin-lock-induced T1-rho-weighted
image
spin-locking
    off-resonance s.-l.
spinning
    variable-angle s. (VAS)
spinning-top
    s.-t. test
    s.-t. urethra
spinocerebellar
    s. degeneration
    s. tract
spinoglenoid
    s. ligament
    s. notch
spinogram
spinographic
    s. angle
    s. line
spinography
    digitized s.
spinolaminar line (SLL)
spinoreticular tract
spinosum
    foramen s.
spinothalamic tract
spinous
    s. foramen
    s. plane
    s. process
    s. process avulsion
    s. process fracture
    s. process impingement syndrome
    s. tarsus ligament
spin-phase
    s.-p. graph
    s. p. phenomenon
spin-spin
    s.-s. coupling
    s.-s. relaxation
    s.-s. relaxation time
spintharicon

S

891

spinthariscope
spin-warp
    s.-w. imaging
    s.-w. method
    s.-w. pulse sequence
SPIO
    superparamagnetic iron oxide
SPIO-enhanced MR imaging
spiperone
SPIR
    selective partial inversion
      recovery
    spectral presaturation with
      inversion recovery
spiral
    s. appearance
    s. arthrosis
    s. band of Gosset
    s. computed tomography (SCT)
    s. computed tomography
      arteriography (SCTA)
    s. CT angiography
    s. CT pitch
    s. CT pitch pit
    s. CT scan
    s. CT scanning
    s. CT, XCT scanner
    s. dissection
    s. echo-planar imaging
    s. echo-planar technique
    s. flow pattern
    s. fold
    s. imaging method
    s. k-space coverage
    s. ligament
    s. multidetector CT
    s. multisplice technology
    s. oblique fracture
    s. pulse sequence
    s. scanning technique
    s. valve
    s. volumetric CT
    s. x-ray computed tomography
      (SXCT)
SPIR-FLAIR
    selective partial inversion recovery-fluid
      attenuated inversion recovery
      SPIR-FLAIR image
      SPIR-FLAIR sequence
spirochete infection
spirometer flow rate
spirometric
    s. acquisition
    s. gating
spirometrically controlled CT lung
  densitometry
spirometry
    full-volume loop s.
splanchnapophysis

splanchnic
    s. aneurysm
    s. AV fistula
    s. blood
    s. vascular imaging
    s. vasculature
    s. venous system
    s. vessel
splanchnography
splanchnoskeleton
SPLATT
    split anterior tibial tendon
splayed cranial suture
splayfoot deformity
splaying
    s. of frontal horn
    s. of pedicle
spleen
    aberrant s.
    absence of s.
    accessory s.
    s. angiosarcoma
    delayed rupture of s.
    s. density
    s. diameter
    s. dimension
    ectopic s.
    epithelial s.
    floating s.
    s. granuloma
    hamartoma s.
    hyperdense s.
    increased density of s.
    s. inflammation
    inflammatory s.
    s. laceration
    large s.
    s. lesion
    liver, kidneys, and s. (LKS)
    long axis of s.
    malpighian body of s.
    microabscess of s.
    multiple accessory s.'s
    nonvisualization of s.
    s. peliosis
    primary cyst of s.
    prolapse of s.
    ruptured s.
    s. sarcoidosis
    s. scan
    s. scintigraphy
    shattered s.
    siderotic nodule in s.
    small s.
    solid lesion s.
    tail of s.
    tip of s.
    s. ultrasonography imaging
    wandering s.

spleen-to-liver ratio
splenatrophy
splenectasis
splenectomy
    traumatic s.
splenectopia, splenectopy
splenectopy (*var. of* splenectopia)
splenelcosis
spleneolus
splenia (*pl. of* splenium)
splenial branch of posterior cerebral artery
splenic
    s. abscess
    s. amyloidosis
    s. angiography
    s. angle
    s. arteriography
    s. artery
    s. artery aneurysm
    s. artery pseudoaneurysm
    s. AV fistula
    s. B-cell lymphoma
    s. bleeding
    s. bump
    s. calcification
    s. capsule
    s. cleft
    s. congestion
    s. epidermoid cyst
    s. flexure
    s. flexure carcinoma
    s. hamartoma
    s. hemangioma
    s. hilum
    s. hyperplasia
    s. infarct
    s. lesion
    s. lobule
    s. lymph node
    s. marginal lymphoma
    s. metastasis
    s. microabscess
    s. neoplasm
    s. notch
    s. perfusion measurement by
    dynamic CT scan
    s. portal venography
    s. portography
    s. pseudocyst
    s. pulp
    s. reagent
    s. rupture
    s. scintigraphy
    s. torsion
    s. trauma
    s. vein
    s. vein thrombosis
    s. vessel
spleniculus

splenium, *pl.* splenia
    s. of corpus callosum
splenization
splenobronchial fistula
splenocaval
splenocolic ligament
splenogastric omentum
splenogonadal fusion
splenography
splenoma
splenomalacia
splenomedullary
splenomegalia (*var. of* splenomegaly)
splenomegaly, splenomegalia,
  megalosplenia
    congenital s.
    congestive s.
    Egyptian s.
    fibrocongestive s.
    Gaucher s.
    hemolytic s.
    infectious s.
    myelophthisic s.
    Opitz thrombophlebitic s.
    persistent s.
    postcardiotomy lymphocytic s.
    siderotic s.
splenomyelomalacia
splenoncus
splenonephric
splenopancreatic
splenophrenic
splenoportal
    s. junction
    s. venography
splenoportogram
splenoportography
    direct s.
    s. imaging
    percutaneous s.
splenorenal
    s. anastomosis
    s. angle
    s. arterial bypass graft
    s. ligament
    s. recess
    s. shunt
splenosis
    abdominal s.
    thoracic s.
splenule
splenunculi (*pl. of* splenunculus)
splenunculus, *pl.* splenunculi
spline curve
splint
    birdcage s.
    semidynamic s.
    shin s.
    thigh s.

S

splintered
    s. bone
    s. fracture
splinting
    serial s.
Spli-Prest
    S.-P. latex
    S.-P. negative control
    S.-P. plate
    S.-P. positive control
split
    s. anterior tibial tendon (SPLATT)
    s. atlas
    s. brain
    s. compression fracture
    s. cord malformation (SCM)
    s. cord syndrome
    s. cranium
    s. foot deformity
    s. heel fracture
    s. image artifact
    s. notochord syndrome
    s. peroneus brevis
    s. pleura sign
    s. renal function decrease
    s. spinal cord
    s. spinal cord malformation
      (SSCM)
    s. water resonance
split-bolus technique
split-brain
    s.-b. imaging
    s.-b. study
split-course
    s.-c. accelerated radiotherapy
    s.-c. hyperfractionated radiation
      therapy
    s.-c. technique
split-function scintigraphy
split-liver transplant
split-screen recording
splitter
    beam s.
splitting
    s. fracture
    plaque s.
    sternal s.
    zero-field s.
SPN
    solitary pulmonary nodule
SPOCS
    Surgical Planning and Orientation
      Computer System
Spofford-Christopher oxygen optimizing
  program (SCOOP)
spoiled
    s. gradient echo
    s. gradient-echo pulse sequence
    s. gradient recall (SPGR)

    s. gradient-recalled echo sequence
    s. GRASS
spoiler
    s. gradient pattern
    Lucite beam s.
spoiling
    radiofrequency s.
    RF s.
    surface s.
spoke bone
spoked wheel pattern
spondylarthritis
spondylitic
    s. change
    s. deformity
spondylitis
    acute pyogenic s.
    ankylosing s.
    bacterial s.
    cryptococcal s.
    s. deformans
    discovertebral s.
    juvenile ankylosing s.
    rheumatoid s.
    staphylococcal discovertebral s.
    tuberculous s.
spondyloarthropathy
    destructive s.
    juvenile s.
spondylocostal dysplasia
spondylodiscitis, spondylodiskitis
    s. drainage
    pyogenic s.
spondylodiskitis (*var. of* spondylodiscitis)
spondyloepiphysial dysplasia
spondylolisthesis
    degenerative s.
    isthmic s.
    sagittal roll s.
    slip-angle s.
    spondylolytic s.
    traumatic s.
spondylolisthetic pelvis
spondylolysis
    traumatic s.
spondylolytic spondylolisthesis
spondylomalacia
spondylosis
    cervical spine s.
    s. deformans
    degenerative s.
    diffuse s.
    Nurick classification of s.
spondylosyndesis
spondylothoracic dysplasia
spondylotic myelopathy
sponge
    blood-filled bone s.
    gelatin s.

Ivalon s.
s. kidney
medullary s.
Ray-Tec x-ray-detectable surgical
    s.
retained surgical s.
surgical s.
Vistec x-ray-detectable s.

Spongel gelatin sponge particle
spongiform
s. change
s. degeneration
s. leukoencephalopathy
s. myelinopathy
spongioblastoma
spongiocytoma
spongiosis
spongiosum
corpus s.
osteoma s.
spongy
s. appearance
s. bone
s. osteoma
s. white matter degeneration
spontaneous
s. carotid dissection
s. cerebrospinal fluid leak
s. closure of defect
s. conversion
s. coronary artery dissection
    (SCAD)
s. detorsion
s. disintegration
s. drainage
s. echo contrast
s. fetal movement
s. fracture
s. hematoma
s. hemodialysis catheter fracture and
    embolization
s. infantile ductal aneurysm
s. intracranial hypotension (SIH)
s. intracranial hypotension syndrome
s. involution
s. lesion
s. osteonecrosis
s. osteonecrosis of knee (SONK)
s. perforation
s. perforation of biliary duct
    (SPBD)
s. perforation of common bile duct
s. pneumomediastinum
s. postural headache
s. radiation
s. regression
s. renal hemorrhage
s. rupture
s. tension pneumothorax

s. transient vasoconstriction
s. urinary extravasation
spoonlike
s. protrusion
s. protrusion of leaflet
spoon-shaped nail
SPOP
sequential paired opposed plaque
    SPOP technique
sporadic
s. Burkitt lymphoma
s. colorectal carcinoma
s. leukodystrophy
s. medullary thyroid carcinoma
s. tumor
spot
blooming focal s.
capitate soft s.
Carleton s.
cold s.
s. compression
s. compression image
s. compression magnification
    mammography
s. compression paddle
s. compression view
cotton-wool s. (CWS)
EIS s.
s. film
s. film device
s. film fluorography
s. film radiography
flying focal s.
focal s. (FS)
focal liver hot s.
hematocystic s. (HCS)
hot s.
hyperechoic splenic s.
s. magnification
s. magnification image
pelvic s.
pituitary bright s.
s. planar image
s. radiograph
Roth s.
scan s.
s. scanning
s. scanography
s. site
soldier's s.
solitary rib hot s.
thermal hot s.
tree-shaped s.
z-flying focal s
SPOT
sonographic planning of oncology
    treatment
    SPOT mobile 3D ultrasound system
    and software

spotted nephrogram
SPPS
> single-photon planar scintigraphy
SPR
> scanned projection radiography
sprain
> acute s.
> chronic s.
> eversion s.
> s. fracture
> inversion s.
> sacroiliac s.
> syndesmosis s.
spray
> resorcinol s.
spread
> s. Bragg peak
> distant s.
> extracapsular s.
> hematogenous s.
> intraocular s.
> lymphatic tumor s.
> s. of tumor
> pattern of s.
> perineural tumor s.
> regional s.
> subependymal s.
> s. suture
> transfascial s.
Sprengel deformity
spring
> s. ligament
> s. onion ureter
spring-driven system
Springer fracture
spring-loaded biopsy needle
sprinter's fracture
Sprint fixed-detector research system
sprodiamide imaging agent
SPS
> sestamibi parathyroid scintigraphy
> superior petrous sinus
> Superpump System
SPT
> selective population transfer
SPTA
> spatial peak-temporal average
SPTL
> subcutaneous panniculitis-like T-cell lymphoma
> SPTL 1b vascular lesion laser
spur
> acromial s.
> anterior s.
> bone s.
> bronchial s.
> calcaneal s.
> calcific s.

> degenerative s.
> drum s.
> s. formation
> heel s.
> impingement s.
> inferior s.
> marginal s.
> medial traction s.
> osteoarthritic s.
> osteocartilaginous s.
> plantar calcaneal s.
> posterior s.
> prominent s.
> retrocalcaneal s.
> traction s.
> uncovertebral s.
spuriae
> costae s.
> vertebrae s.
spurious
> s. aneurysm
> s. ankylosis
> s. finding
> s. pregnancy
Spurling sign
spurring
> bony s.
> degenerative s.
> hypertrophic marginal s.
> marginal s.
> osteophytic s.
> ulnar traction s.
Spyglass angiography catheter
SQFT
> subcutaneous quadriceps fat thickness
squamomastoid suture
squamoparietal suture
squamosal suture
squamosphenoid suture
squamous
> s. cell carcinoma
> s. cell carcinoma of anal canal
> s. cell papilloma
> s. intraepithelial lesion (SIL)
> s. metaphysis
> s. metaplasia
> s. metaplasia with white epithelium
> s. odontogenic tumor
> s. part of frontal bone
> s. part of occipital bone
> s. part of temporal bone
> s. suture
square
> s. brain shift
> s. wave
squared
> s. patella
> s. vertebral body

squared-off
> s.-o. heart
> s.-o. thorax

squatting
> s. facet
> s. maneuver
> s. position

squeeze sign

Squibb system

SQUID
> superconducting quantum interference device

Sr
> strontium

⁸⁹Sr, Sr-89
> strontium 89
> > ⁸⁹Sr bracelet
> > ⁸⁹Sr chloride

⁹⁰Sr, Sr-90
> strontium 90

⁹⁰Sr-loaded eye applicator

Sr-87m
> strontium 87m

SRO
> sagittal ramus osteotomy
> > SRO 2550 x-ray tube

SRS
> somatostatin receptor scintigraphy
> stereotactic radiosurgery

SSA
> subsegmental atelectasis

SSBE
> short-segment Barrett esophagus

SSC
> single-stripe colitis

SSc
> systemic sclerosis

SSCM
> split spinal cord malformation

SSCP
> single-strand conformational polymorphism

SSD
> segmental spinal dysgenesis
> shaded surface display
> source-skin distance
> source-surface distance
> source-to-skin distance
> > SSD imaging

SSFP
> steady-state free precession
> > SSFP magnetization
> > SSFP process
> > SSFP signal

SSFSE
> single-shot fast spin echo

SSH
> spinal subdural hemorrhage

S-shaped
> S-s. gallbladder
> S-s. pouch
> S-s. scoliosis

SShTSE
> SENSE with half-Fourier single-shot turbo spin echo
> single-shot TSE

SSKI
> saturated potassium iodide solution

SSP
> slice sensitivity profile
> stereotactic surface projection

SSPE
> subacute sclerosing panencephalitis

SSQ
> sequential scalar quantization

SSS
> subclavian steal syndrome
> superior sagittal sinus
> > SSS thrombosis

SSST
> superior sagittal sinus thrombosis

St.
> Saint
> > St. Jude Medical aortic valve graft prosthesis

1st
> 1st branchial arch
> 1st branchial cleft cyst
> 1st carpal row
> 1st cuneiform bone
> 1st diagonal branch artery
> 1st digital interosseous (FDI)
> 1st duodenal sphincter
> 1st major diagonal branch
> 1st metatarsal angle
> 1st metatarsal head (FMH)
> 1st obtuse marginal artery
> 1st parallel pelvic plane
> 1st portion of duodenum
> 1st ray instability
> 1st rib
> 1st septal perforator branch
> 1st temporal gyrus
> 1st trimester
> 1st ventricle of cerebrum
> 1st visceral cleft

stability
> bony s.
> magnet s.
> s. of fracture

stabilization
> electronic s.
> s. plate
> spinal column s.

stabilizer
> dynamic s.
> static s.

stabilizing bullet

stable
> s. cavitation
> s. fracture
> s. free radical
> s. isotope
> s. reduction
> s. Xenon CT

stable-state tuberculosis

stacked
> s. ovoid lesion
> s. scan
> s. tomogram

stacked-coins appearance

stacked-foil technique

stacked-scan imaging

stack mode display

stack-of-coins mucosal fold

stack-of-spirals trajectory

Stafne idiopathic bone cavity

stage
> nascent s.
> resolution s.
> Risser s.
> s. 4S neuroblastoma
> T s.

1-stage amputation

2-stage
> 2-s. amputation
> 2-s. fusion
> 2-s. stent implantation
> 2-s. venous cannulation

stage-matched
> s.-m. intervention
> s.-m. intervention on repeat
>   mammography

staghorn
> s. calculus
> s. stone

staging
> distraction-flexion s. (DFS)
> Ficat s.
> invasive surgical s.
> Kadish s.
> lymphoma s.
> malignant melanoma s.
> neuraxis s.
> neuroblastoma s.
> nodal s.
> preslip s.

stagnant loop syndrome

stag wound

stain
> Bielschowsky s.
> congo red s.
> hematoxylin and eosin s.

> hematoxylin-eosin s.
> mucicarmine s.

stained-glass appearance

staining
> alloxan-Schiff s.
> dense capillary s.
> immunocytochemical s.
> tumor s.

stainless
> s. steel coil
> s. steel Greenfield filter
> s. steel mesh stent
> s. steel microsphere
> s. steel plate
> s. steel spider

staircase phenomenon

stairstep
> s. air-fluid level
> s. artifact
> s. fracture

stalk
> body s.
> fibrovascular s.
> infundibular s.
> pituitary s.
> polyp s.
> tumor s.
> yolk s.

standard
> ACR teleradiology s.
> s. atlas
> British S. (BS)
> criterion s.'s
> s. deviation
> s. exchange wire
> s. fixed-core guidewire
> international s.
> s. LITT applicator
> s. multiecho
> s. precaution
> reference s.
> s. single echo
> s. uptake value (SUV)

standard-dose enhanced conventional T1-weighted image

standardization
> International Organization of S. (ISO)

standardized uptake ratio (SUR)

standby rate

standing
> s. dorsoplantar view
> s. false profile view
> s. lateral view
> s. postvoid view
> s. wave
> s. weightbearing view

standoff
> acoustic s.
> s. pad

standstill
    atrial s.
    cardiac s.
    ventricular s.
Stanford
    S. and Wheatstone stereoscope
    S. aortic dissection classification
    S. type B aortic dissection
    S. type B dissection closure
Stanley cervical ligament
stannosis
stannous
    s. chloride
    s. pyrophosphate
stannum (Sn)
stapedes (*pl. of* stapes)
stapedial
    s. artery
    s. nerve anatomy
    s. otosclerosis
stapedius reflex
stapes, *pl.* **stapedes**
staphylococcal discovertebral
  spondylitis
Staphylococcus
    S. aureus
    S. aureus pneumonia
    S. brain abscess
staphyloma
staple
    metallic s.
    orthopaedic s.
    skin s.
    spike s.
    stone s.
    surgical s.
star
    s. artifact
    s. effect
    s. test pattern
Starcam camera
star-cancellation test (SCT)
Starling
    S. curve
    S. force
Starlink software
STARRT
    selective tubal assessment to refine
    reproductive therapy
    STARRT falloposcopy system
star-shaped vessel lumen
starvation
    photon s.
stasis
    antral s.
    bile s.
    bladder s.
    chronic venous s.
    circulation s.

    s. cirrhosis
    complete vascular s.
    s. edema
    s. esophagitis
    s. gallbladder
    intrahepatic biliary s.
    s. liver
    s. of blood flow
    s. ulcer
    ureteral s.
    urinary s.
    vascular s.
    venous s.
state
    cardiac steady s.
    chronic constrictive s.
    3-dimensional Fourier
      transform-constructive interference
      in steady s. (3DFT-CISS)
    double-mode steady s.
    fast adiabatic trajectory in steady s.
      (FATS)
    Fourier-acquired steady s.
    free precession sequence steady s.
    gradient-recalled acquisition in
      steady s. (GRASS)
    ground s.
    high-output s.
    hypoperfused s.
    inducible basal s.
    metastable s.
    s. of equilibrium
    oxidation s.
    post Diamox s.
    vegetative s.
Statham electromagnetic flowmetry
static
    s. blush
    s. bone phase
    s. cervical spine
    s. coupling
    s. 3D FLASH imaging
    s. emission scan
    s. foot deformity
    s. image
    s. image display
    s. liver imaging
    s. lung
    s. magnetic field
    s. nuclear imaging study
    s. rCBF tracer
    s. stabilizer
    s. view
statin-induced myopathy
station
    American Thoracic Society
      node s.
    calf-foot s.
    lower s.

S

station (*continued*)
    lymph node s.
    nodal s.
    oscilloscope tuning s.
stationary
    s. anode
    s. field
    s. focus
    s. spin
    s. zero-order motion
3-station moving table
statistical noise
STATLase-SDL
status
    cardiac s.
    s. epilepticus
    organification s.
Stauffer syndrome
Staunig position
STD
    source-tray distance
1st-degree
    1st-d. AV block
    1st-d. heart block
steady-state
    s.-s. coherence
    s.-s. free precession (SSFP)
    s.-s. free precession imaging
    s.-s. free precession magnetization
    s.-s. free precession sequence
    s.-s. free progression
    s.-s. gradient-echo imaging
    s.-s. projection imaging with
      dynamic echo-train readout
      (SPIDER)
steal
    arterial s.
    s. effect
    false s.
    pelvic s.
    s. phenomenon
    subclavian s.
    s. syndrome
    transmural s.
STEAM
    stimulated echo acquisition mode
    STEAM sequence
steatohepatitis
    nonalcoholic s. (NASH)
steatosis
    hepatic s.
    liver s.
    macrovesicular s.
Stecher position
steel coil
Steele triple innominate osteotomies
steep
    s. left anterior oblique projection
    s. left anterior oblique view

    s. Towne projection
    s. Trendelenburg position
steeple sign
steerable guidewire system
steering
    beam s.
    coaxial s.
    electronic independent beam s.
Steerocath-Dx octapolar valve mapping catheter
Steinberg
    S. classification
    S. sign
Steinbrocker rheumatoid arthritis classification
Steinert epiphysial fracture classification
Stein-Leventhal syndrome
Steinstrasse calculus
Stejskal-Tanner gradient
Stellant dual-head injector
stellate
    s. abnormality
    s. border breast lesion
    s. configuration
    s. confluence
    s. crease
    s. defect
    s. ganglion block
    s. granuloma
    s. ligament
    s. mass
    s. pattern
    s. skull fracture
    s. tear
    s. undepressed fracture
stem
    autologous s.
    s. base plate
    brain s.
    bronchus s.
    s. cell
    s. cell distribution
    s. cell homing
    s. cell implantation
    s. cell therapy
    s. cell tracking
    s. cell transplant
    straight s.
stem-loop structure
Stener gamekeeper's thumb lesion
stenion
stenocardia
Steno duct
stenogyria
stenoobstructive lesion
stenosed aortic valve
stenoses (*pl. of* stenosis)

stenosing
- s. ring of left atrium
- s. tenosynovitis

stenosis, *pl.* **stenoses**
- acquired aortic valve s.
- acquired mitral s.
- acquired spinal s.
- ampullary s.
- anal s.
- anastomotic s.
- antral s.
- aortic s.
- aortic valve s.
- aortoiliac s.
- aqueduct s.
- aqueductal s.
- s. area
- arterial s.
- atheromatous s.
- atherosclerotic s.
- atypical aortic valve s.
- benign papillary s.
- benign tracheobronchial s.
- bicuspid valvular aortic s.
- bilateral carotid stenoses
- bowel s.
- branch pulmonary artery s.
- bronchial s.
- buttonhole mitral s.
- calcific bicuspid valvular s.
- calcific senile aortic valvular s.
- canal s.
- candy-wrapper s.
- carotid s.
- carotid artery s.
- central canal s.
- central spinal s.
- cephalic arch s.
- cerebral artery s.
- cervical s.
- choledochoduodenal junctional s.
- circumferential venous s.
- common pulmonary vein s.
- concentric hourglass s.
- congenital cardiac valve s.
- congenital esophageal s.
- coronary artery s.
- coronary luminal s.
- coronary ostial s.
- critical coronary s.
- critical valvular s.
- cross-sectional area s.
- culprit s.
- s. diameter
- diffuse s.
- discrete focal s.
- discrete subaortic s.
- discrete subvalvular aortic s. (DSAS)
- duodenal hourglass s.
- dynamic subaortic s.
- eccentric s.
- edge s.
- s. encroachment
- esophageal s.
- external iliac s.
- femoropopliteal atheromatous s.
- fibromuscular renal artery s.
- fibromuscular subaortic s.
- fishmouth mitral s.
- fixed-orifice aortic s.
- flow-limiting s.
- focal eccentric s.
- foraminal s.
- graft s.
- granulation s.
- hemodialysis-related venous s.
- hemodynamically relevant s.
- hemodynamically significant s.
- hepatic artery s.
- high-grade proximal s.
- hourglass s.
- hypercalcemic supravalvular aortic s.
- hypertrophic infundibular subpulmonic s.
- hypertrophic pyloric s. (HPS)
- hypertrophic pyloric string-sign s.
- hypertrophic pyloric target-sign s.
- hypertrophic subaortic s.
- idiopathic hypertrophic subaortic s.
- ileal s.
- iliac artery s.
- iliofemoral venous s.
- infrainguinal bypass s.
- infrarenal s.
- infundibular pulmonary s.
- infundibular subpulmonic s.
- innominate artery s.
- in-stent s.
- intragraft s.
- intrarenal s.
- intrinsic vein graft s.
- irislike s.
- juxtaanastomotic s.
- lateral recess s.
- linear s.
- lumbar spinal s.
- luminal s.
- membranous subaortic s.
- membranous subvalvular aortic s.
- midgraft s.
- mitral s. (MS)
- mitral valve s. (MVS)
- multifocal short s.
- multiple small bowel stenoses
- muscular subaortic s.
- napkin-ring anular s.
- native kidney renal artery s.

S

stenosis (*continued*)
    neoplastic s.
    neural foraminal s.
    noncalcified coronary s.
    noncritical s.
    nonrheumatic valvular aortic s.
    s. of aorta
    ostial renal artery s.
    papilla of Vater s.
    papillary bile duct s.
    pedicular renal artery s.
    pelvic venous s.
    peripheral pulmonary artery s.
     (PPAS)
    petrous carotid canal s.
    postangioplasty s.
    postoperative s.
    post PTCA residual s.
    preangioplasty s.
    pulmonary s.
    pulmonary artery s.
    pulmonary valve s.
    pulmonary valvular s.
    pulmonary vein s.
    pyloric s.
    radiation s.
    radionuclide s.
    rectal s.
    relative mitral s.
    renal artery s. (RAS)
    rheumatic aortic valvular s.
    rheumatic mitral s.
    rheumatic tricuspid s.
    saphenous vein s.
    segmental s.
    senescent aortic s.
    silent mitral s.
    spinal s.
    stomal s.
    string-sign s.
    subaortic s.
    subclavian artery s.
    subglottic s.
    subinfundibular s.
    subsonic s.
    subvalvular aortic s.
    subvalvular pulmonary s.
    supraaortic s.
    supraclavicular aortic s.
    suprarenal s.
    supravalvular aortic s. (SAS, SVAS)
    supravalvular mitral s.
    supravalvular pulmonary s.
    tapering s.
    tendon sheath s.
    thoracic outlet s. (TOS)
    TOCU for internal carotid artery s.
    tracheal s.
    tricuspid s.

    true mitral s.
    truncal renal artery s.
    tubular s.
    tunnel subaortic s.
    tunnel subvalvular aortic s.
    uncomplicated supraclavicular s.
    unicuspid aortic valve s.
    unilateral carotid s.
    ureteral s.
    valvular aortic s.
    valvular pulmonic s.
    vein graft s.
    vertebral artery s.

stenotic
    s. change
    s. coronary artery
    s. esophagogastric anastomosis
    s. flow reserve (SFR)
    s. gradient
    s. isthmus
    s. lesion
    s. plaque
    s. tricuspid valve

Stensen
    S. canal
    S. duct
    S. foramen
    S. gland

stent
    Acculink s.
    active MRI s. (AMRIS)
    AneuRx s.
    Aspire covered s.
    Assurant balloon-expanded s.
    AVE Bridge flexible
     balloon-expanded s.
    AVE Bridge SE self-expanding s.
    AVE Bridge stainless steel
     balloon-expandable s.
    balloon-expandable s.
    Bard Saxx s.
    bare-metal s.
    biliary s.
    biodegradable s.
    BiodivYsio s.
    brachiocephalic s.
    Bx Velocity s.
    CardioCoil coronary s.
    Cary-Coon biliary s.
    C-flex s.
    cobalt alloy s.
    coil vascular s.
    compliance matching s. (CMS)
    Conformexx biliary s.
    Cordis Palmaz Corinthian s.
    Cordis Palmaz Schatz long medium s.
    Cordis Smart nitinol s.
    Corinthian stainless steel
     balloon-expandable s.

covered s.
Cragg Endopro System I covered s.
Cypher s.
Dacron s.
deployed s.
s. deployment
detachable balloon-modified reducing s.
double-helix prostatic s.
double-J ureteral s.
drug-eluting s.
Dynalink self-expanding s.
Easy Wallstent s.
electropolished s.
Endeavor drug-eluting s.
EsophaCoil s.
esophageal s.
ev3 premounted balloon-expandable s.
ev3 self-expanding s.
ev3 unmounted balloon-expandable s.
expandable Gianturco metallic s.
s. expansion
Express balloon-expanded s.
Express biliary LD s.
Fabian s.
Flamingo s.
FreeFlo proximal nitinol s.
Genesis s.
Gianturco s.
Gianturco-Rosch biliary s.
gold-marked s.
Guidant Megalink peripheral s.
Hemobahn s.
indwelling s.
internal biliary s.
internal ureteral s.
IntraCoil self-expanding peripheral s.
IntraStent DoubleStrut biliary s.
IntraStent DS, LD, LP balloon-expanded s.
intravascular s.
[192]Ir-loaded s.
Jomed Flexmaster s.
Jomed peripheral s.
Jostent covered s.
Jostent SelfX nitinol s.
kissing s.'s
Luminexx biliary s.
Luminexx self-expanding s.
MedNova s.
Megalink s.
Memotherm nitinol self-expandable s.
s. mesh
metallic s.
s. migration
Miller double mushroom biliary s.
ML-Ultra balloon s.
Monorail Wallstent self-expanding s.

Multi-Link Penta s.
Multi-Link Terra s.
nephroureteral s.
nephroureterostomy s.
NIR s.
NiTi alloy s.
nitinol Symphony s.
Omni Flex biliary s.
Omnilink/Megalink balloon-expanded s.
over-the-wire coronary s.
Palmaz 424, 784 s.
Palmaz Genesis balloon-expanded s.
Palmaz large balloon-expanded s.
Palmaz medium balloon-expanded s.
Palmaz P564, PS424 s.
Palmaz P394 stainless steel balloon-expandable s.
Palmaz-Schatz long medium balloon-expanded s.
pancreatic duct s.
Passager nitinol self-expandable s.
patent s.
Percuflex s.
percutaneous s.
Perflex stainless steel balloon-expandable s.
pigtail s.
platinum-marked s.
polyethylene s.
Polyflex s.
polyurethane s.
porous metallic s.
Precise self-expanding s.
prostatic s.
Protégé GPS s.
Protégé self-expanding s.
Protg GPS self-expanding nitinol s.
s. proximity
PTFE s.
s. pushability
QuaDDS s.
QuaDDS-QP2 s.
QuaDS drug-eluting s.
QueST s.
radioactive s.
radioisotope s.
reducing s.
[188]Re-labeled self-expanding nitinol s.
renovascular s.
rolling membrane Wallstent cobalt-based alloy balloon expandable s.
S7 AVE s.
Schneider enteral s.
self-expandable metal s.
self-expanding covered s.
self-expanding open mesh s.

stent (*continued*)
    S-F Precise s.
    silicone s.
    sirolimus-eluting SMART nitinol s.
    slotted tube s.
    SMART Control self-expanding s.
    SMART nitinol self-expandable s.
    Song covered duodenal s.
    stainless steel mesh s.
    straight s.
    Strecker balloon-expanded s.
    Strecker nitinol self-expandable s.
    Strecker tantalum balloon-expandable
      s.
    s. strut
    Supra G s.
    Symphony nitinol self-expandable s.
    Symphony self-expanding s.
    TAG Excluder s.
    tandem s.
    tantalum s.
    Taxus Express s.
    Temp Tip ureteral s.
    s. thrombosis
    transhepatic biliary s.
    T-tube s.
    Ultraflex s.
    Ultrathane Amplatz ureteral s.
    urethral metallic s.
    urinary s.
    U-tube s.
    vascular s.
    V-Flex Plus s.
    Viabahn covered s.
    Viabil s.
    Vistaflex balloon-expanded s.
    Wallgraft cobalt-based alloy
      balloon-expandable s.
    Wallgraft covered s.
    Wallstent Iliac RP self-expanding
      s.
    XT radiopaque coronary s.
    ZA-stent nitinol self-expandable s.
    Zenith stainless steel self-expandable
      s.
    zigzag s.
    Zilver self-expanding s.
stent-graft
    AneuRx s.-g.
    Cragg EndoPro s.-g.
    Dacron-covered s.-g.
    Excluder s.-g.
    expanded
      polytetrafluoroethylene-covered
      nitinol TIPS s.-g.
    FreeFlo s.-g.
    Gore covered biliary s.-g.
    Hemobahn PTFE-covered
      s.-g.

    Jomed peripheral s.-g.
    Jostent peripheral s.-g.
    modular s.-g.
    Opta balloon s.-g.
    self-expanding s.-g.
    Talent bifurcated abdominal aortic
      s.-g.
    transluminally placed s.-g.
    Viatorr transjugular intrahepatic
      portosystemic shunt s.-g.
    Wallgraft endoprosthesis s.-g.
stenting
    antegrade ureteral s.
    biliary s.
    brachiocephalic artery s.
    bronchial s.
    carotid angioplasty with s. (CAS)
    carotid artery s.
    colon s.
    endobiliary s.
    iliac artery s.
    innominate artery s.
    intracoronary s.
    intravascular s.
    pulmonary artery s.
    subclavian artery s.
    tracheobronchial s.
    ureteral s.
    venous s.
stentless porcine aortic valve
stent-mounted
    s.-m. allograft valve
    s.-m. heterograft valve
stent-related artifact
stent-vessel wall contact
Stenver position
Stenvers
    S. projection
    S. view
step
    modality performed procedure s.
      (MPPS)
    phase-encoding s.
    s. section
    s. wedge
2-step
    2-s. procedure
    2-s. technique
step-and-shoot
    s.-a.-s. IMRT
    s.-a.-s. mode
    s.-a.-s. technique
step-down
    s.-d., step-up phenomenon
    s.-d. transformer
stepladder
    s. appearance
    s. sign
steplike recess

step-oblique mammography
stepoff
    s. of fracture
    orbital rim s.
    s. vertebral body sign
stepping-source position
stepping-table MRA
1-step production
step-up transformer
stepwise
    s. infusion
    s. regression
    s. regression analysis
stercoraceous, stercoral,
  stercorous
stercoral (*var. of* stercoraceous)
    s. ulcer
stercoralis
    Strongyloides s.
stercoroma
stercorous (*var. of* stercoraceous)
stercus
stercocinefluorography
stereocncephalotomy
stereofluoroscopy
stereogram (*var. of* stereoradiograph)
stereograph (*var. of* stereoradiogram,
  stereoradiograph)
stereographic projection
stereography (*var. of* stereoradiography)
StereoGuide
    Lorad S.
    S. prone breast biopsy system
    S. stereotactic core needle biopsy
stereolithography (STL)
StereoLoc upright biopsy system
stereologic method of volume
  estimation
stereomammography
stereometry
stereomicroradiography
stereophotogrammetric
    roentgen s.
StereoPlan stereotactic planning software
stereoradiogram, stereograph,
  stereoroentgenogram
stereoradiograph, stereoroentgenogram,
  stereogram, stereograph
stereoradiography, stereography,
  stereoroentgenography
stereo right lateral projection
stereoroentgenogram (*var. of*
  stereoradiograph)
stereoroentgenography (*var. of*
  stereoradiogram, stereoradiography)
stereosalpingography
stereoscope
    binocular s.
    Stanford and Wheatstone s.

stereoscopic
    s. pelvimetry
    s. radiography
    s. view
    s. vision
    s. zonography
stereoscopy
stereotactic, stereotaxic
    s. ablation
    s. apparatus
    s. automated technique
    s. brachytherapy
    s. breast biopsy system
    s. cerebral angiography
    s. core needle biopsy (SCNB)
    s. CT scan
    s. data
    s. device
    s. external beam irradiation (SEBI)
    s. head frame
    s. localization
    s. localization frame
    s. mammography
    s. needle aspiration
    s. percutaneous lumbar discectomy
    s. percutaneous needle biopsy
    s. procedure
    s. proton irradiation
    s. puncture
    s. radiation therapy
    s. radiosurgery (SRS)
    s. radiotherapy
    s. ring
    s. surface projection (SSP)
    s. surgery
    s. tractotomy
    s. vacuum-assisted breast biopsy
    (SVABB)
stereotactically guided interstitial laser
  therapy
stereotaxic (*var. of* stereotactic)
stereotaxis, stereotaxy
    computer-assisted volumetric s.
    frameless s.
    imaging-based s.
    volumetric minimally invasive s.
stereotaxy (*var. of* stereotaxis)
sterile
    s. barium
    s. bile
    s. vent spike
sterna (*pl. of* sternum)
sternal
    s. abscess
    s. angle
    s. angle of Louis
    s. apex
    s. border
    s. cartilage

sternal (*continued*)
s. clip
s. edge
s. joint
s. lesion
s. lift
s. marrow
s. notch
s. part of diaphragm
s. rib
s. splitting
s. suture
s. vertebra
s. view
sternales
synchondroses s.
sternalis muscle
Sternberg
S. myocardial insufficiency
S. sign
sternebra, *pl.* **sternebrae**
sternebrae (*pl. of* sternebra)
Sterner lesion
sternochondral junction
sternoclavicular
s. angle
s. dislocation
s. hyperostosis
s. joint
s. joint disc
s. ligament
sternocleidomastoid
s.
clavicular head of s.
s. muscle border
s. retraction
s. tumor
sternocostal
s. joint
s. part of diaphragm
s. surface of heart
sternohyoid muscle
sternomanubrial joint
sternopericardial ligament
sternospinal reference
sternothyroid muscle
sternotomy wire
sternoxiphoid plane
sternum, *pl.* **sterna,** *gen.* **sterni**
anterior bowing of s.
corpus sterni
ostitic lesion of s.
s. retraction
tie s.
steroid-induced osteonecrosis
stethoscope
ultrasound s.
Stewart-Hamilton equation
Stewart-Holmes sign

Stewart-Milford traumatic pediatric hip dislocation classification (I-IV)
Stewart-Treves syndrome
Stickler syndrome
1-stick system
Stieda
S. fracture
S. process
Stierlin sign
stiff
s. guidewire
s. lung syndrome
s. man syndrome
s. noncompliant lung
stiffness
acute lung s.
aortic s.
arterial s.
s. coefficient
hepatic s.
lung s.
shear s.
ventricular s.
stigma, *pl.* **stigmas, stigmata**
radiologic s.
stigmas (*pl. of* stigma)
stigmata (*pl. of* stigma)
Still disease
Stiller rib
Stilling canal
Stimucath continuous nerve block catheter
stimulated
s. acoustic emission (SAE)
s. echo
s. echo acquisition mode (STEAM)
s. echo artifact
s. echo-tagging technique
stimulation
alternating hemifield s.
cardiosynchronous s.
electric s.
high-voltage s. (HVS)
high-voltage pulsed galvanic s. (HVPGS)
intraoperative electrocortical s.
magnetic s.
s. mode
noninvasive programmed electrical s. (NIPS)
percutaneous electrical nerve s.
s. scan
transcranial magnetic s. (TMS)
vagus nerve s. (VNS)
stimulator
AME bone growth s.
bone growth s.
DTU-215 cardiac digital s.

transcutaneous electrical nerve s. (TENS)
stimulus-correlated water signal
STING
 subureteric Teflon injection
 STING procedure
stippled
 s. appearance
 s. calcification
 s. mineralization
 s. soft tissue
stippling of lung field
STIR
 short tau inversion recovery
 short TI inversion recovery
 fast STIR
 STIR imaging
 STIR sequence
 STIR slice
 STIR technique
stirrup bone
STL
 stereolithography
1st-line therapy
1st-2nd intermetatarsal angle
stochastic effect
Stoerck loop
Stokes theorem
stoma, *pl.* **stomas, stomata**
 abdominal s.
 anastomotic s.
 bowel s.
 diverting s.
 gastroenterostomy s.
 gastrointestinal s.
 permanent s.
 prolapsed s.
 retracted s.
 silastic collar-reinforced s.
stomach
 s. adenocarcinoma
 air-contrast view of s.
 angulus of s.
 antrum of s.
 s. atony
 s. bed
 bilocular s.
 body of s.
 s. bubble
 s. calculus
 canal of s.
 cardiac s.
 cascade s.
 caterpillar s.
 cobblestone appearance of s.
 contrast-filled s.
 convex border of s.
 coronary artery of s.
 cup-and-spill s.

s. curvature
s. defect incisura
distal blind s.
distended s.
s. diverticulum
dumping s.
s. filling defect
s. fundus
greater curvature of s.
hourglass s.
intrathoracic s.
J-shaped s.
leather bottle s.
s. leiomyoma
s. leiomyosarcoma
lesser curvature of s.
s. margin
miniature s.
mucous lake of s.
s. narrowing
nonvisualization of fetal s.
pit of s.
s. pneumatosis
remnant s.
riding s.
scaphoid s.
sclerotic s.
thoracic s.
trifid s.
s. tube
s. ulcer
upside-down s.
s. varioliform erosion
s. varix
s. volvulus
s. wall
water-bottle s.
waterfall s.
water-trap s.
wet s.
stomal
 s. edema
 s. intussusception
 s. stenosis
stomas (*pl. of* stoma)
stomata (*pl. of* stoma)
stone
 barrel-shaped s.
 bile duct s.
 biliary tract s.
 bilirubinate s.
 black faceted s.
 bladder s.
 bosselated s.
 common bile duct s.
 cystic duct remnant s.
 cystine s.
 dropped s.
 s. extraction

S

stone (*continued*)
    extrahepatic s.
    fecal s.
    gallbladder s.
    gas-containing s.
    s. heart
    high-attenuation s.
    impacted urethral s.
    s. impaction
    intrahepatic s.
    intraluminal s.
    intravesical s.
    kidney s.
    lung s.
    matrix s.
    metabolic s.
    multiple s.'s
    nonopaque s.
    nonradiopaque s.
    opaque s.
    pigment s.
    pituitary s.
    pulp s.
    radiolucent s.
    renal s.
    residual s.
    retained common bile duct s.
    salivary s.
    shadowing s.
    soft pigment s.
    staghorn s.
    s. staple
    ureteral s.
    urinary bladder s.
    vein s.
    womb s.
stone-free rate
stonelike calculus
stony mass
stool
    currant jelly s.
    retention of s.
    s. tagging
stool-tagging agent
stop
    crimp s.
    s. test
stop-action
    s.-a. image
    s.-a. imaging
stopcock
    Accel s.
    3-way s.
3-stopcock manifold
stopping power
1-stop-shop examination
storage
    digital s.
    magnetic tape s.

s. phosphor-based technique
s. phosphor imaging
s. phosphor radiography
s. phosphor radiology
s. phosphor system
1st-order
    1st-o. attenuation correction
    1st-o. chorda
    1st-o. reaction
storiform pattern
storiform-pleomorphic
    s.-p. malignant fibrous histiocytoma
    s.-p. MFH
    s.-p. pattern
storm
    thyroid s.
Storz
    S. infant bronchoscope
    S. thoracoscope
stoved finger
1st-pass
    1st-p. acquisition
    1st-p. cardiac perfusion
    1st-p. contrast bolus perfusion
      image
    1st-p. effect
    1st-p. examination
    1st-p. flow study
    1st-p. function study
    1st-p. MUGA
    1st-p. myocardial perfusion imaging
    1st-p. myocardial perfusion MR
    1st-p. radionuclide angiography
      (FPRNA)
    1st-p. radionuclide exercise
      angiocardiography
    1st-p. radionuclide ventriculography
    1st-p. technique
    1st-p. thallium extraction
    1st-p. view
STR
    skeletal targeted radiotherapy
strabismus convergens alternans
straddle
    s. fracture
    s. injury
straddling
    chondroblastoma s.
    s. embolus
straight
    s. anterior vertebral border
    s. AP pelvic injection
    s. chest tube
    s. cord
    s. endhole catheter
    s. guidewire
    s. guiding sheath
    s. interposition graft
    s. lateral projection

s. sidehole catheter
s. sinus
s. stem
s. stent
s. tubule
s. ureter
straight-line flow
strain
adductor muscle s.
s. fracture
left ventricular hypertrophy with s.
ligamentous s.
lumbosacral spine s.
muscle s.
myotendinous s.
s. pattern
right ventricular s.
shear s.
strain-gauge plethysmography
strain-rate MR imaging
strand
s. of increased density
rabbit car s.
stranding
fascial s.
fat s.
glial s.
mesenteric fat s.
soft tissue s.
strangulated
s. bladder hernia
s. inguinal hernia
s. obstruction
s. small bowel
s. viscus
strangulating obstruction
strangulation
bladder s.
bowel s.
s. necrosis
strap muscle
strata (*pl. of* stratum)
stratification
mural s.
stratified
stratiform
stratigraphy
Stratis II MRI system
stratum, *pl.* **strata**
strawberry gallbladder
strawberry-shaped head
stray
s. light
s. neutron field
s. radiation
1st-3rd ejection fraction
streak
s. artifact
atherosclerotic fatty s.

fatty intima s.
s. of atelectasis
s. of increased density
primitive s.
streaklike
s. artifact
s. configuration
stream
electron s.
regurgitant s.
streaming
s. effect
tram-track s.
streblodactyly (*var. of* camptodactyly)
Strecker
S. balloon-expanded stent
S. nitinol self-expandable stent
S. tantalum balloon-expandable stent
Streeter dysplasia
strength
air Kerma s.
diffusion encoding s.
field s.
high-gradient field s.
hoop s.
magnetic field s.
streptavidin peroxidase technique
streptokinase
stress
adduction s.
biomechanical s.
s. Broden view
s. cystogram
s. echocardiography
s. endpoint
s. eversion view
s. film
s. fracture
hoop s.
s. image acquisition
s. incontinence
s. injury
s. inversion view
mechanical wall shear s.
mediolateral s.
s. myocardial perfusion imaging
s. perfusion and rest function
s. perfusion scintigraphy
pharmacologic s.
s. projection
s. radiograph
s. radiography
s. raiser
resting end-systolic wall s.
shear s.
s. thallium image
s. thallium-201 myocardial imaging
s. thallium scan

S

909

stress (*continued*)
  torque s.
  torsion s.
  s. ulcer
  valgus s.
  varus s.
  wall shear s.
stress-and-rest image
stress-gated blood pool cardiac examination
stress-induced
  s.-i. ischemia
  s.-i. left ventricular dilation
  s.-i. remodeling
stress-injected
stress-only perfusion imaging
stress-redistribution
  s.-r. examination
  s.-r. imaging
stress-rest
  s.-r. reinjection examination
  s.-r. SPECT
stress-strain curve
stretched lung
stretched-out ligament
stria, *pl.* **striae**
  s. diagonalis
  s. laminae granularis externae
  s. laminae granularis internae
  s. laminae pyramidalis internae
  s. longitudinalis lateralis
  s. mallearis
  striae medullares ventriculi quarti
  s. medullaris thalami
  striae olfactoriae
  s. olfactoria lateralis
  s. olfactoria medialis
  s. terminalis
  s. vascularis ductus cochlearis
striae (*pl. of* stria)
striata
  osteopathia s.
striatal
  s. lesion
  s. output pathway
striate
  s. cortex
  s. hemorrhage
  s. vein
striated
  s. angiographic nephrogram
  s. muscle
striation
  s. across image
  fiber-bundle s.
  intermediate signal s.
  paint brush s.
  urothelial s.

striatonigral degeneration
striatothalamic groove
striatum
  corpus s.
Strichman SME-810 camera
Strickler method
strict isolation
stricture
  anal s.
  anastomotic s.
  antral s.
  anular esophageal s.
  benign biliary s.
  benign peptic s.
  bile duct s.
  biliary s.
  bronchial s.
  caustic s.
  choledochojejunostomy s.
  cicatricial s.
  colonic s.
  common bile duct s.
  congenital urethral s.
  contractile s.
  duodenal s.
  enteric s.
  esophageal s.
  esophageal peptic s.
  gastroesophageal junction s.
  irritable s.
  longitudinal esophageal s.
  lye s.
  peptic s.
  pyloric s.
  recurrent s.
  spasmodic s.
  tracheal s.
  ureteral s.
  ureteroenteral anastomotic s.
  urethral s.
string
  s. cell carcinoma
  s. guideline
  navel s.
  s. sign
stringlike band of fibrous tissue
string-of-beads
  s.-o.-b. appearance
  s.-o.-b. sign
string-of-pearls
  s.-o.-p. appearance
  s.-o.-p. nuclear arrangement
  s.-o.-p. sign
string-sign stenosis
strip
  primary motor s.
  s. scan
  sensitometric s.
  sensory s.

stripe

aortopulmonary mediastinal s.
central high signal intensity s.
central intraluminal saturation s.
endometrial s.
esophageal-pleural s.
fat s.
flank s.
Gennari s.
paraspinal pleural s.
paratracheal tissue s.
pleural s.
pleuroesophageal s.
properitoneal flank s.
psoas s.
right paratracheal s.
saturation s.
scaphoid fat s.
s. sign
tracheal wall s.
vertebral s.

striping

horizontal s.

stripped atom

stripping

fibrin sleeve s.

stroke

anterior spinal artery s.
cardiogenic embolic s.
cerebrovascular s.
completed s.
s. count image
s. count ratio
s. ejection rate
embolic s.
s. force
hemisphere s.
hemorrhagic s.
hyperacute s.
hypertensive s.
incomplete s.
s. in evolution (SIE)
ischemic s.
lacunar s.
National Institute of Neurological Disorders and S. (NINDS)
S. Outcome and Neuroimaging of Intracranial Atherosclerosis (SONIA)
S. Outcome and Neuroimaging of Intracranial Atherosclerosis trial
s. output
s. power
progressive s.
s. scale score
slow s.
small-vessel s.
spinal cord s.
thromboembolic s.

vertebrobasilar distribution s.
s. volume (SV)
s. volume image
s. volume index (SVI)
s. volume ratio

stroke-work index (SWI)

stroma, *pl.* **stromata**

bone marrow s.
cartilage s.
cervical s.
extralobular s.
fibrocollagenous s.
gonadal s.
Rollet s.
soft tissue s.
vascular s.

stromal

s. carcinoid tumor of ovary
s. cell tumor
s. matrix
s. necrosis
s. pattern of breast

stromata (*pl. of* stroma)

Strongyloides stercoralis

strongyloidiasis, strongyloidosis

strongyloidosis (*var. of* strongyloidiasis)

strontium (Sr)

s. 89 (^{89}Sr, Sr-89)
s. 90 (^{90}Sr, Sr-90)
s. isotope
s. 87m (^{87m}Sr, Sr-87m)
radioactive s.
s. with yttrium 90

strontium-89

s.-89 chloride
s.-89 imaging agent

structural

s. abnormality
s. anomaly
s. epilepsy
s. lesion
s. pulmonary immaturity
s. support
s. weakness

structurally immature lung

structure

basal forebrain cholinergic s.
biliary s.
bony s.
brain s.
branching linear s.
branching tubular s.
calcified density s.
central hilar s.
cervical s.
collagenous s.
cord s.
cystic s.
demineralized bony s.

S

911

structure (*continued*)
  denture-supporting s.
  3D shape of neuroanatomic s.
  elongated s.
  extracolonic s.
  high-density s.
  hilar s.
  hollow s.
  hypoechoic s.
  intracranial s.
  intratumoral s.
  labyrinthine s.
  linear s.
  low-contrast s.
  low-density s.
  mediastinal s.
  midline cystic s.
  noncolonic s.
  nuclear s.
  onionlike laminar s.
  opaque branching s.
  organoid s.
  osseous s.
  ossification of cartilaginous s.
  parcellation of s.
  periappendiceal s.
  prominent ductal vascular s.
  renal collecting s.
  ringlike s.
  satellite s.
  serpentine s.
  soft tissue density s.
  spheric s.
  stem-loop s.
  superior mediastinal s.
  supraglottic s.
  target parenchymal s.
  test tube s.
  thin linear s.
  treelike airway s.
  tuboreticular s.
  tubular s.
  vascular s.

structured
  s. coil electromagnet
  s. light
  s. noise
  s. platform-independent data entry
    and reporting (SPIDER)
  s. water

struma, *pl.* **strumae**
  multinodular s.
  s. ovarii
  Riedel s.

strumae (*pl. of* struma)
Strümpell sign
Strunsky anterior arch of foot sign
strut
  bone s.

  s. chorda
  corticocancellous s.
  s. fracture
  optic s.
  stent s.
  s. thickness
  tricuspid valve s.
  valve outflow s.

Struthers
  S. arcade
  S. ligament

struvite calculus
Stryker
  S. frame
  S. notch projection
  S. notch view

ST-segment/heart
  ST-s./h. rate
  ST-s./h. rate slope
  ST-s./h. ratio

ST-segment shift
STS-MIP
  sliding thin-slab maximum-intensity
  projection

STT
  scaphotrapeziotrapezoid
  STT joint

1st-5th intermetatarsal angle
1st-trimester
  1st.-t. bleeding
  1st.-t. gestational trophoblastic
    disease
  1st.-t. hemorrhage
  1st.-t. nuchal translucency
  1st.-t. placenta

stuck
  s. without recapture
  s. with recapture

studded fissure
Studer pouch
study
  air-contrast s.
  anatomopathologic s.
  anisotropic volume s.
  antegrade pressure s.
  barium meal s.
  biplane pelvic oblique s.
  bladder contractility s.
  blood flow s.
  bone density s.
  bone length s.
  bone mineral content s.
  brain activation s.
  cardiac gated s.
  carotid and vertebral artery
    transluminal angioplasty s.
    (CAVATAS)
  carotid duplex s.
  cerebral blood flow s.

cerebral perfusion s.
cine s.
complete stress/rest s.
compressibility and phasicity s.
conventional s.
cornflake esophageal motility s.
correlative Doppler s.
Doppler flow probe s.
double-contrast barium s.
double-probe pH s.
DTPA CSF flow s.
dual-contrast s.
dynamic contrast-enhanced
  subtraction s.
dynamic nuclear imaging s.
dynamic supine s.
efficacy s.
electromagnetic blood flow s.
endovascular flow wire s.
factor analysis of dynamic s.
fistula tract s.
flow s.
gallbladder s.
gastrointestinal bleeding localization
  nuclear s.
gas ventilation s.
gated imaging s.
gated planar s.
Gd-DOTA-enhanced subtraction
  dynamic s.
horizontal beam s.
ictal phase s.
imaging s.
inhalation s.
interictal PET FDG s.
interictal SPECT s.
intervention s.
in vivo disposition s.
iodized oil s.
isotopic 3D s.
isotopic volume s.
kidney function s.
kinematic MRI s.
lumbar flexion and extension s.
MAA s.
marker transit s.
minute-sequence s.
morphine-augmented s.
motility s.
MR flow quantification s.
MRI CSF flow s.
multibreath washout s.
multitracer s.
musculoskeletal imaging s.
National Polyp S.
noble gas in magnetic resonance s.
noninvasive imaging s.
paleopathologic and radiologic s.'s
paramagnetic contrast-enhanced MR s.

perfusion s.
peripheral small airway s.
perirenal air s.
phantom s.
3-phase technetium s.
phonation s.
PICCOLO s.
postcaptopril radioisotope s.
precaptopril radioisotope s.
pressure perfusion s.
pullback s.
pulmonary blood flow s.
pulmonary quantitative differential
  function s.
qualitative s.
quantitative regional lung
  function s.
radioaerosol imaging s.
radiochemical s.
radioisotope ventriculography s.
radiolabeled water s.
radiologic-histopathologic s.
radionuclide blood flow s.
radionuclide cardiac perfusion s.
radionuclide cerebrospinal fluid s.
radionuclide gastrointestinal
  bleeding s.
radionuclide voiding s.
RAD-IR s.
reconstruction s.
redistribution s.
renal cyst s.
renal function s.
retrococcygeal air s.
retroperitoneal air s.
salivary gland function s.
scintigraphic s.
simulated equilibrium factor s.
single-contrast s.
sinus tract s.
split-brain s.
static nuclear imaging s.
1st-pass flow s.
1st-pass function s.
swallowing s.
technetium albumin s.
thymidine suicide s.
tracer s.
transmission electron microscopic s.
T1-weighted s.
ureteral reflux s.
urodynamic pressure-flow s.
ventilation s.
videotape s.
voiding s.
wall motion s.
wash-in/washout s.
washout s.
xenon washout s.

S

stump
    appendiceal s.
    biliary s.
    bulbous s.
    s. carcinoma
    cystic duct s.
    duodenal s.
    gastric s.
    s. pregnancy
    s. pressure
    rectal s.
stumped-off appearance
stunned myocardium
stunning
    s. effect
    myocardial s.
    s. phenomenon
    postexercise s.
    poststress s.
    thyroid s.
stunted fetus
Sturge-Weber
    S.-W. syndrome
    S.-W. telangiectasia
Sturge-Weber-Dimitri syndrome
stylet, stylette
    S. esophageal MRI coil
    single-bevel s.
stylette (*var. of* stylet)
styloglossus muscle
stylohyoid
    s. ligament
    s. muscle
styloid
    s. process
    s. prominence
    ulnar s.
styloideum
    os s.
stylomandibular ligament
stylomastoid
    s. foramen
    s. fossa
    s. tumor
stylomaxillary ligament
stylopharyngeus
subacromial
    s. bursa
    s. bursa adhesion
    s. bursitis
    s. enthesophyte
    s. space
subacromial-subdeltoid (SA-SD)
    s.-s. bursa
    s.-s. septic bursitis
subacute
    s. bacterial endocarditis
    s. bronchopneumonia

    s. cardiac tamponade
    s. cerebral infarct
    s. combined spinal cord degeneration
    s. denervation atrophy
    s. encephalitis
    s. extrinsic allergic alveolitis
    s. hemorrhage
    s. hepatic necrosis
    s. inflammation
    s. ischemic brain infarct
    s. myocardial infarct
    s. myositis ossificans
    s. necrotizing encephalomyelopathy
    s. necrotizing lymphadenitis
    s. necrotizing myelitis
    s. necrotizing myelopathy
    s. pneumonitis
    s. renal vein thrombosis
    s. sclerosing panencephalitis (SSPE)
    s. subdural hematoma
    s. testicular torsion
    s. thyroiditis
subadditivity
subadventitial
    s. fibrosis
    s. hyperplasia
    s. plane
    s. tissue
subanular
    s. calcification
    s. placement
subaortic
    s. curtain
    s. gland
    s. muscle
    s. stenosis
subapical bronchus
subaponeurotic abscess
subarachnoid
    s. aneurysm
    s. cavity
    s. cistern
    s. clot
    s. cyst
    s. hemorrhage (SAH)
    s. injection
    s. instillation
    s. metastatic disease
    s. nerve block
    s. phenol block
    s. seeding
    s. septum
    s. space
    s. space disease
subareolar
    s. breast density
    s. carcinoma

s. duct
s. injection
s. lesion
s. lymphatic plexus
s. mass

subarticular
s. bone resorption
s. cyst
s. pseudocyst

subastragalar dislocation
subastrocytic tumor
subatheromatous ulcer
subatmospheric pressure
subband
wavelet s.

subblock
rectifier s.

subbursal rupture
subcallosal gyrus
subcapital fracture
subcapsular
s. bleed
s. hepatic necrosis
s. renal hematoma

subcardinal vein
subcarina
subcarinal
s. angle
s. lymph node

subcecal appendix
subcentimeter node
subchondral
s. bone
s. bone plate
s. bone resorption
s. collapse
s. cyst
s. cystic cavity
s. fracture
s. fracture line
s. insufficiency
s. lesion
s. low signal-intensity sclerosis
s. marrow edema
s. marrow hyperemia
s. microfracture
s. osteosclerosis
s. trabecular compression

subchorionic
s. hematoma
s. hemorrhage

subclavian
s. aneurysm
s. arteriography
s. artery
s. artery obstruction
s. artery occlusion
s. artery stenosis
s. artery stenting

s. flap
s. flap aortoplasty
s. line
s. loop
s. steal
s. steal syndrome (SSS)
s. turndown technique
s. vein (SCV)
s. vein occlusion
s. vein thrombosis
s. vessel
s. vessel thrombosis

subclavian-innominate vein
subclavicular
subclavius muscle
subcollateral gyrus
subcoracoid
s. bursitis
s. dislocation of shoulder

subcortical
s. arteriosclerotic encephalopathy
s. atherosclerotic encephalopathy
s. CNS hamartoma
s. cyst
s. defect
s. gray matter
s. infarct
s. intracerebral hemorrhage
s. intracranial lesion
s. ischemic vascular dementia
s. low-intensity lesion
s. Sudeck osteoporotic atrophy
s. tumor

subcostal
s. artery
s. branch
s. 4-chamber view
s. long-axis view
s. margin
s. nerve
s. plane
s. short-axis view
s. short-axis view echocardiography
s. window

subcritical narrowing
subcutaneous
s. air
s. array electrode
s. arterial bypass graft
s. connective tissue
s. edema
s. emphysema
s. fascia
s. fat
s. fat length
s. fat line
s. fat necrosis
s. fibroma
s. fracture

subcutaneous (*continued*)
  s. hemangioma
  s. implanted injection port
  s. infiltrate
  s. infusion
  s. injection
  s. injection of contrast artifact
  s. metastasis
  s. nodule
  s. panniculitis-like T-cell lymphoma
    (SPTL)
  s. patch
  s. pocket
  s. quadriceps fat thickness
    (SQFT)
  s. sacrococcygeal myxopapillary
    ependymoma
  s. tissue gas
  s. tumor
  s. tunnel
  s. vein
subdeltoid
  s. bursa
  s. bursa adhesion
  s. bursa effusion
  s. bursitis
  s. fat plane obliteration
subdermal injection
subdiaphragmatic
  s. abscess
  s. fat
subdural
  s. abscess
  s. blood
  s. button
  s. cavity
  s. clot
  s. contrast injection
  s. effusion
  s. empyema
  s. hematoma
  s. hemorrhage (SDH)
  s. hygroma
  s. infection
  s. interhemispheric hematoma
  s. space
  s. window
subendocardial
  s. infarct (SEI)
  s. injury
  s. ischemia
  s. myocardial infarct
  s. necrosis
  s. sclerosis
subendometrial halo
subendothelial space
subependymal
  s. cyst
  s. germinolysis

  s. giant cell astrocytoma
  s. hamartoma
  s. hemorrhage
  s. heterotopia
  s. oligodendroglioma
  s. seeding
  s. spread
  s. vein
subependymal/subpial focus
subependymoma
subepicardial fat
suberosis
subeustachian sinus
subfalcine herniation
subfascial
  s. hematoma
  s. transposition
subfascially
subfrontal meningioma
subgaleal
  s. abscess
  s. cerebrospinal fluid
  s. hematoma
  s. hemorrhage
subglandular implant
subglenoid dislocation of shoulder
subglottic
  s. area
  s. carcinoma
  s. edema
  s. hemangioma
  s. narrowing
  s. stenosis
subglottis
subgluteus
  s. maximus bursa
  s. medius bursa
subhepatic
  s. abscess
  s. area
  s. cecum
  s. space
subinfundibular stenosis
subinsular mass
subintimal
  s. cleavage plane
  s. dissection
  s. fibrosis
  s. filling
subject
  s. contrast
  s. placement
sublabral
  s. foramen
  s. recess
subligamentous
  s. disc herniation
  s. extension
  s. vertebral osteomyelitis

sublimis
    flexor digitorum s. (FDS)
    s. tendon
sublingual
    s. gland
    s. varix
sublobar septum
sublux
subluxated (*var. of* subluxed)
subluxation
    anterior tibial s.
    s. articulation
    atlantoaxial s.
    s. complex
    distal radioulnar s.
    element s.
    forward s.
    lateral s.
    occult s.
    s. of patella (SLP)
    patellar s.
    peroneal tendon s.
    posterior s.
    posterolateral rotatory s.
    radial head s.
    radioulnar s.
    recurrent lateral patellar s.
    reduced s.
    sacroiliac s.
    tendon s.
    unilateral facet s.
subluxed, subluxated
    s. facet joint
    s. vertebra
subluxing patella
submandibular
    s. duct
    s. duct calculus
    s. ganglion
    s. gland
    s. gland carcinoma
    s. lymph node
    s. triangle
submassive
    s. hemorrhage
    s. hepatic necrosis
    s. pulmonary embolus
submaxillary
    s. gland
    s. sialography
    s. view
submembranous placental hematoma
submental
    s. lymph node
    s. vertex radiograph
submentovertex, submental vertex
    s. position
    s. projection
    s. view

submentovertical view
submerged segment of esophagus
submetatarsal bursa
submicrometastasis
submicron magnetic particle
submillimeter
    s. collimation
    s. resolution
submucosal
    s. circular fold
    s. colon tumor
    s. esophageal tumor
    s. fibroid
    s. hemorrhage
    s. lesion
    s. lymphangiectasis
    s. malignancy
    s. thickening
    s. venous plexus
submucous myoma
suboccipital shortening
suboccipitobregmatic diameter
suboptimal
    s. detail
    s. effort
    s. examination
    s. film
    s. result
    s. runoff
    s. visualization
suboptimally visualized
subpectoral
    s. implant
    s. pocket
subperiosteal
    s. abscess
    s. bone resorption
    s. cortical abrasion
    s. cortical defect
    s. desmoid
    s. fracture
    s. hematoma
    s. hemorrhage
    s. infection
    s. new bone
    s. osteoid osteoma
subperitoneal space
subphrenic
    s. abscess
    s. biloma
    s. fluid
    s. interposition syndrome
    s. recess
    s. space
subphysial metaphysis
subpial
    s. arteriovenous malformation
    s. lipoma
    s. region

S

subpleural
- s. air cyst
- s. bleb
- s. curvilinear line
- s. dot
- s. effusion
- s. emphysema
- s. honeycombing
- s. interstitium
- s. lymphatics
- s. micronodule
- s. nodule
- s. pulmonary arcade

subpubic arch

subpulmonic
- s. effusion
- s. fluid
- s. obstruction
- s. outflow
- s. pleural space
- s. pneumothorax

subpyloric node

subrectus obstruction

subsartorial
- s. canal
- s. tunnel

subscapular
- s. artery
- s. bursa
- s. echocardiographic view
- s. fossa
- s. lymph node

subscapularis
- s. muscle
- s. recess
- s. tendon

subsecond
- s. FLASH imaging
- s. gantry rotation time
- s. scanning

subsegmental
- s. atelectasis (SSA)
- s. bibasilar atelectasis
- s. bronchus
- s. lower lobe atelectasis
- s. perfusion abnormality
- s. perfusion defect
- s. renal artery branch

subsegment of lung

subselective cannulation

subseptus
- uterus s.

subserosal
- s. fibroid
- s. fibrosis
- s. hemorrhage
- s. lymphangiectasis
- s. tumor

subserous layer

subsite

subsonic stenosis

subspinous dislocation

substance
- bone s.
- brain s.
- diamagnetic s.
- reticular activating s.

substantia, *pl.* **substantiae**
- s. nigra
- s. propria

substantiae (*pl. of* substantia)

substernal
- s. angle
- s. goiter
- s. retraction
- s. thyroid
- s. thyroid gland

substitute
- bone s.
- oxygenated perfluorocarbon blood s.

substrate
- main energy s.
- radiolabeled marker s.

subsystem
- radiofrequency s.

subtalar
- s. angle
- s. articulation
- s. axis
- s. instability
- s. joint
- s. varus
- s. view

subtendinous bursa

subtentorial lesion

subthalamus

subtle
- s. gradation
- s. haziness
- s. malalignment
- s. microcalcification

subtotal
- s. gastric exclusion
- s. gastric resection
- s. lesion
- s. lymphoid irradiation
- s. nodal irradiation
- s. occlusion
- s. overframing
- s. thyroidectomy

subtracted image

subtraction
- s. angiography
- background s.
- s. cloning
- complex s.
- computer-assisted blood background s. (CABBS)

digital s.
dual-energy s.
energy s.
s. film
s. ictal SPECT coregistered to MRI (SISCOM)
s. image
s. imaging
intraoperative digital s. (IDIS)
2nd-order s.
quantitative imaging of perfusion using single s.
s. technique
vector s.
s. venography

subtractive noise
subtrapezial space
subtrochanteric
s. fracture
s. varus deformity
subumbilical space
subungual, subunguial
s. abscess
s. fibroma
s. glomus tumor
subunguial (*var. of* subungual)
subunit
functional s. (FSU)
subureteric Teflon injection (STING)
subvalvular
s. aneurysm
s. aortic obstruction
s. aortic stenosis
s. diffuse muscular obstruction
s. gradient
s. pulmonary stenosis
subvesical duct
subxiphoid
s. implantation
s. paracentesis
s. view
succenturiate placental lobe
succimer
succinate dehydrogenase (SDH)
succinic semialdehyde
sucking
s. muscle
s. pneumothorax
Sucquet-Hoyer
S.-H. anastomosis
S.-H. canal
sucralfate
gadolinium s.
sucrose
s. dosimeter
s. polyester imaging agent
suction
s. polyp trap
s. tube

sudden
s. blockage of coronary artery
s. cardiac death
Sudeck
S. atrophy
S. dystrophy
S. point
SUFE
slipped upper femoral epiphysis
suffocative goiter
sugar
fasting blood s. (FBS)
s. ring
s. tumor
suit
MAST s.
suite
Avantx LC angiography s.
Fuji computed radiography mammography s.
sulcal
s. atrophy
s. dilation
s. enhancement
s. enlargement
s. marking
s. pattern
s. skeleton
sulcation
sulci (*pl. of* sulcus)
sulcocommissural
s. artery
s. branch
sulcus, *pl.* **sulci**
s. angle
s. angularis
atrioventricular s.
basilar s.
blunted posterior s.
s. calcanei
calcarine s.
callosal s.
carotid s.
central s.
cerebral s.
s. chiasmaticus
cingulate s.
collateral s.
coronary s.
cortical s.
costal s.
costophrenic s.
s. dilation
dilation of s.
s. effacement
frontal s.
Harrison s.
hippocampal s.
hypothalamic s.

S

sulcus (*continued*)
    lateral femoral s.
    lateral occipital s.
    lip of lateral s.
    mapping of cerebral s.
    occipitotemporal s.
    olfactory s.
    parietooccipital s.
    perilabral s.
    pontomedullary s.
    postcentral s.
    posterior interventricular s.
    precentral s.
    pulmonary s.
    ramus of lateral s.
    retromalleolar s.
    rolandic s.
    sigmoid s.
    sphenoparietal s.
    superior frontal s.
    superior pulmonary s.
    superior temporal s.
    supracallosal s.
    s. tali
    temporal s.
    ulnar s.
    widened s.
sulfasalazine-induced pulmonary infiltrate
sulfate
    barium s. ($BaSO_4$)
    barium lead s.
    barium strontium s.
    E-Z-CAT Dry barium s.
    manganese s.
    sodium tetradecyl s.
    tetradecyl s.
    Varibar honey barium s.
    Varibar nectar barium s.
    Varibar pudding barium s.
    Varibar thin honey barium s.
    Varibar thin liquid barium s.
sulfide
    tin s.
sulfobromophthalein imaging agent
sulfonate
    sodium-2-mercaptoethane s.
sulfonated polymer
sulfur (S)
    s. 35 (^{35}S, S-35)
    s. colloid
    colloidal s.
    s. colloid imaging agent
    s. colloid scan
    s. colloid scintigraphy
    s. hexafluoride
    radioactive s.

sum
    field-echo s.
    s. of cylinder
    ray s.
summation
    s. of shadows
    s. shadow artifact
summed
    s. difference score (SDS)
    s. image
    s. rest score
    s. stress score
summing correction
summit
    ventricular septal s.
Sumner sign
sump
    s. drain
    s. drainage catheter
    s. tube
sum-peak
    s.-p. coincidence
    s.-p. method
sun
    Brett s.
    s. lamp
    S. SPARCstation system
    S. workstation
sunburst
    s. appearance
    s. brain vascularity
    s. gyral pattern
    s. nephrogram
    s. periosteal reaction
sun-ray appearance
sunrise
    s. knee x-ray view
    s. projection
sunset knee x-ray view
super
    S. Angiorex DSA system
    S. 50 CP high-voltage generator
superabsorbent
    s. polymer embolic material
    s. polymer microsphere (SAP-MS)
superacute
superadditivity
supercam scintillation scanner
superciliary arch
superconducting
    s. magnet
    s. open-magnet system
    s. quantum interference device (SQUID)
superconductive
    s. magnet
    s. MR system

superconductor
    niobium/titanium s.
superdominant left anterior descending artery
Superdup'r left heart system
superfecundation
superfetation
superficial
    s. angioma
    s. basal cell carcinoma
    s. depressed carcinoma
    s. diffuse nephroblastomatosis
    s. dorsal sacrococcygeal ligament
    s. external pudendal artery
    s. femoral artery (SFA)
    s. femoral artery occlusion
    s. femoral vein
    s. hyperthermia treatment
    s. inguinal lymph node
    s. inguinal pouch
    s. inguinal ring
    s. lesion
    s. lymphadenopathy
    s. lymphatic vessel
    s. mucosal space
    s. muscle
    s. necrosis
    s. palmar arterial arch
    s. palmaris longus tendon
    s. parotidectomy
    s. pedal vein
    s. perineal pouch
    s. plexus
    s. pneumonia
    s. posterior compartment
    s. posterior sacrococcygeal ligament
    s. radiation
    s. spreading esophageal carcinoma
    s. spreading stomach carcinoma
    s. temporal artery
    s. temporalis fascia
    s. temporoparietal fascia
    s. tendo Achillis bursa
    s. transitional cell carcinoma
    s. transverse metacarpal ligament
    s. transverse metatarsal ligament
superficialis
    s. arcade
    flexor digitorum s. (FDS)
    s. tendon
superimage
superimposed
    s. acute partial tear
    s. bowel gas
    s. fungal infection
superimposition
    s. artifact

    s. of bowel shadow
    s. of signal
superincumbent spinal curve
superinfection
    bacterial s.
superior
    apertura pelvis s.
    apertura thoracis s.
    s. articular facet
    s. articulating process
    s. aspect
    s. azygoesophageal recess
    s. bilateral vena cava
    s. border
    s. border of heart
    s. border of rib
    s. bronchial artery
    s. caval defect
    s. cerebellar artery (SCA)
    s. cervical ganglion
    s. colliculus
    s. costal facet
    s. costotransverse ligament
    s. duodenal fold
    s. duodenal recess
    s. epigastric artery
    s. extensor retinaculum
    s. frontal axis shift
    s. frontal gyrus
    s. frontal sulcus
    s. genicular artery
    s. gluteal vessel
    s. hypogastric plexus
    s. hypogastric plexus block
    s. intercostal artery
    s. intercostal vein
    s. jugular vein bulb
    s. labral anterior to posterior (SLAP)
    s. labral anterior to posterior tear
    s. labral anteroposterior injury
    s. labral anteroposterior lesion
    s. lobe
    s. lobe bronchus
    s. lobe of lung
    s. longitudinal fasciculus
    s. marginal defect
    s. margin of inferior rib
    s. maxillary foramen
    s. mediastinal structure
    s. mediastinum
    s. mesenteric arteriography
    s. mesenteric artery (SMA)
    s. mesenteric artery syndrome (SMAS)
    s. mesenteric ganglion
    s. mesenteric plexus

S

superior (*continued*)
    s. mesenteric vein (SMV)
    s. oblique
    s. occipitofrontal fasciculus
    s. olivary complex
    s. ophthalmic vein
    s. ophthalmic vein thrombosis
    s. orbital fissure
    s. orbital fissure anatomy
    s. parathyroid adenoma (SPA)
    s. parietal lobule gyrus
    s. peroneal retinaculum
    s. peroneal retinaculum disruption
    s. petrous sinus (SPS)
    s. petrous sinus catheterization
    s. phrenic branch
    s. pole
    s. pubic ligament
    s. pubic ramus
    s. pulmonary artery
    s. pulmonary sulcus
    s. pulmonary sulcus tumor
    s. pulmonary vein
    s. rectal vein
    s. retraction
    s. sagittal sinus (SSS)
    s. sagittal sinus thrombosis (SSST)
    s. segment
    s. segment bronchus
    s. temporal gyrus
    s. temporal sulcus
    s. thoracic aperture
    s. thyroid artery
    s. transverse rectal fold
    s. transverse scapular ligament
    s. triangle sign
    s. turbinate bone
    s. vena cava (SVC)
    s. vena cava obstruction (SVCO)
    s. vena cava pressure
    s. vena cava syndrome
    zygapophysis s.
superioris
    levator palpebrae s.
supernormal
    s. artery
    s. excitation
supernumerary
    s. digit
    s. kidney
    s. parathyroid adenoma
    s. parathyroid gland
    s. sesamoid bone
    s. tooth
superoinferior
    s. flow direction
    s. heart
    s. projection
    s. view

superolateral
    s. aspect
    s. displacement
superolaterally
superomedial
    s. acetabular index (SMAI)
    s. margin
    s. portal
    s. surface
superoxide dismutase
superparamagnetic
    s. iron oxide (SPIO)
    s. iron oxide blood pool agent
    s. iron oxide imaging agent
    s. iron oxide MR imaging
    s. iron oxide particle
    s. microsphere
Superpump System (SPS)
Superscan
superselective
    s. angio-CT
    s. infusion
    s. magnified digital angiography
    s. mesenteric artery catheterization
    s. microcatheter placement
super-stiff
    s.-s. glide wire
    s.-s. guidewire
SuperStitch
    S. closure device
    Sutura 8F S.
supersystemic pulmonary artery pressure
supervoltage
    s. generator
    s. radiation
    s. radiotherapy
    s. technique
supinate
supination-adduction
    s.-a. fracture
    s.-a. injury
supination deformity
supination-eversion fracture
supination-external
    s.-e. rotation (SER)
    s.-e. rotation injury
    s.-e. rotation type IV fracture
supination-outward rotation injury
supinator muscle
supine
    s. bicycle stress echocardiography
    s. film
    s. full view
    s. head-first position
    s. radiograph
supplemental beam filtration
supply
    accessory blood s.

arterial scrotum s.
collateral blood s.
dual blood s.
indirect blood s.
lenticulostriate s.
longitudinal blood s.
3-phase voltage s.
pudendal blood s.
tumor blood s.
vascular s.

support
basic life s. (BLS)
biventricular s. (BVS)
chemoinductive s.
elevated leg s.
lateral lumbar s.
ligamentous s.
structural s.
wedge-shaped s.

suppressed tissue
suppression
ChemSat fat s.
Cytomel s.
DIET method of fat s.
drug-induced bone marrow s.
fat signal s.
FSE-T2 with fat s.
s. of heart pulsation artifact
overdrive s.
paradoxic s.
s. scan
signal s.
solvent s.
spectral-spatial fat s.

suppuration
suppurative
s. ascending cholangitis
s. inflammation
s. pancreatitis
s. pleurisy
s. pneumonia
s. pyelonephritis
s. thyroiditis

supraanal fascia
supraanular constriction
supraaortic
s. lesion
s. ridge
s. stenosis

supracallosal
s. gyrus
s. sulcus

supracardiac total anomalous venous return
supracardinal vein
supraceliac aorta
supracervical hysterectomy
supraclavicular
s. aortic stenosis

s. fossa
s. lymph node
s. node involvement
s. triangle

supraclinoid
s. carotid aneurysm
s. ICA
s. portion
s. segment of internal carotid artery

supracolic compartment
supracollicular spike of cortical bone
supracondylar
s. femoral fracture
s. humeral fracture
s. plate
s. process
s. ridge
s. Y-shaped fracture

supracoronary ridge
supracricoid interval
supracristal
s. plane (SCP)
s. ventricular septal defect

supradiaphragmatic
s. adenopathy
s. aorta
s. extension

supraepicondylar
supraepitrochlear
supraglenoid tubercle
supraglottic
s. carcinoma
s. edema
s. laryngectomy
s. larynx
s. narrowing
s. structure

supraglottis
Supra G stent
suprahepatic
s. caval cuff
s. hypertension
s. inferior vena cava anastomosis
s. vena cava

suprahisian block
suprahyoid
suprailiac aortic mesenteric graft
suprainguinal PTA
suprainterparietal bone
supralevator
s. fistula
s. space

supraligamentous disc herniation
supramalleolar open amputation
supramarginal gyrus
supramesocolic compartment
supranaviculare
os s.

S

supranuclear lesion
supraoccipital bone
supraorbital
 s. artery
 s. canal
 s. fissure
 s. foramen
 s. groove (SOG)
 s. margin (SOM)
 s. ridge
supraorbitomeatal plane
suprapancreatic obstruction
suprapatellar
 s. bursa
 s. plica
 s. pouch
suprapharyngeal bone
suprapubic
 s. area
 s. transabdominal ultrasound
suprapyloric node
suprarenal
 s. aortic aneurysm
 s. extension of aneurysm
 s. gland
 s. impression
 s. stenosis
suprascapular
 s. ligament
 s. nerve entrapment
 s. notch syndrome
suprasellar
 s. adenoma
 s. aneurysm
 s. atypical teratoma
 s. capsule
 s. extension
 s. extension of tumor
 s. hemorrhagic germinoma
 s. low-density lesion
 s. mass
 s. mass calcification
 s. meningioma
 s. subarachnoid cistern
suprasphincteric fistula
supraspinatus
 s. muscle
 s. nerve
 s. tendinosis
 s. tendon
supraspinatus-musculotendinous junction
supraspinous
 s. ligament
 s. ligament disruption
suprasternal
 s. bone
 s. bulge
 s. notch
 s. notch plane

 s. notch view
 s. retraction
 s. scanning
 s. window
suprasyndesmotic fixation
supratentorial
 s. astrocytoma
 s. brain tumor
 s. cerebral blood flow
 s. flow compensation
 s. glioma
 s. gray matter
 s. lesion
 s. neoplasia
 s. primitive neuroectodermal
 tumor
 s. space
 s. volume
 s. white matter
suprathreshold
supratip nasal tip deformity
supratrochlear
 s. artery
 s. node
supratubercular ridge of Meyer
supravalvular
 s. aortic stenosis (SAS, SVAS)
 s. aortography
 s. mitral stenosis
 s. pulmonary stenosis
 s. ring
supravaterian duodenum
supraventricular
 s. crest (SVC)
 s. level
 s. tachyarrhythmia
 s. tachycardia
 s. venous echo
supraventricularis
 crista s.
supravesical obstruction
supreme turbinate bone
SUR
 standardized uptake ratio
suralis
 tensor fasciae s.
sural nerve
SureStart contrast tracking
surface
 acromial articular s.
 anterolateral s.
 anteromedial s.
 s. application of radioelement
 apposing articular s.'s
 articular s.
 articulating s.
 arytenoid articular s.
 attenuated cortical s.
 auricular s.

axial s.
basal s.
bone s.
bosselated s.
buccal s.
calcaneal articular s.
carpal articular s.
cartilaginous joint s.
cerebral s.
s. coil
s. coil localization
s. coil method
s. coil NMR
s. coil rotating-frame spectroscopy
colic s.
s. configuration
s. contamination
contiguous articular s.'s
s. convexity pattern
corrugated fat-pad s.
costal s.
cuboid articular s.
diaphragmatic s.
distal s.
s. distance
s. dose variation
endosteal s.
endothelial s.
epicardial s.
s. epithelium
erosion of articular s.
fibular articular s.
gastric s.
glenoid s.
grooving of articular s.
immunostained s.
joint articular s.
s. matching technique
mediastinal lung s.
metastatic adenocarcinoma in
   serosal s.
s. nodularity
s. normal overlap method
occlusal s.
opposing articular s.'s
opposing pleural s.'s
s. osteosarcoma
s. ovarian epithelium tumor
palmar s.
parallelism of articular s.
pelvic peritoneal s.
permeability s.
plantar s.
posterior s.
s. projection
s. radioelement application
radioulnar s.
s. registration
renal s.

roughened articular s.
serosal s.
s. spoiling
superomedial s.
synovial s.
s. tension of lung
s. variable-attenuation correction
ventral s.
weightbearing s.

surfactant
s. deficiency
s. deficiency disorder (SDD)

surfer's
s. knee
s. knot
s. nodule

surgeon
American Academy of Orthopaedic
   S.'s (AAOS)

surgery
breast-preserving s.
cardiothoracic s.
coronary artery bypass s.
   (CABS)
CT-guided stereotactic s.
cytoreductive s.
debulking s.
gastric bypass s. (GBS)
image-guided s.
larynx-sparing s.
MR-guided focused ultrasound s.
nephron-sparing s.
radioguided s.
radioimmunoguided s. (RIGS)
robotic mitral valve s.
stereotactic s.
telecollaboration s.
video-assisted thoracoscopic s.
voice-sparing s.

surgical
s. anatomy visualization and
   navigation tool (SAVANT)
s. angle
s. artifact
s. asepsis
s. decompression
s. emphysema
s. endarterectomy
s. inspection
s. neck
s. neck fracture
s. neck of humerus
S. Planning and Orientation
   Computer System (SPOCS)
s. simulation CT
s. sponge
s. staple
s. venous interruption
s. wound

S

surgically
- s. corrected transposition of great arteries
- s. created resection cavity

Surgilase
- S. 150 high-powered CO_2 laser
- S. Nd:YAG laser

SurgiScope
Surgitron portable radiosurgical unit
Surgiview laparoscope
Surgi-Vision MRI coil
surveillance
- endoscopic s.
- imaging s.

survey
- bone s.
- s. film
- isotopic skeletal s.
- joint s.
- long-bone s.
- metabolic bone s.
- metastatic bone s.
- osseous s.
- postimplant radiation s.
- preloading radiation s.
- s. radiograph
- s. scan
- serial radiographic s.'s
- skeletal s.
- traumatic bone s.
- 4-view wrist s.

survival
- cause-specific s.
- clinical estimation of s.
- event-free s.
- failure-free s.
- local recurrence-free s.

susceptibility
- s. artifact
- bulk magnetic s. (BMS)
- s. contrast-weighted MRI
- diamagnetic s.
- s. effect
- magnetic s.
- s. mapping

susceptibility-sensitive sequence
susceptibility-weighted
- s.-w. MR imaging
- s.-w. sequence

suspended
- s. heart
- s. inspiration

suspension
- barium s.
- s. characteristic
- chromic phosphate s.
- colloidal s.
- Definity injectable s.
- Enecat CT concentrated rectal s.

- E-Z-Paque barium s.
- fast-exchange cellular s.
- galactose-based s.
- liquid barium s.
- s. of kidney
- perflutren lipid microsphere injectable s.

suspensory
- s. ligament
- s. ligament of ovary
- s. ligament of penis
- s. muscle of duodenum

suspicious
- s. lesion
- s. mass

sustained
- s. anterior parasternal motion
- s. apical impulse
- s. left ventricular heave
- s. tachyarrhythmia

sustentacula (*pl. of* sustentaculum)
sustentacular trauma
sustentaculum, *pl.* **sustentacula**
- s. lienis
- os s.
- s. tali

Sutura 8F SuperStitch
sutural
- s. bone
- s. calcification
- s. ligament
- s. marking

suture
- anterior palatine s.
- apical s.
- basilar s.
- bioabsorbable Dexon s.
- biparietal s.
- bony s.
- bregmatomastoid s.
- s. calcification
- coronal s.
- cranial s.
- delayed closure of s.
- dentate s.
- denticulate s.
- diastasis of s.
- diastatic lambdoid s.
- ethmoidolacrimal s.
- ethmoidomaxillary s.
- false s.
- flat s.
- frontal s.
- frontoethmoidal s.
- frontolacrimal s.
- frontomalar s.
- frontomaxillary s.
- frontonasal s.
- frontoparietal s.

frontosphenoid s.
frontozygomatic s.
Gillies s.
Gruber s.
incisive s.
infiltration s.
infraorbital s.
intermaxillary s.
internasal s.
interpalatine s.
interparietal s.
jugal s.
lacrimoconchal s.
lacrimoethmoidal s.
lacrimomaxillary s.
lacrimoturbinal s.
lambdoid cranial s.
limbus s.
s. line
s. line carcinoma
s. lock
longitudinal s.
malomaxillary s.
mamillary s.
mastoid s.
median palatine s.
metallic s.
metopic s.
middle palatine s.
nasal s.
nasofrontal s.
nasomaxillary s.
nonfusion of cranial s.
occipital s.
occipitomastoid s.
occipitoparietal s.
occipitosphenoid s.
s. of skull
opaque wire s.
overlapping s.
palatine s.
palatoethmoidal s.
palatomaxillary s.
parietal s.
parietomastoid s.
parietooccipital s.
parietotemporal s.
persistent metopic s.
petrobasilar s.
petrosphenobasilar s.
petrosphenooccipital s.
plane s.
posterior palatine s.
prematurely closed s.
premaxillary s.
rhabdoid s.
sagittal cranial s.
serrated s.
silk s.

sphenoethmoidal s.
sphenofrontal s.
sphenomalar s.
sphenomaxillary s.
sphenooccipital s.
sphenoorbital s.
sphenoparietal s.
sphenopetrosal s.
sphenosquamous s.
sphenotemporal s.
sphenovomerine s.
sphenozygomatic s.
splayed cranial s.
spread s.
squamomastoid s.
squamoparietal s.
squamosal s.
squamosphenoid s.
squamous s.
sternal s.
temporal s.
temporomalar s.
temporozygomatic s.
true s.
wide s.
zygomaticofrontal s.
zygomaticotemporal s.

SUV
standard uptake value
SV
sigmoid volvulus
stroke volume
Sv
sievert
SVABB
stereotactic vacuum-assisted breast
biopsy
SVAS
supravalvular aortic stenosis
SVC
superior vena cava
supraventricular crest
SVC syndrome
SVCO
superior vena cava obstruction
SVD
singular valve decomposition
SVG
scatter and veiling glare
SV-5 guidewire
SVI
seminal vesicle invasion
stroke volume index
SvO$_2$
systemic vascular resistance index
SVR
systemic vascular resistance
SVRI
systemic vascular resistance index

S

swallow
>barium s.
>dry s.
>Gastrografin s.
>Hypaque s.
>ice-water s.
>modified barium s.
>video barium s.
>water-soluble contrast esophageal s.
>wet s.

swallowing
>s. artifact
>s. center
>s. dysfunction
>fetal s.
>s. function
>s. mechanism
>s. study

swallowtail
>s. configuration
>s. malformation of scapula

swamp-static artifact
Swan-Ganz balloon catheter
swan-neck
>s.-n. finger deformity
>s.-n. shape of ventricular outflow
>s.-n. tubular lesion

swan neck deformity sign
Swanson finger joint
sweat
>s. duct adenoma
>s. gland carcinoma

sweep
>duodenal s.
>finger s.
>iterative s.
>whole-body s.
>widened duodenal s.

sweet
>S. method
>S. sternal punch

swelling
>ankle s.
>blennorrhagic s.
>brain s.
>bulbar s.
>congestive brain s.
>diffuse cerebral s.
>fusiform s.
>joint s.
>s. of cartilage
>periumbilical s.
>prevertebral soft tissue s.
>soft tissue s.

Swenson colonic pullthrough procedure
SWI
>stroke-work index

swimmer's
>s. position

>s. projection
>s. shoulder
>s. view

swimming pool granuloma
swinging heart
swirl appearance
swirling
>s. motion
>s. smokelike echo

Swiss
>S. Alps appearance
>S. cheese air bronchogram
>S. cheese appearance
>S. cheese nephrogram
>S. cheese ventricular septal defect
>S. lithoclast intracorporeal lithotriptor
>S. roll technique

Swissray scanner
switchable coil
swollen
>s. brain hemisphere
>s. tissue

Swyer-James-Macleod syndrome
Swyer-James syndrome
Swyer syndrome
SXA
>single-energy x-ray absorptiometer

SXCT
>spiral x-ray computed tomography

Syed-Neblett template
Syed-Puthawala-Hedger esophageal applicator
Syed template
sylvian
>s. aqueduct
>s. aqueduct syndrome
>s. candelabrum
>s. cistern
>s. fissure
>s. operculum
>s. point
>s. triangle

sylvian-rolandic junction
Sylvius
>aqueduct of S.
>cistern of S.
>S. fossa
>hereditary stenosis of aqueduct of S. (HSAS)
>S. ventricle

Symbia TruePoint SPECT
symbol
>radiation warning s.

Syme ankle disarticulation amputation
Symington body
symmelia (*var. of* sirenomelia)
Symmers fibrosis
Symmetra I-125 brachytherapy seed

symmetric, symmetrical
s. abnormal increased signal
bilaterally s.
s. chest
s. confluent high signal
intensity
s. consolidation
s. distribution
s. echo
s. heart hypertrophy
s. IUGR
s. loss of DAT
s. narrowing
s. pattern of radiotracer uptake
s. periosteal reaction
s. phased array
s. pulmonary congestion
s. thorax
symmetrical (*var. of* symmetric)
symmetry
architectural s.
bilateral s.
inverse s.
sympathetic
s. block
s. blockade
s. chain
s. denervation
s. discharge
s. dystrophy
s. ganglion
s. ganglion tumor
s. innervation
s. nervous system
s. nervous tissue
s. reinnervation
s. vascular instability
sympathicolysis
MR-guided lumbar s.
sympathogonia
symphony
S. MR imaging system
S. MR unit
S. nitinol self-expandable stent
S. self-expanding stent
symphyseal (*var. of* symphysial)
symphyses (*pl. of* symphysis)
symphysial, symphyseal
symphysis, *pl.* **symphyses**
s. cartilage joint
s. intervertebralis
s. manubriosternalis
s. of mandible
pubic s
s. pubis
symptom
constellation of s.'s
constitutional s.
extrapyramidal s.

segmental bronchus s.
vasomotor s.
symptomatic
s. coarctation of aorta
s. gallstone
s. lateral synovial plica
s. metastatic spinal cord
compression
s. obstructive hydrocephalus
s. vascular ring
symptomatology
synaptic
s. cleft
s. dopamine concentration
s. pathway
s. vesicle
syncephalus
synchondroses (*pl. of* synchondrosis)
synchondrosis, *pl.* **synchondroses**
anterior intraoccipital s.
cartilaginous s.
s. costae primae
cranial synchondroses
synchondroses cranii
disruption of cartilaginous s.
ischiopubic s.
low signal intensity s.
s. manubriosternalis
neurocentral s.
s. of skull
ossifying ischiopubic s.
posterior intraoccipital s.
s. sphenoethmoidalis
sphenooccipital s.
s. sphenopetrosa
synchondroses sternales
s. xiphosternalis
synchronicity
synchronization
s. device
prospective s.
retrospective s.
synchronized retroperfusion
synchronous
s. carotid arterial pulse
s. disease
s. lesion
s. neoplasm
s. primary malignancy
s. transitional cell carcinoma
s. tumor
synchrony
ventricular s.
synchrotron
monochromatic s.
s. radiation
syncinesis (*var. of* synkinesis)
synclitic
synclitism

S

syncytia (*pl. of* syncytium)
syncytium, *pl.* **syncytia**
    circular s.
syncytium-inducing
syndactylization of digit
syndactyly in fetus
syndesmophyte
    marginal s.
    spinal s.
syndesmoses (*pl. of* syndesmosis)
syndesmosis, *pl.* **syndesmoses**
    distal tibiofibular s.
    s. radioulnaris
    s. sprain
    tibiofibular s.
    s. tibiofibularis
    s. tympanostapedialis
syndesmotic
    s. diastasis
    s. impingement
    s. ligament
    s. ligament complex
syndrome
    abdominal muscle deficiency s.
    acquired adult Fanconi s.
    acquired immunodeficiency s.
      (AIDS)
    acute central cord s.
    acute chest s.
    acute compartment s.
    acute radiation s. (ARS)
    acute respiratory distress s.
      (ARDS)
    acute retroviral s.
    Adams-Stokes s.
    adductor canal s.
    adductor insertion avulsion s.
    adenocarcinoma of unknown
      primary s.
    adrenogenital s.
    adult respiratory distress s. (ARDS)
    afferent loop s.
    Aicardi s.
    Aicardi-Goutières s.
    Alagille s.
    Albright s.
    Albright-McCune-Sternberg s.
    Alibert-Bazin s.
    Alpers-Huttenlocher s. (AHS)
    amnionic band s.
    angiomatous s.
    angioosteohypertrophy s.
    anterior compartment s.
    anterior cord s.
    anterior impingement s.
    anterior spinal artery s.
    anterior tarsal tunnel s.
    anterolateral impingement s.
    antiphospholid antibody s.

    aortic s.
    aortitis s.
    apallic s.
    apple-peel s.
    Arnold-Chiari s.
    Asherson s.
    atherosclerotic occlusive s.
    autoerythrocyte sensitization s.
    Avellis s.
    axonopathic neurogenic thoracic
      outlet s.
    Ayerza s.
    Bäfverstedt s.
    Balint s.
    Bannayan-Riley-Ruvalcaba s.
    Banti s.
    Barlow s.
    Barré-Lieou s.
    Bartter s.
    basal cell nevus s.
    basilar artery s.
    battered child s.
    Bazex s.
    beat-knee s.
    Beckwith-Wiedemann s.
    Behçet s.
    Behr s.
    Berdon s.
    Bernard-Horner s.
    Bernard-Soulier s.
    Bertolotti s.
    Beuren s.
    biliary obstruction s.
    Bing-Horton s.
    Blackfan-Diamond s.
    Bland-Garland-White s.
    Blesovsky s.
    blind loop s.
    blind pouch s.
    Bloom s.
    blueberry muffin s.
    blue digit s.
    blue rubber-bleb nevus s.
    blue toe s.
    Boerhaave s.
    bone marrow edema s.
    Bouveret s.
    Brissaud s.
    Brown-Séquard s.
    Brugada s.
    Budd s.
    Budd-Chiari s.
    Caffey s.
    Caffey-Kempe s.
    capillary leak s.
    Caplan s.
    carcinoid s.
    cardiac disturbance s.
    cardiocutaneous s.

cardiosplenic s.
Carney s.
carotid blowout s.
carotid sinus s. (CSS)
carpal tunnel s.
cat's cry s.
cauda equina s. (CES)
caudal regression s.
cavernous sinus s.
Cayler s.
Ceelen-Gellerstedt s.
celiac artery compression s.
celiac axis s.
central cervical cord s.
cerebellar s.
cerebral steal s.
cerebrohepatorenal s. (CHRS)
cervical disc s.
cervical pain s.
cervical rib s.
Cestan-Chenais s.
Chédiak-Steinbrinck-Higashi s.
Chilaiditi s.
CHILD s.
chronic overuse s.
Churg-Strauss s.
Clarke-Hadefield s.
Claude s.
cleft face s.
Clerc-Levy-Cristico s.
clinically isolated s.
COACH s.
coarctation s.
Cobb s.
Cockayne s.
Collet-Sicard s.
compartment s.
complex regional pain s.
compression s.
congenital adrenogenital s.
congenital pulmonary venolobar s.
congenital vascular-bone s. (CVBS)
Conn s.
Conradi-Hünermann s.
constriction band s.
coronary artery steal s.
coronary-subclavian steal s.
costoclavicular s.
Courvoisier-Terrier s.
Cowden s.
craniofacial pain s.
craniomandibular s.
craniosynostosis s.
CRASH s.
CREST s.
cri-du-chat s.
Cronkhite-Canada s.
Crouzon s.
Crow-Fukase s.

crowned dens s.
crush s.
cubital tunnel s.
Cushing paraneoplastic s.
Cyriax s.
Dandy-Walker s.
Davies-Colley s.
defibrination s.
Degos s.
Dejerine-Klumpke s.
de Lange s.
Demons-Mcigs s.
de Morsier s.
Denys s.
Denys-Drash s. (DDS)
Diamond-Blackfan s.
DiFerrante s.
DiGeorge s.
Di Guglielmo s.
disconnected pancreatic duct s.
disseminated intravascular
  coagulation s.
distal intestinal obstruction s.
Down s.
Drash s.
Dressler s.
Dubin-Johnson s.
dumping s.
Dyke-Davidoff-Masson s.
dysarthria-clumsy hand s.
dysmotile cilia s.
Eagle-Barrett s.
ectopic ACTH s.
Edwards s.
Ehlers-Danlos s.
Eisenmenger s.
Ellis-van Creveld s.
empty sella s.
encephalotrigeminal s.
enlarged vestibular vascular
  aqueduct s.
excessive lateral pressure s. (ELPS)
facet s.
facioauriculovertebral s.
FAI s.
failed back s. (FBS)
failed back surgery s. (FBSS)
Fallot s.
familial adenomatous polyposis s.
Fanconi s.
Fanconi-Hegglin s.
fat dissociation s.
fat embolism s. (FES)
Felty s.
feminizing testis s.
fetal alcohol s. (FAS)
fetal cardiosplenic s.
Feuerstein-Mims s.
fibrocystic breast s.

S

syndrome (*continued*)

Fiessinger-Leroy s.
Fiessinger-Leroy-Reiter s.
Fitz-Hugh and Curtis s.
floppy valve s.
Foix-Alajouanine s.
Foix-Chavany-Marie s.
Forney s.
Frey s.
functional bowel s.
Gaisböck s.
Gardner bone s.
gas-bloat s.
Gasser s.
gastrocardiac s.
generalized lymphadenopathy s.
Gerstmann s.
Gianotti-Crosti s.
Goldenhar s.
Goodpasture s.
Gorlin s.
Gorlin-Goltz s.
Graham-Burford-Mayer s.
Grisel s.
Gsell-Erdheim s.
Guillain-Barré s.
Haglund s.
Hajdu-Cheney s.
Hallermann-Streiff-François s.
hamartomatous polyposis s.
Hamman-Rich s.
Hare s.
Hegglin s.
hemisensory s.
hemolytic uremic s.
Hennekam s.
Henoch-Schönlein s.
hepatopulmonary s.
hepatorenal s. (HRS)
hereditary flat adenoma s.
hereditary right heart s. (HRHS)
Hermansky-Pudlak s.
heterotaxia s.
holiday heart s.
Holmes s.
Holt-Oram s.
Horner s.
Howell-Evans s.
Hoyeraal-Hreidarsson s.
Hughes-Stovin s.
Hunter s.
Hurler s.
Hurler-Scheie s.
Hutchinson s.
Hutchinson-Gilford s.
Hutinel-Pick s.
hyperabduction s.
hypereosinophilic s.
hypogenetic lung s.

hypoplastic aortic s.
hypoplastic left heart s. (HLHS)
hypoplastic left parietal s.
hypoplastic right heart s. (HRHS)
ileocecal s.
iliac vein compression s.
iliotibial band friction s.
immature lung s.
impingement s.
inferior vena cava s.
infrapatellar contracture s. (IPCS)
inguinal ligament s.
inhibitory s.
innominate artery compression s.
intermediate coronary s.
intestinal Behçet s.
intestinal hypoperistalsis s.
irritable bowel s. (IBS)
Ivemark CHD s.
Jadassohn-Lewandowsky s.
Jaffe-Campanacci s.
Jarcho-Levin s.
Jeune s.
Joubert s.
jugular foramen s.
juvenile polyposis s. (JPS)
Kallmann s.
Kartagener s.
Kasabach-Merritt s.
Kast s.
Katayama s.
Kearns-Sayre s.
Kimmelstiel-Wilson s.
Kinsbourne s.
Kleffner-Landau s.
Klinefelter s.
Klippel-Feil s.
Klippel-Trenaunay s. (KTS)
Klippel-Trenaunay-Weber s.
Korsakoff s.
Kozhevnikov s.
Lady Windermere s.
Lambert-Eaton myasthenic s.
Landau-Kleffner s.
Langer-Giedion s.
Larsen s.
lateral recess s.
Laubry-Pezzi s.
leaky lung s. (LLS)
left heart s.
Leigh s.
Lemierre s.
Lennox-Gastaut s.
Leriche s.
Léri-Weill s.
Lesch-Nyhan s.
LGL s.
Lhermitte-Duclos s.
Lhermitte-Duclos-Cowden s.

Lightwood s.
linear sebaceous nevus s.
locked-in s.
Löffler s.
Löfgren s.
Louis-Bar s.
low back s.
Lowe s.
low-flow s.
Lown-Ganong-Levine s.
luteinized unruptured follicle s.
Lutembacher s.
luxury perfusion s.
lymphadenopathy s.
lymph node s.
Macleod s.
Maffucci s.
male Turner s.
Mallory-Weiss s.
malperfusion s.
Marchiafava-Micheli s.
Marcus Gunn s.
Marfan s.
Marine-Lenhart s.
Marinesco-Sjögren s.
Maroteaux-Lamy s.
Martin-Bell s.
Martorell aortic arch s.
Mayer-Rokitansky-Küster-Hauser s.
May-Thurner s.
Mazabraud s.
McCune-Albright s.
McKusick-Kaufman s.
Meadows s.
Meckel s.
Meckel-Gruber s.
meconium aspiration s.
meconium plug s.
medial tibial stress s.
median arcuate ligament s.
megacystis-microcolon-intestinal
  hypoperistalsis s.
Meigs s.
Meigs-Cass s.
Meigs-Salmon s.
Melnick-Needles s.
Mendelson s.
Ménière s.
Menkes s.
mermaid s.
metastatic carcinoid s.
midaortic s. (MAS)
middle aortic s.
middle fossa s.
middle lobe s.
Mikity-Wilson s.
Mikulicz s.
milk-alkali s.
milk leg s.

Milkman s.
Miller-Dieker s.
Milwaukee shoulder s.
Minot-von Willebrand s.
Mirizzi s.
Mohr s.
Morgagni s.
Morgagni-Adams-Stokes s.
Morquio s.
Morquio-Brailsford s.
Mosse s.
Mounier-Kuhn s.
moyamoya s.
Moynahan s.
MSA s.
mucocutaneous lymph node s.
  (MCLS)
mucosal prolapse s.
Muir-Torre s.
multiple endocrine neoplasia s.
multiple mucosal neuromas s.
multiple pterygium s.
multiple system atrophy s.
myelodysplastic s. (MDS)
myofascial pain-dysfunction s.
nail-patella s.
Naumoff s.
Nelson s.
neonatal hepatitis/cholestasis s.
neonatal lupus s.
nephrotic s.
neurocutaneous s.
neuroorthopaedic s.
nevoid basal cell carcinoma s.
Nievergelt s.
Nijmegen breakage s.
Noonan s.
Nothnagel s.
nutcracker s.
s. of impending thrombosis
s. of inappropriate antidiuretic
  hormone (SIADH)
Ogilvie s.
Omenn s.
orbital apex s.
organic brain s. (OBS)
orodigitofacial s.
Ortner s.
Osler-Libman-Sacks s.
Osler-Weber-Rendu s.
os peroneum s.
os trigonum s.
ovarian hyperstimulation s.
ovarian remnant s.
ovarian vein s.
overlap s.
Paget-von Schroetter s.
painful osmotic demyelination s.
Pallister-Hall s.

S

syndrome (*continued*)

Pancoast s.
pancreatic cholera s.
pancreaticohepatic s.
pancytopenia-dysmelia s.
Papillon-Lèfevre s.
paraneoplastic s.
Parinaud s.
Parkes-Weber s. (PWS)
parkinsonian s.
Parry-Romberg s.
Pasonage-Turner s.
Patau s.
Pearson s.
pectoralis major s.
PEHO s.
pelvic congestion s.
pelvic spur s.
Pena-Shokeir s.
Pendred s.
Pepper s.
Peutz-Jeghers s.
Pfaundler-Hurler s.
Pfeiffer s.
PHACES s.
phantom limb s.
Pierre-Marie-Bamberger s.
Pierre Robin s.
pinch-off s.
plica s.
Plummer-Vinson s.
POEMS s.
Poland s.
polycystic ovary s. (PCOS, POS)
polysplenia s.
popliteal artery entrapment s.
postcardiac injury s. (PCIS)
postembolization s.
posterior column s.
posterior impingement s.
posterior joint s.
posterior reversible encephalopathy s.
  (PRES)
postmaturity s.
postmyocardial infarction s.
postpericardiotomy s.
postpolio s.
Potter s.
Prader-Willi s.
Proteus s.
proximal loop s.
prune belly s.
pseudo-Meigs s.
pseudothrombophlebitis s.
pseudo-Turner s.
pseudo-Zollinger-Ellison s. (ps-ZES)
pulmonary venolobar s.
quadrilateral space s.
radiation s.

Raeder paratrigeminal s.
Ramsay Hunt s.
Raymond-Cestan s.
Raynaud s.
reactive airway dysfunction s.
Reader paratrigeminal s.
reflex sympathetic dystrophy s.
Reiter s.
respiratory distress s. (RDS)
restrictive hemodynamic s.
Rett s.
reversible posterior
  leukoencephalopathy s. (RPLS)
Richter s.
right middle lobe s.
Riley-Day s.
Roberts s.
Robinow s.
Rokitansky-Mayer-Küster-Hauser s.
Romano-Ward s.
Romberg-Wood s.
Rotor s.
Rundles-Falls s.
Russell-Silver s.
Ruvalcaba-Myhre-Smith s.
Sack-Barabas s.
Saldino-Noonan s.
Sanfilippo s.
SAPHO s.
scalenus anticus s.
scaphocapitate s.
scapulocostal s.
Scheie s.
Schnitzler s.
Schönlein-Henoch s.
Schwartz-Jampel s. (SJS)
scimitar s.
severe acute respiratory s. (SARS)
shaken baby s. (SBS)
Sheehan s.
Shone s.
short gut s.
short rib-polydactyly s.
shoulder-hand s.
shoulder impingement s.
Shprintzen velocardiofacial s.
Shwachman s.
sick sinus s.
silent sinus s.
sinus tarsi s.
Sipple s.
Sjögren s.
Sjögren-Larsson s.
slipping rib s.
slit ventricle s.
sloughed urethra s.
small aorta s.
small left colon s.
Smith-Lemli-Opitz s.

snapping hip s.
snapping triceps s.
Sneddon s.
soleus s.
solitary rectal ulcer s.
Solomon s.
Sotos s.
spastic bowel s.
Spens s.
spinous process impingement s.
split cord s.
split notochord s.
spontaneous intracranial hypotension s.
stagnant loop s.
Stauffer s.
steal s.
Stein-Leventhal s.
Stewart-Treves s.
Stickler s.
stiff lung s.
stiff man s.
Sturge-Weber s.
Sturge-Weber-Dimitri s.
subclavian steal s. (SSS)
subphrenic interposition s.
superior mesenteric artery s.
  (SMAS)
superior vena cava s.
suprascapular notch s.
SVC s.
Swyer s.
Swyer-James s.
Swyer-James-Macleod s.
sylvian aqueduct s.
synovitis, acne, pustulosis,
  hyperostosis, osteitis s.
systemic inflammatory response s.
TAR s.
tarsal tunnel s.
Taussig-Bing s.
Taussig-Snellen-Alberts s.
terminal reservoir s.
tethered cord s. (TCS)
therapy-related myelodysplastic s.
thoracic inlet s.
thoracic outlet s. (TOS)
thrombocytopenia-absent radius s.
Tietze s.
tight filum terminale s.
Tolosa-Hunt s.
Torre s.
Toulouse-Lautrec s.
Touraine-Solente-Golé s.
transient bone marrow edema s.
Treacher Collins s.
trisomy 8 s.
trisomy D, E s.
Trousseau s.
tumor lysis s.

Turcot s.
Turner s.
twiddler's s.
twin embolization s.
twin-to-twin transfusion s. (TTTS)
ulnar impaction s.
ulnar tunnel s.
ulnolunate impaction s.
uncal herniation s.
unroofed coronary sinus s.
urethral s.
VACTERL s.
van Buchem s.
van der Hoeve s.
vanishing lung s.
vanishing testis s.
vascular leak s.
venolobar s.
venous stasis s.
Verner-Morrison s.
vertebral artery s.
vertebrobasilar artery s.
vestibular aqueduct s. (VAS)
Villaret-Mackenzie s.
von Hippel-Lindau s.
Waardenburg s.
Walker-Walburg s.
Wallenberg lateral medullary s.
Weil s.
Weill-Marchesani s.
Wermer s.
Werner s.
Wernicke-Korsakoff s.
West s.
wet lung s.
Widal s.
Wiedemann-Beckwith s.
Wilkie s.
Williams s.
Williams-Beuren s.
Williams-Campbell s.
Wilson-Mikity s.
s. with multiple cortical renal cysts
Wolff-Parkinson-White s.
Wolf-Hirschhorn s.
Wolfram s.
Wyburn-Mason s.
s. X
XY s.
Young s.
Yunis-Varon s.
Zellweger s.
Zieve s.
Zollinger-Ellison s. (ZES)
synechia, *pl.* **synechiae**
  uterine s.
  s. vulvae
synechiae (*pl. of* synechia)
synergic muscle

Synergy ultrasound system
syngeneic
>s. bone marrow transplant
>s. tissue

Syngo Lung CAD software system
syngraft
synkinesia (*var. of* synkinesis)
synkinesis, syncinesis, synkinesia
synophridia
synophrys
synosteosis (*var. of* synostosis)
synostosis, synosteosis
>bicoronal s.
>cervical s.
>congenital radioulnar s.
>coronal suture s.
>cranial s.
>craniofacial s.
>lambdoid s.
>metatarsal s.
>multiple-suture s.
>nonsyndromic bicoronal s.
>nonsyndromic unicoronal s.
>premature suture s.
>radiographically firm s.
>sagittal s.
>single-suture s.
>terminal s.
>tibiofibular s.
>unicoronal s.

synostotic posterior plagiocephaly
synovectomy
>radiation s.
>radioisotope s.
>radionuclide s.
>radiopharmaceutical s.

synovial
>s. bursa
>s. cavity
>s. chondromatosis
>s. cyst
>s. diarthrodial joint
>s. diffuse lipoma
>s. envelope
>s. fluid
>s. fringe
>s. gutter
>s. hemangioma
>s. herniation pit
>s. inflammatory response
>s. ligament
>s. membrane
>s. osteochondromatosis
>s. pannus
>s. plica
>s. proliferation
>s. sarcoma
>s. sheath
>s. shelf

>s. surface
>s. thickening
>s. tissue
>s. tumor

synoviogram
synovioma
synoviorthesis
synovitis
>s., acne, pustulosis, hyperostosis, osteitis syndrome
>s., acne, pustulosis, hyperostosis, osteomyelitis (SAPHO)
>benign transient s.
>boggy s.
>brucellar s.
>s. in active polymyalgia rheumatica
>intraarticular localized nodular s.
>nodular s.
>peripheral s.
>pigmented villonodular s. (PVNS)
>purulent s.
>toxic s.
>transient s.

synovium
>boggy s.
>exuberant s.
>hyperplastic s.
>opaque s.
>pannus of s.

synovium-filled degenerative cyst
synovium-lined fascicle
synpneumonic empyema
synspondylism
>cervical s.

synthesizer
>frequency s.

synthetic
>s. bone implant
>s. graft bypass to ankle
>s. valve
>s. vascular bypass graft

syntropy
syphilis
>bone s.
>meningovascular s.
>tertiary s.

syphilitic
>s. aortic aneurysm
>s. aortic regurgitation
>s. aortitis
>s. node

syringe
>electric s.
>Isovue prefilled s.
>Isovue-370 prefilled s.
>prefilled s.
>tuberculin s.
>Ultraject prefilled s.

syringes (*pl. of* syrinx)
syringobulbia
syringocarcinoma
syringocele
syringoencephalomyelia
syringohydromyelia
    holocord s.
syringohydromyelic cavity
syringoma
    chondroid s.
syringomeningocele
syringomyelia
    ape hand of s.
    cervical s.
    Chiari-associated s.
    communicating s.
    posttraumatic s.
syringopontia
syringosubarachnoid shunting
syrinx, *pl.* **syringes**
    s. cavity
    central spinal cord s.
    fusiform s.
    posttraumatic central spinal cord s.
    spinal cord s.
    traumatic s.
syrup
    diet cola and metoclopramide s.
syssarcosic (*var of* syssarcotic)
syssarcotic, syssarcosic
system
    ABBI s.
    Ablatherm HIFU s.
    AbMap electrophysiologic imaging s.
    accuDEXA bone mineral density assessment s.
    AccuLength arthroplasty measuring s.
    Acuson P10 handheld diagnostic ultrasound s.
    Acuson 128XP ultrasound s.
    Add-On Bucky image acquisition s.
    Advanced Cardiovascular S.'s (ACS)
    Advanced Interventional S.'s
    Advantx-E Legacy s.
    Advantx LC+ cardiovascular imaging s.
    Aegis sonography management s.
    AESOP Hermes-Ready s.
    Agfa ADC 70 storage phosphor s.
    Agfa CR PACS s.
    air-filtration s.
    Airis II MR s.
    Alexa 1000 s.
    Aloka SSD ultrasound s.
    American Medical Association ligament injury classification s.
    Amplatz anchor s.
    AneuRx bifurcated stent-graft s.

    Angioflow meter s.
    Angiomat 3000, 6000 contrast delivery s.
    Angiomat Illumena injector s.
    AngioRad radiation s.
    Angio-Seal s.
    AngioSURF s.
    Ann Arbor staging s.
    anterolateral s.
    aortoiliac inflow s.
    Apogee CX100, CX200 echocardiography s.
    Apogee RX400 diagnostic ultrasound s.
    Apollo DXA bone densitometry s.
    AquaSens fluid monitoring s.
    archival s.
    arrhythmia mapping s.
    arterial port catheter s.
    ArthroProbe laser s.
    Artoscan MRI s.
    Aspen digital ultrasound s.
    Aspire continuous imaging s.
    Atlas diagnostic ultrasound s.
    ATL HDI 3000, 3500, 4000, 5000 ultrasound s.
    Aurora dedicated breast MRI s.
    Aurora diode-based dental laser s.
    automated angle-encoder s.
    automated biopsy s.
    automated cellular imaging s. (ACIS)
    automated infusion s.
    autonomic nervous s.
    Avera breast imaging s.
    Aviva mammography s.
    Axiom Artis dBC magnetic navigation s.
    BAK interbody fusion s.
    Bard CPS s.
    Bard percutaneous cardiopulmonary support s.
    BAT s.
    Batson vertebral brain s.
    Beta-Cath s.
    Biad SPECT imaging s.
    biliary s.
    BiliBed phototherapy s.
    Biodex Venti-Scan III aerosol delivery s.
    biograph molecular imaging s.
    Biosound AU3, AU4, AU5 s.
    BioSpec MR imaging s.
    BioZ s.
    biplane angiographic s.
    biplane image intensifier s.
    Bonopty needle s.
    BrainLAB VectorVision neuronavigation s.

S

system (*continued*)
 Brasfield scoring s.
 Breast Cancer S. 2100
 Breast Imaging Reporting and Data S.
 BreastScan IR s.
 Bremer halo crown s.
 British Engineering S.
 Broselow-Luten pediatric s.
 Brown-Roberts-Wells stereotactic s.
 Bruker CSI Omega MR s.
 BRW stereotactic s.
 CAAS QCA s.
 CADx SecondLook s.
 calyceal s.
 Calypso 4D localization s.
 cardiopulmonary support s.
 cardiovascular s.
 cardiovascular angiography analysis s. (CAAS)
 cardiovascular information s. (CVIS)
 C-arm DSA s.
 carrier-mediated transport s.
 cartesian reference coordinate s.
 Carto EP navigation s.
 cascade s.
 catenary s.
 CathScanner ultrasound imaging s.
 CathTrack catheter locator s.
 CDRPan digital x-ray s.
 Cemax/Icon PACS s.
 Centauri Er:YAG dental laser s.
 central nervous s. (CNS)
 CerASPECT s.
 2-channel phased-array RF receiver coil s.
 Checkmate s.
 Chemo-Port vascular access s.
 circumflex s.
 collateral s.
 collecting s.
 collimating s.
 ColonoSight s.
 2-, 3-compartment s.
 Compass stereotactic s.
 Composite laryngeal recurrence staging s.
 Compton suppression s.
 computer information s.
 computerized thermal imaging s.
 conduction s.
 continuous-wave Doppler ultrasound s.
 continuous-wave laser s.
 Cordis endovascular s.
 Coroskop Plus cardiac angiography s.
 Cotrel-Dubousset s.

 CRYOguide ultrasound guidance s.
 CryoHit tumor ablation s.
 CrystalEyes endoscopic video s.
 Curix Capacity Plus film processing s.
 CyberKnife stereotactic radiosurgery s.
 Cyberware 3D scanning s.
 data acquisition s. (DAS)
 data collection s.
 da Vinci surgical s.
 dedicated mammography s.
 Delta 32 digital stereotactic s.
 DELTAmanager MedImage s.
 Delta 32 TACT 3-dimensional breast imaging s.
 detector s.
 16-detector PET s.
 diffuse neuroendocrine s.
 digestive s.
 Digital Add-On Bucky radiographic detector image acquisition s.
 digital chest imaging s.
 digital equipment s.
 digital flat-panel amorphous silicon detector-radiography s.
 digital holography s.
 digital mammographic s.
 digital medical s.
 digital selenium-based chest imaging s.
 Digital Traumex s.
 Digitron digital subtraction imaging s.
 DirectView CR 900 imaging s.
 Directview CR mammography s.
 Discovery LS imaging s.
 display coordinate s.
 DOBI s.
 Dodick laser photolysis s.
 Doppler S. 97
 drug-delivery s.
 dryer s.
 DryView laser imaging s.
 DSCT s.
 DTU-One UltraSure imaging s.
 dual-head coincidence detection s.
 duplicated renal collecting s.
 Durie-Salmon PLUS staging s.
 3D Viewnix software s.
 dye laser s.
 DynaRad portable x-ray s.
 E.CAM dual-head emission imaging s.
 ECAT Reveal PET/CT imaging s.
 Eccocee CS ultrasound s.
 EchoEye 3D ultrasound imaging s.
 Eclipse MR s.
 Edwards Thrombex PMT s.

electrostatic imaging s.
Elscint Prestige MRI s.
endovascular s.
EndoVasix EPAR laser s.
EnSite 3000 imaging s.
EPAR laser s.
EP2000 electrophysiology imaging s.
Epistar diode laser s.
Evans-D'Angio staging s.
ExAblate 2000 ultrasound s.
excimer laser s.
Exogen 2000+ low-intensity
  ultrasound fracture healing s.
Explorer X70 intraoral radiography s.
Express biliary LD premounted stent
  s.
extracranial carotid s.
extrapyramidal s.
falloposcopy s.
FCR Velocity-U digital imaging s.
femoropopliteal s.
femtosecond laser s.
fetal musculoskeletal s.
Ficat and Axlet staging s.
fiducial alignment s.
FilmFax teleradiology s.
flexible over-wire s.
Flocks and Kadesky s.
FluoroPlus cardiac digital imaging s.
FluoroPlus real-time digital imaging
  s.
fluoroptic thermometry s.
FluoroTrak fluoroscopy-based surgical
  navigation s.
flying spot excimer laser s.
FONAR Standing Ovation MRI s.
Fuji AC2 storage phosphor
  computed radiology s.
Fuji FCR9000 computed radiology
  s.
full-field digital mammography s.
Galen teleradiology s.
Galileo intravascular radiotherapy s.
gasless laparoscopic s.
gated s.
GE CT HiSpeed Advantage CT s.
Generation 6 integrated radiotherapy
  s.
generator s.
genitourinary s.
GentleLASE Plus laser s.
GE OEC Series 9600 cardiac s.
GE Sonographe 2000D digital
  mammography s.
GE Voluson 730 4D ultrasound s.
Given diagnostic imaging s.
GliaSite radiotherapy s.
gradient s.
GRASS s.

gray box s.
greater saphenous s.
Gyrus endourology s.
HDI 1000, 3000, 3500, 4000, 5000
  ultrasound imaging s.
3-head gamma camera-based SPECT
  s.
Helios laser s.
hepatic artery s.
hepatic ductal s.
hepatic venous s.
heterogeneous reasoning and
  mediator s. (HERMES)
Hewlett-Packard phased-array
  ultrasound imaging s.
high-field s.
Hi-Star MRI s.
Hitachi AIRIS II MR s.
Hitachi Altaire Open MRI s.
Hitachi EUB-555 diagnostic
  ultrasound s.
Hitachi 4-head s.
Hitachi rotating detector array s.
homonuclear spin s.
House grading s.
HP Sonos 5500 ultrasound
  echocardiography s.
HP Sonos 5500 ultrasound
  imaging s.
Hunt and Hess aneurysm grading s.
hybrid SPECT/CT s.
Hydra Vision Plus DR, ES, HP
  urologic imaging s.
HydroCoil embolic s.
hydrodynamic thrombectomy s.
Hyperion LTK s.
HyperPACS teleradiology s.
IDIS angiography s.
IDXrad radiology information s.
iLab ultrasound imaging s.
image analysis s.
Imagecast imaging s.
ImageChecker CT CAD software s.
image-forming s.
image-intensifier s.
image recording s.
imaging center information s.
Impax PACS s.
implantable drug delivery s.
Indigo LaserOptic treatment s.
infrared navigation s.
InnerVasc vascular access s.
integrated clinical information s.
  (ICIS)
Integris III-V DSA s.
Integris V3000 digital subtraction s.
intensified radiographic imaging s.
  (IRIS)
internal carotid s.

S

system (*continued*)

Interspec Apogee RX400 diagnostic ultrasound s.

Intrabeam intraoperative radiotherapy s.

intramedullary skeletal kinetic distractor s.

Intra-Op autotransfusion s.

intrarenal collecting s.

IntraStent DoubleStrut ParaMount XS premounted stent biliary s.

INVOS 3100, 3100A cerebral oximeter monitoring s.

iON IntraOperative navigation s.

ISKD s.

Isocam scintillation imaging s.

Isocam SPECT imaging s.

Jackson staging s.

Kadish staging s.

Kaplan PenduLaser 115 laser s.

Kelly-Goerss Compass stereotactic s.

Kretztechnik ultrasound s.

Krigel staging s.

Lagios classification s.

Laitinen CT guidance s.

laser s.

LaTIS endovascular laser s.

left iliac s.

left ventricular support s.

Leksell stereotactic s.

LENT scoring s.

lesser saphenous s.

Liebel-Flarsheim CT 9000 contrast delivery s.

Life-Lung fluorescence endoscopy s.

LightSpeed Ultra CT s.

limbic s.

linear compartmental s.

lipophilic sequestration s.

Litvack Advanced Interventional S.'s (LAIS)

LocaLisa cardiac navigation s.

Lorad full-field digital mammography s.

lower pole collecting s.

low-field MRI s.

LPI laser s.

LP^2 stainless steel delivery s.

LTX3000 lumbar rehabilitation s.

Luma cervical imaging s.

Luxtec fiberoptic s.

LVs s.

LX EchoSpeed 1.5T CV/i, NVi MR s.

LymphoScan nuclear imaging s.

Magnes biomagnetometer s.

magnetic surgery s.

Magnetom Open s.

Magnetom Sonata 1.5T MR s.

Magnetom Trio 3T unlimited MRI s.

Magnetom Vision 1.5T MR imaging s.

Magnex Alpha MR s.

mamillary s.

Mammex TR computer-aided mammography diagnosis s.

Mammo Plus mammography s.

MammoReader computer-aided dectection s.

MammoReader mammography s.

Mammotest breast biopsy s.

Mammotome ultrasound s.

Manchester LDR implant s.

Marex MRI s.

Massachusetts General Hospital utility multiprogramming s.

Meddars cardiac catheterization analysis s.

Medilase angioscope-laser delivery s.

Medi-tech ureteral stent s.

Medspec MR imaging s.

Med-Tec VacLoc immobilization s.

Medweb clinical reporting s.

microscopic angiogenesis grading s.

microSelectron rapid delivery s.

microwave cardiac ablation s.

Millennium VG SPECT s.

mini-balloon s.

MIR s.

MIST therapy s.

Mitsuyasu staging s.

Mobetron electron beam s.

Mobetron intraoperative radiation therapy treatment s.

mobile artery and vein imaging s. (MAVIS)

mucosal mass collecting s.

multichannel RF s.

multicrystal BGO ring s.

multidetector s.

multigated pulsed Doppler flow s.

multileaf collimating s.

multiple-electrode probe s.

multiple-sidehole infusion s.

Multistar Top Plus DSA s.

musculoskeletal s.

MyoSight imaging s.

Myotherm XP cardioplegia delivery s.

Navi Ball guidance s.

Navigus cranial electrode s.

Navitrack computer-assisted surgery s.

needle-wire s.

nephroureteral stent s.

NeuroLink II data acquisition s.

Neurosector ultrasound s.
Nidek EC-5000 excimer laser s.
nondilated s.
Novacor left ventricular assist s.
Novadaq SPY intraoperative imaging s.
Novalis radiosurgery s.
nuclear medicine information s.
Oasis thrombectomy s.
object coordinate s.
OctreoScan s.
ocular magnification s.
Olympus EU-M30 s.
Opdima digital mammography s.
OPD-Scan optical path difference scanning s.
open-architecture s.
open-configuration magnetic resonance s.
open MRI s.
OpenPACS s.
Opmilas 144 Plus laser s.
Optistar MR contrast delivery s.
OR1 electronic s.
OrthOneXT dedicated MRI s.
Oscar ultrasonic bone cement removal s.
OsteoView desktop hand x-ray s.
OsteoView 2000 digital imaging s.
Ostreg spinal marker s.
Ovation falloposcopy s.
Packard Merlin life-monitoring s.
parasympathetic nervous s.
Paris ultrasound s.
Paterson-Parker s.
Peacock s.
pelvicalyceal s.
PenRad mammography clinical reporting s.
Pentax-Hitachi FG32UA endosonographic s.
Perclose PVS suture s.
Performa mammography s.
peripheral nervous s.
PFA-100 s.
3-phase s.
Philips DVI 1 s.
Philips Integris 5000 digital subtraction angiography s.
PhorMax CR desktop workstation s.
photoelectric s.
photon cataract removal s.
photon radiosurgery s. (PRS)
Photopic Imaging ultrasound s.
Picker s.
picture archival communication s. (PACS)
picture archiving and communication s. (PACS)

PiGalileo computer-assisted orthopaedic surgery s.
Pinnacle$_3$ radiotherapy planning s.
plastic Vortex Port s.
PMT robotic fulcrumless tomographic s.
polar coordinate s.
polypoid fibroma collecting s.
portal vein s.
PortalVision radiation oncology s.
port-catheter s.
pressure-gradient wire s.
PrinceStar electrophysiologic imaging study s.
Prism 3-head s.
Probe balloon dilation s.
Profile mammography s.
Prostalase laser s.
Protégé GPS self-expanding nitinol stent-biliary s.
pulmonary venous s.
pulse Holter s.
Pulse-Spray pulsed infusion s.
pyelocalyceal s.
pyramidal s.
Q-catheter catheterization recording s.
QCT bone densitometry s.
quadrature surface coil MRI s.
quantitative image processing s. (QUIPS)
Quick-Core biopsy s.
QuickSeal femoral arterial closure s.
Quimby implant s.
radiation therapy s. (RTS)
radiation therapy planning s.
radioisotope delivery s. (RDS)
radiology information s. (RIS)
radiology telephone access s
radionuclide carrier s.
RadNet radiology information s.
rapid telephone access s. (RTAS)
RatioVision digital fluorescent imaging s.
RDX coronary radiation catheter delivery s.
real-time 2-dimensional Doppler flow imaging s.
real-time 4D ultrasound imaging s.
Redi-Vu teleradiology s.
reference coordinate s.
Refinity Coblation s.
remote afterloading s.
renal collecting s.
respiratory s.
reticuloendothelial s.
Retzius s.
Reveal XVI PET/CT imaging s.
RF coil s.

system (*continued*)
RigiScan Plus rigidity assessment s.
RIGS s.
ring-type imaging s.
Robson modification of
  Flocks-Kadesky s.
Rogan teleradiology s.
Roger s.
Rotablator thrombectomy s.
rotational atherectomy s.
Rotograph Plus panoramic dental
  tomography imaging s.
RPM tracking s.
RTP s.
RX stent delivery s.
Sadowsky breast marking s.
SAMBA imaging s.
saphenous s.
SAVANT imaging s.
SCA s.
Scanditronix MLC s.
scanning-beam digital s.
scattering s.
scavenging s.
scene coordinate s.
Scharff-Bloom-Richardson histologic
  grade s.
Schmidt optics s.
Scintiview nuclear computer s.
Scintron IV nuclear computer s.
ScleroLaser laser s.
ScleroPLUS HP laser s.
Second Look CAD s.
Selectron s.
Selenia imaging s.
selenium-based digital chest s.
selenium drum detector s.
Selvester QRS scoring s.
Senographe 2000D digital
  mammography s.
Senographe DMRt mammography s.
SenoScan full-field digital imaging s.
SenoScan full-field digital
  mammography s.
Sens-A-Ray 2000 dental imaging s.
sequestration s.
Sequoia ultrasound s.
Shape Maker s.
Shimadzu HeadTome s.
side-exiting coaxial needle s.
Siemens AG s.
Siemens HICOR/BICOR x-ray s.
Siemens Mammomat Novation DM
  full-field digital mammography s.
Siemens Somatom Plus-4 CT s.
Siemens 1.5T s.
Signa Advantage s.
Signa Excite MRI s.
Signa Horizon LX MRI s.

Signa MR imaging s.
Silhouette laser s.
Silicon Graphics Reality Engine s.
SimpliCT interventional guidance s.
Simpson Coronary AtheroCath s.
single-photon counting s.
single-stick s.
Site-Rite II ultrasound s.
skeletal s.
slip-ring gantry s.
slot-scan detection s.
SmartSPOT high-resolution digital
  imaging s.
Socrates telementoring s.
Softscan laser mammography s.
Somatom Volume Zoom CT s.
Sonablate 200 ultrasound s.
sonic-accelerated fracture-healing s.
  (SAFHS)
SonicWAVE phacoemulsification s.
Sonifer sonicating s.
Sonoace 6000 II ultrasound s.
SonoHeart Elite personal
  hand-carried ultrasound s.
Sonoline Elegra ultrasound s.
SonoSite 180 ultrasound s.
SPC s.
spiderlike pelvocaliceal s.
splanchnic venous s.
spring-driven s.
Sprint fixed-detector research s.
Squibb s.
STARRT falloposcopy s.
steerable guidewire s.
StereoGuide prone breast biopsy s.
StereoLoc upright biopsy s.
stereotactic breast biopsy s.
1-stick s.
storage phosphor s.
Stratis II MRI s.
Sun SPARCstation s.
Super Angiorex DSA s.
superconducting open-magnet s.
superconductive MR s.
Superdup'r left heart s.
Superpump S. (SPS)
Surgical Planning and Orientation
  Computer S. (SPOCS)
sympathetic nervous s.
Symphony MR imaging s.
Synergy ultrasound s.
Syngo Lung CAD software s.
systemic venous s.
Talairach stereotactic s.
TCD100M digital transcranial
  Doppler s.
Tecmag Libra-S16 s.
TEGwire ST s.
Telocin diagnostic ultrasound s.

Terason Echo ultrasound s.
Tesla s.
thermal dosimetry s.
ThinPrep imaging s.
Thrombex PMT s.
tibioperoneal runoff s.
time of-flight PET imaging s.
titanium Vortex port s.
Tmx-2000 BPH thermotherapy s.
Tomolex tomographic s.
Tomomatic 2-, 3-, 5-slice SPECT
   imaging s.
TomoTherapy Hi-ART s.
Total Recall digital imaging s.
Transonics s.
TransScan TS2000 electrical
   impedance breast scanning s.
treatment planning s.
Trex digital mammography s.
   (TDMS)
Triad SPECT imaging s.
Tron 3 VACI cardiac imaging s.
trumpetlike pelvocaliccal s.
1.5T, 3.0T TwinSpeed s.
3T whole-body s.
1.5T whole-body MR imaging s.
UltraFine erbium laser s.
UltraPACS diagnostic imaging s.
ultrasound s.
UltraSTAR computer-based
   ultrasound reporting s.
UltraSure DTR-One imaging
   ultrasound s.
UMC-I microwave delivery s.
University of Florida staging s.
Univision echocardiographic s.
s. unsharpness
uPACS picture archiving s.
upper pole collecting s.
USCI Probe balloon-on-a-wire
   dilation s.
Vac-Lok patient immobilization s.
vacuum cassette s.
Varian brachytherapy s.
Varian MLC s.
VasoView balloon dissection s.
VAX 4100 s.
Vbeam pulsed-dye laser s.
ventricular s.
VentTrak monitoring s.
Versatome D8 perioperative
   Doppler s.
vertebral artery s.
vertebrobasilar s.
VEST s.
Viatronix virtual colonoscopy s.
view shadow projection
   microtomographic s.
Vingmed CFM ultrasound s.

virtual retinal display s.
Virtuoso portable 3D imaging s.
Vision high-performance gradient s.
Vision MR imaging s.
Visx Star S2 excimer laser s.
Visx WaveScan Wavefront s.
Vitrea 3D s.
Vnus closure s.
Voluson ultrasound s.
Vortex port s.
VoxelView s.
whole-body compact MR s.
widened collecting s.
xenon trap s.
Xillix LIFE-GI fluorescence
   endoscopy s.
Xillix LIFE-Lung fluorescence
   endoscopy s.
XKnife stereotactic radiosurgery s.
Xplorer 1000 digital imaging s.
x-ray shadow projection
   microtomographic s.
Yaglazr s.
Zeus s.
Zlatkin grading s.

systematic
   s. error
   s. noise
   s. relaxation effect
   s. ultrasound-guided biopsy

systemic
   s. adjuvant therapy
   s. arterial circulation
   s. arterial hypertension
   s. arterial vasoconstriction
   s. arteriolar resistance index
   s. blood flow (SBF)
   s. brain lymphoma
   s. diastolic blood pressure
   s. disorder
   s. granulomatous disease
   s. heart
   s. hypoperfusion
   s. inflammatory response syndrome
   s. intravenous infusion
   s. juvenile rheumatoid arthritis
      (S-JRA)
   s. lesion
   s. lupus erythematosus (SLE)
   s. mastocytosis
   s. mean arterial pressure
      (SMAP)
   s. micrometastasis
   s. nodular panniculitis
   s. non-Langerhans cell histiocytosis
   s. output
   s. output flow
   s. output index
   s. oxygen saturation

S

systemic (*continued*)
s. portal shunt
s. sarcoidosis
s. sclerosis (SSc)
s. sclerosis-related myopathy
s. shunt
s. tuberculosis
s. vascular resistance (SVR)
s. vascular resistance index (SvO$_2$, SVRI)
s. vein
s. venous hypertension
s. venous return
s. venous system
systole
atrial s.
cervical CSF s.
CSF ventricular s.
end of atrial s.
ventricular s.
systolic
s. acceleration time
s. anterior motion (SAM)
s. anterior motion of mitral valve
s. anterior movement
s. atrial volume
s. ejection fraction
s. ejection period (SEP)
s. fractional shortening
s. function
s. gating
s. gradient
s. heart failure
s. hypertension
s. impulse
left ventricular s. (LVs)
s. mammary souffle
s. myocardial thickening
s. pressure-time index
s. prolapse
s. prolapse of mitral valve leaflet
pulmonary artery s. (PAS)
s. reconstruction
s. reserve
s. retraction
s. retraction of apex
s. S wave
s. toe/brachial index
s. upstroke time
s. velocity ratio
s. velocity-time integral
s. ventricular overload
systolic-diastolic
s.-d. blood pressure
s.-d. ratio (S/D)
Syvek Patch closure device

T

T artifact
T axis
T condylar fracture
T configuration
T fracture
T loop
T stage
T tubogram
Ultracranio T
T vector

1.5T

1.5T Signa MR unit
1.5T Signa whole-body
  imager/spectrometer
1.5T, 3.0T TwinSpeed system
1.5T whole-body MR imaging
  system

3T

3T Medspec 30/80 MR
  scanner
3T MRI
3T whole-body system

T1

T1 1st field-echo dynamic perfusion
  image
T1, T2 dephasing effect
T1, T2 image
T1, T2 quantitative MRI
T1, T2 relaxation time
T1, T2 shortening
T1, T2 star relaxation
T1, T2 time constant
T1, T2 value

T4

thyroxine
T4 cell
T4 uptake

Ta

tantalum

^{178}Ta, Ta-178

tantalum 178

^{182}Ta, Ta-182

tantalum 182

Tabar pattern

tabes

burned-out t.
t. dorsalis

table

asymmetric lookup t.
binary opacity t.
critical dose t.
Hydradjust IV t.
inner t.

lookup t. (LUT)
MobiTrak automated t.
MobiTrak moving t.
t. movement
t. of radiation doses
pivoting t.
radionuclide t.
resistive exercise t.
3-station moving t.
tilt t.

tabletop

auxiliary CT t.

TAC

transient aplastic crisis

TACE

transarterial chemoembolization
transcatheter arterial
  chemoembolization

tachyarrhythmia

supraventricular t.
sustained t.

tachycardia

atrial ectopic
  automatic t.
atrioventricular nodal
  reentry t.
ischemic sinus t.
nodoventricular t.
noninducible t.
paroxysmal auricular t.
sinuatrial nodal reentry t.
supraventricular t.
ventricular paroxysmal t.

tachycardia-induced cardiomyopathy

tachyphylaxis

tachypnea

transient t.

tackler's exostosis

tacrolimus

TACT

tuned aperture computed
  tomography

tactile disc

TAD

torsional attenuated diameter
TAD steerable guidewire

TAE

transcatheter arterial embolization

taenia

T. solium
t. tissue

TAFI

thrombin-activatable fibrinolysis
inhibitor

T

945

tag
- T. Excluder stent
- t. image file format (TIFF)
- t. of cartilage
- t. plane
- radioactive t.

Tagarno 3SD cine projector for angiography

tagged
- t. atom
- t. magnetic resonance imaging
- radioactively t.
- t. red cell

tagging
- barium-based fecal t.
- bolus t.
- t. cine-magnetic resonance
- cine-magnetic resonance t.
- 2-dimensional cine gradient echo-based t.
- t. material
- myocardial t.
- t. pattern
- segmented k-space cardiac t.
- spin t.
- stool t.

Tagitol V preparation

TAGM
- tris-acryl gelatin microsphere

TAI
- traumatic aortic injury

tail
- t. bone
- dural t.
- hippocampal head, body, and t.
- long dural t.
- t. of breast
- t. of epididymis
- t. of pancreas
- t. of Spence
- t. of spleen
- t. sign
- t. vertebra
- wool t.

tailgut cyst

tail-like segment

tailored
- t. excitation
- t. pulse

tailor's
- t. ankle
- t. muscle

Takayasu
- T. aortitis
- T. arteritis
- T. Arteritis Association
- T. disease

takedown
- Roux-en-Y t.

takeoff
- high t.
- t. of artery
- t. of vessel

Talairach
- T. coordinate
- T. Daemon database
- T. landmark
- T. stereotactic space
- T. stereotactic system
- T. transformation

Talairach-Tournoux atlas

talar
- t. avulsion fracture
- t. beaking
- t. body fusion
- t. dome
- t. dome articular cartilage
- t. dome cyst
- t. dome fracture
- t. dome ischemia
- t. dome osteochondral injury
- t. impingement
- t. neck fracture
- t. osteochondral fracture
- t. tilt angle

talc
- t. plaque
- t. pneumoconiosis
- t. sclerotherapy

talcosis
- lung t.
- pulmonary t.

Talent bifurcated abdominal aortic stent-graft

tali (*pl. of* talus)

talipes
- t. arcuatus
- t. calcaneus
- t. calcaneus calcaneocavus
- t. cavovalgus
- t. cavus
- t. cavus calcaneocavus
- t. equinovarus
- t. valgus
- t. varus

talocalcaneal, talocalcanean
- t. angle
- anteroposterior t. (APTC)
- t. articulation
- t. coalition
- t. index
- t. index classification
- t. joint
- t. ligament

talocalcanean (*var. of* talocalcaneal)

talocalcaneonavicular
- t. articulation
- t. joint

talocrural
  t. angle
  t. fusion
  t. joint
talofibular
  anterior t. (ATF)
  t. impingement
  t. joint
  t. ligament
  t. ligament injury
  posterior t. (PTF)
talohorizontal angle
talometatarsal angle
talonavicular
  t. angle
  t. articulation
  t. beaking
  t. capsule
  t. coalition
  t. joint
  t. ligament
talus, *pl.* **tali**
  beaking of head of t.
  t. bone
  Cedell fracture of t.
  congenital vertical t.
  flat-top t.
  t. foot deformity
  lateral process of t.
  neck of t.
  osteochondral lesion of t.
  Sneppen fracture of t.
  sulcus tali
  sustentaculum tali
  vertical t.
tam-o-shanter appearance
Tamp catheter
tamponade, tamponage
  balloon t.
  cardiac t.
  chronic t.
  esophagogastric t.
  ferromagnetic t.
  florid cardiac t.
  full-blown cardiac t.
  heart t.
  low-pressure cardiac t.
  pericardial t.
  pericardial chyle with t.
  subacute cardiac t.
tamponage (*var. of* tamponade)
tandem
  t. and ovoid
  t. applicator
  external beam with t.
  Fletcher-Suit-Delclos t.
  t. gait
  t. ICA/MCA occlusion
  t. lesion

MIR intrauterine t.
  t. stent
  t. technique
  t. transplant
tangential
  t. breast field
  t. constriction
  t. cut
  t. layer of hand
  t. port
  t. projection
  t. scapular view
tangentially
tangent radiograph
tangle
  intraneuronal neurofibrillary t.
  neurofibrillary t.
tanned red cell (TRC)
tannex
  bisacodyl t.
tantalate
  lutetium t.
tantalum (Ta)
  t. 178 (^{178}Ta, Ta-178)
  t. 182 (^{182}Ta, Ta-182)
  t. bronchogram
  t. imaging agent
  t. mesh
  t. powder
  t. stent
  t. tracer
tantalum-178 contrast medium
tap
  spinal t.
  t. water enema
taper
  fiberoptic t.
tapered-core guidewire
tapered finger
tapered-tip guidewire
tapering
  t. border
  t. dose
  t. occlusion
  t. stenosis
tapetal
tapetoretinal dysplasia
tapetum corporis callosi
tapeworm
tapir mouth
tapiroid
TAPVD
  total anomalous pulmonary venous drainage
TAPVR
  total anomalous pulmonary venous return
TAR
  thrombocytopenia-absent radius
  tissue-air ratio
  TAR syndrome

T

tar
    coal t.
tarda
    osteogenesis imperfecta t.
tardive dyskinesia
tardus-parvus
    t.-p. technique
    t.-p. waveform
target
    angiographic t.
    t. appearance
    t. arch
    t. bone
    t. calcification
    t. canal
    t. coalition
    t. depth
    3D reconstructed t.
    gas t.
    internal cyclotron t.
    t. lung lesion
    t. material
    metal technetium t.
    minimal deformation t. (MDT)
    molybdenum t.
    t. navicular
    t. organ
    t. parenchymal structure
    t. point
    retrogasserian t.
    t. sign
    t. tissue
    tungsten t.
targeted
    t. contrast agent
    t. EIS
    t. monolayer coated microbubble
    t. tissue volume
target-film distance (TFD)
target-filter combination
targeting
    angiographic t.
    t. bead
    B-mode acquisition and t. (BAT)
    pedicle t.
targetoid growth
target-skin distance (TSD)
target-specific
    t.-s. MRI
    t.-s. therapy
target-to-background ratio
target-to-nontarget
    t.-t.-n. ratio
    t.-t.-n. ratio for myocardial imaging
target-trocar distance
Tarlov cyst
TARP
    total atrial refractory period
Tarrant position

tarsal
    t. arch
    t. bone
    t. canal
    t. coalition
    t. cyst
    t. joint
    t. ligament
    t. navicular
    t. plate
    t. sinus
    t. tunnel
    t. tunnel syndrome
tarsoepiphysial aclasis
tarsometatarsal
    t. angle
    t. articulation
    t. joint
    t. ligament
tartrate
    thorium t.
tartrate-resistant acid phosphatase
task
    block motor t.
task-rest pattern
taurodontism
TAUS
    transabdominal ultrasound
Taussig-Bing
    T.-B. anomaly
    T.-B. congenital malformation of
    heart
    T.-B. syndrome
Taussig-Snellen-Alberts syndrome
tautography
taut pericardial effusion
TAV
    transcutaneous aortovelography
Taveras injector
Tawara atrioventricular node
Taxus Express stent
Taybi (type I-III)
Taylor-Blackwood mechanism
Taylor position
Taylor-type dysplasia
TB
    tuberculosis
        HIV-related TB
TBI
    tracheobronchial injury
    traumatic brain injury
TBLB
    transbronchial lung biopsy
TBNA
    transbronchial needle aspiration
TBV
    total brain volume
TBW
    total body water

Tc
  technetium
TCA
  tentorium cerebelli attachment
  transcondylar axis
  tricarboxylic acid
TCAT
  transmission computer-assisted
  tomography
TCBF
  total cerebral blood flow
TCC
  transitional cell carcinoma
TCCS
  transcranial color-coded duplex
  sonography
TCD
  transcranial Doppler
  transverse cerebellar diameter
    TCD measurement
    TCD sonography
    TCD ultrasound
    TCD velocity
TCDD
  threshold contrast detail detectability
TCD-detectable turbulence
**TCD100M digital transcranial Doppler
 system**
T-cell
    T-c. acute lymphoblastic leukemia
    T-c. antigen receptor
    T-c. lymphoblastic lymphoma
    T-c. neoplasia
**T-cell-type acute lymphoblastic
 leukemia**
TcHIDA
  technetium hepatoiminodiacetic acid
Tc-labeled red blood cell scintigraphy
Tc-99m, ^{99m}Tc
  technetium 99m
Tc99m-ECD
  technetium 99m ethyl cysteinate
  dimer
Tc99m-MAG3
  technetium 99m mercapto acetyl
  triglycine
TcO$_4$
  pertechnetate
    TcO$_4$ MIBI subtraction scintigraphy
    TcO$_4$ thyroid scan
T-configuration
T1-contamination artifact
tcPO$_2$
  transcutaneous oxygen pressure
  measurement
TCS
  tethered cord syndrome
  total calcium score
TCT900S helical CT scanner

TDE-derived epsilon (p) and epsilon (m)
TDI
  time delay integration
TDLU
  terminal ductal lobular unit
TDMS
  Trex digital mammography system
TE
  tracheoesophageal
    TE fistula
teacup
    t. breast calcification
    t. fracture
teacup-shaped calcification
Teale amputation
tear
    anular t.
    attritional t.
    Bateman classification of
      full-thickness t.
    bowstring t.
    bucket-handle meniscus t.
    buttonhole t.
    cleavage t.
    complete t.
    concentric anular t.
    degenerative horizontal
      cleavage t.
    dural t.
    entry t.
    esophageal t.
    fishtail t.
    flap t.
    full-thickness t.
    high-grade partial t.
    iatrogenic dural t.
    interstitial meniscal t.
    intimal t.
    intrasubstance cleavage t.
    Johnson-Jahss classification of
      posterior tibial tendon t.
    ligament t.
    Mallory-Weiss esophageal t.
    Mallory-Weiss mucosal t.
    meniscus t.
    mesenteric t.
    parrot-beak labral t.
    parrot-beak meniscus t.
    partial bursal surface t.
    partial-thickness split t.
    peripheral meniscocapsular t.
    posterior longitudinal ligament t.
    quadriceps tendon t.
    radial anular t.
    radial split t.
    rectal t.
    rim-rent t.
    rotator cuff t.
    serosal t.

T

tear (*continued*)
    SLAP t.
    stellate t.
    superimposed acute partial t.
    superior labral anterior to posterior t.
    tendon t. (type I-IV)
    teres minor tendon t.
    tibial tendon t.
    transverse anular t.
    traumatic aortic t.
    tricorn bucket-handle t.
    vertical split nondetached t.

teardrop
    t. appearance
    t. bladder
    t. burst fracture
    t. distance
    t. figure
    t. heart
    pelvic t.
    t. pelvic anatomy
    t. sign
    t. ventriculomegaly

teardrop-shaped
    t.-s. flexion-compression fracture
    t.-s. lesion

tearing
    plaque t.

teat
    pyloric t.

teboroxime
    t. cardiac scan
    t. imaging agent
    t. resting washout (TRW)

tech
    Vena T.

Technegas

TechneLite scan

Techneplex imaging agent

TechneScan
    T. gluceptate
    T. HDP, MAA, MAG3, PYP
      imaging agent
    T. HIDA
    T. MDP
    T. sulfur colloid

technetium (Tc)
    t. albumin study
    t. bond
    t. hepatoiminodiacetic acid
      (TcHIDA)
    hydrolyzed t.
    t. imaging agent
    t. 99m (^{99m}Tc, Tc-99m)
    t. 99m antibody labeling
    t. 99m anti-CEA Fab murine
      monoclonal antibody imaging
    t. 99m antimony sulfur colloid
    t. 99m antimony trisulfide colloid

t. 99m antimyosin Fab fragment
t. 99m bicisate
t. 99m Ceretec
t. 99m ciprofloxacin
t. 99m depreotide
t. 99m dextran
t. 99m diethylenetriamine pentaacetic
    acid (^{99m}Tc-DTPA)
t. 99m dimercaptosuccinic acid
    (^{99m}Tc-DMSA)
t. 99m disofenin
t. 99m DMSA
t. 99m DMSA scintigraphy
t. 99m DTPA
t. 99m DTPA aerosol
t. 99m ethyl cysteinate dimer
    (^{99m}Tc-ECD, Tc99m-ECD)
t. 99m ethylenedicysteine (^{99m}Tc
    EC, Tc-99m EC)
t. 99m ethylenedicysteine-folate
    (^{99m}Tc EC-folate, Tc-99m
    EC-folate)
t. 99m etidronate
t. 99m exametazime
t. 99m fanolesomab
t. 99m ferpentetate
t. 99m filtered sulfur colloid
t. 99m generator
t. 99m glucoheptanoate
t. 99m heat-denatured erythrocyte
t. 99m heat-denatured RBC splenic
    scintigraphy
t. 99m hepatoiminodiacetic acid scan
t. 99m Hepatolite
t. 99m hexamethylpropyleneamine
    oxime (^{99m}Tc-HMPAO)
t. 99m HMPAO mixed leukocyte
    LeukoScan
t. 99m human albumin microsphere
t. 99m human immune globulin
t. 99m hydrazinonicotinyl-
    Tyr3-octreotide
t. 99m hydroxymethylene
    diphosphonate (Tc-99m HMDP)
t. 99m IDA analogue
t. 99m iminodiacetic acid derivative
t. 99m Infecton imaging
t. 99m iron ascorbate DTPA
t. 99m isonitrile radiopharmaceutical
t. 99m leukocyte
t. 99m macroaggregated albumin
    (Tc-99m MAA)
t. 99m MAG3 renography
t. 99m MDP
t. 99m MDP uptake
t. 99m mebrofenin
t. 99m mercapto acetyl triglycine
    (^{99m}Tc-MAG3, Tc99m-MAG3)
t. 99m mertiatide

t. 99m methoxyisobutylisonitrile (^{99m}Tc MIBI, Tc-99m MIBI)
t. 99m methoxyisobutylisonitrile scintimammography
t. 99m methylene diphosphonate (Tc-99m MDP)
t. 99m methylene diphosphonate scan
t. 99m mini-microaggregated albumin
t. 99m minimicroaggregated albumin colloid
t. 99m nanocolloid
t. 99m oxidronate
t. 99m pertechnate/thallium-201 radionuclide subtraction imaging
t. 99m pertechnetate
t. 99m pertechnetate GI bleed
t. 99m pertechnetate sodium
t. 99m phosphate
t. 99m photospectrum
t. 99m phytate scan
t. 99m PIPIDA
t. 99m pyrophosphate (^{99m}Tc-PYP, Tc99m PYP)
t. 99m pyrophosphate imaging
t. 99m red blood cell (^{99m}Tc-RBC)
t. 99m sestamibi dual-phase technique
t. 99m sestamibi parathyroid
t. 99m siboroxime
t. 99m somatostatin analogue SPECT
t. 99m stannous colloid
t. 99m sestamibi
t. 99m sulfur colloid GI bleed
t. 99m tagged red blood cell scan
t. 99m tetrofosmin exercise-rest SPECT myocardial perfusion imaging
t. 99m tin colloid
t. 99m venography
t. polyphosphonate
t. stannous pyrophosphate
t. stannous pyrophosphate imaging
t. sulfur colloid

technetium-99m-labeled (^{99m}Tc-labeled, Tc99m-labeled, ^{99m}Tc-labeled)
t.-99m-l. annexin V
t.-99m-l. damaged red blood cell
t.-99m-l. leukocyte

technetium-99m-2-methoxyisobutyl
dipyridamole t.-99m-2-m.

technetium-99m-tagged red blood cell
technetium-tagged
t.-t. Cardiolite
t.-t. RBC labeling
t.-t. red blood cell

technetium-thallium subtraction imaging
technic (*var. of* technique)
technically induced artifact
Technicare
T. camera
T. Delta 2020 scanner
technician
Association of University Radiologic T.'s (AURT)
technique, technic
acquisition t.
add-on t.
adiabatic fast scanning t.
advanced life support t.
AEC t.
afterloading t.
air-gap t.
algebraic reconstruction t. (ART)
Amplatz coronary catheterization t.
antialiasing t.
antiradial t.
array spatial sensitivity encoding t. (ASSET)
aseptic t.
automatic vessel tracking t.
autoradiographic t.
axial multiplanar reformation t.
background subtraction t.
balanced gradient t.
2 balloon t.
balloon-retriever t.
bayesian t.
best-guess t.
black blood t.
blended beam t.
BLS t.
BOLD t.
bolus-chase imaging t.
bolus triggering t.
bougienage t.
brain surface matching t.
bread loaf t.
breast mammographic t.
breath-hold t.
broad-use linear acquisition speed-up t. (BLAST)
Brown-Roberts-Wells t.
bull's-eye t.
cardiovascular imaging t.
catheter-based intervention t.
catheter-securing t.
cerebral flow image t.
chase bolus imaging t.
chemical-shift imaging t.
chemical-shift selective suppression t.
chromatographic-fluorometric t.
CLEAR t.
coaxial sheath t.
computer subtraction t.

technique (*continued*)

concentric circle t.
continuous suture graft inclusion t. (CSGIT)
contralateral subtraction t.
contrast-enhanced CT with saline flush t.
contrast-enhanced Fourier-acquired steady-state t. (CE-FAST)
contrast-enhanced retrospective electrocardiogram-gated spiral t.
coronal oblique t.
Cr-chromate-labeled red cell t.
Cr-labeled red blood cell t.
cross-correlation t.
cut-film t.
2D t.
3D t.
deblurring t.
deconvolution t.
dephase-rephase magnitude subtraction t.
depth-pulse t.
destructive interference t.
3D gradient-echo acquisition t.
digital subtraction t.
discographic t.
2D multiplanar reformatted t.
DNA microinjection t.
double-contrast t.
double-freeze t.
double-stick t.
double-umbrella t.
double-wire atherectomy t.
3D postprocessing t.
drip infusion t.
driven equilibrium Fourier transform t.
2D time-of-flight t.
dual-isotope subtraction t.
3D volume t.
3D volume-rendering t.
dye injection t.
dynamic bolus tracking t.
echo-tagging t.
EFOV t.
ejection fraction by 1st-pass t.
Eklund t.
elephant trunk aortic graft t.
endofluoroscopic t.
endovascular t.
enzyme-multiplied immunoassay t.
Epistar perfusion t.
equilibrium radionuclide angiocardiography t.
esophageal balloon t.
exclusion-HPLC t.
extended field-of-view t.
external looping t.

fast-FLAIR t.
fast imaging employing steady-state acquisition t.
fat-suppressed T2-weighted FSE t.
fat-suppression t.
4-field t.
field-fitting t.
FIESTA t.
FLAK t.
flow cytometry t.
flow mapping t.
fluoroscopic pushing t.
fluoroscopic road-mapping t.
Fourier-acquired steady-state t. (FAST)
Fourier imaging t.
FRODO t.
FSPGR t.
full-column t.
gadolinium-enhanced venographic t.
gated inflow t.
graded compression sonography t.
gradient-echo cine t.
gradient-echo recall t.
grasping t.
GRE t.
grid t.
Grüntzig PTCA t.
guidewire exchange t.
half-Fourier 3-dimensional t.
half-Fourier transformation t.
half-wedged field t.
Hampton t.
hanging-block t.
HARC-C wavelet compression t.
helical t.
high-kV t.
high-resolution bone algorithm t.
hybridization-subtraction t.
hybrid subtraction t.
image-guided injection t.
immersion t.
inhalation t.
integrated parallel acquisition t. (iPAT)
intercomparison measurement t.
interleaved phase-contrast t.
intraoperative scanning t.
intravascular MRI catheter-based t.
inverse radiotherapy t.
inversion recovery t.
in vivo t.
iron-sensitive imaging t.
Judkins t.
jugular t.
kinematic MR t.
kissing atherectomy t.
kissing balloons t.
Klein t.

large-core t.
loading t.
localization t.
low-angle shot t.
low-dose film mammographic t.
low-dose screen-film t.
lumenographic t.
magnetic resonance hydrographic t.
magnetization transfer t.
mammographic t.
mammography t.
Markov chain Monte Carlo t.
Monte Carlo t.
motion artifact suppression t.
  (MAST)
moving table t.
MPGR t.
MP-RAGE t.
MR colonographic t.
MSCT t.
multiline scanning t.
multimodal image fusion t.
multiphasic multislice MRI t.
multiphasic multislice spin-echo
  imaging t.
multislice spin-echo t.
navigator echo motion correction t.
2-needle biopsy t.
nonaxial beam t.
noncoplanar arc t.
noncoplanar beam t.
noninvasive t.
PACE t.
packing, extraction, and calculation t.
Papillon t.
partial flip-angle fast-scan t.
partial Fourier t.
partial saturation t.
PEI 1-shot t.
PEI 2 shot t.
percutaneous retrograde transfemoral t.
percutaneous transluminal coronary
  recanalization t.
perfusion measurement t.
pinhole t.
3-point Dixon t.
point mutation detection using
  exonuclease amplification couple
  capture t.
point-resolved spectroscopy
  localization t.
presaturation t.
pressure-controlled intermittent
  coronary occlusion t.
pressure half-time t.
projection-reconstruction t.
Propeller FSE t.
pulsed-gradient spin-echo t.
pulse-echo t.

pulse-spray t.
quantitative imaging t.
radial t.
radiofrequency-spoiled
  Fourier-acquired steady-state t.
  (RF-FAST)
radiopharmaceutical volume-dilution t.
radiotracer t.
rapid pull-through t. (RPT)
rapid scan t.
rapid thoracic compression t.
RARE t.
ray-casting t.
recanalization t.
region-of-interest imaging t.
reimplantation t.
relaxation enhancement t.
remodeling t.
respiratory triggered fast SE t.
roadmapping t.
robust registration t.
RODEO imaging t.
rotational therapy t.
sandwich t.
saturation recovery t.
scanning t.
scintillation counting t.
screening t.
Seldinger percutaneous t.
self-reversed parallel-wire balloon t.
semiquantitative t.
sequential extraction-radiotracer t.
serial cut-film t.
SHARP fat saturation t.
silhouette t.
simultaneous multiple-angle
  reconstruction t. (SMART)
single-field hyperthermia t.
single fill/void t.
single-needle biopsy t.
single-sample t.
single-shot imaging t.
single-slice 8-echo t.
SL t.
sliding-slab average-intensity
  projection t.
sliding thin-slab minimum-intensity
  projection t.
Sones cineangiography t.
SPAMM t.
spin-echo t.
spin-label t.
spin-lock imaging t.
spiral echo-planar t.
spiral scanning t.
split-bolus t.
split-course t.
SPOP t.
stacked-foil t.

T

technique (*continued*)
    2-step t.
    step-and-shoot t.
    stereotactic automated t.
    stimulated echo-tagging t.
    STIR t.
    storage phosphor-based t.
    1st-pass t.
    streptavidin peroxidase t.
    subclavian turndown t.
    subtraction t.
    supervoltage t.
    surface matching t.
    Swiss roll t.
    tandem t.
    tardus-parvus t.
    technetium 99m sestamibi
      dual-phase t.
    Tesla system imaging t.
    test bolus t.
    T1-Fourier-acquired steady-state t.
      (T1-FAST)
    time-resolved echo-shared
      angiographic t. (TREAT)
    tissue characterization t.
    toggling-table t.
    tourniquet t.
    transcatheter t.
    transgluteal CT-guided t.
    trephine t.
    triple-pass t.
    trocar-cannula t.
    turbo-spin echo t.
    upgated t.
    ureteral compression t.
    vessel subtraction t.
    volume rendering t. (VRT)
    volumetric mapping t.
    WakiTrak LS t.
    water-suppression MR imaging t.
    wedged-pair t.
    Welin t.
    white matter imaging t.
    woggle t.
    xeroradiographic t.
technologist
    American Society of Radiologic T.'s
      (ASRT)
    American Society of Registered T.'s
    nuclear medicine t.
    radiologic t.
    registered t. (RT)
technology
    acoustic response t.
    adaptive focusing t. (AFT)
    American Registry of Radiologic T.
      (ARRT)
    amorphous silicon filmless digital
      x-ray detection t.

    angiographic contrast injection
      system t. (ACIST)
    ARTMA virtual patient t.
    CellSeek t.
    computer automated scan t. (CAST)
    Emblocker t.
    fused image t.
    Joint Review Committee on
      Education in Radiologic T.
      (JRCERT)
    National Institute of Standards and
      T.
    noncontact imaging t.
    PASV t.
    radiation delivery t. (RDX)
    radiologic t.
    SieScape imaging t.
    single breath-hold dynamic
      subtraction CT with multidetector
      row helical t.
    slip-ring t.
    spiral multisplice t.
    Toshiba Aplio xV tissue Doppler
      and contrast imaging t.
    TruePoint PET-CT t.
    ultrasound imaging t.
Technovit 7210 VLC contact glue
Techtides
Tecmag
    T. Libra-S16 system
    T. Libra-S16 system scanner
TEC-2100 postioning laser
tecta (*pl. of* tectum)
tectal
    t. beaking
    t. cyst
    t. dysplasia
    t. glioma
    t. lesion
    t. plate
tectocerebellar dysraphism
tectoral ligament
tectospinal tract
tectum, *pl.* **tecta**
    t. commissure
TED
    thromboembolic disease
TEDE
    total effective dose equivalent
Tedlar bag
TEE
    transesophageal echocardiography
teeth (*pl. of* tooth)
TEF
    tracheoesophageal fistula
Teflon
    T. bomb
    T. catheter
    T. fascial dilator

T. granulomatous reaction
T. probe
T. prosthesis
Teflon-coated guidewire
tegmen, *pl.* **tegmina**
t. tympani
tegmenta (*pl. of* tegmentum)
tegmental tract
tegmentum, *pl.* **tegmenta**
medullary t.
midbrain t.
t. of brainstem
t. of pons
pontile t.
tegmina (*pl. of* tegmen)
TEGwire ST system
Teichholz
T. ejection fraction
T. equation
T. equation for left ventricular
volume
TEK
total exchangeable potassium
T1EL
type I endoleak
T2EL
type II endoleak
T3EL
type III endoleak
T4EL
type IV endoleak
tela, *pl.* **telae**
t. choroidea
telae (*pl. of* tela)
telangiectases (*pl. of* telangiectasis)
telangiectasia (*var. of* telangiectasis)
ataxia t.
capillary t.
hemorrhagic hereditary t.
hereditary hemorrhagic t.
(HHT)
Osler-Weber-Rendu t.
pulmonary t.
Sturge-Weber t.
telangiectasis, telangiectasia, *pl.*
telangiectases
bilateral juxtafoveal t.
calcinosis cutis, Raynaud
phenomenon, esophageal motility
disorder, sclerodactyly, and t.
(CREST)
telangiectatic
t. angioma
t. brain capillary
t. carcinoma
t. fibroma
t. lesion
t. osteosarcoma
t. vessel

telangiectaticum
Telebrix contrast medium
telecobalt therapy
telecollaboration surgery
telecord
telecurietherapy
telefluoroscopy
telemammography
telemetry
telencephalic
t. malformation
t. ventriculofugal artery
telencephalon
TelePACS
Telepaque imaging agent
teleradiogram, teleroentgenogram
teleradiography, teleroentgenography
teleradiology
diagnostic t.
referral t.
t. videoconferencing
teleradium therapy
teleroentgenogram (*var. of*
teleradiogram)
teleroentgenography (*var. of*
teleradiography)
teleroentgentheraphy (*var. of* teletherapy)
telescopic
t. aerial dilator
t. bougie set
telescoping finger
teletherapy, teleroentgentheraphy
C-60 t.
t. radiotherapy
Telocin diagnostic ultrasound system
telognosis
telomere repeat amplification protocol
(TRAP)
telomeric repeat amplification protocol
(TRAP)
Telos radiographic stress device
Temno II cutting needle
temp
T. Tip drainage catheter
T. Tip ureteral stent
temperature
t. distribution measurement
firing t.
mean perfusate t.
Neel t.
t. sensor
variable t. (VT)
template
deformable t.
t. irradiation
Martinez universal interstitial t.
Syed t.
Syed-Neblett t.
Tempofilter vena cava filter

T

temporal
- t. aliasing
- t. arteritis
- t. artery
- t. artery tap maneuver
- t. average intensity
- t. bone
- t. bone anatomy
- t. bone fracture
- t. bone sclerosis
- t. bone tomogram
- t. bone tumor
- t. canal
- t. diameter
- t. filter
- t. fossa
- t. granulomatous arteritis
- t. gyrus
- t. horn
- t. horn atrophy
- t. horn of lateral ventricle
- t. instability artifact
- t. isthmus
- t. limb of anterior commissure
- t. lobe
- t. lobe epilepsy (TLE)
- t. lobe herniation
- t. lobe infarct
- t. lobe lesion
- t. lobe tumor
- t. meningioma
- t. operculum
- t. orientation
- t. peak
- t. peak intensity
- t. peritumoral enhancement
- t. phase delay
- t. plane
- t. pole
- t. predominance
- t. process
- t. resolution
- t. sawtooth pattern
- t. smoothing
- t. space infection
- t. sulcus
- t. suture

temporalis muscle
temporally
temporary
- t. atrial pacing wire
- t. interstitial implant
- t. pacing catheter

temporoinsular astrocytoma
temporomalar suture
temporomandibular
- t. joint (TMJ)
- t. joint arthrography
- t. joint destruction
- t. joint disc
- t. joint osteolysis
- t. ligament

temporooccipital
- t. artery
- t. glioma
- t. junction

temporoparietooccipital junction
temporopontine tract
temporozygomatic suture
TENa
    total exchangeable sodium
Tenckhoff catheter
tenderness
    skin-rolling scapular t.
tendines (*pl. of* tendo)
tendinitis, tendonitis, tenonitis
- Achilles t.
- calcific t.
- gluteal t.
- popliteal t.
tendinopathy
- patellar t.
tendinosis, tendonosis
- angiofibroblastic t.
- calcific t.
- common extensor t.
- lateral elbow t.
- patellar t.
- supraspinatus t.
tendinous
- t. attachment
- t. band
- t. insertion
- t. part of epicranius muscle
- t. raphe
tendo, *pl.* **tendines**
- t. Achillis
- t. Achillis bursa
- t. calcaneus
tendon
    abductor digiti quinti t.
    abductor hallucis t.
    abductor pollicis brevis t.
    abductor pollicis longus t.
    accessory communicating t.
    Achilles t.
    adductor hallucis t.
    adductor pollicis brevis t.
    adherent profundus t.
    anchoring t.
    anterior tibial t. (ATT)
    t. aponeurosis
    aponeurotic t.
    t. attenuation
    attrition rupture of t.
    biceps brachialis t.
    biceps brachii t.
    biceps femoris t.

bicipital t.
bifid biceps t.
boomerang t.
bowing of t.
brachialis t.
brachial plexus t.
brachioradialis t.
brevis t.
calcaneal t.
carpi radialis brevis t.
carpi radialis longus t.
central perineal t.
common t.
conjoined t.'s
coronary t.
cricoesophageal t.
digital extensor t.
digital flexor t.
elbow extensor t.
extensor carpi radialis brevis t.
extensor carpi radialis longus t.
extensor carpi ulnaris t.
extensor digiti minimi t.
extensor digiti quinti t.
extensor digitorum brevis t.
extensor digitorum communis t.
extensor digitorum longus t.
extensor hallucis longus t.
extensor indicis proprius t.
extensor pollicis brevis t.
extensor pollicis longus t.
extensor quinti t.
flexor carpi radialis t.
flexor carpi ulnaris t.
flexor digitorum communis t.
flexor digitorum longus t.
flexor digitorum profundus t.
flexor digitorum sublimis t.
flexor digitorum superficialis t.
flexor hallucis brevis t.
flexor hallucis longus t.
flexor pollicis brevis t.
flexor pollicis longus t.
flexor profundus t.
flexor sublimis t.
gastrocnemius t.
gastrocnemius-soleus t.
Golgi t.
goose foot t.
gracilis t.
hamstring t.
heel t.
hilum of t.
iliopsoas t.
t. inflammation
infrapatellar t.
infraspinatus t.
interosseous t.
t. irregularity

t. laceration
long head of biceps t. (LHBT)
longitudinal split biceps t.
longitudinal tear of brevis t.
lumbrical t.
membranous t.
midpatellar t.
t. nodularity
t. nodule
obturator internus t.
t. of Hector
palmaris longus t.
patellar t.
patelloquadriceps t.
peroneus brevis t.
peroneus longus t.
peroneus tertius t.
plantaris t.
t. plate
pollicis longus t.
popliteal t.
popliteus fossa muscle t.
posterior tibial t. (PTT)
profundus t.
pronator teres t.
proprius t.
quadriceps t.
rectus femoris t.
rider's t.
t. rupture
sartorius t.
semimembranosus t.
semitendinosus t.
t. sheath
t. sheath giant cell tumor
t. sheath space infection
t. sheath stenosis
t. sheath thickening
t. shortening
t. sling
slip of t.
slipped t.
split anterior tibial t. (SPLATT)
sublimis t.
t. subluxation
subscapularis t.
superficialis t.
superficial palmaris longus t.
supraspinatus t.
t. tear (type I-IV)
thumb extensor t.
thumb flexor t.
tibial t.
tibialis anterior t
tibialis posterior t.
t. tissue
toe extensor t.
triceps brachii t.
Zinn t.

T

tendonitis (*var. of* tendinitis)
tendonosis (*var. of* tendinosis)
tendon-to-bone attachment
tendosynovial (*var. of* tenosynovial)
tendosynovitis (*var. of* tenosynovitis)
tendovaginitis (*var. of* tenosynovitis)
tenesmus
tennis
    t. elbow
    t. leg
    t. shoulder
    t. toe
tenocyte hyperplasia
tenodesis
    band t.
tenography
tenonavicular
tenonitis (*var. of* tendinitis)
tenosynovial, tendosynovial
    t. giant cell tumor
    t. osteochondromatosis
    t. sarcoma
tenosynovitis, tendosynovitis,
tendovaginitis, tenovaginitis
    de Quervain t.
    flexor t.
    LHBT t.
    peroneal t.
    plant thorn t.
    stenosing t.
    tibialis posterior t.
    tuberculous t.
tenovaginitis (*var. of* tenosynovitis)
TENS
    transcutaneous electrical nerve
    stimulator
tense fontanelle
tensile
    t. force
    t. injury
tension
    t. collar
    t. cyst
    diffusion t.
    t. endothorax
    epicardial t.
    t. fracture
    intraventricular systolic t.
    t. pneumothorax
tension-time index (TTI)
tensor, *pl.* **tensores**
    t. diffusion-weighted MR image
    t. fasciae femoris
    t. fasciae latae
    t. fasciae suralis
    t. imaging
    t. tympani
    t. veli palatini
    t. veli palatini muscle

tensores (*pl. of* tensor)
tented up
tenting
    baseline t.
    t. of diaphragm
    t. of hemidiaphragm
tentoria (*pl. of* tentorium)
tentorial
    t. edge
    t. meningioma
    t. notch herniation
    t. ridge
    t. traversal
tentorium, *pl.* **tentoria**
    t. cerebelli
    t. cerebelli attachment
    (TCA)
    t. cerebelli lesion
    t. keyhole configuration
TER
    thermal enhancement ratio
terahertz
    t. ray
    t. wave
TeraRecon software
Terason Echo ultrasound system
teratoblastoma of ovary
teratocarcinoma
    mediastinal t.
    t. of ovary
    pineal gland t.
teratogenic effect
teratogenicity of contrast agent
teratoid
    t. mediastinum
    t. tumor
teratoma
    atypical brain t.
    benign t.
    benign cystic t.
    cardiac t.
    CNS t.
    cystic t.
    embryonal ovary t.
    immature ovarian t.
    malignant t.
    mature mediastinal t.
    mature ovarian cystic t.
    mediastinal t.
    neck t.
    orbital t.
    ovarian cystic t.
    pineal t.
    sacrococcygeal t.
    solid ovarian t.
    spinal t.
    suprasellar atypical t.
    testicular t.
teratomatous mass

teres
- ligamentum t.
- t. major
- t. minor
- t. minor tendon tear
- pronator t.

terminad

terminal
- t. air sac
- t. airspace
- t. aorta
- t. bile duct
- t. bronchiole
- t. carcinoma
- t. cistern
- t. crest
- t. ductal lobular unit (TDLU)
- t. edema
- t. head
- t. ileitis
- t. ileum
- t. inversion
- t. pneumonia
- t. reservoir syndrome
- t. segment of posterior cerebral artery
- t. synostosis
- t. thrombosis
- t. tuft
- t. tuft resorption
- t. ventricle
- t. web

terminale
- fatty filum t.
- filum t.
- os t.
- persistent ossiculum t.
- tight filum t.

terminalis
- cistern of lamina t
- crista t.
- stria t.

terminatio, *pl.* **terminationes** (*var. of* termination)

termination, terminato
- early-phase t.
- late-phase t.
- t. site
- underdrive t.

terminationes (*pl. of* terminatio)

termini (*pl. of* terminus)

terminus, *pl.* **termini**
- duodenal t.
- intrapapillary t.
- rostral t.

terrestrial radiation

territory
- coronary arterial t.
- posterior circulation t.

Terry Thomas sign

tertiary
- t. collimation
- t. hyperparathyroidism (tHPT)
- t. hypothyroidism
- t. sequestrum
- t. syphilis
- t. wave

tertius
- condylus t.
- peroneus t.

Terumo
- T. guidewire
- T. Pinnacle R/OII radiopaque marker introducer sheath

Tesla
- T. field
- T. magnetic resonance imager
- T. superconductive magnet unit
- T. system
- T. system imaging technique

3-tesla neuroimaging

Teslascan

tessellated

test
- abduction stress t.
- acetazolamide vasodilator t.
- Alcock t.
- aluminum ion breakthrough t.
- attached proton t. (APT)
- axial manual traction t.
- t. balloon occlusion
- balloon occlusion tolerance t.
- Barlow pediatric hip instability t.
- bicycle exercise stress t.
- t. bolus
- bolus challenge t.
- t. bolus technique
- carbon-14 urea breath t.
- cardiopulmonary exercise t. (CPET)
- chlormerodrin accumulation t.
- ^{14}C lactose breath test
- coin t.
- colorimetric t.
- conglutinating complement absorption t.
- contraction stress t. (CST)
- costoclavicular t.
- Dicopac t.
- dipyridamole handgrip t.
- duplex screening t.
- dye reduction spot t.
- exercise tolerance t. (ETT)
- false-negative t.
- false-positive t.
- fat absorption t.
- fetal stress t.
- film-screen contact t.
- Finkelstein t.
- flat-hand t.

test (*continued*)
    Fowler t.
    fulcrum t.
    gallbladder function t.
    gastrointestinal protein loss t.
    Graham-Cole t.
    Heaf t.
    hop t.
    t. injection
    internal carotid balloon t.
    intrinsic field uniformity t.
    Kruskal-Wallis t.
    Leclercq t.
    Linsman water t.
    log-rank t.
    lung connectivity t.
    McMurray t.
    t. meal
    Mecholyl t.
    molybdenum-99 breakthrough t.
    Moschcowitz t.
    Müller t.
    NMR LipoProfile t.
    nonstress t. (NST)
    nonstress fetal t.
    O'Connor finger dexterity t.
    Ortolani t.
    Osteo-Gram bone density t.
    pelvic steal t.
    perchlorate washout t.
    peritoneal-venous shunt patency t.
    pivot-shift t.
    positive washout t.
    pulmonary function t.
    quadriceps femoris tendon
      reflex t.
    radioactive renogram t.
    radioimmunoprecipitation t.
    radioiodine t.
    radioisotope renogram t.
    Seidlitz powder t.
    sestamibi ^{99m}Tc with dipyridamole
      stress t.
    Sharp-Purser t.
    Shirmer t.
    Smith orthogonal hole t.
    sniff t.
    Spearman rank t.
    spinal extension t.
    spinning-top t.
    star-cancellation t. (SCT)
    stop t.
    Triboulet t.
    triple-marker screening t.
    tuberculin skin t.
    t. tube structure
    ultrasound dilution t.
    ureteral perfusion t.
    USP XX t.

    vasodilatory hemodynamic stress t.
    Wada t.
    washout t.
    Welch t.
    Wetzel t.
    Whitaker t.
    Whitfield t.
    Wilcoxon signed-rank t.
    Yergason t.
    zinc turbidity t.

testes (*pl. of* testis)

testicle
    undescended t.

testicular
    t. abscess
    t. adrenal rest tissue
    t. appendage torsion
    t. artery
    t. artery avulsion
    t. carcinoma
    t. choriocarcinoma
    t. cyst
    t. cystic lesion
    t. degeneration
    t. ectopia
    t. feminization
    t. gland
    t. infarct
    t. ischemia
    t. metastasis
    t. microlithiasis
    t. parenchyma
    t. posttraumatic edema
    t. relapse
    t. rupture
    t. seminoma
    t. stromal cell tumor
    t. teratoma
    t. torsion appendage
    t. trauma
    t. tubular adenoma
    t. vascular pedicle sign
    t. vein
    t. vein embolization
    t. venography

testiculoma ovarii

testing
    bronchial provocation t.
    constant-load treadmill t.
    Doppler ultrasound segmental blood
      pressure t.
    manual muscle t.
    nuclear gated blood pool t.
    perimetry t.
    pyrogen t.
    radiation sensitivity t.

testis, *pl.* **testes**
    appendix of t.
    burned-out tumor of t.

t. carcinoma
dilated rete t.
t. dysfunction
t. dysplasia
echo-poor t.
ectopic t.
efferent ductule of t.
t. fracture
t. germ cell tumor
hypoechoic t.
infarcted t.
maldescended t.
malpositioned t.
mediastinum t.
occult primary tumor of t.
rete t.
retractile t.
torsed t.
torsion of t.
tubular ectasia of rete t.
undescended t.
vaginal t.
test-retest precision
Tesuloid
tethered
t. cord syndrome (TCS)
t. small bowel fold
t. spinal cord
tethering
spinal cord t.
tetraazacyclododecanetetraacetic acid (DOTA)
tetrabromophenolphthalein sodium
tetracetate
gadolinium benzylopropionic t. (Gd-BOPTA)
tetrad
Fallot t.
tetradecyl sulfate
tetradiploid tumor
tetrahedron chest
tetrahydrobiopterin
tetrahydrouridine
tetraiodophenolphthalein
t. contrast medium
t. sodium
tetralogy
t. of Fallot (TOF)
pink t.
tetraphocomelia
tetraploid tumor
tetrasodium-meso-tetra
manganese t.-m.-t.
tetrasodium pyrophosphate (TSPP)
tetrofosmin
Teutleben ligament
texaphyrin
gadolinium t. (Gd-Tex)

textiloma
texture
ground-glass t.
t. mapping
peripheral t.
t. slice
TFA
thigh-foot angle
tibiofemoral angle
T1-FAST
T1-Fourier-acquired steady-state technique
T-fastener
T-f. delivery needle
T-f. device
TFC
threaded fusion cage
triangular fibrocartilage
TFCC
triangular fibrocartilaginous complex
TFD
target-film distance
TFF3
trefoil factor 3
intestinal peptide TFF3
T1-Fourier-acquired steady-state technique (T1-FAST)
T1FS
T1-weighted fat-suppressed
T1FS image
TFT
thin-film transistor
TGA
transposition of great arteries
TGC
time-gain compensation
TGG
thalamogeniculate group
TGMS
tris-acryl gelatin microsphere
T2-gradient refocused image
4th
4th branchial arch
4th branchial cleft pouch
4th compartment
4th cranial nerve
4th intercostal space
4th parallel pelvic plane
4th turbinate bone
4th ventricle
4th ventricle diverticulum
4th ventricle tumor
5th
5th compartment
5th cranial nerve
5th intercostal space
5th rib
5th ventricle
5th ventricle

T

6th

6th compartment
6th nucleus
6th ventricle

8th

8th cranial nerve complex
8th nerve tumor

THAD

transient hepatic attenuation difference

thalamectomy
thalami (*pl. of* thalamus)
thalamic

t. edema
t. fracture of calcaneus
t. glioma
t. hemorrhage
t. infarct
t. lesion
t. plane
t. syndrome of Dejerine-Roussy
t. vein

thalamic-hypothalamic mass
thalamocaudate artery
thalamogeniculate

t. artery
t. group (TGG)

thalamoperforating

t. artery
t. branch

thalamostriate vein
thalamotegmental involvement
thalamotomy

anterior t.
dorsomedial t.
parafascicular t.

thalamus, *pl.* **thalami**

intralaminar t.
pulvinar of t.
stria medullaris thalami

thallium

t. 201 (^{201}Tl, Tl-201)
t. debris
t. imaging agent
t. myocardial perfusion imaging
t. myocardial scan
t. myocardial scan with SPECT imaging
t. perfusion scintigraphy
t. redistribution phase
t. rest-redistribution imaging
t. scintography imaging
t. single-photon emission computed tomography scan
t. SPECT score
t. stress imaging

thallium-201

t.-201 chloride
t.-201 imaging

t.-201 myocardial scintigraphy
t.-201 scan
t.-201 single-photon emission CT
t.-201 uptake and distribution

thallium-activated

t.-a. sodium iodide
t.-a. sodium iodine detector

thallium-to-scalp ratio
thallous chloride imaging agent
Thal-Quick chest tube
thanatophoric

t. dwarfism
t. dysplasia

Thayer-Doisy unit
THC

transhepatic cholangiogram

THC:YAG

transhepatic cholangiogram:yttrium-aluminum-garnet
THC:YAG laser

thebesian

t. circulation
t. foramen
t. valve
t. vein

theca, *pl.* **thecae**

t. cell ovarian tumor
t. externa
t. interna

thecae (*pl. of* theca)
thecal

t. abscess
t. sac
t. whitlow

theca-lutein ovarian cyst
The Closer arterial puncture site closure device
thecoma of ovary
Theile

T. canal
T. muscle

T-helper cell (type 1)
thenar

t. eminence
t. muscle
t. space
t. space abscess

theophylline attenuation
theorem

Bayes t.
Nyquist sampling t.
Stokes t.

theory

Bohr t.
crystal field t.
Culiner t.
density matrix t.
electron t.

Fourier optical t.
fuzzy set t.
Kubelka-Munk t.
t. of fuzzy connectedness
Planck quantum t.
quantum t.
slider crank t.

therapeutic
t. amniocentesis
t. angiography
t. barium enema
t. cardiac catheterization
t. chemoembolization
t. cordocentesis
t. embolus
t. external radiation
t. gain factor
t. index
t. intervention
t. lymph node dissection
t. pneumothorax
t. radiology
t. range
t. response
t. thrombosis
t. ultrasound

therapist
enterostomal t.

therapy
ablative laser t.
ABMMN cell-based t.
adjunctive t.
adjuvant t.
aggressive tissue-protective t.
5-aminolevulinic acid photodynamic t.
androgen deprivation t.
antiaggregant t.
antiangiogenic t.
antiestrogen radiologic t.
antitubercular t.
antivascular t.
arc t.
beam t.
beta ray ophthalmic plaque t.
boost t.
breast-conserving t.
breast intensity-modulated radiation t.
brisement t.
cardiac shock wave t. (CSWT)
catheter-directed thrombolytic t.
Chaoul t.
combined antiretroviral t.
combined modality t.
compartmental radioimmunoglobulin t.
computer-controlled conformal radiation t. (CCRT)
concomitant boost radiation t.

conformal neutron and photon radiation t.
conformal radiation t. (CRT)
contact radiation t.
continuous hyperfractionated accelerated radiation t.
conventionally fractionated stereotactic radiation t.
coronary radiation t. (CRT)
craniospinal axis radiation t.
crossfire radiation t.
cyclophosphamide t.
3D conformal radiation t.
deep roentgen ray t.
digitalis t.
dynamic conformal t.
dynamic radiation t.
electroconvulsive t.
electron arc t.
electron beam intraoperative radiation t.
embolization transcatheter t.
endocrine ablative t.
endolaser venous t. (ELVT)
enzyme replacement t.
enzyme supplementation t.
Exogen 2000+ noninvasive ultrasound t.
extended-field irradiation t.
external beam radiation t. (EBRT)
external x-ray t.
eye-view 3D conformal radiation t.
fast-neutron radiation t.
4-fiber t.
fibrinolytic t.
Fletcher-Suit system for radium t.
fluoroscopy-guided subarachnoid phenol block t.
focal cranial radiation t.
fractionated external beam radiation t.
fractionated stereotactic radiation t.
fragmentation t.
gallstone dissolution t.
gamma ray t.
gamma-ribbon radiation t.
gene t.
grid t.
hadron t.
half-body radiation t.
heavy-particle t.
high-dose t.
high dose-rate intracavitary radiation t.
highly active antiretroviral t. (HAART)
high-voltage roentgen t.
hyperfractionated accelerated radiation t. (HART)

T

therapy (*continued*)

    hyperperfusion t.
    hypofractionated radiation t.
    hysterectomy and radiation t.
    ^{131}I t.
    I-B1 radiolabeled antibody injection radiation t.
    image-guided radiation t. (IGRT)
    indicator dilution t.
    induction t.
    infusion transcatheter t.
    intensity-modulated arc t.
    intensity-modulated radiation t. (IMRT)
    interferential current t.
    internal radiation t.
    interstitial radiation t.
    interstitial radioactive colloid t.
    interstitial radium t.
    intraarterial t.
    intraarticular radiopharmaceutical t.
    intracavitary radiation t.
    intracavitary radioactive colloid t.
    intracoronary radiation t. (ICRT)
    intracoronary thrombolytic t.
    intradiscal electrothermal t. (IDET)
    intraoperative radiation t.
    intraoperative red light t. (IRLT)
    intravascular radiopharmaceutical t.
    iron chelation t.
    ^{192}Ir seed t.
    large-field radiation t.
    lens-sparing external beam radiation t.
    light t.
    lipid-lowering t.
    low-intensity laser t. (LILT)
    MammoSite radiation t.
    megavolt t.
    megavoltage grid t.
    megavoltage radiation t.
    megavoltage x-ray t.
    microwave coagulation t.
    molecularly targeted t.
    MRI-guided periradicular nerve root infiltration t.
    multimodality t.
    neoadjuvant chemoradiation t.
    neoadjuvant hormonal t.
    neodymium:YAG laser t.
    neuraxis radiation t.
    neutron t.
    neutron/gamma transmission t.
    nonsurgical ablative t.
    ocular radiation t. (ORT)
    orthovoltage radiation t.
    palliative radiation t.
    pamidronate t.
    partial brain radiation t.

    particle beam radiation t.
    percutaneous ethanol injection t.
    percutaneous microwave coagulation t.
    percutaneous transcatheter t.
    peroral cone radiation t.
    photodynamic t. (PDT)
    photon-neutron mixed-beam radiation t.
    photon radiosurgical t.
    PhotoPoint photodynamic t.
    photoradiation t. (PRT)
    plesiocurie t.
    postmenopausal estrogen t.
    postoperative radiation t.
    postorchiectomy paraaortic radiation t.
    proton t.
    pulsed-dye laser t.
    PUVA t.
    radiation t. (RT)
    radiofrequency ablation t.
    radioiodine t.
    radioiodine ablation t.
    radionuclide t.
    radiopharmaceutical t.
    radium beam t.
    reperfusion t.
    reprogramming t.
    rotation t.
    salvage t.
    samarium-153 ethylenediamine tetramethylene phosphonic acid t.
    selective internal radiation t. (SIRT)
    selective tubal assessment to refine reproductive t. (STARRT)
    short-distance radiation t.
    sonodynamic t.
    split-course hyperfractionated radiation t.
    stem cell t.
    stereotactically guided interstitial laser t.
    stereotactic radiation t.
    1st-line t.
    systemic adjuvant t.
    target-specific t.
    telecobalt t.
    teleradium t.
    thrombolytic t.
    tiered t.
    timed sequential t.
    total androgen suppression t.
    transcatheter t.
    transpupillary therma t.
    triple-H t.
    ultraearly thrombolytic t.
    ultrasound ablative t.

ultrasound-guided percutaneous microwave coagulation t.
updraft t.
upper mantle radiation t.
virus-directed enzyme/prodrug t.
virus-mediated gene t.
whole-body radiation t.
whole-brain radiation t. (WBRT)
wide-field radiation t. (WFRT)
x-ray t.
Y-90 silicate t.
yttrium-90 silicate t.
t. zone

therapy-related
t.-r. fibrous tissue
t.-r. myelodysplastic syndrome

TheraSeed
T. imaging agent
T. seeding

TheraSphere

thermal, thermic
t. ablation
t. bioeffect
t. compression
t. conductivity
t. convection pattern
t. diffusion
t. dosimetry system
t. effect
t. energy
t. enhancement ratio (TER)
t. equilibrium
t. hot spot
t. insult
t. mapping
t. modeling
t. neutron
t. noise
t. occlusion
t. radiation
t. relaxation time
t. shape memory
t. spectrum
t. treatment parameter

Thermex
Direx T.

thermic (*var. of* thermal)
thermistor plethysmography
thermoacoustic imaging
thermoacoustics
thermoactinomyces vulgaris
thermocoagulation
thermodilution
t. cardiac output
t. catheter
t. ejection fraction
t. method of cardiac output measurement
t. stroke volume

thermodynamics
thermogram
thermograph
continuous-scan t.
thermography
blood vessel t.
infrared t.
laser-induced t. (LITT)
liquid crystal t. (LCT)
liquid crystal contact t.
thermoluminescence dosimetry
thermoluminescent
t. dosimeter (TLD)
t. dosimeter rod
thermometer
aural t.
disposable t.
glass t.
thermometry
invasive t.
MRI t.
noninvasive t.
thermomostography
thermonic emission
thermonuclear reaction
thermophilic actinomycetes
thermoplacentography
thermoradiosensitization
thermoradiotherapy
simultaneous t.
Thermo-Spheres
thermotherapy
laser-induced t. (LITT)
laser-induced interstitial t.
MR-guided laser-induced t.
MRI-guided laser-induced interstitial t.
thermotolerance
thermotreatment
high frequency-induced t.
thermovision
thesaurosis
THI
tissue harmonic imaging
THI echocardiography
thick
t. bone
t. echo
t. rind sclerosis
thickened
t. airway wall
t. aortic valve
t. bladder
t. bladder wall
t. bowel loop
t. duodenal fold
t. esophageal fold
t. gallbladder wall
t. gastric fold

T

thickened (*continued*)
t. heel pad
t. hypoechoic tissue
t. irregular endometrium
t. irregular small bowel fold dilation
t. nodular irregular small bowel fold
t. septum
t. sinus
t. smooth small bowel fold dilation
t. stomach fold
t. straight small bowel fold

thickening
anterior joint capsule t.
antral mucosal t.
aortic valve t.
aortic wall t.
apical pleural t.
asbestos-related pleural t.
beaded septal t.
breast skin t.
bronchial wall t.
capsular t.
cecal t.
circumferential t.
diffuse gallbladder wall t.
diffuse intimal t.
diffuse pleural t.
disproportionate upper septal t.
facial t.
focal cecal apical t.
focal gallbladder wall t.
focal intimal t.
t. fraction
fusiform t.
gastric wall t.
heel pad t.
inner table t.
interlobular septal t.
interstitial t.
intimal t.
intralobular interstitial t.
irregular gallbladder wall t.
joint capsule t.
ligamentous t.
ligamentum flavum t.
localized pleural t.
mediastinal t.
minimal interstitial t.
mottled t.
mucosal t.
mural t.
myocardial t.
nuchal skin t.
optic excrescentic t.
optic nerve fusiform t.
outer table t.

partial t.
peribronchial t.
peritoneal t.
pleural t.
postlumpectomy skin t.
rindlike t.
sawtoothlike t.
scrotal wall t.
septal t.
skin t.
small bowel wall t.
submucosal t.
synovial t.
systolic myocardial t.
tendon sheath t.
trabecular t.
urinary bladder wall t.
valve t.
visceral t.
wall t.

thickness
antropyloric muscle t.
arterial wall t.
bladder wall t.
effective section t.
endometrial t.
full t.
image slice t.
increased skull t.
interventricular septal t. (IVST)
intimal-medial t. (IMT)
patellar cartilage t.
posterior wall t. (PWT)
postmenopausal endometrial t.
preacinar arterial wall t.
septal wall t.
slab t.
slice t.
strut t.
subcutaneous quadriceps fat t. (SQFT)
urethral t.
ventricular free wall t.
wall t.

thickness-diameter of ventricle ratio
thick-septa collimator
thick-slab 3D multiplanar reformatted image
thick-slice imaging
thick-walled
t.-w. cyst
t.-w. gallbladder
t.-w. ventricle
THID
transient hepatic intensity difference
thigh
t. muscle
t. muscle cross-section
t. splint

thigh-foot angle (TFA)
thin
- t. border
- t. collimation
- t. collimation image
- t. collimation imaging
- t. cylindrical uniform field volume
- t. fibrous cap
- t. linear structure
- t. section
- t. skull

thin-cut axial CT image
thin-film
- t.-f. analysis
- t.-f. transistor (TFT)
- t.-f. transistor array

thinned
- t. cartilage
- t. myocardium

thinning
- apical t.
- cortical t.
- parietal bone t.
- pulmonary interstitial t.
- white matter t.

thin-plate spine
ThinPrep imaging system
thin-section
- t.-s. axial image
- t.-s. CT
- t.-s. dual-phase multidetector-row computed tomography
- t.-s. secondary reformation

thin-septa collimator
thin-slab
- t.-s. coronal acquisition
- t.-s. minimum-intensity projection

thin-slice
- t.-s. CT
- t.-s. imaging

thin-walled
- t.-w. atrium
- t.-w. catheter
- t.-w. cyst
- t.-w. gallbladder
- t.-w. guiding needle
- t.-w. lung cavity

thiol
- t. augmentation
- t. modification

thiosemicarbazide
100th-normal solution
Thom method
Thompson-Epstein femoral fracture classification
Thompson ligament
Thomson scattering
thoracentesis
- misplaced t.

thoraces (*pl. of* thorax)
thoracic
- t. adenopathy
- t. angiography
- t. aorta
- t. aortic aneurysm
- t. aortic coarctation
- t. aortic dissection
- t. arch aortography
- t. asymmetry
- t. bone
- t. cage configuration
- t. cavity
- t. circumference
- t. crush
- t. deformity
- t. disc
- t. disc herniation
- t. duct
- t. duct-cutaneous fistula
- t. duct cyst
- t. duct imaging
- t. duct ligation
- t. duct route
- t. dysplasia
- t. empyema
- t. esophagus
- t. gas volume
- t. gibbus
- t. index
- t. inlet
- t. inlet lesion
- t. inlet soft tissue
- t. inlet syndrome
- t. joint
- t. kidney
- t. kyphosis
- t. lordosis
- t. lymphatics
- t. myelography
- t. neuroblastoma
- t. OPLL
- t. outlet
- t. outlet stenosis (TOS)
- t. outlet syndrome (TOS)
- t. paraganglioma
- t. plane
- t. pulsion diverticulum
- t. root sleeve
- t. root sleeve diverticulum
- t. sarcoidosis
- t. scoliosis
- t. sonography
- t. spinal cord
- t. spine
- t. spine anatomy
- t. spine curve
- t. spine fracture
- t. spine neoplasia

T

thoracic (*continued*)
    t. splenosis
    t. stomach
    t. vent
    t. vertebra
    t. view
    t. wall
thoracoabdominal
    t. aorta
    t. aortic aneurysm
    t. diaphragm
    t. duplication
    t. gradient
    t. venous collateral circulation
    t. wall
thoracoacromial artery
thoracobiliary fistula
thoracodorsal artery
thoracoepigastric vein
thoracofemoral conversion
thoracolumbar
    t. burst fracture
    t. fascia
    t. junction fracture
    t. kyphosis
    t. scoliosis
    t. spine
    t. spine column
    t. vertebral disc
thoracoomphalopagus
thoracopagus twin
thoracoplasty
Thoracoport
thoracoscope
    Boutin t.
    Storz t.
thoracoscopic poudrage
thoracoscopy
    video-assisted t. (VAT)
thoracostomy
    t. tube
    tube t.
thoracotomy
Thoramat
Thoravision selenium x-ray detector
thorax, *pl.* **thoraces**
    t. articulation
    asymmetric t.
    bell-shaped t.
    bony t.
    cylindrical t.
    skeleton thoracis
    squared-off t.
    symmetric t.
Thoreau filter
Thorel
    T. bundle
    T. pathway

thorium
    t. compound
    t. dioxide granuloma
    t. dioxide imaging agent
    t. dioxide radiopaque medium
    t. emanation
    radioactive t.
    t. tartrate
    t. X
thorium-201 SPECT scan
thorn ulcer
Thornwaldt (*var. of* Tornwaldt)
thorny bone radiation
Thorotrast
    T. accumulation
    T. imaging agent
thorotrastosis
Thorpe plastic lens
tHPT
    tertiary hyperparathyroidism
threaded fusion cage (TFC)
threads-and-streaks
    t.-a.-s. sign
    t.-a.-s. vascular channel
threatened vessel closure
threes
    rule of t.
threshold
    above selected t. (AST)
    alpha t.
    attenuation t.
    t. body
    CACS t.
    cell-dose t.
    t. contrast detail detectability (TCDD)
    count-density t.
    detection t.
    erythema t.
    t. erythema dose
    fracture t.
    malignancy t.
    mask t.
    t. of Firooznia
    seizure t.
    signal-to-noise t.
    ultrasound t.
thresholding
    diffusion anisotropy t.
    gray-level t.
    t. method
thrombectomy
    adjunctive mechanical t.
    t. device
    mechanical t.
    percutaneous mechanical t. (PMT)

Thrombex PMT system
thrombi (*pl. of* thrombus)
thrombin
    t. formation
    human t.
thrombin-activatable fibrinolysis inhibitor (TAFI)
thromboangiitis obliterans
thromboaspiration
thrombocythemia (*var. of* thrombocytosis)
thrombocytopenia, thrombopenia
thrombocytopenia-absent
    t.-a. radius (TAR)
    t.-a. radius syndrome
thrombocytosis, thrombocythemia
    essential t.
thromboelastogram
thromboelastograph
thromboelastography
thromboembolic
    t. disease (TED)
    t. lung disease
    t. pontile infarct
    t. stroke
thromboembolism
    aortic t.
    chronic lung t.
    mesenteric t. (MTE)
    paraneoplastic t.
    Prolyse in acute cerebral t. (PROACT)
    pulmonary t.
thromboembolization
    catheter-induced t.
    deep venous t.
    pulmonary t.
    venous t.
thrombogenic coil
thrombokinesis
thrombolysis
    brachiocephalic artery t.
    catheter-directed extremity t.
    clot removal by laser t.
    t. in brain ischemia flow grade
    t. in myocardial infarct (TIMI)
    intracerebral t.
    mechanical t.
    pharmacomechanical t.
    venous t.
thrombolytic therapy
thrombopathy
thrombopenia (*var. of* thrombocytopenia)
thrombophlebitis
    breast t.
    cerebral t.
    septic t.
    venography-related t.
thromboplastinogen
thromboresistance

ThromboScan
    T. imaging
    T. molecular recognition unit
    T. MRU
thrombosed
    t. filter-bearing inferior vena cava
    t. giant vertebral artery aneurysm
    t. intraaortic artery
thromboses (*pl. of* thrombosis)
thrombosis, *pl.* **thromboses**
    abdominal aorta t.
    acute renal vein t.
    aortic t.
    aortoiliac t.
    arterial t.
    ascending medullary vein t.
    atrial t.
    atrophic t.
    axillary vein traumatic t.
    axillosubclavian vein t.
    calf vein t.
    capsular t.
    cardiac t.
    catheter-induced subclavian vein t.
    cavernous sinus t.
    central splanchnic venous t. (CSVT)
    cerebral venous sinus t. (CVST)
    chronic renal vein t.
    common iliac artery t.
    coronary t.
    cortical vein t.
    deep venous t. (DVT)
    dural venous sinus t.
    effort t.
    femoropopliteal t.
    Galen t.
    hepatic artery t.
    hepatic vein t.
    iliofemoral t.
    infective t.
    intentional reversible t.
    intervillous placental t.
    intraarterial t.
    intracranial sinus t.
    intravascular t.
    jugular vein t.
    large-vessel t.
    luminal t.
    mesenteric arterial t.
    mesenteric venous t.
    native kidney renal vein t.
    necrotizing t.
    ovarian vein t.
    pelvic vein t.
    pericatheter t.
    portal vein t. (PVT)
    portomesenteric venous t.
    portosplenic t.
    postangioplasty mural t.

T

thrombosis (*continued*)
    primary subclavian-axillary vein t.
    pulmonary t.
    renal artery transplant t.
    renal vein t. (RVT)
    renal vein transplant t.
    sagittal t.
    secondary central venous t.
    septic t.
    shunt t.
    sinus t.
    splenic vein t.
    SSS t.
    stent t.
    subacute renal vein t.
    subclavian vein t.
    subclavian vessel t.
    superior ophthalmic vein t.
    superior sagittal sinus t. (SSST)
    syndrome of impending t.
    terminal t.
    therapeutic t.
    transverse sinus t.
    upper extremity venous t. (UEVT)
    vascular t.
    vein graft t.
    venous sinus t.
thrombospondin
thrombostasis
Thrombotest
thrombotic
    t. aneurysm
    t. endocarditis
    t. infarct
    t. microangiopathy
    t. obstruction
    t. occlusion
    t. pulmonary artery (TPA)
    t. pulmonary embolism
ThromboView imaging agent
thrombus, *pl.* **thrombi**
    adherent t.
    anechoic t.
    ball-valve t.
    bland t.
    blood plate t.
    t. calcification
    calcified t.
    coral t.
    echogenic intraluminal t.
    t. embolus
    t. extension
    t. formation
    iliocaval t.
    intraaneurysmal t.
    intraarterial t.
    intraatrial t.
    intracardiac t.
    intraluminal t.

    intramural t.
    intravascular tumor t.
    intraventricular t.
    laminar intraluminal t.
    laser desiccation of t.
    mobile t.
    mural t.
    mycotic t.
    t. nidus
    obstructive t.
    occlusive arterial t.
    organized t.
    pedunculated t.
    percutaneous dissolution of t.
    pericatheter t.
    peroneal t.
    platelet-rich t.
    primary t.
    t. propagation
    t. remodeling
    tibial obliterative t.
    traumatic t.
    tumor t.
    ultrasonic lysis of t.
through-and-through
    t.-a.-t. fracture
    t.-a.-t. guidewire
    t.-a.-t. injury
through-plane flow
through-slice motion
through-sound transmission
through-the-scope
through-transfer imaging
through-transmission
thrower's
    t. elbow
    t. fracture
throwing arm injury
thrush breast heart
thrusting ventricle
thulium-holmium-chromium:YAG laser
thulium thumbprinting
thumb
    adducted t.
    adductor sweep of t.
    basal joint of t.
    base of t.
    bowler's t.
    cortical t.
    t. extensor tendon
    t. flexor tendon
    floating t.
    gamekeeper's t.
    hitchhiker's t.
    hypoplastic t.
    skier's t.
    triphalangeal t.
    t. web
thumb-in-palm deformity

thumbprint appearance
thumbprinting
>   t. appearance of colon
>   gastric t.
>   thulium t.

thump
>   wall t.

Thurston
>   T. Holland fracture
>   T. Holland sign

10th-value layer
thymectomy
thymi (*pl. of* thymus)
thymic
>   t. agenesis
>   t. carcinoid
>   t. carcinoma
>   t. cyst
>   t. dysplasia
>   t. enlargement
>   t. epithelial neoplasm
>   t. hyperplasia
>   t. index
>   t. lymphoma
>   t. mass
>   t. neoplasia
>   t. pseudomass
>   t. rebound
>   t. sail sign
>   t. shadow

thymidine
>   t. labeling index (TLI)
>   t. phosphorylase (TP)
>   t. suicide study
>   tritiated t.

thymion
thymokesis
thymokinetic
thymolipoma
thymoma
>   benign t.
>   malignant t.
>   noninvasive t.
>   t. of heart

thymotoxic
thymus, *pl.* **thymi**
>   congenital absence of t.
>   diffuse enlargement of t.
>   ectopic t.
>   t. gland
>   mass t.
>   solid lesion t.
>   t. weight

ThyRex timer
thyroarytenoid
thyrocardiac disease
thyrocervical
>   t. trunk
>   t. trunk of subclavian artery

thyroepiglottic ligament
thyroglossal
>   t. duct
>   t. duct cyst
>   t. duct remnant
>   t. tract

thyrohyoid ligament
thyroid
>   t. abscess
>   t. acropachy
>   t. adenoma
>   t. adenoma calcification
>   t. adenoma nodule
>   t. artery
>   t. bed
>   t. capsule
>   t. carcinoma
>   t. cartilage
>   cold nodule of t.
>   t. colloid nodule
>   t. cyst
>   t. cystadenoma
>   cystic area t.
>   t. degeneration
>   t. disease
>   dual ectopic t.'s
>   t. dysgenesis
>   t. eminence
>   t. follicle
>   t. gland
>   t. gland inflammation
>   t. goiter
>   t. hyperplasia
>   t. incidentaloma
>   t. insufficiency
>   intrathoracic t.
>   iodine-123 t.
>   t. isthmus
>   lingual t.
>   t. lobe
>   t. lymph node
>   t. lymph node scintigraphy
>   t. lymphoma
>   t. mass
>   t. metastasis
> ^{99m}Tc pertechnetate t.
>   multinodular t.
>   multiple ectopic t.'s
>   t. ophthalmopathy
>   t. orbitopathy
>   t. organification defect
>   papillary microcarcinoma of t.
>   t. plasmacytoma
>   t. primordium
>   t. psammoma body
>   t. radioiodine treatment
>   t. radioiodine uptake
>   t. remnant
>   retrosternal t.

T

thyroid (*continued*)
- t. scintigraphy
- t. stimulation scan
- t. storm
- t. stunning
- substernal t.
- t. suppression scan
- t. trapping defect
- t. ultrasonography imaging
- t. uptake measurement
- t. whole-body scan

thyroid-associated orbitopathy
thyroidectomy
- completion t.
- subtotal t.
- total t.

thyroiditis
- acute suppurative t.
- aspecific lymphocytic t.
- chronic lymphocytic t.
- de Quervain t.
- Hashimoto t.
- nonspecific lymphocytic t.
- painless t.
- Riedel t.
- subacute t.
- suppurative t.

thyroid-stimulating hormone (TSH)
thyrolingual cyst
thyrotoxicosis medicamentosa
thyrotoxic periodic paralysis (TPP)
thyrotroph cell adenoma
thyrotropin-releasing hormone (TRH)
thyroxin (*var. of* thyroxine)
thyroxine, thyroxin (T$_4$, T4)
- t. iodine (TI)
- labeled t.
- radioactive t.
- radiolabeled t.

TI
- inversion time
- thyroxine iodine
  - dual-isotope TI 201

TIA
- transient ischemic attack
- carotid distribution TIA
- crescendo TIA
- ipsilateral hemispheric carotid TIA

tibarius
- torsus t.

tibia, *pl.* **tibiae**
- anterior bowing of t.
- t. bone
- focal fibrocartilaginous dysplasia of t.
- posteromedial t.
- proximal t.

repetitive anterior subluxation of t.
- t. vara

tibiae (*pl. of* tibia)
tibial
- t. artery
- t. artery disease
- t. bending fracture
- t. bone marrow development
- t. collateral ligament
- t. collateral ligament bursa
- t. condyle
- t. condyle fracture
- t. crest
- t. diaphysial fracture
- t. epiphysis
- t. flare
- t. hallux sesamoid
- t. intercondylar eminence
- t. medullary canal
- t. node
- t. obliterative thrombus
- t. open fracture
- t. pilon fracture
- t. plafond
- t. plafond fracture
- t. plateau
- t. plateau depression
- t. plateau fracture
- t. pseudarthrosis
- t. sesamoid bone
- t. sesamoid ligament
- t. sesamoid position
- t. shaft fracture
- t. spine
- t. stress fracture
- t. tendon
- t. tendon tear
- t. torsion
- t. translation
- t. triplane fracture
- t. tubercle
- t. tubercle ossification center
- t. tubercle prominence
- t. tuberosity
- t. tuberosity fracture
- t. varus
- t. vein

tibialis
- t. anterior
- t. anterior tendon
- t. posterior
- t. posterior tendon
- t. posterior tenosynovitis
- t. sign

tibiocalcaneal
- t. angle
- t. fusion
- t. joint complex
- t. ligament

tibiofemoral
 t. angle (TFA)
 t. joint dislocation
tibiofibular
 t. articulation
 t. diastasis
 t. fracture
 t. joint
 t. ligament
 t. syndesmosis
 t. synostosis
tibiofibularis
 syndesmosis t.
tibioligamentous fascicle
tibionavicular ligament
tibioperoneal
 t. occlusive disease
 t. runoff system
 t. trunk
tibiotalar
 t. angle
 t. joint
 t. rotation
tibiotalocalcaneal fusion
tibiotarsal dislocation
TIC
 time-intensity curve
TICA
 traumatic intracranial aneurysm
ticlopidine
tidal
 t. breathing
 t. inspiratory flow volume
 t. wave of carotid arterial
 pulse
tiered therapy
tie sternum
Tietze syndrome
TIFF
 tag image file format
tight
 t. dural sac
 t. filum terminale
 t. filum terminale syndrome
 t. lesion
 t. spinal canal
tigroid
 t. demyelination
 t. pattern
Tikhonov regularization
tile mode display
Tillaux-Chaput anterolateral tibial epiphysis fracture
Tillaux fracture
Tillaux-Kleiger fracture
tilt
 bent-knee pelvic t.
 caudal t.
 gantry t.

infundibular t.
lunate t.
palmar t.
patellar t.
t. table
valgus t.
varus t.
volar t.
tilted
 t. optimized nonsaturating excitation (TONE)
 t. sacrum
tilting-disc valve
time
 acceleration t.
 acquisition t.
 activated partial thromboplastin t.
 arm-lung t.
 asymmetric appearance t.
 atrial activation t.
 atrioventricular t.
 bolus arrival t. (BAT)
 calculated clearance t.
 capillary filling t.
 carotid ejection t.
 cerebral circulation t.
 chromoscopy t.
 circulation t.
 colonic transit t.
 concentration times t. (C × T)
 t. constant
 conventional ultrashort echo t.
 corrected sinus node recovery t.
 correlation t.
 t. correlation function
 cycle t.
 data acquisition t.
 dead t.
 decay t.
 deceleration t.
 delayed transit t.
 t. delay integration (TDI)
 diastolic perfusion t.
 diffusion t.
 t. domain
 doubling t.
 echo delay t.
 echo-train echo t.
 effective transverse relation t.
 efficient relaxation t.
 ejection t.
 emptying t.
 esophageal transit t.
 fat and long T2-suppressed ultrashort echo t. (FLUTE)
 fat-suppressed ultrashort echo t. (FUTE)
 fixing t.
 fluoroscopy t.

time (*continued*)
t. following inversion pulse
gantry rotation t.
gastric transit t.
half emptying t. (T 1/2)
image acquisition t.
image reconstruction t.
imaging t.
increased left ventricular ejection t.
interecho t.
interpulse t.
inversion t. (TI)
ischemic t.
isovolumic contraction t.
isovolumic relaxation t. (IVRT)
lattice relaxation t.
left ventricular ejection t. (LVET)
left ventricular fast filling t.
left ventricular slow filling t.
longitudinal recovery t.
longitudinal relaxation t.
long ultrashort T2-suppressed
   echo t.
maximum inflation t.
maximum walking t.
mean circulation t. (MCT)
mean examination t.
mean pulmonary transit t.
mean transit t. (MTT)
membrane closure t.
t. motion (TM)
myocardial contrast appearance t.
   (MCAT)
^{23}Na MR imaging with short
   echo t.
t. of formation of RF spin-echo
   when adjusted to be different
   from gradient spin-echo
overall treatment t.
perfusion t.
phasing-in t.
t. point
prolonged ejection t.
proton spin-lattice relaxation t.
pulse reappearance t.
pulse repetition t.
pulse transit t. (PTT)
pyelographic appearance t.
radionuclide esophageal dead t.
ramp t.
reaction recovery t.
receiver dead t.
recovery t.
regional mean transit t. (rMTT)
relaxation t.
repetition t. (RT)
resolving t.
retinocortical t.
right ventricle-to-ear t.

rise t.
rotational correlation t.
scan t.
sequence t.
short echo t.
short T1 relaxation t.
sinuatrial conduction t. (SACT)
sinus node recovery t. (SNRT)
small bowel transit t.
sojourn t.
spin-lattice relaxation t.
spin-spin relaxation t.
subsecond gantry rotation t.
systolic acceleration t.
systolic upstroke t.
thermal relaxation t.
t. to local failure
t. to peak (TTP)
t. to peak activity
t. to peak contrast (TPC)
t. to peak filling (TTPF)
t. to peak filling rate (TPFR)
t. to peak intensity
t. to peak value
t. to PME
transit t.
transverse relaxation t.
trigger delay t.
T1, T2 relaxation t.
tumor sojourn t.
venous filling t. (VFT)
venous refill t. (VRT)
venous return t.
ventricular activation t. (VAT)
ventricular isovolumic
   relaxation t.
t. without symptoms and toxicity
time-action analysis
time-activity curve
time-adaptive SENSE (TSENSE)
time-attenuation curve
time-averaged flow
time-compensated gain
time-course fracture scintigraphy
timed
t. bolus delivery
t. imaging
t. sequential therapy
time-density curve
time-dependent
t.-d. metabolic cascade
t.-d. xenon concentration
time-efficient T2 relaxometry
time-gain compensation (TGC)
time-insensitive
time-intensity curve (TIC)
**time-lapse quantitative computed
   tomographic lymphography**
time-motion mode (M-mode)

time-of-flight (TOF)
t.-o.-f. echo-planar imaging
t.-o.-f. effect
electron t.-o.-f. (E-TOF)
t.-o.-f. enhancement
t.-o.-f. flow measurement
t.-o.-f. magnetic resonance
angiography (TOF-MRA)
t.-o.-f. method
t.-o.-f. PET imaging system
t.-o.-f. signal loss

time-out
ventriculoatrial t.-o.

time-proportional phase incrementation (TPPI)

timer
ThyRex t.

time-resolved
t.-r. CE MRA
t.-r. 3D imaging
t.-r. echo-shared angiographic
technique (TREAT)
t.-r. imaging by automatic data
segmentation (TRIADS)
t.-r. imaging of contrast kinetics
(TRICKS)

time-reversal method of focal reconstruction

time-sensitive

time-to-distant failure

time-to-repetition (TR)

time-to-treatment
t.-t.-t. bias
t.-t.-t. failure (TTF)

time-varied
t.-v. gain (TVG)
t.-v. gain control

time-varying magnetic field

time-velocity
t.-v. integral
t.-v. measurement

time-weighted average

TIMI
thrombolysis in myocardial
infarct

timing
bolus t.
gradient t.
t. parameter
urographic scan t.

tin (Sn)
t. 113 (^{113}Sn, Sn-113)
t. oxide inhalation
t. sulfide
t. with indium 113m

tine

Tinel sign

tinnitus

tiny ventricle

tip
active needle t.
t. angle
catheter t.
conus t.
t. deflector
t. dispersion characteristic
hockey-stick appearance of catheter
t.
mitral valve leaflet t.
occipital t.
t. of spleen
petrous t.
pole t.
radiopaque distal t.
rectal t.
t. trauma
valve t.

tip-deflecting guidewire

TIPS
transjugular intrahepatic portosystemic
shunt
elective TIPS
TIPS failure
TIPS imaging

TIRP
transcatheter intravascular ring platform

tissue
aberrant t.
abnormal t.
t. adhesive
adipose t.
adventitial t.
aerated t.
anisotropic t.
apical t.
arcolar connective t.
bony t.
breast t.
bronchus-associated lymphoid t.
(BALT)
brown adipose t. (BAT)
cancellous t.
t. capsule
cartilaginous t.
cavernous t.
t. characterization
t. characterization technique
chondroid t.
chorionic t.
collagenous t.
t. conductivity
connective t.
t. contrast
t. cooling
cortical t.
crushed t.
dartoic t.
dead t.

T

tissue (*continued*)

t. deficit compensator
degenerated t.
dense connective t.
t. density
destruction of t.
devitalized t.
diamagnetic t.
disc t.
t. Doppler imaging
ectopic endometrial t.
ectopic thyroid t.
edematous t.
engorged t.
escape of air into lung
  connective t.
extraadrenal chromaffin t.
extralobular connective t.
exuberant granulation t.
fascial connective t.
fast-exchange soft t.
fatty prostatic t.
fetal lymphoid t.
fibroadipose t.
fibroareolar t.
fibrocartilaginous t.
fibrocollagenous connective t.
fibrofatty breast t.
fibroglandular t.
fibroinflammatory t.
fibromuscular t.
fibrosing t.
fibrotic t.
fibrous connective t.
fibrous scar t.
fibrovascular t.
t. flow
gangrenous t.
gastrointestinal-associated
  lymphoid t.
gelatinous t.
granulation t.
grumous t.
gut-associated lymphoid t.
  (GALT)
t. harmonic imaging (THI)
t. harmonic sonography
hyalinized fibrocollagenous t.
hypermetabolic brown adipose t.
  (HBAT)
hyperplastic t.
hypertrophic t.
hypervascular granulation t.
hypoechoic t.
hypoenhanced t.
t. imprint
indurated t.
t. inhibitor of metalloproteinase
t. inhomogeneity factor

interlobular t.
interstitial t.
intertrabecular soft t.
intralobular connective t.
intrasplenic t.
t. island
island of t.
isointense soft t.
isotropic t.
joint t.
late effect of normal t. (LENT)
lipomatous t.
loose mesenchymal t.
lymphatic t.
lymph node t.
lymphoreticular t.
t. magnetization
mammary t.
t. mass
mediastinal thyroid t.
mesenchymal t.
mesenteric t.
t. migration
mucosa-associated lymphoid t.
  (MALT)
muscle t.
necrotic t.
neoplastic t.
neural crest t.
nodal t.
noncontractile scar t.
noncritical soft t.
nonviable t.
t. of fetus
osseous tumor of soft t.
osteocartilaginous t.
t. outflow valve
t. oxygenation
paraffin-embedded t.
paratracheal soft t.
paravaginal soft t.
parenchymatous t.
passively congested lung t.
t. perfusion
periarticular t.
peribronchial connective t.
perilobular connective t.
peritumoral t.
t. plasminogen activator
t. plate
postcricoid soft t.
postoperative scar t.
postpharyngeal soft t.
preepiglottic soft t.
prevertebral soft t. (PVST)
proliferation of fibrous t.
regeneration of t.
regressed adenoidal t.
regular connective t.

t. relaxometry
residual ductal t.
reticular connective t.
retrodiscal t.
retropharyngeal soft t.
retrosternal soft t.
retrotracheal soft t.
revascularized t.
scar t.
t. sequela
t. signature
t. slice
slow-exchange soft t.
soft t.
t. space
stippled soft t.
stringlike band of
  fibrous t.
subadventitial t.
subcutaneous connective t.
suppressed t.
swollen t.
sympathetic nervous t.
syngeneic t.
synovial t.
taenia t.
target t.
tendon t.
testicular adrenal rest t.
therapy-related fibrous t.
thickened hypoechoic t.
thoracic inlet soft t.
t. tolerance dose (TTD)
t. tolerance to radiation
tongue of t.
tuberculosis granulation t.
underlying t.
vascular t.
vascularized granulation t.
t. veil
ventricular soft t.
t. viability
visceral adipose t.
  (VAT)
t. water content
t. weighting factor
white adipose t.
white cottonlike fibrous t.

tissue-air
  t.-a. interface
  t.-a. ratio (TAR)
tissue-based T2 relaxation
tissue-equivalent detector
tissue-maximum ratio (TMR)
tissue-phantom ratio (TPR)
tissue-specific imaging agent
tissue-type plasminogen activator
titanate
  barium t.

titanium
  t. compound
  t. dioxide
  t. Greenfield filter
  t. plate
  t. Vortex port system
titrate
  gallium t.
Titterington position
TIV
  total intracranial volume
TJLB
  transjugular liver biopsy
TKA
  total knee arthroplasty
^{201}Tl, T1-201
  thallium 201
    Tl-201 chloride
TLA
  translumbar aortography
    TLA needle
TLB
  transjugular liver biopsy
TLD
  thermoluminescent
    dosimeter
  tumor lethal dose
    TLD rod
TLE
  temporal lobe epilepsy
    refractory TLE
TLI
  thymidine labeling index
TM
  time motion
    TM ultrasound
TMA
  transmetatarsal amputation
  true metatarsus adductus
TME
  trapezium-metacarpal eburnation
    TME ratio
TMJ
  temporomandibular joint
TMR
  tissue-maximum ratio
  topical magnetic resonance
  transmyocardial revascularization
TMS
  transcranial magnetic stimulation
**Tmx-2000 BPH thermotherapy
  system**
TMZ
  transformation zone
TNB
  transthoracic needle biopsy
TNM
  tumor, nodal involvement,
    metastasis

T

TNR
>tumor-to-normal tissue ratio

TOA
>tuboovarian abscess

to-and-fro flow

tobacco
>t. heart
>t. nodule

tocolysis

tocopherol
>alpha t.
>gamma t. (gamma-T)

TOCU
>transoral carotid ultrasonography
>TOCU for internal carotid artery stenosis

Todani classification

Todani-type cyst

Todaro triangle

Todd cirrhosis

toddler's fracture

TODE
>total organ dose equivalent

Tod muscle

toe
>base of t.
>claw t.
>t. extensor tendon
>monophalangic great t.
>Morton t.
>overriding t.
>tennis t.

TOF
>tetralogy of Fallot
>time-of-flight
>TOF imaging
>TOF sequence
>TOF signal loss

TOF-MRA
>time-of-flight magnetic resonance angiography

toggle sign

toggling-table technique

Toldt
>white line of T.

tolerance
>drug t.
>Fletcher rule of irradiation t.
>irradiation t.
>narrow gating t.

Tolosa-Hunt syndrome

tombstone
>t. pelvis
>t. pelvis configuration

Tomocat imaging agent

tomogram, planogram, planigram
>blurred-image t.
>Bucky t.
>coned panoramic t.

plain t.
sagittal t.
single-slice long-axis t.
stacked t.
temporal bone t.

tomograph
>Heidelberg retina t. (II) (HRT-II)

tomographic
>t. brain scan
>t. cut
>t. emission image
>t. imaging
>t. modality
>t. multiplane scanner
>t. section
>t. skull immobilizer
>t. slice
>t. view

tomography, planigraphy, planography
>automated computed axial t. (ACAT)
>axial transverse t.
>bone computed t.
>cardiac gated quantitative computed t.
>cardiac multidetector row computed t.
>^{11}C-methionine positron emission t. (MET-PET)
>coincidence detection positron emission t.
>computed t. (CT)
>computed axial t. (CAT)
>computed tomography-positron emission t. (CT-PET)
>computed tomography/single-photon emission computed t. (CT/SPECT)
>computed transmission t.
>computerized axial t. (CAT)
>computerized cranial t.
>computerized transverse axial t. (CTAT)
>contrast-enhanced computed t. (CECT)
>conventional t.
>cranial computed t. (CCT)
>digital axial t. (DAT)
>direct imaging of local gradients by group echo selection t. (DIGGEST)
>dual-energy contrast-enhanced computed t.
>dual-phase helical computed t. (DHCT)
>dual-source computed t. (DSCT)
>dynamic computed t. (DCT)
>dynamic computerized t.
>electrical impedance t. (EIT)
>electrocardiogram-gated high-speed x-ray computed t.
>electron beam t. (EBT)

electron beam computed t. (EBCT)
emission t.
emission computed t. (ECT)
emission computer-assisted t.
emission computerized axial t.
  (ECAT)
endoscopic optical coherence t.
  (EOCT)
exercise thallium-201 t.
expiratory computed t.
FDG positron emission t.
^{18}F-fluorodeoxyglucose positron
  emission t. (^{18}FDG-PET)
flat-panel detector-based volumetric
  computed t.
flat-panel volume computed t.
  (FPVCT)
flow-mode ultrafast computed t.
fluoride ion positron emission t.
fluorine-18
  fluorodeoxyglucose-positron
  emission t.
fluorodeoxyglucose positron emission
  t. (FDG-PET)
focal plane t.
focused appendix computed t.
  (FACT)
gated single-photon emission
  computed t. (GSPECT)
gradient-echo single-photon
  emission-computed t.
helical biphasic computed t.
  (HBCT)
high-resolution computed t. (HRCT)
high-resolution 3D microcomputed t.
high spatial resolution cine
  computed t. (HSRCCT)
high temporal resolution cine
  computed t. (HTRCCT)
H2-150 positron emission t.
hypercycloidal t.
hypocycloidal t.
indirect computed t.
intravascular contrast-enhanced
  computed t.
kidney t.
lateral t.
limited-slice computed t.
linear t.
longitudinal section t.
low-dose hepatic multidetector
  computed t.
magnetic resonance t. (MRT)
metrizamide myelography computed t.
microcomputed t.
multidetector computed t.
multidetector-row helical computed t.
multiphasic perfusion computed t.
multiphasic renal computerized t.

multislice spiral computed t.
myocardial perfusion t.
NewTom VG cone beam t.
nonenhanced computed t. (NECT)
nuclear magnetic resonance t.
optic coherence t. (OCT)
optic Doppler t. (ODT)
panoramic t.
peripheral quantitative computed t.
  (pQCT)
phase-contrast x-ray computed t.
  (PCCT)
2-phase helical computed t.
plesiosectional t.
pluridirectional t.
polycycloidal t.
polydirectional t.
portal-enhanced computed t.
positron emission t. (PET)
positron emission transaxial t.
  (PETT)
positron emission transverse t. (PETT)
process t.
quadruple-phase helical computed t.
quantitative computed t. (QCT)
quantitative contrast-enhanced
  computed t. (QECT)
radionuclide emission t.
rapid-acquisition computed t.
rectilinear t.
reformatted computed t.
rotational t.
sellar t.
simultaneous multifilm t.
single-detector computed t. (SDCT)
single-photon emission t. (SPET)
single-photon emission computed t.
  (SPECT)
skip t.
spiral computed t. (SCT)
spiral x-ray computed t. (SXCT)
thin-section dual-phase
  multidetector-row computed t.
transmission computed t.
transmission computer-assisted t.
  (TCAT)
transverse t.
trispiral t.
tuned aperture computed t. (TACT)
UHR optical coherence t.
ultrafast computed t. (UFCT)
ultrafast CT electron beam t.
ultrasonic t.
ultrasound computed t. (UCT)
ultrasound diffraction t.
volumetric computed t.
water-contrast computed t.
whole-body computed t.
wide-angle t.

T

tomography (*continued*)
    xenon computed t.
    xenon-enhanced computed t. (XeCT)
    x-ray computed t. (XCT)
Tomolex tomographic system
Tomomatic 2-, 3-, 5-slice SPECT
   imaging system
tomomyelography
Tomoscan
    T. AVEU spiral CT scanner
    T. SR 7000 scanner
tomoscintigraphy
tomoscopy
tomosynthesis
    circular t.
    digital t.
tomotherapy
    T. Hi-ART system
    nomosSTAT serial t.
TomTec
TONE
   tilted optimized nonsaturating excitation
   TONE sequence
tone
    vascular t.
tongue
    t. carcinoma
    t. fasciculation
    t. fracture of calcaneus
    t. of tissue
    t. stud artifact
    venous malformation of t.
tongue-shaped villus
tongue-type intraarticular fracture
tonically contracted sphincter
tonic-clonic seizure
tonography
    carotid compression t.
tonometric blood pressure monitor
tonsil
    adenoid t.
    buried t.
    cerebellar t.
    eustachian t.
    faucial t.
    hypertrophic lingual t.
    lingual t.
    t. of torus tubarius
    palatine t.
    pharyngeal t.
    tubal t.
tonsillar, tonsillary
    t. carcinoma
    t. ectopia
    t. fossa
    t. herniation
    t. papilloma
    t. pillar
tonsillary (*var. of* tonsillar)

tonsillitis
tonus
    arterial t.
tool
    automatic registration t.
    Quant-X color quantification imaging
     t.
    surgical anatomy visualization and
     navigation t. (SAVANT)
tooth, *pl.* **teeth**
    connate t.
    fibroosteoma of t.
    floating t.
    Hutchinson teeth
    incisor t.
    milk t.
    molar t.
    premolar t.
    primary t.
    secondary t.
    t. sign
    supernumerary t.
    wisdom t.
toothed vertebra
toothpaste shadow
top
    Bicor T.
    t. normal limits of size
    t. of carotid T occlusion
Topaz CO$_2$ laser
tophaceous gout
tophi (*pl. of* tophus)
tophus, *pl.* **tophi**
    t. formation
    gouty t.
topical
    t. magnetic resonance (TMR)
    t. water-soluble contrast medium
topo
    topoisomerase
    topo II
topodermatography
topogram
topographic
    t. identification
    t. measurement
topography
    arterial t.
    balloon t.
    ocular globe t.
    scintigraphic balloon t.
    vessel t.
    x-ray t.
topoisomerase (topo)
    t. II (topo II)
torch
    saline t.
Torcon blue catheter
torcular herophili

torcular-lambdoid inversion
tori (*pl. of* torus)
Tornado coil
torn meniscotibial ligament
Tornwaldt, Thornwaldt
    T. bursitis
    T. cyst
torque
    high t.
    t. stress
torqueable guidewire
torque-control guidewire
Torre syndrome
torr pressure
torsed
    t. ovarian mass
    t. testis
torsion
    t. abnormality
    acute testicular t.
    adnexal t.
    t. alignment
    chronic testicular t.
    t. deformity
    external tibial t.
    extravaginal testicular t.
    t. fracture
    gallbladder t.
    t. impaction force
    internal tibial t. (ITT)
    internal tibiofibular t.
    intravaginal t.
    lung t.
    missed testicular t.
    t. of fracture fragment
    t. of testis
    ovarian t.
    painless t.
    spermatic cord t.
    splenic t.
    t. stress
    subacute testicular t.
    testicular appendage t.
    tibial t.
    t. wedge nonunion
torsional attenuated diameter (TAD)
torso phased-array coil (TPAC)
torsus tibarius
torticollis
tortuosity
    elongation and t.
    t. of cervical vessel
    t. of ureter
    vessel t.
tortuous
    t. aorta
    t. aortic arch
    t. emptying
    t. esophagus

    t. vein
    t. vein dilation
    t. vessel
toruloma
torus, *pl.* **tori**
    t. fracture
    t. hyperplasia
    t. mandibularis
    t. pylorus
    t. tubarius
TOS
    thoracic outlet stenosis
    thoracic outlet syndrome
Toshiba
    T. Aplio xV tissue Doppler and
      contrast imaging technology
    T. Aspire continuous imaging
    T. GGA 9300 camera
    T. MR scanner
    T. 900S helical CT scanner
    T. 900S/XII scanner
    T. TCT-80 CT scanner
    T. Xpress SX helical CT scanner
    T. X-Vigor scanner
    T. Xvision scanner
total
    t. ablation
    t. androgen suppression therapy
    t. anomalous pulmonary venous
      connection
    t. anomalous pulmonary venous
      drainage (TAPVD)
    t. anomalous pulmonary venous
      return (TAPVR)
    t. artificial heart
    t. atrial refractory period (TARP)
    t. body irradiation
    t. body scan imaging
    t. body scanning
    t. body water (TBW)
    t. brain volume (TBV)
    t. calcium score (TCS)
    t. cerebral blood flow (TCBF)
    t. condylar depression fracture
    t. effective dose equivalent (TEDE)
    t. exchangeable potassium (TEK)
    t. exchangeable sodium (TENa)
    t. image noise
    t. intracranial volume (TIV)
    t. knee arthroplasty (TKA)
    t. knee implant
    t. lesion
    t. liver perfusion
    t. lung capacity
    t. lymphoid irradiation
    t. lymphoid radiation
    t. mesorectal excision
    t. necrosis
    t. occlusion

T

total (*continued*)
- t. organ dose equivalent (TODE)
- t. parenteral nutrition (TPN)
- t. peripheral resistance (TPR)
- t. placenta previa
- t. pulmonary resistance (TPR)
- t. radiation dose
- T. Recall digital imaging system
- t. reference air Kerma (TRAK)
- t. resorption
- t. saturation recovery (TSR)
- t. stroke volume (TSV)
- t. suppression of sideband
- t. thoracic esophagectomy
- t. thyroidectomy

totalis
- situs inversus t.

totipotential stem cell

toto
- in t.

touch preparation

Toulouse-Lautrec syndrome

Touraine-Solente-Golé syndrome

tourniquet
- caval t.
- t. technique

tourniquet-directed approach

towering cerebellum

Towne
- T. position
- T. projection radiograph
- T. view

toxic
- t. adenoma
- t. autonomous nodule
- t. cardiomyopathy
- t. cirrhosis
- t. demyelination
- t. leukoencephalopathy
- t. lung disease
- t. megacolon
- t. multinodular goiter
- t. nodular goiter
- t. nodule
- t. pneumonia
- t. synovitis

toxicity
- bone marrow t.
- carbon monoxide t.
- desferrioxamine t.
- dose-limiting t.
- late central nervous system t.
- pulmonary t.
- radiation-induced pulmonary t.
- time without symptoms and t.

toxin
- bacterial t.

toxoabscess

Toxocara canis

toxoplasmosis
- cerebral t.
- CNS t.
- t. encephalitis

Toynbee muscle

TP
- thymidine phosphorylase

TPA
- thrombotic pulmonary artery

TPAC
- torso phased-array coil

TPBS
- 3-phase bone scintigraphy

TPC
- time to peak contrast

TPFR
- time to peak filling rate

TPN
- total parenteral nutrition

T-portagram

TPP
- thyrotoxic periodic paralysis

TPPI
- time-proportional phase incrementation

TPR
- tissue-phantom ratio
- total peripheral resistance
- total pulmonary resistance

TR
- time-to-repetition
- ultralong TR
- variable TE, TR

trabecula, *pl.* **trabeculae**
- bony t.
- septomarginal t.

trabeculae (*pl. of* trabecula)

trabecular
- t. architecture
- t. bone
- t. bone detail
- t. bone resorption
- t. carcinoma
- t. degeneration
- t. destruction
- t. disruption
- t. fracture
- t. microfracture
- t. osteoma
- t. pattern
- t. thickening
- t. weakening

trabeculated
- t. atrium
- t. bone
- t. bone lesion
- t. osteolysis
- t. outline

trabeculation
    endocardial t.
trabeculectomy
    argon laser t.
trabeculoplasty
trace
    t. amount of radiopharmaceutical
    t. edema
    t. element distribution
    t. map
tracer
    t. abnormality
    t. accumulation
    t. activity
    t. bolus
    t. concentration equation
    delayed transport of t.
    deposition of t.
    diffusible t.
    t. dose
    extravasated t.
    focal pooling of t.
    gold-195m t.
    t. horseradish peroxidase
    t. kinetic modeling
    T. microcatheter
    ^{13}N ammonia radioactive t.
    neutron-rich biomedical t.
    patchy distribution of t.
    t. principle
    radioactive t.
    radioisotope-labeled t.
    radiolabeled t.
    radiopharmaceutical t.
    shunted t.
    static rCBF t.
    t. study
    tantalum t.
    transependymal uptake
      of t.
    tumor-specific t.
    t. uptake
trachea, *pl.* **tracheae**
    anular ligament of t.
    bifurcatio tracheae
    carina of t.
    carrot-shaped t.
    intrathoracic t.
    lunate-shaped t.
    napkin-ring t.
    saber-sheath t.
    scabbard t.
tracheae (*pl. of* trachea)
tracheal
    t. anastomosis
    t. aspiration
    t. band
    t. bifurcation
    t. bifurcation angle

    t. bronchus
    t. button
    t. caliber
    t. cartilage
    t. deviation
    t. displacement
    t. diverticulosis
    t. fracture
    t. granuloma
    t. lumen
    t. lymph node
    t. mass effect
    t. narrowing
    t. neoplasm
    t. ring
    t. shift
    t. stenosis
    t. stricture
    t. triangle
    t. tube
    t. tumor
    t. wall stripe
trachelocele (*var. of*
 tracheocele)
tracheobiliary fistula
tracheobronchial
    t. angle
    t. aspiration
    t. fistula
    t. foreign body
    t. hypersensitivity
    t. injury (TBI)
    t. lymph node
    t. mucosal necrosis
    t. papillomatosis
    t. rupture
    t. stenting
    t. tree
tracheobronchoesophageal fistula
tracheobronchography
    CT t.
tracheobronchomalacia
    acquired t.
tracheobronchomegaly
    congenital t.
tracheobronchopathia
  osteochondroplastica
tracheobronchoscopy
    CT-based virtual t.
tracheocele, trachelocele
tracheoesophageal (TE)
    t. fistula (TEF)
    t. junction
    t. voicing
tracheomalacia
    congenital t.
tracheopathia, tracheopathy
    t. osteochondroplastica
    t. osteoplastica

tracheopathy (*var. of* tracheopathia)
tracheopulmonary aspiration
tracheostomy tube
trachomatis
    Chlamydia t.
tracing
    carotid pulse t.
    electrocardiogram t.
    paper strip t.
    pulmonary capillary wedge t.
    ray t.
    vessel t.
track
    t. cone length
    deep white matter t.
    t. dilation
    t. etching
    ionization t.
    nephrostomy t.
    t. of pin
    t. valve
trackability
tracker
    T. 10 catheter
    T. Excel catheter
    T. 10 microcatheter
tracking
    abnormal t.
    anterior t.
    automatic peak t. (APT)
    bolus t.
    brain fiber t.
    fiber t.
    focal spot t.
    t. limit
    magnetic bolus t.
    magnetic resonance needle t.
    MR imaging-guided endovascular
      device t.
    periportal t.
    presaturation bolus t.
    real-time biplanar needle t.
    real-time magnetic resonance
      imaging t.
    sheet t.
    stem cell t.
    SureStart contrast t.
    vessel t.
    wall motion t.
tract
    aerodigestive t.
    alimentary t.
    anterior corticospinal t.
    anterior spinocerebellar t.
    anterior spinothalamic t.
    apple-peel appearance of GI t.
    ascending t.
    atriofascicular t.
    atrio-His bypass t.

atrioventricular nodal bypass t.
biliary t.
brainstem pyramidal t.
bronchial t.
bulbar t.
carcinoid GI t.
central tegmental t. (CTT)
cerebellar t.
corticobulbar t. (CBT)
corticopontine t.
corticorubral t.
corticospinal t. (CST)
cuneocerebellar t.
dentatothalamic t.
dermal sinus t.
descending t.
digestive t.
dorsal spinocerebellar t.
dorsolateral t.
extrapyramidal t.
fascial t.
fasiculoventricular bypass t.
fetal urogenital t.
fistulous t.
flow t.
frontopontine t.
frontotemporal t.
gastrointestinal t.
geniculocalcarine t.
genital t.
genitourinary t.
GI t.
hepatic outflow t.
hypothalamohypophysial t.
ileal inflow t.
iliotibial t.
intermediolateral t.
intersegmental t.
intestinal t.
intrahepatic biliary t.
lateral corticospinal t.
lateral lemniscus t.
lateral spinothalamic t.
left ventricular outflow t. (LVOT)
Lissauer t.
long t.
lower t.
mesencephalic t.
motor t.
nucleus of solitary t.
occipitopontine t.
olfactory t.
outflow t.
pancreaticobiliary t.
pilonidal t.
posterior spinocerebellar t.
pyramidal t.
respiratory t.
reticulospinal t.

right ventricular outflow t. (RVOT)
seminal t.
sensory t.
sinus t.
spinocerebellar t.
spinoreticular t.
spinothalamic t.
tectospinal t.
tegmental t.
temporopontine t.
thyroglossal t.
trigeminothalamic t.
upper aerodigestive t.
upper gastrointestinal t.
urinary t.
urogenital t.
ventral spinocerebellar t.
ventral spinothalamic t.
ventricular outflow t.
vestibulospinal t.

traction
    t. anchor
    breast t.
    t. bronchiectasis
    t. bronchiolectasis
    t. diverticulum
    t. epiphysis
    t. exostosis
    t. fracture
    t. radiography
    t. spur

tractogram

tractography
    diffusion-tensor t. (DTT)
    3-dimensional t.

tractotomy
    stereotactic t.

tragi (*pl. of* tragus)

tragus, *pl.* **tragi**

train
    dual-interval echo t. (DIET)
    echo t.
    spin-echo t.

trainer
    virtual endoscopic surgery t. (VEST)

training
    velocity-enhanced resistance t. (VERT)

trajectory
    k-space t.
    stack-of-spirals t.

TRAK
    total reference air Kerma

Trak Back pullback device

TRAM
    transverse rectus abdominis myocutaneous
      TRAM flap

tramline
    t. cortical calcification
    t. effect in liver
    t. shadow

trampoline fracture

tram-track
    t.-t. appearance
    t.-t. ductus arteriosus calcification
    t.-t. gyral calcification
    t.-t. pattern
    t.-t. renal cortical necrosis calcification
    t.-t. streaming

transabdominal
    t. catheterization of thoracic duct
    t. cholangiography
    t. color Doppler sonography
    t. imaging
    t. left lateral retroperitoneal maneuver
    t. pneumoperitoneum
    t. scanning
    t. sonogram
    t. ultrasound (TAUS)
    t. ultrasound scan

transactivator

transanular patch reconstruction

transaortic
    t. radiofrequency ablation
    t. systolic gradient

transapical endocardial ablation

transarterial chemoembolization (TACE)

transaxial
    t. annihilation photon pair
    t. CT scan
    t. fat-saturated 3D image
    t. imaging
    t. joint scan
    t. maximum-intensity projection
    t. PET scan
    t. scan plane
    t. slice
    t. thoracic inlet

transaxillary lateral view

transbrachial arch aortogram

transbronchial
    t. lung biopsy (TBLB)
    t. needle aspiration (TBNA)

transcaphoid fracture

transcapitate fracture

transcarpal amputation

transcatheter
    t. ablation
    t. arterial chemoembolization (TACE)
    t. arterial embolization (TAE)
    t. filter placement
    t. hepatic arterial chemoembolization
    t. intravascular ring platform (TIRP)
    t. oily chemoembolization

T

transcatheter (*continued*)
    radiofrequency modification t.
    t. stent-graft treatment
    t. technique
    t. therapy
transcerebral medullary vein
transcervical
    t. balloon tuboplasty
    t. catheterization of fallopian tube imaging
    t. fallopian tube recanalization
    t. femoral fracture
transchelation
transchondral talar dome fracture
transcondylar
    t. amputation
    t. axis (TCA)
    t. fracture
    t. line
transcoronal STIR image
transcortical
transcranial
    t. color-coded Doppler
    t. color-coded Doppler sonography
    t. color-coded duplex sonography (TCCS)
    t. color-coded duplex ultrasound
    t. Doppler (TCD)
    t. Doppler ultrasound
    t. Doppler velocity
    t. examination
    t. lateral view
    t. magnetic stimulation (TMS)
    t. radiograph
    t. real-time color Doppler imaging
    t. real-time color-flow Doppler sonography
transcutaneous
    t. angiogenesis gene delivery
    t. aortovelography (TAV)
    t. broadband sector transducer
    t. crush injury
    t. electrical nerve stimulator (TENS)
    t. extraction catheter atherectomy
    t. oxygen pressure measurement ($tcPO_2$)
transducer
    Acuson linear-array t.
    Acuson V5M multiplane transesophageal echocardiographic t.
    Acuson 128XP t.
    Aloka SSD-1700 t.
    anular array t.
    ART t.
    t. beam pattern
    biopsy t.

    biplanar t.
    broadband t.
    catheter-borne sector t.
    curved-array t.
    diffracting Doppler t.
    electronic linear-array t.
    endfire t.
    endviewing t.
    epicardial Doppler flow sector t.
    Gaeltec catheter-tip pressure t.
    Gould Statham pressure t.
    high-frequency t.
    high-resolution linear-array t.
    linear t.
    linear-array t.
    Logic 700 MR t.
    magnetic resonance imaging-guided focused ultrasound sector t.
    Millar catheter-tip t.
    M-mode sector t.
    Mountain View t.
    MRI-guided focused ultrasound t.
    multiplanar t.
    phased-array t.
    piezoelectric t.
    PSH-25GT transcranial imaging t.
    puncture t.
    rectal multiplane t.
    sector t.
    signal t.
    sonicating t.
    transcutaneous broadband sector t.
    transesophageal t.
    Ultramark 8 t.
    ultrasound t.
    V510B Biplane TEE t.
    V5M Multiplane t.
transducer-skin interface
transducer-tipped catheter
transduction
    signal t.
transduodenal
    t. endoscopic decompression
    t. endosonography
    t. fiberscopic duct injection
transdural fistula
transection, transsection
    aortic t.
    t. of spinal cord
    spinal cord t.
    traumatic aortic t.
Transend steerable guidewire
transependymal uptake of tracer
transepiphysial fracture
transesophageal
    t. Doppler color-flow imaging
    t. echocardiography (TEE)
    t. echocardiography probe
    t. transducer

transethmoidal encephalocele
transfascial spread
transfemoral
    t. arteriography
    t. cerebral angiography
transfer
    energy t.
    fluorescence resonance energy t.
      (FRET)
    Fourier t.
    gradient-echo MR with
      magnetization t.
    Haas trapezius muscle t.
    t. imaging
    interhemispheric t.
    inversion t.
    t. lesion
    linear energy t. (LET)
    magnetization t. (MT)
    quantitative magnetization t.
    rapid image t.
    saturation t.
    selective population t. (SPT)
    sliding board t.
    ultrafast video t.
    ultrasound guidance during
      embryo t.
transference
transferrin
    indium t.
transfibular fusion
transfixing screw
transforaminal
    t. examination
    t. insonation
    t. window
transform
    automated Hough t.
    cosine t.
    2D Fourier t.
    3-dimensional Fourier t.
      (3DFT)
    2-dimensional Fourier t. (2DFT)
    discrete cosine t.
    discrete Fourier t. (DFT)
    driven equilibrium Fourier t.
    fast Fourier t. (FFT)
    fast inversion-recovery Fourier t.
      (FIRFT)
    Fourier t.
    Fourier discrete t.
    Hough t. (HT)
    t. imaging
    inverse Fourier t. (IFT)
    nuclear magnetic resonance
      Fourier t.
    partially relaxed Fourier t. (PRFT)
    water eliminated Fourier t. (WEFT)
    wavelet t.

transformation
    blastic t.
    cavernous portal vein t.
    t. constant
    enthesopathic t.
    fast Talairach t.
    hemorrhagic t.
    malignant t.
    t. matrix
    photo t.
    rho t.
    Talairach t.
    vascular t.
    t. zone (TMZ)
transformer
    closed-core t.
    Coolidge t.
    distribution t.
    doughnut t.
    t. equation
    filament t.
    high-voltage t.
    t. law
    t. loss
    ratio t.
    real-time chirp Z t.
    step-down t.
    step-up t.
transfusional iron overload
transgastric
    t. echocardiographic view
    t. endosonography
transgluteal CT-guided
  technique
transgression
    cortical t.
transhamate fracture
transhepatic
    t. biliary stent
    t. catheter
    t. cholangiogram (THC)
    t. cholangiogram:yttrium-aluminum-
      garnet (THC:YAG)
    t. drainage
    t. portography
    t. variceal embolization
transhiatal esophagectomy
transient
    t. aplastic crisis (TAC)
    t. AV block
    t. bone marrow edema
    t. bone marrow edema syndrome
    t. cavitation
    t. cerebral ischemia
    t. chyle leak
    t. equilibrium
    t. gallbladder hydrops
    t. hepatic attenuation difference
      (THAD)

T

transient (*continued*)
t. hepatic intensity difference (THID)
t. hiatal hernia
t. intussusception
t. invagination
t. ischemic attack (TIA)
t. ischemic carotid insufficiency
t. left ventricular dilation
t. myocardial ischemia
t. osteoporosis of hip
t. paralysis
t. perfusion defect
t. peritumoral enhancement
t. pleural effusion
t. pseudomass
t. punctate cortical hyperintensity on T1-weighted image
t. regional osteoporosis
t. shunt obstruction
t. sinus arrest
t. 1st-pass effect
t. symmetric pulmonary infiltrate
t. synovitis
t. synovitis of hip
t. tachypnea
t. tricuspid regurgitation
transiliac fracture
transillumination
multispectral diffuse t.
t. of head
transistor
metal oxide semiconductor field effect t. (MOSFET)
thin-film t. (TFT)
transit
biliary-to-bowel t.
bolus t.
delayed small bowel t.
impaired tubular t.
parenchymatous t.
t. scintigraphy
small bowel delayed t.
t. time
tubular t.
t. volume
transition
allowed beta t.
beta t.
t. delay
t. electron
isobaric t.
isomeric t.
t. metal
t. zone (TZ)
transitional
t. carcinoma in situ
t. cell carcinoma (TCC)
t. cell neoplasia
t. kidney cell carcinoma

t. meningioma
t. rhythm
t. ureteral cell carcinoma
t. urethral cell papilloma
t. urinary bladder cell carcinoma
t. vertebra
t. zone fissure
transjugular
t. cholangiogram
t. intrahepatic portosystemic shunt (TIPS)
t. intrahepatic portosystemic shunt gradient
t. intrahepatic portosystemic shunt imaging
t. liver biopsy (TJLB, TLB)
t. portography
t. portosystemic stent-shunt placement
t. venography
translation
condylar t.
parallel mean t.
perpendicular mean t.
radioulnar proximodistal t.
tibial t.
translational
t. diffusion
t. motion
translation-invariant filter
translesional pressure gradient
translocation
t. of coronary artery
robertsonian t.
translucency
nuchal t. (NT)
1st-trimester nuchal t.
translucent
t. depression
t. silicone tube
translumbar
t. amputation
t. aortic route
t. aortography (TLA)
t. aortography needle
transluminal
t. aortic endograft implantation
t. atherectomy
t. balloon angioplasty
t. coronary artery angioplasty complex
t. dilation
t. endarterectomy
t. endografting
t. endovascular stent-graft placement
transluminally placed stent-graft
transmalleolar
t. ankle
t. axis-thigh angle

transmantle dysplasia
transmedial plane
transmesenteric plication
transmetallation assessment
transmetatarsal amputation (TMA)
transmetatarsal-thigh angle
transmissible venereal tumor
transmission
    airborne t.
    t. block
    t. computed tomography
    t. computer-assisted tomography (TCAT)
    t. data
    direct-contact t.
    t. dosimetry
    t. electron microscopic study
    indirect-contact t.
    neutron/gamma t.
    parallel t.
    t. scan
    t. silhouette image
    sound t.
    through-sound t.
transmission-based precaution
transmitral
    t. flow
    t. gradient
transmit-receive coil
transmitter coil
transmural
    t. colitis
    t. fibrosis
    t. inflammation
    t. invasion
    t. match
    t. myocardial infarct
    t. necrosis
    t. steal
transmyocardial
    t. perfusion pressure
    t. revascularization (TMR)
transnasally
transonic
Transonics
    T. flow probe
    T. system
transoral carotid ultrasonography
  (TOCU)
transorally
transorbital window
transosseous venography
transpapillary placement
transparent rendering
transparietal biopsy
transpedicular
    t. decompression
    t. vertebroplasty
transpeptidase
    r-glutamyl t. (r-GT)

transperineal
    t. implant
    t. ultrasonography
    t. ultrasound
transphysial bone bridge
transplant, transplantation
    adult-to-adult liver t.
    allogeneic bone marrow t.
    allogeneic peripheral cell t.
    allogeneic stem cell t.
    antigen-modulated mini-stem
     cell t.
    arteriovenous fistula t.
    autologous bone marrow t. (ABMT)
    autologous hematopoietic progenitor
     cell t.
    autologous peripheral blood stem
     cell t.
    autologous stem cell t.
    bone marrow t.
    cadaveric renal t.
    enteric drained pancreas t.
    heart t.
    heart-lung t.
    hemopoietic stem cell t.
    hepatic t.
    intraarterial ABMMN cell t.
    kidney t.
    kidney-pancreas t.
    liver t.
    living-donor liver t. (LDLT)
    lung t.
    marrow t.
    organ t.
    orthotopic heart t.
    orthotopic liver t.
    pancreas t.
    renal t.
    single-lung t.
    solid organ t.
    split-liver t.
    stem cell t.
    syngeneic bone marrow t.
    tandem t.
transplantation (*var. of* transplant)
transplantectomy
transplutonium radioisotope
transporionic axis
transport
    forward t.
    iodide t.
    Monte Carlo photon t.
     (MCPT)
    mucociliary t.
    reverse t.
transporter
    ATP-binding cassette t.
    dopamine t. (DAT)
    vesicular amine t.

T

transposed
t. adnexa
t. aorta
transposition
atrial t.
carotid-subclavian t.
t. cipher
t. complex
congenitally corrected t.
gastric t.
great vessel t.
inferior vena cava t.
Jatene t.
t. of great arteries (TGA)
t. of great vessels
t. of inferior vena cava
t. of ovaries
subfascial t.
ventricular t.
transpulmonary pressure (Ptp)
transpulmonic gradient
transpupillary therma therapy
transpyloric plane
**transradial styloid perilunate
dislocation**
transradiancy
transradiant
t. air
t. zone
transrectal
t. echography
t. sonography
t. ultrasound (TRUS)
t. ultrasound-guided biopsy of
prostate
transrenal ureteric occlusion
transsacral fracture
**TransScan TS2000 electrical impedance
breast scanning system**
transscaphoid
t. dislocation fracture
t. perilunate dislocation
transscapular view
transsection (*var. of* transection)
transseptal
t. angiocardiography
t. angiography
t. perforation
t. radiofrequency ablation
t. sheath
transspatial disease
transsphincteric anal fistula
transstenotic gradient
transsyndesmotic screw fixation
transtemporal
t. insonation
t. window
transtentorial herniation
transtentorially

transthoracic
t. 3-dimensional echocardiography
t. esophagectomy
t. imaging
t. lateral view
t. needle aspiration biopsy
(TTNAB)
t. needle biopsy (TNB)
t. projection
t. ultrasound
transthyretin
transtrabecular plane
transtracheal aspiration
transtricuspid valve diastolic gradient
transtriquetral fracture
transtubercular plane (TTP)
transudate
transudation of fluid
transudative
t. pericardial fluid
t. pleural effusion
transumbilical plane (TUP)
transureteroureterostomy
transurethral
t. incision of prostate
t. needle ablation (TUNA)
t. resection (TUR)
t. resection of bladder
t. resection of prostate (TURP)
t. ultrasound-guided laser-induced
prostatectomy (TULIP)
transvaginal
t. cone
t. echography
t. hysterosonography (TVHS)
t. implant
t. oocyte retrieval
t. sonography (TVS)
t. ultrasound (TVUS)
t. ultrasound-guided drainage
transvalvular pressure gradient
transvenous
t. digital subtraction angiography
t. implantation
t. occlusion
transversalis fascia
transversarium
foramen t.
transverse
t. acoustic wave
t. anular tear
t. aortic arch
t. atlantal ligament
t. axial ligament
t. band
t. breath-hold gradient-echo
cine-magnetic resonance imaging
t. carpal ligament
t. cerebellar diameter (TCD)

t. cervical ligament
t. colon
t. colon carcinoma
t. colon loop
t. comminuted fracture
t. cord lesion
t. costal facet
t. cranial area
t. crural ligament
t. diameter between ischia
t. ECD brain SPECT image
t. esophageal fold
t. fissure of lung
t. genicular ligament
t. heart
t. humeral ligament
t. hypoplasia
t. intertarsal ligament
t. lie
t. ligament of atlas
t. lucent metaphysial line
t. magnetization
t. maxillary fracture
t. mesocolon
t. metacarpal ligament
t. metatarsal ligament
t. myelitis
t. orientation
t. oval pelvis
t. pelvic diameter
t. pericardial sinus
t. perineal ligament
t. plane
t. plane alignment
t. plane force
t. plane vectorcardiography
t. presentation
t. process
t. process fracture
t. process of vertebra
t. rectus abdominis myocutaneous (TRAM)
t. relaxation
t. relaxation of proton spin
t. relaxation rate
t. relaxation time
t. relaxivity
t. ridge
t. scan
t. section
t. section imaging
t. sinus thrombosis
t. slice
t. suture of Krause
t. tarsal joint
t. temporal gyrus
t. testicular ectopia
t. tibiofibular ligament
t. tomography
t. ultrasound
t. vaginal septum
t. view
transversely oriented endplate compression fracture
transverse/neutral view
transverse-plane PET image
transversum
   septum t.
transversus
   t. abdominis muscle
   situs t.
transvesical oocyte retrieval
Transwell membrane
TRAP
   telomere repeat amplification protocol
   telomeric repeat amplification protocol
trap
   duodenum water t.
   metastable t.
   suction polyp t.
TrapEase
   T. inferior vena cava filter
   T. permanent IVC filter
trapezia (*pl. of* trapezium)
trapeziometacarpal joint
trapezioscaphoid joint
trapeziotrapezoid joint
trapezium, *pl.* **trapezia, trapeziums**
   t. bone
   t. fracture
trapezium-metacarpal
   t.-m. eburnation (TME)
   t.-m. eburnation ratio
trapeziums
trapezius muscle
trapezoid
   t. body
   t. bone
   t. bone of Henle
   t. bone of Lyser
   t. ligament
trapping
   air t.
   gas t.
   t. of aneurysm
   t. of radioisotope
   t. thyroid defect
Traube
   T. heart
   T. sign
trauma, *pl.* **traumata, traumas**
   abdominal blunt t.
   acoustic t.
   asphyxial renal t.
   balloon-related t.
   bladder contusion t.
   blunt chest t.
   blunt gastrointestinal t.

T

trauma (*continued*)
    blunt pancreatic t.
    brain t.
    cardiothoracic t.
    carotid artery dissection t.
    chest wall t.
    craniofacial t.
    eye t.
    facial t.
    focused assessment by sonography
      for t. (FAST)
    focused assessment with sonography
      in t.
    gallbladder t.
    genitourinary tract t.
    GI tract t.
    handheld focused assessment with
      sonography for t. (HHFAST)
    head t.
    hepatic t.
    high-energy t.
    hypovolemia t.
    iatrogenic t.
    kidney t.
    ligamentous t.
    liver t.
    multiple t.'s
    t. oblique view
    ocular t.
    orbital t.
    osseous t.
    pancreatic t.
    pelvic vascular t.
    penetrating t.
    t. register image
    renal t.
    splenic t.
    sustentacular t.
    testicular t.
    tip t.
    urethral t.
    urinary bladder t.
    vascular t.
    vessel t.
traumas (*pl. of* trauma)
traumata (*pl. of* trauma)
traumatic
    t. amputation
    t. aortic disruption
    t. aortic injury (TAI)
    t. aortic pseudoaneurysm
    t. aortic rupture
    t. aortic tear
    t. aortic transection
    t. arthritis
    t. avulsion
    t. bone cyst
    t. bone survey
    t. brain injury (TBI)

    t. clinodactyly
    t. degeneration
    t. diaphragmatic hernia
    t. dislocation
    t. emphysema
    t. fat necrosis
    t. head injury
    t. infarct
    t. intracranial aneurysm (TICA)
    t. lipid cyst
    t. lung cyst
    t. meningeal hemorrhage
    t. meningocele
    t. osteoarthritis
    t. pneumatocele
    t. pneumomediastinum
    t. pneumonia
    t. pneumothorax
    t. rhabdomyolysis
    t. rupture of diaphragm (TRD)
    t. spleen laceration
    t. splenectomy
    t. spondylolisthesis
    t. spondylolysis
    t. syrinx
    t. thrombus
    t. tricuspid incompetence
traumatica
    diplegia spinalis brachialis t.
    myositis ossificans t.
traumatogenic occlusion
traversal
    k-space t.
    tentorial t.
traverse
traversing the fracture
Trax catheter
t-ray
tray
    Müller t.
TRC
    tanned red cell
TRD
    traumatic rupture of diaphragm
    penetrating TRD
Treacher Collins syndrome
TREAT
    time-resolved echo-shared angiographic
    technique
treatment
    allocation of t.
    breast-conservation t.
    cobalt-60 Gamma knife
      radiosurgical t.
    crossfire t.
    early endovascular t.
    endovenous laser t. (EVLT)
    t. energy
    equivalent t.

ferromagnetic microembolization t.
fibrinolytic t.
intensity-modulated radiotherapy t.
(IMRT)
interstitial hyperthermia t.
intracavitary hyperthermia t.
iodine-131 antiferritin t.
low-energy radiofrequency conduction
hyperthermia t.
maintenance immunosuppressive t.
(MIST)
microwave hyperthermia t.
microwave nonsurgical t.
percutaneous tumor t.
t. planning system
t. port
refractory to t.
sonographic planning of oncology t.
(SPOT)
superficial hyperthermia t.
thyroid radioiodine t.
transcatheter stent-graft t.
ultrasound hyperthermia t.

tree
airway t.
arterial t.
t. artifact
bile t.
biliary t.
bronchial t.
coronary artery t.
hepatobiliary t.
iliocaval t.
intrahepatic biliary t.
lower extremity arterial t.
tracheobronchial t.
vascular t.
tree-barking kidney
tree-in-bud
t.-i.-b. bronchiole
t.-i.-b. opacity
t.-i.-b. pattern
t.-i.-b. sign
tree-in-winter bile duct appearance
treelike airway structure
tree-shaped spot
trefoil
t. appearance
t. deformity
t. factor 3 (TFF3)
Treitz
T. fossa
T. hernia
ligament of T.
T. muscle
tremor
Holmes t.
midbrain t.
rubral t.

Trendelenburg
T. position
T. radiograph
trephine
t. biopsy
t. technique
treppe phenomenon
Trerotola thrombectomy device
Trevor disease
Trex digital mammography system
(TDMS)
TRH
thyrotropin-releasing hormone
triad
acute compression t.
Beck t.
Carney t.
Charcot t.
Currarino t.
Cushing t.
Garland t.
Kartagener t.
O'Donoghue unhappy t.
Osler t.
Phemister t.
portal t.
Rigler t.
Saint t.
T. SPECT imaging system
wall-echo shadow t.
Whipple t.
TRIADS
time-resolved imaging by automatic
data segmentation
trial
carotid revascularization
endarterectomy stent t.
CAVATAS t.
European Carotid Surgery T.
Malmo mammographic screening t.
North American Symptomatic
Carotid Artery Endarterectomy T.
PROACT I, II t.
randomized clinical t. (RCT)
SONIA t.
Stroke Outcome and Neuroimaging
of Intracranial Atherosclerosis t.
WASID t.
triamine
triangle
aponeurotic t.
auricular t.
axillary t.
Bolton t.
Bryant t.
Burger scalene t.
Calot t.
cardiohepatic t.
carotid t.

triangle (*continued*)
  cephalic t.
  cervical t.
  clavipectoral t.
  Codman t.
  t. configuration
  crural t.
  cysticohepatic t.
  deltoideopectoral t.
  digastric t.
  Einthoven t.
  facial t.
  femoral t.
  Garland t.
  Gerhardt t.
  Grynfeltt t.
  Henke t.
  Hesselbach t.
  iliofemoral t.
  inguinal t.
  insular t.
  internal jugular t.
  Kager Achilles tendon t.
  Koch t.
  Korányi-Grocco t.
  Labbé t.
  Langenbeck t.
  Lesgaft t.
  Livingston t.
  lumbocostoabdominal t.
  mandibular t.
  mesenteric t.
  t. of Capener
  t. of Laimer
  paramedian t.
  Pawlik t.
  posterior cervical t.
  Raider t.
  Rauchfuss t.
  scalene t.
  Scarpa t.
  submandibular t.
  supraclavicular t.
  sylvian t.
  Todaro t.
  tracheal t.
  urogenital t.
  vertebrocostal t.
  Ward t.
triangular
  t. area of dullness
  t. bone
  t. defect
  t. disc
  t. external ankle fixation
  t. fibrocartilage (TFC)
  t. fibrocartilaginous complex (TFCC)
  t. fontanelle
  t. ligament

    t. muscle
    t. ridge
triangulation
    interactive t.
    t. method
triatrial heart
triatriatum
    cor t.
Triboulet test
tributary
    t. collateral
    extrahepatic portal vein t.
    large venous t.
tricarboxylic
    t. acid (TCA)
    t. acid cycle
triceps, *pl.* **triceps, tricepses**
    t. brachii
    t. brachii tendon
tricepses (*pl. of* triceps)
trichinous embolus
trichloroacetic acid
trichobezoar
trichoptysis
trichorhinophalangeal (TRP)
TRICKS
    time-resolved imaging of contrast
      kinetics
    TRICKS method
tricompartmental chondromalacia of knee
tricorn bucket-handle tear
tricuspid, tricuspidal, tricuspidate
    t. aortic valve
    t. atresia
    t. incompetence
    t. insufficiency
    t. orifice
    t. orifice regurgitation
    t. stenosis
    t. valve anomaly
    t. valve anulus
    t. valve area
    t. valve atresia
    t. valve closure
    t. valve cusp
    t. valve deformity
    t. valve dysplasia
    t. valve flow
    t. valve gradient
    t. valve prolapse
    t. valve regurgitation
    t. valve strut
    t. vertebra
tricuspidal (*var. of* tricuspid)
tricuspidate (*var. of* tricuspid)
tricyclic
trident
    t. hand
    t. pelvis

Tridrate bowel preparation
trifascicular block
trifid
    t. precordial motion
    t. stomach
triflanged nail
trifurcation
    t. of artery
    patency t.
    popliteal artery t.
trigeminal
    t. cavernous fistula
    t. cavity
    t. cistern
    t. ganglion
    t. hemangioma
    t. nerve
    t. nerve anatomy
    t. pattern
    t. rhizotomy
    t. schwannoma
    t. trigonal hypertrophy
trigeminothalamic tract
trigeminy
    ventricular t.
trigger
    t. delay
    t. delay time
    ECG t.
    electrocardiogram t.
    t. finger
    t. finger deformity
    t. point injection
    respiratory t.
triggered
    t. flow mode
    t. pacing mode
triggering
    electrocardiograph t.
    fluoroscopic t.
    navigator echo-based real-time
      respiratory gating and t.
    respiratory t.
triglycine
    technetium 99m mercapto acetyl t.
      (^{99m}Tc-MAG3, Tc99m-MAG3)
trigonal
    t. hypertrophy
    t. muscle
    t. process
trigone
    angle of t.
    collateral t.
    deltoideopectoral t.
    fibrous t.
    Henke t.
    hypertrophied t.
    hypoglossal t.
    inguinal t.

    lateral ventricle t.
    Lieutaud t.
    t. of bladder
    t. of ventricle
    Pawlik t.
    vertebrocostal t.
trigonocephaly
trigonum
    t. calcis
    os t.
    unfused os t.
triiodinated imaging agent
triiodobenzoic
    t. acid
    t. acid contrast medium
triiodothyronine
trilaminar appearance
trilateral retinoblastoma
trilayer appearance
trileaflet aortic valve
trilinear interpolation
trilobate, trilobed
trilobed (*var. of* trilobate)
trilobulation
trilocular heart
trilogy of Fallot
trimalleolar ankle fracture
trimester
    1st t.
    2nd t.
    3rd t.
triode tube
triolein
    iodine-131 t.
Trionix
    T. camera
    T. scanner
    T. SPECT
Trionix-Triad camera
Triosil contrast medium
tripartite duodenal carcinoma
triphalangeal
    t. thumb
    t. thumb deformity
triphasic
    t. spiral CT
    t. waveform
Triphasix generator
triphenyltetrazolium chloride (TTC)
triphosphate
    adenosine t.
    arabinsylguanosine t.
    cyclic guanosine t.
    deoxyguanosine t.
    nucleoside t. (NTP)
triplane fracture
triple
    t. bubble sign
    t. contrast

T

triple (*continued*)
    t. inversion recovery-prepared FSE imaging
    t. label
    t. match
    t. match defect
    t. rule-out protocol
    t. signal pattern
    t. track sign
triple-dose
    t.-d. gadolinium-enhanced MR imaging without MT
    t.-d. gadolinium imaging
    t.-d. MR angiogram
triple-head
    t.-h. coincidence imaging
    t.-h. gamma camera
triple-H therapy
triple-leaf collimator
triple-marker screening test
triple-pass technique
triple-peak cerebellum configuration
triple-phase
    t.-p. bone scan
    t.-p. bone scan imaging
triple-resonance NMR probe circuit
triplet
    t. gestation
    ghost reduction by equalized acquisition t.'s (GREAT)
triple-voiding
    t.-v. cystogram
    t.-v. cystography
triplex-mode Doppler sonography
triplex scanning
tripod
    t. fracture
    t. position
tripoint bullet
Tripter
    Direx T.
triquetral
    t. bone
    t. fracture
    t. impingement
triquetrohamate
    t. helicoid slope
    t. joint
    t. ligament
triquetrolunate dislocation
triquetropisiform articulation
triquetroscaphoid
    t. fascicle
    t. ligament
triquetrotrapezoid fascicle
triquetrum
triradiate cartilage
tris-acryl gelatin microsphere (TAGM, TGMS)

trisegmental image reconstruction
trisodium
    gadofosveset t.
    mangafodipir t.
trisomic fetus
trisomy
    t. D, E syndrome
    t. 8 syndrome
TriSpan
    T. aneurysm neck bridge device
    T. detachable coil
trispiral tomography
tristimulus
    t. value
    t. value flip
tritiated
    t. thymidine
    t. thymidine labeling index
tritium
triton tumor
trocar-cannula technique
trochanter
    greater t.
    lesser t.
trochanterian (*var. of* trochanteric)
trochanteric, trochanterian
    t. bursa
    t. bursitis
    t. flare
    t. spine
trochlea, *pl.* **trochleae**
    peroneal t.
trochleae (*pl. of* trochlea)
trochlear
    t. defect
    t. groove
    t. nerve
    t. nerve neoplasia
    t. notch
    t. process
trochleocapitellar groove
troika
    aponeurotic t.
Troisier
    T. node
    T. sign
Trolard
    vein of T.
trolley track sign
Tron 3 VACI cardiac imaging system
Tronzo intertrochanteric fracture classification (1-3)
trophedema
trophic
    t. fracture
    t. lesion

trophoblastic
- t. material
- t. ring

tropical
- t. pancreatitis
- t. ulcer osteoma

tropic ulcer

tropism
- facet t.
- negative t.
- positive t.

tropolone

tropomyosin

trough
- t. line
- t. line sign
- t. of venous pulse
- X t.
- Y t.

trousers
- military antishock t. (MAST)

Trousseau
- T. sign
- T. syndrome

TRP
- trichorhinophalangeal

TR-TE
- short TR-TE

TR/TE
- repetition time to echo time ratio
- long TR/TE

true
- t. aortic aneurysm
- t. apex
- t. back muscle
- t. channel
- t. conjugate measurement
- t. dynamic joint imaging
- t. event
- t. fast imaging and steady progression
- t. fast imaging with steady-state precession (trueFISP)
- t. heart aneurysm
- t. hermaphroditism
- t. histiocytic lymphoma
- t. intersex
- t. lateral view
- t. lumen
- t. metatarsus adductus (TMA)
- t. mitral stenosis
- t. negative
- t. pelvis
- t. porencephaly
- t. positive
- t. rib
- t. short-axis orientation
- t. suture

- t. umbilical cord knot
- t. unilateral hyperlucent lung
- t. ventricular aneurysm
- t. vertebra
- t. vocal cord

trueFISP
- true fast imaging with steady-state precession
- blood-to-myocardium contrast of trueFISP

true-negative
- t.-n. lesion
- t.-n. mammogram

TruePoint PET-CT technology

true-positive result

TruFill n-BCA surgical glue

Trümmerfeld
- T. scurvy line
- T. zone

trumpeting

trumpetlike pelvocaliceal system

truncal
- t. artery
- t. instability
- t. renal artery stenosis
- t. rhabdomyosarcoma
- t. shortening
- t. valve

truncated
- t. arch index
- t. atrial appendage
- t. NMR probe

truncation
- t. band artifact
- t. error
- t. phenomenon

truncus arteriosus

trunk
- aortopulmonary t.
- arterial brachiocephalic t.
- atrioventricular t.
- bifurcation of t.
- brachiocephalic t.
- bronchomediastinal lymph t.
- celiac t.
- celiomesenteric t.
- cordlike t.
- costocervical t.
- dilated pulmonary t.
- joint of t.
- lumbosacral t.
- lymphatic t.
- meningohypophysial t.
- nerve t.
- neuromeningeal t.
- posterior vagal t.
- pulmonary t.
- sinus of pulmonary t.
- thyrocervical t.

trunk (*continued*)
  tibioperoneal t.
  twin t.
  vagal t.
Trunkey pelvic fracture classification (I-III)
TruPulse CO$_2$ laser
TRUS
  transrectal ultrasound
TRW
  teboroxime resting washout
T-Scan 2000
T-score measurement of bone mineral density
TSD
  target-skin distance
TSE
  turbo-spin echo
    TSE image
    single-shot TSE (SShTSE)
TSENSE
  time-adaptive SENSE
TSE-relaxometry
TSH
  thyroid-stimulating hormone
T-shaped
  T-s. fracture
  T-s. uterus
TSPP
  tetrasodium pyrophosphate
    TSPP imaging
TSR
  total saturation recovery
TSV
  total stroke volume
TTC
  triphenyltetrazolium chloride
  T-tube cholangiogram
TTD
  tissue tolerance dose
TTF
  time-to-treatment failure
TTI
  tension-time index
TTNAB
  transthoracic needle aspiration biopsy
TTP
  time to peak
  transtubercular plane
TTPF
  time to peak filling
1.0T, 1.5T superconducting magnet
TTTS
  twin-to-twin transfusion syndrome
T-tube
  T-t. cholangiogram (TTC)
  T-t. cholangiography
  French T-t.
  T-t. stent

tubal
  t. canal
  t. fimbrial opening
  t. insufflation
  t. mass
  t. obstruction
  t. occlusion
  t. pregnancy
  t. ring
  t. tonsil
tubarius
  tonsil of torus t.
  torus t.
tube, tubing
  Angio-Seal carrier t.
  angled pleural t.
  anode t.
  anteroposterior t.
  apically directed chest t.
  atretic t.
  auditory t.
  bilateral pleural t.'s
  blocked shunt t.
  bronchial t.
  calyx t.
  Cantor t.
  capillary t.
  carrier t.
  cathode ray t. (CRT)
  Celestin t.
  Chaoul voltage x-ray t.
  chest t.
  collecting t.
  Coolidge x-ray t.
  corked tracheostomy t.
  corneal t.
  Crookes t.
  Crookes-Hittorf t.
  cuffed endotracheal t.
  t. current
  t. decompression
  decompression t.
  Dennis t.
  t. device
  dialysis t.
  digestive t.
  discharge t.
  Dotter t.
  t. drainage
  electron multiplier t.
  endobronchial t.
  endotracheal t. (ETT)
  eustachian t.
  fallopian t.
  feeding t.
  fenestrated t.
  field emission t.
  fMR t.
  Frederick-Miller t.

functional MR t.
gastrostomy t.
Geiger-Müller t.
t. geometry module
glow modular t.
Harris t.
Herring t.
high heat-capacity x-ray t.
hot cathode x-ray t.
image-intensifier t.
interstitial afterloading nylon t.
intestinal t.
J-shaped t.
large-caliber t.
Lenard ray t.
Lester Jones bypass t.
Levine t.
mediastinal t.
metallic distal end of t.
MIC gastroenteric t.
MIC-Key low-profile transgastric
  jejunal feeding t.
microfocal direct magnification
  in vitro x-ray t.
MIC transgastric jejunal
  feeding t.
Miller-Abbott t.
Minnesota t.
Miser t.
molybdenum target t.
Moss gastrostomy t.
muscular t.
nasoenteric t.
nasogastric t. (NGT)
nasojejunal feeding t.
nasotracheal t.
neural t.
Newvicon camera t.
Nutriflex t.
obstructed shunt t.
Olshevsky t.
oroendotracheal t.
orogastric t.
Orthicon t.
overcouch t.
pharyngotympanic t.
photomultiplier t. (PMT)
pickup t.
pleural t.
polyethylene t.
t. position rotation
pull-type gastrostomy t.
rectifier t.
right-angled chest t.
roentgen t.
rotating anode t.
Salem sump t.
self-quenched counter t.
Sengstaken-Blakemore t.

separator t.
Shiner radiopaque t.
shunt t.
solid-phase extraction t.
SRO 2550 x-ray t.
stomach t.
straight chest t.
suction t.
sump t.
Thal-Quick chest t.
thoracostomy t.
t. thoracostomy
tracheal t.
tracheostomy t.
translucent silicone t.
triode t.
uterine t.
vacuum t.
valve t.
Vidicon camera t.
t. voltage waveform
Westergren t.
x-ray t.
tuber, *pl.* **tubera**
brain t.
t. cinereum
t. cinereum hamartoma
cortical t.
tubera (*pl. of* tuber)
tubercle
accessory t.
acoustic t.
adductor t.
amygdaloid t.
articular t.
auricular t.
calcaneal t.
carotid t.
Chaput t.
conoid t.
corniculate t.
costal t.
crown t.
cuneiform t.
darwinian t.
dental t.
dissection t.
dorsal t.
epiglottic t.
fibrous t.
genial t.
Gerdy t.
Ghon t.
greater t.
iliac t.
intercondylar t.
jugular t.
lesser t.
Lister t.

tubercle (*continued*)
  Lower t.
  noncaseating t.
  t. of Morgagni
  olfactory t.
  Parsons t.
  peroneal t.
  prominent t.
  pubic t.
  rib t.
  Rolando t.
  scalene t.
  supraglenoid t.
  tibial t.
  ulnar t.
tubercula (*pl. of* tuberculum)
tubercular
  t. bone disease
  t. bone infection
  t. sinus
tuberculation
tuberculin
  t. skin test
  t. syringe
tuberculoid
tuberculoma
  brain t.
  calcified myocardial t.
  cerebral t.
  intracranial t.
  intraparenchymal t.
  lung t.
  noncavitary t.
  pulmonary t.
tuberculosis (TB)
  abdominal t.
  acinar t.
  adrenal t.
  airway t.
  anorectal t.
  anthracotic t.
  atypical t.
  basal t.
  bone t.
  cavitary t.
  cervical t.
  cestodic t.
  t. cutis indurativa
  t. cutis lichenoides
  t. cutis miliaris disseminata
  cystic t.
  Delmege sign of t.
  disseminated t.
  endobronchial t.
  extrapulmonary t.
  extraskeletal t.
  exudative t.
  fibroproductive t.
  fulminant t.

gastrointestinal t.
genitourinary t.
GI tract t.
t. granulation tissue
GU tract t.
hematogenous t.
inhalation t.
laryngeal t.
t. lichenoides
lymphatic t.
meningeal t.
mesenteric t.
t. miliaris disseminata
miliary pulmonary t.
multidrug-resistant t.
multifocal systemic t.
neural t.
open t.
peritoneal t.
postprimary pulmonary t.
primary pulmonary t.
progressive primary t.
pulmonary t.
reactivation t.
recrudescent t.
renal t.
Schick sign of t.
skeletal t.
soft tissue t.
spinal t.
stable-state t.
systemic t.
urinary tract t.
t. verrucosa cutis
tuberculous
  t. abscess
  t. arthritis
  t. bone
  t. bronchiectasis
  t. bronchopneumonia
  t. cystitis
  t. dactylitis
  t. effusion
  t. empyema
  t. granuloma
  t. infiltrate
  t. lesion
  t. lymphadenitis
  t. lymphadenopathy
  t. mediastinal adenopathy
  t. meningitis
  t. nodule
  t. osteomyelitis
  t. peritonitis
  t. pneumonia
  t. pneumothorax
  t. salpingitis
  t. spondylitis
  t. tenosynovitis

tuberculum, *pl.* **tubercula**
    t. sellae
    t. sellae meningioma
tuberosis
tuberosity
    bicipital t.
    calcaneal t.
    coracoid t.
    costal t.
    deltoid t.
    femoral t.
    greater t.
    iliac t.
    infraglenoid t.
    ischial t.
    lesser t.
    navicular t.
    omental t.
    radial t.
    tibial t.
    ulnar t.
    unguiculate t.
tuberous sclerosis
tubing (*var. of* tube)
tuboabdominal pregnancy
tubogram
    T t.
tuboligamentary pregnancy
tuboovarian
    t. abscess (TOA)
    t. mass
    t. pregnancy
tuboplasty
    balloon t.
    transcervical balloon t.
    ultrasound transcervical t.
tuboreticular structure
tubotympanic canal
tubouterine pregnancy
tubular
    t. aneurysm
    t. aortic hypoplasia
    t. bone
    t. breast carcinoma
    t. bronchiectasis
    t. cavity
    t. dilation
    t. dysgenesis
    t. ectasia
    t. ectasia of rete testis
    t. fertility index
    t. fluid-density adnexal mass
    t. function
    t. gas pattern
    t. hiatal hernia
    t. kidney secretion
    t. lesion
    t. lung density
    t. magnet

    t. necrosis
    t. nephrogram
    t. opacity
    t. polyp
    t. shadow
    t. signal void
    t. stenosis
    t. structure
    t. transit
    t. ventricle
    t. wire mesh
tubule
    collecting t.
    connecting t.
    convoluted t.
    dentinal t.
    discharging t.
    distal convoluted t.
    proximal convoluted t.
    renal t.
    seminiferous t.
    straight t.
tubuloacinar
tubulointerstitial nephritis
tubulovillous
    t. colon adenoma
    t. polyp
Tuffier inferior ligament
tuft
    t. fracture
    osteolysis t.
    osteosclerosis t.
    penciling of terminal t.
    silk t.
    terminal t.
    ungual t.
    vascular t.
tug, tugging
    lateral t.
tugging (*var. of* tug)
tularemic pneumonia
TULIP
    transurethral ultrasound-guided
    laser-induced prostatectomy
tulip
    t. bulb aorta
    t. sheath
tumbling bullet sign
tumefactive
    t. biliary sludge
    t. multiple sclerosis
    t. synovial osteochondromatosis
tumeur d'emblée mycosis fungoides
tumor
    abdominal wall desmoid t.
    t. ablation
    Abrikosov t.
    acidophilic pituitary t.
    acinic cell t.

T

tumor (*continued*)
    acoustic nerve sheath t.
    ACTH-producing t.
    acute splenic t.
    adenoid t.
    adenomatoid odontogenic t.
    adipose t.
    adrenal t.
    adrenocortical t.
    amelanotic t.
    ameloblastic adenomatoid t.
    ampulla t.
    amyloid t.
    anaplastic t.
    androgen-producing t.
    angiogenesis t.
    t. angiogenesis factor
    angiomatoid t.
    aortic body t.
    apple-core t.
    Askin thoracopulmonary
      neuroepithelial t.
    astrocytic t.
    astroglial t.
    atypical teratoid/rhabdoid t. (ATRT)
    Azzopardi t.
    ball-valve t.
    basiocciput t.
    B-cell t.
    t. bed
    Bednar t.
    benign congenital Wilms t.
    benign duodenal t.
    benign fibrous bone t.
    benign lung t.
    benign lymphoepithelial parotid t.
    benign osteogenic t.
    benign ovarian t.
    benign small bowel t.
    benign teratoid mediastinal t.
    benign urethral t.
    biphasic breast t.
    bladder t.
    t. blood supply
    blood vessel t.
    t. blush
    t. blush on angiography
    bone t.
    bone-forming bone t.
    t. boundary
    brain t.
    Braun t.
    breast phyllode t.
    Brenner t.
    bright signal intensity t.
    bronchial carcinoid t.
    bronchopulmonary carcinoid t.
    Brooke t.
    brown t.

    t. bulk
    bulky t.
    t. burden
    burned-out t.
    Buschke-Löwenstein t.
    calcaneal t.
    calcaneal t.
    calcified t.
    calcified amorphous t.
    t. capillary permeability
    t. capsule
    carcinoid t.
    cardiac t.
    carotid body t.
    cartilage-containing giant cell t.
    cartilage-forming bone t.
    cartilaginous soft tissue t.
    catecholamine-producing t.
    cavernous t.
    cell t.
    t. cell-host bone relationship
    cellular t.
    central nervous system t.
    cerebellopontine angle t.
    cervical t.
    choline t.
    chondrogenic t.
    chondroid-origin t.
    chromaffin t.
    t. cleavage plane
    clivus meningioma t.
    CNS ghost t.
    CNS multifocal t.
    Codman t.
    collision t.
    colloid cystic t.
    combined germ cell t.
    congenital cardiac t.
    connective tissue fibrous t.
    t. conspicuity
    cranial nerve sheath t.
    cystic t.
    deep t.
    deep-seated t.
    t. defect
    Denys-Drash t.
    dermal duct t.
    dermoid t.
    desmoid t.
    desmoplastic small round-cell t.
      (DSRCT)
    destructive t.
    discrete t.
    disseminated t.
    t. dormancy
    drug-resistant t.
    ductectatic mucinous t.
    dumbbell t.
    duodenal malignant t.

dysembryoplastic neuroepithelial t. (DNET)
dyssynchronous primary t.
echogenic t.
t. embolus
embryonal t.
embryonic t.
endobronchial t.
endocrine t.
endodermal sinus ovarian t.
endodermal sinus testis t.
endolymphatic sac t.
endometrioid t.
t. entity
epidermoid t.
epidural t.
epithelial t.
Erdheim t.
t. erosion
esophageal t.
essential t.
estrogen-producing t.
Ewing sarcoma family of t.'s
Ewing sarcoma-Wilms t. 1 (EWS-WT1)
exfoliating t.
t. extension
t. extirpation
extraaxial t.
extracompartmental t.
extradural t.
extrahepatic primary malignant t.
extramedullary myeloid t.
extramedullary plasma cell t.
extratesticular t.
exuberant t.
fatty soft tissue t.
fecal t.
feign t.
feminizing adrenal t.
fetal mesenchymal t.
fibrohistiocytic t.
fibroid t.
fibrous connective tissue t.
finger of t.
flocculonodular t.
focal t.
focus of t.
friable t.
frontal lobe t.
fungating t.
galeal extension of t.
ganglion cell t.
gastric t.
gastroesophageal junction t.
gastrointestinal fibrous t. (GIFT)
gastrointestinal glial/schwannoma t.
gastrointestinal leiomyogenic t. (GILT)

gastrointestinal stromal t. (GIST)
germ cell t.
gestational trophoblastic t.
ghost t.
giant cell t.
Glazunov t.
glial brain t.
globular t.
glomus body t.
glomus bone t.
glomus jugulare t.
glomus jugulotympanicum t.
glomus neck t.
Godwin t.
gonadal steroid-dependent benign smooth muscle t.
gonadal stromal t.
granulosa-theca cell t.
Grawitz t.
gross t.
growth hormone-releasing factor t.
Gubler t.
heart t.
hepatic t.
high-grade t.
highly vascular t.
hilar t.
Hodgkin t.
hourglass t.
HPV16-associated t.
HPV18-associated t.
hypermetabolic t.
hypervascular pancreatic t.
hypodiploid t.
hypoechogenic t.
hypoechoic solid t.
hypopharyngeal t.
hypothalamus t.
t. hypoxia
t. imaging
t. implant
incomplete t.
t. inflammation
inflammatory myofibroblastic t.
infratentorial Lindau t.
infundibular t.
inoperable brain t.
intestinal carcinoid t.
intraarticular t.
intraaxial brain t.
intracardiac t.
intracavitary extension of t.
intracerebral t.
intracompartmental t.
intracranial t.
intraductal mucin-producing t.
intraductal papillary mucinous t. (IPMT)
intradural extramedullary t.

T

tumor (*continued*)

intradural intramedullary t.
intramedullary spinal cord t.
intramural t.
intraosseous desmoid t.
intraparenchymal lung t.
intraperitoneal t.
intrasellar t.
intraspinal t.
intraventricular brain t.
invasive malignant sheath t.
islet cell t.
jugular bulb t.
juxtaglomerular t.
Klatskin t.
Krukenberg t.
laryngeal giant cell t.
t. lethal dose (TLD)
Leydig cell t.
lipogenic t.
lipomatous t.
lobulated t.
localized pleura t.
locally invasive t.
low signal intensity t.
lung t.
lymphocyte-rich t.
lymphoepithelial parotid t.
lymphoid t.
t. lysis syndrome
main t.
malignant duodenal t.
malignant giant cell t.
malignant mediastinal teratoid t.
malignant mesenchymal t.
malignant ovarian germ cell t.
malignant ovarian teratoma t.
malignant peripheral nerve sheath t.
  (MPNST)
malignant salivary gland t.
malignant small bowel t.
malpighian cell t.
t. margin
t. marker
masculinizing t.
t. mass
t. matrix
mediastinal teratoid t.
melanin-containing t.
melanotic neuroectodermal t.
meningeal cell t.
mesenchymal t.
metastatic myocardial t.
metasynchronous t.
microcystic pancreatic t.
t. microembolus
micropapillary t.
mixed müllerian t.

mucinous ovarian t.
mucosal esophageal t.
müllerian mucinous borderline t.
multicentric carcinoid t.
multifocal brain t.
musculoskeletal t.
myxomatous t.
napkin-ring anular t.
2nd primary t.
neck germ cell t.
t. necrosis
necrotic t.
t. neovascularity
t. neovasculature
nerve root t.
nerve sheath t.
neural-origin bone t.
neuroectodermal t.
neuroendocrine t.
neurogenic t.
neuroglial t.
neuronal cell-origin t.
t. nidus
t., nodal involvement, metastasis
  (TNM)
nonechogenic t.
nonfunctioning islet cell t.
nonglial brain t.
nonneoplastic t.
nonseminomatous testicular germ
  cell t.
occult phosphaturic mesenchymal t.
odontogenic t.
t. of infundibulum
t. of liver scar
t. of surface epithelium
optic complex t.
oral cavity t.
orbital childhood t.
osteoblastic t.
osteocartilaginous t.
t. osteoid
osteoid-origin t.
ovarian epithelial t.
ovarian germ cell t.
ovarian mesonephroid t.
Pancoast t.
pancreatic islet cell t.
papillary t.
paracardiac t.
parasellar dermoid t.
paraspinous t.
parasympathetic ganglion t.
paratesticular t.
parathyroid t.
parotid t.
paucilocular t.
pearlescent solid t.

pearly CNS t.
pediatric primary brain t.
pediatric solid t.
pedunculated vesical t.
Pepper t.
periampullary duodenal t.
perineural fibroblastoma t.
peripheral neuroectodermal t.
peritoneal desmoid t.
phantom breast t.
phantom lung t.
phosphate-inducing t.
phosphate-wasting t.
phosphaturic mesenchymal t.
phyllodes t.
pilar t.
pilocytic t.
Pindborg t.
pineal germ cell t.
pineal gland t.
pineal parenchymatous t.
pineal region t.
pituitary t.
placenta t.
pontile angle t.
poorly circumscribed t.
poorly differentiated embryonal
  cell t.
posterior fossa t.
Pott puffy t.
pregnancy t.
primary benign liver t.
primary implanted t.
primary intracranial germ cell t.
primary malignant liver t.
primary renal t.
primitive neuroectodermal t. (PNET)
primitive neuroepithelial t.
prolapsed t.
pseudomalignant t.
pseudoorbital t.
pseudosarcomatous fibromyxoid t.
pulmonary t.
pulmonary carcinoid t.
radiation-associated papillary t.
radiation-induced peripheral nerve t.
radiosensitive t.
Rathke pouch t.
3rd ventricle t.
Recklinghausen t.
t. recurrence
refractory t.
t. regression grade
renal t.
renal pelvis t.
renin-secreting t.
Response Evaluation Criteria in
  Solid T.'s (RECIST)

reticuloendothelial t.
retinal anlage t.
retromolar trigone t.
retroperitoneal t.
rhabdoid t.
round bone cell t.
Rous t.
sacral bone t.
sacrococcygeal remnant t.
sand t.
scannable t.
Schmincke t.
Schwann t.
scirrhous t.
sclerosing stromal t.
Scully t.
secondary ovarian t.
t. seeding
seminomatous t.
serous ovarian t.
Sertoli cell t. (SCT)
Sertoli-Leydig cell t.
sessile t.
t. shrinkage
t. signature
sinonasal t.
skull base t.
small adrenal t.
small bowel benign t.
small bowel malignant t.
smooth-muscle t.
soft tissue t.
t. sojourn time
solid and cystic pancreatic t.'s
solid ovarian t.
solid primary t.
solid pseudopapillary t.
solitary pleura t.
sphenoid ridge t.
t. spheroid
spinal axis t.
spinal cord t.
sporadic t.
spread of t.
squamous odontogenic t.
t. staining
t. stalk
sternocleidomastoid t.
stromal cell t.
stylomastoid t.
subastrocytic t.
subcortical t.
subcutaneous t.
submucosal colon t.
submucosal esophageal t.
subserosal t.
subungual glomus t.
sugar t.

tumor (*continued*)
  superior pulmonary sulcus t.
  suprasellar extension of t.
  supratentorial brain t.
  supratentorial primitive
    neuroectodermal t.
  surface ovarian
    epithelium t.
  sympathetic ganglion t.
  synchronous t.
  synovial t.
  temporal bone t.
  temporal lobe t.
  tendon sheath giant cell t.
  tenosynovial giant cell t.
  teratoid t.
  testicular stromal cell t.
  testis germ cell t.
  tetradiploid t.
  tetraploid t.
  theca cell ovarian t.
  8th nerve t.
  t. thrombus
  4th ventricle t.
  tracheal t.
  transmissible venereal t.
  triton t.
  turban t.
  ulcerative t.
  umbilical t.
  unifocal t.
  unilocular t.
  unknown primary t.
  urethral t.
  urinary bladder t.
  uroepithelial t.
  vaginal t.
  vanishing lung t.
  t. vascularity
  t. vascularization
  vascular origin bone t.
  vasoactive intestinal polypeptide t.
    (VIPoma)
  ventricular t.
  vertebral body bone t.
  viable t.
  villous t.
  t. volume
  t. volumetry
  von Hippel retina t.
  Warthin t.
  well-circumscribed t.
  well-differentiated polycystic
    Wilms t.
  Wharton t.
  Wilms t.
  yolk sac ovary t.
  Zollinger-Ellison t.

tumoraffin
tumoral
  t. calcification
  t. calcinosis
  t. callus
  t. fat
  t. hemorrhage
  t. invasion
tumor-associated
  t.-a. macrophage
  t.-a. tissue eosinophilia
tumor-bearing
  t.-b. bone
  t.-b. lymph node
tumor-feeding vessel
tumorigenesis
  mammary t.
tumorigenic
tumor-induced osteomalacia
tumorlet
tumorlike
  t. lesion
  t. shadow
tumor-mimicking breast lesion
tumorous
tumor-related spontaneous
  bleed
tumor-specific tracer
tumor-to-background ratio
tumor-to-gray matter ratio
tumor-to-normal
  t.-t.-n. brain ratio
  t.-t.-n. tissue ratio
    (TNR)
tumor-to-white matter ratio
TUNA
  transurethral needle ablation
tuned aperture computed tomography
  (TACT)
tungstate
  calcium t.
tungsten
  t. 188 (^{188}W, W-188)
  t. anode
  t. bead
  t. carbide pneumoconiosis
  t. eye shield
  t. powder
  t. syringe shield
  t. target
tungstosilicates
tunica, *pl.* **tunicae**
  t. albuginea
  t. albuginea cyst
  t. intima
  t. medium
  t. propria
  t. vaginalis

tunicae (*pl. of* tunica)
tunnel
    aortic-left ventricular t.
    baffled t.
    carpal t.
    cross-trigonal t.
    cubital t.
    fibroosseous t.
    intramural t.
    t. projection
    t. radiograph
    retropancreatic t.
    retroperitoneal t.
    t. subaortic stenosis
    subcutaneous t.
    subsartorial t.
    t. subvalvular aortic stenosis
    tarsal t.
    t. view
tunneled catheter
Tuohy aortography needle
Tuohy-Borst
    T.-B. adaptor
    T.-B. introducer
TUP
    transumbilical plane
TUR
    transurethral resection
turban tumor
turbidimetric detection
turbinate
    t. bone
    nasal t.
    paradoxic middle t.
turbinated
turbo
    t. fast low-angle shot
    (turboFLASH)
    t. gradient-refocused echo
    (turboGRE)
    t. inversion recovery sequence
    t. short tau inversion recovery
    t. short tau/T1 inversion recovery
turboFLAIR imaging
turboFLASH
    turbo fast low-angle shot
    turboFLASH imaging
    turboFLASH sequence
turboGRE
    turbo gradient-refocused echo
turbohaler
turbo-IR sequence
turbo-pulse sequence
turbo-SE sequence
turbo-spin
    t.-s. echo (TSE)
    t.-s. echo technique
    t.-s. echo T2-weighted sequence

turboSTIR image
turbulence
    TCD-detectable t.
turbulent
    t. blood flow
    t. intraluminal flow
    t. signal
turcica
    sella t.
Turcot syndrome
turn
    insufficient cochlear t.
turned-up pulp deformity
Turner
    T. marginal gyrus
    T. syndrome
turnover
    bone t.
    erythrocyte iron t.
    plasma iron t.
    red blood cell iron t.
TURP
    transurethral resection of
    prostate
turret exostosis
turricephaly
Turyn back pain sign
tutamen, *pl.* **tutamina**
tutamina (*pl. of* tutamen)
TVG
    time-varied gain
TVHS
    transvaginal hysterosonography
TVS
    transvaginal sonography
TVUS
    transvaginal ultrasound
T-wave
    asymmetric negative T-w.
T1-weighted
    T1-w. acquisition
    T1-w. axial image
    T1-w. axial image with fat
    saturation
    T1-w. axial localizer
    T1-w. conventional spin echo
    T1-w. coronal fat-suppressed fast
    spin-echo sequence
    T1-w. coronal image
    T1-w. coronal imaging
    T1-w. FAST
    T1-w. fat-suppressed (T1FS)
    T1-w. fat-suppressed gadolinium-
    enhanced SE image
    T1-w. image (T1WI)
    T1-w. magnetic resonance
    T1-w. sagittal imaging
    T1-w. study

T

T2-weighted
 T2-w. axial image
 T2-w. combination sequence
 T2-w. fast spin-echo coronal
  oblique
 T2-w. fat-saturated sequence
 T2-w. image (T2WI)
 T2-w. pulse sequence
 T2-w. sagittal oblique image
 T2-w. scan
 T2-w. shortening
 T2-w. signal
 T2-w. spin-echo image
 T2-w. spin-echo sequence
 T2-w. turbo SE image
T1WI
 T1-weighted image
T2WI
 T2-weighted image
twiddler's syndrome
twig
 cutaneous t.
 muscular t.
 t. of artery
twin
 conjoined t.'s
 craniopagus t.
 dichorionic-diamniotic t.
 discordant t.
 dizygotic t.
 donor t.
 t. ectopic pregnancy
 t. embolization syndrome
 fraternal t.
 ischiopagus t.
 monochorionic-monoamniotic t.
 monozygotic t.
 omphalopagus t.
 t. peak sign
 perfused t.
 t. pregnancy discordant
  growth
 pygopagus t.
 t. reversed arterial perfusion
  sequence
 thoracopagus t.
 t. trunk
 vanishing t.
twin-beam CT
TwinCath
 Arrow T.
twining
 t. line
 T. position
 t. recess
 T. view
twinkling artifact
twin-peak

twin-peaked pulse
twin-to-twin transfusion syndrome
 (TTTS)
twist
 myocardial t.
twisted
 t. ankle
 t. body habitus
 t. pedicle sign
 t. ribbonlike rib
 t. small bowel ribbon
  appearance
twister gradient
twist-release coil
twofold accelerated parallel imaging
twos
 rule of t.
tylectomy
tyloses (*pl. of* tylosis)
tylosis, *pl.* **tyloses**
 t. palmaris et plantaris
tympani
 apertura tympanica canaliculi
  chordae t.
 chorda t.
 tegmen t.
 tensor t.
tympanic
 t. bone
 t. cavity
 t. plexus
tympanicum
 glomus t.
tympanography
tympanosclerosis
tympanostapedialis
 syndesmosis t.
type
 t. A carotid cavernous fistula
 t. B aortic dissection
 centrocyte-like t.
 diffuse fibrosis t.
 t. I endoleak (T1EL)
 epidermolysis bullosa, dermal t.
 epidermolysis bullosa, epidermal t.
 epidermolysis bullosa,
  junctional t.
 t. II collagen C-telopeptide
 t. II endoleak (T2EL)
 t. III endoleak (T3EL)
 t. I, II muscle fiber
 IPMT of branch duct t.
 t. IV endoleak (T4EL)
 pleomorphic t.
 reticular t.
 sonographic hip t.
typhlenteritis (*var. of* cecitis)
typhlitis (*var. of* cecitis)

typhoid
- t. nodule
- t. pleurisy

typhus nodule

typical
- t. carcinoid
- t. cobblestone pattern
- t. medullary carcinoma

tyropanoate sodium
Tyropaque imaging agent
tyrosinase
tyrosinemia
tyrphostin radiotracer for PET
TZ
- transition zone

T-zone lymphoma

U
uranium
^{235}U, U-235
^{235}uranium
UA
umbilical artery
uterine artery
UA to OA anastomosis
UA velocimetry
UAE
uterine artery embolization
UAL
ultrasound-assisted lipoplasty
ubiquinone
UBIS
ultrasound bone imaging scanner
UBIS 5000 ultrasound bone
sonometer
UBM
ultrasound backscatter
microscopy
ultrasound biomicroscopy
UBM imaging
UBO
unidentified bright object
UC
ulcerative colitis
UCG
ultrasonic cardiogram
UCL
ulnar collateral ligament
UCLA
University of California Los Angeles
UCLA imaging protocol
UCLA pouch
U-clip
nitinol U-c.
UCT
ultrasound computed tomography
UES
upper esophageal sphincter
UEVT
upper extremity venous
thrombosis
UFCT
ultrafast computed tomography
UFE
uterine fibroid embolization
U-fiber damage
UGI
upper gastrointestinal
Uhl
U. anomaly
U. disease

UHMM
ultrahigh-magnification mammography
UHR
ultrahigh resolution
UHR optical coherence tomography
Uhthoff sign
UIP
usual interstitial pneumonia
UIQ
upper inner quadrant
ulcer
acid-peptic u.
active duodenal u.
acute peptic u.
anastomotic u.
anterior wall antral u.
antral u.
aortic penetrating u.
aphthoid u.
aphthous stomach u.
apical duodenal u.
arteriolar ischemic u.
atheromatous u.
atherosclerotic aortic u.
Barrett u.
u. base
bear's claw u.
benign gastric u.
bleeding u.
bulbar peptic u.
channel pyloric u.
chronic peptic u.
collar-button u.
colonic u.
u. crater
craterlike u.
Cruveilhier u.
Curling u.
Cushing u.
Cushing-Rokitansky u.
decubitus u.
u. disease
duodenal u.
esophageal u.
flask-shaped u.
focal u.
frontier u.
gastric u.
gastrointestinal u.
giant duodenal u.
giant peptic u.
greater curvature u.
healed gastric u.
healing u.

ulcer (*continued*)
    Hunner u.
    hypertensive ischemic u.
    indolent radiation-induced rectal u.
    intestinal u.
    intractable u.
    ischemic u.
    jejunal u.
    juxtapyloric u.
    kissing u.'s
    Kocher dilation u.
    lesser curvature u.
    linear u.
    malignant gastric u.
    marginal u.
    Martorell hypertensive u.
    minute bleeding u.
    mucosal u.
    multiple small bowel u.'s
    necrotic u.
    u. osteoma
    patchy colonic u.
    penetrating aortic u.
    penetrating atherosclerotic u.
      (PAU)
    peptic u.
    perforated u.
    u. perforation
    phagedenic u.
    postbulbar u.
    postsurgical recurrent u.
    prepyloric u.
    punched-out u.
    punctate u.
    puncture u.
    pyloric channel u.
    radiation-induced u.
    rake u.
    recurrent u.
    rodent u.
    Rokitansky-Cushing u.
    round u.
    ruptured u.
    Saemisch u.
    secondary u.
    serpiginous u.
    sloughing u.
    solitary rectal u.
    stasis u.
    stercoral u.
    stomach u.
    stress u.
    subatheromatous u.
    thorn u.
    tropic u.
    urinary u.
    venous u.
    V-shaped u.
    u. with heaped-up edges

ulcerated
    u. atheromatous plaque
    u. carotid artery plaque
ulcerating
    u. adenocarcinoma
    u. granuloma of pudenda
ulcerative
    u. colitis (UC)
    u. esophageal carcinoma
    u. jejunitis
    u. jejunoileitis
    u. lesion
    u. lymphoma
    u. tumor
ULDR
    ultralow-dose rate
ulegyria
Ullmann line
ulna, *pl.* **ulnae**
    capitulum ulnae
    coronoid of u.
    fetal biometry of u.
    sigmoid cavity of u.
ulnae (*pl. of* ulna)
ulnar
    u. bursa
    u. chondromalacia
    u. collateral ligament (UCL)
    u. deviation
    u. deviation view
    u. digital artery
    u. drift deformity
    u. extensor
    u. facing of metacarpal head
    u. fracture
    u. groove
    u. hand
    u. head
    u. impaction syndrome
    u. inclination
    u. nerve entrapment
    u. nerve lesion
    u. notch
    u. ridge
    u. sesamoid bone
    u. styloid
    u. styloid process
    u. styloid process index (USPI)
    u. sulcus
    u. traction spurring
    u. translocation of carpus
    u. tubercle
    u. tuberosity
    u. tunnel syndrome
    u. variance
ulnaris
    extensor carpi u. (ECU)
    flexor carpi u.
ulnocarpal ligament

ulnolunate
 u. impaction syndrome
 u. impingement
 u. ligament
ulnotriquetral
 u. distance
 u. ligament
ULP
 ultralow profile
ULQ
 upper left quadrant
ultimobranchial pouch
ultra
 Bolus Pro U.
 U. ICE catheter
 U. Tag kit
 U. Vision Rapid screen
UltraCision ultrasonic knife
Ultracranio T
ultraearly thrombolytic therapy
UltraEase ultrasound pad
ultrafast
 u. computed tomography (UFCT)
 u. computed tomography scanner
 u. contrast-enhanced MRA
 u. CT
 u. CT electron beam tomography
 u. CT imaging
 u. CT scan
 u. 3D MR digital subtraction
 angiography
 u. FLASH 2D sequence
 u. MRI
 u. video transfer
ultrafiltration
UltraFine erbium laser system
Ultraflex stent
Ultra-Fluid
 Lipiodol U.-F.
ultrahigh
 u. field-strength whole-body MR
 scanner
 u. magnification
 u. resolution (UHR)
**ultrahigh-energy parallel-hole
 collimator**
ultrahigh-field magnetic resonance
**ultrahigh-magnification mammography
 (UHMM)**
**ultrahigh-resolution parallel-hole
 collimator**
Ultraject prefilled syringe
ultralong TR
ultralow-dose rate (ULDR)
ultralow profile (ULP)
Ultramark
 ATL U. 8, 9
 U. 9 HDI ultrasound
 U. 9 scanner

 U. 8 transducer
 U. 4 ultrasound
UltraPACS diagnostic imaging system
UltraPulse CO$_2$ laser
ultrascan
 B-mode u.
Ultraseed brachytherapy
ultrashort method
**ultrasmall superparamagnetic iron oxide
 (USPIO)**
UltraSoft GDC
ultrasonic
 u. aortography
 u. aspiration
 u. assessment
 u. assessment of injury
 u. atherolysis
 u. attenuation
 u. cardiogram (UCG)
 u. cardiography
 u. cephalometry
 u. guidance
 u. hysterography
 u. hysterosalpingography
 u. lithotresis
 u. lithotripsy
 u. lithotripter cannula
 u. lysis
 u. lysis of thrombus
 u. pachymetry
 u. probe
 u. tomographic image
 u. tomographic imaging
 u. tomography
 u. wave
ultrasonically activated scalpel
ultrasonogram
ultrasonograph
ultrasonographer
ultrasonographic
 u. echo
 u. finding
 u. modeling
ultrasonographically guided injection
ultrasonography (US)
 advanced u.
 axillary u.
 color Doppler u. (CDUS)
 compression u.
 Doppler u.
 duplex u. (DUS)
 endorectal u.
 endovaginal u.
 endovascular u.
 gray-scale u.
 infant cranial Doppler u.
 intracaval endovascular u. (ICEUS)
 intraductal u.
 intraoperative u.

U

ultrasonography (*continued*)
 intraportal endovascular u. (IPEUS)
 laparoscopic contact u. (LCU)
 periorbital directional Doppler u.
 pulsed-wave Doppler u.
 real-time u.
 rectal endoscopic u.
 transoral carotid u. (TOCU)
 transperineal u.
 venous u.
 vertebrobasilar transcranial
  color-coded duplex u.
ultrasonometer
 QUS-2 calcaneal u.
ultrasonometry
ultrasound
 abdominal u.
 u. aberration correction
 u. ablative therapy
 ACM u.
 Acuson 128 Doppler u.
 ADR Ultramark 4 u.
 AI 5200 diagnostic u.
 Aloka linear u.
 Aloka sector u.
 A-scan u.
 automated cardiac flow measurement
  u.
 u. backscatter microscopy (UBM)
 u. backscatter microscopy imaging
 u. biomicroscopy (UBM)
 BladderScan u.
 B-mode u.
 u. bone imaging scanner (UBIS)
 breast u.
 Bruel-Kjaer u.
 carbon dioxide microbubble u.
 u. cardiography
 carotid duplex u.
 color-coded duplex u.
 color-coded real-time u.
 color Doppler u.
 color duplex u.
 color power transcranial Doppler u.
 u. computed tomography (UCT)
 contact B-scan u.
 contrast-enhanced u.
 cranial u.
 CT-guided u.
 1D u.
 2D B-mode u.
 3D freehand u.
 u. diagnosis
 diagnostic range u.
 u. diagnostic yield
 Diasonics u.
 diathermy u.
 u. diffraction tomography
 u. dilution

u. dilution test
Doppler u.
duplex B-mode u.
duplex carotid u.
duplex pulsed Doppler u.
u. echocardiography
EchoGen-enhanced u.
u. echogenicity
endoanal u.
endorectal u. (ERU, ERUS)
endoscopic u. (EUS)
endovaginal u. (EVUS)
endovascular u.
entertainment u.
Eye Cubed u.
FDI u.
fetal u.
FloWire Doppler u.
focused u.
freehand interventional u.
full bladder u.
gallbladder u.
gastrointestinal endoscopic u.
u. gel
graded compression u.
gray-scale endorectal u.
u. guidance during embryo transfer
Hewlett-Packard u.
high-frequency Doppler u.
high-frequency therapeutic u.
high-intensity focused u. (HIFU)
high-resolution u.
Hitachi u.
u. hyperthermia treatment
hypoechoic area of u.
u. imaging technology
immersion B-scan u.
intracaval endovascular u. (ICEUS)
intracoronary u. (ICUS)
intraluminal u. (ILUS)
intraoperative u. (IOUS)
intrarectal u.
intravascular u. (IVUS)
in utero u.
Irex Exemplar u.
laparoscopic u. (LUS)
laparoscopic intracorporeal u. (LICU)
level I obstetric u.
limitation of u.
low-frequency u. (LFUS)
low-intensity pulsed u.
M-mode u.
u. monitoring
multiplanar endorectal u.
neonatal adrenal u.
neonatal transfontanellar brain u.
Neurosector u.
Nicolet Elite Doppler u.
noninvasive u.

obstetric u.
Olympus endoscopic u.
u. pad
pancreaticobiliary u.
pelvic u.
photoacoustic u.
postnatal u.
power Doppler u.
PowerVision u.
u. probe
ProSound SSD-5500 u.
pulsed Doppler u.
pulsed therapeutic low-intensity u.
pulse-inversion harmonic u.
quantitative u. (QUS)
real-time scan u.
renal u.
RT 6800 u.
RT 3200 Advantage u.
sagittal u.
SieScape u.
Sonicator portable u.
Sonolayer u.
SonoSite digital u.
SonoSite hand-carried u.
SonoSite iLook 24 u.
SonoSite MicroMaxx laptop u.
SonoSite 180Plus u.
SonoSite Titan u.
spectral u.
u. stethoscope
suprapubic transabdominal u.
u. system
TCD u.
therapeutic u.
u. threshold
TM u.
transabdominal u. (TAUS)
u. transcervical tuboplasty
transcranial color-coded duplex u.
transcranial Doppler u.
u. transducer
transperineal u.
transrectal u. (TRUS)
transthoracic u.
transvaginal u. (TVUS)
transverse u.
Ultramark 4 u.
Ultramark 9 HDI u.
u. venography
Vingmed u.
ultrasound-assisted lipoplasty (UAL)
ultrasound-augmented mammography
ultrasound-based strain rate and strain imaging
ultrasound-guided
u.-g. anterior subcostal liver biopsy
celiac plexus neurolysis, endoscopic
u.-g.

u.-g. core biopsy
u.-g. cyst aspiration
u.-g. large-core needle biopsy
u.-g. methotrexate injection
u.-g. nephrostomy puncture
u.-g. percutaneous cholecystostomy
u.-g. percutaneous interstitial laser ablation
u.-g. percutaneous microwave coagulation therapy
u.-g. pseudoaneurysm compression
u.-g. reduction of spigelian hernia
u.-g. stereotactic biopsy
u.-g. transthoracic needle aspiration
u.-g. vacuum-assisted biopsy
UltraSTAR computer-based ultrasound reporting system
ultrastructural abnormality
UltraSure DTR-One imaging ultrasound system
UltraTag RBC
Ultrathane Amplatz ureteral stent
ultratherm
Ultrathin Diamond balloon
ultraviolet (UV)
u. A, B, C
extravital u.
u. fluorescent dosimeter
intravital u.
u. irradiation
u. lamp
u. radiation
u. ray
u. spectrophotometry
u. spectrum
Ultravist 150, 240, 300, 370 contrast agent
Umbau zone
umbilical
aberrant u.
u. artery (UA)
u. artery velocimetry
u. canal
u. cord
u. cord anatomy
u. cord angiomyxoma
u. cord cyst
u. cord edema
u. cord hemangioma
u. cord hematoma
u. cord lesion
u. cord pseudocyst
u. fissure
u. granuloma
u. hernia
u. ligament
u. mass
u. plane

U

umbilical (*continued*)
  u. portography
  u. ring
  u. tumor
  u. vein
  u. vein varix
umbilicalis
  anulus u.
umbilical-urachal sinus
umbilici (*pl. of* umbilicus)
umbilicovesical fascia
umbilicus, *pl.* umbilici
umbo, *pl.* umbones
  u. of tympanic membrane
umbonate
umbones (*pl. of* umbo)
UMC-I microwave delivery system
UM4 real-time sector scanner
unaccelerated 2D cine SSFP imaging
U1-NA cephalometric measurement
unattached fraction
unbalanced hemivertebra
uncal
  u. gyrus
  u. herniation
  u. herniation syndrome
uncalcified pleural plaque
uncertainty principle
unci (*pl. of* uncus)
unciform bone
uncinate
  u. aura
  u. gyrus
  u. process
  u. process fracture
  u. process mass
  u. process of pancreas
uncoiling
  u. ascending aorta
  u. descending aorta
  u. of great vessel
uncommitted metaphysial lesion
uncompensated rotary scoliosis
uncomplicated
  u. myocardial infarct
  u. myoma
  u. pneumothorax
  u. supraclavicular stenosis
uncoupled spin
uncoupler
  mitochondrial u.
uncovering
  lateral meniscal u.
uncovertebral
  u. joint
  u. spur
uncus, *pl.* unci
  arachnoid of u.
  u. of temporal lobe

undefined lymphoma
undepressed skull fracture
undercalling disease
undercorrection
underdamping
underdetection
underdrainage
underdrive
  u. mode
  u. termination
underexposed image
underfilled submentovertical projection
underinflation
  lung u.
underloading
  ventricular u.
underlying
  u. disorder
  u. tissue
underperfusion
under-scan
  u.-s. method
  u.-s. method projection
undersurface
  u. of liver
  u. of patella
underventilated lung
underventilation
undescended
  u. testicle
  u. testis
undifferentiated
  u. liver sarcoma
  u. nasopharyngeal carcinoma
  u. non-Hodgkin lymphoma
undifferentiation
undisplaced fracture
Undritz anomaly
undulant impulse
undulating, undulatory
  u. contour
  u. course
undulatory (*var. of* undulating)
unenhanced
  u. magnetic resonance imaging
    scan
  u. MR imaging
unequal pulmonary blood flow
uneven
  u. air expansion
  u. exposure
  u. recruitment of alveolar population
  u. ventilation
unfavorable neutron-to-proton ratio
unfolding
  incomplete u.
unfused
  u. os trigonum
  u. physis

ungual
>　u. fibroma
>　u. tuft

unguiculate tuberosity
uniaxial
unibasal
unicalyceal kidney
unicameral, unicamerate
>　u. bone cyst
>　u. brain

unicamerate (*var. of* unicameral)
unicentral
unicentric angiofollicular lymph node
hyperplasia
unicollis
>　uterus bicornis u.

unicommissural aortic valve
unicondylar fracture
unicornate (*var. of* unicornous)
unicornis
>　uterus u.

unicornous, unicornuate, unicornate
>　u. uterus

unicornuate (*var. of* unicornous)
unicoronal synostosis
unicortical screw
unicuspid, unicuspidate
>　u. aortic valve stenosis
>　u. with aortic valve
>　u. with central raphe

unicuspidate (*var. of* unicuspid)
unidentified bright object (UBO)
unidirectional
>　u. block
>　u. current
>　u. lead configuration

unifascicular block
unified Parkinson disease rating scale
unifocalization
unifocal tumor
uniform
>　u. attenuation coefficient
>　u. distribution
>　u. loading
>　u. phantom scan
>　u. sensitivity
>　u. TR excitation
>　u. uptake

uniformity
>　differential u.
>　extrinsic field u.
>　field u.
>　image u.
>　intervertebral disc space u.
>　intrinsic field u.
>　scintillation camera field u.
>　SPECT u.

uniformly hyperechoic
Uni-Fuse infusion catheter

uniglandular
unigravida
unilateral
>　u. adrenal mass
>　u. bronchogram
>　u. carotid stenosis
>　u. consolidation
>　u. diaphragmatic elevation
>　u. facet dislocation
>　u. facet subluxation
>　u. fetal chest mass
>　u. flow restriction
>　u. fracture
>　u. fragmentation
>　u. hallux valgus
>　u. hilar enlargement
>　u. hydrocephalus
>　u. hyperlucent lung
>　u. hypertrophy
>　u. interfacetal dislocation
>　u. intrafacetal dislocation
>　u. kidney mass
>　u. large smooth kidney
>　u. lesion
>　u. lobar emphysema
>　u. locked facet injury
>　u. lung perfusion
>　u. megaloencephaly
>　u. mesial temporal sclerosis
>　u. obstructive emphysema
>　u. occlusion
>　u. ossification
>　u. overinflation
>　u. pleural effusion
>　u. pulmonary agenesis
>　u. pulmonary edema
>　u. pulmonary hyperlucency
>　u. pulmonary vein atresia
>　u. Raynaud phenomenon
>　u. small kidney

unilobar
unilobular cirrhosis
unilocular
>　u. cyst
>　u. cystic lesion
>　u. disc
>　u. osteolysis
>　u. tumor
>　u. well-demarcated bone defect
>　　expansile lesion

unimalleolar fracture
uninfected infarct
uninhibited bladder
union
>　bony u.
>　delayed fracture u.
>　faulty u.
>　fibrous u.
>　nonbony u.

U

union (*continued*)
    u. of fracture fragments
    osseous u.
    secondary u.
    solid bony u.
unipapillary kidney
unipara
unipediculate approach
unipennate muscle
uniphasic imaging agent
unipolar pacing mode
unirhinal phantosmia
uniseptate
unit
    adapted standard mammography u.
    add-on stereotactic u.
    AdvanTeq II TENS u.
    Angström u.
    Aspen sonography u.
    atomic mass u. (amu)
    Bart abdominoperipheral angiography u.
    Behnken u.
    Bethesda u.
    BICAP u.
    biplane DSA u.
    British thermal u. (BTU)
    burst-forming u.
    C-arm portable x-ray u.
    cobalt-60 beam therapy u.
    colony-forming u.
    Cox sterilizer and incinerator u.
    CT u.
    Dent-X intraoral x-ray u.
    depicted Hounsfield u.
    dry heat sterilizer and incinerator u.
    Eclipse TENS u.
    electromagnetic u. (emu, EMU)
    EMI u.
    fibrinogen equivalent u.
    gamma u.
    gray u.
    Gyroscan ACS-NT MR u.
    Hampson u.
    heat u.
    Hercules 7000 mobile x-ray u.
    Holzknecht u.
    Hounsfield u. (HU)
    Hounsfield calcium density
      measurement u.
    Intelect Legend Combo stimulator
      and ultrasound u.
    International Commission on
      Radiation U.'s (ICRU)
    JACE-Stim electrotherapy u.
    Kienböck u.
    Leksell gamma u.
    linear accelerator u.
    Magnetom Espree open MRI u.
    Magnetom Vision MR u.

    Mammotest u.
    Maxima II TENS u.
    molecular recognition u. (MRU)
    monitor u.
    Multistar angiographic u.
    musculotendinous u.
    Odelca camera u.
    u. of radioactivity
    u. of wavelength
    Optiplanimat automated u.
    Orbix x-ray u.
    orthopantomograph panoramic digital
      radiography u.
    ostiomeatal u.
    photodisplay u.
    Picker Eclipse MR u.
    pilosebaceous u.
    Plasma 1000 ICP-AES u.
    pressor u.
    quantum u.
    radiation effect u.
    radiologic u.
    reflectometer tuning u.
    roentgen u. (RU)
    rutherford u.
    sector u.
    Sheffield gamma u.
    Siemens Somatom nonhelical u.
    sonography u.
    Sonos 2000 ultrasound u.
    Surgitron portable radiosurgical u.
    Symphony MR u.
    terminal ductal lobular u. (TDLU)
    Tesla superconductive magnet u.
    Thayer-Doisy u.
    ThromboScan molecular recognition u.
    1.5T Signa MR u.
    video display u. (VDU)
    whole-body u.
    Wood u.
    X u.
    x-ray u.
United States Catheter and Instrument (USCI)
uniting canal
univentricular heart
universalis
    calcinosis u.
university
    U. of California Los Angeles
      (UCLA)
    U. of Florida linear accelerator
    U. of Florida staging system
Univision echocardiographic system
Unix/X11 workstation
unknown
    u. primary
    u. primary site
    u. primary tumor

unleveling
    pelvic u.
unloading
    bone u.
unmitigated
unmodulated radiofrequency current
unmyelinated nerve fiber
unneurulated neural placode
unopacified bowel loop
unopposed image
unossified cartilage
unpaired
    u. parietal branch
    u. visceral branch
unplicated sheath
unraveling
    digital u.
unresectable
    u. colorectal carcinoma
    u. lesion
unresolved pneumonia
unroofed coronary sinus syndrome
unruptured follicle
unsaturated
    u. compound
    u. spin
unsegmented vertebral bar
unsharp
    u. masking
    u. mask-type contrast
unsharpness
    absorption u.
    geometric u.
    motion u.
    system u.
unshunted hydrocephalus
unstable
    u. fracture
    u. joint
    u. lesion
    u. mucosa
    u. plaque
unsuppressed
    u. examination
    u. imaging
    u. water signal
untethered
untransformed nadir
ununited fracture
unusual
    u. fetal lie
    u. interstitial pneumonitis
    u. marrow distribution
    u. occurrence report (UOR)
unwinding of aorta
unwrapping
    Dixon method of phase u.
UOQ
    upper outer quadrant

UOR
    unusual occurrence report
up
    ramp u.
    tented u.
uPACS picture archiving system
updraft therapy
UP7 film
upfront delay
upgated technique
uphill varix
UPJ
    ureteropelvic junction
    UPJ obstruction
upper
    u. aerodigestive tract
    u. airway obstruction
    u. esophageal sphincter (UES)
    u. extremity
    u. extremity venous thrombosis (UEVT)
    u. gastrointestinal (UGI)
    u. gastrointestinal endoscopy
    u. gastrointestinal hemorrhage
    u. gastrointestinal series
    u. gastrointestinal tract
    u. GI with small bowel followthrough
    u. inner quadrant (UIQ)
    u. jaw bone
    u. left quadrant (ULQ)
    u. limits of normal
    u. lobe
    u. lobe of lung
    u. lobe vein prominence
    u. lung disease
    u. lung field
    u. mantle radiation therapy
    u. moiety ureter
    u. motor neuron
    u. motor neuron lesion
    u. outer quadrant (UOQ)
    u. pole
    u. pole collecting system
    u. pole moiety
    u. pole of ureter
    u. pulmonary lobe atelectasis
    u. rate interval
    u. respiratory tract disease
    u. right quadrant (URQ)
    u. sternal border
    u. thoracic esophagus
    u. thoracic spine fracture
upregulated AQP4 expression
upregulation
    radiation-induced u.
upright
    u. chest film
    u. compression spot film

U

upright (*continued*)
    u. position
    u. postvoid view
UPSC
    uterine papillary serous carcinoma
upscanning
upside-down stomach
upsloping curve of kidney
upstairs-downstairs heart
upstream blood
upstroke
    carotid pulse u.
    u. pattern on apexcardiogram (dP/dt)
    u. phase of cardiac action potential
    weak carotid u.
uptake
    abnormal tissue u.
    absence of u.
    absent radiotracer u.
    u. and excretion
    u. and retention
    asymmetric limb u.
    atherosclerotic u.
    bilateral diffuse increased u.
    bilateral reduction of tracer u.
    cell preparation bone marrow u.
    contrast u.
    decreased thyroid radiotracer u.
    diffuse lung u.
    diffuse pulmonary u.
    dye u.
    extracardiac focal u.
    extracerebral soft tissue u.
    extraosseous u.
    extrapulmonary u.
    extraskeletal u.
    ^{18}F 2-deoxyglucose u.
    FDG u.
    fluorescein u.
    focal decreased radiotracer u.
    focal pulmonary u.
    ^{67}Ga u.
    gallium u.
    hepatocyte tracer u.
    heterogeneous u.
    u. in bone marrow
    incidental lung u.
    increased isotope u.
    increased thyroid u.
    increased tracer u.
    Infecton u.
    u. in supraclavicular adipose (USA)
    intense u.
    iodine u.
    isotope u.
    laryngeal musculature
      fluorodeoxyglucose u.
    leukocyte u.
    localized u.

    mediastinal u.
    metabolic tracer u.
    mottled hepatic u.
    mottled liver u.
    ^{99m}Tc HMPAO u.
    ^{99m}Tc MDP u.
    muscle u.
    myocardial u.
    ^{13}N ammonia u.
    near-normal radiotracer u.
    normal variant of Ga-67 u.
    observed maximal u.
    u. of radioactive material
    u. of radionuclide
    papillary muscle u.
    periprosthetic u.
    physiologic u.
    predicted maximal u.
    progressive u.
    prominent u.
    radioactive iodine u. (RAIU)
    radioiodine u.
    radioisotope u.
    radiopharmaceutical u.
    radiotracer u.
    u. ratio
    regional tracer u.
    symmetric pattern of radiotracer u.
    T4 u.
    technetium 99m MDP u.
    thyroid radioiodine u.
    tracer u.
    uniform u.
    variable u.
    V-like pattern of u.
uptilted cardiac apex
upward
    u. and backward dislocation
    u. lens dislocation
    u. retraction
urachal
    u. abnormality
    u. anomaly
    u. carcinoma
    u. cyst
    u. diverticulum
    u. ligament
    u. remnant disease
    u. sinus
urachus
    patent u.
uracil
uranium (U)
    u. imaging agent
^{235}**uranium** (^{235}**U, U-235**)
urate
    u. arthropathy
    u. calculus
    u. nephropathy

urceiform, urceolate
urceolate (*var. of* urceiform)
uremia
uremic
    u. amaurosis
    u. lung
    u. medullary cystic disease
    u. myopathy
ureter
    atonic u.
    beaded u.
    bifid u.
    champagne glass u.
    circumcaval u.
    cobra-head u.
    corkscrew u.
    curlicue u.
    u. diameter
    dilated u.
    dilation of u.
    ectopic u.
    extravesical infrasphincteric ectopic u.
    hockey-stick appearance of u.
    hood-shaped u.
    intestinal u.
    intramural portion of distal u.
    intravesical u.
    J-hook deformity of distal u.
    J-shaped u.
    kinked u.
    lower moiety u.
    lower pole of u.
    moderately dilated u.
    notching u.
    orthotopic u.
    pipestem u.
    postcaval u.
    redundant u.
    retrocaval u.
    retroiliac u.
    rigid u.
    saddle peristalsis of u.
    sawtooth u.
    seesaw peristalsis of u.
    spring onion u.
    straight u.
    tortuosity of u.
    upper moiety u.
    upper pole of u.
ureteral, ureteric
    u. achalasia
    u. adenomyosis
    u. artery
    u. bud
    u. bud bifurcation
    u. calculus
    u. carcinoma
    u. clipping
    u. compression technique

    u. deviation
    u. dilation
    u. distention
    u. diverticulum
    u. division
    u. duplication
    u. endometriosis
    u. filling
    u. filling defect
    u. fistula
    u. jet
    u. kinking
    u. notching
    u. occlusion
    u. orifice
    u. perforation
    u. perfusion test
    u. reflux study
    u. renal transplant obstruction
    u. seesaw peristalsis
    u. spindle
    u. stasis
    u. stenosis
    u. stenting
    u. stone
    u. stricture
ureterectasis
ureteric (*var. of* ureteral)
ureteritis cystica
ureterocele
    ectopic u.
    orthotopic u.
    pyoureter ectopic u.
    simple u.
ureterocutaneous fistula
ureterocystography
ureteroenteral anastomotic stricture
ureterogram
    retrograde u.
ureterography
    bulb u.
    retrograde u.
ureterohydronephrosis
ureteroileostomy
ureterointestinal fistula
ureterolysis
ureteroneocystostomy
ureteropelvic
    u. junction (UPJ)
    u. junction obstruction
ureteroperitoneal fistula
ureteropyelogram
    retrograde u.
ureteropyelography
ureteropyelostomy
ureterorenal junction
ureterorenoscopy
ureteroscope
    solid-rod u.

U

ureteroscopy
ureterostomy
ureteroureteral anastomosis
ureterovaginal fistula
ureterovesical
    u. anastomosis
    u. junction
    u. junction obstruction
urethra
    angle of inclination
     of u.
    anterior u.
    bulbous u.
    cavernous u.
    female u.
    male u.
    membranous u.
    pendulous u.
    penile u.
    posterior u.
    prostatic u. (PU)
    ragged u.
    spinning-top u.
urethral
    u. amyloidosis
    u. angle
    u. atresia
    u. calculus
    u. condyloma acuminatum
    u. crest
    u. diverticulum
    u. fish-hooking
    u. gland
    u. groove
    u. inclination
    u. length
    u. metallic stent
    u. obstruction
    u. orifice
    u. papilla
    u. ridge
    u. straddle injury
    u. stricture
    u. syndrome
    u. thickness
    u. trauma
    u. tumor
    u. uterus
    u. valve
    u. warming
urethritis
urethrocystogram
urethrocystography
    u. imaging
    retrograde u.
    voiding u.
urethrocystometry
urethrogram
    excretory u.

    normal fold u.
    retrograde u. (RUG)
urethrography
urethroplasty
    prostatic u.
    retrograde transurethral prostatic u.
urethroscopy
urethrotome
urethrotomy
    internal u.
urethrovaginal fistula
urethrovesical angle (UVA)
uric
    u. acid calculus
    u. acid nephropathy
urinary
    u. bladder adenocarcinoma
    u. bladder atony
    u. bladder calculus
    u. bladder capacity
    u. bladder contusion
    u. bladder cuff
    u. bladder diverticulum
    u. bladder exstrophy
    u. bladder extrinsic mass
    u. bladder fundus
    u. bladder hemangioma
    u. bladder leiomyoma
    u. bladder lymphoma
    u. bladder rupture
    u. bladder stone
    u. bladder trauma
    u. bladder tumor
    u. bladder wall calcification
    u. bladder wall mass
    u. bladder wall thickening
    u. blunt trauma bladder
    u. conduit
    u. diversion
    u. excretion
    u. excretory route
    u. extravasation
    u. fistula
    u. glucosyl-galactosyl-pyridinoline
    u. obstruction
    u. stasis
    u. stent
    u. tract
    u. tract anomaly
    u. tract calculus
    u. tract fibroepithelioma
    u. tract gas
    u. tract infection (UTI)
    u. tract obstruction
    u. tract tuberculosis
    u. ulcer
urine
    u. ascites
    postvoid residual u.

radiopaque u.
residual u.
retained u.

urinoma
perinephric u.

urinothorax

uriposia

urodynamic pressure-flow study

uroepithelial
u. malignancy
u. tumor

urogenital
u. canal
u. diaphragm
u. embryology
u. malignancy
u. sinus
u. tract
u. triangle

Urografin imaging agent

urogram
constant-infusion excretory u.
diuresis u.
excretory u.
retrograde u. (RU)

urographic
u. density
u. scan timing

urography
antegrade u.
ascending u.
cystoscopic u.
descending u.
diuretic radionuclide u.
drip infusion u.
excretion u.
u. imaging
intravenous u. (IVU)
magnetic resonance u. (MRU)
multidetector computed tomography
u. (MDCTU)
oral u.
percutaneous antegrade u.
retrograde u.

urokinase
catheter-directed u.
u. imaging agent

Urolase
U. fiber laser
U. fiber laser ablation

urolithiasis

Uromiro contrast medium

uropathy
chronic obstructive u.
obstructive u.

uroradiologic procedure

uroradiology

Uroselectan

urostealith calculus

urothelial
u. carcinoma
u. striation

urothelium

Urovision

Urovist
U. Cysto imaging agent
U. meglumine Diu/CT imaging
agent
U. sodium 300 imaging agent

URQ
upper right quadrant

urticate

urtication

US
ultrasonography

USA
uptake in supraclavicular adipose
USA fat

USCI
United States Catheter and Instrument
USCI PET balloon
USCI probe
USCI Probe balloon-on-a-wire
dilation system

useful
u. beam
u. beam radiation

user
service class u.

USP
uterine stimulating potency
USP XX test

USPI
ulnar styloid process index

USPIO
ultrasmall superparamagnetic iron oxide
USPIO imaging agent

usual
u. interstitial pneumonia (UIP)
u. interstitial pneumonia of
Liebow
u. interstitial pneumonitis

uteri (*pl. of* uterus)

uteric fold

uterinae
ampulla tubae u.
ostium abdominale tubae u.

uterine
u. adenomyosis
u. agenesis
u. anatomy
u. artery (UA)
u. artery embolization (UAE)
u. artery pseudoaneurysm
u. artery waveform
u. blood volume flow
u. blush
u. body

U

uterine (*continued*)
  u. canal
  u. cavity
  u. cervical ganglion
  u. cervical lymphoma
  u. cervix
  u. cervix carcinoma
  u. cirsoid aneurysm
  u. contraction
  u. corpus carcinoma
  u. didelphia
  u. duplication anomaly
  u. fibroid
  u. fibroid embolization (UFE)
  u. fibroid polyp
  u. fundus
  u. horn
  u. hypoplasia
  u. insufficiency
  u. isthmus
  u. leiomyoma
  u. leiomyosarcoma
  u. ligament
  u. mass
  u. myoma
  u. myometrium
  u. opacity
  u. papillary serous carcinoma
   (UPSC)
  u. peristalsis
  u. retroflexion
  u. sarcoma metastasis
  u. size
  u. stimulating potency (USP)
  u. synechia
  u. tube
  u. venography
  u. wry neck

utero
  fetal death in u.
  fetal echocardiography
   in u.
  in u.

uteroabdominal pregnancy
uterocervical canal
uterogram
uterography
uteropelvic
uteroplacental
  u. circulation
  u. insufficiency
uterosacral ligament
uterosalpingogram
uterosalpingography
uterotubal pregnancy
uterotubography
uterovaginal
  u. canal
  u. plexus

uterovesical
  u. fossa
  u. junction
  u. ligament
  u. pouch
uterus, *pl.* **uteri**
  adenocarcinoma of u.
  anteflexed u.
  anteverted u.
  aplastic u.
  arcuate u.
  u. arcuatus
  bicameral u.
  u. bicornis unicollis
  bicornuate u.
  biforate u.
  bilocular u.
  bipartite u.
  bleeding u.
  body of u.
  cervix uteri
  cochleate u.
  cornu of u.
  corpus uteri
  Couvelaire u.
  didelphic u.
  u. didelphys
  double u.
  double-mouthed u.
  duplex u.
  empty u.
  enlargement of u.
  fetal u.
  fibroid u.
  fundus uteri
  gas gangrene of u.
  gravid u.
  heart-shaped u.
  horn of u.
  infantile u.
  isthmus of u.
  large-for-dates u.
  nonpregnant horn of bicornuate u.
  outer border of u.
  pear-shaped u.
  postpartum u.
  pregnant u.
  pubescent u.
  retroflexed u.
  retroverted u.
  ribbon u.
  round ligament of u.
  saddle-shaped u.
  septate u.
  u. subseptus
  T-shaped u.
  u. unicornis
  unicornous u.
  urethral u.

UTI
 urinary tract infection
utilization
 radioiron red cell u.
utricle
 large u.
 prostatic u.
utriculosaccular canal
utriculus prostaticus
U-tube stent
U-1100 UV-Vis spectrophotometer
UV
 ultraviolet
UVA
 urethrovesical angle

uveitis
 granulomatous u.
 sarcoid u.
uviofast, uvioresistant
uviometer
uvioresistant (*var. of* uviofast)
uviosensitive
uvula, *pl.* **uvuli**
 cerebellar u.
 u. of bladder
 u. palatina
uvulae
 musculus u.
uvuli (*pl. of* uvula)
uvulopalatoplasty
 laser-assisted u. (LAUP)

U

V

V pattern
V peak of jugular venous pulse
technetium 99m-labeled annexin V

V18

V18 Control Wire guidewire
V18 micro guidewire

VΛ, V-Λ

ventriculoatrial
VA shunt

va

volt-ampere

VABES

vasoablative endothelial sarcoma

Vac-Lok patient immobilization system

VACTERL

vertebral, anal, cardiac, tracheal, esophageal, renal, limb
VACTERL spectrum
VACTERL syndrome

vacuo

hydrocephalus ex v.

vacuolating myelinopathy

vacuole

vacuolization

vacuum

v. arthrography
v. cassette system
v. cleaner effect
v. cleft
v. disc phenomenon
v. extraction
facet joint v.
v. phenomenon sign
v. tube

vacuum-assisted

v.-a. core biopsy
v.-a. imaging-guided biopsy

vagale

glomus v.

vagal trunk

vagatomy effect

vagi (*pl. of* vagus)

vagina, *pl.* **vaginae**

aditus vaginae
anterior fornix of v.
azygos artery of v.
double v.
vestibule of v.

vaginae (*pl. of* vagina)

vaginal

v. agenesis
v. bleeding

v. canal
v. carcinoma
v. code irradiation
v. cuff
v. cylinder
v. endosonography
v. fistula
v. fornix
v. fundus
v. intraepithelial neoplasia
v. ligament
v. orifice
v. plexus
v. testis
v. tumor
v. wall

vaginalis

portio v.
processus v.
tunica v.
vestigium processus v.

vaginitis emphysematosa

vaginogram

vaginography

barium v.

vaginoperineoplasty

vagotomy

vagus, *pl.* **vagi**

v. nerve-stimulated functional magnetic resonance imaging (VNS-fMRI)
v. nerve stimulation (VNS)
v. nerve stimulation-synchronized blood oxygen level-dependent functional MRI

Valdini method

valence, valency

v. band
v. bond
v. electron
electron v.
ionic polar v.

valency (*var. of* valence)

valga

coxa v.

valgum

genu v.

valgus

adolescent hallux v.
anatomic genu v.
v. angulation
bilateral hallux v.
v. carrying angle
cubitus v.
v. deviation

V

valgus (*continued*)
    digitus v.
    v. foot
    hallux v. (HV)
    v. heel deformity
    hindfoot v.
    v. index
    metatarsus v.
    pes malleus v.
    v. stress
    talipes v.
    v. tilt
    unilateral hallux v.
valgus-external rotation injury
vallecula, *pl.* **valleculae**
    v. cerebelli
valleculae (*pl. of* vallecula)
vallecular
    v. cyst
    v. dysphagia
    v. narrowing
valley-to-peak dose rate
Valsalva
    coronary sinus of V.
    V. maneuver
    V. muscle
    sinus of V.
valsalviana
    dysphagia v.
value
    ADCav v.
    attenuation v.
    bright pixel v.
    comparative v.
    CT attenuation v.
    dark pixel v.
    echo-train v.
    v. flip
    maximal standardized uptake v.
    negative predictive v. (NPV)
    pixel v.
    positive predictive v. (PPV)
    S v.
    soft tissue attenuation v.
    standard uptake v. (SUV)
    time to peak v.
    tristimulus v.
    T1, T2 v.
    velocity encoding v. (VENC)
    venous blood gas v.
valve
    absent v.
    afferent nipple v.
    Ahmed glaucoma v.
    anterior semilunar v.

    v. anulus
    aortic v.
    aortocoronary v.
    v. area
    artificial cardiac v.
    atrioventricular nodal v.
    v. attenuation
    ball occluder v.
    ball-type v.
    Bauhin v.
    Beall v.
    bicommissural aortic v.
    bicuspid aortic v.
    bicuspid atrioventricular v.
    bileaflet v.
    billowing mitral v.
    biologic tissue v.
    Björk-Shiley heart v.
    blunting of v.
    Braunwald-Cutter v.
    Bunsen-type v.
    calcified aortic v.
    capillary v.
    Carbomedics v.
    cardiac v.
    caval v.
    C-C heart v.
    central caged ball occluder v.
    central caged disc occluder v.
    v. cinefluoroscopy
    cleft mitral v.
    v. closure
    Codman Medos programmable v.
    v. commissure
    competent ileocecal v.
    composite aortic v.
    conduit v.
    congenital absence of pulmonary v.
    congenital anomaly of mitral v. (CAMV)
    convexoconcave heart v.
    coronary sinus v.
    v. cusp
    v. dehiscence
    v. diameter
    disc-type v.
    doming of v.
    dysplastic pulmonary v.
    early opening of v.
    eccentric monocuspid disc v.
    echodense v.
    ectatic aortic v.
    efferent nipple v.
    E-to-F slope of v.
    eustachian v.
    failed v.
    fibroelastoma of heart v.
    fishmouth configuration of mitral v.
    flail mitral v.

flaplike v.
floppy mitral v.
flow-controlled v.
foramen ovale v.
frenulum of v.
globular v.
gradient across v.
Harken v.
heart v.
hockey-stick deformity of tricuspid v.
hypoplastic v.
ileocecal v.
incompetent ileocecal v.
incompetent lymph v.
v. leaflet
leaky v.
low-profile mitral v.
lymphatic v.
v. malformation
mechanical v.
Medos Hakim programmable v.
midsystolic buckling of mitral v.
miniaturized mitral v.
mitral v.
monocuspid tilting-disc v.
M-shaped pattern of mitral v.
mural leaflet of mitral v.
narrowed v.
native aortic v.
neoaortic v.
nonfunctioning heart v.
notching of pulmonic v.
v. of Heister
v. of Houston
v. of navicular fossa
Omniscience v.
v. opening slope
v. outflow strut
parachute deformity of mitral v.
v. plane
v. pocket
posterior urethral v. (type I-IV)
  (PUV)
premature middiastolic closure of
  mitral v.
preservation of native aortic v.
pressure-activated safety v.
  (PASV)
programmable ventricular
  shunt v.
v. prolapse
prolapsed mitral v. (PMV)
prolapse of aortic v.
prosthetic heart v.
prosthetic mitral v.
pullback across aortic v.
pulmonary v. (PV)
pyloric v.
quadricuspid aortic v.

quadricuspid pulmonary v.
rectal v.
regurgitant v.
v. replacement
retrograde blood flow across v.
rheumatic heart v.
v. ring
Rosenmüller v.
rotating hemostatic v.
sail-like tricuspid v.
semilunar v.
shunt v.
sigmoid v.
Smelloff-Cutter v.
Sophy programmable v.
spiral v.
stenosed aortic v.
stenotic tricuspid v.
stentless porcine aortic v.
stent-mounted allograft v.
stent-mounted heterograft v.
synthetic v.
systolic anterior motion of
  mitral v.
thebesian v.
thickened aortic v.
v. thickening
tilting-disc v.
v. tip
tissue outflow v.
track v.
tricuspid aortic v.
trileaflet aortic v.
truncal v.
v. tube
unicommissural aortic v.
unicuspid with aortic v.
urethral v.
v. vegetation
venous v.
Vieussens v.
v. wrapping
xenograft v.
4-valve tube rectification
valviform
valvoplasty, valvuloplasty
  balloon mitral v.
valvotome
  spade-shaped v.
valvotomy, valvulotomy
  balloon v.
valvula, *pl.* **valvulae**
  valvulae conniventes
valvulae (*pl. of* valvula)
valvular
  v. aortic insufficiency
  v. aortic stenosis
  v. apparatus
  v. atresia

valvular (*continued*)
v. cardiac defect
v. damage
v. disease
v. dysfunction
v. efficiency
v. heart disease
v. incompetence
v. leaflet calcification
v. opening
v. orifice
v. pneumothorax
v. pulmonic stenosis
v. regurgitant lesion
v. regurgitation (VR)
v. scarring
v. sclerosis
valvuloplasty (*var. of* valvoplasty)
valvulotomy (*var. of* valvotomy)
van
V. Aman pulmonary pigtail catheter
v. Buchem disease
v. Buchem syndrome
V. de Graaf generator
v. der Hoeve syndrome
V. Neck disease
V. Nuys prognostic index for DCIS
V. Rosen view
V. Sonnenberg chest drain set
V. Sonnenberg sump catheter
vanadium
vanishing
v. bone disease
v. lung
v. lung syndrome
v. lung tumor
v. testis syndrome
v. twin
v. white matter
Vanzetti sciatica sign
vaporization
plaque v.
Vaquez disease
vara
adolescent tibia v.
Blount tibia v.
congenital tibia v.
coxa v.
epiphysial coxa v.
infantile tibia v.
tibia v.
variability
anatomic v.
beat-to-beat v.
interpretive v.
intertumoral v.
intratumoral v.
peak flow v.
ventricular rate v.

variable
v. cerebral dysplasia
v. energy
v. flip-angle excitation
v. intensity
v. number tandem repeat
v. projection (VARPRO)
v. projection method
quantitative exercise thallium-201 v.
v. response rate
v. segment
v. temperature (VT)
v. TE, TR
v. tube current
v. tube potential
v. uptake
variable-angle
v.-a. gamma camera
v.-a. spinning (VAS)
v.-a. uniform signal excitation (VUSE)
variable-density SMASH
variable-stiffness guidewire
Varian
V. accelerator
V. Associates spectrometer
V. brachytherapy system
V. CT scanner
V. LINAC
V. MLC system
V. NMR spectrometer
variance
Hulten v.
v. image
negative ulnar v.
neutral ulnar v.
positive ulnar v. (PUV)
ulnar v.
variant
anatomic bile duct v.
blastic v.
congenital mediastinal arterial v.
v. Creutzfeldt-Jakob disease (vCJD)
Dandy-Walker v.
electrocardiographic v.
fibrosarcoma v.
Heidenhain v.
high-riding v.
labral v.
mediastinal arterial v.
normal v.
ossification v.
pancreaticobiliary function v.
variation
anatomic v.
area/hemidiameter v.
biologic v.
BO field v.
circadian v.

coefficient of v.
exposure v.
field v.
v. in density
interobserver v.
intraobserver v.
low interobserver v.
normal anatomic v.
observer v.
positional v.
pulse width v.
surface dose v.
view-to-view v.

Varibar
V. honey barium sulfate
V. nectar barium sulfate
V. oral contrast agent
V. pudding barium sulfate
V. thin honey barium sulfate
V. thin liquid barium sulfate

varication
variceal
v. column
v. decompression
v. hemorrhage
v. sclerosis
v. wall

varicella pneumonia
varicella-zoster
varices (*pl. of* varix)
varicocele
idiopathic v.
v. tumor of breast

varicography
varicoid esophageal carcinoma
varicose
v. aneurysm
v. bronchiectasis
v. vein

varicosity
parovarian v.
reticular v.

variegated pattern
varioliform erosion
VariTone
Varivas loop graft
varix, *pl.* **varices**
arterial v.
arteriovenous v.
colonic v.
Dagradi classification of esophageal v.
downhill v.
duodenal v.
ectopic v.
esophageal v.
gastric v.
intraaxial v.
lung v.
v. of aneurysm

Okuda transhepatic obliteration of v.
orbital v.
paraesophageal v.
pericholedochal v.
pulmonary v.
ruptured pelvic v.
saphenous v.
stomach v.
sublingual v.
umbilical vein v.
uphill v.

VARPRO
variable projection

varum
genu v.

varus
v. angulation
cubitus v.
v. deformity
v. deviation
digitus v.
v. foot
hallux v.
v. heel
mechanical genu v.
v. metatarsophalangeal angle
metatarsus v.
pes v.
rearfoot v.
v. rerotation
v. stress
v. stress laxity
subtalar v.
talipes v.
tibial v.
v. tilt

varus-valgus
v.-v. instability
v.-v. plane

varying degrees of obliquity
VAS
variable-angle spinning
vestibular aqueduct syndrome

vas, *pl.* **vasa,** *gen.* and *pl.* **vasorum**
aortic vasa vasorum
vas deferens
vasa deferentia
vasa differentia calcification

vasa (*pl. of* vas)
vascular
v. abdominal calcification
v. abnormality
v. access device
v. access safety kit
v. and airway modeling
v. aneurysm
v. anomaly
v. assessment
v. attenuation

vascular (*continued*)
v. band
v. bed
v. blood
v. blood pool
v. blush
v. bone
v. brachytherapy
v. brain occlusion
v. bud
v. bundle
v. bypass graft
v. catastrophe
v. cell adhesion molecule-1 (VCAM-1)
v. channel
v. cirrhosis
v. colon ectasia
v. compartment
v. compromise
v. congestion
v. contour
v. cord damage
v. dementia
v. encasement
v. esophageal compression
v. fibrous polyp
v. flask
v. flow imaging
v. goiter
v. graft infection
v. groove
v. hamartoma
v. hemangioma
v. hemostatic device (VHD)
v. hydraulic conductivity
v. hydraulics
v. impedance
v. insufficiency
v. insult
v. invasion
v. jejunization
v. kidney anatomy
v. leak syndrome
v. leiomyoma
v. lesion
v. lumen
v. malformation
v. marking
v. MR contrast enhancement
v. myxoma
v. necrosis
v. neoplasm
v. network
v. obstruction
v. occlusive disease
v. origin bone tumor
v. parkinsonism
v. patency
v. pedicle

v. perforation
v. phase
v. phenomenon
v. plexus
v. protrusion
v. pterygoid attachment
v. redistribution
v. reflection
renal v.
v. renal anatomy
v. reserve
v. ring
v. sarcoma
v. sclerosis
v. segmentation
v. segmentation and extraction
v. shadow
v. sheath
v. sling
v. smooth muscle
v. space of placenta
v. spasm
v. stasis
v. stent
v. stroma
v. structure
v. supply
v. systemic resistance
v. thrombosis
v. tissue
v. tone
v. tracheal compression
v. transformation
v. trauma
v. tree
v. tuft
v. villous atrophy
v. wall
v. xenograft
v. zone
vascularity
decreased pulmonary v.
femoral head v.
increased pulmonary v.
moyamoya v.
overcirculation v.
pulmonary v.
sunburst brain v.
tumor v.
vascularization
graft v.
hand v.
tumor v.
vascularized granulation tissue
vasculature
brain tumor v.
cardiac v.
cerebral v.
depiction of v.

extracranial cerebral v.
increased pulmonary v.
interlobular v.
meningeal v.
peripheral v.
pruned appearance of pulmonary v.
pulmonary v.
splanchnic v.

vasculitic lesion
vasculitis
large-vessel v.
mesenteric v.
small-vessel v.

vasculopathy
lenticulostriate v. (LSV)
radiation v.
radiation-induced v.

vasoablative endothelial sarcoma (VABES)
vasoactive
v. intestinal polypeptide tumor (VIPoma)
v. response

vasoconstriction
hypoxic pulmonary v.
peripheral circulatory v.
peripheral cutaneous v.
pulmonary arteriolar v.
spontaneous transient v.
systemic arterial v.

vasoconstrictor response
vasodepressor response
vasodilatation (*var. of* vasodilation)
vasodilating agent
vasodilation, vasodilatation
breakthrough v.

vasodilator administration
vasodilatory
v. capacity
v. effect
v. hemodynamic stress test
v. response

vasoepididymography
vasogenic
v. edema
v. impotence
v. shock

vasography
vasomotor
v. change
v. reaction
v. symptom

vasoocclusive
v. angiotherapy (VAT)
v. crisis

vasoreactivity
cerebral v.
pulmonary v.

vasoregulation

vasorelaxation of epicardial vessel
vasorum (*gen.* and *pl. of* vas)
VasoSeal
V. diagnostic device
V. Elite
V. Elite vascular closure
V. ES, VHD arterial puncture site closure device
V. therapeutic device

vasospasm
catheter-induced v.
cerebral v.
primary v.

vasospastic vessel
vasovagal reaction
VasoView balloon dissection system
Vasovist
vastus
v. intermedius
v. lateralis
v. medialis
v. medialis advancement (VMA)
v. medialis muscle
v. medialis obliquus (VMO)

VAT
vasoocclusive angiotherapy
ventricular activation time
video-assisted thoracoscopy
visceral adipose tissue

VATER
vertebral, anal, tracheal, esophageal, renal
VATER association
VATER complex

Vater
ampulla of V.
V. diverticulum
V. duct
V. fold
papilla of V.

vaterian segment
vault
cranial v.
plantar v.
rectal v.

Vaxcel
V. peripherally inserted catheter
V. PICC

Vax 4100 system
VB
virtual bronchoscopy

V510B Biplane TEE transducer
Vbeam
V. pulsed-dye laser
V. pulsed-dye laser system

VBI
vertebrobasilar insufficiency

VBR
ventricle-brain ratio

V

V/C
  vermis-cerebellum
    V/C ratio
VCA
  vertical-center-anterior
VCAM-1
  vascular cell adhesion molecule-1
VCB
  ventricular capture beat
VCE
  vein contrast enhancer
VCF
  ventricular contractility function
  vertebral compression fracture
VCG
  vectorcardiogram
vCJD
  variant Creutzfeldt-Jakob disease
    pulvinar sign of vCJD
VCMG
  videocystometrography
VCU
  voiding cystourethrogram
  voiding cystourethrography
VCUG
  vesicoureterogram
  voiding cystourethrogram
VDI
  venous distensibility index
VDR
  vessel density ratio
VDS
  ventral derotating spinal
    VDS implant
VDU
  video display unit
VE
  virtual endoscopy
VEA
  ventricular ectopic activity
VEB
  ventricular ectopic beat
VEC
  velocity-encoded cine
    VEC imaging
VEC-MR
  velocity-encoded cine-magnetic
    resonance
vector
    bulk magnetization v.
    electrocardiographic angle between
      QRS and T v.'s (QRS-T)
    expression v.
    v. loop
    v. loop vectorcardiography
    macroscopic magnetization v.
    v. magnitude
    mean cardiac v.
    net magnetization v.

    nonviral v.
    QRS v.
    v. quantization
    spin v.
    v. subtraction
    T v.
vectorcardiogram (VCG)
vectorcardiography
    Frank v.
    frontal plane v.
    v. imaging
    sagittal plane v.
    spatial v.
    transverse plane v.
    vector loop v.
vegetation
    cardiac v.
    dendritic v.
    friable v.
    heart valve v.
    valve v.
vegetative
    v. lesion
    v. state
veil
    tissue v.
veiling glare
vein, vena
    absent peripheral v.
    accessory cephalic v.
    accessory hemiazygos v.
    accessory hepatic v.
    accessory saphenous v.
    accessory vertebral v.
    accompanying v.
    adrenal v.
    anal v.
    anastomotic v.
    aneurysmal v.
    angular v.
    anonymous v.
    antebrachial v.
    antecubital v.
    anterior cardiac v.
    anterior internal vertebral v. (AIVV)
    anterior jugular v.
    anterior terminal v. (ATV)
    aplasia of deep v.
    appendicular v.
    aqueous v.
    arcuate v.
    arterial v.
    ascending lumbar v.
    auditory v.
    auricular v.
    autogenous v.
    axillary v.
    azygos v.
    basal placenta v.

basilic v.
basivertebral v.
blind percutaneous puncture of subclavian v.
Boyd perforating v.
brachial v.
brachiocephalic v.
brain bridging v.
branch of v.
bronchial v.
bulb of v.
Burrow v.
cannulated central v.
capacious v.
capillary v.
cardiac v.
cardinal v.
carotid v.
caudate v.
cavernous transfer of portal v.
cavernous transformation of portal v.
central v.
cephalic v.
cerebral v.
cervical v.
choroid v.
chronic insufficiency of v.
ciliary v.
circumaortic left renal v.
circumflex v.
colic v.
common basal v.
common cardinal v.
common facial v.
common femoral v.
communicating v.
companion v.
condylar emissary v.
congenital stenosis of pulmonary v.
conjunctival v.
v. contrast enhancer (VCE)
coronary v.
cortical v.
costoaxillary v.
cutaneous v.
cystic v.
deep v.
dense abdominal v.'s
digital v.
dilated collateral v.
dilated spinal v.
v. dilation
diploic v.
distended v.
dorsal penile v.
dorsispinal v.
dual popliteal v.'s
duodenal v.

embryonal v.
embryonic umbilical v.
emissary v.
engorged v.
epigastric v.
episcleral v.
esophageal v.
ethmoidal v.
external jugular v. (EJV)
external pudendal v.
extirpation of saphenous v.
extradural vertebral plexus of v.
facial v.
familial varicose v.
feeder v.
femoral v.
fibular v.
flat neck v.
frontal v.
gastric v.
gastroepiploic v.
v. graft
v. graft occlusion
v. graft stenosis
v. graft thrombosis
great cardiac v.
greater saphenous v.
harvested v.
hemiazygos v.
hemispheric v.
hepatic v.
ileocolic v.
iliac v.
iliofemoral v.
inferior mesenteric v.
inferior ophthalmic v.
inferior pulmonary v.
inferior rectal v.
inferior thyroid v.
v. inflammation
infradiaphragmatic v.
innominate v.
intercostal v.
internal cerebral v. (ICV)
internal jugular v. (IJV)
internal thoracic v.
intraforaminal v.
intrahepatic umbilical v.
v. intussusception
jugular v.
Labbé v.
labial v.
leaking v.
left hepatic v. (LHV)
left pulmonary v. (LPV)
left retroaortic renal v.
lesser saphenous v.
lobe of azygos v.
v. mapping

V

vein (*continued*)
    marginal v.
    Marshall v.
    median antebrachial v.
    mediastinal v.
    medullary v.
    meningeal v.
    mesencephalic v.
    mesenteric v.
    middle cardiac v.
    middle hepatic v. (MHV)
    middle rectal v.
    v. nodularity
    oblique v.
    v. of Galen fistula
    v. of Galen malformation
    v. of Trolard
    ophthalmic v.
    orbital varix of ophthalmic v.
    ovarian v.
    palmar cutaneous v.
    pancreatic v.
    paraspinal v.
    parathyroid v.
    paraumbilical v.
    parent v.
    v. patency
    patency and valvular reflux of deep v.
    penile v.
    perforating v.
    pericallosal v.
    pericardiacophrenic v.
    pericardial v.
    perithyroid v.
    peroneal v.
    petrosal v.
    pontomesencephalic v.
    popliteal v.
    portal v.
    posterior auricular v.
    posterior cardinal v.
    posterior interventricular v.
    posterior terminal v.
    posterior tibial v. (PTV)
    precentral cerebellar v.
    prepyloric v.
    pudendal v.
    pulmonary v.
    pulsating v.
    quadrigeminal v.
    ranine v.
    renal v.
    retroaortic renal v.
    Retzius v.
    reversed greater saphenous v.
    right hepatic v. (RHV)
    right pulmonary v. (RPV)
    saphenous v.
    Sappey inferior v.
    sausaging of v.
    Schlesinger v.
    Schwartz test for patency of deep saphenous v.
    scimitar v.
    scrotal v.
    segmental v.
    septal v.
    Servelle v.
    simultaneous acquisition of artery and v. (SAAV)
    single popliteal v.
    sludging of retinal v.
    small cardiac v.
    small saphenous v.
    soleal v.
    spermatic v.
    splenic v.
    v. stone
    striate v.
    subcardinal v.
    subclavian v. (SCV)
    subclavian-innominate v.
    subcutaneous v.
    subependymal v.
    superficial femoral v.
    superficial pedal v.
    superior intercostal v.
    superior mesenteric v. (SMV)
    superior ophthalmic v.
    superior pulmonary v.
    superior rectal v.
    supracardinal v.
    systemic v.
    testicular v.
    thalamic v.
    thalamostriate v.
    thebesian v.
    thoracoepigastric v.
    tibial v.
    tortuous v.
    transcerebral medullary v.
    umbilical v.
    v. valve wrapping
    varicose v.
    vermian v.
    vertebral v.
vela (*pl. of* velum)
velamenta (*pl. of* velamentum)
velamentous, veliform
    v. insertion
    v. insertion of cord
    v. placenta
velamentum, *pl.* **velamenta**
velar
Velcro strap immobilizer
veliform (*var. of* velamentous)
vellus

velocimetry
 laser Doppler v.
 particle image v. (PIV)
 UA v.
 umbilical artery v.
velocity
 acoustic v.
 angular v.
 v. artifact
 average peak v.
 blood flow v.
 v. calculation
 carotid v.
 closing v.
 v. compensation
 coronary blood flow v. (CBFV)
 decreased closing v.
 diastolic regurgitant v.
 v. distribution function
 v. encoding on brain MR
  angiography
 v. encoding value (VENC)
 v. evaluation phantom
 fiber-shortening v.
 flow v.
 forward v.
 v. gradient
 high v.
 v. imaging
 impact v.
 intrasac spectral Doppler flow v.
 main portal vein peak v. (MPPv)
 v. mapping
 maximum transaortic jet v.
 mean aortic flow v.
 mean posterior wall v.
 mean pulmonary flow v.
 midshunt peak v. (MSPv)
 mitral inflow v.
 modal v.
 muzzle v.
 peak aortic flow v.
 peak early diastolic filling v.
 peak late diastolic filling v.
 peak pulmonary flow v.
 peak regurgitant flow v.
 peak systolic v. (PSV)
 peak transmitted v.
 portal vein v.
 v. profile
 prostate-specific antigen v. (PSAV)
 regurgitant v.
 retrograde blood v.
 v. spectrum
 TCD v.
 transcranial Doppler v.
 v. waveform (VWF)
velocity-compensating gradient pulse
velocity-density imaging

velocity-encoded
 v.-e. cine (VEC)
 v.-e. cine-magnetic resonance
  (VEC-MR)
 v.-e. cine MRI
 v.-e. cine-MR imaging
 v.-e. color Doppler signal
 v.-e. color Doppler sonography
 v.-e. image
 v.-e. sequence
velocity-enhanced resistance training
 (VERT)
velocity-induced phase shift
velocity-time graph
velolaryngeal endoscopy
velopharyngeal
 v. closure
 v. insufficiency
velopharynx
Velpeau
 V. axillary view
 V. deformity
velum, *pl.* **vela**
vena (*var. of* vein), *pl.* **venae**
 v. cava
 v. cava anomaly
 v. cava filter
 v. comitans
 V. Tech
 V. Tech LGM vena cava filter
 V. Tech low-profile filter
 V. Tech LP vena cava filter
venacavogram
 inferior v. (IVCV)
venacavography
 inferior v. (IVCV)
venae (*pl. of* vena)
VENC
 velocity encoding value
venereal lymphogranuloma
venereum
 lymphogranuloma v.
venetian blind artifact
venoarterial cannulation
venobiliary fistula
venodilator
venofibrosis
venogram
 magnetic resonance v. (MRV)
 renal v.
venography
 adrenal v.
 antegrade v.
 ascending contrast v.
 cerebral CT v.
 computed tomography pulmonary v.
  (CTPV)
 computed tomography v. (CTV)
 contrast v.

V

venography (*continued*)
    conventional v.
    descending v.
    digital free hepatic v.
    direct spiral computed tomography v.
    epidural v.
    extradural v.
    free hepatic v.
    gonadal v.
    hepatic v.
    iliac v.
    v. imaging
    impedance v.
    intraosseous v.
    isotope v.
    limb v.
    lower extremity CT v. (LE-CTV)
    lower limb v.
    magnetic resonance v. (MRV)
    ovarian v.
    peripheral v.
    phase-contrast v.
    portal v.
    radionuclear v.
    radionuclide v.
    renal v.
    selective v.
    spermatic v.
    splenic portal v.
    splenoportal v.
    subtraction v.
    technetium 99m v.
    testicular v.
    transjugular v.
    transosseous v.
    ultrasound v.
    uterine v.
    vertebral v.
    wedged hepatic v.
venography-related
    v.-r. air embolism
    v.-r. arrhythmia
    v.-r. thrombophlebitis
venolobar syndrome
venolymphatic
Venoscope
    Landry vein light V.
venospasm
venostasis
venosum
    foramen v.
venosus
    ductus v.
    sinus v.
venotomy
venous
    v. access device
    v. anatomy
    v. aneurysm

v. angiocardiography
v. angioma
v. angioplasty
v. angiosarcoma
v. anomaly
v. aortography
v. avulsion
v. backflow
v. blood
v. blood gas value
v. brain angiography
v. brain angle
v. bypass graft
v. calcification
v. cannulation
v. capillary
v. circulation
v. collateral
v. contamination
v. decompression
v. defect
v. distensibility index (VDI)
v. distention
v. Doppler examination
v. drainage
v. edema
v. embolism
v. filling time (VFT)
v. fistulogram
v. groove
v. heart congestion
v. hemangioma
v. hemorrhage
v. hyperemia
v. hypertension
v. imaging
v. infarct
v. injection
v. insufficiency
v. interposition graft
v. intraplacental lake
v. intravasation
v. intussusception
v. junction
v. ligament
v. malformation of tongue
v. motion
v. neck angle
v. network
v. occlusion
v. occlusive disease
v. outflow obstruction
v. overlay
v. oxygen content
v. phase
v. plethysmography
v. plexus
v. pooling
v. pouch

v. pressure
v. refill time (VRT)
v. return
v. return time
v. scan
v. sclerosis
v. segment
v. sheath
v. sinus
v. sinus flow void
v. sinus thrombosis
v. skull lake
v. spasm
v. stasis
v. stasis syndrome
v. stenting
v. thromboembolic disease (VTED)
v. thromboembolization
v. thrombolysis
v. thrombosis embolus
v. thrombotic disease
v. ulcer
v. ultrasonography
v. valve
v. vascular malformation
v. ventricle
v. waveform
v. web

venovenous cannulation
vent
pulmonary arterial v.
thoracic v.
ventilation
airway pressure release v.
alveolar v.
v. defect
high minute v.
v. image
v. lung scan
v. map
mask v.
maximum voluntary v. (MVV)
mechanical v.
minute v.
partial liquid v.
v. pneumonitis
pulmonary perfusion and v.
v. radionuclide
reduced alveolar v.
regional v.
v. scintigraphy
v. scintigraphy equilibrium phase
v. study
uneven v.
volume-controlled inverse ratio v.
volume-cycled v.
ventilation-perfusion (V/Q)
v.-p. defect
v.-p. imaging

impaired v.-p.
v.-p. inequality
v.-p. lung scan
v.-p. mismatch
v.-p. pulmonary scintigraphy
v.-p. ratio
ventilator
babyPAC v.
MR-compatible v.
SLE2000 v.
ventilatory
v. capacity-demand imbalance
v. dysfunction
v. effort
v. failure
venting of heart
ventosa
spina v.
ventrad
ventral
v. aorta
v. aspect
v. branch
v. bridge
v. cochlear nucleus
v. decubitus position
v. derotating spinal (VDS)
v. derotating spinal implant
v. duct of Wirsung
v. epidural abscess
v. epidural fat
v. hernia
v. hernia defect
v. horn
v. mesentery
v. muscle
v. occipitotemporal visual cortex
v. pancreas
v. pancreatic anlage
v. pancreatic bud
v. pontile infarct
v. primary ramus
v. root
v. sacrococcygeal ligament
v. sacroiliac ligament
v. spinocerebellar tract
v. spinothalamic tract
v. surface
v. venous pressure line
ventralis
funiculus v.
ventralward
ventricle
absent v.
akinetic left v.
aortic vestibule of v.
Arantius v.
atrialized v.
augmented filling of right v.

V

ventricle (*continued*)
    auxiliary v.
    backrush of blood into left v.
    ballooned floor of v.
    batwing appearance of v.
    batwing configuration of v.
    bulb of occipital horn of lateral
      v.
    bulb of posterior horn of lateral
      v.
    cephalic v.
    cerebral v.
    colloid cyst of 3rd v.
    compensatory enlargement of v.
    dilated v.
    dilation of v.
    double-inlet left v. (DILV)
    double-inlet single v.
    double-outlet both v.'s (DOBV)
    double-outlet left v. (DOLV)
    double-outlet right v. (DORV)
    dual v.'s
    v. effacement
    elongation of v.
    enlargement of v.
    floor of v.
    fractional shortening of left v.
    frontal horn of lateral v.
    Galen v.
    high-riding 3rd v.
    hourglass v.
    hyperdynamic 4th v.
    hypokinetic left v.
    hypoplastic heart v.
    hypoplastic left v.
    hypoplastic right v.
    v. impedance adapter
    inflow tract of left v.
    ipsilateral lateral v.
    laryngeal v.
    lateral v.
    left v.
    loculated v.
    Morgagni v.
    morphologic left v.
    native v.
    v. of larynx
    outflow of v.
    papilloma of 4th v.
    parchment right v.
    partial obliteration of lateral v.
    pineal v.
    primitive v.
    3rd v.
    right v.
    roof of 4th v.
    v. root
    rudimentary v.
    shift of v.

    single v.
    slit v.
    Sylvius v.
    temporal horn of lateral v.
    terminal v.
    4th v.
    5th v.
    6th v.
    thick-walled v.
    thrusting v.
    tiny v.
    trigone of v.
    tubular v.
    venous v.
    Verga v.
ventricle-brain ratio (VBR)
1-ventricle heart
ventricose
ventricular
    v. aberration
    v. activation time (VAT)
    v. apex
    v. aqueduct
    v. assist device
    v. atresia
    v. atrium
    v. block
    v. branch
    v. canal
    v. capture beat (VCB)
    v. catheter blockage
    v. cavity
    v. cineangiogram
    v. cleft
    v. contractility function
      (VCF)
    v. contraction pattern
    v. decompensation
    v. depression
    v. disproportion
    v. D-loop
    v. drainage
    v. dysfunction
    v. dysplasia
    v. echo
    v. ectopic activity (VEA)
    v. ectopic beat (VEB)
    v. effective refractory period
      (VERP)
    v. ejection fraction
    v. electrical instability
    v. encasement
    v. end-diastolic volume
    v. endomyocardial biopsy
    v. enlargement
    v. escape mechanism
    v. failure
    v. filling
    v. free wall

v. free wall rupture
v. free wall thickness
v. function curve
v. function equilibrium image
v. function parameter
v. gradient
v. horn
v. hypertrophy
v. index
v. intracerebral hemorrhage
v. inversion
v. irritability
v. isovolumic relaxation time
v. left-handedness
v. ligament
v. loop
v. mass
v. muscle necrosis
v. myocardium
v. myxoma
v. obstruction
v. outflow tract
v. outlet
v. output
v. paroxysmal tachycardia
v. perforation
v. preexcitation
v. premature beat (VPB)
v. premature complex (VPC)
v. premature contraction (VPC)
v. premature contraction couplet
v. premature depolarization (VPD)
v. pressure
v. pseudoperfusion beat
v. rate
v. rate variability
v. reflux
v. repolarization (T wave)
v. reserve
v. response
v. rhythm
v. right-handedness
v. segmental contraction
v. septal aneurysm
v. septal defect
v. septal rupture
v. septal summit
v. septum
v. shift
v. size
v. soft tissue
v. space
v. span
v. standstill
v. stiffness
v. synchrony
v. system
v. systole
v. transposition

v. trigeminy
v. tumor
v. underloading
v. view
v. wall dilation
v. wall motion
v. wall motion echocardiography
ventricularis
    sacculus v.
ventricularization of pressure
ventriculitis
ventriculoarterial
    v. conduit
    v. connection
ventriculoatrial (VA, V-A)
    v. block
    v. conduction
    v. interval
    v. shunt
    v. time-out
ventriculocele
ventriculocisternostomy
ventriculofugal artery
ventriculogram
    axial left anterior oblique v.
    bicycle exercise radionuclide v.
    biplane v.
    cine left v.
    contrast v.
    digital subtraction v.
    dipyridamole thallium v.
    exercise radionuclide v.
    gated blood pool v.
    gated nuclear v.
    gated radionuclide v.
    intraoperative v.
    iohexol CT v.
    left v. (LVG)
    left anterior oblique projection v.
    metrizamide v.
    radionuclide v. (RNV, RNVG, RVG)
    retrograde left v.
    right anterior oblique position v.
    xenon-133 v.
ventriculography
    bubble v.
    cardiac v.
    v. catheter
    cerebral v.
    equilibrium radionuclide v.
    isotope v.
    planar gated radionuclide v.
    radionuclide v. (RNV, RNVG, RVG)
    1st-pass radionuclide v.
ventriculoinfundibular fold
ventriculomegaly
    ex vacuo v.
    fetal v.
    teardrop v.

V

ventriculoperitoneal (VP)
    v. diversion
    v. shunt
ventriculoradial dysplasia
ventriculostomy
ventriculotomy
    map-guided partial endocardial v.
ventriculus cordis
ventricumbent
ventriduct
ventriduction
ventriflexion
ventrimesal
ventrimeson
ventrodorsad, ventrodorsal
ventrodorsal (*var. of* ventrodorsad)
ventroinguinal
ventrolateral
ventromedial hypothalamic hamartoma
ventromedian
ventroposterior
ventrose
VentTrak monitoring system
Venturi effect
venule
    high endothelial v.
    postcapillary v.
venulitis
    cutaneous necrotizing v.
vera
    vertebra v.
verae
    costae v.
Verga
    V. lacrimal groove
    V. ventricle
vergae
    septum cavum v.
verge
    anal v.
vergence
    downward v.
Verluma diagnostic imaging agent
vermes (*pl. of* vermis)
vermetoid
vermian
    v. agenesis
    v. hypoplasia
    v. medulloblastoma
    v. pseudotumor
    v. vein
vermian-cerebellar hypoplasia
vermicular
    v. appendage
    v. appendix
vermiform
    v. appendix
    v. process
verminous aneurysm

vermis, *pl.* vermes
    cerebellar v.
    v. cerebelli
    folia v.
    v. hypoplasia
vermis-cerebellum (V/C)
vermis-splenium (V/S)
vermography
vernal edema
Verner-Morrison syndrome
Verneuil canal
vernix membrane
Verocay body
VERP
    ventricular effective refractory period
verruciform
verrucose, verrucous
verrucosus
    nevus v.
verrucous (*var. of* verrucose)
    v. carcinoma
    v. hemangioma
Versadopp ultrasonic Doppler probe
VersaLight laser
VersaPulse holmium laser
Versatome
    V. D8 perioperative Doppler
      system
    V. laser
versive motor
VERT
    velocity-enhanced resistance training
    VERT software
vertebra, *pl.* vertebrae
    abdominal v.
    accordion v.
    anterior scalloping of v.
    articular process of v.
    basilar v.
    beaked v.
    biconcave v.
    block v.
    body of v.
    bone-within-bone v.
    bony projection from v.
    bullet-shaped v.
    butterfly v.
    butterfly-wing v.
    caudal v.
    cervical v.
    cleft v.
    coccygeal v.
    codfish v.
    coin-on-edge v.
    cold v.
    coronal cleft v.
    cranial v.
    v. dentata
    displaced v.

dorsal v.
facet surface of v.
false v.
fishmouth v.
fishtail v.
focal subluxation of v.
fractured v.
fused v.
great terminal v.
honeycomb v.
hooked v.
hourglass v.
H-shaped v.
ivory v.
last normal v. (LNV)
limbus v.
v. lumbales
lumbar v.
v. magnum
mature v.
midbody of v.
movable v.
non-rib-bearing v.
notched v.
odontoid v.
pedicle of v.
picture-frame v.
v. plana
posterior scalloping of v.
primitive v.
prominent v.
rib-bearing v.
rugger jersey v.
sacral v.
sandwich v.
saucerization of v.
solitary collapsed v.
vertebrae spuriae
sternal v.
subluxed v.
tail v.
thoracic v.
toothed v.
transitional v.
transverse process of v.
tricuspid v.
true v.
v. vera
wedge-shaped v.

vertebrae (*pl. of* vertebra)

vertebral

    v., anal, cardiac, tracheal, esophageal, renal, limb (VACTERL)
    v., anal, tracheal, esophageal, renal (VATER)
    v. angiography
    v. ankylosis
    v. arch

v. arch ligament ossification
v. arterial dissection
v. arteriography
v. artery
v. artery fenestration
v. artery occlusion
v. artery of Henry
v. artery segment V0-V4
v. artery stenosis
v. artery syndrome
v. artery system
v. articular sinus
v. body alignment
v. body bone tumor
v. body collapse
v. body endplate
v. body fracture
v. body height
v. body index
v. body line
v. body margin
v. body marrow signal intensity
v. body ossification center
v. body overgrowth
v. body plate
v. body ratio method
v. body retrolisthesis
v. body retropulsion
v. body shape
v. body size
v. border abnormality
v. canal
v. chordoma
v. column
v. compression fracture (VCF)
v. cross-section
v. disc
v. disc interspace
v. endplate abnormality
v. epiphysitis
v. expansile lesion
v. foramen
v. fusion
v. groove
v. hemangioma
v. hyperostosis
v. lamina
v. marrow cavity
v. osteochondrosis
v. osteomyelitis
v. part of diaphragm
v. plana fracture
v. process
v. rib
v. scalloping
v. segmentation anomaly
v. spine
v. steal phenomenon
v. stripe

V

vertebral (*continued*)
    v. vein
    v. venography
    v. venous plexus
    v. wedge compression fracture
    v. wedging
vertebrobasilar
    v. artery
    v. artery occlusion
    v. artery syndrome
    v. circulation
    v. complex
    v. disease
    v. distribution stroke
    v. dolichoectasia
    v. insufficiency (VBI)
    v. ischemia
    v. occlusion
    v. system
    v. transcranial color-coded duplex
    ultrasonography
vertebrocostal
    v. rib
    v. triangle
    v. trigone
vertebrojugular fistula
vertebromammary diameter
vertebropelvic ligament
vertebrophrenic angle
vertebroplasty
    percutaneous v.
    transpedicular v.
vertebrospinous process
vertebrosternal rib
vertebrovertebral fistula
vertex, *pl.* **vertices**
    V. camera
    v. corneae
    v. cranii
    v. cranii ossei
    cube v.
    v. of bony cranium
    v. presentation
vertical
    v. axis
    v. diameter
    v. generation
    v. heart
    v. long axis
    v. long-axis slice
    v. muscle
    v. partial laryngectomy
    v. plane
    v. ray
    v. shear fracture
    v. split nondetached tear
    v. synchronization pulse
    v. talus
    v. talus foot deformity

vertical-center-anterior (VCA)
    v.-c.-a. angle
vertices (*pl. of* vertex)
verticillate
verticomental
verticosubmental
    v. position
    v. projection
    v. view
vertigo/orthostatic
  dysregulation
vertigraphy
vesalianum
    v. bone
    v. of vertebral body
Vesalius
    foramen of V.
vesical
    v. calculus
    v. carcinoma
    v. distention
    v. diverticulum
    v. fascia
    v. fistula
    v. injury
    v. neck
    v. outlet obstruction
    v. stone formation
    v. venous plexus
vesicalis
    extrophia v.
vesical-urachal diverticulum
vesicant
vesicle
    acoustic v.
    acrosomal v.
    air v.
    allantoic v.
    auditory v.
    brain region v.
    cerebral v.
    cervical v.
    cutaneous chylous v.
    encephalic v.
    graafian v.
    grapelike v.
    malpighian v.
    metanephric v.
    pulmonary v.
    seminal v.
    synaptic v.
vesicocolic fistula
vesicorectal
vesicosacral ligament
vesicoumbilical ligament
vesicoureteral
    v. reflux (VUR)
    v. scintigraphy
vesicoureterogram (VCUG)

vesicourethral
    v. angle
    v. canal
vesicouterine
    v. ligament
    v. pouch
vesicovaginal fistula
vesicula, *pl.* **vesiculae**
vesiculae (*pl. of* vesicula)
vesicular
    v. amine transporter
    v. block
    v. bronchiolitis
    v. emphysema
    v. lymph node
    v. pattern
vesiculogram
vesiculography
    v. imaging
    seminal v.
vesiculosa
    appendix v.
vessel
    abdominal great v.
    aberrant v.
    absorbent v.
    afferent lymph v.
    angiographically occult v.
    anomalous v.
    antegrade filling of v.
    arcuate v.
    atraumatic occlusion of v.
    axillary v.
    beading of v.
    blood v.
    brachiocephalic v.
    bronchial v.
    v. caliber
    capillary v.
    cephalized v.
    cerebral blood v.
    chyle v.
    chyliferous v.
    circumflex v.
    codominant v.
    collateral v.
    collecting v.
    commencement of v.
    complex of v.'s
    contralateral v.
    corkscrew v.
    coursing v.
    cranial v.
    cross-pelvic collateral v.
    culprit v.
    curved v.
    v. cutoff of contrast material
    deep lymphatic v.
    v. density ratio (VDR)

    v. diameter
    diminutive v.
    disease-free v.
    v. displacement brain infection
    displacement of brain v.
    distal runoff v.
    dominant v.
    eccentric v.
    efferent lymph v.
    end-on v.
    enlarged pulmonary v.
    extracranial v.
    feeding v.
    femoropopliteal v.
    fenestrated v.
    v. filling
    gastroepiploic v.
    great v.
    hairpin v.
    heart and great v.
    hilar v.
    ileocolic v.
    iliac v.
    increased prominence of pulmonary
      v.'s
    infrapopliteal v.
    in-plane v.
    intercostal v.
    interlobular v.
    internal pudendal v.
    intimal attachment of diseased v.
    intracranial v.
    intradural v.
    intraosseous v.
    kidney v.
    lacteal v.
    lenticulostriate v.
    v. loop
    lymphatic collecting v.
    lymphocapillary v.
    mesenteric v.
    mesocolic v.
    minute v.
    musculophrenic v.
    native v.
    nondominant v.
    occipital v.
    v. occlusion
    origin of v.
    parent v.
    patency of v.
    patent v.
    pelvic collateral v.
    penile v.
    perforator v.
    perfusate v.
    pericallosal v.
    peripelvic collateral v.
    peripheral v.

V

vessel (*continued*)
 peroneal v.
 pial v.
 plump v.
 pole of v.
 portosystemic collateral v.
 posterior lumbar v.
 proximal and distal portions of v.
 pulmonary v.
 radicular v.
 reduced prominence of pulmonary v.
 renal hilar v.
 v. reshaping by angioplasty
 retroesophageal v.
 retroperitoneal lymphatic v.
 retrotracheal v.
 v. runoff
 v. rupture
 saccular blood v.
 splanchnic v.
 splenic v.
 subclavian v.
 v. subtraction technique
 superficial lymphatic v.
 superior gluteal v.
 takeoff of v.
 telangiectatic v.
 v. topography
 v. tortuosity
 tortuosity of cervical v.
 tortuous v.
 v. tracing
 v. tracking
 transposition of great v.'s
 v. trauma
 tumor-feeding v.
 uncoiling of great v.
 vasorelaxation of epicardial v.
 vasospastic v.
 vestigial v.
 v. wall abnormality
 Windkessel v.
 wraparound v.
2-vessel
 2-v. runoff
 2-v. umbilical cord
3-vessel
 3-v. coronary disease
 3-v. multiple-projection biplane angiography
 3-v. runoff
 3-v. umbilical cord
4-vessel
 4-v. arteriography
 4-v. cerebral angiography
 4-v. multiple-projection biplane angiography
vessel-to-background contrast

VEST
 virtual endoscopic surgery trainer
 VEST system
vest
 Bremer AirFlo v.
 halo v.
 immobilizing v.
vestibula (*pl. of* vestibulum)
vestibular
 v. apparatus
 v. aqueduct
 v. aqueduct syndrome (VAS)
 v. canal
 v. division of 8th cranial nerve
 v. ganglion
 v. labyrinth
 v. ligament
 v. schwannoma
 v. window
vestibule
 anatomic esophageal v.
 esophageal v.
 inner ear v.
 large v.
 laryngeal v.
 nasal v.
 v. of larynx
 v. of vagina
vestibuli
 apertura externa aqueductus v.
vestibulocochlear nerve
vestibulogenic
vestibulospinal tract
vestibulum, *pl.* vestibula
vestige
 coccygeal v.
vestigia (*pl. of* vestigium)
vestigial
 v. commissure
 v. fold
 v. left sinuatrial node
 v. vessel
vestigium, *pl.* vestigia
 v. processus vaginalis
V-Flex Plus stent
VFT
 venous filling time
VHD
 vascular hemostatic device
 VHD closure
Viabahn
 V. covered stent
 V. endoprosthesis
Viabil
 V. biliary endoprosthesis
 V. stent
viability
 myocardial tissue v.
 tissue v.

viable
- v. fetus
- v. myocardium
- v. tumor

vial
- multidose v.
- reaction v.

Viatorr
- V. endoprosthesis
- V. transjugular intrahepatic portosystemic shunt stent-graft

Viatronix virtual colonoscopy system

VIBE
- volumetric interpolated breath-hold examination
- VIBE sequence

vibex, *pl.* vibices
vibices (*pl. of* vibex)
vibrating-reed electrometer
vibration
- v. frequency
- lattice v.
- molecular v.

vibratory motion
vibroacoustography
vicarious contrast excretion
Victoreen dosimeter
Vidar scanner
video
- v. barium swallow
- v. digital gastrointestinal radiography
- v. display camera
- v. display unit (VDU)
- v. electroencephalography monitoring
- v. fluoroscopy
- v. pill
- v. pill camera
- v. proctogram
- v. signal generator

videoangiography
- digital v.

video-assisted
- v.-a. thoracoscopic surgery
- v.-a. thoracoscopy (VAT)

videocamera
- Circon v.

videoconferencing
- teleradiology v.

videocystometrography (VCMG)
videocystourethrography
videodensitometer
videodensitometric
videodensitometry
videodensity curve
videofluoroscopic imaging
videofluoroscopy
- spinal v.

videognosis

videolaparoscope
- EL2-LS2 flexible v.

videolaseroscopy
videometry
videomicroscopy
videoradiography
video-rate 2-photon laser scanning microscope
videotape study
videothoracoscopy
vidian
- v. artery
- v. canal
- v. nerve

Vidicon camera tube
Vieussens
- ansa of V.
- V. anulus
- circle of V.
- isthmus of V.
- limbus of V.
- V. loop
- ring of V.
- V. valve

view
- abdominal v.
- afferent v.
- air-contrast v.
- Alexander acromioclavicular joint v.
- amputated foot v.
- angiographic system for unlimited rolling field of v. (AngioSURF)
- angled craniocaudal v.
- anterior foot v.
- anterior oblique v.
- anteroposterior v.
- anteroposterior-posteroanterior v.
- apical and subcostal 4-chamber v.'s
- apical lordotic v.
- AP inversion stress vaginal v.
- AP supine portable v.
- Arcelin petrous temporal v.
- axial sesamoid v.
- axillary tail v.
- ball-catcher v.
- basal short-axis v.
- base v.
- baseline v.
- beam's-eye v.
- Beath v.
- bicipital groove v.
- biplane orthogonal v.
- bird's-eye v.
- v. box
- Broden subtalar joint (I-II) v.
- brow-down skull v.
- brow-up skull v.
- Bucky abdominal v.
- bull's-eye v.

V

view (*continued*)

Caldwell occipitofrontal v.
cardiac long-axis v.
cardiac short-axis v.
carpal tunnel v.
Carter Rowe shoulder v.
caudad v.
caudocranial tangential v.
cephalic tilt v.
cerebellar v.
cervical spine dens v.
4-chamber apical v.
Chamberlain-Towne v.
change-of-angle v.
Chassard-Lapiné v.
Chausse v.
Chaussier v.
chest v.
cine v.
cineradiographic v.
classic carpal tunnel v.
clenched fist v.
Cleopatra v.
closed-mouth v.
close-up v.
coalition v.
comparison v.
coned-down compression v.
cone spot compression v.
contact lateral v.
coronal bending v.
coronal reconstruction v.
couch v.
cranial angled v.
craniocaudal v.
cross-table lateral v. (CTLV)
decubitus v.
3D endoluminal v.
dens v.
dorsal v.
dorsiflexion v.
dorsoplantar v.
Dunlop-Shands v.
efferent v.
Eklund v.
endoluminal v.
en face v.
equilibrium v.
erect v.
exaggerated craniocaudal v.
expiration v.
expiratory v.
extension v.
external rotation v.
fan-shaped v.
fast spin-echo v.
FCS v.
femoral v.
Ferguson sacroiliac v.

fetal echocardiographic v.
field of v. (FOV)
Fleckinger v.
flexion and extension v.'s
fluoroscopic v.
followthrough v.
frogleg lateral v.
frontal v.
Fuchs odontoid v.
full cervical spine v.
full column v.
full-length v.
Garth shoulder v.
gated v.
Granger v.
Grashey shoulder v.
great vessel v.
half-axial v.
Hampton v.
Harris v.
Harris-Beath axial hindfoot v.
heavily penetrated v.
Heinig v.
hemiaxial v.
hepatoclavicular v.
hip-to-ankle v.
Hobb sternoclavicular joint v.
Hughston patella v.
ice-pick v.
infrapatellar v.
inspiration and expiration v.'s
inspiratory v.
v. insufficiency artifact
internal and external rotation v.'s
intraoperative v.
inversion ankle stress v.
Jones v.
Jude pelvic v.
Judet v.
knee v.
KUB v.
kyphotic v.
large field of v. (LFOV)
lateral anterior drawer stress v.
lateral bending v.
lateral decubitus v.
lateral extension v.
lateral flexion v.
lateral oblique v.
lateral tilt stress ankle v.
lateromedial oblique v.
Laurin x-ray v.
Law v.
Lawrence lateral proximal humerus v.
left anterior oblique v.
limited v.
long axial oblique v.
long-axis parasternal v.

longitudinal ultrasound v.
lordotic v.
Low-Beers v.
lumbar spine v.
magnification v.
Mayer v.
medial oblique v.
mediolateral oblique v.
Merchant patella v.
v. microtomography
mortise v.
MPR v.
multiplanar reformatting v.
navicular v.
Neer lateral shoulder v.
Neer transscapular v.
nonforeshortened angiographic v.
nonstanding lateral oblique v.
nonweightbearing v.
normal anteroposterior v.
notch v.
oblique v.
occipital v.
odontoid v.
open-mouth odontoid v.
optimally positioned v.
orthogonal v.
outlet v.
overcouch v.
overhead oblique v.
Owen v.
panoramic v.
Panorex v.
pantomographic v.
parallax v.
parasternal long-axis v.
parasternal short-axis v.
patellar skyline v.
pelvic v.
v.'s per segment (VPS)
pillar v.
pinhole v.
plain v.
planar v.
2-plane v.
plantar axial v.
plantar flexion stress v.
plumbline v.
portable v.
posterior skull v.
posteroanterior v.
posterooblique v.
postevacuation v.
postoperative v.
postreduction v.
postvoid v.
preliminary v.
preoperative v.
prereduction v.

profile ray v.
prone angled v.
prone lateral v.
push-pull ankle stress v.
push-pull hip v.
ray-sum v.
rear endoluminal v.
reconstruction v.
reconstruction field of v. (RFOV)
rectangular field of v.
recumbent v.
replacing oblique v.
retroflexed v.
retromammary space v.
Rhese v.
rib v.
right anterior oblique v.
right lateral decubitus v.
right ventricular inflow v.
Rokus v.
rolled v.
room's-eye v. (REV)
rotated craniocaudal v.
routine magnification v.
Rumstrom v.
sagittal and coronal reconstruction
   v.'s
sagittal magnetization transfer v.
scan field of v. (SFOV)
Schatzki v.
Schüller v.
scotty dog v.
scout v.
selective coronary arteriography v.
semiupright v.
serendipity v.
v. shadow projection
   microtomographic system
short-axis parasternal v.
single-breath v.
sitting-up v.
ski jump v.
skyline v.
spider x-ray v.
spot compression v.
standing dorsoplantar v.
standing false profile v.
standing lateral v.
standing postvoid v.
standing weightbearing v.
static v.
steep left anterior oblique v.
Stenvers v.
stereoscopic v.
sternal v.
1st-pass v.
stress Broden v.
stress eversion v.
stress inversion v.

V

view (*continued*)
Stryker notch v.
subcostal 4-chamber v.
subcostal long-axis v.
subcostal short-axis v.
submaxillary v.
submentovertex v.
submentovertical v.
subscapular echocardiographic v.
subtalar v.
subxiphoid v.
sunrise knee x-ray v.
sunset knee x-ray v.
superoinferior v.
supine full v.
suprasternal notch v.
swimmer's v.
tangential scapular v.
thoracic v.
tomographic v.
Towne v.
transaxillary lateral v.
transcranial lateral v.
transgastric echocardiographic v.
transscapular v.
transthoracic lateral v.
transverse v.
transverse/neutral v.
trauma oblique v.
true lateral v.
tunnel v.
Twining v.
ulnar deviation v.
upright postvoid v.
Van Rosen v.
Velpeau axillary v.
ventricular v.
verticosubmental v.
virtual endoscopic v.
von Rosen hip v.
washout v.
Waters v.
weeping willow v.
weightbearing dorsoplantar v.
West Point v.
White leg-length v.
whole-body imaging with magnified v.
x-ray v.
Zanca acromioclavicular joint v.

2-view
2-v. chest x-ray
2-v. film-screen mammography

4-view
4-v. chest x-ray
4-v. wrist survey

view-box luminance
5-view chest x-ray
viewer
dedicated v.
Mammo Mask dedicated v.
viewing
cine-based v.
film-based v.
fly-through v.
group v.
PVR fly-through v.
v. wand
ViewMax software
view-to-view variation
vignetting
vigorous achalasia
Villaret-Mackenzie syndrome
villi (*pl. of* villus)
villoglandular polyp
villose (*var. of* villous)
villotubular adenoma
villous, villose
v. adenoma
v. atrophy
v. carcinoma
v. frond
v. hypertrophy
v. papilloma
v. placenta
v. proliferation
v. stomach polyp
v. tumor
villus, *pl.* **villi**
anchoring v.
arachnoid v.
atrophic v.
duodenal v.
fingerlike v.
floating v.
gallbladder v.
hydropic v.
intestinal v.
leaflike v.
placental v.
ridged convoluted v.
tongue-shaped v.
vinculum breve
Vingmed
V. CFM ultrasound system
V. ultrasound
violaceous presternal eruption
violation
articular cartilage v.
violin string appearance
VIPoma
vasoactive intestinal polypeptide tumor

viral
   v. esophagitis
   v. gastroenteritis
   v. infusion
   v. meningitis
   v. myositis
   v. particle
   v. pleuritis
   v. pneumonia
   v. vector delivery
Virchow
   V. gland
   V. hydatid
   V. law of skull growth
   V. metastasis
   V. plane
   V. psammoma
   V. sentinel node
Virchow-Robin
   V.-R. perivascular space
   V.-R. space dilation
   V.-R. space of brain
Virchow-Troisier node
viremia
   primary v.
   secondary v.
virtual
   v. angioscopy
   v. array
   v. arterial endoscopy
   v. bone biopsy
   v. bronchoscopy (VB)
   v. colonoscopy
   v. CT colonography
   v. cystoscopy
   v. dissection imaging
   v. endoscope
   v. endoscopic surgery trainer (VEST)
   v. endoscopic view
   v. endoscopy (VE)
   v. enteroscopy
   v. fly-through
   v. reality flexible cystoscopy
   v. reality imaging
   v. reality simulator
   v. reality view box
   v. retinal display system
Virtuoso portable 3D imaging system
virulent atherosclerosis
virus, *pl.* **viruses**
   Epstein-Barr v. (EBV)
   herpes v. (type 1, 2)
   herpes simplex v. (HSV)
   herpes simplex v. 1 (HSV1)
   human immunodeficiency v. (type 1, 2) (HIV)
   human mammary tumor v.
   human T-cell leukemia v.
   parainfluenza v.

   parenterally acquired human immunodeficiency v.
   prion v.
   West Nile v. (WNV)
virus-directed enzyme/prodrug therapy
viruses (*pl. of* virus)
virus-mediated gene therapy
viscera (*pl. of* viscus)
visceral
   v. adipose tissue (VAT)
   v. angiography
   v. angiomatosis
   v. aortography
   v. arteriography
   v. artery
   v. catheter
   v. edema
   v. embolus
   v. fat
   v. heterotaxia
   v. layer
   v. lesion
   v. lymph node
   v. metastasis
   v. muscle
   v. pelvic fascia
   v. pericardial calcification
   v. pericardium
   v. peritoneum
   v. pleura
   v. pleurisy
   v. situs solitus
   v. skeleton
   v. space
   v. surface of liver
   v. thickening
viscerocranium
   cartilaginous v.
   membranous v.
viscerography
visceromegaly
visceroparietal
visceroperitoneal
visceropleural
visceroptosia (*var. of* visceroptosis)
visceroptosis, visceroptosia
viscerosomatic
viscerum
   situs inversus v.
viscid
viscosity coefficient
viscous
viscus, *pl.* **viscera**
   abdominal v.
   abdominopelvic v.
   hollow v.
   intraabdominal v.
   intraperitoneal v.

V

viscus (*continued*)
    mediastinal v.
    pelvic v.
    perforated hollow v.
    retroperitoneal v.
    ruptured hollow v.
    solid v.
    strangulated v.
VISI
    volar intercalated segment instability
    VISI deformity
visibility of foramen magnum
visible
    v. anterior motion
    v. peristalsis
vision
    V. camera
    V. high-performance gradient system
    V. MR imaging system
    stereoscopic v.
    V. Ten V-scan scanner
    V. 1.5T Siemens MRI scanner
Visipaque 270, 320 contrast agent
Vistaflex balloon-expanded stent
Vistec x-ray-detectable sponge
visual
    v. alexia
    v. cortex
    v. inspection
    v. laser ablation of prostate (VLAP)
    v. object agnosia
    v. shimmering
    v. word form area
visualization
    breakthrough v.
    delayed v.
    direct v.
    double-contrast v.
    endoluminal v.
    genital v.
    inadequate v.
    intraoperative x-ray v.
    needle v.
    object-based v.
    v. of Z line
    optimal v.
    poor v.
    scene-based v.
    selective v.
    suboptimal v.
    volume-mode v.
visualized
    suboptimally v.
Visulas Nd:YAG laser
Visx
    V. Star 3 excimer laser
    V. Star S2 excimer laser
    V. Star S2 excimer laser system
    V. WaveScan Wavefront system

vita glass
vital capacity
vitelline
    v. duct
    v. fistula
vitellointestinal duct
Viterbi decoding
Vitesse Cos laser
Vitrea
    V. 2 computer workstation
    V. 2 3D CT angiographic software
    V. 3D imaging
    V. 3D system
    V. workstation (version 1.1, 1.2)
vitreous
    v. hemorrhage
    v. lymphoma
    primary v.
vivo
    DAI in v.
    hydrolysis in v.
    in v.
    measurement in v.
    micron-resolution retinal image
      in v.
    water diffusion in v.
Vladimiroff-Mikulicz amputation
VLAP
    visual laser ablation of prostate
V-like pattern of uptake
VMA
    vastus medialis advancement
V5M Multiplane transducer
VMO
    vastus medialis obliquus
VNS
    vagus nerve stimulation
      VNS epoch
VNS-fMRI
    vagus nerve-stimulated functional
      magnetic resonance imaging
VNS-synchronized BOLD fMRI
Vnus
    V. closure system
    V. radiofrequency generator
vocal
    v. cord
    v. cord carcinoma
    v. cord paralysis
    v. cord paresis
    v. ligament
    v. muscle
vocalis muscle
Vogele-Bale-Hohner head holder
Vogt
    V. bone-free projection
    V. cephalosyndactyly
VOI
    volume of interest

voice-sparing surgery
voicing
    tracheoesophageal v.
void
    color v.
    v. determination
    flow v.
    serpentine signal v.
    signal v.
    tubular signal v.
    venous sinus flow v.
voiding
    v. cystogram
    v. cystourethrogram (VCU,
      VCUG)
    v. cystourethrography (VCU)
    v. sequence
    v. study
    v. urethrocystography
volar
    v. angulation
    v. capsule
    v. carpal ligament
    v. dislocation
    v. inclination
    v. intercalated segment instability
      (VISI)
    v. plate
    v. radiocarpal ligament disruption
    v. rim
    v. rim distal radial fracture
    v. tilt
    v. wrist
volar-flexed intercalated segment
 instability
volarward
Volkmann
    V. canal
    V. deformity
    V. fracture
    V. ischemic contracture
volt
    billion electron v.'s (BeV)
    electron v. (eV)
    kiloelectron v. (keV)
    megaelectron v. (MeV)
    million electron v.'s (MeV)
Volta effect
voltage
    v. amplifier
    operating v.
    pulse v.
    ripple v.
volt-ampere (va)
volume
    v. acquisition
    adaptive cardiac v. (ACV)
    adequate stroke v.
    alveolar v.

amnionic fluid v.
amygdala v.
v. analysis
aortic flow v.
aqueductal CSF stroke v.
articular cartilage v.
v. artifact
Arvidsson dimension-length method
  for ventricular v.
atomic v.
atrial emptying v.
augmented stroke v.
v. averaging
back stroke v.
biologic target v.
bladder v.
blood v.
brain v.
capillary blood v.
cardiac v.
caudate v.
cavity v.
central blood v.
cerebellar v.
cerebral blood v.
  (CBV)
cerebrospinal fluid v.
chamber v.
circulating blood v.
circulation v.
clinical target v.
  (CTV)
clinical tumor v.
closing v.
v. coil
3D v.
decreased stroke v.
decreased tidal v.
determination of lung v.
diastolic atrial v.
diminished lung v.
Dodge area-length method for
  ventricular v.
v. element (voxel)
end-diastolic v.
end-expiratory lung v.
endocardial v.
end-systolic v. (ESV)
end-systolic pressure to end-systolic
  v. (ESP/ESV)
end-systolic residual v.
epicardial v.
v. estimation
expiratory reserve v. (ERV)
extracellular fluid v.
fetal aortic flow v.
flow v.
fluid v.
forced expiratory v.

volume (*continued*)
forward stroke v. (FSV)
fractional moving blood v.
fractional vascular v.
gas v.
gland v.
gross tumor v. (GTV)
heart stroke v.
heart-to-thorax v.
hippocampal v.
v. histogram
image v.
v. imaging
v. implant calculation
increased extracellular fluid v.
inspiratory reserve v. (IRV)
interstitial lung disease with
  increased lung v.
intracranial v.
ipsilateral lung v.
left atrial maximal v.
left ventricular chamber v.
left ventricular end-diastolic v.
left ventricular inflow v. (LVIV)
left ventricular maximal v.
left ventricular outflow v. (LVOV)
left ventricular stroke v.
v. loss
low lung v.
lung v.
mean corpuscular v.
minimal v.
minute v.
v. mode
molar v.
v. of interest (VOI)
ovarian v.
v. overload
patient v.
pericardial reserve v.
ping-pong heart v.
planning target v. (PTV)
plasma v.
postvoid residual urine v.
prism method for ventricular v.
pulmonary blood v. (PBV)
pyloric v.
pyramid method for ventricular v.
quantitative amnionic fluid v.
radioactivity per v.
radionuclide stroke v.
reduced lung v.
reduced plasma v.
reduced stroke v.
regional cerebral blood v. (rCBV)
v. regulation
regurgitant stroke v. (RSV)
relative cerebral blood v. (rCBV)
v. rendered

v. rendering
v. rendering of helical CT data
v. rendering technique (VRT)
residual v. (RV)
respiratory v.
right ventricular end-diastolic v.
  (RVEDV)
right ventricular end-systolic v.
  (RVESV)
right ventricular stroke v.
scan v.
v. score
sensitive v.
Simpson rule method for ventricular
  v.
skull v.
slice v.
stroke v. (SV)
supratentorial v.
systolic atrial v.
targeted tissue v.
Teichholz equation for left
  ventricular v.
thermodilution stroke v.
thin cylindrical uniform field v.
thoracic gas v.
tidal inspiratory flow v.
total brain v. (TBV)
total intracranial v. (TIV)
total stroke v. (TSV)
transit v.
tumor v.
ventricular end-diastolic v.
voxel v.
whole-brain parenchymal v.
volume-controlled inverse ratio
  ventilation
volume-cycled ventilation
volume-mode
v.-m. EBCT
v.-m. visualization
volume-ratio method
volume-rendered
v.-r. CT angiogram
v.-r. CT colonography
v.-r. 3D image
v.-r. mode
v.-r. MR angiogram
volume-selective excitation
volumetric
v. acquisition
v. analysis
v. computed tomography
v. dataset
v. expiratory HRCT
v. function
v. image
v. image data
v. imaging

v. interpolated breath-hold examination (VIBE)
v. interstitial hyperthermia
v. magnetic resonance brain mapping
v. mapping technique
v. minimally invasive stereotaxis
v. multiplexed transmission holography
v. resampling
v. scan

volumetry
CT-aided v.
3D ultrasound v.
hippocampal magnetic resonance v.
v. of ventilated airspace
tumor v.

voluntary
v. effort
v. muscle

Voluson ultrasound system
volute
volvulus
cecal v.
colonic v.
gastric v.
mesenteroaxial v.
midgut v.
organoaxial v.
sigmoid v. (SV)
sigmoid colon v.
small bowel v.
stomach v.

Volz wrist implant
vomer bone
vomerine canal
vomerorostral canal
vomerovaginal canal
von
v. Hippel-Lindau
v. Hippel-Lindau syndrome
v. Hippel retina tumor
v. Meyenburg complex
v. Recklinghausen disease
v. Rosen hip view
v. Willebrand disease

Voorhoeve disease
vortex, *pl.* **vortices**
v. coccygeus
v. cordis
vortices pilorum
V. port system

vortices (*pl. of* vortex)
vorticity
VortXX coil
Vostal radial fracture classification
Voxar Plug-n-View 3D imager
voxel
volume element

adjacent voxel
voxel array
cubic voxel
voxel gradient
isotropic voxel
voxel localization
proton brain exam-single voxel (PROBE-SV)
seed voxel
voxel size
spectroscopic voxel
voxel volume

voxel-based coregistration
voxel-by-voxel analysis
Voxel-Man software
VoxelView
V. software
V. system

Voxgram multiple-exposure holography
voyager
Brain V.

VP
ventriculoperitoneal
VP shunt

VPB
ventricular premature beat

VPC
ventricular premature complex
ventricular premature contraction

VPD
ventricular premature depolarization

VPS
views per segment

V/Q
ventilation-perfusion
V/Q imaging
V/Q lung segment scan
V/Q mismatch

VR
valvular regurgitation

Vrolik disease
VRT
venous refill time
volume rendering technique

V/S
vermis-splenium
V/S ratio

VScore with AutoGate cardiac imaging
V-shaped
V-s. fracture
V-s. ulcer

V-sign of Naclerio
VT
variable temperature
VT multinuclear spectrometer

VTED
venous thromboembolic disease

vulgaris
thermoactinomyces v.

V

vulnerability
 selective v.
vulnerable coronary plaque
vulva, *pl.* **vulvae**
 preinvasive disease of cervix,
  vagina, and v.
 synechia vulvae
vulvae (*pl. of* vulva)
vulval (*var. of* vulvar)
vulvar, vulval
 v. adenoid cystic adenocarcinoma
 v. carcinoma
 v. intraepithelial neoplasia
 v. malignancy

vulvectomy
 radical v.
vulvouterine canal
vulvovaginal carcinoma
VUR
 vesicoureteral reflux
VUSE
 variable-angle uniform signal excitation
V0-V4
 vertebral artery segment V0-V4
V-wave pressure
VWF
 velocity waveform
  Doppler VWF

¹⁸⁸W, W-188
  tungsten 188
Waardenburg syndrome
Wada test
Waddell nonorganic back pain sign
wafer
  Gliadel w.
  w. of endocardium
waferlike appearance
wafer-shaped injury
Wagner line
Wagstaffe fracture
waist
  cardiac w.
  w. immobilizer
  w. in balloon
waistlike constriction
waiter's tip palsy
WakiTrak
  wide-aperture kinematic table with
    isotropic resolution
  WakiTrak LS technique
Walcher position
Waldeyer
  W. fascia
  W. fossa
  W. ring
  W. ring lymphoma
  W. throat ring lesion
walker
  W. carcinoma
  W. carcinosarcoma
  W. magnet
Walker-Walburg syndrome
walking
  w. pneumonia
  w. saturation band
walking-stick appearance
wall
  aneurysmal w.
  anterior abdominal w.
  anterolateral abdominal w.
  apical w.
  arterial w.
  axial w.
  bladder w.
  body w.
  bowel w.
  bullous edema of bladder w.
  w. calcification
  capillary w.
  carotid w.
  cavity w.
  chest w.
  cystic w.

dorsal abdominal w.
fetal abdominal w.
w. filter
friable w.
full-thickness button of
  aortic w.
gallbladder w.
w. hypokinesis
inferior w.
inferoapical w.
intestinal w.
left anterior chest w.
left ventricular w. (LVW)
left ventricular free w. (LVFW)
left ventricular posterior w.
  (LVPW)
linear focus within cyst w.
luminal w.
midabdominal w.
w. motion
w. motion abnormality (WMA)
w. motion imaging
w. motion score
w. motion score index
w. motion study
w. motion tracking
multiple bull's-eye lesions of
  bowel w.
myocardial w.
nasal cavity w.
orbital w.
paraumbilical anterior abdominal w.
pelvic w.
posterior w.
posterior abdominal w.
posterior free w.
posterolateral w.
septal w.
w. shear stress
stomach w.
thickened airway w.
thickened bladder w.
thickened gallbladder w.
w. thickening
w. thickness
thoracic w.
thoracoabdominal w.
w. thump
vaginal w.
variceal w.
vascular w.
ventricular free w.
wall-echo
  w.-e. shadow (WES)
  w.-e. shadow triad

W

walled-off abscess
Wallenberg lateral medullary syndrome
wallerian degeneration
Wallgraft
    W. cobalt-based alloy
      balloon-expandable stent
    W. covered stent
    W. endoprosthesis
    W. endoprosthesis stent-graft
Wallstent
    W. biliary endoprosthesis
    W. Iliac RP self-expanding
    stent
    Magic S/P W.
    self-expanding Easy W.
Walt Disney dwarfism
Walther
    W. hip fracture
    W. oblique ligament
Waltman loop
wand
    programmer w.
    viewing w.
wandering
    w. gallbladder
    w. goiter
    w. heart
    w. kidney
    w. liver
    w. spleen
Wang
    W. applicator
    W. biopsy
Wang-Binford edge detector
Warburg
    W. disease
    W. effect
Ward triangle
warfarin
    w. embryopathy
    w. sodium
warfarin-aspirin symptomatic intracranial
  disease (WASID)
warming
    urethral w.
warm nodule
warping
    atlas w.
    brain w.
Wartenberg sign
Warthin tumor
washboard effect
wash-in
    w.-i. effect
    w.-i. phase
wash-in/washout study
washout
    contrast medium w.
    w. curve

delayed w.
differential w.
w. effect
w. gradient
kidney w.
w. kinetics
lung w.
MIBG w.
nitrogen w.
w. phase
w. pyelography
rapid tracer w.
w. study
teboroxime resting w. (TRW)
w. test
w. view
washout-phase ventilation scan
WASID
  warfarin-aspirin symptomatic
  intracranial disease
    WASID trial
wasp-tail deformity
Wassel classification of thumb
  polydactyly (I-VI)
wastage
    pregnancy w.
wasting
    cerebral salt w.
    muscle fiber w.
Watanabe discoid meniscus classification
watch
    Yperwatch gamma control w.
water
    w. bolus
    coexistent intravoxel fat and w.
    w. density
    w. density area
    w. density line
    w. density mass
    diffusion characteristic of w.
    w. diffusion in vivo
    doped w.
    w. eliminated Fourier transform
    (WEFT)
    glucose w.
    heavy w.
    intracellular w.
    ion-bound w.
    w. on brain
    oxygen-supersaturated w.
    w. path
    w. path scan
    w. perfusable tissue index
    polar-bound w.
    w. proton resonance frequency
    radioactive w.
    w. range
    w. retention
    w. seal

w. signal on magnetic resonance
  imaging scan
structured w.
total body w. (TBW)

water-bottle
w.-b. configuration
w.-b. heart
w.-b. stomach

water-contrast computed tomography
waterfall
w. appearance
w. hilum
w. stomach

water-infusion catheter
waterlike signal intensity
Waters
W. position
W. positioner
W. projection
W. view
W. view radiograph

water-sealed drainage
water-selective spin-echo imaging
watershed
w. area
w. brain infarct
w. mechanism
w. zone in brain

water-soluble
w.-s. contrast enema
w.-s. contrast esophageal swallow
w.-s. contrast medium (WSCM)
w. s. iodinated imaging agent
w.-s. myelography
w.-s. nonionic imaging agent

Waterston
W. groove
W. shunt

Waterston-Cooley shunt
water-suppressed proton spectrum
water-suppression
w.-s. MR imaging technique
w.-s. pulse sequence

water-trap stomach
**Watson-Jones tibial tubercle avulsion
fracture classification**
watt
wave
abdominal fluid w.
acoustic w.
aperiodic w.
circular polarization w.
constant tilt w.
continuous w.
electrocardiographic w. (QRS)
electromagnetic w.
energy w.
extracorporeal shock w.
fluid w.

longitudinal acoustic w.
motion-sensitive spin-echo sequence
  mechanical w.
w. of excitation
periodic sharp w. (PSW)
peristaltic w.
pressure w.
primary peristaltic w.
pulsed w.
radiofrequency w.
rapid filling w. (RFW)
reference w.
secondary w.
sine w.
slice excitation w. (SEW)
slow filling w.
sound w.
square w.
standing w.
systolic S w.
terahertz w.
tertiary w.
transverse acoustic w.
ultrasonic w.

waveform
apiculate w.
arterial w.
cerebrospinal fluid flow w.
dampened w.
Doppler spectral w.
flow velocity w.
w. generator
gradient w.
low-resistance spectral w.
parvus et tardus w.
pressure w.
pulsed Doppler w.
pulse volume w.
segmental bronchus-renal artery w.
sinusoidal w.
spectral w.
tardus-parvus w.
triphasic w.
tube voltage w.
uterine artery w.
velocity w. (VWF)
venous w.

wavelength
Compton w.
de Broglie w.
energy w.
readout w.
unit of w.

wavelet
w. compression
w. encoding
w. scalar quantization (WSQ)
w. subband
w. transform

W

wavelet-encoded magnetic resonance imaging
WaveWire angioplasty guidewire
wax phantom
waxy liver
3-way stopcock
WBC
    white blood cell
    white blood count
      ^{111}In WBC
      ^{111}In oxine WBC
      ^{99m}Tc-labeled WBC
      radiolabeled WBC
WBR
    whole-body radiation
WBRT
    whole-brain radiation therapy
    whole-brain radiotherapy
WDFA
    well-differentiated fetal adenocarcinoma
weak
    w. carotid upstroke
    w. signal
weakened artery
weakening
    trabecular w.
weakness
    respiratory muscle w.
    structural w.
wear-and-tear degeneration
web
    antral w.
    w. contracture
    duodenal w.
    esophageal w.
    fibrous w.
    finger w.
    hepatic w.
    intestinal w.
    laryngeal w.
    lateral w.
    postcricoid w.
    terminal w.
    thumb w.
    venous w.
webbed
    w. finger
    w. neck
    w. penis
Weber C fracture
Weber-Christian mesentery
weblike appearance
Weck Hem-o-lock clip
wedge
    w. arteriography
    w. bond
    w. compression fracture
    45-degree spinal w.
    55-degree tomography w.

dynamic w.
w. factor
w. filter
w. flexion-compression fracture
w. fracture of spine
w. hepatic venous pressure (WHVP)
w. isodose angle
matchline w.
mediastinal w.
w. resection
step w.
wedged hepatic venography
wedged-pair
    w.-p. beam
    w.-p. technique
wedge-shaped
    w.-s. defect
    w.-s. density
    w.-s. infarct
    w.-s. lesion
    w.-s. lobe
    w.-s. mass
    w.-s. support
    w.-s. vertebra
    w.-s. zone
wedging
    anterior w.
    w. deformity
    keystone w.
    w. of vertebral interspace
    vertebral w.
week
    gestational w.
weeping willow view
WEFT
    water eliminated Fourier transform
Wegener granulomatosis
Wegner
    W. line
    W. sign
Weibel-Palade body
weight
    body w.
    estimated fetal w. (EFW)
    fetal w.
    mean body w.
    normal spleen w.
    thymus w.
weight-adjusted dosing protocol
weightbearing
    w. acetabular dome
    w. axis
    w. bone
    w. dorsoplantar view
    w. film
    w. joint
    w. rotation injury
    w. surface

weighted
w. computed tomography dose index
w. CT dose index
w. spin-echo column
weighting
exponential w.
human visual sensitivity w.
multislice spiral w.
Weill-Marchesani syndrome
Weill sign
Weil syndrome
Weiner spatially varying filter
Weiss sign
Weitbrecht
W. cord
W. foramen
W. ligament
Welcher basal angle
Welch test
Welcker angle
weld
callus w.
welder's lung
welding
laser w.
Welin technique
well
w. circumscribed
w. counter
well-circumscribed
w.-c. breast mass
w.-c. lesion
w.-c. neoplasia
w.-c. tumor
well-defined
w.-d. appearance
w.-d. border
w.-d. lesion
w.-d. mass
well-demarcated scar
well-differentiated
w.-d. adenoma
w.-d. astrocytoma
w.-d. fetal adenocarcinoma (WDFA)
w.-d. liposarcoma
w.-d. papillary mesothelioma
w.-d. polycystic Wilms tumor
well-inflated lung
well-preserved ejection fraction
96-well scanning fluorometer
well-type ionization chamber
Wenckebach
W. AV block
W. cardioptosis
W. phenomenon
Werdnig-Hoffmann disease
Wermer syndrome

Werner
W. classification
W. classification of thyroid eye disease
W. syndrome
Wernicke
W. area
W. encephalopathy
Wernicke-Korsakoff syndrome
Wertheim hysterectomy
WES
wall-echo shadow
west
W. lacuna skull
W. Nile virus (WNV)
W. Point view
W. syndrome
zone 1-4 of W.
Westcott needle
West-Engstler skull
Westergren tube
Westermark sign
western boot in open fracture
Westphal-Strümpell disease
Westphal zone
wet
w. bowel preparation
w. brain
w. laser imaging
w. lung
w. lung disease
w. lung syndrome
w. pleurisy
w. reading
w. stomach
w. swallow
wet/dry generator
Wetzel test
WFRT
wide-field radiation therapy
Wharton
W. duct
W. gland
W. tumor
wheal
Wheatstone bridge
wheelchair artifact
W3000 helical CT
whiplash injury
Whipple
W. disease
W. operation
W. radical pancreatoduodenectomy procedure
W. triad
whirl
w. appearance
w. sign

W

whirllike pattern
whirlpool
    w. appearance
    w. sign
whistling deformity
Whitacre spinal needle
Whitaker test
white
    w. adipose tissue
    w. asbestos
    black and w.
    w. blood cell (WBC)
    w. blood cell imaging
    w. blood cell with indium-111
      scintigraphy
    w. blood count (WBC)
    w. branching linear pattern
    w. cerebellum sign
    w. commissure of spinal
      cord
    w. cottonlike fibrous tissue
    w. echo writing
    w. epidermoid
    w. epithelium
    W. leg-length view
    w. light pattern projector
    w. line
    w. line of Toldt
    w. masking
    w. matter
    w. matter abnormality
    w. matter buckling
    w. matter commissure
    w. matter demyelination
    w. matter diffusivity
    w. matter disease
    w. matter edema
    w. matter hypodensity
    w. matter imaging technique
    w. matter infarct
    w. matter lambda
    w. matter lesion
    w. matter shearing injury
    w. matter signal hyperintensity
    w. matter thinning
    w. matter tract direction
    w. metastasis
    w. noise artifact
    w. pneumonia
    w. point
    w. pupil reflex
    w. radiation
    w. shuttering
    w. star breast lesion
Whitehead deformity
whiteout
Whitfield test
whitlow
    herpetic w.

    melanotic w.
    thecal w.
whole-body
    w.-b. bone scan
    w.-b. compact MR system
    w.-b. computed tomography
    w.-b. counter
    w.-b. counting
    w.-b. dose monitoring
    w.-b. echo-planar MR imaging
    w.-b. ^{29}FDG scanning
    w.-b. GI Signa MRI scanner
    w.-b. imaging with magnified view
    w.-b. inflammatory response
    w.-b. irradiation
    w.-b. MRA
    w.-b. nuclear physical examination
    w.-b. PET scan
    w.-b. protein
    w.-b. radiation (WBR)
    w.-b. radiation therapy
    w.-b. radiotherapy
    w.-b. scan imaging
    w.-b. screening examination
    w.-b. sweep
    w.-b. 1.5-Tesla scanner
    w.-b. thallium imaging
    w.-b. 3T MRI system scanner
    w.-b. transmission scan
    w.-b. 1.5T Siemens Vision scanner
    w.-b. unit
whole-brain
    w.-b. acquisition
    w.-b. irradiation
    w.-b. magnetization transfer
      measurement
    w.-b. parenchymal volume
    w.-b. radiation therapy (WBRT)
    w.-b. radiotherapy (WBRT)
whole-breast sonography
whole-lung opacity
whole-volume coil
Wholey steerable guidewire
whorl
    coccygeal w.
whorled appearance
whorling
WHVP
    wedge hepatic venous pressure
Wiberg
    W. angle
    CE angle of W.
    center-edge angle of W.
    W. patellar-type classification
Wickham-Miller nephroscope
Widal syndrome
wide
    w. caliber
    w. rib

w. suture
w. tortuous aorta
w. window setting
wide-angle tomography
wide-aperture kinematic table with isotropic resolution (WakiTrak)
wide-based, blunt-ended, right-sided atrial appendage
wide-beam scanning
wide-field
w.-f. lesion
w.-f. radiation therapy (WFRT)
wide-latitude film
widely
w. invasive follicular carcinoma
w. patent
wide-mouth sac
wide-neck carotid cavernous aneurysm
widened
w. anterior meningeal index
w. cardiac silhouette
w. collecting system
w. duodenal sweep
w. heart shadow
w. joint space
w. mediastinum
w. optic canal
w. sacroiliac joint
w. sulcus
w. superior orbital fissure
w. symphysis pubis
w. teardrop distance
w. thoracic outlet
widening
acute mediastinal w.
ankle mortise w.
crural cistern w.
diffuse mediastinal w.
growth plate w.
infundibulum w.
interpediculate distance w.
interspinal w.
joint w.
mediastinal w.
w. of aorta
sacroiliac joint w.
scapholunate w.
widespread
w. hyperattenuating mediastinal adenopathy
w. metastasis
width
aryepiglottic fold w.
collimated slice w.
collimation w.
contrast window w.
intracranial w. (ICW)
isodose w.
line w.

metatarsal head w. (MHW)
prevertebral w.
pulse w. (PW)
radial w.
spectral w.
window w.
Wiedemann-Beckwith syndrome
Wiener
W. MRI filter
W. spectrum
Wigby-Taylor position
Wigle scale for ventricular hypertrophy
Wilcoxon signed-rank test
Wilkie syndrome
Wilkins radial fracture classification
Williams-Beuren syndrome
Williams-Campbell syndrome
Williams syndrome
Willis
W. antrum
arterial circle of W.
artery of W.
circle of W.
W. pouch
willisii
chordae w.
willow fracture
Wilms tumor
Wilson
W. block
W. cloud chamber
W. disease
W. fracture
W. muscle
Wilson-Mikity syndrome
Wiltse angle
Wimberger
W. bilateral metaphysial sign
W. ring
Winchester disc
windblown deformity
winding
wire w.
Y w.
zero-pitch solenoid w.
Windkessel vessel
window
acoustic w.
acquisition w.
aortic w.
aortopulmonary w.
apical w.
beryllium mammography x-ray tube w.
biologic w.
bone w.
brain w.
w. center
coincidence-resolving w.

window (*continued*)
    cortical w.
    CT bone w.
    cycle-length w.
    w. duct
    w. efficiency
    energy w.
    esophageal w.
    gastric w.
    w. level
    localization w.
    lung w.
    mediastinal w.
    oval w.
    parasternal w.
    pericardial w.
    w. period
    pulmonary parenchymatous w.
    radiation w.
    sampling w.
    short acquisition w.
    soft tissue w.
    spectral w.
    subcostal w.
    subdural w.
    suprasternal w.
    transforaminal w.
    transorbital w.
    transtemporal w.
    vestibular w.
    w. width
    xenon energy w.
windowed balloon
windowing
    intensity w.
window-level setting
windsock
    w. aneurysm
    w. appearance
    w. appearance of duodenum
    w. diverticulum
    w. sign
windswept
    w. deformity
    w. hand
    w. pelvis
windup injury
wine
    w. glass
    w. glass appearance
    w. glass pelvis
    w. glass shape
wing
    absent greater sphenoid w.
    champagne glass iliac w.
    greater sphenoid w.
    iliac w.

    w. of sphenoid bone
    sphenoid w.
winged
    w. configuration
    w. scapula
winging
    scapular w.
Winiwarter-Buerger disease
Winquist-Hansen femoral fracture (0-IV) classification
Winslow
    foramen of W.
    W. ligament
Winston-Lutz for LINAC-based radiosurgery
Winter-King-Moe scoliosis
wire
    w. fixation
    guide w.
    heavy-duty standard exchange w.
    ^{192}Ir w.
    iridium w.
    J-tipped w.
    Kirschner w. (K-wire, K wire)
    w. localization
    pacemaker w.
    platinum w.
    Rosen w.
    standard exchange w.
    sternotomy w.
    super-stiff glide w.
    temporary atrial pacing w.
    w. winding
wire-fixation buckle
wireless
    w. capsule endoscopy
    w. handheld Web pad
wire-loop lesion
wire-related defect
wiring
    cheese w.
    intraosseous w.
Wirsung
    W. dilation
    W. duct
    ventral duct of W.
wisdom tooth
Wiseman classification
Wishart-Lee-Abbott NF2
wispy connection
withdrawal pressure
within-slice filtering process
within-view motion
Wits measurement
WMA
    wall motion abnormality
WNV
    West Nile virus

woggle
> w. device
> w. technique

Wolf
> W. method
> W. Piezolith 2200 lithotriptor

Wolfe
> W. DY, NI, P1, P2 pattern
> W. mammogram classification
> W. mammographic parenchymatous
> pattern

Wolff-Chaikoff effect

wolffian
> w. cyst
> w. duct
> w. duct carcinoma

Wolff law

Wolff-Parkinson-White syndrome

Wolf-Hirschhorn syndrome

Wolfram syndrome

Wolin meniscoid lesion

Wolman xanthomatosis

womb stone

wood
> W. lamp
> W. light
> W. unit
> W. unit index
> W. unit index of resistance

wooden-shoe
> w.-s. configuration
> w.-s. heart

woody mass

wool
> w. coil
> w. tail

work
> lattice w.
> left ventricular stroke w. (LVSW)
> myocardial w.
> right ventricular stroke w. (RVSW)

working
> w. film
> W. Formulation classification
> w. sheath

workspace
> Extended Brilliance W.

workstation
> AccuView computer w.
> Advantage W.
> Alpha 21064 microprocessor w.
> Argus image processing w.
> DIMAQ integrated ultrasound w.
> eNTEGRA w.
> freestanding w.
> Fuji QA 771 w.
> image processing w.
> imaging w.

> ISG medical imaging w.
> J-Vision w.
> Leonardo software fusion w.
> MacSpect real-time NMR w.
> MagicView w.
> Navigator computer w.
> Octane postprocessing w.
> PACS w.
> Pegasys w.
> postprocessing w.
> POWERstation LNX w.
> RADstation radiology w.
> Renaissance 3D w.
> Shebele physician reporting w.
> Siemens e.soft w.
> Sun w.
> Unix/X11 w.
> Vitrea 2 computer w.
> Vitrea w. (version 1.1, 1.2)

worm aneurysm

wormian bone

wormy appearance

wound
> w. dehiscence
> exit w.
> gunshot w. (GSW)
> high-velocity gunshot w.
> missile w.
> penetrating w.
> perforating w.
> stag w.
> surgical w.

woven bone

wrap
> aneurysmal w.
> aortic w.
> no frequency w.

wraparound
> w. ghosting artifact
> w. vessel

wrapped
> w. aneurysmal sac
> w. artifact

wrapping
> valve w.
> vein valve w.

Wratten 6B filter

W ray

wrenched knee

wrestler's elbow

wrinkle artifact

wrinkled pleura

wrinkler muscle

Wrisberg
> W. cardiac ganglion
> intermediate nerve of W.
> W. ligament
> ligaments of Henry and W.

W

wrist
  w. capsule
  w. dislocation
  w. extensor compartment
  w. fracture
  gymnast's w.
  w. joint
  palmar w.
  w. quadrature phased-array surface
    coil
  SLAC w.
  w. triquetrum bone
  volar w.

wristdrop
writing
  black echo w.
  white echo w.
WSCM
  water-soluble contrast medium
W-shaped ileal pouch
WSQ
  wavelet scalar quantization
Wuchereria bancrofti
Wyburn-Mason
  W.-M. arteriovenous malformation
  W.-M. syndrome

X

Xanthosine
X axis
X gradient
histiocytosis X
monosomy X
syndrome X
thorium X
X trough
X unit
Xanar 20 Ambulase CO₂ laser
xanthelasma
xanthic calculus
xanthoastrocytoma
pleomorphic x. (PXA)
xanthogranuloma
bone x.
juvenile x.
xanthogranulomatous
x. cholecystitis
x. pyelonephritis
xanthoma
Achilles tendon x.
gastric x.
x. tuberosum simplex
xanthomatosis
cerebrotendinous x.
primary familial x.
Wolman x.
xanthomatous
x. granuloma
x. pseudotumor
xanthosarcoma
xanthosine (X)
X-band LINAC
X-CBF
xenon-enhanced cerebral blood
flow
XCCL
exaggerated craniocaudal lateral
XCT
x-ray computed tomography
Xe
xenon
¹²⁷Xe, Xe-127
xenon 127
¹²⁹Xe, Xe-129
xenon 129
¹³³Xe, Xe-133
xenon 133
X-Echo-Speed
Signa Horizon X-E.-S.
XeCl
xenon chloride
XeCl excimer

XeCT
xenon-enhanced computed tomography
xenon-enhanced CT
Xenetix 250, 300, 350 contrast medium
xenograft
bovine heart x.
porcine heart x.
x. valve
vascular x.
xenon (Xe)
x. 127 (¹²⁷Xe, Xe-127)
x. 129 (¹²⁹Xe, Xe-129)
x. 133 (¹³³Xe, Xe-133)
x. arc photocoagulator
x. arc lamp
x. chloride (XeCl)
x. computed tomography
x. CT measurement
x. CT scanning
x. energy window
x. imaging agent
x. trap system
x. washout study
xenon-133
x.-133 SPECT imaging
x.-133 ventriculogram
xenon-chloride laser
xenon-enhanced
x.-e. cerebral blood flow
(X-CBF)
x.-e. computed tomography
(XeCT)
x.-e. CT (XeCT)
xenotransplantation
xerogram (*var. of* xeroradiograph)
xerography (*var. of* xeroradiography)
xeromammogram
chest wall lateral x.
xeromammography
xeroradiograph, xerogram
xeroradiographic
x. selenium plate
x. technique
xeroradiography, xerography
xerorhinia
xerosialography
xerostomia
xerotomography
x-height
Xillix
X. LIFE-GI fluorescence endoscopy
system
X. LIFE-Lung fluorescence
endoscopy system
Ximatron simulator

X

XIP
    x-ray in plaster
xiphisternal joint
xiphocostal ligament
xiphoid
    x. angle
    x. appendix
    x. bone
    x. cartilage
    x. ligament
    x. process
xiphopagus
xiphopubic area
xiphosternalis
    synchondrosis x.
x-irradiation
XKnife stereotactic radiosurgery system
X-linked adrenoleukodystrophy
XOP
    x-ray out of plaster
Xplorer 1000 digital imaging system
X-Prep bowel preparation
X-Press suture-mediated closure device
Xpress/SW helical CT scanner
Xpress/SX helical CT scanner
XRA
    x-ray arteriography
x-ray
    x-r. arteriography (XRA)
    x-r. attenuation
    baseline chest x-r.
    x-r. beam
    x-r. beam size
    x-r. burn
    cast-off x-r.
    characteristic x-r.
    chest x-r. (CXR)
    x-r. computed tomography (XCT)
    x-r. crystallography
    x-r. detector
    x-r. diffraction
    x-r. diffraction analysis
    x-r. dosimetry
    echoeSystem digital x-r.
    x-r. energy
    E sign on x-r.
    x-r. film

    x-r. generator
    hard x-r.
    x-r. image
    x-r. in plaster (XIP)
    inside-out x-r.
    Jude pelvic x-r.
    x-r. mammogram
    x-r. mammography
    mobile mass x-r. (MMR)
    monochromatic x-r.
    x-r. out of plaster (XOP)
    polychromatic x-r.
    portable x-r.
    postreduction x-r.
    prereduction x-r.
    scanning-beam digital x-r. (SBDX)
    x-r. shadow projection
      microtomographic system
    x-r. spectrometer
    x-r. spectrum
    x-r. therapy
    x-r. thickness gauge
    x-r. tomographic microscope (XTM)
    x-r. topography
    x-r. tube
    x-r. tube housing
    x-r. tube rating chart
    x-r. unit
    x-r. view
    2-view chest x-r.
    4-view chest x-r.
    5-view chest x-r.
x-shaped guidewire
X-terminal
XTM
    x-ray tomographic microscope
XT radiopaque coronary stent
X-Vigor CT scanner
X-wave pressure
XY
    normal male sex chromosome
    XY plane
    XY syndrome
X, Y, and Z coordinates for target lesion
xylenol orange imaging agent
xylol pulse indicator

Y
  yttrium
    Y axis
    Y bone plate
    Y cartilage
    Y configuration
    Y fracture
    Y trough
    Y winding
^{50}Y, Y-50
  yttrium-50
^{90}Y, Y-90
  yttrium-90
    ^{90}Y microsphere
    Y-90 silicate therapy
YAG
  yttrium-aluminum-garnet
  YAG laser
Yaglazr system
Yb
  ytterbium
yellow
  y. cartilage
  y. marrow
yellow-out
Yergason test
Yersinia
  Y. enterocolitis
  Y. pestis
yield
  y. comparison
  diagnostic y.
  low y.
  ultrasound diagnostic y.
ying-yang (var. of yin-yang)
yin-yang, ying-yang
  y.-y. appearance
  y.-y. sign
Y-jaws
YLF
  yttrium lithium fluoride

Y-line
yolk
  y. sac
  y. sac diameter
  y. sac ovary tumor
  y. stalk
Young syndrome
yo-yo
  y.-y. esophageal peristalsis
  y.-y. ureteral peristalsis
Yperwatch gamma control
  watch
Y-shaped
  Y-s. acetabulum
  Y-s. distortion
  Y-s. ligament
Y-T fracture
ytterbium (Yb)
  y. pentetate sodium
ytterbium-169 DTPA
ytterbium-90 microsphere
yttrium (Y)
  ferritin-labeled y.
  y. lithium fluoride (YLF)
  y. radioactive source
  strontium with y. 90
yttrium-50 (^{50}Y, Y-50)
yttrium-90 (^{90}Y, Y-90)
  y.-90 ibritumomab
  y.-90 microsphere
  y.-90 silicate therapy
yttrium-aluminum-garnet (YAG)
  y.-a.-g. laser
yttrium-90-labeled
Y-tube
Yueh centesis needle
Yuge
  oculosubcutaneous syndrome
    of Y.
Yunis-Varon syndrome
Y-wave pressure

Z

Z axis
Z axis field
Z band
Z gradient
Z line of esophagus
Z score in bone mineral density measurement

Zaglas ligament
Zahn

Z. anomaly
pocket of Z.

Zanca acromioclavicular joint view
Zanelli position
ZA-stent nitinol self-expandable stent
Z-dependent CT
zebra

z. stripe appearance
z. stripe artifact
z. stripe image
z. stripe pattern

Zeeman hamiltonian function
Zeiss

Z. EndoLive endoscope
Z. Visulas 690s laser

Zellballen
Zellweger syndrome
Zener diode
Zenith

Z. AAA endovascular graft
Z. stainless steel self-expandable stent

Zenker

Z. degeneration
Z. diverticulum
Z. necrosis
Z. pouch

zeolite pneumoconiosis
zero

z. exposure
z. filling
z. line
z. net flow
z. padding
z. phase
z. reference level
z. time of x-ray apparatus

zero-field splitting
zero-filling interpolation scheme
zero-fill interpolation
zero-pitch solenoid winding
ZeroRad MRI scan
zeroth moment

ZES

Zollinger-Ellison syndrome

zetacrit
Zetafuge
zeugmatography

Fourier transform z.
rotating-frame z.

zeugopodium
Zeus system
Zevalin
Z-filtering
z-flying focal spot
Zickel supracondylar nail
Zielke derotation level
Zieve syndrome
zigzag stent
Zilver self-expanding stent
Zilverstent
Zimmerman

Z. arch
Z. cell

Zimmermann elementary particle
Zimmer method
zinc (Zn)

z. 65 (^{65}Zn, Zn-65)
z. deficiency
irradiated z.
z. turbidity test

Zinn

Z. anulus
Z. ligament
Z. tendon

zipper artifact
zirconium (Zr)

z. granuloma
z. with niobium 95

Zlatkin grading system
ZMC

zygomaticomaxillary complex
ZMC fracture

Z-Med balloon catheter
Z-MIVE

methoxy-17-alpha-iodovinyl estradiol
^{123}I-labeled Z-MIVE

Zn

zinc

^{65}Zn, Zn-65

zinc 65

Zollinger-Ellison

Z. E. syndrome (ZES)
Z.-E. tumor

zona, *pl.* **zonae**

z. fasciculata
z. glomerulosa

zona (*continued*)
    z. orbicularis
    z. reticularis
zonae (*pl. of* zona)
zonal
    z. gastritis
    z. prostate anatomy
    z. sampling
    z. uterine anatomy
zonary
zone
    airtrapping z.
    arrhythmogenic border z.
    basal z.
    bilaminar z.
    border z.
    clear z.
    convergence z.
    cross-sectional z.
    detection z.
    dorsal root entry z.
      (DREZ)
    echo-free central z.
    entry z.
    epileptogenic z.
    esophageal transition z.
    focal z.
    focal high-intensity z.
    z. focusing
    fracture z.
    Fraunhofer z.
    Fresnel z.
    high-intensity z. (HIZ)
    high signal intensity z.
    hypoechogenic retroplacental
      myometrial z.
    hypoechoic z.
    hypovascular z.
    ischemic z.
    junctional z.
    lipid z.
    Looser transformation z.
    lung z.
    marginal z.
    midlung z.
    noninfarct z.
    z. of partial preservation
      (ZPP)
    z. of slow conduction
    z. 1-4 of West
    patchy z.
    penumbra z.
    periinfarcted z.
    periinfarction z.
    peripheral z. (PZ)
    posterior root entry z.
    prostatic transition z.
    pyramidal hemorrhagic z.

    Rolando z.
    root entry z.
    root exit z. (REZ)
    rough z.
    sonolucent z.
    therapy z.
    transformation z. (TMZ)
    transition z. (TZ)
    transradiant z.
    Trümmerfeld z.
    Umbau z.
    vascular z.
    wedge-shaped z.
    Westphal z.
zonifugal
zonipetal
zonogram
zonography
    stereoscopic z.
zonoskeleton
zonula ciliaris
zoom imaging
zoonosis
    respiratory z.
Z-point pressure
ZPP
    zone of partial preservation
Zr
    zirconium
Z-stent
    Gianturco biliary Z-s.
zuckerguss
Zuckerkandl
    Z. body
    Z. convolution
    Z. fascia
    Z. organ
Zurich growth centile diagram
Zuska disease
zwitterion
zygal
zygapophyseal (*var. of* zygapophysial)
zygapophyses (*pl. of* zygapophysis)
zygapophysial, zygapophyseal
    z. articulation
    z. joint
zygapophysis, *pl.* **zygapophyses**
    z. inferior
    z. superior
zygoma
zygomatic
    z. arch
    z. bone
    z. complex
    z. process
zygomaticofacial
    z. canal
    z. foramen

zygomaticofrontal suture
zygomaticomalar
    z. area
    z. reconstruction
zygomaticomaxillary, zygomaxillary
    z. complex (ZMC)
    z. fracture

zygomaticotemporal
    z. canal
    z. suture
zygomaxillary (*var. of*
  zygomaticomaxillary)
ZY plane

Z

Contents: The Appendices

1. Anatomical Illustrations A1
2. Contrast Media, Imaging Agents, and Related Substances A25
3. Common Radiation Oncology Terms A29
4. Sample Reports A34
5. Common Terms by Procedure A49
6. Common Breast Imaging Terms A55
7. Common Radiographic Imaging Techniques A59

Anatomical Illustrations

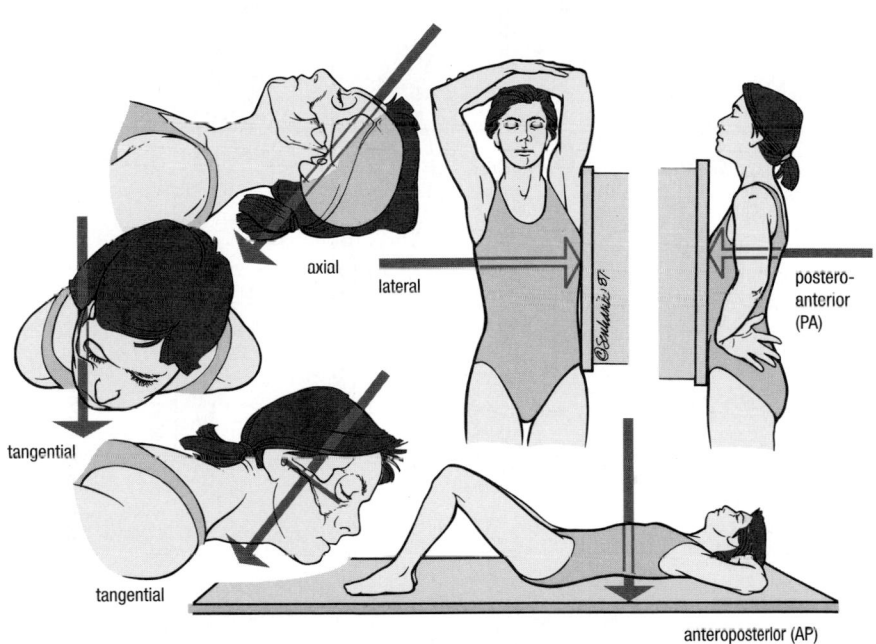

axial

lateral

tangential

postero-
anterior
(PA)

tangential

anteroposterior (AP)

radiographic projections: x-rays pass through body parts with the denser structures absorbing
more x rays, resulting in the lighter areas on the radiograph

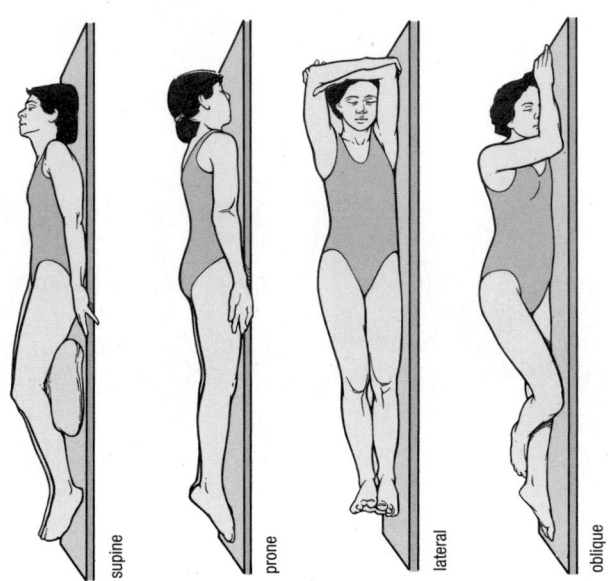

supine

prone

lateral

oblique

patient positions

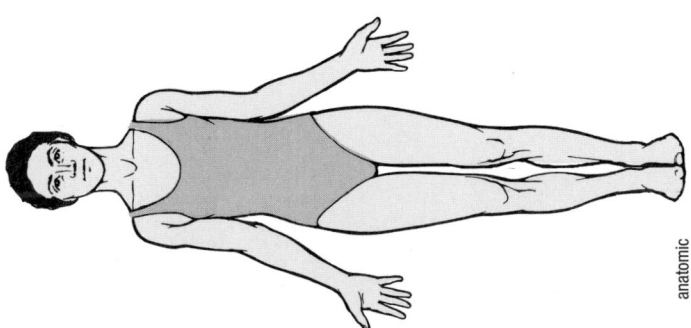

anatomic

Anatomical Illustrations

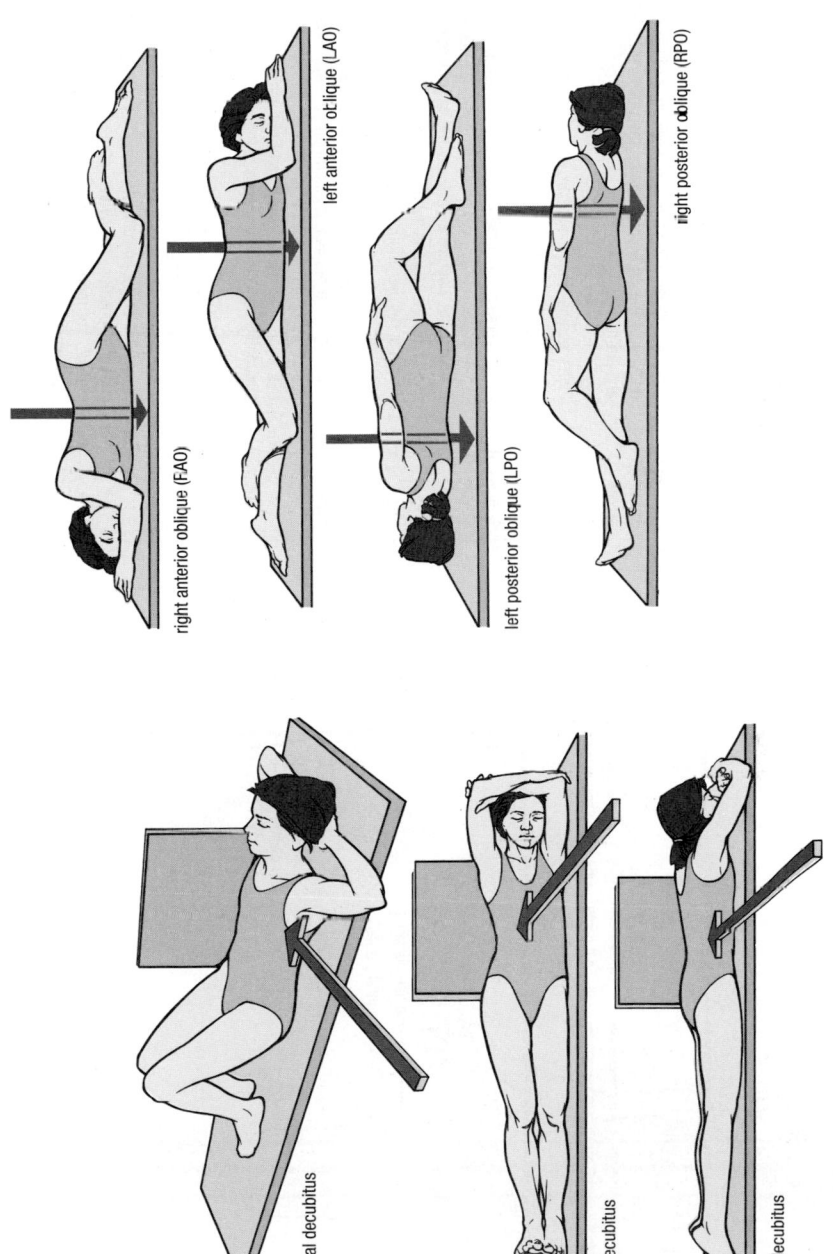

right anterior oblique (RAO)

left anterior oblique (LAO)

left posterior oblique (LPO)

right posterior oblique (RPO)

dorsal decubitus

lateral decubitus

ventral decubitus

patient positions

Anatomic Planes

Frontal (coronal) plane:	A vertical plane at right angles to a sagittal plane, dividing the body into anterior and posterior portions, or any plane parallel to the central coronal plane.
Longitudinal plane:	Running lengthwise; in the direction of the long axis of the body or any of its parts.
Median (midsagittal) plane:	A plane vertical in the anatomic position, through the midline of the body that divides the body into right and left halves.
Sagittal plane:	Plane parallel to the median plane; sagittal planes are vertical planes in the anatomic position.
Subcostal plane:	A transverse plane passing through the inferior limits of the costal margin, i.e., the 10th costal cartilages; it marks the boundary between the hypochondriac and epigastric regions superiorly and the lateral and umbilical regions inferiorly.
Transpyloric plane:	A transverse plane midway between the superior margins of the manubrium sterni and the symphysis pubis; the pylorus may be located on this plane in the supine or prone positions, but in the erect (anatomic) position it descends to the lower level.
Transverse plane:	A plane across the body at right angles to the frontal and sagittal planes; transverse planes are perpendicular to the long axis of the body or limbs, regardless of the position of the body or limb; in the anatomic position, transverse planes are horizontal planes; otherwise the two terms are not synonymous.

terms of relationship, anatomic planes

transverse plane

transpyloric plane (9th costal cartilage)

subcostal plane (10th costal cartilage)

transverse plane

median plane

sagittal planes

frontal planes

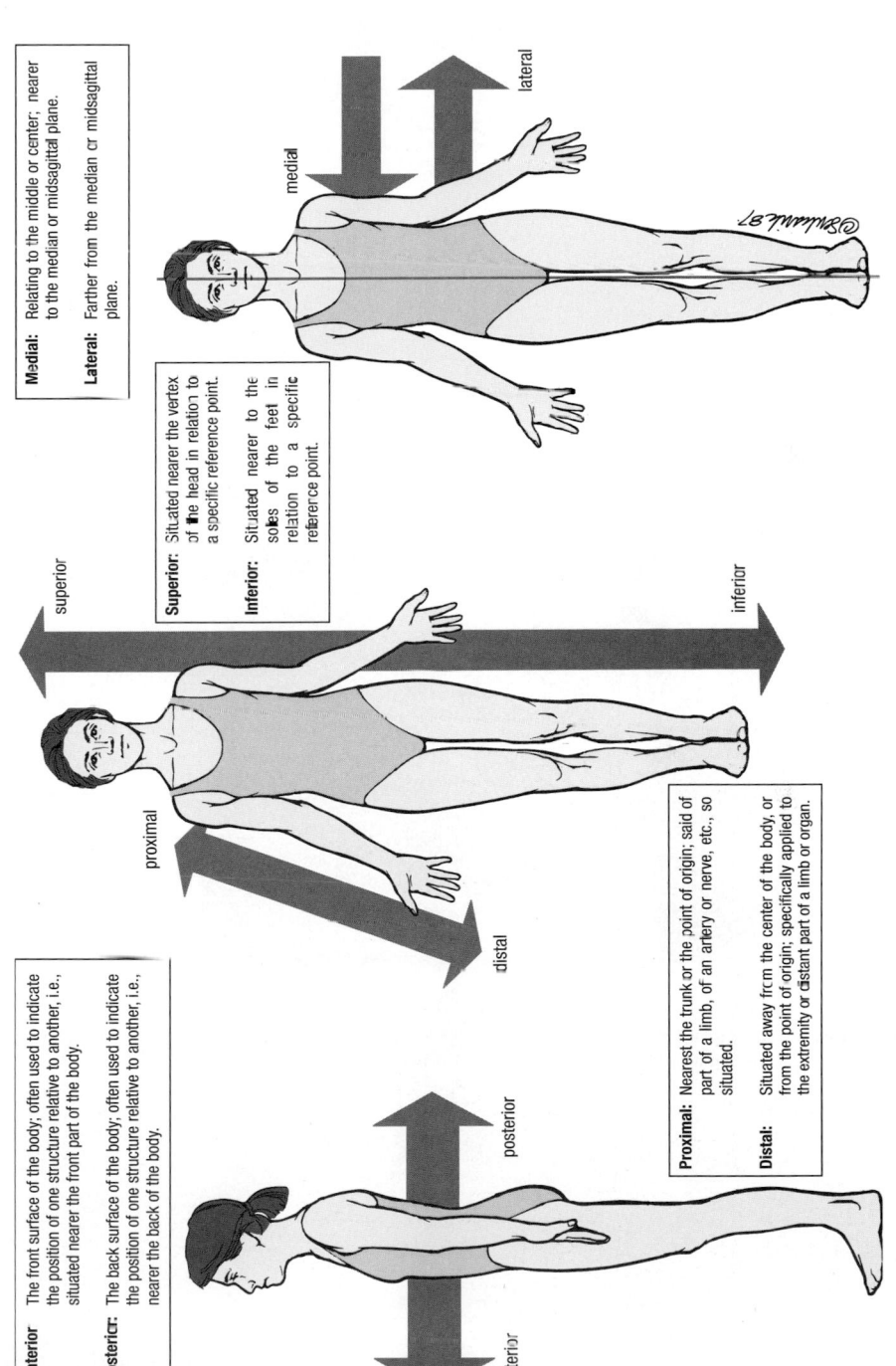

terms of relationship, body part terminology

Medial: Relating to the middle or center; nearer to the median or midsagittal plane.

Lateral: Farther from the median or midsagittal plane.

Superior: Situated nearer the vertex of the head in relation to a specific reference point.

Inferior: Situated nearer to the soles of the feet in relation to a specific reference point.

Anterior The front surface of the body; often used to indicate the position of one structure relative to another, i.e., situated nearer the front part of the body.

Posterior: The back surface of the body; often used to indicate the position of one structure relative to another, i.e., nearer the back of the body.

Proximal: Nearest the trunk or the point of origin; said of part of a limb, of an artery or nerve, etc., so situated.

Distal: Situated away from the center of the body, or from the point of origin; specifically applied to the extremity or distant part of a limb or organ.

superior

inferior

proximal

distal

posterior

anterior

medial

lateral

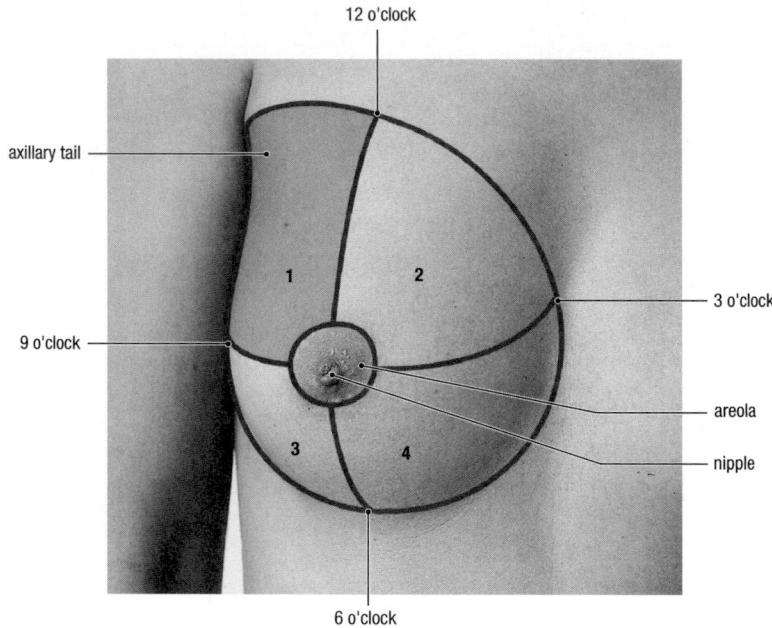

12 o'clock

axillary tail

9 o'clock

1 2

3 o'clock

areola

nipple

3 4

6 o'clock

quadrants of the right breast: (1) upper outer (50% of cancerous breast tumors are found in the quadrant), (2) upper inner, (3) lower outer, (4) lower inner

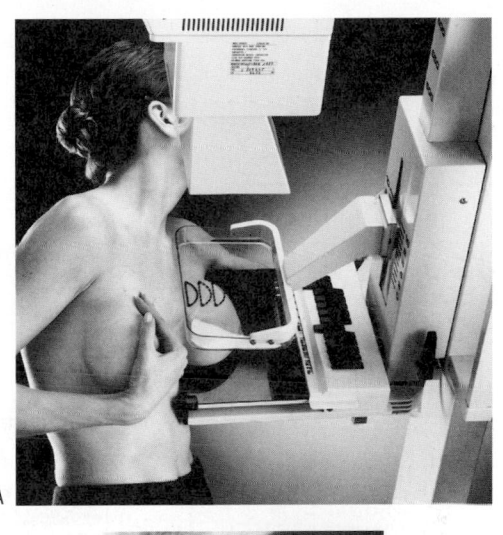

A

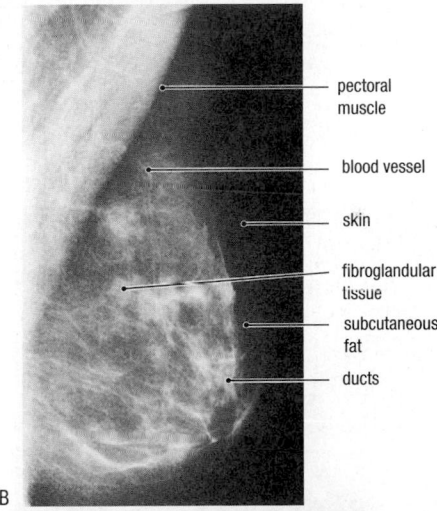

pectoral muscle

blood vessel

skin

fibroglandular tissue

subcutaneous fat

ducts

B

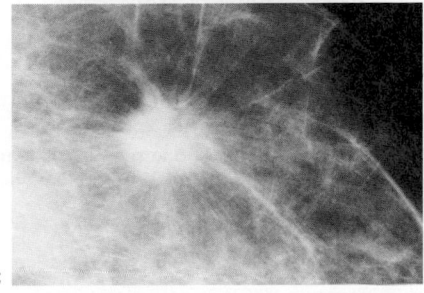

C

mammography: (A) patient positioning for a mediolateral oblique (MLO) view, (B) normal mammogram of left breast, (C) infiltrating duct carcinoma

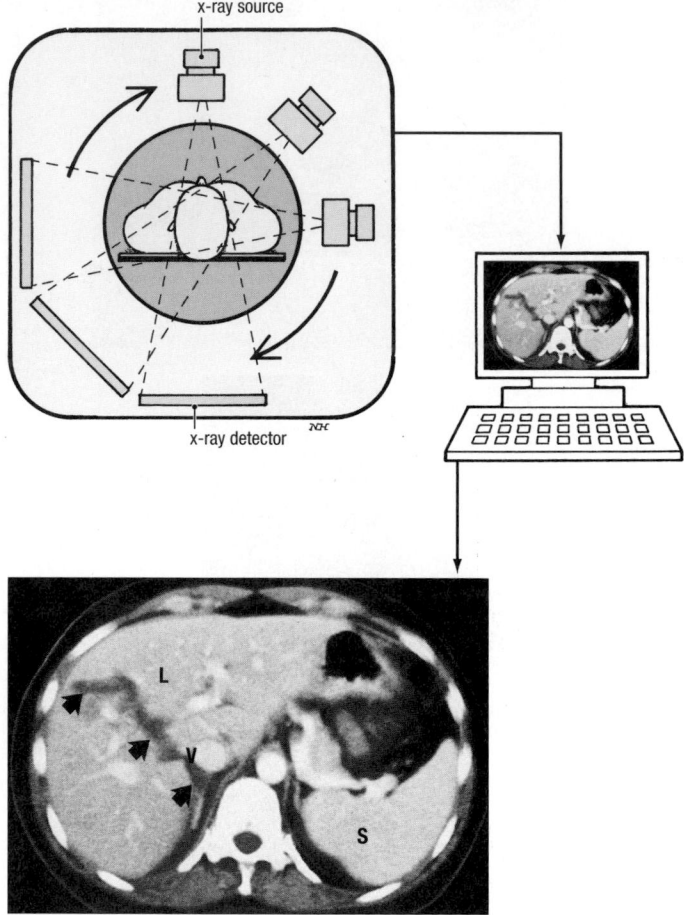

CT scan: patient involved in a motor vehicle accident demonstrates a jagged laceration (arrows) extending from posterior to inferior vena cava (V) through right lobe of the liver (L); (S), spleen

computed tomography (CT): a radiologic procedure using a scanner to examine the body site by taking a series of cross-sectional images one slice at a time in a full-circle rotation; a computer then calculates and converts the rates of absorption and density of the x-rays into a picture on a screen

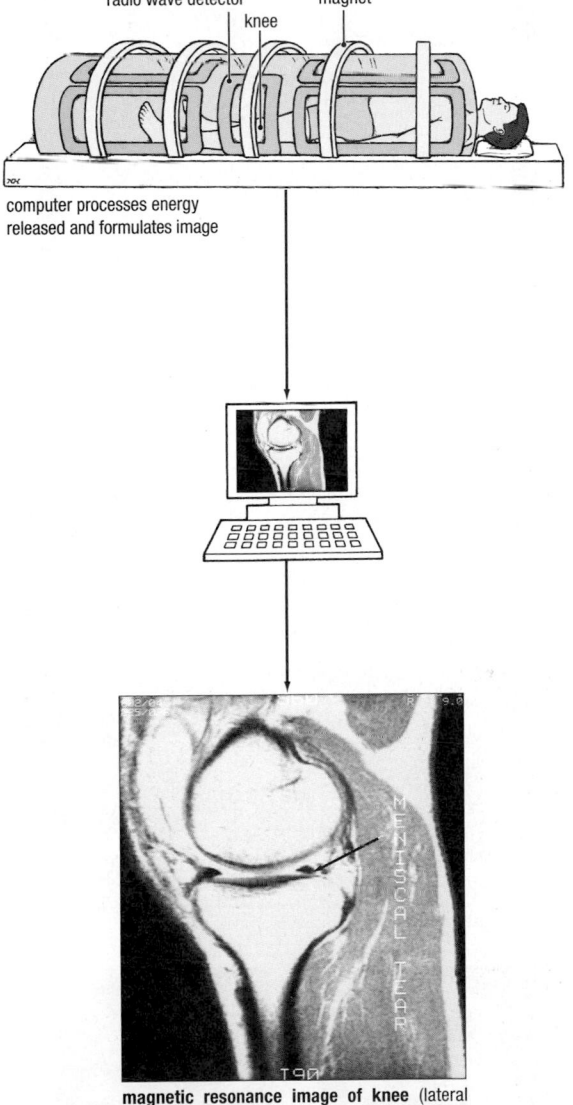

magnetic resonance image of knee (lateral view): torn meniscus

magnetic resonance imaging (MRI): a nonionizing (non-x-ray) technique using magnetic fields and radiofrequency waves to visualize anatomic structures; it is useful in detecting joint, tendon, and vertebral disorders; the patient is positioned within a magnetic field as radio wave signals are conducted through the selected body part; energy is absorbed by tissues and then released

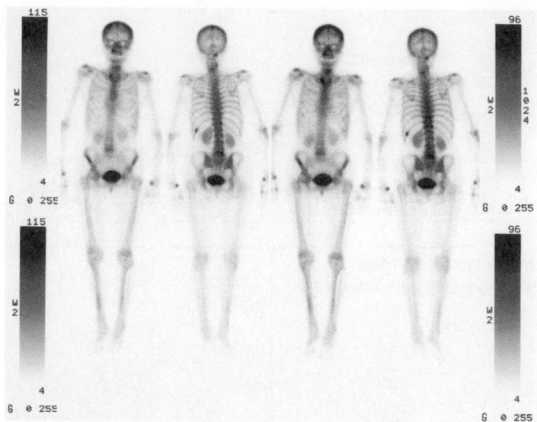

full-body bone scan: nuclear scan of bone tissue to detect abnormalities such as tumors and malignancies

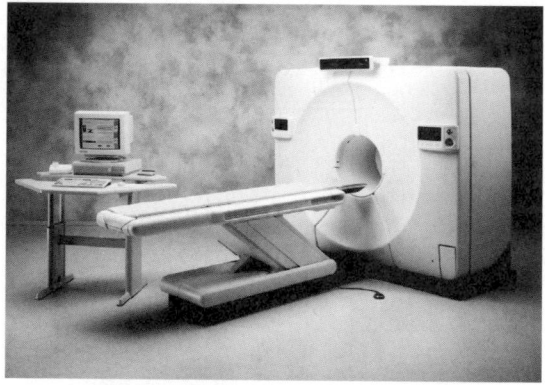

positron emission tomography (PET): combination of nuclear medicine and computed tomography produces images of brain anatomy and corresponding physiology, and is used to study conditions and diseases, including stroke, Alzheimer disease, epilepsy, and metabolic brain disorders

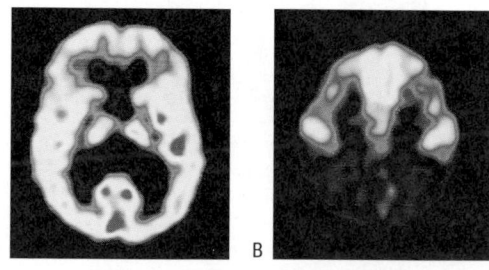

A   B

PET scan: (A) normal brain, (B) Alzheimer disease

nuclear medicine imaging: a diagnostic technique using injected or ingested radioactive isotopes and a gamma camera for determining size, shape, location, and function of various body parts

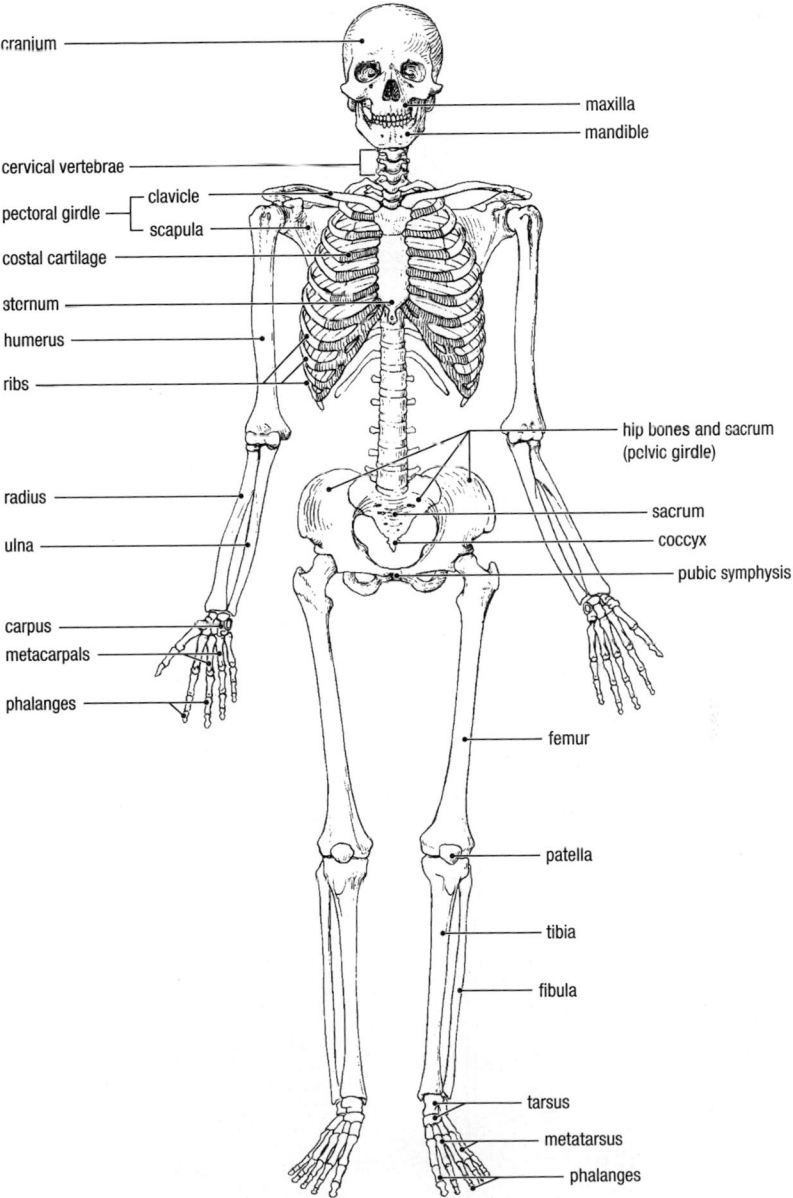

cranium

maxilla

mandible

cervical vertebrae

pectoral girdle — clavicle

scapula

costal cartilage

sternum

humerus

ribs

hip bones and sacrum
(pelvic girdle)

sacrum

coccyx

pubic symphysis

radius

ulna

carpus

metacarpals

phalanges

femur

patella

tibia

fibula

tarsus

metatarsus

phalanges

skeleton, adult, anterior view

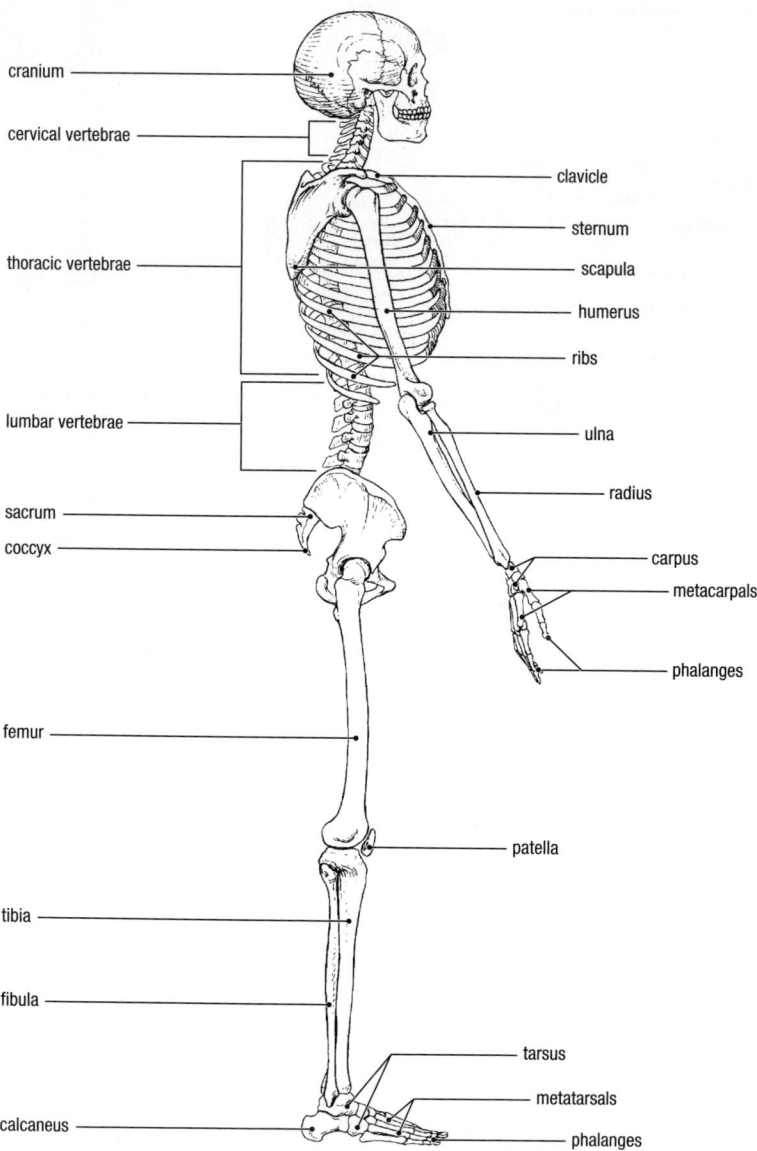

cranium

cervical vertebrae

clavicle

sternum

scapula

thoracic vertebrae

humerus

ribs

lumbar vertebrae

ulna

radius

sacrum

coccyx

carpus

metacarpals

phalanges

femur

patella

tibia

fibula

tarsus

metatarsals

calcaneus

phalanges

skeleton, adult, lateral view

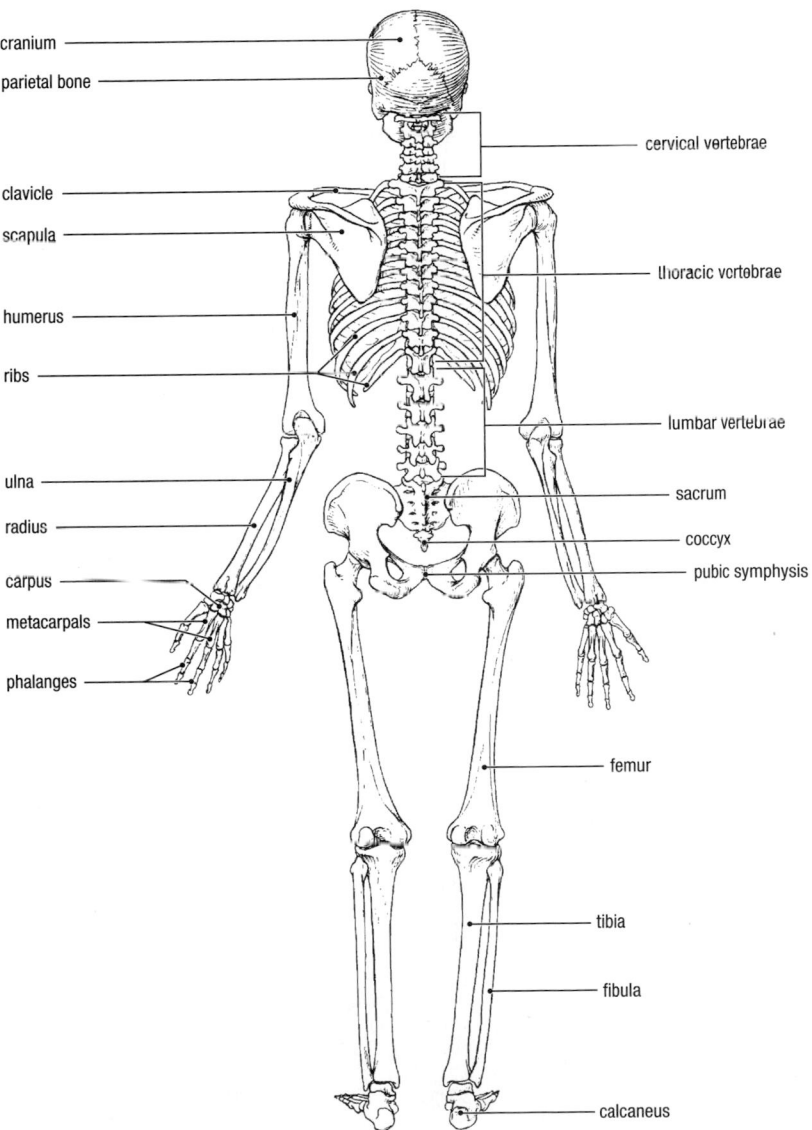

cranium

parietal bone

cervical vertebrae

clavicle

scapula

thoracic vertebrae

humerus

ribs

lumbar vertebrae

ulna

sacrum

radius

coccyx

pubic symphysis

carpus

metacarpals

phalanges

femur

tibia

fibula

calcaneus

skeleton, adult, posterior view

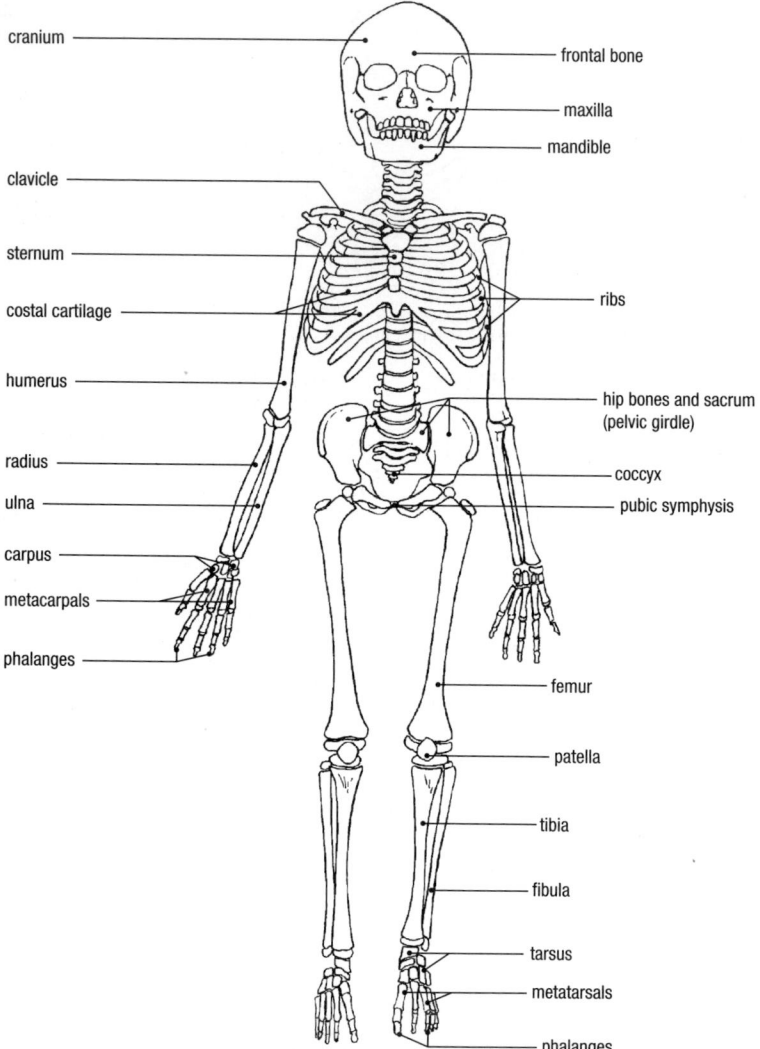

cranium

frontal bone

maxilla

mandible

clavicle

sternum

costal cartilage

ribs

humerus

hip bones and sacrum
(pelvic girdle)

radius

coccyx

ulna

pubic symphysis

carpus

metacarpals

phalanges

femur

patella

tibia

fibula

tarsus

metatarsals

phalanges

skeleton, child, anterior view

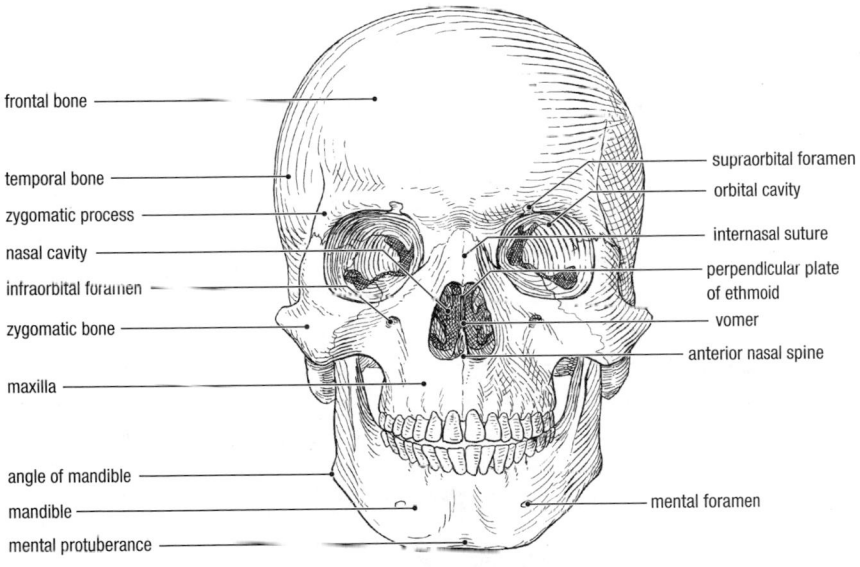

frontal bone

temporal bone

zygomatic process

nasal cavity

infraorbital foramen

zygomatic bone

maxilla

angle of mandible

mandible

mental protuberance

supraorbital foramen

orbital cavity

internasal suture

perpendicular plate
of ethmoid

vomer

anterior nasal spine

mental foramen

skull, frontal view

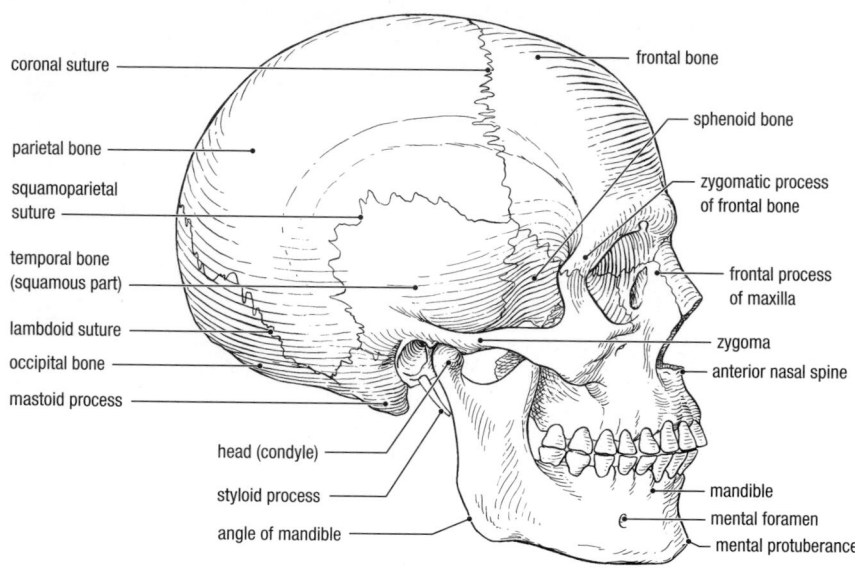

coronal suture — frontal bone

parietal bone — sphenoid bone

squamoparietal suture — zygomatic process of frontal bone

temporal bone (squamous part) — frontal process of maxilla

lambdoid suture — zygoma

occipital bone — anterior nasal spine

mastoid process —

head (condyle) — mandible

styloid process — mental foramen

angle of mandible — mental protuberance

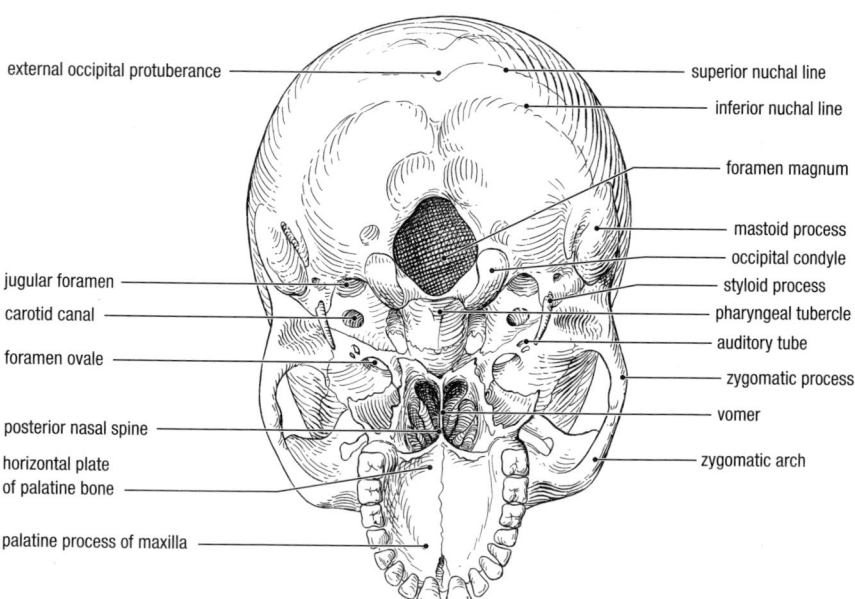

external occipital protuberance — superior nuchal line

— inferior nuchal line

— foramen magnum

— mastoid process

— occipital condyle

jugular foramen — styloid process

carotid canal — pharyngeal tubercle

foramen ovale — auditory tube

— zygomatic process

posterior nasal spine — vomer

horizontal plate of palatine bone — zygomatic arch

palatine process of maxilla —

skull, lateral (top) and inferior (bottom) views

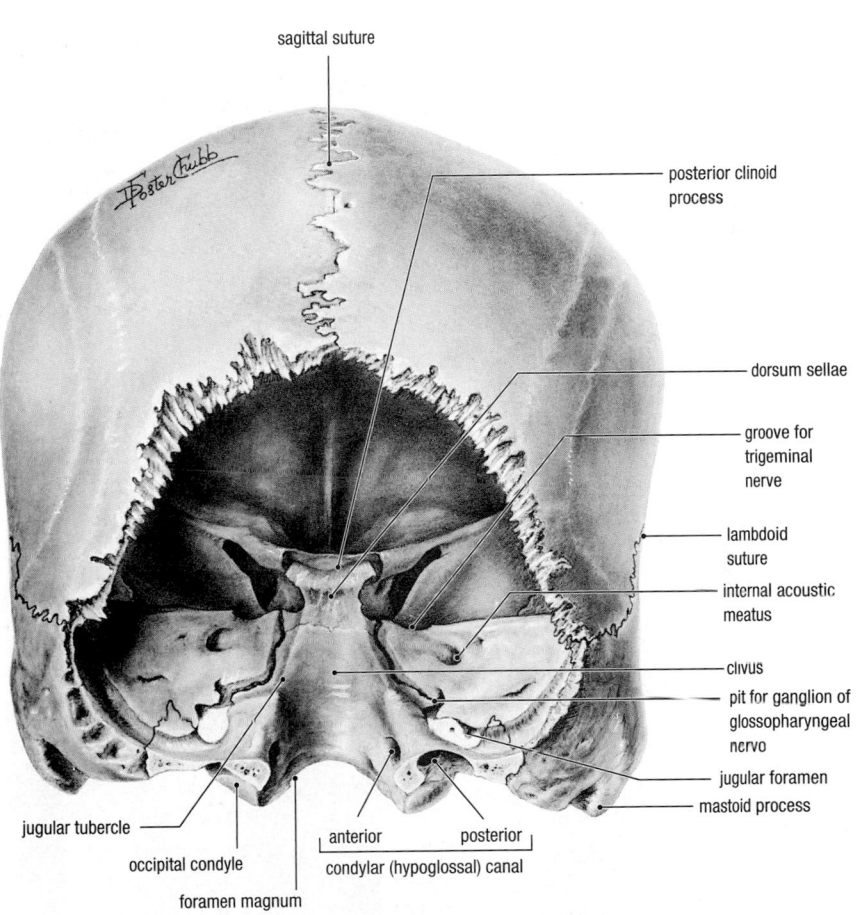

sagittal suture

posterior clinoid process

dorsum sellae

groove for trigeminal nerve

lambdoid suture

internal acoustic meatus

clivus

pit for ganglion of glossopharyngeal nerve

jugular foramen

mastoid process

jugular tubercle

occipital condyle

foramen magnum

anterior   posterior
condylar (hypoglossal) canal

skull: bony features of posterior cranial fossa

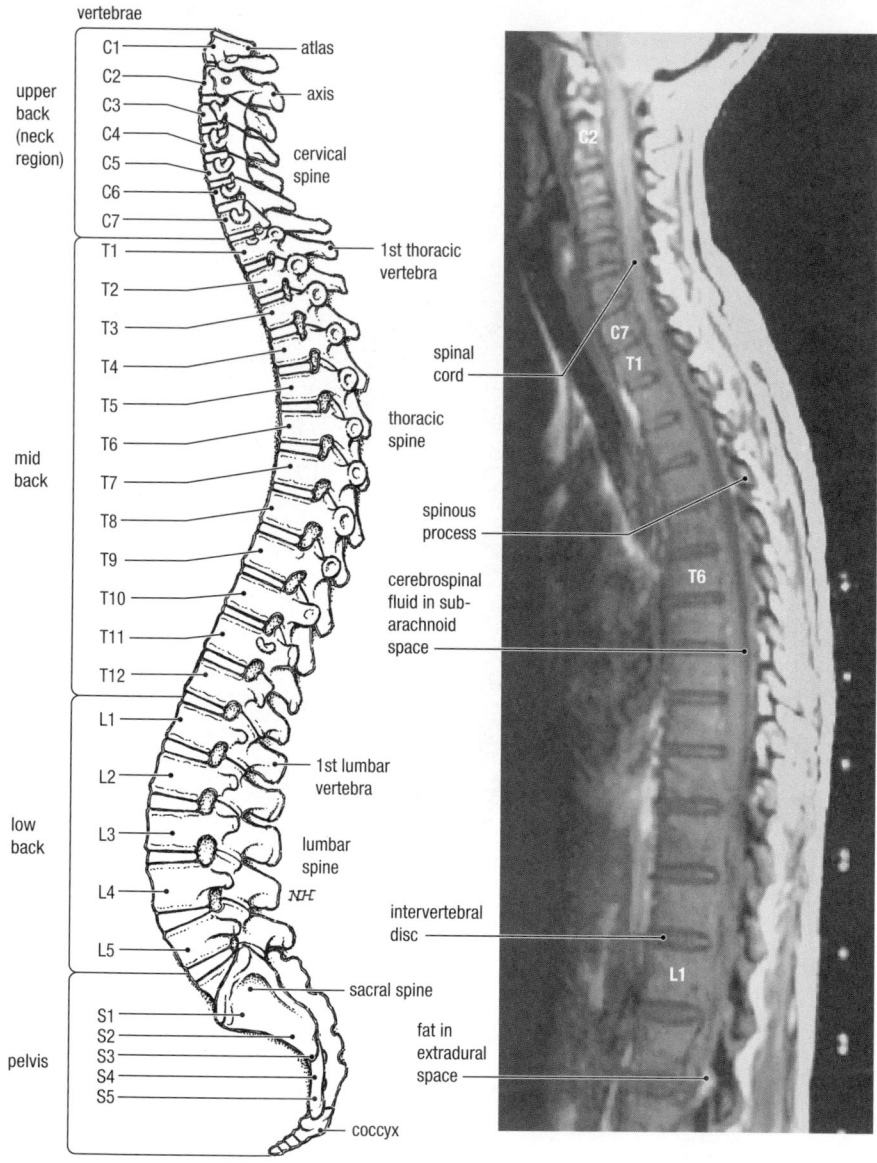

vertebral column, lateral view (radiograph courtesy of Dr. D. Salonen, University of Toronto, Toronto, Ontario, Canada)

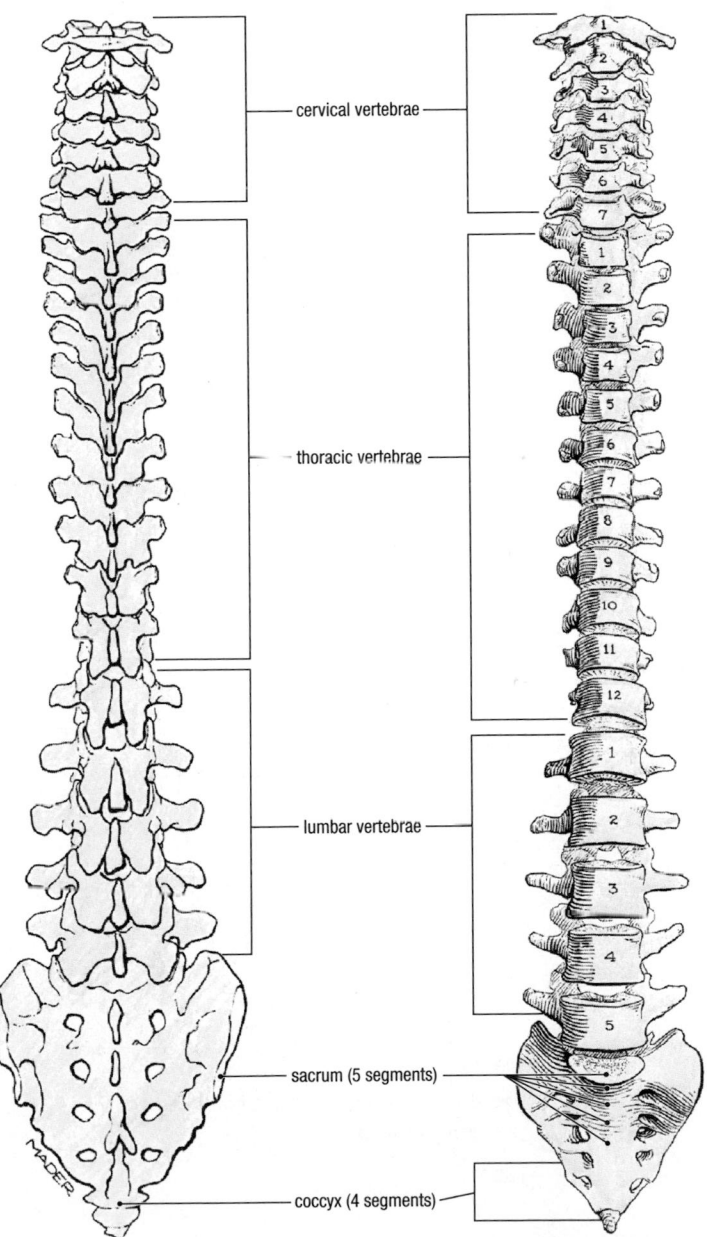

cervical vertebrae

thoracic vertebrae

lumbar vertebrae

sacrum (5 segments)

coccyx (4 segments)

vertebral column, posterior (left) and anterior (right) views

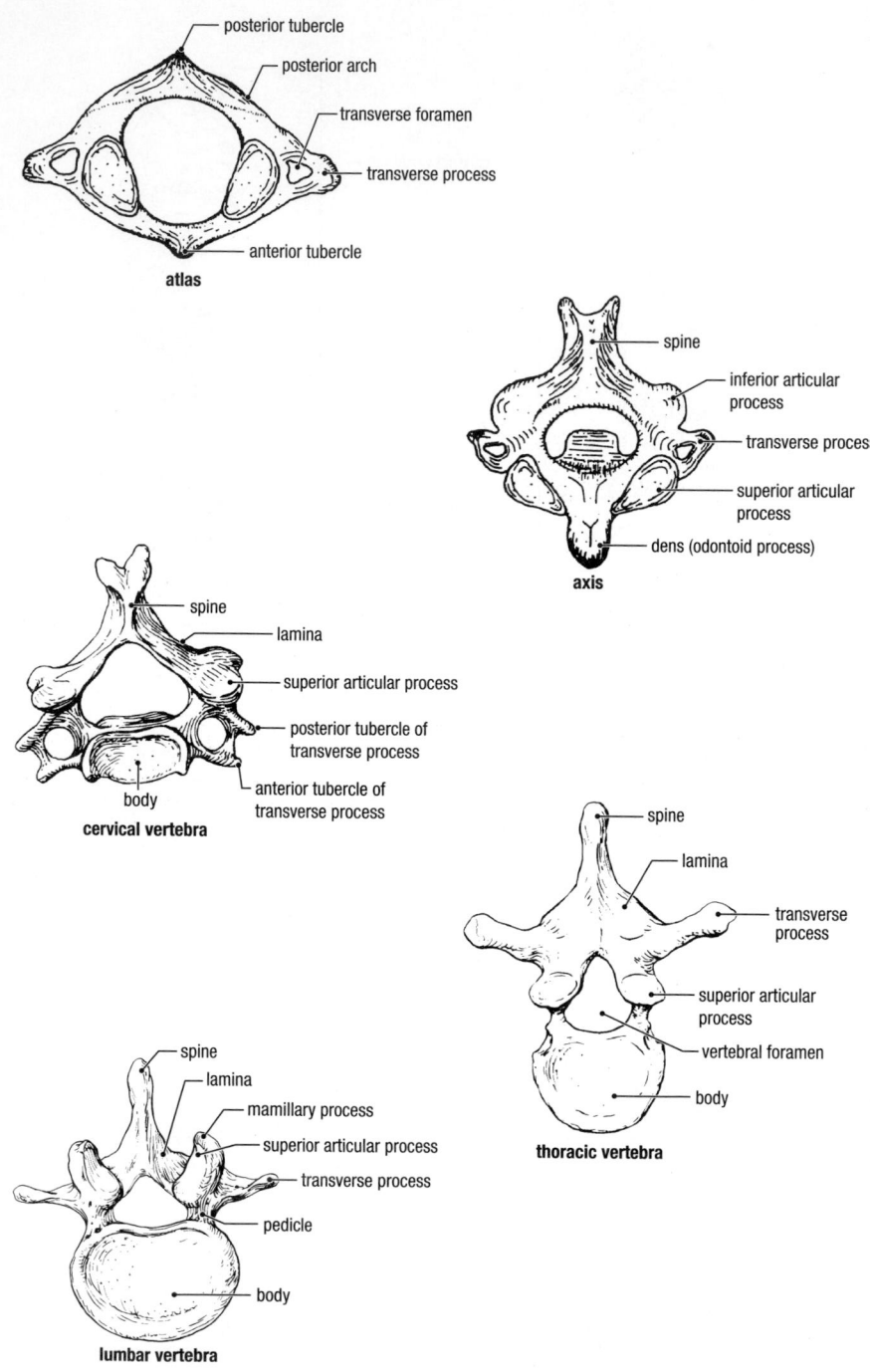

— posterior tubercle

— posterior arch

— transverse foramen

— transverse process

— anterior tubercle

atlas

— spine

— inferior articular process

— transverse process

— superior articular process

— dens (odontoid process)

axis

— spine

— lamina

— superior articular process

— posterior tubercle of transverse process

— anterior tubercle of transverse process

body

cervical vertebra

— spine

— lamina

— transverse process

— superior articular process

— vertebral foramen

— body

thoracic vertebra

— spine
— lamina
— mamillary process
— superior articular process
— transverse process
— pedicle
— body

lumbar vertebra

typical atlas, axis, cervical, thoracic, and lumbar vertebrae

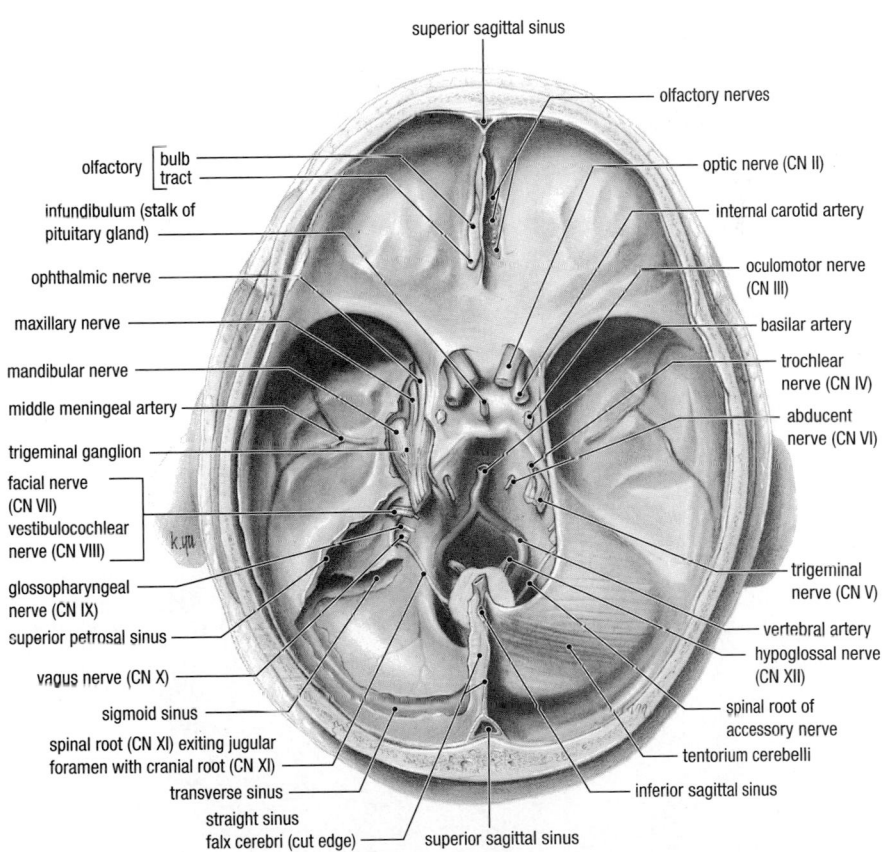

superior sagittal sinus

olfactory nerves

olfactory [bulb / tract]

optic nerve (CN II)

infundibulum (stalk of pituitary gland)

internal carotid artery

ophthalmic nerve

oculomotor nerve (CN III)

maxillary nerve

basilar artery

mandibular nerve

trochlear nerve (CN IV)

middle meningeal artery

abducent nerve (CN VI)

trigeminal ganglion

facial nerve (CN VII)
vestibulocochlear nerve (CN VIII)

trigeminal nerve (CN V)

glossopharyngeal nerve (CN IX)

vertebral artery

superior petrosal sinus

hypoglossal nerve (CN XII)

vagus nerve (CN X)

spinal root of accessory nerve

sigmoid sinus

spinal root (CN XI) exiting jugular foramen with cranial root (CN XI)

tentorium cerebelli

transverse sinus

inferior sagittal sinus

straight sinus
falx cerebri (cut edge)

superior sagittal sinus

nerves and vessels of the interior base of the skull, superior view

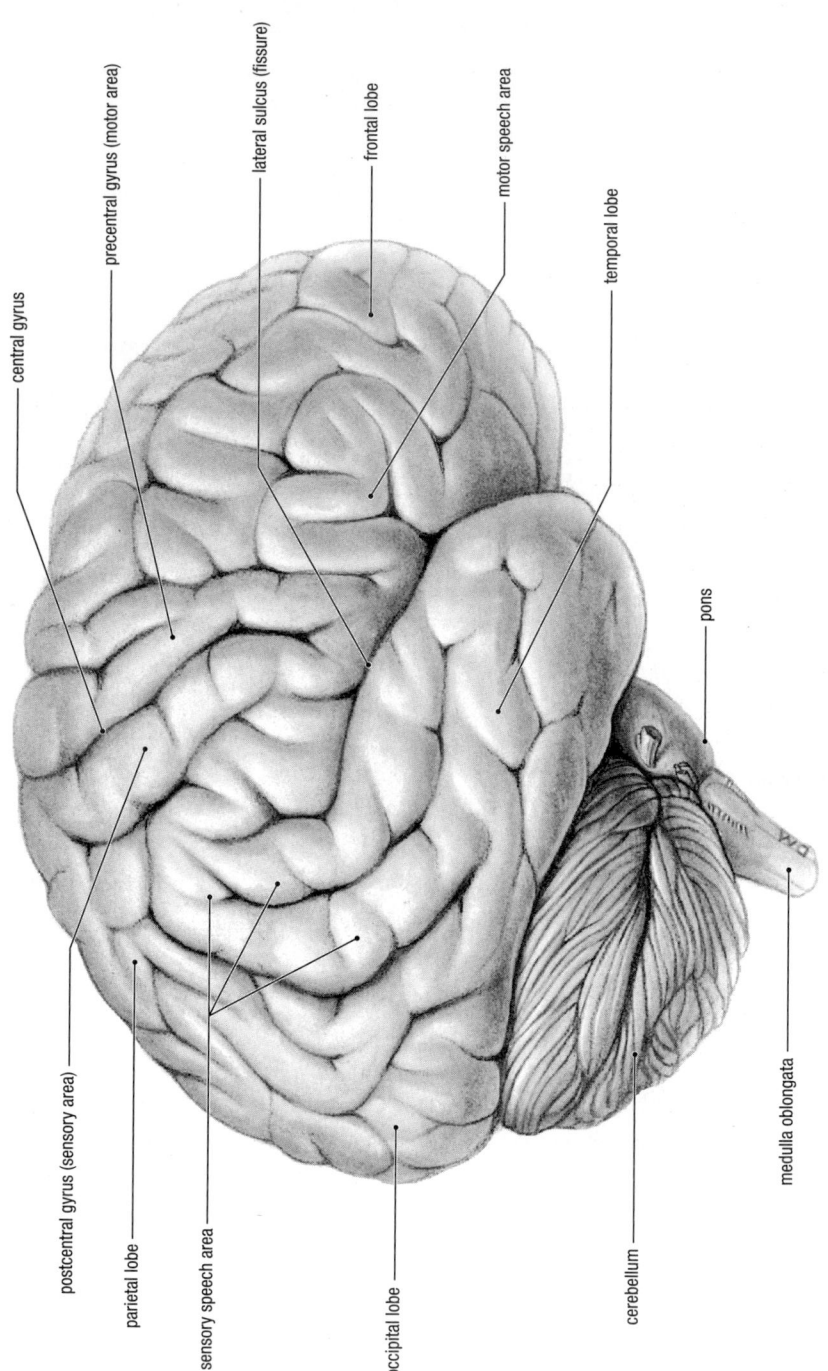

central gyrus

precentral gyrus (motor area)

lateral sulcus (fissure)

frontal lobe

motor speech area

temporal lobe

pons

postcentral gyrus (sensory area)

parietal lobe

sensory speech area

occipital lobe

cerebellum

medulla oblongata

brain, lateral view:

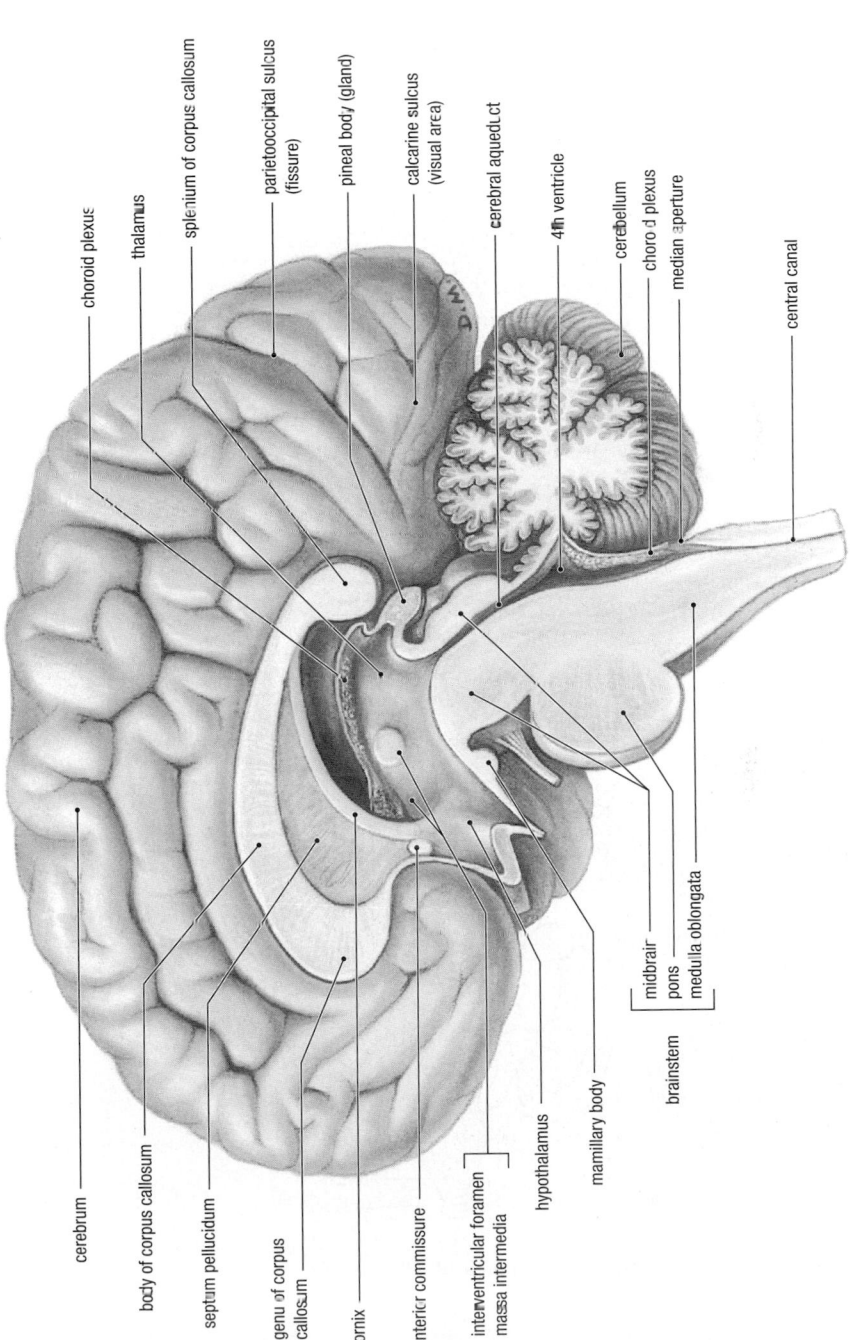

choroid plexus

thalamus

splenium of corpus callosum

parietooccipital sulcus (fissure)

pineal body (gland)

calcarine sulcus (visual area)

cerebral aqueduct

4th ventricle

cerebellum

choroid plexus

median aperture

central canal

cerebrum

body of corpus callosum

septum pellucidum

genu of corpus callosum

fornix

anterior commissure

interventricular foramen
massa intermedia

hypothalamus

mamillary body

midbrain
pons
medulla oblongata

brainstem

brain, median section

A23

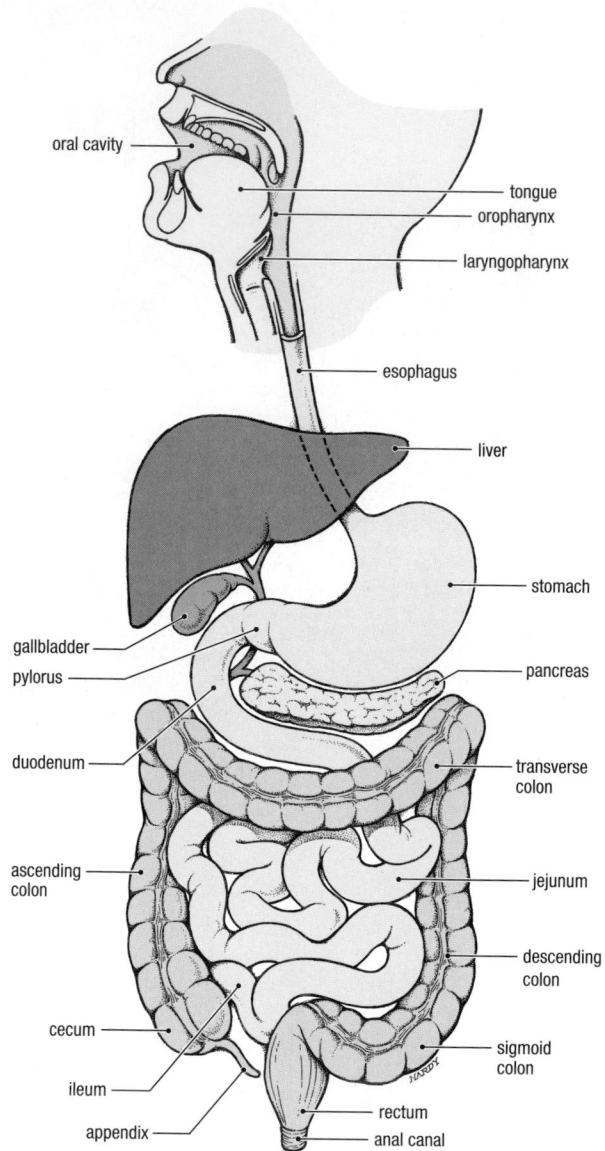

oral cavity

tongue

oropharynx

laryngopharynx

esophagus

liver

stomach

gallbladder

pylorus

pancreas

duodenum

transverse colon

ascending colon

jejunum

descending colon

cecum

sigmoid colon

ileum

appendix

rectum

anal canal

digestive system and adjacent organs

Appendix 2
Contrast Media, Imaging Agents, and Related Substances

^{11}Cu-TETA octreotide
5-iodo-2-deoxyuridine
  (IUdR)
acetrizoate
AcuTect
Adenoscan
Altropane
AMI 121
AMI 227
amidotrizoic acid
Amipaque
Amiscan
Anatrast
Angiografin
AngioMARK
Apomate
arcitumomab
Baricon
barium sulfate
Barobag enema kit
Baro-Cat
Baros effervescent
  granules
Barosperse
benzamide
benzoic acid
Biliscopin
Biloptin
bismuth
calcium 45 (^{45}Ca)
calcium 47 (^{47}Ca)
calcium ipodate
carbon 11 (^{11}C)
carbon 11-labeled
  cocaine
carbon 11-labeled fatty
  acid
carbon-11 acetate
carbon-11 butanol

carbon-11 carfentanil
carbon-11 flumazenil
carbon-11 N-methyl-
  spiperone
carbon-11 nomifensine
carbon-11 raclopride
carbon-11 thymidine
CardioGen-82
Cardiolite
Cardiotec
CEA-Scan
CEA-Tc 99m (^{99m}Tc
  CEA)
CentoRx
Ceretec
cerium
cesium chloride
CheeTah
Cholebrine
Choletec
Cholografin meglumine
Cholografin Dilute
Chromitope sodium
chromium
Clariscan
Cobatope-57
Combidex
Conray 30, 43, 60, 400
copper 64 (^{64}Cu)
cyanocobalamin
Cysto-Conray
Cysto-Conray II
Cystografin Dilute
d,1-HMPAO
Definity
deuterium
dextrose 5% in water
Diaginol
diatrizoate meglumine

diatrizoate sodium
diatrizoic acid
diazepam
diethylenetriaminepenta-
  acetic acid (DTPA)
Digibar 190
Digital HD
Dionosil Oily
dobutamine
dodecafluoropentane
  (DDFP)
Dopascan
dysprosium
EchoGen
Echovist
Enecat CT enema
EneMark rectal marker
  kit
Enhancer
Entero Vu
Entrobar
Entrocel
EntroEase
Entrokit
Eovist
Esopho-Cat
ethiodized oil
Ethiodol
etidronate disodium
Evans blue
exametazime
E-Z-AC
E-Z-Cat
E-Z-Cat Dry
E-Z-HD
E-Z-Paque
E-Z-Paste
F-18 fluoro-2-deoxy-
  glucose

F-18 sodium fluoride
Feridex IV
feruglose
ferumoxsil
Fibrimage
Flo-Coat
fluorine
fluorine-18-dihydroxy-
   phenylalanine
   (^{18}F-DOPA)
fluorodeoxyglucose
   (FDG)
FS-069
furosemide
gadobenate
   dimeglumine
   (Gd-BOPTA)
gadobenic acid
gadobutrol
gadodiamide
gadolinium (Gd)
gadolinium chelate
gadolinium oxide
gadopentetate
   dimeglumine
   (Gd-DTPA)
gadoterate meglumine
   (Gd-DOTA)
gadoteridol (Gd-D03A)
gadoversetamide
gadoxetic acid
   (Gd-EOB-DTPA)
galactose
gallium
Gastrografin
GastroMARK
Gastromiro
Gastrovist
Gd-DTPA with mannitol
Glofil-125
glucagon
glucarate
HD 200 Plus
HD 85

Hepatolite
Hexabrix
Hippuran
holmium
human serum albumin
   (HSA)
hydrogen peroxide
hyoscine butylbromide
Hypaque meglumine
Hypaque sodium
Hypaque-76
Hypaque-Cysto
Imagent GI
Imavist
ImmuRAIT
indium 111 (^{111}In)
indium-111
   pentetreotide
Indium-Oxine
indocyanine green (ICG)
Intropaste
iobitridol
iocetamic acid
iodamide
iodide
iodine-123 MIBG
iodine-131 MIBG
iodipamide meglumine
iodixanol
iodized oil
iodohippurate sodium
   I-123, I-131
iodopyracet
Iodotope
ioglunide
iohexol
Iomeron 150, 250, 300,
   350
iopamidol
iopanoate
iopanoic acid
iophendylate
iopromide
iothalamate meglumine

iothalamate sodium
iothalamic acid
iotrolan
iotroxamide
ioversol
ioxaglate meglumine
ioxaglate sodium
ioxaglic acid
ioxilan
ioxithalamate
ipodate sodium
iridium
iridium 192 (^{192}Ir)
Isopaque
isosulfan blue
Isovue Multipack-250,
   -300, -370
Isovue-200, -250, -300,
   -370
Isovue-M 200, 300
Kinevac
LeukoScan
LeuTech
Levovist
Lipiodol
Liqui-Coat HD
Liquid Barosperse
L-tyrosine
Lymphazurin
LymphoScan
macroaggregated
   albumin
Macrotec
magnesium
magnetite albumin
Magnevist
mangafodipir trisodium
manganese chloride
mannitol and saline
MD-76R
MD-Gastroview
MDP-Bracco
Medebar Plus
Medescan

meglumine diatrizoate
meglumine iocarmate
meglumine iodipamide
meglumine iothalamate
meglumine iotroxate
Metastron
methyl methacrylate
methylglucamine
metrizamide
metrizoate
Micropaque
mineral oil
Miraluma
MS-325
MultiHance
Myoscint
Myoview
naloxone
NeoSpect
NeoTect
Neurolite
nicotinamide
nimodipine
Niopam
nitrogen-13 ammonia
nofetumomab
OctreoScan
octreotide
Omnipaque 140, 180,
   240, 300, 350
Omniscan
OncoScint CR/OV
OncoSeed
OptiMARK
Optiray 160, 240, 300,
   320, 350
Optison
Oragrafin calcium
Oragrafin sodium
Oxilan
palladium
Pantopaque
pentagastrin
pentetreotide

peppermint oil
Perchloracap
perflubron
perfluorocarbon
Persantine
pertechnetate
phosphoric acid
phosphorus
Phosphotec
Polibar
Polibar Plus
potassium perchlorate
Prepcat
ProHance
propyliodone
ProstaScint
Quadramet
radiopaque polyvinyl
   chloride
RAPID strand
Readi-Cat
Readi-Cat 2
recombinant thyrotropin
Reno-60
Renocal-76
Reno-DIP
Renografin-60
Reno-M 30
Reno-M Dip
Renovist
Renovist II
Renovue-65
Renovue-Dip
rhenium
RIGScan CR49
rubidium chloride
Rubratope-57
samarium
samarium-153
   ethylenediamine
   tetramethylene
   phosphoric acid
   (^{153}Sm-EDTMP)
satumomab pendetide

Scan C
selenium
sestamibi
Sethotope
sincalide
Sinografin
Sitzmarks
sodium bicarbonate
sodium chloride
sodium diatrizoate
sodium iodide
sodium iodipamide
sodium iodohippurate
sodium iothalamate
sodium ipodate
sodium meglumine
   ioxaglate
sodium methiodal
sodium metrizoate
sodium pertechnetate
sodium tartrate
sodium tyropanoate
Sol-O-Pake
Solu-Biloptin
Solutrast
somatostatin
Sonazoid
SonoRx
SonoVue
sorbitol
sprodiamide
strontium
sucrose polyester
sulfobromophthalein
sulfur colloid
tantalum
tantalum 178 (^{178}Ta)
teboroxime
Techneplex
TechneScan HDP,
   MAA, MAG3, PYP
technetium 99m (^{99m}Tc)
mtechnetium stannous
   pyrophosphate (TSPP)

technetium-99m
albumin
technetium-99m
albumin aggregated
technetium-99m
albumin colloid
technetium-99m
albumin microsphere
technetium-99m
biciromab
technetium-99m bicisate
technetium-99m
depreotide
technetium-99m
dimercaptosuccinic
acid
technetium-99m
disofenin
technetium-99m
exametazime
technetium-99m
furifosmin
technetium-99m
galactosyl human
serum albumin
technetium-99m
glucarate
technetium-99m
gluceptate
technetium-99m
hepatoiminodiacetic
acid (Tc-HIDA)
technetium-99m
Hepatolite
technetium-99m human
serum albumin
technetium-99m
lidofenin
technetium-99m
macroaggregated
albumin

technetium-99m MAG 3
technetium-99m
mebrofenin
technetium-99m
medronate
technetium-99m
mertiatide
technetium-99m
N-para-isopropyl-
acetanilide-
iminodiacetic acid
(Tc-PIPIDA)
technetium-99m
oxidronate
technetium-99m
pentetate
technetium-99m
pentetate calcium
trisodium
technetium-99m
pertechnetate sodium
technetium-99m
polyphosphate
technetium-99m
pyrophosphate
technetium-99m
sestamibi
technetium-99m
siboroxime
technetium-99m sodium
technetium-99m sodium
pertechnetate
technetium-99m
succimer
technetium-99m sulfur
colloid
technetium-99m
teboroxime

technetium-99m
tetrofosmin
Telebrix
Telepaque
Teslascan
tetrabromophenolphthalein
tetraiodophenolphthalein
thallium 201
thallous chloride
TheraSeed
thorium dioxide
Thorotrast
Tomocat
Tomocat 1000
Tonojug
Tonopaque
Top-Cat
triiodobenzoic acid
Triosil
tyropanoate
Ultra-R
UltraTag
Ultravist 150, 240, 300,
370
uranium
Urografin
Uromiro
Urovist Cysto
Urovist meglumine
Urovist sodium 300
UroVysion
Varibar
Verluma
Visipaque 270, 320
Xenetix 250, 300, 350
xenon
xylenol orange

Common Radiation Oncology Terms

abscopal effect
absolute dose
absorbed dose
accelerated radiation
accelerator
acute exposure
adjacent field
adjuvant therapy
afterloading technique
algorithm
alloy
alopecia
alpha cradle immobilization device
alpha particle
amygdaloid complex
anesthesia
angle
antiemetic
applicator
Aquaplast immobilization device
arc therapy
asymmetric collimation
attenuation
backpointer
backscatter
beam film
beam modifier
beam quality
beam shaping
beam's eye view
becquerel (Bq) LC
belly board
beta particle
beta plaque
beta radiation
betatron
bite block block
bolus
boost
brachytherapy
Bragg peak

breast board
breast bridge
Bremsstrahlung x-ray
buildup region
calcification
calculation
calipers
cast
catheter
centigray (cGy)
central axis
central axis depth dose
central plane
Cerrobend
cesium teletherapy unit
cesium 137 (^{137}Cs, Cs-137)
chemoradiotherapy
chemotherapy regimen
Clinac linear accelerator
clinical target volume (CTV)
cobalt teletherapy unit
cobalt 60 (^{60}Co, Co-60)
cobalt-60 teletherapy
cold spot
collimator angle
collimator leaf
compensator
composite plan
computer assisted tomography (CAT)
coned down
conformal radiation therapy (CRT)
conformal radiotherapy
contact therapy
contour preparation
conventional therapy
convergence
coplanar beam arrangement
couch angle
couch kick
craniospinal irradiation
CT simulator

curative intent care
curative radiotherapy
curie (Ci)
cyclotron
decay
Delclos applicator depth dose
desquamation
digitally composited radiograph (DCR)
digitally reconstructed radiograph
 (DRR)
diode
divergence
divergent beams
dose calculation
dose distribution
dose escalation
dose-volume histogram
dosimetrist
dosimetry
dwell position
dynamic multileaf collimator (DMLC)
dynamic wedge
electromagnetic radiation
electron beam radiation therapy
electron cone
Ellis filter
entrance port
equal weighting
extended distance
external beam radiation therapy
 (EBRT, XRT)
external radiation
eye shield
facial mask
field arrangement
field block
field weighting
film digitizer
filter
Fletcher-Suit applicator
fluid-attenuated inversion recovery
 (FLAIR)
fluorodeoxyglucose positron emission
 tomography (FDG PET)

fraction
fractionated external beam radiation
 therapy
fractionation
frontocentral
Gamma knife
gamma radiation
gamma ray
gantry
gap calculation
geometry
gold 198 (^{198}Au, Au-198)
gray (Gy) LC
gross tumor volume (GTV)
half beam block
half-life
half-value layer (HVL)
half-value thickness
hand block
headrest (sizes range from A to F)
helical tomotherapy
Heyman capsule
high dose
high dose rate (HDR)
high linear energy transfer (LET)
 radiation
high dose rate remote afterloading
 machine
high dose rate remote brachytherapy
high dose rate remote radiation therapy
high-energy proton therapy
hindbrain
hot spot
hyperfractionated radiation
hyperfractionation
hyperthermia
hypofractionated radiation
image fusion
image-guided radiation therapy
immobilization device
immunotherapy
implant radiation
independent collimator
informed consent

intensity modulated radiation therapy (IMRT)
interaortocaval lymphadenopathy
internal radiation
interpeduncular cistern
interstitial brachytherapy
interstitial implant
interstitial radiation therapy
intracavitary irradiation
intracavitary radiation
intracavitary therapy
intracavity brachytherapy
intraluminal implant
intraoperative radiation therapy
iodine 125 (^{125}I, I-125)
ionization chamber
iridium
iridium 192 (^{192}Ir, Ir-192)
irradiated volume
irregular fields
isocenter
isocentric
isodose curve
isodose distribution
isodose plan
isotherm
isotope
Karnofsky Performance Status (KPS)
kilovolt (kV)
laser alignment system
LD 50/30
lead
lesion length
lethal dose (LD)
linear accelerator (LINAC)
linear energy transfer (LET)
localization film
local-regional
low dose rate (LDR)
lucite filter
lumen
magnetic resonance imaging (MRI)
mantle field
megavoltage

megavolt (MV)
minimum target dose
missing tissue compensator
mold
monitor unit (MU)
monoclonal antibody
mucositis
multileaf collimator (MLC)
multiplanar reconstruction
neutron beam therapy
noncoplanar beam arrangement
nuclide
oblique
off-axis factor
orthogonal pair
orthovoltage x-ray therapy
ovoid
oxygen enhancement ratio (OER)
palladium
palliation
palliative intent care
paraaortic field
parallel opposed fields
parenchymal hyperlucency
particle beam treatment
penumbra
percentage depth dose (PDD)
perimesencephalic cistern
permanent interstitial implant seed
phosphorus 32
photon beam radiation therapy
pin and arc
piriform sinus
planning target volume (PTV)
point calculation
port film
portal imaging
positron emission tomography (PET)
prescription point
primary beam
prostate seed implant
proton beam therapy
pterygoid process
punctate foci

radiation absorbed dose (RAD)
radiation biology
radiation field
radiation oncologist
radiation physicist
radiation physics
radiation portal
radiation therapist
radiation therapy planning (RTP)
radiation therapy technologist (RTT)
radiation treatment planning (RTP)
radioactive implant
radiobiology
radiocolloid
radioimmunotherapy (RIT)
radioiodine seeds
radiolabeled antibody
radiologist
radionuclide
radiopharmaceutical
radioprotector, radiation protector
radioresistance
radiosensitivity
radiosensitizer
radiotherapy
radium implant
radium 226
radon
reference depth
relative biologic effect (RBE)
remote brachytherapy
removable implant
ribbon
roentgen (R)
roentgen-equivalent-man (REM)
rotational therapy
separation
sestamibi
shield
short tau inversion recovery (STIR)
    image
simulated annealing
simulation
simulator

single-photon emission computed
    tomography (SPECT) imaging
skin sparing
source-axis distance (SAD)
source-film distance (SFD)
source-surface distance (SSD)
source-to-skin distance (SSD)
spiculated margin
split course
stereotactic external beam
    radiation
stereotactic head frame
stereotactic injection
stereotactic radiation therapy
stereotactic radiosurgery (SRS)
stereotactic radiotherapy (SRT)
stereotaxic radiosurgery
stereotaxis
strontium 89 (^{89}Sr, Sr-89)
strontium 90 (^{90}Sr, Sr-90)
superficial machine
superficial therapy
supervoltage range
supervoltage therapy
surface mold
systemic radiation therapy
T1 fat-saturated
tandem
target localization
tattoo
teletherapy
testicular shield
thermoluminescent dosimeter (TLD)
thermoplastic
3-dimensional conformal radiation
    therapy (3DRT)
3-dimensional radiotherapy treatment
    planning (3DRTP)
tolerance dose
total body irradiation (TBI)
total skin electron (TSE) irradiation
treatment beam
treatment field
treatment plan

treatment time
tumor localization
tumor volume
tungsten
2-dimensional radiotherapy treatment
   planning (2DRTP)
unequal weighting
unsealed internal radiation therapy

vaginal cylinder
verification film
volumetric calculation
Von de Graaf generator
wedge filter
wing board
X-knife
x-ray therapy

Sample Reports

ABDOMINAL ULTRASOUND

HISTORY: Elevated liver enzymes.

TECHNIQUE: Sonographic evaluation of the complete abdomen.

COMPARISON: No prior studies for comparison.

FINDINGS: The liver is borderline increased in echogenicity. Elliptical 3-cm hypodense structure is seen in the right hepatic lobe on image 17. This may be volume averaging with vascular or biliary structure; this is not specifically labeled by the technologist. The liver is somewhat echodense, and this is likely due to fatty infiltration.

The pancreas is not seen due to bowel gas shadowing, but the aorta and inferior vena cava appear normal.

The gallbladder is without gallbladder wall thickening. No gallstones. No pericholecystic fluid. There is no dilation of the intrahepatic or extrahepatic biliary ductal system, and the common duct measures 3.7 mm.

Spleen measures 11.0 x 10.5 x 4.9 cm and is structurally normal.

Right kidney measures 11.9 cm, and left kidney measures 11.5 cm. There is good preservation of corticomedullary demarcation. No hydronephrosis, mass, or abnormal calcification.

IMPRESSION: Echogenic liver potentially correlating with fatty infiltration and the elevated liver enzymes. All other findings noted above are incidental.

ARTERIOVENOUS GRAFT FISTULOGRAM AND DECLOTTING PROCEDURE WITH PLACEMENT OF DIALYSIS CATHETER

PROCEDURES:
1. Left arm arteriovenous graft fistulogram and failed declotting
2. Placement of new dialysis access in the right upper chest.

INDICATIONS: The patient is a middle-aged female with stage 4 chronic kidney disease, on hemodialysis. She has been noted to have a clotted left arm AV graft that needs declotting. Alternatively, she will need a new dialysis access.

ANESTHESIA: Local anesthesia with 1% lidocaine.

DESCRIPTION OF PROCEDURE: Informed written consent was obtained from the patient after explaining the procedure as well as its risks and alternatives. The patient understood the discussion and expressed her wish to proceed.

The patient was placed supine on the x-ray table, and the left arm was prepped in the usual sterile fashion. Skin and subcutaneous tissues in the left cubital fossa were infiltrated with 1% lidocaine, and proximal portion of the graft was accessed using 4-French micropuncture kit. This was exchanged for a 4-French micropuncture sheath over a 0.018 wire. Subsequently a fistulogram was obtained which revealed prominent collaterals in the proximal portion of the vein between the left brachial artery and the AV graft; however, the graft portion of the fistula was thrombosed. Then a 4-French sheath was exchanged for a 6-French short sheath over a 0.035 angled Glidewire. We traversed the thrombosed graft using the 0.035 angled Glidewire; however, multiple and persistent attempts to traverse the venous anastomosis of the graft were unsuccessful, so declotting effort was aborted. All catheters and wires were removed. Hemostasis was obtained with manual pressure. The patient tolerated the procedure well. There were no procedural complications. Given the failed attempt in traversing the venous anastomosis and patient's need for dialysis, the decision was made to place a right upper chest tunneled dialysis catheter.

Right lower neck and upper chest were prepped in the usual sterile fashion. Skin and subcutaneous tissues were infiltrated with 1% lidocaine. Right jugular vein was accessed using 4-French micropuncture kit under sonographic guidance and exchanged for a 4-French micropuncture sheath over a 0.018 wire. Subsequently the skin in the infraclavicular region was infiltrated with 1% lidocaine, and a 2-mm skin incision was made in the lateral aspect of the infraclavicular region. A 14.5-French dual-lumen tunneled dialysis catheter, 23 cm, was placed into the subcutaneous tunnel using a metallic tunneler. It was pulled out through the venotomy access site. Subsequently a 4-French sheath in the internal jugular venous access was exchanged for a 0.035 J-wire, 3 mm in length, in the upper inferior vena cava. The skin and subcutaneous tissues were then dilated using 10-French and 12-French fascial dilators, and a 15-French peel-away sheath was placed over the wire with its tip in the upper right atrium. The free end of the dialysis catheter was placed with its tip in the upper right atrium; however, during the procedure I noted the preferential entry of the venous portion of the dialysis catheter entered into the left brachiocephalic vein. The catheter was subsequently pulled back and repositioned in the upper right atrium. However, at that point I was unable to get the arterial port into the upper right atrium, so I performed a venogram which revealed a focal 50% stenosis of the distal superior vena cava. A 0.035 angled Glidewire was then negotiated and placed via the arterial access into the upper right atrium. The catheter was repositioned into the upper right atrium. Both ports of the catheter were aspirated and flushed freely. The catheter was secured to the skin using 2-0 Prolene suture. The skin entry site closure was obtained using 3-0 Vicryl suture. Both ports were flushed free of blood, and a heparin lock was placed. Radiograph of the upper chest was obtained.

FINDINGS

1. The sonography of the lower neck revealed widely patent and compressible right jugular vein.
2. An image documenting the entry of the needle into right internal jugular vein was obtained.
3. Right brachiocephalic venogram revealed 50% stenosis of the distal right superior vena cava.
4. Final radiograph showed a dual-lumen tunneled dialysis catheter, 23 cm, with its tip in the upper right atrium.

CONCLUSIONS

1. Successful sonography of the right lower neck and sonographic guidance for access into right jugular vein.
2. Successful placement of a dual-lumen tunneled dialysis catheter with its tip in the upper right atrium under fluoroscopic guidance, without incident.

BILATERAL DIGITAL SCREENING MAMMOGRAM WITH COMPUTER-AIDED DETECTION

HISTORY: Twelve months ago the patient underwent needle localization biopsy of the left breast for malignancy. This is a 1-year followup. The right breast has not been previously studied here.

TECHNIQUE: Images obtained include 2 digitally acquired images of the right breast along with a cleavage view as well as 4 digitally acquired views of the left breast. Computer-aided detection was applied.

FINDINGS: Secretory calcifications are seen. Vascular calcifications are identified on the right side. No dominant masses are present. No microcalcification clusters are present.

Left breast has dense vascular calcifications. Surgical clips are located in 3 of the 4 quadrants. No mass is identified, although there is parenchymal scarring.

IMPRESSION: Scattered vascular calcifications. Previous left breast surgery. No evidence of malignancy on either side. BIRADS-2, benign findings only. The next routine study will be in 1 year.

BILATERAL LOWER EXTREMITY ARTERIAL ULTRASOUND BEFORE AND AFTER EXERCISE

HISTORY: The patient has bilateral lower extremity claudication with a claudication distance of a 7-minute walk and has been symptomatic for the past 4 years with progressive worsening. The patient also has bilateral lower extremity pain at rest, and this needs additional evaluation. History is also positive for peripheral vascular disease, hypertension and hyperlipidemia. The patient reports a 10-pack-year smoking history.

TECHNIQUE: Bilateral lower extremity ankle-brachial indices and duplex interrogation of the pedal arteries obtained. Postexercisem ankle-brachial indices obtained after exercising for 2 minutes 16 seconds, with calf raises.

FINDINGS
1. Prior to exercise, ankle-brachial indices measure 1.18 on the right and 1.07 on the left.
2. After exercise, the ankle-brachial indices measure 1.19 on the right and 1.05 on the left.
3. On duplex interrogation, the patient has triphasic waveforms in both posterior tibial arteries and monophasic waveforms in both dorsalis pedis arteries.

IMPRESSION
1. No significant peripheral vascular disease to explain the patient's symptoms. The patient has mild tibioperoneal disease.
2. Consider neurogenic etiology for the patient's symptoms.

BILATERAL UPPER EXTREMITY VEIN MAPPING FOR DIALYSIS ACCESS PLACEMENT

HISTORY: Need for dialysis access placement.

TECHNIQUE: Gray-scale, color Doppler, and duplex sonography of both upper extremity venous and arterial systems performed with additional compression maneuvers.

FINDINGS

Right Upper Extremity

Arterial: Right radial artery 1.5 mm, right ulnar artery 1.4 mm, and brachial artery 3.9 mm in anteroposterior dimension, showing triphasic waveforms.

Venous system: Veins of the right forearm are too small to be of use in hemodialysis access placement. Cephalic vein at the level of the elbow measures 2.8 mm, at the level of midhumerus measures 3.4 mm, at the level of the upper humerus measures 4.1 mm, at the level of the shoulder measures 3.8 mm, and shows normal compressibility. The basilic vein measures 2.7 mm at the level of the elbow, 3.6 mm at the level of the midhumerus, and 4.9 mm at the level of the upper humerus. Brachial vein measures 2.6 mm at the level of the elbow, 3.6 mm at the level of the midhumerus, and 3.3 mm at the level of the upper humerus. Axillary vein measures 6.1 mm. Right subclavian vein shows normal respiratory phasicity. No deep venous thrombosis seen in right upper extremity venous system. The patient would be a candidate for right brachiocephalic fistula at the level of the cubital fossa.

Left Upper Extremity

Arterial: Radial artery 1.7 mm and ulnar artery 1.2 mm in anteroposterior dimension. Left brachial artery 3.9 mm in anteroposterior dimension with triphasic waveforms.

Venous system: Left cephalic vein measures 3.2 mm at the level of the shoulder, 2.6 mm at the level of the upper humerus, 2.2 mm at the level of the midhumerus, and 2.2 mm at the level of the elbow. Basilic vein measures 3.7 mm at the level of the upper humerus, 2.2 mm at the level of the midhumerus, and 2.1 mm at the level of the elbow. The brachial vein measures 3.8 mm at the level of the elbow, 3.6 mm at the level of the midhumerus, and 4.1 mm at the level of the upper humerus. Axillary vein measures 7 mm at the level of axilla. Left subclavian vein shows normal respiratory phasicity. No deep venous thrombosis seen in left upper extremity venous system.

Impression

1. The patient would be a candidate for right brachial artery to cephalic vein fistula in right cubital fossa.
2. In left upper extremity, the patient would be a candidate for left brachial artery to brachial vein arteriovenous fistula with transposition of the brachial vein. The other option would be left brachial artery to left axillary vein arteriovenous graft.

BILATERAL UTERINE ARTERY EMBOLIZATION

Procedure: Bilateral uterine artery embolization.

Indications: The patient has had progressively worsening severe menorrhagia, history of multiple large uterine fibroids, and history of prior myomectomy which failed to relieve her symptoms. She needs uterine-preserving therapy to control her menorrhagia.

MEDICATIONS
1. Versed 7 mg IV.
2. Fentanyl 200 mcg IV.
3. Clindamycin 600 mg IV.

DESCRIPTION OF PROCEDURE: Informed written consent was obtained from the patient after explaining the procedure, risks and alternatives. The patient understood the discussion and expressed her wish to proceed.

The patient was placed supine on the x-ray table. Right groin was prepped in the usual sterile fashion. Skin and subcutaneous tissues were infiltrated with 1% lidocaine. A 2-mm skin incision was made over the right common femoral pulse using a #11 scalpel, and subcutaneous dissection was performed using the tip of the hemostat. Right common femoral artery was accessed under real-time sonographic guidance using 4-French micropuncture kit and exchanged for 4-French micropuncture sheath over a 0.018 wire. A 4-French micropuncture sheath was exchanged for a 4-French 11 cm sheath over a 3-mm 0.035 J-wire. A 4-French Omni Flush catheter was placed above the aortic bifurcation and exchanged for a 4-French C1 Glide catheter with its tip in the proximal portion of the left common iliac artery. Subsequently, under digital road map arteriogram guidance, the left uterine artery was cannulated. The tip of the catheter was advanced to the horizontal segment of the left uterine artery over a 0.035 angled Glidewire. A left uterine arteriogram was obtained selectively in a frontal projection. Under oblique fluoroscopic guidance, the left uterine artery embolization was performed initially using 300 to 500 micron Embosphere particles, and special attention was given to antegrade flow and presence of any retrograde reflux. Subsequently, a total of 3 syringes of 300 to 500 Embosphere particles were injected. This was followed by 4 additional syringes of 500 to 700 micron Embosphere particles. Upon slowing of the antegrade flow, injection was stopped and final left uterine arteriogram was obtained selectively in a frontal projection. The catheter was then removed, and a new 4-French C1 Glide catheter was placed over the 0.035 angled Glidewire, and the right uterine artery was cannulated selectively under fluoroscopic guidance using digital road map arteriogram. The selective right uterine arteriogram was obtained with the tip of the catheter in the horizontal section in frontal projection. After confirming its optimal position, a right uterine artery embolization was performed using 500 to 700 micron Embosphere particles. After near stasis of antegrade flow, injection was stopped, and a final right uterine arteriogram was obtained which revealed lack of adequate antegrade flow and reflux retrograde. Following this, all catheters and wires were removed, and right groin hemostasis was obtained with manual pressure.

The patient tolerated the procedure well. There were no procedural complications. She was given education about the use of a Demerol PCA pump.

Total sedation time during the procedure was 60 minutes. Appropriate physiologic monitoring was performed throughout the procedure including skilled nursing supervision of conscious sedation.

FINDINGS

1. Selective left uterine arteriogram shows markedly enlarged hypertrophic left uterine artery with multiple enlarged branches supplying myometrium and multiple fibroids showing evidence of neovascularization but without evidence of arteriovenous shunting. Successful embolization of the left uterine artery, initially with 300 to 500 micron particles and subsequently with 500 to 700 micron particles.
2. Successful right uterine artery cannulation and embolization using 500 to 700 micron Embosphere particles with stasis of flow.

IMPRESSION: Successful bilateral uterine artery embolization using 300 to 500 micron and subsequently 400 to 700 micron Embosphere particles, without incident.

CT AND CTA OF THE ABDOMEN

HISTORY: The patient has secondary renovascular hypertension and high blood pressure.

TECHNIQUE: Abdominal CTA to include collimated reformatted multiplanar images through the bilateral renal artery ostia.

After uneventful injection of 100 mL of Isovue-370, 1.25-mm postcontrast multiphase images were performed through the abdominal aorta, reformatted images through the abdominal aorta, sagittal and coronal, with collimated images to the renal arteries.

COMPARISON: There is no prior study available for comparison.

FINDINGS: Scout is unremarkable. Lung bases are clear. Prior to contrast injection there is no evidence of abdominal aortic calcifications or mural hematoma. There is no nephrolithiasis. The patient is status post cholecystectomy. No abnormal fluid is seen in the gallbladder fossa. On this technique the liver is normal, as is the spleen. Accessory Riedel lobe is noted and is a normal variant. No dilation of the intrahepatic or extrahepatic biliary ductal system seen. Normal pancreas and adrenal glands. There is no free fluid. No evidence of abnormal lymphadenopathy. The examination does not include the pelvis.

The abdominal aorta is normal on enhancement. There is no aneurysm. No evidence of mural thickening. The ostia of the celiac, superior mesenteric, inferior mesenteric, and renal arteries are all normal without evidence of stenosis from any cause or fibromuscular dysplasia. There is no evidence of congenital anomaly or evidence of adverse sequelae. The patient's history of coarctation and postprocedural changes to the bladder is noted, but the urinary bladder is not collimated into this examination.

The bilateral renal arteries are solitary. There is hydronephrosis/pyelectasis about both kidneys with mixed cortical thinning and irregular attenuation about both kidneys, with the left kidney diminutive, measuring 8.5 cm in major axis, whereas the right kidney measures 12.1 cm. There is ectasia, cortical scarring about both kidneys, pyelectasis right greater than left, and ureteromegaly noted, right greater than left, with right ureteral tortuosity throughout the course in the retroperitoneum. An indeterminate node is noted adjacent to the right kidney on image 34 of series 5, which measures just under 1 cm.

IMPRESSION

1. No evidence of renovascular anomaly.
2. No evidence of aortic disease with major ostia normal. Renal arteries are solitary and there is no evidence of vascular disease, vasculitis, or fibromuscular dysplasia.
3. The patient's renal hypertension may arise from chronic reflux nephropathy, but in any case there is diffuse renal scarring, hydronephrosis, atrophy of the left kidney, and lobular ectasia of the thinned renal cortices, although portions of the renal cortices enhance symmetrically.
4. A 1-cm nodule is present adjacent to the lower pole of the right kidney, of uncertain significance. This is potentially postinflammatory or reactive.

CT HEAD UNENHANCED

HISTORY: Hemorrhagic stroke.

TECHNIQUE: Contiguous transaxial images at intervals of 5 mm, without intravenous contrast.

FINDINGS: When compared with prior study, we again see the hemorrhagic infarct in the right frontal lobe with surrounding edema. There is mass effect with leftward shift of midline. The region of hemorrhage, the surrounding edema, and the degree of midline shift have not increased when compared to the prior study.

There is blood in the dependent portions of the lateral ventricles. The left lateral ventricle is mildly dilated but unchanged from the earlier film. There is a geographic region of encephalomalacia in the occipital lobe on the right, residua of a prior infarct.

An intracranial shunt is seen traversing the left frontal calvaria and coursing posteriorly to terminate in the right posterior fossa.

IMPRESSION

1. No increase in the size of the hemorrhagic infarct, surrounding edema, or leftward shift of midline structures is seen in comparison with prior study.
2. Encephalomalacia, right occipital lobe, from prior infarct.
3. Dilation of left lateral ventricle, without interval change.
4. Intracranial shunt.

ENDOVAGINAL PELVIC ULTRASOUND

HISTORY: Acute pelvic pain.

TECHNIQUE: Transabdominal and endovaginal sonography was used to examine the uterus and adnexa.

FINDINGS: The uterus is 8.7 cm in length by 6.0 cm by 6.8 cm. The endometrial stripe is 17 mm. This included the junctional zone. No myometrial masses are seen. No endometrial nodules or masses. The patient is status post cesarean section.

The right ovary is 3.5 x 2.6 x 2.3 cm. It has a smooth contour. A small amount of free fluid is seen in the cul-de-sac.

The left ovary is 2.8 x 1.8 x 1.9 cm. No adnexal masses or dominant cysts are seen.

IMPRESSION

1. No uterine masses are seen. Endometrial stripe is 17 mm.
2. Unremarkable left and right ovaries.

L2 VERTEBROPLASTY USING LEFT INTERPEDICULAR ROUTE UNDER FLUOROSCOPIC GUIDANCE

HISTORY: The patient has severe low back pain which is rated 10/10 with any activity. Over the past 2 months, the patient has had progressively worsening pain in spite of the use of narcotic medications. Nuclear medicine bone scan and CT scan of the lumbar spine revealed anterior wedge compression fracture of L2. Given the severity of the pain and lack of improvement over the last 8 weeks, the patient is now here for vertebroplasty.

MEDICATIONS

1. Local anesthesia with 1% lidocaine.
2. Versed 2.5 mg IV.
3. Fentanyl 100 mcg IV.
4. Ancef 1 g IV.

DESCRIPTION OF PROCEDURE: Informed written consent was obtained from the patient after explaining the procedure, risks and alternatives. The patient understood the discussion and expressed a wish to proceed.

The patient was placed prone on the x-ray table. Site for L2 vertebroplasty was localized at the upper outer portion of the left pedicle. The skin was prepped in the usual sterile fashion. Skin and subcutaneous tissues and periosteum over the left pedicle were infiltrated with 1% lidocaine. A 2-mm skin incision was made with a #11 scalpel. A 13-gauge vertebroplasty needle was advanced to the upper outer portion of the left pedicle. After advancement of the needle tip to the anterior third, bone cement prepped in the usual sterile fashion was injected using percutaneous cement delivery kit. The bone cement was injected until opacification of the anterior two-thirds of the vertebral body was accomplished. The injection was then stopped, and the needle was removed. Hemostasis was obtained with manual pressure. Frontal and lateral radiographs of the lumbar spine were obtained.

The patient tolerated the procedure well. There were no procedural complications. There was no change in lower extremity neurologic status after the procedure and no adverse drug reactions. Total sedation time during the procedure was 45 minutes. Appropriate physiologic monitoring was performed throughout the procedure, including skilled nursing supervision of conscious sedation.

FINDINGS
1. Lateral radiograph of the lumbar spine shows anterior wedge compression fracture with about 60% loss of height anteriorly and 50% loss of height centrally.
2. Successful L2 vertebroplasty without incident.

IMPRESSION: Successful L2 vertebroplasty using left interpedicular route without incident.

LEFT FOOT X-RAY

HISTORY: The patient has left foot pain and swelling.

TECHNIQUE: Three views of the left foot.

COMPARISON: None.

FINDINGS: No definitive fracture or dislocation is found. Probable bony osteopenia is noted. No bone lesions are identified.

IMPRESSION: Probable bony osteopenia without fracture or dislocation. No significant arthritic change noted.

LEFT L3 ROOT BLOCK

HISTORY: The patient has left L3 radiculopathy and history of previous L4, L5, and S1 lower lumbar posterior spinal fusion. She needs left L3 root block.

MEDICATIONS
1. Local anesthesia with 1% lidocaine.
2. Isovue-200, a total of 1 mL.
3. Mixture of 1 mL each of bupivacaine 0.25%, lidocaine 1%, and Kenalog 40 mg.

DESCRIPTION OF PROCEDURE: Informed written consent was obtained from the patient after explaining the procedure, its risks, and the alternatives. The patient understood the discussion and expressed her wish to proceed.

The patient was subsequently placed in the right anterior oblique position on the x-ray table. Site for the left total lumbar root block was localized at the 6 o'clock position of the left L3 pedicle. Skin was prepped in the usual sterile fashion. Skin and subcutaneous tissues were infiltrated with 1% lidocaine. A 22-gauge, 6-inch spinal needle was advanced to the 6 o'clock position of the left L3 pedicle. During the needle advancement, the patient noted severe radicular pain down the left leg similar to her usual pain. At that point the tip of the needle was slightly withdrawn, and 1 mL of Isovue-200 was injected, revealing perineural spread of contrast. The above-mentioned mixture of local anesthetics and Kenalog was injected, and the needle was removed.

The patient tolerated the procedure well. There were no procedural complications. The patient noted complete resolution of the left-sided radicular symptoms after the injection. There were no adverse drug reactions.

IMPRESSION: Successful left L3 root block under fluoroscopic guidance without incident.

MRI LEFT FOOT WITHOUT AND WITH GADOLINIUM

HISTORY: Pain along the bottom of the left foot with a focal lump. The patient's symptoms are located at the 5th MTP joint.

TECHNIQUE: Multiplanar MR imaging was performed through the left forefoot before and after IV gadolinium.

COMPARISON: No prior relevant comparison available.

FINDINGS: There is marked circumferential soft tissue thickening or mass surrounding the distal aspect of the 5th metatarsal head that involves the 5th metatarsophalangeal joint. This area is predominantly decreased on T1 and has mixed but predominantly increased STIR signal intensity. There is irregular contrast enhancement within this mass. This mass measures approximately 8.4 mm in maximum thickness and extends approximately 26 mm in length. This is best seen on series 12 of image 14 and series 13 of image 9. Within the 5th metatarsal head is a small 2.5-mm focus of increased STIR signal intensity with mild enhancement, suggesting erosion. A 2nd erosion may be present within the base of the proximal phalanx of the 5th toe. There seems to be mild malalignment of the 5th metatarsophalangeal joint, suggesting mild subluxation. Overall imaging findings are most suspicious for severe erosive arthropathy of the 5th MTP joint, likely with severe associated synovitis. An infectious arthropathy cannot be excluded. Consider needle aspiration of the joint to rule out this possibility. A soft tissue sarcoma such as a synovial cell sarcoma is also a possibility for the mass as described above. Because of this possibility, a biopsy should be considered. Of note, there is a small joint effusion involving the 1st MTP joint.

IMPRESSION

1. Irregular partially enhancing soft tissue mass encircling the 5th metatarsophalangeal joint as described above. In view of the possibility of 2 erosions and subluxation of the 5th metatarsophalangeal joint, this mass is most likely a severe synovitis. I would suggest consideration of an erosive arthropathy, possibly infectious. I would also consider a needle aspiration of the joint to rule out the possibility of a septic joint. A soft tissue sarcoma such as a synovial cell sarcoma is also a possibility, and therefore a biopsy of the mass should be considered.
2. Small effusion of the 1st metatarsophalangeal joint.

REMOVAL AND REPLACEMENT OF TUNNELED HEMODIALYSIS CATHETER

INDICATIONS: Nonfunctioning and infected dialysis catheter, sepsis, and need for new catheter.

MEDICATIONS

1. Lidocaine 1% for local anesthesia.
2. Ancef 1 g IV.

DESCRIPTION OF PROCEDURE: Informed written consent was obtained after explaining the procedure and its risks and alternatives. The patient understood the discussion and expressed a wish to proceed.

The patient was placed supine on the x-ray table. Skin and subcutaneous tissues around the catheter were infiltrated with 1% lidocaine. Imaging of the old catheter position was obtained. Heparin locks in both ports of the catheter were removed. Under fluoroscopy a 0.035 angled Glidewire and 0.035 Amplatz wire were placed in each port of the catheter with the tips in upper right atrium. Catheter cuff was separated from adjacent soft tissues. The catheter was removed over the wire under fluoroscopic guidance. Following this a new 23-cm dual-lumen tunneled dialysis catheter was placed over the wire with its tip in the upper portion of right atrium.

Both ports of the catheter were aspirated and flushed freely. The new catheter was sutured to the skin using 2-0 Prolene suture. Chest x-ray was obtained.

FINDINGS

1. Initial radiograph of the upper chest revealed tip of the tunneled left internal jugular hemodialysis catheter in the right atrium.
2. Successful removal of the nonfunctioning catheter and placement of new tunneled dialysis catheter. Radiograph shows a functioning catheter with its tip in the upper right atrium.

IMPRESSION

1. Successful removal of a nonfunctioning tunneled hemodialysis catheter in the left upper chest.
2. Successful placement under fluoroscopic guidance of a functioning 23-cm dual-lumen tunneled hemodialysis catheter in the left upper chest.

3-VIEW LUMBOSACRAL SPINE X-RAY

HISTORY: The patient has low back pain; ICD-9 code 721.3 and 724.2.

TECHNIQUE: Three views of the lumbosacral spine were obtained.

COMPARISON: None.

FINDINGS: The patient has undergone previous L4 and L5 laminectomy and posterior metallic fusion with transpedicular screws at L4, L5 and S1. These are linked by vertical paraspinal rods and a crosslink device at the L4-5 disc space level. Bone graft material is seen at the L4-5 and L5-S1 disc space levels.

The vertebral bodies of the lumbosacral spine demonstrate normal height and alignment. The disc spaces are well preserved at most levels, with the exception of disc space narrowing at the L3-4 level with posterior disc osteophyte noted. The neural foramina are patent at most levels, with the exception of the L3-4 level where there is encroachment by the superior articular facets of L4 into the neural foramen which may be compressing the exiting L4 nerve roots. Canal stenosis at the L3-4 level cannot be entirely excluded as this would be the most common area for canal stenosis after a fusion of this type.

Surgical clips are seen in the left upper quadrant of the abdomen. The bowel gas pattern is nonobstructive. The psoas margins are intact. A few pelvic phleboliths are identified. The sacroiliac joints and hip joints appear normal. The pedicles of the lumbar spine are intact. No evidence of pneumoperitoneum or pneumatosis intestinalis is demonstrated.

IMPRESSION

1. No evidence of fracture or hardware failure in the lumbosacral spine.
2. Canal narrowing may be present at the L3-4 level as well as bilateral neural foraminal narrowing at the L3-4 level. This may be affecting the exiting L3 nerve roots. If detailed evaluation of this region is required clinically, an MRI of the lumbosacral spine could be performed for more detailed evaluation of any potential nerve root compression.

THYROID ULTRASOUND

HISTORY: A patient with 2 small nonspecific nodules visualized in the right and left thyroid lobes on prior examination 9 months ago. The patient presents for followup.

TECHNIQUE: A pulsed Doppler duplex transducer with color mapping was utilized.

FINDINGS: The right thyroid lobe measures 4.7 x 1.8 x 2.1 cm. There are 2 small nodules noted in the right thyroid lobe, the largest measuring approximately 7 mm, similar to description on the prior examination. Neither nodule shows significant growth, and the nodules are nonspecific.

The left thyroid lobe measures 4.6 x 2.1 x 2.2 cm with 2 nonspecific nodules, the largest measuring 10 mm. The largest nodule measured 11 mm on previous exam. The 2nd nodule is smaller and appears stable. There may be a 3rd smaller nodule measuring 4 mm in the right thyroid lobe that was not mentioned on prior exam.

The thyroid isthmus is normal.

CONCLUSION: Multiple stable, small thyroid nodules that probably indicate multinodular goiter. No dominant nodule noted at this time.

ULTRASOUND ANKLE-BRACHIAL INDICES RESTING

HISTORY: The patient has a history of diabetes, hypertension, and hyperlipidemia. The patient complains of discoloration to both lower extremities and also has pain in the right lower extremity, suggesting rest pain. Additional evaluation is needed to determine the severity of the peripheral vascular disease.

TECHNIQUE: Bilateral lower extremity ankle-brachial indices and duplex interrogation of the pedal arteries obtained.

FINDINGS: Ankle-brachial indices measure 1.53 on the right and 1.51 on the left. On duplex interrogation, the patient has triphasic waveforms in both posterior tibial and dorsalis pedis arteries.

Great toe pressures measure 1.08 on the right and 1.03 on the left.

IMPRESSION: The patient has significant calcific peripheral vascular disease but no significant disease to explain the symptoms. Consideration should be given to venous or neurogenic etiology for these symptoms.

Common Terms by Procedure

ABDOMINAL ULTRASOUND
abdomen
aorta
biliary structure
bowel gas shadowing
calcification
common duct
corticomedullary demarcation
dilation
echodense
echogenic
echogenicity
elliptical
extrahepatic biliary ductal system
fatty infiltration
gallbladder wall thickening
gallstone
hepatic lobe
hydronephrosis
hypodense structure
image
inferior vena cava
intrahepatic biliary ductal system
kidney
liver
liver enzyme
mass
pancreas
pericholecystic fluid
sonographic evaluation
spleen
vascular

ARTERIOVENOUS GRAFT FISTULOGRAM AND DECLOTTING PROCEDURE WITH PLACEMENT OF DIALYSIS CATHETER
0.018 wire
0.035 angled Glidewire
0.035 J-wire
1% lidocaine
10-French fascial dilator
12-French fascial dilator
14.5-French dual-lumen tunneled
    dialysis catheter
15-French peel-away sheath
2-0 Prolene suture
3-0 Vicryl suture
4-French micropuncture kit
4-French micropuncture sheath
6-French short sheath
arterial port
arteriovenous graft
atrium
AV graft
brachial artery
brachiocephalic vein
catheter
chest
cubital fossa
declotting
dialysis access
dialysis catheter
distal superior vena cava
dual-lumen tunneled dialysis catheter
fistula
fistulogram
fluoroscopic guidance
graft
hemostasis
heparin lock
image
inferior vena cava
infraclavicular region
jugular vein
manual pressure
metallic tunneler
radiograph
sonographic guidance sonography
stenosis

subcutaneous tunnel
supine
thrombosed graft
tunneled dialysis catheter
vein
venogram
venotomy access site
venous anastomosis
wire
x-ray table

BILATERAL DIGITAL SCREENING MAMMOGRAM WITH COMPUTER-AIDED DETECTION

benign
BIRADS-2
cleavage view
computer-aided detection
digitally acquired image
dominant mass
malignancy
microcalcification cluster
parenchymal scarring
secretory calcification
vascular calcification

BILATERAL LOWER EXTREMITY ARTERIAL ULTRASOUND BEFORE AND AFTER EXERCISE

ankle-brachial index
calf raise
claudication distance
dorsalis pedis artery
duplex interrogation
exercise
monophasic waveform
neurogenic etiology
pedal artery
peripheral vascular disease

postexercise
posterior tibial artery
tibioperoneal disease
triphasic waveform

BILATERAL UPPER EXTREMITY VEIN MAPPING FOR DIALYSIS ACCESS PLACEMENT

anteroposterior dimension
arterial system
arteriovenous fistula
arteriovenous graft
axillary vein
basilic vein
brachial artery
brachiocephalic fistula
cephalic vein
color Doppler
compressibility
compression maneuver
cubital fossa
deep venous thrombosis (DVT)
dialysis access placement
duplex sonography
elbow
fistula
gray-scale Doppler
hemodialysis access placement
humerus
radial artery
respiratory phasicity
shoulder
subclavian vein
triphasic waveforms
ulnar artery
vein
venous system

BILATERAL UTERINE ARTERY EMBOLIZATION

#11 scalpel
0.018 wire

0.035 angled Glidewire
0.035 J-wire
1% lidocaine
300 to 500 micron Embosphere particles
4-French 11-cm sheath
4-French C1 Glide catheter
4-French micropuncture kit
4-French micropuncture sheath
4-French Omni Flush catheter
500 to 700 micron Embosphere particles
antegrade flow
aortic bifurcation
arteriogram
arteriovenous shunting
cannulated
cannulation
catheter
Clindamycin IV
common femoral pulse
common iliac artery
conscious sedation
Demerol PCA pump
digital road map arteriogram guidance
embolization
Fentanyl IV
fibroid
fluoroscopic guidance
frontal projection
groin
hemostasis
hemostat
hypertrophic
manual pressure
menorrhagia
myometrium
neovascularization
physiologic monitoring
real-time sonographic guidance
retrograde reflux
sonographic guidance
stasis
subcutaneous dissection
supine
syringe

uterine arteriogram
uterine artery
uterine artery embolization
uterine fibroid
uterine-preserving therapy
Versed IV
x-ray table

CT AND CTA OF THE ABDOMEN

abdominal aorta
abdominal aortic calcification
abdominal CTA
accessory Riedel lobe
adrenal gland
aneurysm
aortic disease
atrophy
bilateral renal artery ostia
celiac
chronic reflux nephropathy
collimated image
collimated reformatted multiplanar image
congenital anomaly
coronal image
cortical
dilation
diminutive
ectasia
enhancement
extrahepatic biliary ductal system
fibromuscular dysplasia
fluid
free fluid
gallbladder fossa
hydronephrosis
image
indeterminate node
inferior mesenteric artery
intrahepatic biliary ductal system
irregular attenuation
Isovue-370

kidney
liver
lobular ectasia
lymphadenopathy
major axis
mixed cortical thinning
mural hematoma
mural thickening
nephrolithiasis
nodule
ostium
pancreas
postcontrast multiphase image
pyelectasis
reformatted image
renal artery
renal cortex
renal hypertension
renal scarring
renovascular anomaly
retroperitoneum
sagittal image
scout
sequela
spleen
stenosis
superior mesenteric artery
ureteral tortuosity
ureteromegaly
urinary bladder
vascular disease
vasculitis

CT HEAD UNENHANCED
blood
contiguous transaxial image
dilated
edema
encephalomalacia
frontal calvaria
frontal lobe
hemorrhagic infarct
hemorrhagic stroke
infarct

intracranial shunt
lateral ventricle
mass effect
midline shift
occipital lobe
posterior fossa
residua

ENDOVAGINAL PELVIC ULTRASOUND
adnexa
adnexal mass
cul-de-sac
cyst
endometrial stripe
endovaginal sonography
free fluid
junctional zone
mass
myometrial mass
nodule
ovary
pelvic pain
transabdominal sonography
uterine mass
uterus

L2 VERTEBROPLASTY USING LEFT INTERPEDICULAR ROUTE UNDER FLUOROSCOPIC GUIDANCE
#11 scalpel
1% lidocaine
13-gauge vertebroplasty needle
Ancef IV
anterior wedge compression fracture
bone cement
conscious sedation
Fentanyl IV
hemostasis
interpedicular route
L2

low back pain
lumbar spine
manual pressure
opacification
pedicle
percutaneous cement delivery kit
periosteum
physiologic monitoring
radiograph
Versed IV
vertebral body
vertebroplasty
x-ray table

LEFT FOOT X-RAY
arthritic change
bone lesion
bony osteopenia
dislocation
foot pain
fracture
swelling

LEFT L3 ROOT BLOCK
1% lidocaine
spinal needle
bupivacaine 0.25%
fluoroscopic guidance
Isovue-200
Kenalog
L3 pedicle
lidocaine 1%
needle advancement
radicular pain
radiculopathy
root block
spinal fusion
total lumbar root block
x-ray table

MRI LEFT FOOT WITHOUT AND WITH GADOLINIUM
biopsy
contrast enhancement

effusion
erosion
erosive arthropathy
focal lump
forefoot
image
infectious arthropathy
IV gadolinium
malalignment
mass
metatarsal head
metatarsophalangeal joint
MTP joint
multiplanar MR imaging
needle aspiration
proximal phalanx
septic joint
soft tissue mass
soft tissue sarcoma
soft tissue thickening
STIR signal intensity
subluxation
synovial cell sarcoma
synovitis
T1
toe

REMOVAL AND REPLACEMENT OF TUNNELED HEMODIALYSIS CATHETER
0.035 Amplatz wire
0.035 angled Glidewire
1% Lidocaine
2-0 Prolene suture
dual-lumen tunneled dialysis catheter
Ancef IV
aspirated
atrium
catheter cuff
dialysis catheter
fluoroscopic guidance

fluoroscopy
flushed
hemodialysis catheter
heparin lock
infected
port
radiograph
sepsis
wire
x-ray table

3-VIEW LUMBOSACRAL SPINE X-RAY

abdomen
alignment
bone graft material
bowel gas pattern
canal narrowing
canal stenosis
cross-link device
disc osteophyte
disc space narrowing
encroachment
exiting nerve root
fracture
fusion
hardware failure
hip joint
laminectomy
low back pain
lumbar spine
lumbosacral spine
metallic fusion
nerve root compression
neural foramen
neural foraminal narrowing
nonobstructive

patent
pedicle
pelvic phlebolith
pneumatosis intestinalis
pneumoperitoneum
psoas margin
sacroiliac joint
superior articular facet
surgical clip
transpedicular screw
vertebral body
vertical paraspinal rod

THYROID ULTRASOUND

color mapping
multinodular goiter
nodule
pulsed Doppler duplex transducer
thyroid isthmus
thyroid lobe

ULTRASOUND ANKLE-BRACHIAL INDEX RESTING

ankle-brachial index
calcific peripheral vascular disease
discoloration
dorsalis pedis artery
duplex interrogation
great toe pressure
neurogenic etiology
pedal artery
peripheral vascular disease
posterior tibial artery
rest pain
triphasic waveform
venous etiology

Common Breast Imaging Terms

90-degree lateral view
abscess
accessory nipple
acinar space
adenocarcinoma
adenoma
adrenocortical tumor
amorphous calcification
androgen
anechoic
angiolipoma
angioma
angiosarcoma
anterior compression view
artifact
aspiration
ataxia-telangiectasia
atypical ductal hyperplasia (ADH)
automated gun-needle device
axial resolution
axillary adenopathy
axillary dissection
axillary lymph node
axillary lymphadenopathy
axillary tail
bacterial mastitis
baseline
beam intensity
benign
biopsy
biopsy change
biopsy marker
branch pattern
bullet
calcification
callback
cancer
capsular calcification
carcinogenic
carcinoma

cassette
change-of-angle view
chest wall
circumscribed mass
cleavage view
comedo mastitis
complex cystic mass
complex sclerosing lesion (CSL)
compression paddle
computed tomography (CT)
computer-aided detection
computerized axial tomography (CAT)
contrast resolution
core
coupling gel
craniocaudal view
cross-linked silicone gel
cryptorchism
curvilinear lucency
cyst
Dacron central line cuff
dendritic gynecomastia
density
dermatofibrosarcoma protuberans
diabetic mastopathy
diagnostic imaging
diffuse change
digital mammography
dilated lymphatic channel
dilated vasculature
dimpling
Doppler ultrasound
double-spot compression
double-spot compression magnification
  view
draining sinus
duct cannulation
duct ectasia
ductal calcification
ductal carcinoma in situ (DCIS)

ductal lavage
ductography
dynamic range
dystrophic calcification
ecchymosis
echogenicity
edema
eggshell
electromagnetic field radiation
elevation resolution
epithelial hyperplasia
exaggerated craniocaudal view
   (XCCL)
extensive intraductal component
   (EIC)
extramammary metastasis
fat necrosis
fat-containing lesion
fatty lobulation
fenestrated alphanumeric
fibroadenolipoma
fibroadenoma
fibrous mastopathy
filariasis
filling defect
fine-needle aspiration (FNA)
floating echo
focal fibrosis
focal parenchymal asymmetry
focal zone
follicular center cell
follicular center cell lymphoma
geometric unsharpness
giant cell arteritis
global area
granulomatous disease
grid malfunction
gross finding
gun-needle device
gurgling cyst
halo sign
hamartoma
hematoma

Hickman catheter Dacron cuff
high-grade
histiocytoid feature
histoplasmosis
hyalinized
hyperechoic
hypoechoic band
hypoechoic mass
imaging-guided biopsy
inframammary fold (IMF)
internal echo
intracystic calcification
invasive ductal carcinoma
ipsilateral axilla
kilovoltage
kyphosis
labeling
lactational
lactiferous
lateral resolution
lateral tug
leiomyosarcoma
Lexan
lexicon
linear
lipoma
lobular carcinoma in situ (LCIS)
low-grade
lumpectomy site
lymphatic channel
magnetic resonance imaging (MRI)
magnification view
malignant
mammogram
mammography-guided wire
   localization
margin
marker
mass
matrix determination
mediolateral oblique view
metastasis
metastatic pattern

microcyst
microlobulated
milk of calcium
milliamperage output
mishandling crimp
mixed-density mass
moderately differentiated
motion
mucinous feature
multicentric cancer
needle biopsy
needle-wire system
negative-density artifact
neurofibroma
nipple ring
oil cyst
opacified
orthogonal ultrasound
orthogonal view
outlining mole crevice
outlining skin lesion
pancake breast
papilloma
parenchyma
peak kilovoltage
peau d'orange
pectoral muscle
pectoralis minor muscle
phantom image
photocell positioning
phyllodes tumor
pleomorphic liposarcoma
pneumocystogram
pneumocystography
poor contrast
poorly differentiated
popcorn calcification
popcorn-like
positron emission tomography
  (PET)
posterior nipple line (PNL)
postlumpectomy fluid collection
psammoma body

pseudoangiomatous stromal hyperplasia
  (PASH)
pseudolesion
punctate calcification
radial scar
radiolucent
radiopathologic concordance
retroglandular fat
reverberation artifact
rim
rodlike
rolled view
round mass
scanning technique
scatter radiation
scintimammography
screening mammography
sebaceous cyst
sentinel lymph node
septation
shadowing
skinfold simulating
skin mass
smudgy
spatial resolution
specular echo
spiculated mass
spicule
spot compression view
spot tangential view
standoff pad
stereotactic-guided biopsy
sternalis muscle
subject contrast
suboptimal contrast
synchronous lesion
talc
tissue-air interface
touch prep
trabecular marking
transducer orientation
triangulation
tubular

tumor sojourn time
tumor-marking clip
ultrasound-guided biopsy
ultrasound-guided core biopsy
underexposed image
uneven exposure
upside-down cassette

vacuum-assisted imaging-guided
  biopsy
vascular lesion
water-density mass
well differentiated
wire localization
x-ray attenuation

Appendix 7
Common Radiographic Imaging Techniques

angiography

Angiography is accomplished by passing a catheter through an artery to the area of the body being investigated. A contrast material is injected into the vessels highlighting them, and x-rays are taken. The procedure is used to determine if blood vessels, including those in the brain, heart, kidneys, and other parts of the body, are diseased, enlarged, blocked, narrowed, or otherwise abnormal.

computed tomography (CT)

The CT scan is also referred to as a CAT scan (computerized axial tomography). CT scans can image both hard and soft tissues, including bones, organs, muscles, and tumors. Three-dimensional images are generated by computer graphics software using x-ray data obtained from multiple cross-sections of an area in any given plane.

magnetic resonance imaging (MRI)

MRIs align the magnetic nuclei of a patient. Radiofrequency pulses are then used to produce signals that are converted into 3-dimensional tomographic images of any given plane.

mammography

Mammography uses low-dose x-rays to examine the breasts to enable early detection of breast cancers and other breast diseases. The screening mammogram is a tool capable of detecting breast cancers up to 2 years before they can be felt by self-examination or by a physician. Diagnostic mammograms are used to evaluate abnormal or suspicious areas of the breast, such as lumps found by the patient or physician.

myelography

Myelography is used to visualize the spinal column and its contents. Contrast media are is used to help identify spinal lesions resulting from disease or trauma.

positron emission tomography (PET)

The PET scan is a diagnostic tool used to obtain physiologic images through the detection of radiation from the emission of positrons, tiny particles emitted from a radioactive substance administered to the patient. The level of organ or tissue function can be determined by interpreting the degree of brightness and/or colors on the PET images.

ultrasonography (Doppler ultrasound)

Diagnostic Doppler ultrasound detects movement of blood cells and other moving structures in the body, measuring both direction and speed of movement. By measuring changes in frequency of the echoes reflected from moving structures, arteries and veins can be viewed in motion. Ultrasound is also widely used for fetal monitoring.

x-rays

X-rays utilize high-energy radiation to produce images to assist in the diagnosis of diseases and structural abnormalities in the body. High-dose x-rays are used to treat cancer.